SCANDINAVIAN JOURNAL OF Infectious Diseases

Editors

Vol. 26, 1994

Datapage International Ltd, Dublin, Ireland 1994

Scand J Infect Dis 26: 1–6, 1994

REVIEW ARTICLE

Does Vitamin C Alleviate the Symptoms of the Common Cold? – A Review of Current Evidence

HARRI HEMILÄ

From the Department of Public Health, University of Helsinki, Helsinki, Finland

Since 1971, 21 placebo-controlled studies have been made to establish whether vitamin C at a dosage of ≥1 g/day affects the common cold. These studies have not found any consistent evidence that vitamin C supplementation reduces the incidence of the common cold in the general population. Nevertheless, in each of the 21 studies, vitamin C reduced the duration of episodes and the severity of the symptoms of the common cold by an average of 23%. However, there have been large variations in the benefits observed, and clinical significance cannot be clearly inferred from the results. Still, the consistency of the results indicates that the role of vitamin C in the treatment of the common cold should be reconsidered.

H. Hemilä, PhD, Department of Public Health, University of Helsinki, Haartmaninkatu 3, P.O. Box 21, FIN-00014 Helsinki, Finland

INTRODUCTION

There has been a long-standing controversy about whether vitamin C is effective against the common cold. From 4 placebo-controlled studies carried out before 1971, Pauling concluded that vitamin C reduces the incidence and severity of the common cold (1, 2). The greatest benefit was observed by Ritzel (3, 4), who used the largest dose (1 g/day). This led Pauling to propose such amounts for the prevention and treatment of the common cold. Pauling's claims were not generally accepted, yet they inspired a number of intervention studies to determine whether vitamin C has any actual effect.

In the present study the placebo-controlled studies published since 1971 in which at least 1 g/day of vitamin C has regularly been given to test subjects are briefly reviewed. If vitamin C has any effect on the incidence of, or morbidity due to, the common cold it should be observed most clearly in these studies. Moreover, these studies test whether Pauling's conclusions (1, 2) were correct, since none of the studies on which his claims were based are included.

MATERIALS AND METHODS

The literature was thoroughly searched to find all placebo-controlled studies published since 1971, in which at least 1 g/day of vitamin C had been regularly given to the study subjects. The search of the literature consisted of several database searches using various search strategies (SCISEARCH, EMBASE, MEDLINE) and inspection of the reference lists of all relevant articles and reviews. 18 publications (5–22) and 1 correction (23) were found, describing studies falling under the specifications of the search. Two other extensive literature searches of "vitamin C and the common cold" have also been carried out previously (21, 24). The studies found by this author are consistent with the studies found in the 2 other literature searches (21, 24).

The data shown in Fig. 1 are derived from 18 publications (5–22), 3 of which contain results with 2 vitamin groups (9, 10, 17). Thus, the total number of vitamin groups has been 21. For a concise summary of the original results, see Table I in ref. 25. The total number of subjects in the studies has been 6,600. All studies except 1 (6) were double-blind. Some of the placebo groups were given 10–70 mg/day of vitamin C to ensure that the effects of the larger doses were not due to alleviation of dietary deficiency (17, 19, 21). The group of twins living together in the study by Carr et al. (19) has not

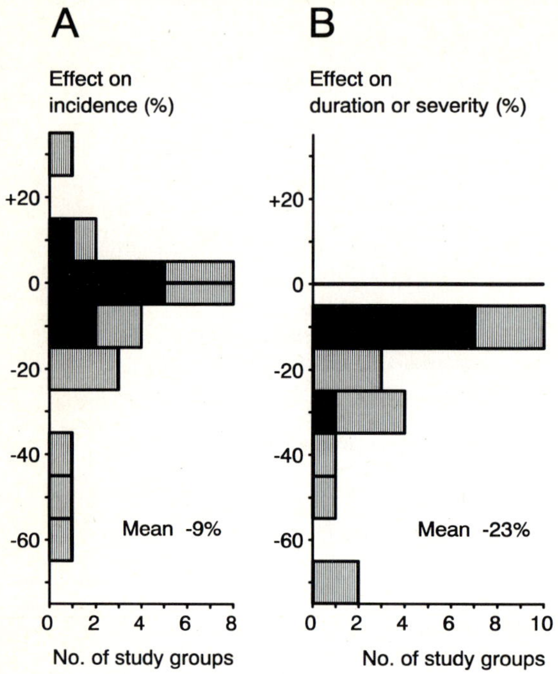

Fig. 1. Effect of vitamin C on the common cold. (A) Relative effect on incidence. (B) Relative effect on the duration of episodes or on the severity of symptoms. A horizontal bar indicates the number of studies recording a relative change in the vitamin group which falls within the vertical region of the bar. Black bars indicate the studies in which at least 400 subjects have been used (test and control group combined). A horizontal line is added to visualize the level of the control group.

been included, for reasons previously discussed (25). The D-ascorbic acid group in the study by Clegg and Macdonald (12) is not included, even though a benefit from the D-isomer was observed, since the physiological form of vitamin C is L-ascorbic acid. Some studies have used several parameters to quantify the duration of the episode or the severity of the symptoms (25). As regards alternative outcome parameters, days off from work, absence from school, days in bed (5, 16, 17), general malaise and fever (11), and severity of symptoms (18) have been chosen as measures of morbidity due to the common cold for Fig. 1B.

The probability that the distribution of results in Fig. 1B was due to chance was calculated with the formula for binomial distribution. Provided that the vitamin C and placebo groups are well matched, and that vitamin C does not affect the common cold, a vitamin group has a 50% probability of showing an increase and a 50% probability of showing a decrease in morbidity, when compared with a placebo group. Consequently, the probability that all 21 groups, purely by chance, experienced a decrease in morbidity is $(0.5)^{21} = 0.0000005$. However, this is a very conservative estimate of the statistical significance of all the evidence, since several studies have found a statistically significant difference ($p \leq 0.05$) between vitamin and placebo groups (25). The probabilities of individual studies could be combined by using Fisher's method (26), but it would not be worthwhile, since the null hypothesis that vitamin C does not differ from placebo, can already be rejected by the simple binomial distribution analysis.

RESULTS AND DISCUSSION

No marked effect on incidence

Vitamin C has no marked effect on the incidence of the common cold (Fig. 1A). The mean decrease in incidence has been −9%. 10 study groups out of 21 found a decrease in incidence (−7% and over), while 8 groups found no effect on incidence (range −3% to +2%) and 3 groups found an increase in incidence (+9% and over). Apart from 4 studies, all the results are quite symmetrically grouped around zero. Of the 4 outliers, 2 contained fewer than 25 subjects (16, 22), the third was poorly described and not published in a regular scientific forum (11), and the fourth was the only non-double-blind study of the entire group (6).

It is noteworthy that the studies with the largest numbers of subjects have not shown any consistent decrease in incidence (black bars in Fig. 1A). If the results are weighted with the number of subjects used in each study, the mean change in incidence becomes quite insignificant (−4%). Thus, the studies do not support the practice of regular ingestion of vitamin C with the purpose of reducing the incidence of the common cold in the general population.

It is possible that vitamin C reduces the incidence of common cold in certain subgroups, but the intervention studies indicate that such subgroups may not be very large or numerous. Still, it is interesting that 2 studies which found a significant decrease in incidence were conducted using Canadian military troops undergoing Arctic exercises (11), and students at a ski school in the Swiss mountains (3), which may suggest that vitamin C has some effect on the common cold incidence under conditions of great stress.

Symptoms are alleviated

Each one of the 21 vitamin C groups showed a decrease in the duration or the severity of symptoms, of common cold episodes (Fig. 1B). The probability that, purely by chance, none of the vitamin groups would find an increase in morbidity is extremely small ($p = 0.0000005$). Hence, it is very unlikely that the pattern of results emerging was due to chance (Fig. 1B). Moreover, the possibility of a systematic bias seems to be excluded, since all studies, with the exception of a single one (6), were conducted with the double-blind method. Several of the individual studies, though not all of them, have observed a decrease in morbidity that has been statistically significant (5–8, 11, 17–20, 22). Accordingly, there is very strong evidence which indicates that vitamin C alleviates the symptoms of the common cold. The next question is to assess the magnitude of the benefit.

Estimation of the benefit

In most of the studies the decrease in morbidity has been between 5% and 35% (Fig. 1B). The mean decrease in duration or severity of the common cold has been 23%, which is not negligible, even though it does not promise total relief from symptoms. A large number of factors have varied between the studies: types of subject, geographical location and climate, types of respiratory viruses infecting the subjects, definition of disease and calculation of the duration and severity, etc. Furthermore, the intake of vitamin C in the control groups may be an important variable; in some of the studies the control subjects had received quite large doses of the vitamin in their diet (25). Thus, the large variation in the effects of vitamin C supplementation may depend on several factors and, consequently, certain subgroups may benefit much more than the calculated average.

Dose of vitamin C

What is the best dose of vitamin C for the treatment of the common cold? Most of the studies have used 1 g/day. Six study groups were given 2 g/day (7, 9, 10, 18, 20, 22) and 2 groups were given 3 g/day (8, 13). Anderson et al. gave 1 g/day regularly, but increased the dose to 4 g/day during a cold episode (5). The mean decrease in severity was 19% in studies that used 1 g/day of the vitamin, and 29% in studies that used 2–4 g/day of the vitamin during the cold episode (25). This difference suggests that maximal benefit is not obtained with 1 g/day of the vitamin, even though one must be cautious when comparing the quantitative results, since there are large experimental variations in the studies.

Some of the studies have contained 2 or 3 vitamin groups that were given different doses. In such studies the definition of disease and several other factors have been constant and therefore the results of the different vitamin groups are comparable. Karlowski et al. gave

1 group 3 g vitamin C/day regularly, a second group 3 g/day during the cold episode, and a third group 3 g/day regularly plus 3 g/day during a cold episode (i.e. 6 g/day during an episode). The average decrease in the duration of symptoms was 5% and 8% in the 3 g/day groups, and 17% in the 6 g/day group (13). Coulehan et al. gave 1 group of children 1 g/day and another group 2 g/day of the vitamin. The decrease in duration of the episode in these 2 groups was 12% and 29%, respectively (10). Anderson et al. compared the effect of 4 and 8 g/day when given, in several doses, only on the first day of illness. The larger dose was consistently more effective when 8 classes of symptoms were followed to determine the duration of the episodes (9). Thus, these three studies also suggest that the maximal benefit is not obtained with 1 g/day of the vitamin.

Certain physicians have treated their common cold patients with doses still larger than those used in the intervention studies (27, 28). Cathcart observed that patients with common cold infection can ingest over 30 g/day of vitamin C without getting diarrhea, in contrast to healthy subjects who get diarrhea with 4–15 g/day (28). Based on his observations, Cathcart has proposed that the best dose may be one that is slightly smaller than the dose that causes stomach problems. He suggests that the dose is first increased to a level that causes minor stomach ailments, in order to find the upper limit, and thereafter smaller doses are used for therapy (28).

Placebo effect does not explain the results

It has been suggested that the effect of vitamin C on the common cold could be due to the placebo effect (29). This suggestion was based on the study by Karlowski et al., in which the subjects who could correctly identify vitamin C reported, on average, greater benefit from the vitamin than those who could not identify it (13). In this study the placebo consisted of lactose, which could easily be distinguished from ascorbic acid by taste. However, it has been explicitly reported in a number of studies that the placebo tablets were indistinguishable from the vitamin C tablets (4, 5, 7, 9, 10, 12, 14, 15, 17–20). It is unlikely that the placebo effect could explain the benefits observed in these studies. Furthermore, provided that vitamin C does afford some benefit, it is probable that certain subjects can identify whether they get the vitamin or the placebo on the basis of the physiological effects. For example, Asfora initiated a double-blind study to test the effect of 6 g/day of vitamin C on the common cold, but subjects receiving the vitamin could be identified due to their clinical progress (30).

Physiological effects of vitamin C

The beneficial effects of vitamin C against the common cold may be caused by its antioxidant properties (25). Vitamin C is one of the major biological antioxidants (31). It appears that neutrophils play a significant role in producing the symptoms of the common cold (32); in an infection they release large amounts of oxidizing compounds that are toxic to other cells (33–35). Activation of neutrophils promotes an efficient consumption of extracellular vitamin C, which suggests that high concentrations of the vitamin may provide protection against the harmful effects of the oxidants released (36). Furthermore, a common cold episode causes a significant decrease in vitamin C concentration in leukocytes, and this decrease can be prevented by giving the subjects 6 g/day of the vitamin (37).

It is a common assumption that the only physiological role of vitamin C is to prevent scurvy. For example, the purpose of the nutritional recommendation for vitamin C (60 mg/day) is the prevention of deficiency (25, 38–42). However, the diet of our ancestors contained 0.4–2 g/day of vitamin C (40, 43, 44), which indicates that such amounts are not unfamiliar to human physiology, i.e. they are not pharmacological. Furthermore, the nutritional recommendations are based on the concept of 'nutrient need', which appears to lack a sound biochemical basis (41, 42). Vitamin C is a cheap and safe nutrient; several of the suspected side effects of fairly large amounts are unfounded (40, 45, 46). For example, none of the intervention trials has revealed any significant side effects of the vitamin (3–22). Furthermore, in a recent epidemiological study the men who had been taking vitamin C supplements, on their own initiative, had a standardized mortality rate 30% lower than the control group (47). Accordingly, there are good reasons for reconsidering the potential role of vitamin C in the treatment of the common cold.

REFERENCES

1. Pauling L. The significance of the evidence about ascorbic acid and the common cold. Proc Natl Acad Sci USA 68: 2678–2681, 1971.
2. Pauling L. Ascorbic acid and the common cold. Am J Clin Nutr 24: 1294–1299, 1971.
3. Ritzel G. Critical analysis of the role of vitamin C in the treatment of the common cold [in German]. Helvetica Medica Acta 28: 63–68, 1961.
4. Ritzel G. Ascorbic acid and the common cold. JAMA 235: 1108, 1976.
5. Anderson TW, Reid DB, Beaton GH. Vitamin C and the common cold: a double-blind trial. Can Med Assoc J 107: 503–508, 1972.
6. Charleston SS, Clegg KM. Ascorbic acid and the common cold. Lancet 1: 1401–1402, 1972.
7. Elliott B. Ascorbic acid; efficacy in the prevention of symptoms of respiratory infection on a Polaris submarine. International Research Communications System/Medical Science 1(3): 12, 1973.
8. Schwartz AR, Togo Y, Hornick RB, Tominaga S, Gleckman RA. Evaluation of the efficacy of ascorbic acid in prophylaxis of induced rhinovirus 44 infection in man. J Infect Dis 128: 500–505, 1973.
9. Anderson TW, Suranyi G, Beaton GH. The effect on winter illness of large doses of vitamin C. Can Med Assoc J 111: 31–36, 1974.
10. Coulehan JL, Reisinger KS, Rogers KD, Bradley DW. Vitamin C prophylaxis in a boarding school. N Engl J Med 290: 6–10, 1974.
11. Sabiston BH, Radomski MW. Health problems and vitamin C in Canadian northern military operations. DCIEM Report no. 74-R-1012. Downsview, Ontario: Defence Research Board, 1974.
12. Clegg KM, Macdonald JM. L-ascorbic acid and D-isoascorbic acid in a common cold survey. Am J Clin Nutr 28: 973–976, 1975.
13. Karlowski TR, Chalmers TC, Frenkel LD, Kapikian AZ, Lewis TL, Lynch JM. Ascorbic acid for the common cold. A prophylactic and therapeutic trial. JAMA 231: 1038–1042, 1975.
14. Coulehan JL, Eberhard S, Kapner L, Taylor F, Rogers K, Garry P. Vitamin C and acute illness in Navajo schoolchildren. N Engl J Med 295: 973–977, 1976.
15. Elwood PC, Lee HP, Leger AS, Baird IM, Howard AN. A randomized controlled trial of vitamin C in the prevention and amelioration of the common cold. British Journal of Preventive and Social Medicine 30: 193–196, 1976.
16. Miller JZ, Nance WE, Norton JA, Wolen RL, Griffith RS, Rose RJ. Therapeutic effect of vitamin C. A co-twin control study. JAMA 237: 248–251, 1977.
17. Ludvigsson J, Hansson LO, Tibbling G. Vitamin C as a preventive medicine against common colds in children. Scand J Infect Dis 9: 91–98, 1977.
18. Pitt HA, Costrini AM. Vitamin C prophylaxis in marine recruits. JAMA 241: 908–911, 1979.
19. Carr AB, Einstein R, Lai LYC, Martin NG, Starmer GA. Vitamin C and the common cold: A second MZ co-twin control study. Acta Genet Med Gemellol (Roma) 30: 249–255, 1981.
20. Bancalari A, Seguel C, Neira F, Ruiz I, Calvo C. Prophylactic value of vitamin C in acute respiratory infections of schoolchildren [in Spanish]. Rev Med Chil 112: 871–876, 1984.
21. Briggs M. Vitamin C and infectious disease: a review of the literature and the results of a randomized, double-blind, prospective study over 8 years. In: Briggs MH, ed. Recent Vitamin Research. Boca Raton, Fla: CRC Press, 39–82, 1984.
22. Mink KA, Dick EC, Jennings LC, Inhorn SL. Amelioration of rhinovirus colds by vitamin C (ascorbic acid) supplementation. Medical Virology 7: 356, 1988.
23. Anderson TW, Reid DB, Beaton GH. Vitamin C and the common cold (correction). Can Med Assoc J 108: 133, 1973.
24. Kleijnen J, Riet G, Knipschild PG. Vitamin C and the common cold [in Dutch]. Ned Tijdschr Geneeskd 133: 1532–1535, 1989.
25. Hemilä H. Vitamin C and the common cold. Br J Nutr 67: 3–16, 1992.

26. Fisher RA. Statistical Methods for Research Workers. 7th ed. London: Oliver and Boyd, 104–106, 1938.
27. Regnier E. The administration of large doses of ascorbic acid in the prevention and treatment of the common cold. Part II. Review of Allergy 22: 948–956, 1968.
28. Cathcart RF. Vitamin C, titrating to bowel tolerance, anascorbemia, and acute induced scurvy. Med Hypotheses 7: 1359–1376, 1981.
29. Chalmers TC. Effects of ascorbic acid on the common cold. An evaluation of the evidence. Am J Med 58: 532–536, 1975.
30. Asfora J. Vitamin C in high doses in the treatment of the common cold. Int J Vitam Nutr Res Suppl 16: 219–234, 1977.
31. Halliwell B, Gutteridge JMC. The antioxidants of human extracellular fluids. Arch Biochem Biophys 280: 1–8, 1990.
32. Turner RB. The role of neutrophils in the pathogenesis of rhinovirus infections. Pediatr Infect Dis J 9: 832–835, 1990.
33. Anderson BO, Brown JM, Harken AH. Mechanisms of neutrophil-mediated tissue injury. J Surg Res 51: 170–179, 1991.
34. Maeda H, Akaike T. Oxygen free radicals as pathogenic molecules in viral diseases. Proc Soc Exp Biol Med 198: 721–727, 1991.
35. Ward PA. Mechanisms of endothelial cell killing by H_2O_2 or products of activated neutrophils. Am J Med 91: Suppl 3C, 89S–94S, 1991.
36. Hemilä H, Roberts P, Wikström M. Activated polymorphonuclear leucocytes consume vitamin C. FEBS Lett 178: 25–30, 1984.
37. Hume R, Weyers E. Changes in leucocyte ascorbic acid during the common cold. Scott Med J 18: 3–7, 1973.
38. National Research Council. Recommended Dietary Allowances. 10th ed. Washington DC: National Academy Press, 115–124, 1989.
39. Levine M. New concepts in the biology and biochemistry of ascorbic acid. N Engl J Med 314: 892–902, 1986.
40. Pauling L. How to live longer and feel better. San Francisco: Freeman, 1986.
41. Hemilä H. Nutritional need versus optimal intake. Med Hypotheses 14: 135–139, 1984.
42. Hemilä H. Is there a biochemical basis for 'nutrient need'? Trends in Food Science and Technology 2: 73, 1991.
43. Pauling L. Evolution and the need for ascorbic acid. Proc Natl Acad Sci USA 67: 1643–1648, 1970.
44. Eaton SB, Konner M, Shostak M. Stone agers in the fast lane: chronic degenerative diseases in evolutionary perspective. Am J Med 84: 739–749, 1988.
45. Rivers JM. Safety of high-level vitamin C ingestion. Ann NY Acad Sci 498: 445–454, 1987.
46. Bendich A. Safety issues regarding the use of vitamin supplements. Ann NY Acad Sci 669: 300–312, 1992.
47. Enstrom JE, Kanim LE, Klein MA. Vitamin C intake and mortality among a sample of the United States population. Epidemiology 3: 194–202, 1992.

Scand J Infect Dis 26: 7–13, 1994

Nephropathia Epidemica in Finland: A Retrospective Study of 126 Cases

JUKKA MUSTONEN[1], MARKUS BRUMMER-KORVENKONTIO[2], KLAUS HEDMAN[2], AMOS PASTERNACK[1], KARI PIETILÄ[1] and ANTTI VAHERI[2]

From the [1]Department of Clinical Medicine, University of Tampere, Tampere and the [2]Department of Virology, University of Helsinki, Helsinki, Finland

A total of 126 (99 males, 27 females) serologically confirmed hospital-treated adult cases of nephropathia epidemica (NE) were studied. The initial diagnosis suggested by the referring physician was correct in only 28%. Some rare clinical manifestations of NE were observed; acute myopericarditis in 3 patients and encephalitis in 1. Pulmonary involvement due to vascular congestion was observed in 16% and liver involvement in 34% of the patients. Thrombocytopenia was present in 75%, leukocytosis in 50% and anemia in 50%. Erythrocyte sedimentation rate (ESR) was 2–108 (mean 38) mm/h and C-reactive protein (CRP) 0–126 (mean 52) mg/l. Proteinuria was observed in 94%, hematuria in 58% and pyuria in 28%. Electrolyte abnormalities (hyponatremia, hypokalemia, hypocalcemia, hyperphosphatemia) were all common but rarely serious. Serum lipid changes caused by the acute infection and renal failure included very low total and HDL-cholesterol as well as high triglyceride levels. Renal function was transiently impaired in 94% of the patients and 7 needed transient dialysis therapy. All recovered.

J. Mustonen, MD, Department of Clinical Medicine, University of Tampere, P.O. Box 607, FIN-33101 Tampere, Finland

INTRODUCTION

Nephropathia epidemica (NE) is a mild type of hemorrhagic fever with renal syndrome (HFRS) which is caused by Puumala virus and found widely in Finland, elsewhere in Scandinavia and in many other parts of Europe (1). In 1980 it was found that bank voles (Clethrionomys glareolus) serve as a virus reservoir, and since that time serologic diagnosis of NE has been possible (2). NE is serologically related to Korean hemorrhagic fever, the severe form of HFRS caused by Hantaan virus and endemic in many parts of Asia (3).

Certain clinical, histological and epidemiological findings on NE have previously been reported in studies from Scandinavia (4, 5) and Western Europe (6). The diagnosis of NE in these reports was based on the clinical picture (4) or on serologic verification (5, 6). The present paper constitutes a retrospective analysis of a large, uniformly studied material of patients with a serologically confirmed diagnosis of NE.

MATERIALS AND METHODS

The study group was selected from patients treated at Tampere University Hospital and serologically tested for Puumala virus during the years 1982 to 1990. In 126 patients a recent Puumala virus infection was confirmed by demonstration of a 4-fold or greater rise in antibody titer against Puumala virus (indirect immunofluorescence antibody test) (2) and/or detection of low avidity of the IgG antibodies to Puumala virus (7). The avidity testing was performed retrospectively using sera stored at –70°C.

Clinical data were available for all patients and the results of routine laboratory blood and urine tests in 110 to 126 cases. Serum lipid values were studied in 90 patients.

We calculated correlation coefficients by either parametric or non-parametric methods as appropriate. The calculations were made using the Stagraphics^{R} (version 5.0) statistical package.

Table I. *The initial diagnoses of 119 patients with serologically verified nephropathia epidemica*

Initial diagnoses	Number of patients (%)
Nephrologic disease	69 (58)
Nephropathia epidemica	33 (28)
Unclassified nephritis	16
Pyelonephritis	7
Glomerulonephritis	2
Others	11
Infectious diseases	25 (21)
Acute febrile infection	22
Septicemia	2
Endocarditis	1
Neurologic diseases	10 (8)
Headache	4
Meningitis	4
Others	2
Gastroenterologic diseases	9 (8)
Acute abdomen	5
Acute gastroenteritis	2
Others	2
Miscellaneous	6 (5)
Respiratory tract disease	2
Dehydration	2
Acute cononary infarction	1
Hyperglycemia	1

RESULTS

Clinical data

The material comprised 99 (79%) males and 27 (21%) females, mean age 37 (range 16–75) years. Symptoms of the present acute illness had lasted from 1 to 10 (mean 5) days before admission to hospital.

Of the 126 patients who during the hospital examinations turned out to have NE, 119 had been sent to the hospital by a primary care doctor. The diagnoses suggested in the dispatches are presented in Table I. In more than half of the cases the initial diagnosis was nephrologic and in 28% it was correct, i.e. NE. Eight percent came to hospital because of acute abdominal symptoms, but a surgical approach was not undertaken in any case.

Clinical symptoms and findings are shown in Table II. The most common symptoms were fever, headache, nausea, vomiting, backache, abdominal pain and visual disturbances. One-third of the patients had myalgia. Respiratory tract symptoms or findings were recorded in about one-fifth of the cases. There were clinical findings of increased bleeding diathesis in one-tenth, including conjunctival or retinal bleeding, petechial rash, visible hematuria, melena, hematemesis, epistaxis, or bleeding from puncture sites.

Encephalitis was diagnosed in 1 patient with confusion, aggressiveness, lethargy, depression of consciousness and convulsions. The protein level in the cerebrospinal fluid was increased, being 1.09 g/l.

Acute myopericarditis was found in 3 patients, the diagnosis being based on the following findings: pericardial friction rub, cardiac enlargement on chest X-ray, pericardial effusion or

Table II. *Clinical symptoms and findings observed in 126 patients with nephropathia epidemica*

Symptom/finding	Presence (%)
General symptoms	
Fever	98
Nausea	58
Vomiting	51
Smarting of eyes/sensitivity to light	10
Edema	9
Conjunctival bleeding	9
Lymphadenopathy	6
Petechial rash	2
Pain	
Backache	54
Abdominal pains	43
Myalgia	27
Arthralgia	1
Thoracic pains	1
Neurologic	
Headache	62
Visual disturbance	36
Dizziness	9
Confusion	2
Convulsions	1
Meningism	1
Nephrologic	
Tenderness in kidney area	48
Anamnestic oliguria/anuria	34
Visible hematuria	7
Dysuria	3
Gastroenterologic	
Diarrhea	18
Constipation	8
Melena	2
Hematemesis	1
Respiratory	
Red throat/tonsil exudates	19
Cough	14
Sore throat	6
Cold	4

impaired contractility of the left ventricle on echocardiography, as well as transient abnormalities in the electrocardiogram. These abnormalities included depression of the ST-interval, inversion of T-waves and first-degree atrioventricular block.

Only a minority of the patients were hypotensive on admission. Systolic blood pressure was <100 mmHg in 11% and diastolic blood pressure <60 mmHg in 15% of the cases.

Laboratory data

Laboratory findings are shown in Table III. Thrombocytopenia was present in 75%, leukocytosis in 50% and anemia in 50% of the patients. The level of liver enzymes did not correlate with

Table III. *Laboratory findings of the patients*

	Mean value (Range)
Hematologic parameters	
Leukocyte count – maximum	11.425 (4.500–50.300) × 10^9 /l
Thrombocyte count – minimum	117 (10–489) × 10^9/l
Inflammatory parameters	
ESR – maximum	38 (2–108) mm/h
CRP – maximum	52(0–126) mg/l
Liver enzymes	
ALT[a]	56(3–1323) μkat/l
GGT[b]	39(9–161)μkat/l
Renal function	
Creatinine	439(80–1537) μmol/l
Lipids	
Total cholesterol	3.6(1.9–6.0) mmol/l
HDL cholesterol	0.42(0.1–0.8) mmol/l
Triglycerides	3.3(0.9–8.2) mmol/l

[a]ALT = alanine amonitransferase, [b]GGT = gammaglutamyltransferase.

ESR or CRP values. The severity of the renal disease as determined by the highest serum creatinine values was not statistically related to the age of the patients.

Transient electrolyte abnormalities were common: hypocalcemia in 89%, hyponatremia in 58%, hyperphosphatemia in 50% and hypokalemia in 31%. Hyperkalemia, observed in 12%, was rarely severe; in only 1 patient was a maximum serum potassium >6.0 mmol/l noted. Hypoproteinemia due to hypoalbuminemia was present in half of the patients; the lowest protein levels were observed on admission. An elevated total serum protein concentration was found in 1 patient only.

Proteinuria was the most common urinary abnormality; the dipstick test for albumin was positive in 83% of the patients. The maximum daily urine protein loss was >200 mg in 94% of the cases and in the nephrotic range (>3.5 g/day) in 25%. Hematuria defined as a positive dipstick for hemoglobin was observed in 58% of the cases and when defined as 3 or more erythrocytes per high-power field, in 42%. Leukocyturia (3 or more leukocytes per high-power field) was detected in 28%, and glucosuria (dipstick test for glucose) in 9% of patients.

Samples for serum lipid levels were obtained mostly on the second day of hospitalization. Total and HDL-cholesterol values were of depressed and triglyceride levels elevated in the acute phase of the disease (Table III). The levels of total serum cholesterol or triglycerides did not correlate with the severity of renal failure (the highest serum creatinine) or with inflammatory parameters (ESR or CRP values). Triglyceride levels correlated positively with the blood leukocyte counts ($r = 0.34$, $p < 0.01$).

Chest X-ray

During the acute phase of the disease a chest X-ray was taken in 94 patients. In 15 cases an abnormal finding related to the present illness was recorded: pleural effusion in 9, parenchymal infiltrations in 6, pulmonary edema in 3 and cardiac enlargement in 2. Both patients with enlarged heart had acute myopericarditis. All but 1 of the 15 patients with an abnormal chest

X-ray had received antibiotics during the course of the disease. In no patient could bacterial pneumonia be documented.

Course of the disease

The treatment time in hospital ranged from 3 to 66 days (mean 11 days). Polyuria was observed in most patients: the maximum daily urine volume was >2000 ml in 97% and >3000 ml in 83%. The highest urine volume measured was 9.8 l/day. During the polyuric phase the weight of the patients decreased by a mean of 3.2 kg, maximum decrease was 13 kg.

Dialysis therapy was needed in 7 patients. All patients recovered. During the oliguric phase a minority of the patients were hypertensive. The highest systolic blood pressure measured was >160 mmHg in 11% and the highest diastolic blood pressure >100 mmHg in 5% of the cases.

DISCUSSION

The initial diagnosis made by the referring physicians was correct in less than one-third of the NE cases. The patients were usually believed to have some acute nephrologic or infectious disease. It would appear that NE is seldom diagnosed as an acute respiratory tract disease. As the most common symptoms of the patients were rather unspecific, it is quite understandable that the initial diagnosis was commonly incorrrect.

As rare manifestations of NE, 1 patient suffered from encephalitis and 3 from acute myopericarditis. Some patients with encephalitis have been recorded (4, 8), but acute myopericarditis has not previously been reported during NE.

Chest X-ray revealed pulmonary involvement in some patients, most commonly a pleural effusion. Pulmonary involvement was most probably due to increased vascular congestion. Bacterial pneumonia was not observed. During Korean hemorrhagic fever, bacterial infections often involve the lungs (9). Lähdevirta (4) considered that pulmonary infiltrations in NE are due to uremia, whereas Swedish authors have suggested that the lung may be a site for viral replication (10).

Thrombocytopenia was found during the acute phase in most patients. However, 25% of the patients did not have thrombocytopenia, but its absence does not rule out NE. It is clinically important to note that the leukocytosis and thrombocytopenia often found in NE are also often present during acute bacterial infections such as septicemia. The maximal values of ESR and CRP found during NE were lower than those usually observed during bacterial infections. There is, however, an overlap between groups of patients with viral and bacterial infections (11). In some viral infections, complicated cases present higher levels than uncomplicated ones (12).

Transient impairment of renal function was noted in most patients. Morphologically the renal lesion seen during NE is acute tubulointerstitial nephritis (13). In renal transplant patients with acute nephritic syndrome, NE must be taken into account in the differential diagnosis of acute graft rejection (14).

There are many reasons for the electrolyte abnormalities in NE, such as vomiting, diarrhea and dehydration during the early illness. Later, renal failure, retention of fluid and disturbances in its distribution, as well as polyuria are seen during the polyuric phase. Hyperkalemia very rarely seems to be severe during NE. Hypocalcemia, often present in NE, is due to renal failure and hypoproteinemia.

The lowest serum protein values were recorded on admission. Clinically the serum protein level, however, cannot be used as an indicator of the fluid balance, since hypoproteinemia in NE is caused by a universally increased capillary permeability, resulting in protein leakage from the circulation (9). This causes laboratory findings such as hypoproteinemia, proteinuria and hypocalcemia and secondarily clinical manifestations such as cardiovascular, pulmonary, ophthalmologic and central nervous symptoms.

The serum lipid profile was highly abnormal during the acute phase of NE. These changes were probably caused by both the acute infection and acute renal failure. The alterations were more profound in our patients than those previously observed during other viral infections (15). There was no correlation between lipid levels and the severity of renal failure. The severity of infection as determined by the degree of leukocytosis, however, was related to the changes in lipid levels. The release of cytokines during the acute infection is one mechanism possibly responsible for the changes noted in the lipid metabolism (16).

Dialysis therapy was given in 6% of the cases. All patients recovered. In a recent series, 1% of the patients needed dialysis (17). NE is known to be a more benign disease than Korean hemorrhagic fever (1). Nevertheless, serologically verified lethal cases of NE have recently been reported from Finland and Sweden (18, 19).

In summary, the clinical diagnosis made by the referring physicians was correct in less than one-third of cases of NE. Our patients included some cases with rare manifestations of NE, such as encephalitis and acute myopericarditis. Pulmonary involvement was observed in 16% and elevated aminotransferases levels in 34% of cases. Dialysis therapy was performed in 7/126 patients. No deaths occurred.

ACKNOWLEDGEMENTS

This study was financially supported by the Finnish Kidney Foundation and the Sigrid Juselius Foundation. The technical assistance of Virpi Rauta and Heidi Hällström is greatly appreciated.

REFERENCES

1. Lee HW, van der Groen G. Hemorrhagic fever with renal syndrome. Prog Med Virol 36: 62–102, 1989.
2. Brummer-Korvenkontio M, Vaheri A, Hovi T, von Bonsdorff C-H, Vuorimies J, Manni T, Penttinen K, Oker-Blom N, Lähdevirta J. Nephropathia epidemica: detection of antigen in bank voles and serologic diagnosis of human infection. J Infect Dis 141: 131–134, 1980.
3. Lee HW, Lee PW, Lähdevirta, J, Brummer-Korvenkontio M. Etiological relation between Korean hemorrhagic fever and nephropathia epidemica Lancet 1: 186–187, 1979.
4. Lähdevirta J. Nephropathia epidemica in Finland. A clinical, histological and epidemiological study. Ann Clin Res 3 (Suppl 8): 1–154, 1971.
5. Settergren B, Juto P, Trollfors B, Wadell G, Norrby SR. Clinical characteristics of nephropathia epidemica in Sweden: prospective study of 74 cases. Rev Infect Dis 11: 921–927, 1989.
6. Van Ypersele de Strihou C, Mery JP. Hantavirus-related acute interstitial nephritis in Western Europe. Expansion of a world-wide zonoosis. Q J Med 73: 941–950, 1989.
7. Hedman K, Vaheri A, Brummer-Korvenkontio M. Rapid diagnosis of hantavirus disease with an IgG avidity assay. Lancet 338: 1353–1356, 1991.
8. Launes J, Hautanen A. Nephropathia epidemica encephalitis. Acta Neurol Scand 78: 234–235, 1988.
9. Cosgriff TM. Mechanisms of disease in hantavirus infection: pathophysiology of hemorrhagic fever with renal syndrome. Rev Infect Dis 13: 97–107, 1991.
10. Linderholm M, Billström Å, Settergren B, Tärnvik A. Pulmonary involvement in nephropathia epidemica as demonstrated by computed tomography. Infection 20: 263–266, 1992.
11. Shaw AC. Serum C-reactive protein and neopterin concentrations in patients with viral and bacterial infection. J Clin Pathol 44: 596–599, 1991.
12. Lindbäck S, Hellgren U, Julander I, Hansson L-O. The value of C-reactive protein as a marker of bacterial infection in patients with septicemia/endocarditis and influenza. Scand J Infect Dis 21: 543–549, 1989.
13. Mustonen J, Helin H, Pietilä K, Brummer-Korvenkontio M, Hedman K, Vaheri A, Pasternack A. Renal biopsy findings and clinicopathologic correlations in nephropathia epidemica. Clin Nephrol [in press].

14. Mustonen J, Saha H, Pasternack A, Brummer-Korvenkontio M. Nephropathia epidemica in a patient with renal transplant. Clin Nephrol 35: 233, 1991.
15. Sammalkorpi K, Valtonen V, Kerttula Y, Nikkilä E, Taskinen M-R. Changes in serum lipoprotein pattern induced by acute infections. Metabolism 37: 859–865, 1988.
16. Ehnholm C, Aho K, Huttunen JK, Kostiainen E, Mattila K, Pakkarainen J, Cantell K. Effect of interferon on plasma lipoproteins and on the activity of postheparin plasma lipases. Arteriosclerosis 2: 68–73, 1982.
17. Settergren B, Juto P, Trollfors B, Wadell G, Norrby SR. Hemorrhagic complications and other clinical findings in nephropathia epidemica in Sweden. A study of 355 serologically verified cases. J Infect Dis 157: 380–382, 1988.
18. Forslund T, Saltevuo J, Anttinen J, Auvinen S, Brummer-Korvenkontio M, Korhonen A, Poutiainen M. Complications of nephropathia epidemica: three cases. J Intern Med 232: 87–90, 1992.
19. Linderholm M, Settergren B, Ahlm C, Burman L-Å, Träff S, Bäcklund U, Juto P. A Swedish fatal case of nephropathia epidemica. Scand J Infect Dis 23: 501–502, 1991.

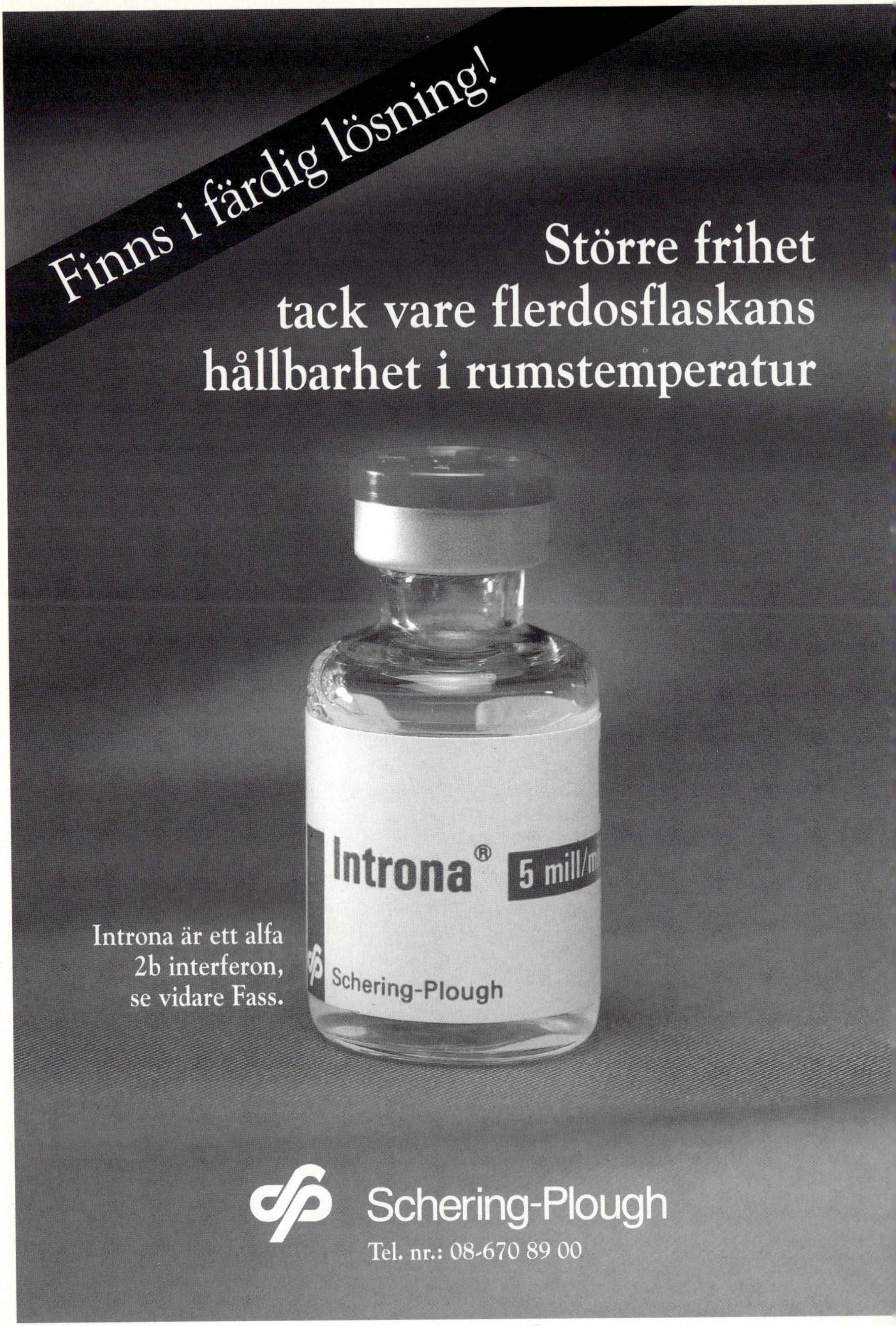
Finns i färdig lösning!
Större frihet
tack vare flerdosflaskans
hållbarhet i rumstemperatur
Introna®
5 mill/m
Schering-Plough
Introna är ett alfa
2b interferon,
se vidare Fass.
Schering-Plough
Tel. nr.: 08-670 89 00

Scand J Infect Dis 26: 15–18, 1994

Intrafamilial Spread of Hepatitis C Virus Infection

MANUEL GARCÍA-BENGOECHEA[1], ALICIA CORTÉS[2], PILAR LÓPEZ[1], JOSÉ L. VEGA[1], JOSÉ I. EMPARANZA[3], ANGEL SARRIUGARTE[1], EVA SANTOS[1] and JUAN I. ARENAS[1]

From the Services of [1]Gastroenterology, [2]Haematology and [3]Unit of Clinical Epidemiology, Hospital Nuestra Señora de Aránzazu, San Sebastián, Basque Country, Spain

We assessed the prevalence of antibodies to hepatitis C virus (anti-HCV) among 401 household contacts of 161 persons with chronic hepatitis C (index patients). None of the index patients had antibodies against HIV. The overall prevalence of anti-HCV was 3.2% (2.5% in the absence of previous parenteral exposure). Sexual partners had a seroprevalence of 4.7% and non-sexual contacts, 2.5%. Among non-sexual contacts, parents showed the highest rate (4.2%). The mean duration of exposure in the anti-HCV-positive sexual partners was 17.3±8.5 years, vis-à-vis 9.2±7.4 years in the anti-HCV-negative sexual partners. We conclude that there is little risk of HCV infection through household contact. Although the form of transmission is not well identified, the duration of sexual activity suggests that the time needed to become infected is long.

M. García-Bengoechea, MD, Podavines 6 9º-A, E-20010 San Sebastián, Guipúzcoa, Spain

INTRODUCTION

Although there is epidemiological evidence that sexual contact is a risk factor for acute non-A, non-B hepatitis, the intrafamilial spread of hepatitis C virus (HCV) through sexual or household contact with chronic carriers has not been clearly defined. We assessed the prevalence of antibodies to hepatitis C virus (anti-HCV) among family members of anti-HCV-positive index patients.

MATERIALS AND METHODS

There were 161 index patients (103 men and 58 women, mean age 42.4 ± 13.5 years) with chronic hepatitis C. Parenteral transmission was identified as the soruce of infection in 72 (45%) subjects (transfusion 50, intravenous drug abuse 20, tattoo 2). The mean (± SD) timespan from the parenteral exposure was 13.6 ± 10.1 years. A total of 401 household contacts were interviewed to identify a possible history of parenteral exposure and the duration of sexual activity with an index patient.

Blood specimens from each contact were tested for anti-HCV by second generation ELISA (Ortho Diagnostic System, Raritan, NJ). Specimens found to be above the calculated cut-off in the test were further examined by a 4-antigen recombinant immunoblot assay (4-RIBA) (Ortho Diagnostic System). Serum samples of anti-HCV index patients were retested with 4-RIBA. Antibodies to HIV (anti-HIV) were determined by using a recombinant-derived viral protein-based enzyme immunoassay (Abbott HIV-1/HIV-2 EIA, Abbott Laboratories, North Chicago, IL, USA) according to the manufacturer's instructions.

Fisher's exact test and Mann-Whitney test were used for statistical comparisons. Results are expressed as the percent positive, with 95% confidence intervals (CI).

RESULTS

The group of 401 household contacts of 161 anti-HCV-positive patients consisted of 188 men and 213 women whose mean age was 39.1 years (range 1 to 79 years). Family members included 127 sexual partners (39 men and 88 women, mean age 45.6 years) with a mean duration of sexual activity with an index patient of 19.2 years (range 1 to 42 years), and 274 other non-sexual household contacts (parents 48, offspring 177, siblings 37, others 12).

Table I. *Exposure time among 54 sexual partners and 116 nonsexual household contacts of 72 index patients with known onset date of their HCV infection*

Family members	No.	Exposure time mean years (range)
Anti-HCV negative	165	10.2 (1–35)[a]
Sexual partners	51	9.3 (1–32)[b]
Non-sexual household contacts	114	10.5 (1–35)[c]
Anti-HCV positive	5	12.8 (6–27)[a]
Sexual partners	3	17.3 (11–27)[b]
Non-sexual household contacts	2	6.0 (6–6)[c]

Mann-Whitney test, $^{a}p=0.385$; $^{b}p=0.085$; $^{c}p=0.338$.

Of the 401 household contacts, 13 (3.2%) were anti-HCV positive in the 4-RIBA assay: 6 of 127 sexual partners (4.7%, 95% CI 2–10) and 7 of 274 non-sexual contacts (2.5%, 95% CI 0.9–5.2) (Fisher's exact test, $p=0.20$) parents 6.2% (3/48), offspring 1.1% (2/177), siblings 2.7% (1/37), others 8.3% (1/12). The mean age of sexual partners (45.6 years) and parents (55.9) was significantly higher than that of the remaining non-sexual contacts (31.3 years) (Mann-Whitney test, $p<0.01$).

The history of parenteral exposure was recorded in 3 relatives: 1 parent (transfusion), 1 sibling (intravenous drug abuse) and 1 offspring (tattooing). In the absence of previous parenteral exposure, the overall prevalence of anti-HCV was 2.5% (10/401). The seroprevalence was 4.7% (6/127) in sexual partners and 1.5% (4/274) in non-sexual contacts (Fisher's exact test, $p=0.08$) parents 4.2% (2/48), offspring 0.6% (1/177), siblings 0%, others 8.3% (1/12).

In the 72 index patients in whom parenteral transmission was the source of infection, 54 sexual partners were analysed (mean duration of sexual activity 9.7 ±7.6 years), where of 3 were anti-HCV positive. The mean duration of exposure in the anti-HCV-positive sexual partners was 17.3 ±8.5 years, compared with 9.3 ±7.4 years in the anti-HCV-negative sexual partners (Mann-Whitney test, $p=0.085$). No statistical significant difference in the duration of exposure between anti-HCV positive and anti-HCV negative household contacts to the index patients was found, either for the whole group or for the sexual contacts (Table I).

The occurrence of anti-HCV positivity among household contacts of index patients with elevated ASAT/ALAT values was 2.7% (9/336) vis-à-vis 6.1% (4/65) among household contacts of index patients with normal ASAT/ALAT values (Table II). Histopathological findings in 42 index patients with elevated ASAT/ALAT who underwent liver biopsy were as follows: chronic active hepatitis, 23 cases; chronic persistent hepatitis, 13 cases; and cirrhosis, 6 cases.

None of the participants in the study was anti-HIV-positive.

Table II. *Prevalence of anti-HCV in 401 family members of index patients with chronic HCV infection with or without elevated aminotransferases values*

Aminotransferases	Index patients *n*	Household contacts *n*	Anti-HCV positive *n*	%
Normal values	36	65	4	6.1
Elevated	125	336	9	2.7
With liver biopsy	42	100	3	3.0
No liver biopsy	83	236	6	2.5

DISCUSSION

The transmission of HCV via sexual contact has been studied in sexual partners of intravenous drug users (1–3) and preliminary data are controversial. Whereas Tedder et al. (4) and Tor et al. (5) have reported that the presence of antibodies to HIV was associated with a greater risk of transmission of HCV, Pachucki and associates (6) found a prevalence of only 4% among female sex partners who did not use intravenous drugs. On the other hand, Everhart and colleagues (7) failed to demonstrate conclusive evidence of HCV transmission to sexual contacts or family members of adult patients with well-documented non-A, non-B hepatitis. The low transmission rate is supported by the study by Hsu et al. (8) who failed to detect HCV RNA in secretions from patients with HCV RNA readily detectable in the blood.

In the present study, the overall prevalence of HCV infection among household contacts was 3.2%, and in the absence of previous parenteral exposure, 2.5%. These figures are higher than the seroprevalence found among blood donors in our country (0.7%), and support the observations of other authors (9, 10). Buscarini et al. (10) have recently reported significantly higher prevalences of anti-HCV positivity in family members of index patients than in blood donors (14.9% vs 1.7%).

In our study, the seroprevalence was greater among sexual partners than among non-sexual contacts; in the group of non-sexual contacts, parents accounted for the highest seroprevalence rate. Sexual partners and parents were older than the remaining categories of family members. The mean duration of sexual activity in the anti-HCV-positive sexual partners was higher than the duration of exposure in the anti-HCV-negative sexual partners. HCV transmission through household and sexual contact, however, is much less efficient than for hepatitis B virus.

Although it has been suggested that a relationship between the severity of the liver disease in the index patient and the risk of HCV transmission exists, we did not find this. Thus the prevalence of anti-HCV among family members of the 42 index patients with chronic liver disease diagnosed by liver biopsy (3%) was similar to that found in the whole group (3.2%).

We conclude that, in the absence of parenteral transmission, there is little risk of HCV infection via non-sexual household contact. Although the form of transmission is not well identified, the duration of sexual activity suggests that the time needed to become infected is long.

ACKNOWLEDGEMENTS

We thank Ms Celina Pariente and the nursing staff of the haematology and haemotherapy laboratory for their valuable help, and Marta Pulido, MD, for editorial assistance.

Supported by a grant from the Department of Health of the Basque Government.

REFERENCES

1. Benamouzig R, Ezratty V, Chaussade S. Risk for type C hepatitis through sexual contact. Ann Intern Med 113: 638, 1990.
2. Cilla G, Pérez-Trallero E, Iturriza M, Arrizabalaga J, Iribarren JA. Possibility of heterosexual transmission of hepatitis C virus. Eur J Clin Microbiol Infect Dis 10: 533–534, 1991.
3. Pérez-Romero M, Sánchaz-Quijano A, Lissen E. Transmission of hepatitis C virus. Ann Intern Med 113: 411, 1990.
4. Tedder RS, Gilson RJC, Briggs M, Loveday C, Cameron CH, Garson JA, Kelly GE, Weller IVD. Hepatitis C virus: evidence for sexual transmission. BMJ 302: 1299–1302, 1991.
5. Tor J, Llibre JM, Carbonell M, Muga R, Ribera A, Soriano V, Clotet B, Sabriá M, Foz M. Sexual transmission of hepatitis C virus and its relation with hepatitis B virus and HIV. BMJ• 301: 1130–1133, 1990.

6. Pachucki CT, Lentino JR, Schaaff D, Schaefer MR, Heynen CA, Holzer TJ, Dawson GJ, Dous W. Low prevalence of sexual transmission of hepatitis C virus in sex partners of seropositive intravenous drug users. J Infect Dis 164: 820–821, 1991.
7. Everhart JE, Di Bisceglie AM, Murray LM, Alter HJ, Melpolder JJ, Kuo G, Hoofnagle JH. Risk for non-A, non-B (type C) hepatitis through sexual or household contact with chronic carriers. Ann Intern Med 112: 544–545, 1990.
8. Hsu HH, Wright TL, Luba D, Martin M, Feinstone SM, Garcia G, Greenberg HB. Failure to detect hepatitis C virus genome in human secretions with the polymerase chain reaction. Hepatology 14: 763–767, 1991.
9. Riestra S, Suárez A, Rodrigo L. Transmission of hepatitis C virus. Ann Intern Med 113: 411–412, 1990.
10. Buscarini E, Tanzi E, Zanetti AR, Sbolli G, Civardi G, Di Stasi M, Fornari F, Buscarini L. High prevalence of antibodies to hepatitis C virus among family members of patients with anti-HCV-positive chronic liver disease. Scand J Gastroenterol 28: 343–346, 1993.

Scand J Infect Dis 26: 19–22, 1994

Substantial Decline of Notified Hepatitis B in Major Parts of Europe After 1985

STEN IWARSON[1], WOLFGANG JILG[2] and TOMMASO STROFFOLINI[3]

From the [1]Department of Infectious Diseases, University of Göteborg, Östra Hospital, Göteborg, Sweden, [2]Institut für Medizinische Mikrobiologie und Hygiene, University of Regensburg, Regensburg, Germany and [3]Laboratorio di Epidemiologica Biostatistica, Instituto Superior di Sanità, Rome, Italy

A decline in the incidence of notified hepatitis B cases has been observed in major parts of Europe since the mid-1980s. Sweden may be taken as an example of a low prevalence area in the north where notifications of acute hepatitis B declined from 6 cases/100,000 inhabitants in 1985 to only 3/100,000 annually in 1988–91.

Choosing W. Germany as an example from central Europe, the notification rate of acute hepatitis B declined from 11 cases/100,000 inhabitants in 1984 to 6–8/100,000 in 1988–91. In Italy, a dramatic decline in hepatitis B infections has occurred since 1985, according to the national hepatitis surveillance system (SEIEVA), from 12 cases/100,000 inhabitants in 1985 to 5/100,000 in 1988–91. A similar trend has also been observed in the USA which seems to be unrelated to vaccination, since only limited vaccination programs have been initiated in high-risk groups. Also in Europe, changed sexual and needle-usage practices in risk groups such as drug addicts and male homosexuals have probably contributed to the observed decline. In southern Europe, rapidly improving socio-economic conditions and improved medical precautions against hepatitis B have probably also been important factors.

S. Iwarson, MD, PhD, Department of Infectious Diseases, University of Göteborg, Östra Hospital, S-416 85 Göteborg, Sweden

INTRODUCTION

Available data speak in favour of substantial decline in the incidence of notified hepatitis B virus infections in major parts of Europe since 1985. This is probably only partially attributable to the effect of vaccination against hepatitis B, since only limited success has been achieved with vaccination programs introduced in the countries concerned.

To study the changing epidemiology of hepatitis B in Europe, 3 countries have been examined, representing different types of epidemiological patterns of hepatitis B infection. Sweden represents the Nordic, low-prevalence pattern, the former W. Germany illustrates the central European pattern, while Italy represents the high-prevalence pattern found in southern Europe.

MATERIALS AND METHODS

Official statistics from national health authorities have been the basis for this report. In Sweden it is mandatory to report hepatitis cases to the National Bacteriological Laboratory, which publishes monthly reports on the number of cases notified from different parts of the country.

Italian data were obtained through the national hepatitis surveillance system, the Sistema Epidemiologico Integrato dell'Epatite Virale Acuta (SEIEVA), which was established in Italy in 1984. SEIEVA relies on information provided by approximately 150 health departments scattered all over the country, covering approximately 27% of the Italian population.

Figures from Germany are based on cases of hepatitis B notified to the Bundesgesundheitsamt and published in Bundesgesundheitsblatt. Only cases occurring in the former West German Republic are included in this report.

Table I. *Incidence of hepatitis B (per 100,000 inhabitants) in Italy, West Germany and Sweden 1985 and 1991, respectively*

	Notifications (per 100,000)		Reduction in incidence
	1985	1991	1985–91
Italy	12	5	58%
W. Germany (FRG)	10	8	20%
Sweden	6	3	50%

RESULTS

Hepatitis B in Northern Europe (Sweden)

The annual rates of notifications of acute hepatitis B in Sweden have declined from 6 cases/100,000 inhabitants in 1984–85 to only 3/100,000 annually in 1990–91 (Table I, Fig. 1). During the same period the number of chronic HBsAg carriers increased from 5 newly diagnosed carriers per 100,000 inhabitants in 1982–84 to 20/100,000 in 1991–92, the main reason being increased immigration from high-prevalence areas of hepatitis B.

Hepatitis B in Central Europe (W. Germany)

The notification rate for acute hepatitis B in W. Germany has declined from 10–12 cases/100,000 inhabitants year in 1984–85 to 6–8/100,000 per year in 1988–91 (Table I, Fig. 1).

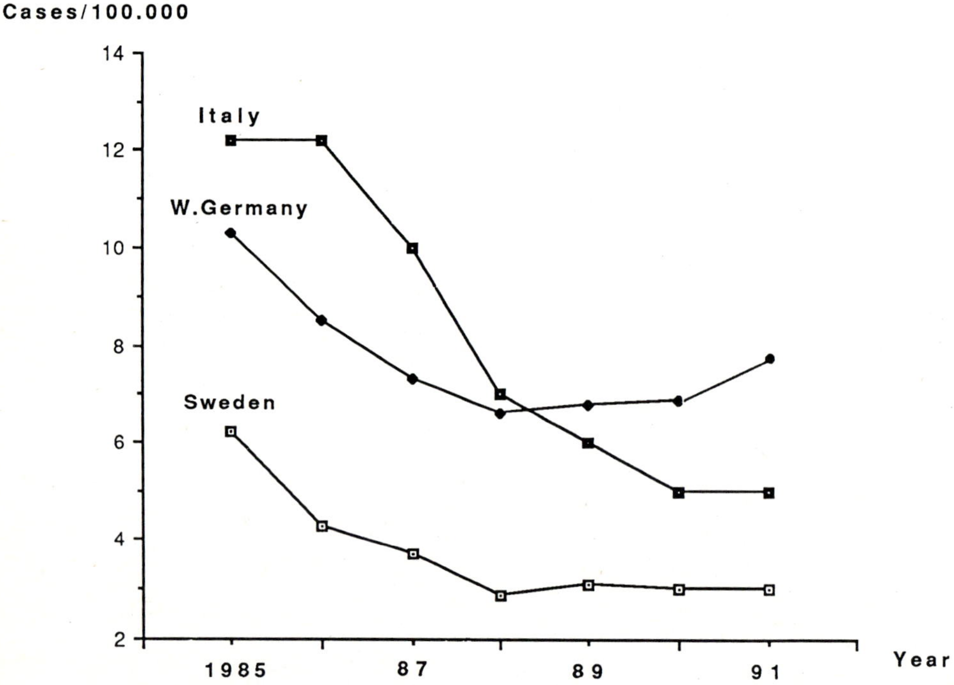

Fig. 1. Annual incidence of hepatitis B in some European countries 1985–1991.

In 1992 the incidence of hepatitis B in the western part of the unified Germany was 9.2 cases/100,000 inhabitants.

Hepatitis B in Southern Europe (Italy)

Hepatitis B notification rates declined in Italy according to the national hepatitis surveillance system (SEIEVA) from 12 cases/100,000 inhabitants in 1985 to only 5/100,000 in 1990–91 (Table I, Fig. 1).

DISCUSSION

Since the mid-1980s the European countries studied in this report have all experienced a decline in the incidence of notified hepatitis B cases. Recent data from the USA indicate a decline in the incidence of hepatitis B during 1988–91 in the order of 40%, a reduction being seen in male homosexuals as a result of changes in high-risk sexual behaviour and in i.v. drug users because of changed needle-usage practices (personal communication, M. Alter, 1993).

In Sweden, close to 250 cases of hepatitis B in i.v. drug addicts were notified in 1985, while in 1989 fewer than 100 cases were reported. In Swedish male homosexuals too a decline in the reported incidence of hepatitis B has been observed since the mid-1980s (1). As in the USA, changed sexual and needle-usage practices have probably contributed most to the declining incidence of hepatitis B in these groups in Sweden.

Also in Norway a substantial decline in the incidence of hepatitis B occurred during the 1980s. In 1991–92 only 1 case of hepatitis B/100,000 inhabitants was notified. In Britain a substantial reduction in the incidence of hepatitis B during the 1980s was reported by Polakoff in 1990 (2).

In Sweden the total number of notified new carriers of HBsAg (mainly immigrants from high-prevalence areas) has increased substantially, from approximately 350 new notified carriers/year in 1983–84 to over 3,000 in 1992. Interestingly, the increased number of carriers has so far not had any negative impact on the very low reported incidence of acute hepatitis B cases.

Of course, notification data may vary considerably in completeness and constancy. It is also difficult to compare such data between countries due to differences in reporting propensity. This is why the present report mainly compares trends within the countries studied. Also, the study period is rather short and it is well known that the epidemiology of hepatitis B displays a cyclical pattern. However, it seems unlikely that different parts of Europe as Sweden and Italy should have a synchronisation of their epidemic waves.

A substantial decline in the HBsAg prevalence among Italian military recruits in the eighties was reported by d'Amelio et al. (3). In 1981, 2.3% of recruits from northern Italy presented with HBsAg in serum as compared with 0.8% in 1990 when comparable samples of recruits were studied. In recruits from southern Italy the corresponding figures were 4.3% (1981) and 2.0% (1990), respectively. These Italian prevalence figures tally with the results of a population-based survey of 7,400 healthy subjects 3–13 years of age, carried out during the period May 1987 to November 1989 by Stroffolini et al. (4). In that study the prevalence of HBsAg was 0.6%.

In Italy the national surveillance system (SEIEVA) has shown that the age of maximum incidence of hepatitis B infection has changed from early childhood, when the risk of becoming a chronic carrier after infection is very high, to late adolescence (15–24 years) (4). The reduced circulation of HBV with little virus exposure in children has the drawback of increasing the number of clinical cases in the adolescent and adult populations. In Italy however, general vaccination against hepatitis B was passed as law in late 1991, and is now compulsory at both 3 months and 12 years of age.

In southern European countries like Italy and Greece, an improvement in socioeconomic conditions during the 1980s with smaller families, better education, etc., as well as improved medical precautions against hepatitis B, has probably also contributed to the observed decline of hepatitis B.

The observation of a halt in the declining incidence in Germany during 1991–92 disturbs the general picture, but may at least in part be due to an impact of the unification with the eastern part. Also, immigrants coming from countries such as Russia, Poland and Romania may have had an impact. The reason for the decline seen in the 1980s in W. Germany probably has a similar background to that in the USA, Sweden and Italy.

The dynamic epidemiological situation concerning hepatitis B in Europe will have to be considered when new vaccination programs against hepatitis B are designed (5). It also has to be discussed whether general immunization against hepatitis B of all newborns, as suggested by WHO representatives (6), is the best possible option in areas where the current incidence of hepatitis B is extremely low, as in Scandinavia. Finally, it is important to note the downward trends in the incidence of hepatitis B in major parts of Europe when vaccination programs are started and being followed-up.

REFERENCES

1. Struve J. Hepatitis B virus infection among Swedish adults: aspects on seroepidemiology, transmission, and vaccine response. Scand J Infect Dis Suppl 82: 1–57, 1992.
2. Polakoff, S. Reports of clinical hepatitis B from Public Health and hospital microbiology laboratories to the PHLS Communicable Disease Surveillance Centre during the period 1980–85. J Infect Dis 21: 111–117, 1990.
3. D'Amelio R, Matricardi PM, Biselli R, Stroffolini T, Mele A, Spada E, Chionne P, Rapicetta M, Ferrigno L, Pasquini P. Changing epidemiology of hepatitis B in Italy: public health implications. Am J Epidemiol 135: 1012–1018, 1991.
4. Stroffolini T, Chiaramonte M, Craxi A, Franco E, Rapicetta M, Trivello R, de Mattia D, Mura I, Giammanco A, Rigo G, Scarpa B. Baseline seroepidemiology of hepatitis B virus infection in children and teenagers in Italy. A survey before mass hepatitis B vaccination. J Infect Dis 22: 191–199, 1991.
5. Iwarson S. Strategies for immunization against hepatitis B in western Europe. Vaccine 11 (Suppl 1): 18–20, 1993.
6. Schatz GC, Kane MA. A Global Portrait of Hepatitis B Virus Demographics and Programs. 8th International Symposium on Viral Hepatitis and Liver Disease, Tokyo, 1993 (Poster).

Scand J Infect Dis 26: 23–26, 1994

HTLV-I and -II in Intravenous Drug Users from Sweden and Denmark

JONAS BLOMBERG[1], TORKIL MOESTRUP[2], JAN FRIMAND[3], BENGT-GÖRAN HANSSON[1], KIM KROGSGAARD[4], LENA GRILLNER[5] and ERIK NORDENFELT[1]

From the [1]Section of Virology, Department of Medical Microbiology, University of Lund, Lund, the [2]Department of Infectious Diseases, Malmö General Hospital, Malmö, the [3]Health Department, Fosie Penitentiary, Malmö, Sweden, the [4]Department of Infectious Diseases, Hvidovre Hospital, Copenhagen, Denmark and the [5]Section of Virology, Department of Clinical Microbiology, Karolinska Hospital, Stockholm, Sweden

693 IVDU (intravenous drug user) sera from Copenhagen, Malmö and Stockholm were tested, 247 retro- and 446 prospectively, for antibodies to human T-lymphotropic virus (HTLV), types I and II, by means of a commercial whole-virus EIA and/or an HTLV-I/-II peptide-based EIA. Positive EIA reactions were checked and typed by electrophoretic immunoblotting, a differential peptide-based EIA and nucleic acid amplification/hybridization with HTLV-I and -II specific primers and probes. 3 (0.7%) of the prospectively tested IVDUs from Malmö, none of 100 from Stockholm and none of 45 from Copenhagen were HTLV-seropositive. The 3 Malmö IVDU cases were a female immigrant from South America, her male native Swedish spouse (both HTLV-I), and a male immigrant Italian heroinist (HTLV-II). We conclude that HTLV was uncommon among intravenous drug users, a sentinel population, in Sweden and Denmark during 1986 and 1989. However, the occurrence of 3 HTLV-positive cases in Malmö 1993 indicates that the situation can change rapidly.

J. Blomberg, MD, Section of Virology, Department of Medical Microbiology, Sölvegatan 23, S-223 62 Lund, Sweden

INTRODUCTION

Although human T-lymphotropic virus (HTLV-II) infections are rare in the general population, intravenous drug users (IVDUs) are not infrequently infected in the U.S.A. (1). Likewise, HTLV is not a common infection in Europe (2), although endemic foci of HTLV-II among IVDUs do occur, e.g. in Milan, Italy (e.g. (3)). The epidemiology in Northern Europe is not well known (cf. (4)). Although giving a less dramatic infection than HIV, HTLV creates life-long risks of developing neurological (HTLV-I and -II; (5)) and hematological (mainly HTLV-I) disease, and of further transmission via sex, blood and breast milk (for a review, see (6)). We have searched for HTLV infection among IVDUs in Sweden and Denmark with serum samples collected between 1986 and 1993.

MATERIALS AND METHODS

Sera

(*a*) *Retrospective study*: 102 sera were collected between 1986 and 1988 from IVDUs in Malmö, as part of a hepatitis surveillance program. 100 IVDU sera were collected in 1988–89 for HIV screening at the Karolinska Hospital, Stockholm. 45 sera from IVDUs attending the Department of Infectious Diseases, Hvidovre Hospital as outpatients were also collected 1988–89. These 247 sera were screened with the Abbott HTLV-I antibody test.

(*b*) *Prospective study*: 342 sera were from IVDUs participating in a needle exchange program at the Department of Infectious Diseases, Malmö General Hospital and 104 sera from IVDUs attending the Health care section of the Fosie Penitentiary, Malmö, January–June 1993. The patients gave informed consent to HTLV antibody testing. These 446 sera were screened with a synthetic peptide-based test (see below).

 ISSN 0036-5548

Immunoassays and serotyping

The sera were screened either with an HTLV-I whole-virus lysate antibody test (Abbott, Chicago, IL, USA) utilizing a cutoff value half of that prescribed by the manufacturer, or with an HTLV-I/-II peptide EIA employing a mixture of HTLV-I and -II *gag* and *env* peptides, which was validated against a panel of known HTLV-I and -II positive sera. The test was designed to detect weakly reactive HTLV-II positive sera too (J. Blomberg et al., data not shown). The peptides and their antigenicity were described recently (7). Peptide-reactive sera were further tested in the HTLV whole-virus lysate antibody test, using the low cutoff value mentioned above. Sera which were still reactive were subjected to an HTLV-I western blot (Diagnostic Biotechnologies, Singapore; version 2.3 was used with sera from 1993; version 2.2 with earlier sera) and a differential HTLV peptide antibody test (7). Those which reacted with p19, p24, recombinant gp21 (rgp21) and rgp46 (from either type -I or -II) in EIB and showed characteristic peptide reactivity were considered HTLV-I or -II positive.

PCR verification

Lymphocytes were obtained from the 3 seropositive IVDUs, and analysed with the Roche HTLV-I and -II PCR tests (Roche Molecular systems, New Jersey, USA).

RESULTS

Immunoassays

In the retrospective study, 1 serum from 1988, 5 1988–89 sera from Hvidovre, and none of the 1988–89 sera from Stockholm reacted in the whole-virus lysate test. Of these 6, 3 gave only p19 bands and 3 were blank in HTLV EIB. Thus, none of the sera collected between 1986 and 1989 proved HTLV antibody positive. In contrast, 3 of the Malmö sera tested prospectively during the spring of 1993 were positive (Table I). Two reacted as HTLV-I, and 1 as HTLV-II in both EIB and differential peptide EIA (Table II). The diagnosis was further corroborated with type-specific PCR from leukocytes. Leukocytes from patients 1 and 2 harboured HTLV type I sequences, while those from patient 3 harboured HTLV type II sequences.

Description of the three HTLV positive cases

Patient 1. A 28-year-old female born in South America who came to Sweden in 1986. She is a drug addict and commercial sex worker. She started using heroin intravenously in 1990, when she met patient 2, who is now her steady sex partner. She was negative for HBsAg and positive for anti-HBc and anti-HCV (Ortho II) in December 1992.

Patient 2. A 26-year-old male with Swedish parents who has taken drugs from the age of 13, starting with haschisch, going on to amphetamine and finally to heroin. He is a steady sexual

Table I. *HTLV serology with IVDU sera*

1) R = Retrospective, P = Prospective.

Place	Year of collection	No.	Positive	Type of investigation (1)
Malmö	1986–88	102	0	R
Stockholm	1988–89	100	0	R
Copenhagen	1988–89	45	0	R
Malmö, Dept Infectious Dis.	1993	342	2	P
Malmö, penitentiary	1993	104	1	P
Sum		693	3	

Table II. *Serotyping of the 3 HTLV positive sera*

	Western blot		Peptide EIA			
	rgp46		p19 (gag)		rgp46 (env)	
Patient	Type I	Type II	Type I	Type II	Type I	Type II
1	+	−	+	−	+	−
2	+	−	+	−	+	−
3	−	+	−	+	−	+

and syringe-sharing partner of patient 1 at least since 1992. He was HBsAg negative, anti-HBc negative and anti-HCV positive (Ortho II test) in November 1992.

Patient 3. A 28-year-old male of Italian origin who arrived in Sweden 3 years ago. He started using heroin intravenously several years before arriving in Sweden. He travels much in south Sweden. He was HBsAg negative, anti-HBc positive and anti-HCV positive in January 1993. All 3 patients were HIV negative.

DISCUSSION

The 3 cases are the first known HTLV cases among Swedish IVDUs. The finding of so few cases among 693 south Scandinavian sera attests to the low seroprevalance of HTLV reported earlier from the area (4).

The patient histories suggest that the HTLV underlying all 3 cases was brought into Sweden by immigration a few years before the positive serological test. We found no evidence of HTLV-associated disease in the 3 positive persons. The degree of spread of HTLV varies widely among IVDU communities (3). The low prevalence described here contrasts with the much higher frequency recently found among IVDUs in Oslo, Norway (8).

In the age of AIDS, informing someone of his/her HTLV infection raises special problems. The serious consequences of HIV-1 make the physician's information task relatively straightforward. On the other hand, it is hard to capture the patient's attention with a more innocuous infection like HTLV-I/-II without turning alarmist. The patient's take-home message easily becomes "I do not have AIDS" rather than "I have HTLV". Yearly follow-up visits to the Department of Infectious Diseases in Malmö, needle exchange, condom use and, for the female IVDU, abstinence from any breast feeding in the future, were recommended to the 3 HTLV-positive patients.

ACKNOWLEDGEMENTS

We are indebted to Elzbieta Vincic for skilful technical assistance, and to Dr Rüdiger Pipkorn for supplying the synthetic peptides. This work was supported by the Swedish Medical Research Council, grant no. B09933-03A.

REFERENCES

1. Robert-Guroff M, Weiss SH, Giron JA, Jennings AM, Ginzburg HM, Margolis IB, Blattner WA, Gallo RC. Prevalence of antibodies to HTLV -I, -II and -III in intravenous drug abusers from an AIDS endemic region. JAMA 255: 3133–3137, 1986.
2. Mayer V, Ebbesen P. HTLV-I virus in Europeans: the continuous spread. A meta-analysis. Acta Virol 35: 472–95, 1991.

3. Zanetti AR, Zehender G, Tanzi E, Galli C, Rezza G, Cargnel A, Boschini A, Mari D, Pizzocolo G, Mazzotta F. HTLV-II among Italian intravenous drug users and hemophiliacs. Eur J Epidemiol 8: 702–707, 1992.
4. Blomberg J, Fäldt R. Antibodies to human adult T cell leukemia virus type I associated antigens in Swedish leukaemia patients and blood donors. Br J Haematol 60: 555–557, 1985.
5. Harrington WJ Jr, Sheremata W, Hjelle B, Dube DK, Bradshaw P, Foung SK, Snodgrass S, Toedter G, Cabral L, Poiesz B. Spastic ataxia associated with human T-cell lymphotropic virus type II infection. Ann Neurol 33: 411–414, 1993.
6. Cann AJ, Chen ISY. Human T-Cell leukemia virus types I and II. In: Fields BN, et al. eds. Virology. 2nd ed. New York: Raven Press, 1501–1527, 1990.
7. Blomberg J, Robert-Guroff M, Blattner WA, Pipkorn R. Type- and group-specific continuous antigenic determinants of HTLV. Use of synthetic peptides for serotyping of HTLV-I and -II infection. J Acquir Immune Defic Syndr 5: 294–302, 1992.
8. Holm-Samdahl H, Haukenes G, Kalland KH. HTLV-infeksjon i Norge. (HTLV infection in Norway.) MSIS-rapport 21: 1, 1993 [in Norwegian].

Scand J Infect Dis 26: 27–31, 1994

HIV Infection among Seafarers in Denmark

HENRIK L. HANSEN[1,2], LARS BRANDT[1], JANNE JENSEN[3], ULLA BALSLEV[4], SIGURDUR SKARPHEDINSSON[5], ANDERS F. JØRGENSEN[6], KIM DAVID[7] and FINN T. BLACK[2]

From the Departments of [2]Infectious Diseases, Marselisborg Hospital, Aarhus, [3]Internal Medicine, Central Hospital, Esbjerg, [4]Infectious Diseases, Rigshospitalet, Copenhagen, [5]Infectious Diseases, Hvidovre Hospital, Copenhagen, [6]Internal Medicine, Odense University Hospital, Odense, [7]Internal Medicine, Frederiksberg Hospital, Copenhagen, and the [1]Institute of Maritime Medicine, South Jutland University Centre, Esbjerg, Denmark

The purpose of this study was to estimate the minimal magnitude of the HIV problem among seafarers in Denmark. The material is based on case records from the 6 medical departments in Denmark that undertake treatment of HIV patients. Retrospectively, all case records of HIV infection among seafarers - and of their sexual contacts - have been identified. 33 seafarers with HIV infection or AIDS were identified; 17 had no other known risk factor than heterosexual contacts in high-endemic areas. These results show that HIV infections have entered into the heterosexual group of seafarers. HIV-infected seafarers are a risk group for carrying HIV infection into the heterosexual population in non-endemic areas. In 5 known cases, this has actually taken place in Denmark. The majority of the heterosexually infected seafarers were probably infected early in the AIDS era. We do not know if Danish seafarers are still acquiring HIV abroad.

H. L. Hansen, MD, Institute of Maritime Medicine, South Jutland University Centre, Niels Bohrs Vej 9, DK-6700 Esbjerg, Denmark

INTRODUCTION

Sexually transmitted diseases have been a scourge of seafarers for centuries (1). Therefore, not long after the recognition of HIV as the cause of AIDS, it was pointed out that seafarers, like other travellers to areas with a high prevalence of HIV infection, ran an increased risk of contracting HIV infection (2).

HIV infection and AIDS among seafarers is not a new phenomenon. In 1959 an English seaman from Manchester died of pulmonary infection with Pneumocystis carinii and cytomegalovirus (3). By means of PCR-technique, HIV was identified in frozen samples taken from the man (4). In the late 1960s, a Norwegian seaman in the merchant navy, his wife and their child became immunodeficient and all died. In this case too, it was possible to prove that they were all immunodeficient due to HIV (5). Both index cases had visited ports in central Africa at a time when HIV has been proved to have been present in that area (6). These were the first known cases of AIDS in Europe. Later, heterosexually acquired HIV infection has become known among seafarers from several maritime countries in Europe (7).

Screening for HIV antibody has been carried out among seafarers in different countries (Table I). Only 1 survey, the one from the former Soviet Union (9), covers a random sample of the seafarers in the populations studied. From Spain, HIV-2 infection has been reported among seafarers (12). The remaining studies report only on HIV-1 infection.

The purpose of this study was to estimate the magnitude of the HIV problem among seafarers from Denmark.

MATERIALS AND METHODS

Denmark has, in comparison with its size, a large merchant navy, accounting for approximately 1.35% of

Table I. *Selected published investigations concerning HIV prevalence among seafarers*

Author	Country of origin	Numbers screened	Year	Results/comments
1. Vuksanovic, P. et al. (2)	W. Germany	2,051	1985–87	Performed among seafarers of all nationalities visiting a port health clinic in Hamburg. Nine (0.5%) were HIV-positive, among these 5 from Western Europe and 4 from Africa.
2. Goethe, W. H. et al. (7)	W. Germany	873	1987–88	Performed like the above-mentioned. Five (0.57%) positive, 3 from Western Europe and 2 from Africa.
3. van Damme, J. et al. (8)	Belgium	321	1988	Seafarers in Belgian merchant ships. One Belgian was positive and 14 out of 124 Africans were positive.
4. Gold, E. et al. (9)	USSR	20,000	1988	The survey was performed among Soviet seafarers who had been employed in international trade. All negative.
5. Verhaert, P. (10)	Belgium	300	1989–90	Performed among seafarers of all nationalities visiting a port health clinic in Antwerp, Belgium. All negative.
6. Estebanez, P. et al. (11)	Spain	521	1990	Spanish seafarers from the merchant fleet and the overseas fishing fleet. Six were HIV-positive. Four of the 6 had other risk factors than sexual contacts abroad.

the world's merchant navy, measured in gross tonnage. Most merchant ships are engaged in foreign trade all over the world. At any one time approximately 5,000 Danes are employed on board ships engaged in foreign trade, but due to vacations it is estimated that approx. 10,000 are employed during a whole year. The majority are men.

It has been estimated, on the basis of the few available sources, that in 1991 the total number of HIV-positive persons in Denmark was between 4,500 and 5,300. Of these about 600 had acquired the infection heterosexually (13), half of them being men.

The material presented here is based on medical records from all 6 departments in Denmark which treat HIV patients. By checking all case records of HIV patients who had attended their out-patient clinics, been admitted, or who had died because of AIDS, the cases of HIV infection among seafarers and their sexual contacts in Denmark could be identified retrospectively.

Information about occupation is generally not recorded in Danish hospital medical records, but with few exceptions, it is noted in all records, the way in which the individual acquired the infection. Therefore, in the case of heterosexual transmission, it would be mentioned that the patient was a seafarer in the merchant navy. On the other hand, in the case of a homosexual seafarer, the occupation would not necessarily be recorded.

RESULTS

Up to the end of 1992, 33 seafarers with HIV infection or AIDS had been identified. 16 men and 1 woman had no other known risk factor except heterosexual contacts outside Denmark. Of the remaining 16 seafarers, 9 had homosexual experience and 7 had used intravenous drugs. All had HIV-1 infection.

The 17 seafarers with probable heterosexually-acquired HIV infection had a mean age of 37 years (range 23–55) at the time of diagnosis. All kinds of maritime professions were represented in this subgroup, including able seamen, deck and engine room officers and catering crew. No single group predominated. All were permanent residents in Denmark and 15 out of the 17 born in Denmark. The remaining 2 were of Finnish and Spanish origin, respectively.

At the end of 1992, 7 out of the 17 had developed AIDS and 3 had died. All AIDS cases were men.

Two of the seafarers with heterosexually-acquired HIV infection stated that they had been infected in South America. One was infected on board by a colleague. The remaining 14 did not state where they thought they had been infected, but 10 reported visits to African ports. The remaining 4 seafarers had all sailed "world wide".

Most of those with heterosexually-acquired HIV infection were not identified until they got HIV-related symptoms or a partner was identified as HIV-positive.

Two seafarers were identified when they enrolled as voluntary blood donors, 1 when tested on his own initiative. The reason for the test is unknown among the remaining 4 seafarers.

In most cases, the time of infection is unknown. 11 out of the 17 seafarers with heterosexually-acquired HIV stated that they probably were infected before 1986, when they were unaware of the risk of acquiring HIV infection.

The 17 seafarers with probable heterosexually-acquired HIV infection had had several sexual contacts in Denmark. We are aware of 8 Danish contacts, among whom 2 have sero-converted. One of the secondary cases transmitted the disease further to a new partner and to their child.

One further woman has been infected by a seafarer, but of unknown identity.

Altogether, a minimum of 23 people have contracted HIV infection as a direct or indirect consequence of seafarers' heterosexual contacts abroad.

A very rough estimate of seafarers' risk during the last 10 years, of acquiring HIV infection heterosexually can be made by comparing the number of known HIV infections among male seafarers and the estimated number of cases among the general population. Estimating that there has been a mean of 10,000 male seafarers for the last 10 years, the risk is 0.00016 cases/person-year. For the general male population between 20 and 59 years, the estimated number of cases has been 300 during 14,500,000 person-years, giving a risk of 0.00002 cases/person-year or one-eighth of the estimated risk for seafarers.

DISCUSSION

Our figures show that Danish seafarers, like other travellers to endemic areas, have contracted HIV infection early in the AIDS era. In contrast to the general pattern in Denmark, a large proportion of the HIV-positive seafarers have acquired the infection heterosexually.

The estimated risk should be considered an absolute minimum due to the method used. It is not taken into account that a considerable number of the known cases of heterosexually acquired HIV in Denmark are among persons from high prevalence areas. Finally, the occupation might not have been recorded in some cases and therefore some seafarers might have been missed.

The majority of the seafarers with heterosexually-acquired HIV infection presented here were infected at a time when there was no or very limited knowledge of HIV, which is why they were unaware of the risk.

That there are only a few known cases from the last couple of years might have several explanations. Sexual behaviour has probably changed since the public recognition of HIV and, viewed from that aspect, the problem should diminish. On the other hand, we know from a recently completed study in Denmark that the Danish population still has risky sexual practices (14). We do not know whether some seafarers still practice 'unsafe sex' while abroad. Venereal diseases are still diagnosed among Danish seafarers, but as no exact statistics exist we do not know if or to what extent the incidence of other sexually transmitted diseases has diminished.

Even with changed sexual behaviour, the risk of acquiring HIV infection abroad might increase because of the rapid spread of HIV in Asia within the last few years (15), Asia being a much more important area for Danish shipping than Africa.

A noteworthy point is that the majority of the identified seafarers with heterosexually acquired HIV infection were diagnosed when they - or a sexual contact - developed HIV-related symptoms. Therefore, it appears that very few seafarers, despite risky sexual behaviour, have used the free and anonymous HIV-testing service available in Denmark; hence it can be expected that more HIV-positive seafarers will turn up when they develop symptoms. A recent study from Sweden, where the pattern of HIV transmission is similar to that of Denmark, has shown that it can be estimated that there are probably twice as many HIV-positives among heterosexuals as the actually known number (16).

Our group of HIV-positive seafarers seem to have infected only a few secondary cases. However, most of them are still alive and potentially infectious, and an unknown number of seafarers are undiagnosed. These may be more infectious, since they are unaware of their HIV infection. Further investigation into the sexual behaviour of this group is needed in order to deal with the problem of heterosexual spread of HIV.

REFERENCES

1. Arya OP, Plumb JB. Seamen's dispensary, Liverpool 1924–1991. Genitourin Med 68: 84–89, 1992.
2. Vuksanovic P, Goethe WH, Burchard U, Schmitz H, Backhaus A, Koeppen M. Seamen and AIDS. Travel Medicine International 6: 18–20, 1988.
3. Williams G, Streeton TB, Leonard JC. Cytomegalic inclusion disease and Pneumocystis carinii infection in an adult. Lancet 1: 951–955, 1960.
4. Corbitt G, Bailey AS, Williams G. HIV infection in Manchester, 1959. Lancet 336: 51, 1990.
5. Frøland SS, Jenum P, Lindboe CF, Wefring KW, Linnestad PJ, Bohmer T. HIV-1 infection in Norwegian family before 1970. Lancet 1: 1344–1345, 1988.
6. Nahmias AJ, Weiss J, Yao X, Lee F, Kodsi R, Schanfield M, Matthews T, Bolognesi D, Durack D, Moyulsky A, Kanki P, Essex M. Evidence for human infection with an HTLV III/LAV-like virus in Central Africa, 1959. Lancet 1: 1279–1280, 1986.
7. Goethe WH, Schmitz H, Vuksanovic P, Perisic S. State of knowledge about AIDS among seamen as well as the spreading of HIV in this occupational group. Bull Inst Marit Trop Med Gdynia 40: 57–66, 1989.
8. Van Damme J, Van Damme P. Incidence of HIV infection in a seafarers' population. In: Proceedings of the 7th European Nautical Meeting. Hamburg 243–283, 1989.
9. Gold E. Yu, Boschenko YA, Korobov LI, Ryzchko VO, Mantura AA. Sailors as a potential source of importation of HIV infection. In: Proceedings from XI International Symposium on Maritime Medicine, Gdynia. 208, 1989.
10. Verhaert P. HIV-seroprevalence study and epidemiologic investigation among seafarers in the port of Antwerp. In: Proceedings of The International Conference on Maritime Medical Care. Maryland, USA, 1990.
11. Estebanez P, Sarasqueta C, Najera R, Contreras G, Perez L, Fitch K, Vicente A. Prevalence of HIV-1, HIV-2, and HTLV-I/II in Spanish seamen. J Acquir Immune Defic Syndr 5: 316–317, 1992.
12. Soriano V, Gutierrez M, Fernandez JL, Aguilera A, Gonzalez A, Bernal A. HIV-2 infection in Spain: report of the first 34 cases. The HIV-2 Spanish Study Group. AIDS 6: 1222–1223, 1992.

13. Foldspang A, Smith E. Overvågning af HIV og AIDS i Danmark. Status og perspektiver. Sundhedsstyrelsen, Copenhagen, 1992. [in Danish]
14. Melbye M, Biggar RJ. Interactions between persons at risk for AIDS and the general population in Denmark. Am J Epidemiol 135: 593–602,1992.
15. Anderson R, May R. Understanding the AIDS pandemic. Sci Am 266: 20–26, 1992.
16. Blaxhult A, Svensson Å. Assessing the extent of the HIV epidemic in Sweden, using information on the extent to which people who develop AIDS are already known to be HIV infected. Int J Epidemiol 21: 784–791, 1992.

Scand J Infect Dis 26: 33–40, 1994

Seroreactivity to Pneumocystis carinii in Patients with AIDS versus Other Immunosuppressed Patients

KERSTIN ELVIN[1], ANDERS BJÖRKMAN[2], NADJA HEURLIN[3], BRITT-MARIE ERIKSSON[5], LISBETH BARKHOLT[4] and EWERT LINDER[1]

From the [1]Laboratory of Parasitology, Microbiology and Tumorbiology Center, Karolinska Institute, Swedish Institute for Infectious Disease Control, Stockholm, Sweden, the Departments of [2]Infectious Diseases, [3]Pulmonary Diseases, and [4]Transplantation Surgery, Karolinska Institute, Huddinge University Hospital, Stockholm, and the [5]Department of Infectious Diseases, University Hospital, Uppsala, Sweden

The aim was to study the humoral response to Pneumocystis carinii and its diagnostic use in patients with P. carinii pneumonia (PCP). The antibody response was measured by indirect immunofluorescence in AIDS patients versus other immunosuppressed patients with 122 episodes of confirmed PCP. During the early acute stage of the pneumonia, anti-P. carinii antibodies were found in 17% of AIDS and 24% of other immunosuppressed patients. In the second serum sample, antibodies were still found in 17% of the AIDS patients but in as many as 56% of the otherwise immunosuppressed patients. Antibodies were also found in 17% of HIV-positive and 15% of other immunosuppressed control patients, but only in 3% of immunocompetent controls ($p < 0.001$). Paired sera were available from 55 patients during 58 PCP episodes. Seroconversion or a fourfold rise in titre was detected in only 1/36 (3%) AIDS patients but in 10/22 (45%), (95% c.i.: 24–66%) other immunosuppressed patients ($p < 0.001$). We conclude that AIDS patients seem to have lost their ability to develop a humoral response to P. carinii during pneumonia, whereas many other immunosuppressed patients do respond. In these patients the serological test against P. carinii was of no diagnostic value in the acute phase of the infection, whereas when analysing paired sera it was a useful complement to the clinical diagnosis.

K. Elvin, Laboratory of Parasitology, Swedish Institute for Infectious Disease Control, S-105 21 Stockholm, Sweden

INTRODUCTION

Definitive diagnosis of P. carinii pneumonia (PCP) is dependent on finding the organism in lung-derived samples. This has become increasingly feasible thanks to improved methods of specimen collection, viz. bronchoalveolar lavage (1) and induced sputum in particular (2, 3), and with better detection methods by staining with monoclonal anti-P. carinii antibodies (4–6). However, bronchoscopy and sputum induction are not always available, and clinicians often prefer to send a simple serum sample for diagnosis. This is especially the case in children, infants and severely ill patients. Although assays for the detection of circulating antigen have been reported (7, 8) the results have not been reproducible, their specificity has been questioned, and their clinical utility is doubtful (9–12).

Exposure to P. carinii stimulates a humoral immune response in immunocompetent experimental animals (13, 14). The diagnostic use of serology for P. carinii is often considered unreliable, however, since antibodies are present in the healthy population and reported seroprevalences vary from 0 to 100% (15, 16). Furthermore, the humoral immune response may not be adequate in immunocompromised patients (17). Studies on seroreactivities to P. carinii have been performed in patients with lymphoma and leukaemia, in transplant recipients (15, 18, 19), and in HIV patients (12, 20). The results are difficult to compare, since the antigens employed as well as the patient populations included have varied. The PCP diagnosis has not always been verified by microscopical demonstration and PCP not excluded in the immunosuppressed controls. A few studies of anti-P. carinii

 ISSN 0036-5548

antibodies in serial serum samples from immunosuppressed patients have been conducted in the 1970s, before the HIV epidemic. Collection intervals were irregular however or not mentioned at all, and no distinct pattern was found (15, 18).

We present here a comparative study of the humoral responses to P. carinii in HIV versus otherwise immunosuppressed patients (non-HIV) with verified PCP.

PATIENTS AND METHODS

Inclusion criteria for patients

Patients with an acute clinical PCP confirmed by silver methenamine staining (21) at the Department of Pathology, Huddinge Hospital in 1983–85 (15 episodes), or by immunofluorescence (4) at the Department of Parasitology, NBL, in 1986–89 (107 episodes) from whom sera were available were included. Immunosuppressed patients with other acute respiratory diseases but no detectable P. carinii in BAL by immunofluorescence ($n = 64$) 1986–89 were used as controls. Patients with PCP within 6 months before the registered episode. Clinically or laboratory suspected – but not confirmed – PCP episodes were excluded from the study.

Patients with PCP

66 AIDS patients with 83 episodes of PCP (63 men, 3 women, age 23–74 years, mean age 41) and 39 non-HIV patients with PCP (17 men, 22 women, age 7–73 years, mean age 50) fulfilled the inclusion criteria (Table I). The non-HIV patients included organ transplant recipients ($n = 23$), patients with lymphoma or leukaemia ($n = 7$), chronic alcohol abusers ($n = 2$), patients receiving immunosuppressive drugs for breast cancer ($n = 2$), brain tumour ($n = 2$), Wegeners granulomatosis ($n = 1$), haemolytic anaemia ($n = 1$) and rheumatoid arthritis ($n = 1$).

Patients with other respiratory infections (non-PCP)

PCP was not clinically diagnosed nor was P. carinii detected by bronchoscopy in 12 AIDS patients (11 men, 1 woman, age 25–59 years, mean age 38) or in 52 immunosuppressed non-HIV patients (28 men, 24 women; age 18–77 years, mean age 49) with respiratory symptoms (Table I). The non-HIV patients comprised transplant recipients ($n = 22$), patients with lymphoma or leukaemia ($n = 17$), myelodysplastic syndrome ($n = 2$), chronic alcohol abuse ($n = 2$), patients receiving high doses of steroids and/or cytostatic drugs due to tumours or various disorders; lung cancer ($n = 2$), Wegener's granulomatosis ($n = 1$), Systemic lupus erythematosus nephritis ($n = 2$), vasculitis ($n = 1$), diabetes and sarcoidosis ($n = 1$), sarcoidosis ($n = 1$) and pulmonary fibrosis with chronic bronchitis ($n = 1$).

Serum samples from patients: Serum 1: The first serum sample was collected during clinical symptoms (within 30 days before and 7 days after diagnostic bronchoscopy or sputum sampling). *Serum 2:* A second serum sample was collected some 8–31 days after serum 1 (or 8–31 days after diagnostic respiratory sampling when serum 1 was missing). *Paired serum samples:* Serum 1 and serum 2 collected within an 8–31-day interval.

Table I. *Numbers of episodes of P. carinii pneumonia (PCP) and other respiratory infections (non-PCP) in each patient group evaluated for antibodies to P. carinii*

	No. of episodes				
	AIDS		Otherwise immunosuppressed		Immuno-competent
	PCP ($n = 66$)	Non-PCP ($n = 12$)	PCP ($n = 39$)	Non-PCP ($n = 52$)	Non-PCP ($n = 55$)
Serum 1	77	12	34	48	55
Serum 2	42	3	27	22	55
Paired sera	36	3	22	18	55

Controls with respiratory symptoms

Paired sera were obtained from 55 immunocompetent patients (Table I) with X-ray-verified pneumonia (26 men, 29 women, age 12–93 years, mean age 55). The first serum was collected 1–14 days and the second serum 15–73 days after the first day of symptoms. The interval between the 2 samples was 12–68 days. The etiologies of the pneumonias were: Streptococcus pneumoniae ($n = 14$), Mycoplasma pneumoniae ($n = 11$), Chlamydia species ($n = 3$), Haemophilus influenzae ($n = 4$), Influenza virus ($n = 2$), a combination of 1–3 of these agents ($n = 8$) and pneumonia of unknown origin ($n = 12$).

Controls with no respiratory symptoms

Routine sera were obtained from HIV antibody-positive patients with persistent lymphadenopathy (PGL) (80 men, age 20–48 years). A matched control for the serum 1 from the non-HIV PCP patients was selected: A serum sample was obtained 8 weeks–8 months (mean 3.6 months) after transplantation from transplant recipients ($n = 21$) matched for grafts, age (<20, 20–39, 40–59, >60 years) and immunosuppression (rejection treatment). Sera were obtained as part of the routine medical care from adult patients (>40 years old) with leukaemia ($n = 6$), lymphoma ($n = 6$), and breast cancer ($n = 4$). Stored serum samples were analysed from 127 randomly selected healthy 18-year-old boys ($n = 84$) and girls ($n = 43$).

Control antisera to fungi. Polyclonal rabbit or goat antisera to Candida albicans, Aspergillus fumigatus, Cryptococcus neoformans and Histoplasma capsulatum. Patients antisera to Candida albicans and Aspergillus fumigatus.

Assay for P. carinii detection. P. carinii was demonstrated by microscopy after silver-methenamine staining (21) or indirect immunofluorescence using monoclonal 3F6 as described previously (22, 4).

Assay for antibodies to P. carinii

Paraffin sections of human autopsy lung tissue from individuals with PCP were used as antigen in an indirect immunofluorescence assay (23, 19, 24). The tissue was fixed in Rossman's fixative and embedded in paraffin wax. Paraffin sections (μm) on microscopic slides were deparaffinized in xylene, rehydrated in ethanol, and incubated with 50 μl of patients serum in 2-fold serial dilutions starting from 1/10. Bound antibodies to P. carinii were detected with sheep antihuman immunoglobulin conjugated to fluorescein isothiocyanate (fluorescein:protein molar ratio 3.4, NBL). Evans' blue 1/10,000 was used as counter stain. The slides were examined under a fluorescence microscope. A bright yellow-green fluorescence of P. carinii cysts filling up the alveoli was considered positive. A seroconversion or a 4-fold titre increase was considered as a significant antibody response in paired serum samples.

Quantitation of serum immunoglobulins. Serum immunoglobulin levels were measured by the radial immunodiffusion method.

Assay for antibodies to measles. To control the specificity of reactive antibodies in paired sera we looked for presence of polyclonal activation represented by measles antibodies which are present in the vast majority of the Swedish population. Anti-measles antibodies were determined by the EIA using purified measles virus coated on solid phase microtitre plates and incubated with serial dilutions of patient's serum essentially as described (25). Serum sample dilutions giving absorbance values over 0.2 were regarded as positive.

Statistics. The frequencies of serum antibodies to P. carinii among different groups were compared by the χ^2-test.

RESULTS

During the acute stage of PCP, anti-P. carinii antibodies were found in 17% (13/77) of AIDS patients, versus 24% (8/34) of non-HIV patients (N.S.) (Table II). At this stage no significant difference was found between PCP and non-PCP patients. Detectable antibodies to P. carinii were more frequent in the HIV-positive and the otherwise immunosuppressed patients without PCP (16%) (29/177) as compared with the immunocompetent controls (3%) (6/182) ($\chi_1^2 = 22.79$, $p < 0.001$) (Fig. 1).

Table II. *Seropositivity to P. carinii in HIV and other immunosuppressed patients with P. carinii pneumonia (PCP) compared with patients with other respiratory diseases (non-PCP)*

	HIV		Other immunosuppressed	
	PCP	Non-PCP	PCP	Non-PCP
Serum 1	17% (13/77)	17% (2/12)	24% (8/34)	16% (8/48)
Serum 2	17% (7/42)	(0/3)[a]	56% (15/27)	18% (4/22)

[a] Only 3 sera available.

In the patients with PCP, when a second serum sample was obtained 8–31 days later, the seropositivity in the non-HIV immunosuppressed patients had increased to 56% (15/27) (95% c.i.: 37–74%) whereas in the AIDS patients it remained at 17% (7/42) ($\chi_1^2 = 11.44$, $p < 0.001$). When studying individual paired serum samples in PCP patients, almost half the non-HIV patients (45%) (10/22) (95% c.i.: 24–66%) but only 1 AIDS patient (3%) (1/36) were found to have seroconverted, or showed a 4-fold increase in titres ($\chi_1^2 = 16.18$, $p < 0.001$) (Table III). In individuals with bacterial, viral or non-specific pneumonia or other respiratory disorder, a titre increase was observed in only 1/18 (6%) immunosuppressed non-HIV patients and 1/55 (2%) immunocompetent subjects. A titre decrease was even observed in 3/18 non-HIV patients with other respiratory disorders. There was no additional seroconversion or titre increase in sera obtained after 1–3 months in 22 AIDS PCP patients or in 14 non-HIV PCP patients.

The antibody titres were generally low (range 10–320), with 40 being the most prevalent positive titre found (38%) (mean titre 36.22). The distribution of titres did not differ between the study groups.

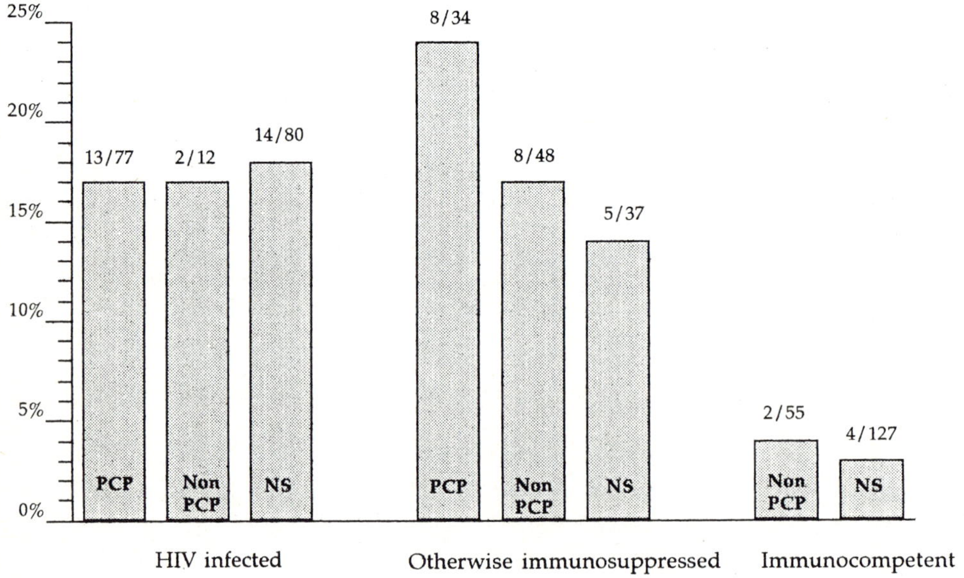

Fig. 1. Seropositivity (%) to P. carinii in serum 1 in the HIV-infected and otherwise immunosuppressed groups, compared with the immunocompetent controls. Non-PCP: respiratory disorder other than PCP. NS: No respiratory symptoms.

Table III. *Humoral response to P. carinii pneumonia as defined by seroconversion or 4-fold rise in titre in HIV and other immunosuppressed patients (non-HIV)*

	Immunocompetent control	Immunosuppressed	
		HIV	Non-HIV
P. carinii pneumonia	–	3% (1/36)	45% (10/22)
Other respiratory disease	2% (1/55)	(0/3)[a]	6% (1/18)

[a] Only 3 sera available.

Table IV. *Comparison of antibody titres to P. carinii, measles and total IgG in paired sera from 7 immunosuppressed patients with an apparent humoral response to confirmed PCP*

Patient no.	P. carinii titre		IgG		Measles titre	
	1st	2nd	1st	2nd	1st	2nd
1	neg	40	4.6	4.9	4,400	5,800
2	40	160	6.5	6.5	9,900	5,800
3	neg	40	8.9	7.7	5,800	9,900
4	neg	40	9.8	8.9	76,000	58,000
5	neg	40	7.3	11.7	47,000	37,500
6	neg	40	9.8	12.6	83,000	99,000
7	neg	40	5.4	16.6[a]	11,000	34,000[a]

[a] Possible polyclonal activation.

In 14 patients, seroreactivity to P. carinii had been routinely determined 1–10 months before the observed PCP episode. A significant rise in titre in serum 1 vis-à-vis the previous titre was seen in all of 4 non-HIV patients versus none of 10 AIDS patients. No patient showed a reduction in titre.

To investigate the possible role of polyclonal reactivation, e.g. due to withdrawal of immunosuppressive therapy, paired samples from the first 7 PCP patients in whom a titre rise or seroconversion occurred were checked for total IgG and IgG antibodies to measles. Polyclonal activation was considered in only 1 of the patients (Table IV). Furthermore, control antisera to Candida albicans, Aspergillus fumigatus, Histoplasma capsulatum, and Cryptococcus neoformans showed no cross-reaction to P. carinii at the lowest serum dilution tested (1/10).

DISCUSSION

Seroreactivity to P. carinii was found in only 3% of healthy adults. This may reflect a truly low seroprevalence in the population, or a low sensitivity of the test. In the literature, the reported seroprevalences have shown a wide variation even within a single country (England, USA). Low seroprevalences, 0–17% in healthy population groups, as measured by immunofluorescence, have been reported in the USA, Scotland and Japan, using human or rat P. carinii cysts as antigen (26, 15, 12, 27, 28). Higher seroprevalences, 57–96%, were reported from the UK and The Netherlands, using human or rat P. carinii cysts or sections of P. carinii infected lung tissue as antigen in immunofluorescence (18, 19, 29). Rat-derived antigen applied in EIA or immunoblotting assays have resulted in seroprevalences of 70–100% in

Britain, Gambia and USA (5, 16, 30). The various results may reflect differences between populations, but may also be due to the various sources of antigens (rat and human), as well as different preparation methods and assays used. Some of the antigens recognized by antibodies in other assays may have been destroyed by the antigen preparation in the picric acid-formol fixation used in this study.

The specificities of the different serological assays may be questioned. However, a number of specificity tests have suggested the immunoblotting assays to be truly P. carinii specific (31, 16). The specificity of our assay is supported by the fact that the fixation procedure leaves mainly carbohydrates intact (32) and that carbohydrates are the major P. carinii antigens according to cytochemical staining and immunoblotting studies (23, 33). The specificity of the immunofluorescence test is further supported by the results discussed below.

Immunosuppressed individuals without PCP were significantly more often positive (16%) than were healthy ones (3%). A similar difference has been reported in a previous study using immunofluorescence (28). In contrast, in another study with immunoblotting, all healthy blood donors were positive, versus only 71% of immunosuppressed patients (16). The antibodies we found in the immunosuppressed patients may represent a true humoral response to a latent or subclinical P. carinii infection. However, polyclonal antibody production, which is known to occur in HIV patients, or passive transfer of antibodies by transfusions, or antirejection treatment using polyclonal anti thymocyte/lymphocyte globulins in transplant recipients cannot be excluded.

In 111 verified episodes of PCP seroprevalence in the early acute phase did not differ from that of the non-PCP patients or the controls (Fig. 1). However, in the convalescent sera, 56% of the non-HIV patients with confirmed PCP proved seropositive, which was significantly more than in the other groups tested and which is comparable to previous studies where antibodies were detected in 44–70% (26, 15, 19, 28). When studying individual responses in paired sera, significant antibody responses to P. carinii were detected in only 1 AIDS patient, in contrast to almost half of the non-HIV immunosuppressed patients. The detected humoral responses seem to be due to stimulation by P. carinii rather than to polyclonal reactivation, since only 1/7 of responding patients showed a significant increase in IgG levels and measles titres. AIDS patients' failure to respond to P. carinii corresponds to their inability to respond to various other protozoa or to viruses, fungi and bacteria (17, 34–36). Paired sera have previously been examined in a few studies. Seroconversion or a rise in titres after confirmed PCP was found in 4/10 non-HIV patients (19), in 5/15 combined non-HIV and AIDS patients (28), in 2/26 AIDS patients (37) and recently in 10/20 AIDS patients (38). Other studies on serial samples from HIV patients with PCP have shown a significant loss of IgG (29) or a selective loss of IgM class (not IgG or IgA) antibodies to P. carinii (39, 37) prior to the PCP, or else inconclusive results (12). However, using Western blots, Peglow et al. (16) showed that AIDS patients over a longer period of time (months to year) and with recurrent infections can develop antibodies to a 40 kD band which may not be detectable by immunofluorescence. The 8–31-day interval between paired samples was chosen at the beginning of the study on the basis of 2 previous studies in humans recording maximum titres at 10–14 days and within 1 month respectively (19, 27), and one study in mice in which maximum titres were found 2–3 weeks after experimental infection (40). The interval chosen seems to have been appropriate, since no additional rise in titres were seen up to 3 months after the acute infection.

Absence of a detectable immune response in many of the PCP patients in our study could have been due not only to a possible low sensitivity of the test, but also to a true unresponsiveness in the patients due to continuous heavy immunosuppression. Experimental P. carinii infection in rats has shown the antibody response to be low during immunosuppression but high titres develop within 6–8 weeks after withdrawal of steroids (13).

We conclude that serology, using picric acid and formalin-fixed paraffinized sections of P. carinii-infected human lung tissue as antigen in an immunofluorescence test, seems to have a high specificity even if it lacks in sensitivity. The assay can support the clinical PCP diagnosis in immunosuppressed patients other than AIDS, but may not be of diagnostic value in the early acute stage of PCP. The clinical value of P. carinii serology can probably be further improved using more sensitive assays based on specific defined antigens.

ACKNOWLEDGEMENTS

We gratefully acknowledge the helpful suggestions and comments of Inger Julander, Jonas Jonsson, Eva Fridell, and Michael Willcox; the technical assistance of Kerstin Helmer, Aija Lassfolk, and Marjatta Karlsson; the generous help in search of sera of Elisabeth Eklund, Margit Halvarsson and Ann-Margret Pettersson; and the kind and efficient cooperation of Håkan Mellstedt, Madeleine von Sydow, Aud Krook, Åsa Bergström and Monica Nyström.

REFERENCES

1. Broaddus C, Dake MD, Stulbarg MS, Blumenfeld W, Hadley WK, Golden JA, Hopewell PC. Bronchoalveolar lavage and transbronchial biopsy for the diagnosis of pulmonary infections in the acquired immunodeficiency syndrome. Ann Intern Med 102: 747–752, 1985.
2. Bigby TD, Margolskee D, Curtis JL, Michael PF, Sheppard D, Hadley WK, Hopewell PC. The usefulness of induced sputum in the diagnosis of Pneumocystis carinii pneumonia in patients with the acquired immunodeficiency syndrome. Am Rev Respir Dis 133: 515–518, 1986.
3. Leigh TR, Hume C, Gazzard B, Parsons P, Husain OAN, Collins JV. Sputum induction for diagnosis of Pneumocystis carinii pneumonia. Lancet 2: 205–206, 1989.
4. Elvin KM, Björkman A, Linder E, Heurlin N, Hjerpe A. Pneumocystis carinii pneumonia: detection of parasites in sputum and bronchoalveolar lavage fluid by monoclonal antibodies. BMJ 297: 381–384, 1988.
5. Kovacs JA, Ng VL, Masur H, Leoung G, Hadley WK, Evans G, Lane HC, Ognibene FP, Shelhamer J, Parrillo JE, Gill VJ. Diagnosis of Pneumocystis carinii pneumonia: improved detection in sputum with use of monoclonal antibodies. N Engl J Med 318: 589–593, 1988.
6. Ng VL, Virani NA, Chaisson RE, Yajko DM, Sphar HT, Cabrian K, Rollins N, Charache P, Krieger M, Hadley WK, Hopewell PC. Rapid detection of Pneumocystis carinii using a direct fluorescent monoclonal antibody stain. J Clin Microbiol 28: 2228–2233, 1990.
7. Pifer LL, Hughes WT, Stagno S, Woods D. Pneumocystis carinii infection: evidence for high prevalence in normal and immunosuppressed children. Pediatrics 61: 35–41, 1978.
8. Tanabe K, Fuchimoto M, Egawa K, Nakamura Y. Use of Pneumocystis carinii genomic DNA clones for DNA hybridization analysis of infected human lungs. J Infect Dis 157: 593–596, 1988.
9. Meyers JD, Pifer LL, Sale GE, Thomas ED. The value of Pneumocystis carinii antibody and antigen detection for diagnosis of Pneumocystis carinii pneumonia after marrow transplantation. Am Rev Respir Dis 120: 1283–1287, 1979.
10. Milder JE, Walzer PD, Coonrod JD, Rutledge ME. Comparison of histological and immunological techniques for detection of Pneumocystis carinii in rat bronchial lavage fluid. J Clin Microbiol 11: 409–417, 1980.
11. Maddison SE, Hayer GV, Slemenda SB, Norman LG, Ivey MH. Detection of specific antibody by enzyme-linked immunosorbent assay and antigenemia by counterimmunoelectrophoresis in humans infected with Pneumocystis carinii. J Clin Microbiol 15: 1036–1043, 1982.
12. Maddison SE, Walls KW, Haverkos HW, Juranek DD. Evaluation of serologic tests for Pneumocystis carinii antibody and antigenemia in patients with acquired imunodeficiency syndrome. Diagn Microbiol Infect Dis 2: 69–73, 1984.
13. Walzer PD, Rutledge ME. Humoral immunity in experimental Pneumocystis carinii infection. Serum and bronchial lavage fluid antibody response in rats. J Lab Clin Med 97: 820–833, 1981.
14. Walzer PD, Kim CK, Linke MJ, Pogue CL, Huerkamp MJ, Chrisp CE, Lerro AV, Wixson SK, Hall E, Shultz LD. Outbreaks of Pneumocystis carinii pneumonica in colonies of immunodeficient mice. Infect Immun 57: 62–70, 1989.
15. Normal L, Kagan IG. Some observations on the serology of Pneumocystis carinii infections in the United States. Infect Immun 8: 317–321, 1973.
16. Peglow SL, Smulian AG, Linke MJ, Pogue CL, Nurre S, Crisler J, Phair J, Gold JW, Armstrong D, Walzer PD. Serologic responses to Pneumocystis carinii antigens in health and disease. J Infect Dis 161: 296–306, 1990.

17. Roberts CJ. Coccidiodomycosis in Acquired Immune Deficiency Syndrome. Am J Med 76: 734–736, 1984.
18. Meuwissen JHET, Tauber I, Leeuwenberg ADEM, Beckers PJA, Sieben M. Parasitologic and serologic observations of infection with Pneumocystis in humans. J Infect Dis 136: 43–49, 1977.
19. Shepherd V, Jameson B, Knowles GK. Pneumocystis carinii pneumonitis: a serological study. J Clin Pathol 32: 773–777, 1979.
20. Hofmann B, Ødum N, Platz P, Ryder LP, Svejgaard A, Nielsen PB, Holten-Andersen W, Gerstoft J, Nielsen JE, Mojon M. Humoral responses to Pneumocystis carinii in patients with acquired immunodeficiency syndrome and in immunocompromised homosexual men. J Infect Dis 152: 838–840, 1985.
21. Musto L, Flanigan M, Elbadawi A. Ten-minute silver stain for Pneumocystis carinii and fungi in tissue sections. Arch Pathol Lab Med 106: 292–294, 1982.
22. Linder E, Lundin, L, Vorma H. Detection of Pneumocystis carinii in lung-derived samples using monoclonal antibodies to an 82 kDa parasite component. J Immunol Methods 98: 57–62, 1987.
23. Brzosko WJ, Nowoslawski A. Identification of Pneumocystis carinii antigens in tissues. Bulletin de l'Académie Polonaise des Sciences 13: 49–54, 1965.
24. Gerrard MP, Eden OB, Jameson B, Craft W. Serological study of Pneumocystis carinii infection in the absence of immunosuppression. Arch Dis Child 62: 177–179, 1987.
25. Pauksen K, Duraj V, Ljungman P, Sjölin J, Öberg G, Lönnerholm G, Fridell E, Smedmyr B, Simonsson B. Immunity and immunization against measles, rubella and mumps in patients after autologous bone marrow transplantation. Bone Marrow Transplantation 9: 427–432, 1992.
26. Norman L, Kagan IG. A preliminary report of an indirect fluorescent antibody test for detecting antibodies to cysts of Pneumocystis carinii in human sera. Am J Clin Pathol 58: 170–176, 1972.
27. Tanabe K, Furuta T, Ueda K, Tanaka H, Shimada K. Serological observations of Pneumocystis carinii infection in humans. J Clin Microbiol 22: 1058–1060, 1985.
28. Chatterton JMW, Joss AW, Williams H, Ho-Yen DO. Pneumocystis carinii antibody testing. J Clin Pathol 42: 865–868, 1989.
29. Burns SM, Read JA, Yap PL, Brettle RP. Reduced concentrations of IgG antibodies to Pneumocystis carinii in HIV-infected patients during active Pneumocystis carinii infection and the possibility of passive immunisation. J Infect 20: 33–39, 1990.
30. Wakefield AE, Stewart TJ, Moxon ER, Marsh K, Hopkin JM. Infection with Pneumocystis carinii is prevalent in healthy Gambian children. Trans R Soc Trop Med Hyg 84: 800–802, 1990.
31. Kovacs JP, Halpern JL, Swan JC, Moss J, Parrillo JE, Masur H. Identification of antigens and antibodies specific for Pneumocystis carinii. Immunology 140: 2023–2031, 1988.
32. Nairn RC. Cytological and histological methods. In: R. C. Nairn, ed. Fluorescent protein tracing, 4th edn. London: Churchill Livingstone, 131–153, 1961.
33. Graves DC, Scott JN, Worley MA, Downs TD, Ivey MH. Analyses of rat pneumocystis carinii antigens recognized by human and rat antibodies by using western immunoblotting. Infect Immun 54: 96–103, 1986.
34. Carne CA, Weller JW, Briggs M, Pearce F, Adler MW, Tedder RS. Impaired responsiveness of homosexual men with HIV antibodies to plasma derived hepatitis B vaccine. BMJ 294: 866–868, 1987.
35. Janoff ED, Douglas JM, Gabriel JM, Blaser MJ, Davidson AJ, Cohn DL, Judson FN. Class-specific antibody response to pneumococcal capsular polysachharides in men infected with human immunodeficiency virus type 1. J Infect Dis 158: 983–990, 1988.
36. Janoff ED, Smith PD, Blaser MJ. Acute antibody responses to Giardia lamblia are depressed in patients with AIDS. J Infect Dis 157: 798–804, 1988.
37. Laursen AL, Andersen PL. Serum antibodies directed against Pneumocystis carinii in patients with AIDS. Immunology and Infectious Diseases 2: 275–280, 1992.
38. Lundgren B, Lundgren JD, Nielsen T, Mathiesen L, Nielsen JO, Kovačs JA. Antibody responses to A major Pneumocystis carinii antigen in human immunodeficiency virus-infected patients with and without Pneumocystis carinii pneumonia. J Infect Dis 165: 1151–1155, 1992.
39. Hofmann B, Nielsen PB, Ødum N, Gerstoft J, Platz P, Ryder LP, Poulsen A-G, Mathiesen L, Dickmeiss E, Norrild B, Andersen HK, Westergaard BF, Møller Nielsen C, Holten-Andersen W, Mojon M, Nielsen JO, Svejgaard A. Humoral and cellular responses to Pneumocystis carinii, CMV, and Herpes simplex in patients with AIDS and in controls. Scand J Infect Dis 20: 389–394, 1988.
40. Furuta T, Fujiwara K, Yamanouchi K, Ueda K. Detection of antibodies to Pneumocystis carinii by enzyme-linked immunosorbent assay in experimentally infected mice. J Parasitol 71: 522–523, 1985.

Scand J Infect Dis 26: 41–47, 1994

Clinical Significance of Neutrophil Functional Activity in HIV Infection

DMITRY GABRILOVICH, LARISA IVANOVA, LIDIA SEREBROVSKAYA, GALINA SHEPELEVA and VADIM POKROVSKY

From the Laboratory of AIDS Epidemiology and Prevention, Central Institute of Epidemiology, Moscow, Russia

Functional activity of polymorphonuclear neutrophils (PMN) was tested in 63 HIV-1 infected patients. PMN chemiluminescence (CL) and intracellular enzyme activity were both depressed in patients at all stages of infection, though this depression was more pronounced in AIDS patients. We found no such depression when cells were incubated in the presence of autologous serum. PMN phagocytosis in the presence of serum was reduced in the early stage of HIV infection (LAS) but was in the normal range in AIDS patients. No differences in PMN functional activity between patients with LAS and those with dermatological disorders were found. The appearance of recurrent upper respiratory tract infection was associated with reduced PMN CL. The most pronounced changes in PMN activity were observed in patients with severe, recurrent bacterial pneumonia and Pneumocystis carinii pneumonia. A lower level of PMN activity was found in patients with infection progressing rapidly towards AIDS than in patients with a relatively stable course of infection. Thus, PMN CL may be regarded as a predictive factor for the progression of HIV infection.

D. Gabrilovich, MD, Antigen Presentation Group, Clinical Research Centre, Watford Road, Harrow, Middlesex, HA1 3UJ, England

INTRODUCTION

Polymophonuclear neutrophils (PMN), an important element of antibacterial defence, play an important role in immunoregulation. PMN produce highly reactive oxygen metabolites following appropriate stimulation which suppress the functional activity of lymphocytes (1–4). Moreover, the release of some cytokines by PMN was recently shown (5, 6). There is evidence that PMN may be involved in the pathogenesis of HIV infection (7, 8). Impairment of PMN activity may be an important factor facilitating various opportunistic infections in patients with HIV infection. However, the role of PMN in the development of various clinical manifestations of HIV infection is still unclear.

In this study we analysed the relationship between the PMN functional activity and the clinical manifestations of HIV infection, the duration of infection, and immunodeficiency. We found that the PMN activity was closely associated with disease progression.

MATERIALS AND METHODS

Patients

63 HIV-1-infected adults (22 females and 41 males, aged 18–44 years) were studied. All patients had antibodies to HIV, as determined by ELISA (Behringwerke AG, Marburg, Germany) and confirmed by Western blot (DuPont, Wilmington, DE). The suspected routes of infection were: homosexual intercourse (19 cases) and heterosexual intercourse (44 cases). Clinical data were evaluated according to the classification proposed by the Centres for Disease Control (CDC): 34 HIV-1-seropositive subjects with lymphoadenopathy syndrome (LAS) (class III); 21 with ARC (5 class IV subgroup A and 16 subgroup C, category C-2); 8 with AIDS (5 class IV subgroup C; category C-1, and 3-subgroup D). Eight patients with AIDS and 7 patients with ARC were being treated with AZT (3'-azido-3' deoxythimidine) at the time of the study. Five patients with AIDS and 6 with ARC were given antibacterial therapy. 20 clinically healthy HIV-seronegative donors (8 females and 12 males, aged 18–32) served as a control group. Seven HIV-seronegative healthy homosexuals were included in the other control group.

 ISSN 0036-5548

Granulocyte isolation

PMN were isolated from 10 ml heparinized blood by centrifugation in a double gradient of Percoll having specific weights of 1.077 and 1.120. After 3 washing procedures the granulocytes were adjusted to 5×10^6/ml in phosphate-buffered saline solution (PBS).

Chemiluminescence of PMN

Chemiluminescence of PMN (PMN CL) was determined with a chemiluminometer "LKB Wallac 1251" (Sweden). Five different series of experiments were carried out. In the first, PMN (5×10^5 cells) were treated with luminol (2×10^{-6} M) (Sigma, St. Louis, MO, USA) without presense of autologous serum (CL). In the second, autologous sera (10% of final volume) were added to the reaction mixture (CL ser.). In the third and fourth series, 10^{-7} M N-formyl-L-methionyl-L-leucyl-L-phenylalanine (FMLP) (Sigma) was used as a supplementary activator (CL st. and CL ser. st.). In these cases, PMN were pre-incubated with PBS or serum at 37°C for 30 min prior to stimulation by FMLP. In the fifth, non-opsonized particles of Candida albicans (5×10^5 cells) were used as stimulator (CLst. y.). Chemiluminescence was recorded for 30 min, and the maximum peak of CL was detected.

Assessment of phagocytosis by granulocytes

Assay of phagocytosis was performed as described (9). To assess the number of PMN with engulfed yeast cells, FITC-labelled yeast cells (C. albicans) (5×10^5 cells) were incubated with PMN (10^5 cells) with or without autologous serum (Phag. or Phag. ser.) for 1 h at 37°C. The number of PMNs showing green fluorescence (i.e. phagocytosing cells) was determined in the FL1 channel (FITC filter transmission 530 ± 30 nm) of a FACScan flow cytometer (Becton Dickinson, Mountain View, CA, USA). FACScan gates were set around the PMN cluster in a cytogram, simultaneously evaluating both forward and right-angle diffraction properties of the cell passing through the focused laser beam.

To determine the proportion of yeast cells killed after phagocytosis by granulocytes, 10^5 yeast cells were incubated with 10^5 PMN in presence of autologous serum (10% v/v) for 1 h at 37°C. Tubes containing yeast cells and serum – but without PMN – were used as a control. After this incubation, PMN were lysed with Triton X-100 (Serva). DNA released from the lysed granulocytes was removed with DNAse (Serva) and, after adding propidium iodide, the proportion of yeast cells showing red fluorescence (i.e. killed cells) was determined in the FL3 channel of the FACScan (red pass filter, transmission 650 ± 30 nm). Calculation of the killed yeast cells was performed using the following formula: % cells killed in test sample – % cells killed in control = % yeast cells killed.

Activity of intracellular enzymes in PMN

The activity of alkaline phosphatase (AP) in neutrophils was estimated using naphthol-AS-MX-phosphate (Serva), non-specific esterase (EST) using naphthol-AS-acetate (Serva). Myeloperoxidase activity was measured according to Graham-Knoll. Glycogen content was determined by the periodic acid-Shiff reaction. All cytochemical studies were carried out as described in (10). The cytochemical coefficient (CC) was determined as described by Kaplow (11). It is defined as $CC = 100 \times (0 \times N_0 + 1 \times N_1 + 2 \times N_2 + 3 \times N_3)/(N_0 + N_1 + N_2 + N_3)$,where N_0 is the number of cells lacking enzyme activity, N_1 is the number of cells containing single enzyme-positive granules, N_2 is the number of cells with a considerable number of enzyme-positive granules (covering approximately half the cytoplasm), and N_3 is the number of cells with considerable enzyme content (covering the entire cytoplasm).

Assay of lymphocyte subsets

Two-colour FACS analysis was performed with the Becton Dickinson flow cytometer FACScan using the whole-blood lysis procedure. Monoclonal antibody was purchased from Becton Dickinson, including Simultest Control (mouse IgG1-FITC, mouse IgG2-PE for non-specific mouse Ig binding), anti-Leu-3a (CD4)-FITC, anti-Leu-2a (CD8)-PE, anti-Leu-4 (CD3)-FITC, anti-Leu-12 (CD19)-PE, anti-HLA-DR-PE, anti-Leu-11c (CD16)-PE, and anti-Leu-19-PE.

The statistical analysis was performed using parametric and non-parametric methods on an IBM PC by means of the "Statgrafics" program (CTSC Inc., USA). Correlation analysis was performed using a coefficient of Spearman's rank correlation (Rs).

RESULTS

Relationship between PMN functional activity and stage of HIV infection

The functional activity of PMN was shown to be considerably depressed in patients with HIV

Table I. *Indices of PMN functional activity in patients with HIV infection (average ± stand. dev.)*

Indices	Controls $n = 20$	LAS $n = 34$	ARC $n = 21$	AIDS $n = 8$
Polymorphonuclear chemoluminescence, mV (PMN-CL)	861.6±155.7	215.3±241.5[a]	182.3±217.3[a]	134.8±132.2[a]
PMN-CL stimulated with f MLP, mV	2520.1±362.7	943.2±929.8[a]	708.5±790.9[a]	392.2±414.7[a]
PMN-CL stimulated with yeast cells, mV	1485.6±342.7	721.2±411.3[a]	442.4±292.7[a]	227.7±161.9[a]
PMN-CL with autologous serum, mV	261.2±98.6	193.3±189.2	193.6±180.8	640.7±681.1
Ditto stimulated with f MLP, mV	500.6±122.7	263.5±233.8	338.4±365.5	856.0±387.5
PMN phagocytosis, %	40.3±6.2	37.2±17.2	40.3±20.7	37.7±18.7
Ditto with autologous serum, %	39.1±7.1	16.6±9.9[a]	28.5±14.4	43.7±5.5
PMN killing of Candida cells, %	25.2±2.7	14.3±9.2[a]	13.3±6.4[a]	8.0±1.0[a]
Myeloperoxidase, u	196.7±8.9	115.9±36.4[a]	104.2±27.6[a]	119.7±68.5[a]
Alkaline phosphatase, u	119.1±11.0	52.3±18.0[a]	50.0±13.8[a]	50.3±20.4[a]
Esterase, u	139.1±8.1	90.3±19.1[a]	94.6±19.7[a]	85.3±11.2[a]
Glycogen, u	221.2±12.3	178.9±29.6[a]	186.6±16.8[a]	189.7±27.9[a]

[a] = $p < 0.05$.

infection when cells were incubated without autologous serum (Table I). We found no statistically significant differences in PMN activity between patients at different stages of infection, although a tendency to deeper suppression in patients with AIDS was evident. No depression in PMN CL was found when cells were incubated in presence of autologous serum. Moreover, enhanced PMN CL was found in AIDS patients.

In order to examine the association between sexual behaviour and PMN activity, we have studied groups of healthy homosexual and heterosexual men and groups of HIV-infected homosexuals and heterosexuals. The latter 2 groups were formed only of patients with asymptomatic HIV-infection (LAS) in order to avoid the influence of other factors on PMN activity. No differences in PMN activity between groups of homosexuals and heterosexuals were found (data not shown).

PMN functional activity in patients with different clinical manifestations of HIV infection

Patients with symptomatic infection were divided into 4 groups according to main clinical symptoms of HIV infection. The first group was formed of patients with only various minor dermatological disorders (seborrheic dermatitis, folliculitis, pruritis, fungal nail infection, recurrent oral ulceration); patients with oral candidiasis formed the second group, patients with recurrent upper respiratory tract infection, bronchitis and non-disseminated herpes zoster comprised the third group; and patients with severe recurrent bacterial pneumonia and Pneumocystis carinii pneumonia formed the fourth group. We found no differences in PMN functional activity between patients with LAS and those from the first and second groups (patients with minor dermatological disorders and oral candidia) (data not shown). PMN killing was markedly reduced in patients with bacterial pneumonia (data not shown). Identical results were obtained when testing PMN CL (Fig. 1). In the presence of autologous serum, enhanced PMN CL was obtained from patients in this group. The same tendency was found in PMN phagocyte activity. No difference was evident in the activity of intracellular enzymes, between patients with different clinical manifestations of HIV infection.

We performed an analysis of the relationship between the approximate duration of HIV infection and PMN functional activity. Since the level of PMN activity was linked with clinical manifestations of infection, we analysed data from patients with asymptomatic HIV infection.

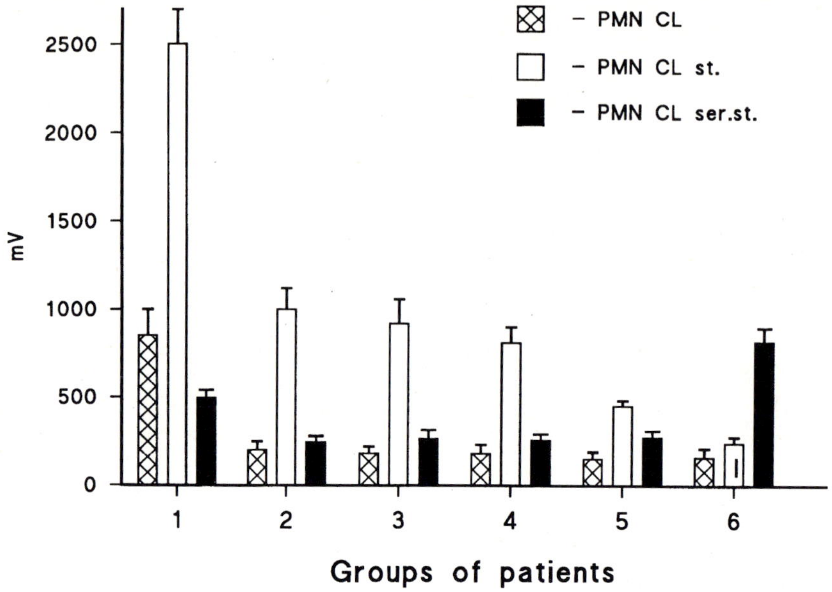

Fig. 1. Relationship between PMN activity and clinical manifestations of HIV infection.
Groups of patients:
1 – healthy donors ($n=20$);
2 – patients with lymphoadenopathy syndrome ($n=34$);
3 – patients with minor dermatological disorders ($n=8$);
4 – patients with oral candidiasis ($n=6$);
5 – patients with recurrent upper respiratory tract infection ($n=6$);
6 – patients with recurrent bacterial pneumonia, or with Pneumocystis carinii pneumonia ($n=6$).
All results are expressed as average ± standard error.

The date of the first HIV-positive blood sample was chosen as the starting point. Patients with a stable course of HIV infection also had a stable level of PMN functional activity over the first 5 years (data not shown). The initial level of PMN activity was found to be related to the progression of HIV infection. We compared the values of PMN activity in 2 groups of patients with LAS. The first group was composed of patients with symptomatic infection developing within a year after testing. The second was composed of patients with a stable course of

Table II. *PMN functional activity in patients with differing progression of HIV infection (average ± SD)*
All patients had LAS at the moment of testing.

Indices	Control $n=20$	Group 1[a] $n=8$	Group 2[b] $n=14$	p
PMN-CL, mV	861.6±155.7	134.8±116.5	368.6±145.6	< 0.05
PMN-CL with f MLP, mV	2520.1±362.7	657.8±492.1	1524.9±512.4	< 0.05
PMN-CL with serum, mV	261.2±98.6	144.2±133.1	359.8±126.9	< 0.05
PMN-CL with serum and f MLP, mV	500.6±122.7	175.4±125.9	422.6±166.8	< 0.05
Myeloperoxidase, u	196.7±8.9	107.5±23.9	130.2±18.4	< 0.05

[a]Patients with development of symptomatic HIV infection over the year after testing.
[b]Patients with stable course of HIV infection.

Table III. *Relationship between the level of some immunological parameters and PMN functional activity*

Immunological indices [a]		PMN-CL with f MLP	PMN-CL with serum and f MLP
	< 300/μl ($n=23$)	366.8±146.1[b,c]	259.1±114.5[c]
CD4 cells	300–500/μl ($n=16$)	1431.3±610.4	419.8±196.9
normal level[b]	> 500/μl ($n=24$)	1187.9±690.2	392.8±46.9
	< 0.6 ($n=42$)	713.8±534.6[c]	287.5±195.3
CD4/8	0.6–1.0 ($n=12$)	1300.5±497.4	304.4±126.7
normal level	> 1.0 ($n=9$)	1412.3±523.5	327.8±211.3

[a]Average ± S.D.
[b]Values of PMN-CL in patients with normal level of immunological indices.
[c] $= p < 0.05$.

infection. Patients from the first group had significantly lower levels of PMN CL and activity of MP than patients from second group (Table II).

Patients with severe immunodeficiency (concentration of $CD4^+$ cells < 300 cells/μl and CD4/8 ratio < 0.6) had significantly lower values of stimulated PMN CL than patients with a normal number of CD4 cells and CD4/8 ratio (Table III). No statistically significant correlation has been found between neutropenia and impairment of PMN functional activity.

DISCUSSION

This study shows that PMN functional activity (phagocytosis, bactericidal activity, superoxide anion production and activity of intracellular enzymes) is reduced in patients with HIV infection. Impaired PMN functional activity in HIV patients has been demonstrated by several groups of researchers. PMN phagocytosis, bactericidal activity against Staphylococcus aureus and chemiluminescence of PMN have been reported to be depressed in patients with HIV infection (7, 12–14). Depressed PMN chemotaxis in patients with HIV infection has also been found (8, 14–16). On the other hand, Baldwin et al. found neutrophil superoxide generation, neutrophil antibody-dependent cell-mediated cytotoxicity, PMN phagocytosis and intracellular killing to be normal in most AIDS patients (17). Normal neutrophil superoxide anion release in HIV-infected patients was found by Nielsen et al. (18). A high level of PMN phagocytosis, oxidative burst and F-actin formation in patients with intraoral candidiasis and HIV infection was reported by Ryder et al. (19). Increased phagocytosis and generation of reactive oxygen products by neutrophils were shown recently by Bandres et al. (20). The nature of these contradictions is not clear. It can be explained by different clinical manifestations of HIV infection in the patients studied. For instance, both groups of researchers, Nielsen with co-workers (18) and Ellis with co-workers (13), studied patients with AIDS. However, the main clinical manifestation of AIDS in the first investigation was various opportunistic infections (17/18 patients). The main clinical feature of AIDS patients in the second study was Kaposi's sarcoma and only 33% of patients with AIDS and 18% with ARC had significant bacterial infections. Unfortunately, in some of the other papers there was no information about the clinical manifestation of HIV infection in patients.

The differences in experimental protocols used in these studies could be another possible explanation. All authors who reported on the decrease in PMN activity in patients with HIV infection used fractions of PMN which were free from autologous sera. However, in some studies on the enhancement of PMN activity, PMN were not serum-free. For instance, Bandres et al. (20) used non-separated peripheral blood cells to determine phagocytosis and oxidative burst of PMNs. Apparently the presence of autologous serum plays a crucial role in changes in PMN activity in HIV infection.

In this study we did not find significant changes in PMN CL when PMN were incubated with autologous serum. Moreover, enhanced PMN CL in the presence of autologous serum was observed in AIDS patients. These findings confirm data published by Ellis et al. (13), who reported that chemotaxis of control neutrophils incubated with serum from patients with AIDS or ARC was significantly greater than chemotaxis of neutrophils incubated with autologous serum. PMN from patients with AIDS had normal chemotaxis when incubated with autologous serum, whereas chemotaxis of a pure fraction of PMN was suppressed in those patients.

The role of serum in the impairment of PMN in patients with HIV infection has not yet been clarified. Previously we have reported enhanced PMN CL from healthy donors in the presence of sera from HIV-infected patients. We have obtained some data showing that this phenomenon is partly due to the influence of HIV antigens on PMN (21). Recently, augmentation of PMN CL from healthy donors by a fragment of HIV-1 was also shown (22). Augmentation of neutrophil superoxide anion release under the influence of serum may be mediated by various cytokines and soluble factors (23–26).

In our study, we have attempted to assess the relationship between the various clinical manifestations of HIV infection and PMN functional activity. No difference was found in PMN functional activity between groups of patients with LAS and dermatological disorders. This tallies with data obtained by Foppa et al. (8). These investigators did not find any differences in PMN activity between a group of patients with ARC, having no candida infection and a group of patients with candidiasis. The emergence of recurrent upper respiratory tract infection was linked with decreased PMN CL. The most pronounced changes in PMN activity (low level of intracellular killing of yeast cells, PMN CL and activity of esterase) were observed in patients with severe recurrent bacterial pneumonia, including Pneumocystis carinii pneumonia. Thus, deficiency in PMN functional activity may be closely associated with clinical manifestations of HIV infection.

When analysing these results, an important question should be answered, namely: what role does the treatment of patients with various medicines play in the effects described above? Our study did not give a definite answer to this question. However, we did not find any statistically significant differences between the group of patients with LAS (without medication) and AIDS patients (all had received AZT and some of them antibacterial treatment too). We also did not find any differences in PMN functional activity between groups of patients with ARC who received and those who did not receive antibacterial treatment (data not shown). All these data may constitute indirect evidence that AZT and antibacterial therapy do not have a significant influence on PMN functional activity in patients with HIV infection.

A lower level of PMN activity was found in infected patients rapidly progressing towards AIDS than in patients with a relatively stable course of infection. PMN chemiluminescence may be regarded as having a predictive value in estimating the progress of HIV infection.

REFERENCES

1. Shau H, Golub SH. Inhibition of lymphokine-activated killer- and natural killer-mediated cytotoxicities by neutropils. J Immunol 143: 1066–1072, 1989.
2. Zoschke DC, Staite ND. Suppression of human lymphocyte proliferation by activated neutrophils or H_2O_2: surviving cells have an altered T helper/T suppressor ratio and an increased resistance to secondary oxidant exposure. Clin Immunol Immunopathol 42: 160–170, 1987.
3. El-Hag A, Clark RA. Immunosuppression by activated human neutrophils. Dependence on the myeloperoxidase system. J Immunol 139: 2406–2413, 1987.
4. Gabrilovich DI, Shepeleva GK, Serebrovskaya LV, Avdeeva LA, Pokrovsky VV. Polymophonuclear neutrophils modify functional activity of lymphocyte and monocyte in HIV infection. Scand J Immunol 37: 459–467, 1993.

5. Djeu JY, Serbousek D, Blanchard DK. Release of tumor necrosis factor by polymorphonuclear leukocytes. Blood 76: 1405–1409, 1990.
6. Bazzoni F, Cassatella MA, Rossi F, Ceska M, Dewald B, Baggiolini M. Phagocytosing neutrophils produce and release high amounts of the neutrophil-activating peptide 1/interleukin 8. J Exp Med 173: 221–224, 1991.
7. Murphy PM, Lane HC, Fauci AS, Galli JI. Impairment of neutrophil bactericidal capacity in patients with AIDS. J Infect Dis 158: 627–630, 1988.
8. Foppa UC, Franzetti F, Negri C, Novati R, Cinque P, Privitera G, Farente F, Crocchiolo P, Lazzarin A. Role of PMN's candidicidal activity in the pathogenesis of AIDS-related systematic candidiasis. Boll Ist Sieroter Milan 66: 471–478, 1987.
9. Buschmann H, Winter M. Assesment of phagocytic activity of granulocytes using laser flow cytometry. J Immunol Meth 124: 231–234, 1989.
10. Hayhoe FGJ, Quaglino D. Haematological cytochemistry. Edinburgh: Churchill Livingstone, 1980.
11. Kaplow LS. A histochemical procedure for localization and evaluating leukocytes alkaline phosphatase activity in smears of blood and marrow. Blood 10: 1023–1029, 1955.
12. Stohr L, Altmeyer P, Sessler MJ, Scharrer I, Helm EB, Holzmann H. Chemiluminescence measurement in AIDS, lymphoadenopathy and hemophilia patients. Z Hautkr 60: 1214–1223, 1985.
13. Ellis M, Gupta S, Galant S, Hakim S, Van den Ven C, Toy C, Cairo MS. Impaired neutrophil function in patients with AIDS or AIDS-related complex: a comprehensive evaluation. J Infect Dis 158: 1268–1276, 1988.
14. Antonanci S, Jirillo E, Stasi D, De Mitrio V, La Via MF, Bonomo L. Immunoresponsiveness in hemophilia: lymphocyte- and phagocyte-mediated function. Diagn Clin Immunol 5: 318–325, 1988.
15. Ras GI, Anderson R, Lukey PT. Defective polymorphonuclear leukocyte migration in AIDS. S Afr Med J 68: 292–293, 1985.
16. Martin LS, Spira TJ, Orloff SL, Holman RC. Comparison of methods for assessing chemotaxis of monocytes and polymorphonuclear leukocytes isolated from patients with AIDS or AIDS-related conditions. J Leukoc Biol 44: 361–366, 1988.
17. Baldwin GC, Gasson JC, Quan SG, Fleischmann J, Weisbart R, Oette D, Mitsuyasi RT, Golde DW. Granulocyte-macrophage colony-stimulation factor enhances neutrophil function in acquired immunodeficiency syndrome patients. Proc Natl Acad Sci USA 85: 2763–2766, 1988.
18. Nielsen H, Kharazmi A, Faber V. Blood monocyte and neutrophil functions in the acquired immune deficiency syndrome. Scand J Immunol 24: 291–296, 1986.
19. Ryder MI, Winkler JR, Weinreb RN. Elevated phagocytosis, oxidative burst, and F-actin formation in PMNs from individuals with intraoral manifestation of HIV infection. J Acquir Immune Defic Syndr 1: 346–353, 1988.
20. Bandress JC, Trial J, Musher DM, Rossen RD. Increased phagocytosis and generation of reactive oxygen products by neutrophils and monocytes of men with stage I human immunodeficiency virus infection. J Infect Dis 168: 75–83, 1993.
21. Gabrilovich DI, Avdeeva LA, Serebrovskaya LV, Shepeleva GK, Suvorova ZK, Buravcova EV, Oganezov VK, Platonov AE, Habarova VV, Rosly IM, Pokrovsky VV. Impact of HIV positive sera on functional activity of polymorphonuclear neutrophils from healthy donors. Scand J Immunol 37: 159–164, 1993.
22. Gabrolovich DI, Kozhich AT, Rosly IM, Suvorova ZK, Ivanov VS, Moshnikov SA, Tchikin LD, Melikhov VI, Pokrovsky VV. The synthetic peptide from HIV increases functional activity of granulocytes in healthy subjects. AIDS 5: 889–892, 1991.
23. Kharazim A, Nielsen H, Rechnitzer C, Bendtzen K. Interleukin 6 primes human neutrophils and monocyte oxidative burst response. Immunol Lett 21: 177–182, 1989.
24. Shalaby MR, Aggarwal BB, Rinderknecht E, Svedersky LP, Finkle BS, Palladino MAJr. Activation of human polymorphonuclear neutrophil functions by interferon gamma and tumor necrosis factor. J Immunol 135: 2069–2074, 1985.
25. Djeu JI, Matsushima K, Oppenheim JJ, Shiotsuki K, Blanchard DK. Functional activation of human neutrophils by recombinant monocyte-derived neutrophil chemotactic factor/IL-8. J Immunol 44: 2205–2211, 1990.
26. Gabrilovich DI, Shepeleva GK, Serebrovskaya LV, Avdeeva LA, Suvorova ZK, Rosly IM, Oganezov VK, Saidov MZ, Panyutich AV, Pokrovsky VV. Mononuclear cells from HIV-infected patients produce factors which enhance functional activity of polymorphonuclear neutrophils from healthy subjects. Clin Exp Immunol 89: 663–667, 1992.

Scand J Infect Dis 26: 49–54, 1994

Safety of Alternating Ganciclovir and Foscarnet Maintenance Therapy in Human Immunodeficiency Virus (HIV)-related Cytomegalovirus Infections. An Open-labeled Pilot Study

MALTE PETERS[1], DIRK SCHÜRMANN[1], FRANK BERGMANN[1], THOMAS GRÜNEWALD[1], HARALD TIMM[2], HANS D. POHLE[1] and BERNHARD RUF[1]

From the [1]Department of Medicine, Rudolf Virchow University Hospital, Freie Universität Berlin, and the [2]Department of Virology, Robert Koch Institute, Berlin, Germany

In the treatment of cytomegalovirus (CMV) disease in patients with AIDS, a life-long suppression therapy following an induction therapy consisting of ganciclovir or foscarnet is essential. Due to drug-related toxicities, anti-CMV therapy frequently has to be discontinued. To determine whether toxicities and side effects may be reduced with an alternating combination therapy consisting of ganciclovir and foscarnet (ganciclovir: 5 mg/kg every other day; foscarnet: 120 mg/kg every other day), 10 AIDS patients with CMV disease received this maintenance therapy for a median time of 18.5 weeks (5–51 weeks). Side effects were reported from 5 patients (nausea 5, malaise/fatigue 2, penile ulcers 1). Hematological or renal toxicities were mild, 1-week discontinuation of therapy due to neutropenia was necessary in 1 patient. Progression of CMV disease was observed in 3 patients at 2, 6, and 30 weeks of maintenance therapy. Median relapse-free interval for all patients was 105 days. We conclude that combination therapy with ganciclovir and foscarnet can be used safely for induction and maintenance therapy. Therefore, this regimen should be assessed in further trials to evaluate safety, efficacy, and the development of resistance in comparison to ganciclovir or foscarnet monotherapy.

B. Ruf, MD, II. Department of Medicine, Rudolf Virchow University Hospital, Freie Universität Berlin, Augustenburger Platz 1, D-13353 Berlin, Germany

INTRODUCTION

Cytomegalovirus (CMV) infection is the most serious opportunistic viral infection in patients with AIDS (1). Almost all patients with AIDS are seropositive for CMV and active disease involves most commonly the retina, intestine, adrenal glands, the brain or the lungs, occurring late during the course of HIV infection (1).

Two drugs are currently available for the treatment of CMV disease: ganciclovir and foscarnet. Each drug is administered intravenously initially in high doses (induction therapy: usually 2–3 weeks) and then continuously in lower doses (maintenance therapy: life-long). Despite treatment, CMV retinitis has been reported to recur frequently in patients receiving maintenance therapy: in one study, the median time to progression of retinitis was 24.5 days in foscarnet-treated patients, and 42 days in ganciclovir-treated patients compared to 16 days for patients who did not receive maintenance therapy (2). In another trial, patients receiving ganciclovir maintenance therapy developed progression of retinitis at a median of 105 days compared to 47 days in patients who received induction therapy only (3).

Ganciclovir, a nucleoside analogue, inhibits CMV replication. Its main toxicity is related to myelosuppressive effects, causing neutropenia during chronic ganciclovir therapy in 30–40% of the patients (2), which limits its concomitant use with optimal doses of zidovudine (1). Moreover, ganciclovir seems to antagonize the anti-HIV activity of zidovudine and didanosine in vitro (4).

Foscarnet, a pyrophosphate analogue, inhibits not only the DNA polymerase of CMV and other herpes viruses, but, in contrast to ganciclovir, also the reverse transcriptase and the

 ISSN 0036-5548

replication of HIV in vitro (5) and in vivo (6). Its toxicity consist primarily of renal impairment and electrolyte disturbances. Although these toxic effects can be severe and life-threatening, there is little overlap with those of zidovudine, which makes it a candidate for simultaneous therapy. Indeed, foscarnet and zidovudine have synergistic activity against HIV in vitro (7), and there may be additive benefit of both drugs in vivo (8).

Since severe toxicities of both drugs frequently limit their use, alternative regimens have to be established to reduce the frequency of side effects. A combination therapy consisting of alternating ganciclovir and foscarnet in the maintenance treatment phase was administered to 10 AIDS patients with CMV disease in order to evaluate tolerance and safety of this regimen.

MATERIALS AND METHODS

Patients

11 consecutive white men diagnosed as having AIDS entered the study. The diagnosis of CMV colitis, esophagitis, and pharyngeal ulcer was documented by biopsy confirming the presence of giant cells with cytomegalic inclusion bodies. Patients with isolated CMV retinitis had typical retinal opacifications in the absence of any other cause and a positive CMV culture from at least one site within 4 weeks of entry. CMV encephalitis was diagnosed if altered mental status, personality changes, headaches, confusion or somnolence were present in the absence of any other causes typically affecting the central nervous system (CNS) in HIV infections (9). Patients were excluded if they had serum creatinine levels >2.0 mg/dl, absolute neutrophil counts $<0.7 \times 10^9$/l, levels of serum aspartate aminotransferase greater than 3 times the upper limits of normal, or had received previous anti-CMV therapy or concomitant zidovudine treatment.

Therapy

Combination induction therapy: 6 patients were treated with a 3-week induction therapy consisting of both ganciclovir (5 mg/kg twice daily) and foscarnet (60 mg/kg three times daily). **Ganciclovir induction therapy:** 5 patients received a 3-week induction therapy with ganciclovir only at 5 mg/kg twice daily. The decision as to whether patients received combination induction therapy or ganciclovir induction therapy was left to the discretion of the attending physicians in accordance with severe manifestations of CMV disease, i.e. macula-near retina lesions, severe life-threatening diarrhea, or severe encephalitis. Patients were hospitalized during induction therapy and observed mostly on an outpatient basis during maintenance therapy. All patients were switched to maintenance therapy consisting of ganciclovir 5 mg/kg every other day alternating with foscarnet 120 mg/kg every other day, which was planned to be administered lifelong.

Laboratory and clinical evaluation

Laboratory studies performed before therapy, every 3 days during induction therapy and once a week during maintenance therapy, included complete blood count with differential, platelet count, biochemistry profile, and a complete urinalysis with microscopy. Samples of urine and blood were cultured for CMV at study entry, at the end of the induction phase, and at 2-week intervals according to previously described methods (10). T-lymphocyte subsets were counted according to standard flow cytometry methods (11).

Patients were questioned daily during induction treatment and weekly during maintenance treatment for symptoms of headache, malaise, fatigue, nausea, anorexia, tremors, lethargy, frequency and consistency of stools, pain, and any other symptoms pertinent to their manifestations of CMV. Indirect ophthalmoscopy was performed at least once weekly during the study period. Cultures of urine and blood for virus culture was collected once a week.

Three categories of invasive CMV disease were present: retinitis, gastrointestinal disease, and encephalitis. Pneumonitis was not seen in the patients studied. Response to therapy for each organ system was defined as improvement, stabilization, or progression (12). For retinitis, improvement was considered to be present if there was at least 50% regression of the retinal lesions and if vision improved or did not deteriorate; stabilization was defined as no new retinal lesions and <50% regression and no deterioration in vision; progression was defined as progressive loss of vision in combination with new retinal lesions. For gastrointestinal disease, a patient was considered to have improved if there was at least a 50% decrease in the number of stools and increased consistency and firmness in the stool specimens; to have stabilized if there was a <50% decrease in the number of stools; to have progressed if no change or worsening in severity, frequency, or consistency of stools. The patient with pharyngitis responded rapidly to therapy; the initially present ulcer healed and finally disappeared. The patient with encephalitis had a rapidly improving course.

RESULTS

The median duration of maintenance therapy was 18.5 weeks (range, 5–51 weeks). Of the 11 patients, 5 had retinitis alone, 3 had gastrointestinal disease alone, 1 had pharyngeal ulcer only, 2 had multi-organ involvement (retinitis and colitis; colitis and encephalitis). The mean patient age was 33 years, the median CD4 cell count was 20/μl at entry. Concomitant AIDS-defining conditions are listed in Table I. One patient with retinitis developed an acute renal failure at day 9 of ganciclovir induction therapy with a rise of his creatinine level to 4.4 mg/dl, and was withdrawn from the study.

Induction phase

Clinical improvement was observed in 8/10 evaluable patients. Stabilization was achieved in 2 patients with retinitis, 1 receiving ganciclovir induction therapy, the other combination induction therapy. Blood and urine cultures at study entry were available from 9/10 patients, respectively, and were positive in all at the beginning of the study. Clearance of viremia and viruria was observed in 8/9 patients by the end of the induction period. In 1 patient, CMV was cultured repeatedly from his blood and urine during follow-up. However, he stayed free of relapse.

Maintenance phase

Relapses occurred in 3 patients (no 1, no 7, and no 9) who had retinitis alone at 2, 6 and 30 weeks of maintenance therapy (patients no 1 and no 9 received combination induction therapy, patient no 7 ganciclovir induction therapy). Patient no 1 responded well to a second course of ganciclovir/foscarnet combination therapy with regression of retinitis; thereafter, maintenance therapy was continued. Patient no 7 could not tolerate another course of induction therapy due to concomitantly developed progressive multifocal leukencephalopathy (PML); he died shortly after the relapse had been diagnosed. In patient no 9, retinal detachment was observed at week 6 of maintenance therapy, probably being a result of progression of CMV disease. A second course of ganciclovir/foscarnet combination therapy could not stop the progression of detachment. Gastrointestinal disease improved in all 3 patients, and no relapses were seen. The patient with the pharyngeal ulcer responded well: the ulcer healed and relapses were not noted. One patient with encephalitis and gastrointestinal disease and another with retinitis and colitis responded well, relapses did not occur. Four patients died from CMV-unrelated causes, 2 of whom received combination induction therapy. Median survival was 18.5 weeks.

Laboratory parameters at study entry were compared with the last recorded value. Three out of 10 patients had a decline of their absolute leukocyte counts by at least 50%, 2 of whom were treated with the combined induction therapy. One patient had an absolute granulocyte count of below 0.5×10^9/l which normalized after therapy was discontinued for 1 week. Thereafter, maintenance therapy was continued at the same dosage and no further hematological toxicity was noted. None of the patients developed infections or episodes of fever during the time in which neutropenia was present. In none of these patients G-CSF or GM-CSF was administered. In 1 patient, the platelet count decreased from 172×10^9/l to 70×10^9/l. Significant changes of hemoglobin or hematocrit were not observed. However, 29 packs of red blood cells had to be given to 6 patients. Two of these had disseminated mycobacterial infections. No important electrolyte disturbances were seen. In 1 patient, a rise of the creatinine level from 1.3 mg/dl to 2.3 mg/dl was observed in the maintenance phase; a

Table I. *Patient characteristics and results of acute and maintenance treatment*

Patient no	Age	CD4+ cells[a] /µl	Diagnoses[b] before entry	Diagnoses[b] during study	Duration of maintenance (weeks)	Manifestation (response)[c]	Relapse on maintenance therapy (week)	Induction therapy[d]	Clearance of virus	Transfusion requirement (number)[e]	Outcome	Adverse reactions
1	33	139	CMV	MAI	33	retinitis (+)	yes (30)	G/F	blood: yes urine: yes	3	dead	penile ulcer, nausea
2	51	40	Candida esophagitis		5	colitis (+)	no	G/F	blood: yes urine: yes		dead	nausea
3	42	14	Candida esophagitis Cerebral Toxoplasmosis		38	esophagitis (+)	no	G	blood: yes urine: yes	2	alive	nausea, malaise
4	23	1	PCP		51	retinitis (+) colitis (+)	no	G/F	blood: yes	2	dead	nausea, malaise
5	28	3	Candida esophagitis		15	colitis (+), encephalitis (+)	no	G/F	urine: yes		dead	nausea
6	41	25	Candida (oral)		15	duodenitis (+) gastritis	no	G	blood: yes urine: yes	5	dead	
7	25	20	MAI, Toxoplasmosis	PML	6	retinitis (0)	yes (2)	G	blood: yes urine: yes		dead	
8	29	43	CMV	MAI	8	pharyngitis (+)	no	G	blood: no urine: no		dead	
9	46	9	Cryptococcal meningitis PCP	MAI	46	retinitis (0)	yes (6)	G/F	blood: yes urine: yes	16	dead	
10	40	11	Toxoplasmosis	PCNSL	22	retinitis (+)	no	G	blood: yes urine: yes	1	alive	

[a] At entry.
[b] Cytomegalovirus infection as first manifestation of AIDS; PCP, pneumocystis carinii pneumonia; MAI, disseminated mycobacterium avium-intracellulare infection; PCNSL, primary CNS lymphoma; PML, progressive multifocal leukencephalopathy.
[c] Response to induction therapy: (+), improvement; (0), stabilization; (−), progression.
[d] G, Ganciclovir only; G/F, Ganciclovir/Foscarnet combination induction therapy.
[e] Number of transfusions during maintenance therapy.

dose reduction was not necessary, since no further increase was observed. He received ganciclovir induction therapy.

Side effects were reported from 5 patients during maintenance therapy, 4 of whom were treated with the combination induction therapy. Nausea with occasional vomiting was observed in 5 patients. Malaise and fatigue were reported from 2 patients. One patient developed repetitive penile ulcers that healed after short interruption of foscarnet therapy.

DISCUSSION

Since active retinitis recurs in almost all patients treated with any available maintenance regimen, the efficacy of the drugs may be measured by their ability to extend the time to disease progression. In this study, 10 patients with AIDS-related CMV disease were treated with a combination therapy consisting of ganciclovir and foscarnet on a daily alternating basis. Relapses occurred in 3 patients with retinitis alone at 2, 6, and 30 weeks of maintenance therapy (median time to progession of retinitis: 42 days), which is in line with results reported from others (2, 9). Two patients who relapsed, responded well to the second course of induction therapy. One patient could not receive induction therapy due to the presence of PML and worsening condition. The median relapse-free interval for all patients was 105 days.

The combined and alternating ganciclovir/foscarnet maintenance therapy was safe and well tolerated in our patients with AIDS-related CMV disease. Discontinuation of therapy or dose reduction due to hematological side effects were not necessary. In 1 patient a 1-week interruption of therapy resolved neutropenia. The high number of transfusions required in our patients may be attributed to some extent to concomitant opportunistic AIDS-related diseases, but also to the hematologic potency of foscarnet; 2 of the 6 patients requiring transfusions had disseminated mycobacterium avium-intracellulare (MAI) infection. In both induction therapy groups, transfusions were required with equal frequency. In view of the essential life-long anti-CMV therapy and the absence of significant hematological or renal toxicities during this combination maintenance therapy, we believe that this regimen may be a potential alternative to established monotherapy with ganciclovir or foscarnet alone to control CMV disease in AIDS patients on a chronic basis.

Nausea and vomiting were the most frequently reported side effects, and were reported from 5 patients during maintenance therapy. Four out of 5 received a combination induction therapy. It may be speculated whether a prolonged administration of foscarnet is associated with a higher frequency of side effects, and whether the concomitant use of both drugs during acute therapy should be limited to severe manifestations. Since CSF concentrations of both drugs are highly variable and CSF drug levels often represent only small fractions of serum levels (13, 14), in patients with CNS-involvement, both drugs may be more effective if they are administered simultaneously. Severe macula-near retinitis or life-threatening CMV-related diarrhea may also resolve more rapidly with a combination induction therapy (unpublished observation).

Given the small number of patients enrolled in this study, the question as to whether this combination regimen may be superior to a maintenance therapy of either drug alone will not be answered until larger studies are performed. Also, the emergence of resistance to either drug should be addressed in further trials. Primary ganciclovir-resistant strains may be found, as well as initially sensitive strains becoming resistant during therapy (8, 15, 16). Also, the development of a CMV isolate resistant to both ganciclovir and foscarnet has been reported (17).

In conclusion, the combination of ganciclovir and foscarnet can safely be used for induction and maintenance therapy. The rate of relapse and the relapse-free interval during maintenance therapy seem to be in line with previous data (2). However, further studies are needed to compare safety, efficacy and development of resistance of this combination therapy with ganciclovir or foscarnet monotherapy.

REFERENCES

1. Hochster H, Dieterich D, Bozzette S, Reichmann RC, Connor JD, Liebes L, Sonke RL, Spector SA, Valentine F, Pettinelli C, Richman DD. Toxicity of combined ganciclovir and zidovudine for cytomegalovirus disease associated with AIDS: an AIDS Clinical Trial Group Study. Ann Intern Med 113: 111–117, 1990.
2. Jacobson MA, O'Donnell JJ, Mills J. Foscarnet treatment of cytomegalovirus retinitis in patients with the acquired immunodeficiency syndrome. Antimicrob Agents Chemother 33: 736–741, 1989.
3. Buhles WC, Mastre BJ, Tinker AJ, Strand V, Koretz SH. Ganciclovir treatment of life- or sight-threatening cytomegalovirus infection: experience in 314 immunocompromized patients: Rev Infect Dis 10: S495–S506, 1988.
4. Medina DJ, Hsiung GD, Mellors JW. Ganciclovir antagonizes the anti-human immunodeficiency virus type 1 activity of zidovudine and didanosine in vitro. Antimicrob Agents Chemother 36: 1127–1130, 1992.
5. Sandstrom EG, Kaplan JC, Byington RE, Hirsch MS. Inhibition of human T-cell lymphotropic virus type III in vitro by phophonoformate. Lancet 1: 1480–1482, 1985.
6. Palestine AG, Polis MA, De Smet MD, Baird BF, Falloon J, Kovacs JA, Davey RT, Zurlo JJ, Zunich KM, Davis M, Hubbard L, Brothers R, Ferris FL, Chew E, Davis JL, Rubin BI, Mellow SD, Metcalf JA, Manischewitz J, Minor JR, Nussenbladt RB, Masur H, Lane HC. A randomized, controlled trial of foscarnet in the treatment of cytomegalovirus retinitis in patients with AIDS. Ann Intern Med 115: 65–673, 1991.
7. Eriksson BF, Schinazi RF. Combinations of 3′-azido-3′deoxythymidine (zidovudine) and phosphonoformate (foscarnet) against human immunodeficiency virus type 1 and cytomegalovirus replication in vitro. Antimicrob Agents Chemother 33: 663–669, 1989.
8. Jacobson MA, von der Horst C, Causey DM, Dehlingder M, Hafner R, Mills J. In vivo additive antiretroviral effect of combined zidovudine and foscarnet therapy for human immunodeficiency virus infection (ACTG protocol 053). J Infect Dis 163: 1219–1222, 1991.
9. Drew WL. Cytomegalovirus infection in patients with AIDS. Clin Infect Dis 14: 608–615, 1992.
10. Quinnan GV, Masur H, Gelmann EP. Herpesvirus infection in the acquired immunodeficiency syndrome. JAMA 252: 72–77, 1984.
11. Stites DP, Casavant CH, McHugh TM. Flow cytometric analysis of lymphocyte phenotypes in AIDS using monoclonal antibodies and simultaneous dual immunofluorescence. Clin Immunol Immunopathol 38: 161–177, 1986.
12. Laskin OL, Stahl-Bayliss CM, Kalman CM, Rosecan LR. Use of ganciclovir to treat serious cytomegalovirus infections in patients with AIDS. J Infect Dis 155: 323–327, 1987.
13. Fletcher C, Sawchuk R, Chinnock B, de Miranda P, Balfour HH. Human pharmacokinetics of the antiviral drug DHPG. Clin Pharmacol Ther 1: 281–286, 1986.
14. Sjövall J, Bergdahl S, Movin G, Ogenstad S, Saarimäki M. Pharmakokinetics of foscarnet and distribution to cerebrospinal fluid after intravenous infusion in patients with human immunodeficiency virus infection. Antimicrob Agents Chemother 33: 1023–1031, 1989.
15. Erice A, Chou S, Biron KK, Stanat SC, Balfour HH, Jordan MC. Progressive disease due to ganciclovir-resistant cytomegalovirus in immunocompromized patients. N Engl J Med 320: 289–293, 1989.
16. Drew WL, Miner RC, Busch DF, Follansbee SD, Gullett J, Mehalko SG, Gordon SM, Owen Jr WF, Matthews TR, Buhles WR, DeArmond B. Prevalence of resistance in patients receiving ganciclovir for serious cytomegalovirus infection. J Infect Dis 163: 716–719, 1991.
17. Knox KK, Drobyski WR, Carrigan DR. Cytomegalovirus isolate resistant to ganciclovir and foscarnet from a marrow transplant patient. Lancet 337: 1292–1293, 1991.

Scand J Infect Dis 26: 55–57, 1994

Vasoactive Intestinal Polypeptide (VIP) Secretion and Refractory Diarrhea in Patients with AIDS or AIDS-Related Complex (ARC)

ROBERTO MANFREDI[1], PAOLO VEZZADINI[2], MARIA PIA FANTI[2] and FRANCESCO CHIODO[1]

From the Departments of [1]Infectious Diseases and [2]Medicine and Gastroenterology, University of Bologna, Bologna, Italy

Elevated plasma levels of vasoactive intestinal polypeptide (VIP) (as assessed by a radio-immunoassay), were found in 7/11 patients with AIDS or AIDS-related Complex (ARC), evaluated because of prolonged intractable diarrhea with either an infectious (6 cases) or a non-infectious (5 cases) etiology. Six subjects have been treated with the somatostatin analogue octreotide, which gave both a favourable clinical response and a significant reduction in plasma VIP concentrations. Evaluation of plasma VIP levels may provide a pathophysiological basis for explaining the efficacy of octreotide therapy in HIV-infected patients suffering from both infectious and non-infectious refractory diarrhea.

R. Manfredi, MD, Istituto Malattie Infettive, Università di Bologna, Via Massarenti 11, I-40138 Bologna, Italy

INTRODUCTION

Octreotide, long-acting somatostatin prescribed on several therapeutic indications in gastroenterology, particularly in the treatment of some gastroenteropancreatic tumours (including VIPomas associated with secretory diarrhea) (1), has recently been used as symptomatic therapy for AIDS-related refractory diarrhea, a common disease often leading to severe nutritional impairment and electrolyte abnormalities. Following octreotide treatment for chronic refractory HIV-related diarrhea, a response rate ranging from 40–70% is seen. It is, however, still difficult to identify subjects who will respond to this therapy. According to recent reports, non-infectious (idiopathic) diarrhea seems to have a more favourable outcome (2–4).

Even though the most important mechanism of action of octreotide is to directly inhibit the release of gastrointestinal peptide hormones, the role of the gastroenteropancreatic endocrine system has not been studied extensively in HIV-infected patients with infectious and non-infectious chronic diarrhea (2–6).

We have previously described 3 AIDS patients with chronic idiopathic diarrhea associated with an abnormal VIP secretion (5). In the present report, we evaluate a series of HIV-infected subjects suffering from both infectious and non-infectious refractory diarrhea.

MATERIALS AND METHODS

11 HIV-infected patients (8 intravenous drug abusers and 3 homosexuals, aged 27–41 years (mean 31.4 ± 5.3 years)) have been evaluated for severe intractable large-volume diarrhea of 1–6 months' duration, by a complete diagnostic work-up, including repeated microbiological evaluation and radiological, ultrasonographic, endoscopic and histopathologic studies (with both light and electron microscopy examination). Five patients had a previous diagnosis of AIDS (due to major opportunistic infections in all cases), while 6 subjects had AIDS-related complex (ARC). In all cases, profuse, watery diarrhea also occurring during the night (4–15 liquid stools/day with a stool volume always larger than one liter per day), was complicated by progressive weight loss (3–10 kg), severe fatigue and anorexia, and fluid and electrolyte abnormalities. Hypokalemia was diagnosed in 9/11 subjects, with values ranging from 3.0–3.7 mEq/l, while hypochloridemia was present in 6/11 patients (89–96 mEq/l). Cryptosporidiosis

had been recognized in 6 subjects (in 2 associated with Salmonella group D and Campylobacter jejuni infection, respectively) while in the remaining 5 patients a diagnosis of idiopathic diarrhea had been established, since no clinically significant results had been obtained from the diagnostic work-up. No significant response was obtained with standard antimicrobial and symptomatic antidiarrheal treatment. Laxative use and steatorrhea were also ruled out.

Plasma levels of VIP were evaluated (as previously described) (5) by a radio-immunoassay using synthetic human VIP (Peninsula Laboratories, Belmont, CA, USA), the rabbit anti-VIP antiserum V9 and [3-iodotyrosyl-^{125}I]VIP (Amersham International, Amersham, England) as labelled tracer, and compared with those of 12 HIV-infected subjects (7 with AIDS, 5 with ARC) with no gastrointestinal disorders and a comparable immunological status (mean CD4+ lymphocyte count $98 \pm 46/mm^3$, compared with $104 \pm 39/mm^3$ in patients suffering from diarrhea), and with values obtained in a control group of 23 healthy volunteers.

RESULTS

Elevated plasma concentrations of VIP were found in 4/6 patients with infectious diarrhea (mean 13.87 ± 2.21 pmol/l; range 11.5–16.0 pmol/l), and in 3/5 subjects with idiopathic disease (mean 12.83 ± 4.16 pmol/l; range 9.5–17.5 pmol/l), while all HIV-infected patients with no diarrhea showed normal plasma VIP levels (mean 4.42 ± 2.28 pmol/l; range 2.0–7.5 pmol/l), comparable with those obtained in healthy controls (values below 8.8 pmol/l).

Six patients (3 suffering from infectious diarrhea and 3 with idiopathic disease) have been treated with octreotide alone, 50–100 µg 2–3 times a day subcutaneously, over a period ranging from 3–33 (mean 12.2 ± 8.7) weeks. Cure or a relevant improvement of the clinical picture during the treatment was seen in all cases. In particular, recovery of intestinal functions (1–2 bowel movements/day) was accompanied by an improvement in stool consistency, a significant gain in body weight (2–5 kg), complete resolution of fluid and electrolyte abnormalities, and consequently a better quality of life for the patients (resolution of anorexia and weakness). Clinical response was associated with a significant reduction of plasma VIP concentrations, observed in all treated patients, when compared with pretreatment values (from a mean level of 11.92 ± 3.32 pmol/l to 7.25 ± 3.56 pmol/l; $p < 0.001$, Student's t-test for paired data). No significant adverse effect occurred during octreotide treatment.

Plasma VIP concentrations evaluated in each examined subject are presented in Fig. 1.

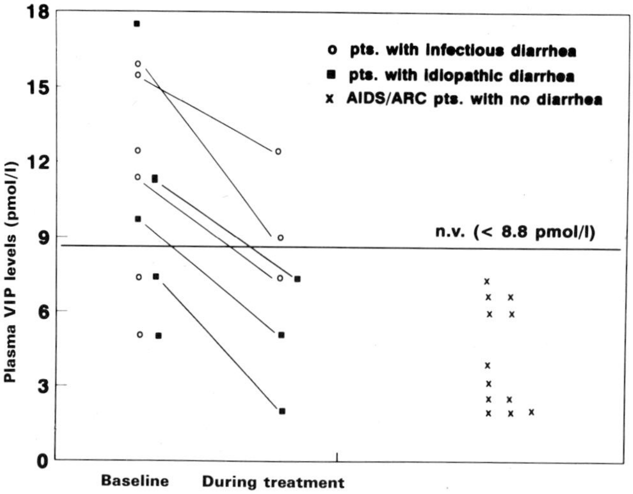

Fig. 1. Plasma VIP levels (pmol/l) measured in AIDS/ARC patients with infectious and non-infectious diarrhea, before and after octreotide treatment, compared with values observed in a group of subjects with AIDS or ARC and a similar immunological status, but without gastrointestinal disorders.

DISCUSSION

Successful treatment of secretory diarrhea with octreotide relies on multifactorial mechanisms, including specific inhibition of the release of hormone mediators of the gastroenteropancreatic endocrine system, and multiple non-specific effects on intestinal functions (such as motility, secretion and absorption) (1). Furthermore, the efficacy of octreotide in HIV-related diarrhea may depend on other hypothesized mechanisms: HIV-induced damage of intestinal enterochromaffin cells, the possible direct activation of gut VIP receptors by HIV itself, and the proposed immunomodulating properties of the drug (5–8).

According to our data, both infectious and non-infectious intractable diarrhea in HIV-infected patients appears to show a frequent association with abnormally elevated plasma VIP levels, corrected by octreotide administration.

Since in patients evaluated for chronic diarrhea of varying etiology, elevated plasma VIP concentrations usually show a good correlation with potential neuroendocrine tumours, and an abnormal VIP secretion can very rarely be attributed to inflammatory bowel disease or other non-specific intestinal pathological findings (9), a local imbalance of VIP secretion and/or activity may be conjectured as a major mechanism leading to chronic diarrhea in patients with AIDS.

Although a definitive treatment for AIDS-associated chronic diarrhea remains a persistent clinical problem in the management of HIV-infected patients, evaluation of VIP concentrations may identify the pathophysiological basis for explaining the efficacy of octreotide therapy in the majority of treated subjects. A diagnosis of secretory-like diarrhea, associated with an abnormal secretion of VIP, will help to recognize, in advance, patients who may present a better clinical response to this treatment.

REFERENCES

1. Grossman I, Simon D. Potential gastrointestinal uses of somatostatin and its synthetic analogue octreotide. Am J Gastroenterol 85: 1061–1072, 1990.
2. Fanning M, Monte M, Sutherland LR, Brodhead M, Murphy GF, Harris AG. Pilot study of sandostatin (octreotide) therapy of refractory HIV-associated diarrhea. Dig Dis Sci 36: 476–480, 1991.
3. Romeu J, Mirò JM, Sirera G, Mallolas J, Arnal J, Valls ME, Tortosa F, Clotet B, Fox M. Efficacy of octreotide in the management of chronic diarrhoea in AIDS. AIDS 5: 1495–1499, 1991.
4. Cello JP, Grendell JH, Basuk P, Simon D, Weiss L, Wittner M, Rood RP, Wilcox M, Forsmark CE, Read AE, Satow JA, Weikel CS, Beaumont C. Effect of octreotide on refractory AIDS-associated diarrhea. A prospective, multicenter clinical trial. Ann Intern Med 115: 705–710, 1991.
5. Manfredi R, Vezzadini P, Costigliola P, Ricchi E, Fanti MP, Chiodo F. Elevated plasma levels of vasoactive intestinal peptide in AIDS patients with refractory idiopathic diarrhoea. Effects of treatment with octreotide. AIDS 7: 223–226, 1993.
6. Kreinik G, Burstein O, Landor M, Bernstein L, Weiss LM, Wittner M. Successful management of intractable cryptosporidial diarrhea with intravenous octreotide, a somatostatin analogue. AIDS 5: 765–767, 1991.
7. Bigornia E, Simon D, Weiss L, Tanowitz H, Wittner M, Lyman W. Detection of HIV-1 viral protein and genomic sequences in enterochromaffin cells of HIV-1 seropositive patients. Am J Gastroenterol 85: 1188, 1990.
8. Moore TC, Spruck CH, Said SI. In vivo depression of lymphocyte traffic in sheep by VIP and HIV (AIDS)-related peptides. Immunopharmacology 16: 181–189, 1988.
9. Koch TR, Michener SR, Go VL. Plasma vasoactive intestinal polypeptide concentration determination in patients with diarrhea. Gastroenterology 100: 99–106, 1991.

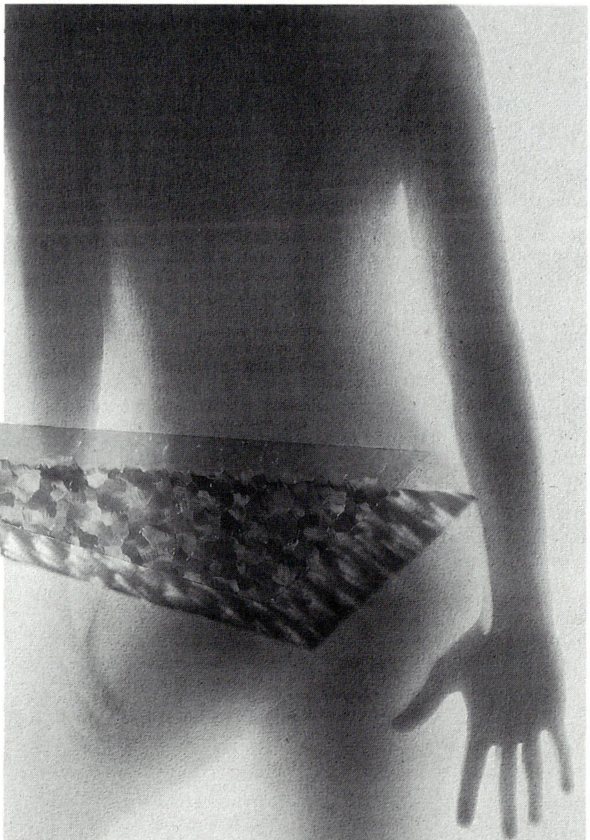

Scand J Infect Dis 26: 59–66, 1994

Five Versus Ten Days Treatment of Streptococcal Pharyngotonsillitis: A Randomized Controlled Trial Comparing Cefpodoxime Proxetil and Phenoxymethyl Penicillin

HENRI PORTIER[1], PASCAL CHAVANET[1], ANNE WALDNER-COMBERNOUX[1], JEAN PAUL KISTERMAN[1], PETER CORNÉLIUS GREY[2], FRANÇOISE ICHOU[3] and CHRISTINE SAFRAN[4]

[1]*Hôpital Universitaire, Dijon, France,* [2]*Waterkloof Pretoria, South Africa, the* [3]*Laboratoires Diamant, Paris-la-Défense and* [4]*Roussel Uclaf, Romainville, France*

A total of 220 adults and children >10 years old (mean 29.5 ± 11.7 years) with pharyngitis/tonsillitis were randomized to receive either cefpodoxime proxetil 100 mg bid for 5 days ($n = 113$) or phenoxymethyl penicillin, 600 mg tid for 10 days ($n = 107$). At the end of treatment of the 166 evaluable patients, a satisfactory clinical response was obtained in 85/88 (96.6%) patients treated with cefpodoxime proxetil and in 75/78 (96.1%) treated with phenoxymethyl penicillin. Group A β-hemolytic streptococci (GABHS) eradication was similar in both groups: 79/82 (96.3%) patients in the cefpodoxime proxetil group and 64/68 (94.1%) patients in the phenoxymethyl penicillin group. At follow-up (20–30 days after the end of treatment) the GABHS eradication persisted in 67/72 (93.1%) patients treated with cefpodoxime proxetil and in 56/61 (91.8%) patients treated with phenoxymethyl penicillin. Significantly better compliance ($p < 0.01$) was noticed with the cefpodoxime proxetil regimen compared with the phenoxymethyl penicillin regimen, with only 2/110 (2%) poorly compliant patients in the cefpodoxime proxetil group vs 17/104 (16%) in the phenoxymethyl penicillin group. Thus, the shorter duration of therapy, in conjunction with demonstrated clinical and bacteriological efficacy that is equivalent to standard therapy, makes cefpodoxime proxetil an acceptable alternative for the treatment of GABHS pharyngitis/tonsillitis.

H. Portier, MD, Hôpital Universitaire, F-21034 Dijon, France

INTRODUCTION

The success of an antibiotic regimen is greatly influenced by the ease of administration. Phenoxymethyl penicillin, the conventional therapy for streptococcal pharyngitis/tonsillitis, is prescribed for thrice daily dosing for 10 days, as recommended by the American Heart Association (1).

Studies have shown that shortening the duration of penicillin therapy results in decreased eradication rates (2–5). As streptococcal pharyngitis/tonsillitis can lead to severe complications, such as acute rheumatic fever, eradication of the organism is critical.

Cefpodoxime proxetil, the isopropyloxy-carbonyl-oxyethyl ester of cefpodoxime, is a prodrug that is suitable for oral administration. Cefpodoxime, the active compound is a third generation oral cephalosporin which is highly active against the main bacteria commonly involved in pharyngitis/tonsillitis (Group A, C, and G streptococci). The MIC_{90} of cefpodoxime for Group A streptococci ranges from ≤0.01 mg/l to ≤0.06 mg/l (6–9).

The peak concentration of cefpodoxime in serum following a 100 mg oral dose is 1.4 mg/l with a serum half-life of 2.1 h and a trough level of 0.07–0.09 mg/l (12 h after intake) (10). Serum protein binding is about 40%, and approximately 40% of the administered dose is recoverable from the urine. The mean tonsillar tissue concentration of cefpodoxime 4 h after administration of a 100 mg oral dose is 0.24 mg/kg (11).

Cefpodoxime proxetil has been shown to be effective in the treatment of streptococcal pharyngitis when administered for 10 days (12).

Recent studies on second and third generation cephalosporins administered for 4 or 5 days in pharyngitis/tonsillitis have proved to be effective (13–17). One pilot study of 66 patients demonstrated comparable efficacy between cefpodoxime proxetil and cefuroxime axetil after 5 days of administration (13).

Therefore, this study was undertaken to investigate the efficacy of a 5 day course of cefpodoxime proxetil, compared with a standard regimen of 10 days of phenoxymethyl penicillin in the treatment of streptococcal infections. Results of an interim analysis after enrolment of 160 patients have already been briefly described in an article summarizing the overall experience gained with cefpodoxime administered to patients suffering from tonsillitis/pharyngitis during 1989–90 (13).

MATERIALS AND METHODS

This study was conducted as a multicentre, comparative, open-label, randomized clinical trial.

Patients were recruited (after informed consent had been obtained) from 44 investigational sites located in France and South Africa from July 1989 to September 1990. The trial was conducted in accordance with the Declaration of Helsinki and the protocol was approved by local medical ethics committees.

Eligible adults or children >10 years with a suspected bacterial pharyngitis/tonsillitis on the basis of clinical signs and/or symptoms were enrolled in the study after the presence of group A β-hemolytic streptococci (GABHS) was presumed from a positive Strep A test (Hybritec®) for which the specificity and positive predictive value are expected to be around 95%. Patients were excluded for the following reasons: pregnancy or lactation; severe infection requiring parenteral antibiotic administration; obesity; pharyngitis/tonsillitis of suspected viral origin in the presence of associated cough, common cold or laryngitis; associated sinusitis; past history of allergy to β-lactams; renal or liver impairment; immunosuppression; CDC III or IV HIV infection; malabsorption syndrome; terminal neoplasia; grave psychiatric disorder; or currently receiving probenecid or anti-vitamin K treatment. Patients were not to have participated in a therapeutic trial within 15 days prior to entering this study and were not to have received another antibiotic regimen within 48 h preceding this trial, except in the case of resistance of the causative pathogen to that antibiotic.

Assuming that cefpodoxime proxetil would not demonstrate a superiority over phenoxymethyl penicillin in terms of bacteriological eradication, these 2 antibiotics were compared for equivalence. Equivalence was defined as a difference (△) not exceeding 10%. A sample size of 112 patients in each group would provide a power of 80% (type II error risk of 20%) when using a 1-sided test for a type I risk of α = 5%, with an expected 90% success rate with both antibiotics. Therefore it was planned to include 224 patients in order to obtain 154 patients evaluable for efficacy (77 in each group).

On admission, each patient underwent a complete anamnesis and physical examination, including associated signs and symptoms of pharyngitis/tonsillitis. Patients were started on study drug treatment before the results of throat cultures were known, provided the Strep A test was positive. Patients with a clear clinical presentation consistent with GABHS pharyngitis/tonsillitis, but a negative Strep A test, were allowed to proceed in the study and were retained for the clinical and bacteriological efficacy assessment *only* if GABHS was isolated from the throat culture. Throat swabs were taken and preserved on Difco medium at inclusion.

A throat culture including isolation, identification and susceptibility testing of GABHS to cefpodoxime and penicillin was performed on each patient at inclusion in each centre and later checked in a central laboratory.

Patients were randomized to receive either cefpodoxime proxetil, 100 mg bid orally for 5 days, or phenoxymethyl penicillin, 600 mg tid orally for 10 days.

Post-treatment evaluations were performed 2–3 days (end of treatment) and 20–30 days (follow-up) after completion of therapy.

Unused drugs were collected at the end of the treatment visit to assess patient compliance with the prescribed therapeutic regimen. Poor compliance was defined as an intake of less than 80% of the total dose prescribed.

The clinical response to therapy was assigned at the end of treatment evaluation using the following definitions:

Table I. *Demographic and admission variables in the overall population*

Variables	Cefpodoxime (n = 113)	Phenoxymethyl penicillin (n = 107)
Age (years)		
Mean (SD)	30.4(12.1)	28.6(11.2)
Range	11–82	11–70
Sex		
Male	61	53
Female	52	54

(1) *Satisfactory* meant that the infection was cleared, with disappearance or improvement of clinical symptoms, and

(2) *Unsatisfactory* meant that the clinical symptoms remained unchanged or worsened. A *satisfactory* or *unsatisfactory* response to therapy was also assigned at the follow-up evaluation depending upon the continued absence or reappearance of clinical signs and symptoms of pharyngitis/tonsillitis.

Bacteriological response at the end of treatment evaluation was assigned using the following definitions: (1) *eradication* meant that no GABHS were isolated at the end of treatment throat culture, and (2) *persistence* meant that GABHS were isolated at the end of treatment culture. At the follow-up evaluation, a satisfactory response meant that no GABHS were isolated from the follow-up throat culture. An unsatisfactory response meant that the GABHS were eradicated at the end of therapy, but were re-isolated from the follow-up throat culture.

All patients who received any trial medication were considered evaluable for tolerance.

Demographic characteristics of the patient population were summarized for each treatment group. Overall clinical and bacteriological response rates were summarized according to treatment group and compared using χ^2 test or Fisher's exact test. 95% confidence intervals of the success rates were calculated for both treatment groups.

RESULTS

More than 700 adults or children >10 years of age with clinical signs of pharyngotonsillitis were screened with a Strep A test. Of these, 220 patients were enrolled in the study with a range of 2–30 patients recruited by each centre. Both treatment groups were comparable for each of the demographic and admission variables analysed (Table I).

175 (80%) of the 220 enrolled patients had GABHS isolated from the pre-treatment throat culture. It was noticed that GABHS were not isolated from 45 of the 220 patients enrolled

Table II. *Resolution of clinical signs and symptoms present on admission: end of treatment evaluation*

Clinical signs	Day 5 Cefpodoxime	Day 10 Phenoxymethyl penicillin
Dysphagia	80/81(98.8%)	71/74(95.9%)
Sore throat	83/86(96.5%)	70/75(93.3%)
Inflamed throat	83/86(96.5%)	72/76(94.7%)
Headache	73/74(98.6%)	66/69(95.6%)
Adenopathy	73/78(93.6%)	66/73(90.4%)
Temperature on admission >38°C, ≤37°C at end of treatment	58/59(98.3%)	52/53(98.1%)

Table III. *Clinical responses at end of treatment and follow-up evaluations*

	Cefpodoxime	Phenoxymethyl penicillin
End of treatment evaluation	(*n* = 88)	(*n* = 78)
Satisfactory	85(96.6%)	75(96.1%)
Unsatisfactory	3 (3.4%)	3 (3.8%)
Follow-up evaluation	(*n* = 80)	(*n* = 68)
Satisfactory	77(96.3%)	67(98.5%)
Unsatisfactory	3 (3.7%)	1 (1.5%)

despite a positive strep A test at enrollment (24 in the cefpodoxime proxetil group and 21 in the phenoxymethyl penicillin group).

Positive culture rates were comparable between the treatment groups; 78.8% for the cefpodoxime proxetil group and 80.4% for the phenoxymethyl penicillin group. All GABHS isolates were sensitive to cefpodoxime and to penicillin using the disk diffusion method.

Of the 220 patients enrolled in the study, 166 (88 cefpodoxime proxetil and 78 phenoxymethyl penicillin) were evaluable for clinical efficacy at the end of treatment and 150 (82 cefpodoxime proxetil and 68 phenoxymethyl penicillin) were evaluable for bacteriological efficacy. The primary reason for non-evaluability for both treatment groups was non-isolation of GABHS in the pretreatment culture.

Among the evaluable patients, no difference was observed in the regression of clinical signs between the treatment groups, at the end of treatment (Table II).

For evaluable compliant patients, there were no statistically significant differences between the treatment groups regarding clinical response either at the end of treatment or at follow-up (Table III), with both groups demonstrating excellent clinical response rates. In addition, both treatment groups demonstrated equally high bacteriological eradication rates (Table IV).

10/143 patients (5 in each group) who showed GABHS eradication at the end of treatment had become culture positive by follow-up and these patients were considered as relapses (Table IV).

29/220 (13.1%) patients were suffering from recurrent tonsillitis, 14 in the cefpodoxime proxetil group and 15 in the penicillin group. Among them, 18 patients were evaluable for bacteriological response at the end of treatment. The GABHS eradication was similar in both groups, with 8/9 (88.8%) satisfactory responses in the cefpodoxime proxetil group and 9/9 in the penicillin group. Of the 16 patients evaluable for the bacteriological response at the

Table IV. *Bacteriological responses at end of treatment and follow-up evaluations*

	Cefpodoxime	Phenoxymethyl penicillin
End of treatment evaluation	(*n* = 82)	(*n* = 68)
Eradication	79(96.3%)	64(94.1%)
Persistence	3 (3.7%)	4 (5.9%)
Follow-up evaluation	(*n* = 72)	(*n* = 61)
Satisfactory	67(93.1%)	56(91.8%)
Unsatisfactory (relapse)	5 (6.9%)	5 (8.2%)

Table V. *Clinically relevant biological abnormalities*

Clinically relevant abnormality	Cefpodoxime (*n*)	Phenoxymethyl penicillin (*n*)
Possibly or probably related to study drug		
Diaorrhea	2	0
Gastrointestinal pain	0	2
Urticaria	1	1
Anemia ↘ haemoglobin	2	2
Neutropenia	2	0
Hyperleukocytosis	0	1
Thrombocytosis	2	0
S. creatinine increase	4	3
↗ Alk. phosphatase	8	7
↗ Transaminase	1	3

follow-up visit, a satisfactory response was observed in 7/8 (87.5%) patients in each treatment group.

Among the clinically evaluable patients, the mean duration of treatment was 5.0 ± 0.2 days for the cefpodoxime proxetil group and 9.6 ± 0.8 days for the phenoxymethyl penicillin group.

Among the clinically evaluable patients, the mean duration of treatment was 5.0±0.2 days for the cefpodoxime proxetil group and 9.6±0.8 days for the phenoxymethyl penicillin group.

Compliance data were not available for 3/113 patients in the cefpodoxime proxetil group and from 3/107 patients in the penicillin group.

Poor compliance was documented for 2/110 (1.8%) patients in the cefpodoxime proxetil group and 17/104 (16.3%) patients in the phenoxymethyl penicillin group; this difference in compliance between the treatment groups was statistically significant ($p<0.01$).

218/220 patients enrolled were evaluable for tolerance; the 2 remaining patients never returned to the study centre after the enrollment visit and were excluded from all evaluations. 13 patients (7 in the cefpodoxime proxetil group and 6 in the penicillin group) experienced a total of 16 adverse events (8 in each group). Adverse events possibly or probably related to the study medication were noted in 6 patients (3 in each group).

These events were mainly gastrointestinal or cutaneous in nature. No treatment discontinuation due to adverse events occurred in the cefpodoxime proxetil group, whereas 2 patients in the phenoxymethyl penicillin group discontinued treatment due to gastralgia. Only 1 severe adverse event (diarrhea) possibly or probably related to the antibiotic treatment was recorded in the cefpodoxime proxetil group, vs. 3 such events in the phenoxymethyl penicillin group (1 urticaria and 2 gastralgia).

Clinically relevant biological abnormalities were equally distributed between the 2 groups (Table V).

DISCUSSION

Phenoxymethyl penicillin, 600 mg tid for 10 days, has been the standard therapy for treating pharyngitis/tonsillitis for the past 45 years in many countries (1, 18–20). Despite the recommended 10-day course of treatment, many patients discontinue their penicillin medication before completing the prescribed regimen. The 10-day course of penicillin for the treatment of pharyngitis/tonsillitis has not been altered since previously published trials showed decrease in GABHS eradication rates, both at the end of treatment and at follow-up when the duration of penicillin treatment was shortened. A review of the literature by Scheimberg (21) showed that non-eradication rates increased by up to 30% when penicillin courses were shortened. Mohler et al. (22) demonstrated that the proportion of positive follow-up cultures varied inversely with the number of treatment days for patients receiving penicillin. A recent study by Strömberg et al. (5) has shown that cumulative rates of recurrence, 2 months after the beginning of phenoxymethyl penicillin treatment, were 24% in the 10-day group and 55% in the 5-day group. Thus, shortening the 10-day course of penicillin therapy to increase compliance is not a practical alternative.

Cephalosporins have been successfully used in the treatment of GABHS pharyngitis for the past 20 years; a meta-analysis combining the results of 19 comparative trials evaluating the relative efficacy of various cephalosporins vs. penicillin reported in the literature showed significantly higher bacteriologic and clinical cure rates for the cephalosporins vis-à-vis the penicillin groups (3). The effectiveness of the cephalosporins in the treatment of pharyngitis may be related to their resistance to degradation by β-lactamases and/or ability to eradicate strains of Staphylococcus aureus, Haemophilus influenzae and Moraxella catarrhalis in the presence of synergistic infections or their ability to diffuse better into the tonsil tissues (23).

Promising results have recently been obtained with oral cephalosporins when shortening the duration of treatment: Cerstelotte found in children that a 7-day course of cefetamet-pivoxil 20 mg/kg/day was as effective as a 10-day course of phenoxymethyl penicillin 12 mg/kg/day tid (14) and Gehanno & Chiche reported in 1991 (15) that a 4-day course of cefuroxime axetil appeared to be just as effective as a 10-day course of phenoxymethyl penicillin.

After an initial study demonstrating the equivalence of a 10-day course cefpodoxime proxetil with amoxicillin for tonsillitis/pharyngitis of adults (12), the efficacy of a 5-day course of treatment had therefore to be evaluated first in adults and teenagers, since no pediatric formula was available in 1989–90.

In the current trial involving 220 adults and children >10 years of age who came for medical care, showing signs and/or symptoms of pharyngotonsillitis, were enrolled as soon as they showed a positive Strep A test. Only 175 (80%) patients had GABHS isolated in the pretreatment throat culture, but these patients were distributed equally between the 2 treatment groups.

No clear explanation could be given for this high rate of apparent false-positive results, using the Strep A test. However, some authors have observed that, to ensure clinical efficaciousness, a Group A streptococcal antigen detection test should have both a sensitivity and a positive predictive value of 95%. They found in reviewing 10 kits from 8 manufacturers that none of the test kits met those criteria, despite the manufacturers' own claims (24, 25). Furthermore, 2 recent publications have also mentioned 20% false-positive results when using Strep A test as a rapid diagnostic test for GABHS pharyngotonsillitis (17, 26).

The results of this study demonstrate that twice-daily cefpodoxime proxetil administered for 5 days was just as effective in compliant patients as thrice daily phenoxymethyl penicillin for 10 days in the treatment of GABHS pharyngitis/tonsillitis, using only conventional per-protocol analysis. No intent-to-treat analysis is available for this trial, which was conducted in 1989–90. At this date, no guidelines requesting intent-to-treat evaluations were available (27). Nevertheless, one should emphasize that in the specific case of GABHS/tonsillitis pharyngitis, the eradication of the GABHS through a per-protocol analysis must be the primary analysis, since the persistence of the causative organism can lead to acute rheumatic fever.

Overall compliance with the cefpodoxime proxetil regimen was significantly better than that with the phenoxymethyl penicillin regimen. Thus, a 5-day course of cefpodoxime proxetil ensures greater security in terms of GABHS eradication in patients who generally fail to comply with a prescribed treatment. No significant side effects were noted with either treatment regimen.

We conclude that cefpodoxime proxetil can offer a shorter duration of therapy without sacrificing clinical and bacteriologic effectiveness. The demonstrated efficacy, combined with increased compliance, suggests that cefpodoxime proxetil is an acceptable alternative to penicillin for the treatment of pharyngitis/tonsillitis and could be recommended specially for uncompliant patients.

ACKNOWLEDGEMENTS

We thank Antoine Kazmierczak for central susceptibility testing, and Roussel-Uclaf and Laboratoires Diamant for supplying and coordinating the trial.

REFERENCES

1. Dajani AS, Bisno AL, Chung KJ, Durack DT, Gerber MA, Kaplan EL, Miliard HD, Randolph MF, Shulman ST, Watanakunakorn C. Prevention of rheumatic fever: a statement for health professionals by the committee on rheumatic fever, endocarditis and Kawasaki Disease of the council on cardiovascular disease in the young, the American Heart Association. Pediatr Infect Dis J 8: 263–266, 1989.
2. Gerber MA, Randolph MD, Chanatry J, Wright LL, De Meo K, Kaplan EL. Five vs ten days of penicillin V therapy for streptococcal pharyngitis. Am J Dis Child 141: 224–227, 1987.
3. Pichichero M, Margolis P. A comparison of cephalosporins and penicillins in the treatment of group A beta-hemolytic streptococcal pharyngitis: a meta-analysis supporting the concept of microbial copathogenicity. Pediatr Infect Dis J 10: 275–281, 1991.
4. Schwartz RH, Wientzen RL Jr, Pedreira F, Feroli EJ, Mella GW, Guandolo VL. Penicillin V for group A streptococcal pharyngitis: a randomized trial of seven versus ten days therapy. JAMA 246: 1790–1795, 1981.
5. Strömberg A, Schwan A, Cars O. Five versus ten days treatment of group A streptococcal pharyngotonsillitis: a randomized controlled clinical trial with phenoxymethylpenicillin and cefadroxil. Scand J Infect Dis 20: 37–46, 1988.
6. Utsui Y, Inoue M, Mitsuhashi S. In vitro and in vivo antibacterial activities of CS-807, a new oral cephalosporin. Antimicrob Agents Chemother 31: 1085–1092, 1987.
7. Chin NX, Neu HC. In vitro activity of an oral iminomethoxy aminothiazolyl cephalosporin, R-3746. Antimicrob Agents Chemother 32: 671–677, 1988.
8. Fass RJ, Helsel VL. In vitro activity of U-76, 252 (CS-807), a new oral cephalosporin. Antimicrob Agents Chemother 32: 1082–1085, 1988.
9. Jones R, Barry AL. Antimicrobial activity and disk diffusion susceptibility testing of U-76253 A (R-3746), the active metabolite of the new cephalosporin ester, U-76252 (CS-807). Antimicrob Agents Chemother 32: 443–449, 1988.
10. Tremblay D, Dupront A, Ho C, Coussediere D, Lenfant B. Pharmacokinetics of cefpodoxime in young and elderly volunteers after single doses. J Antimicrob Chemother 26: 21–28, 1990.
11. Gehanno P, Andrews JM, Ichou F, Sultan E, Lenfant B. Concentration of cefpodoxime in plasma and tonsillar tissue after a single oral dose of cefpodoxime proxetil. J Antimicrob Chemother 26: 47–51, 1990.
12. Portier H, Waldner-Combernoux A, Clarysse C, Kurzeja AH, Rostand A. Cefpodoxime proxetil vs amoxycillin in the treatment of pharyngitis or tonsillitis in adult out-patients, abstr. 631. International Congress for Infectious Diseases, Montreal, 1990.
13. Portier H, Chavanet P, Gouyon JB, Guetat F. Five day treatment of pharyngotonsillitis with cefpodoxime proxetil. J Antimicrob Chemother 26: 79–85, 1990.
14. Cerstelotte E, Vandenberghe P, Bradbury F, Murphy N, Käsnänen T, Germano G, Kissling M. Cefetamet pivoxil and penicillin V in the treatment of group A beta-hemolytic streptococcal pharyngitis. Acta Therapeutica 16: 163–173, 1990.
15. Gehanno P, Chiche D. Traitement des angines à streptocoque bêta hémolytique du groupe A par le céfuroxime axétil pendant 4 jours: étude comparative à la pénicillin V pendant 10 jours. Médecine et Maladies Infectieuses 21: 66–70, 1991.
16. Hebblethwaite EM, Brown GW, Cox DM. A comparison of the efficacy and safety of cefuroxime axetil and Augmentin® in the treatment of upper respiratory tract infections. Drugs Exp Clin Res 2: 91–94, 1987.
17. Peyramond D, Tigaud S, Darchy L, Bremard-Oury C. Etude multicentrique comparant l'efficacité du

céfixime pendant 4 jours à la phénoxyméthylpénicilline pendant 10 jours chez des patients ayant une angine à streptocoque bêta-hémolytique du groupe A (SBHGA). Médecine et Maladies Infectieuses 23: 419–424, 1993.
18. Dillon HC. Antibiotic therapy: influence of duration frequency, route of administration and compliance. In: Schulman ST, ed. Pharyngitis: management in an era of declining rheumatic fever. New York: Prager, 133–151, 1984.
19. Gerber MA, Markowitz M. Management of streptococcal pharyngitis reconsidered. Pediatr Infect Dis J 4: 518–526, 1985.
20. Vaudaux B. Traitement antibiotique de l'angine streptococcique. Médecine et Hygiéne 45: 2916–2922, 1987.
21. Scheimberg A. Pharyngite streptococcique à streptocoque β-hémolytique du groupe A. Revue de la litterature. La Lettre de l'Infectiologue 5: 462–465, 1990.
22. Mohler DN, Wallin DG, Dreyfus EG, Bakst AJ. Studies in the home treatment of streptococcal disease. A comparison of the efficacy of oral administration of penicillin and intramuscular injection of benzathine penicillin in the treatment of streptococcal pharyngitis. N Engl J Med 254: 45–50, 1956.
23. Pichichero M. Controversies in the treatment of streptococcal pharyngitis. Am Fam Physician 42: 1567–1575, 1990.
24. Radetsky M, Solomon JA, Todd JK. Identification of streptococcal pharyngitis in the office laboratory: reassessment of new technology. Pediatr Infect Dis J 46: 556–563, 1987.
25. Kellogg JA, Manzella JP. Detection of group A streptococci in the laboratory or physicians office. Culture vs antibody methods. JAMA 255: 2638–2642, 1986.
26. Carbon C, Chatelain A, Orvain J, Zuck P, Rio Y, Bingen E. Comparative efficacy and safety of 5-day cefotiam-hexetil and 10-day penicillin V for treatment of Streptococci pharyngitis. A double-blind trial. Abstract 1675. ICAAC, Anaheim, 1992.
27. Beam TR, Gilbert DN, Kunin CM. Guidelines for the evaluation of antiinfective drug products. Clin Infect Dis 15: S1, 1–32, 1992.

Scand J Infect Dis 26: 67–75, 1994

Sensitivity of 880 Blood Culture Isolates to 24 Antibiotics

MATS WALDER, EVA KARLSSON and BERIT NILSSON

From the Department of Medical Microbiology, Lund University, Malmö General Hospital, Malmö, Sweden

Blood culture isolates ($n = 880$) collected during 2.5 years (period I $n = 515$, July 1988 to December 1989; period II $n = 365$, January 1992 to December 1992) were analysed with the agar dilution method to ascertain their sensitivity to 24 antibiotics. The susceptibility of bacteria was classified according to MIC values and susceptibility grouping used in the SIR system (sensitive-S, intermediate-I, resistant-R). Comparison of percentage S + I values for the 2 periods revealed no major development of resistance. Co-trimoxazole and some cephalosporins (cefpirom, cefepime and cefotaxime) were active (S + I) against 88–92% of the strains. Imipenem and the combination piperacillin–tazobaclam were active against 95% of the strains. A very large number of strains (98.2 to 98.6%) were inhibited (S + I) by the quinolones tested, ciprofloxacin and ofloxacin. Comparison of the present results with those of our 1980–81 study yielded no evidence of resistance development, except for an increase in betalactamase-producing S. aureus strains, from 67% to 85%.

M. Walder, MD, Department of Medical Microbiology, Lund University, Malmö General Hospital, S-214 01 Malmö, Sweden

INTRODUCTION

In cases of bacteraemia/sepsis it is crucial that adequate antibiotic treatment is initiated as soon as possible. Since in most cases it is not known which micro-organism is responsible for the disease, the choice of antibiotic will be based on several factors, including best guess of microbial agent, patient's age, history of the disease and the prevailing antibiotic sensitivity situation in the region. Reports of antibiotic sensitivity i.e., based on pattern for bacteraemia strains should be regularly updated and should preferably be regional (1, 2), e.g. Northern Europe, if that is where treatment is to be administered (3, 4).

The aim of this study was to answer the following questions. What is the sensitivity to commonly used antibiotics and to newer drugs? Which antibiotic would kill most strains in cases of bacteraemia of unknown origin? Has the resistance pattern changed in our hospital during the last decade (5)?

MATERIALS AND METHODS

The city of Malmö (pop. 235,000) is served by 3 hospitals: Malmö General Hospital with 1,028 beds for acute cases, and 2 other hospitals, 1 geriatric, the other psychiatric (both also providing long-term care) with together 2,029 beds.

The Department of Clinical Microbiology, Malmö General Hospital, receives a total of approximately 185,000 samples for culture annually, of which approximately 10,000 are blood culture samples. About 12% of these 10,000 blood-cultures yield significant growth of bacteria (on average 2–3 positive blood cultures/patient), i.e. representing about 500 patients with sepsis/bacteraemia.

Blood culture. From most patients 5 ml blood from the cubital vein was transferred into each of 2 blood culture bottles (Bactec, Becton-Dickinson) containing broth and anticoagulant, one for aerobic culture, the other for anaerobic culture, which is the recommended routine procedure. The culture bottles were incubated at 37°C and analysed in a Bactec machine twice a day for 2 days, and then once a day from day 3 to day 5. Bacteria were identified with conventional methods (6). The strains were stored in glycerol broth at −20°C until antibiotic sensitivity testing.

Strains. *Period I.* During an 18-month period from July 1988 to December 1989, 515 aerobic strains were isolated in blood cultures at the Department of Clinical Microbiology, Malmö General Hospital. *Period II.* During 1 year from January 1992 to December 1992, a further 365 strains were isolated. Altogether 880/896 strains originally isolated and stored were available for testing.

The strains were: 151 Staphylococcus aureus, 58 Staphylococcus epidermidis (either strains isolated at least twice from the same patient or from compromised hosts), 23 Streptococci group A, 15 Streptococci group B, 41 Enterococcus faecalis (enterococci), 78 Pneumococci, 46 Streptococcus species, 267 E. coli, 72 Klebsiella (64 K. pneumoniae and 8 K. oxytoca), 19 Enterobacter (16. E. cloacae, 2 E. agglomerans and 1 E. aerogenes), 35 Proteus mirabilis, 16 Proteus vulgaris and Morganella morganii, 21 Pseudomonas aeruginosa, 10 Acinetobacter (either A. calcoaceticus, DNA group 1, or A. bowmannii complex, DNA group 2) (7). The number of strains for each species were proportionally distributed between period I and period II.

28 strains were not included in Fig. 1 as their occurrence was too rare for analytical purposes: 1 Yersinia, 7 Salmonella, 3 Shigella, 2 Listeria, 4 Citrobacter, 2 Serratia, 2 Xanthomonas maltophilia, 5 Moraxella and 2 Neisseria meningitidis.

In addition, 84 strains from an earlier similar study (1980–81) were also included in this study: 10 Staphylococcus aureus, 10 Staphylococcus epidermidis, 10 Enterococcus faecalis, 10 E. coli, 10 Klebsiella (7 K. pneumoniae, 3 K. oxytoca), 10 Enterobacter (7 E. cloacae, 2 E. aerogenes, 1 E. agglomerans), 10 Proteus mirabilis, 5 Proteus vulgaris and Morganella morganii and 9 Acinetobacter (these Acinetobacter were identified as A. lwoffi, DNA group 8) (7).

Antibiotics. In all, 24 antibiotics were tested: benzylpenicillin (PB 1033, Astra, Sweden); cloxacillin (MC 209, Astra, Sweden); ampicillin (OM 659, Astra, Sweden); mecillinam (J 13, Leo, Denmark); piperacillin (W 9F 1213, Lederle, USA); piperacillin-tazobactam (MRWO 1389-0129, Lederle, USA); gentamicin (BE-9-9-GMF-02, AB Biodisk, Sweden); tobramycin (F 10370, Lilly, USA); netilmicin (USQ-NLMN-600, Essex, Belgium); amikacin (MP 6404, Bristol-Myers, USA); co-trimoxazole (93557-01, Astra, Sweden); clindamycin (810 × PY, Upjohn, USA); choramphenicol (129C-0128, Sigma, USA); tetracycline (636-58021, Pfizer, USA); ciprofloxacin (204212 H, Bayer, Germany); ofloxacin (000U 232, Hoechst, Germany); cephalothin (S1-146-63, Lilly, USA); cefoxitin (ABF 998, Merck Sharp and Dohme KB, USA); cefuroxime (Vnr 059030, Glaxo, GB); cefotaxime (U 538, Hoechst, Germany); ceftazidime (CRZ 0051, Glaxo, GB); cefpirom (U87, Hoechst, Germany); cefepime (D 87040, Bristol-Myers, USA) and imipenem (C 2250, MSD, USA).

Susceptibility testing (MIC). Before susceptibility testing, all strains were cultivated on blood–agar plates. Most of the strains were enriched in Mueller-Hinton broth (Oxoid), but for pneumococci, streptococci group A and group B and other streptococcal species, Todd-Hewitt broth (Difco) was used. Susceptibility testing was done with the agar dilution method (8). The test medium used for most strains was PDM-ASM no. II agar (AB Biodisk). For pneumococci, streptococci groups A and B and other streptococcal species, PDM-ASM no. II with addition of 5% horse blood was used. For all Proteus species, PDM-ASM no. II with added PNFG (1-(4-nitrophenyl)-1, 2, 3-propanetriol, Merck 820902) was used. Antibiotics were added to the agar in freshly prepared solutions at concentrations ranging from 0.03 to 32 mg/l. All concentrations and breakpoints used corresponded to the recommendations in Sweden by the SIR-system (sensitive, intermediate, resistant) for antibiotic sensitivity testing (9).

The inoculum consisted of a 4 h-culture, except for pneumococci, streptococci groups A and B, other streptococcal species, Pseudomonas and Acinetobacter which were grown overnight. Using a multipoint inoculator, 2-μl aliquots of bacterial suspension in saline at a concentration of 10^7 colony forming units (cfu)/ml (10^3 cfu/spot) were applied to the surface of the agar, 22 tests being applied per plate as well as 3 control strains: (Enterococcus faecalis ATCC 29212, Staphylococcus aureus ATCC 29213, E. coli ATCC 25922). All plates were incubated for 18 h at 37°C, pneumococci, streptococci group A and other streptococcal species in CO_2 atmosphere. By recording the lowest concentration of antibiotics giving complete inhibition of growth (as judged by the naked eye), the bacteria were classified according to MIC values or the susceptibility groups, Sensitive (S), Intermediate (I) or Resistant (R) (Table I) used in Sweden (9) revised 1990. The proportion of strains inhibited by each antibiotic was calculated from the number of strains in the susceptibility groups S + I divided by the total number of strains, 880.

For S. aureus, betalactamase production was tested with the clover-leaf method (10). The susceptibility of S. epidermidis to methicillin and isoxacillin (1 μg paper disc) was tested at 30°C on PDM medium with 3.5% NaCl added.

Table I. *Breakpoints used for sensitivity testing (mg/l). RAF ref. 9, revised 1990*

	S ≤	R ≥
Benzylpenicillin	1	8
Ampicillin	1	16
Ampicillin/mecillinam	2	16
Piperacillin/tazobactam	8	32
Cloxacillin	1	2
Cephalothin	1	16
Cefoxitin	4	16
Cefuroxime	4	16
Cefotaxime	4	16
Ceftazidime	4	16
Cefpirom	4	16
Cefepime	4	16
Imipenem	4	16
Clindamycin	2	8
Tetracycline	1	4
Chloramphenicol	8	16
Gentamicin	4	8
Tobramycin	4	8
Netilmicin	4	8
Amikacin	8	16
Co-trimoxazole	32	64
Ciprofloxacin	1	8
Ofloxacin	1	8

RESULTS AND DISCUSSION

During the 18-month period, July 1988–December 1989, 12,573 blood cultures were performed. From 532 patients whose specimens were positive in culture during the period, 515 isolates were available for MIC tests. During the 12-month period II, January 1992–December 1992, 8,432 blood cultures were performed. From 378 patients with positive blood cultures, 365 isolates were available for MIC tests. When comparing values of MIC_{50}, MIC_{90} and % S + I for periods I and II, we found almost identical results, which enables presentation in the same figure. In Fig. 1, all betalactamase-producing staphylococci have been given an MIC value of 64 mg/l for benzylpenicillin, ampicillin and piperacillin, while all methicillin-resistant staphylococci MRS (1 MRSA, 29 MRSE) have been given an MIC value of 64 mg/l for all betalactam-antibiotics due to a presumed treatment failure with betalactam-antibiotics.

A. Gram-positive isolates (Fig. 1)

Penicillins

Of the 151 S. aureus strains isolated, 83% produced betalactamase, a frequency 15% higher than that of 1980–81. One strain was methicillin resistant (MRSA), and no borderline S. Aureus (BORSA) (11) was found. Methicillin-resistant S. aureus is not endemic in Sweden, but is sometimes imported from abroad. A few borderline methicillin-resistant S. aureus strains have been isolated at our laboratory during the last decade, but not during the periods covered by this study.

All 58 coagulase-negative staphylococci (CNS) were identified as S. epidermidis. 44 (76%) of the isolates produced betalactamase, and 29 (50%) were resistant to methicillin (MRSE).

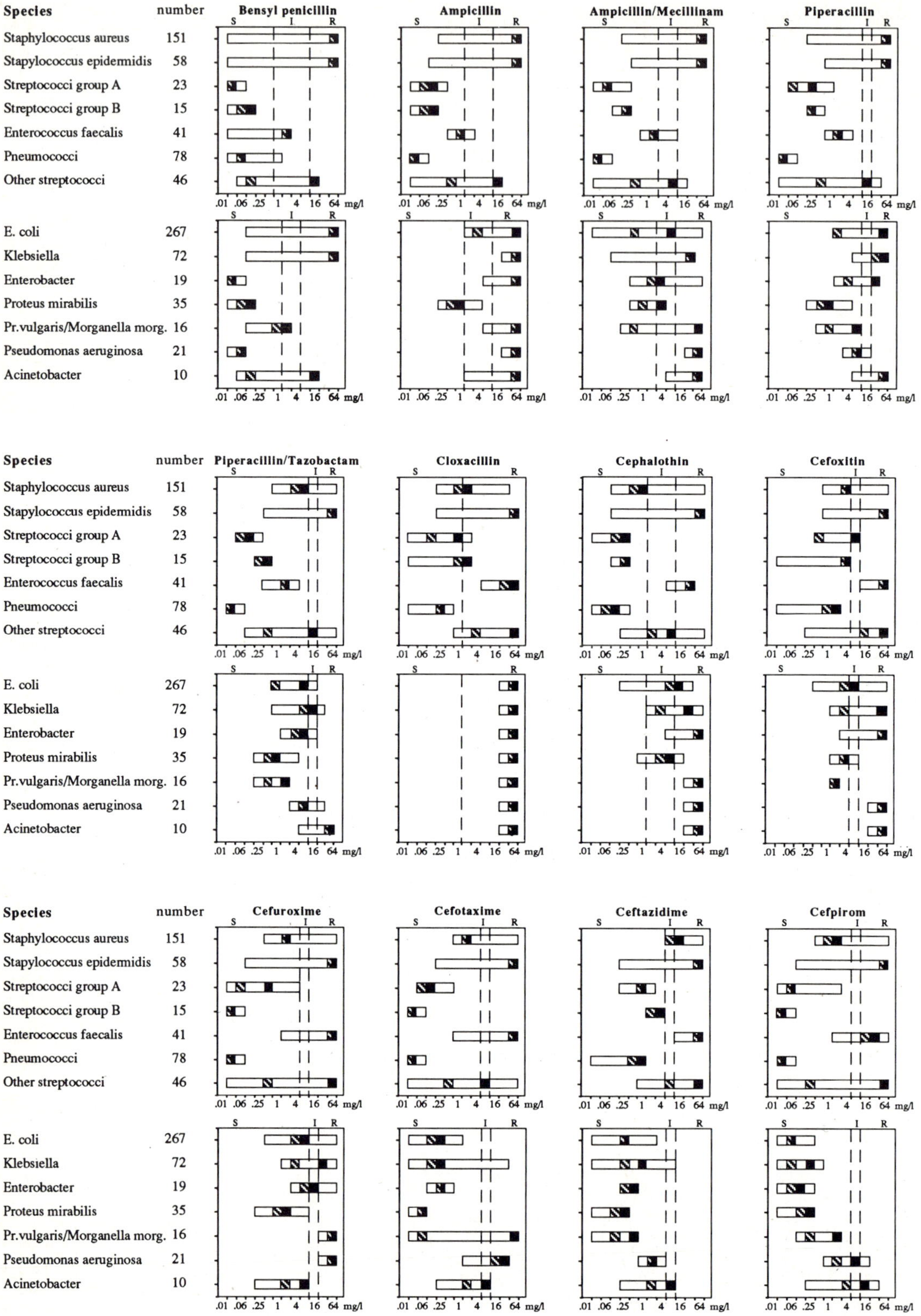
Species
number
Staphylococcus aureus 151
Stapylococcus epidermidis 58
Streptococci group A 23
Streptococci group B 15
Enterococcus faecalis 41
Pneumococci 78
Other streptococci 46
E. coli 267
Klebsiella 72
Enterobacter 19
Proteus mirabilis 35
Pr.vulgaris/Morganella morg. 16
Pseudomonas aeruginosa 21
Acinetobacter 10
Bensyl penicillin
Ampicillin
Ampicillin/Mecillinam
Piperacillin
Piperacillin/Tazobactam
Cloxacillin
Cephalothin
Cefoxitin
Cefuroxime
Cefotaxime
Ceftazidime
Cefpirom
S
I
R
.01 .06 .25 1 4 16 64 mg/l

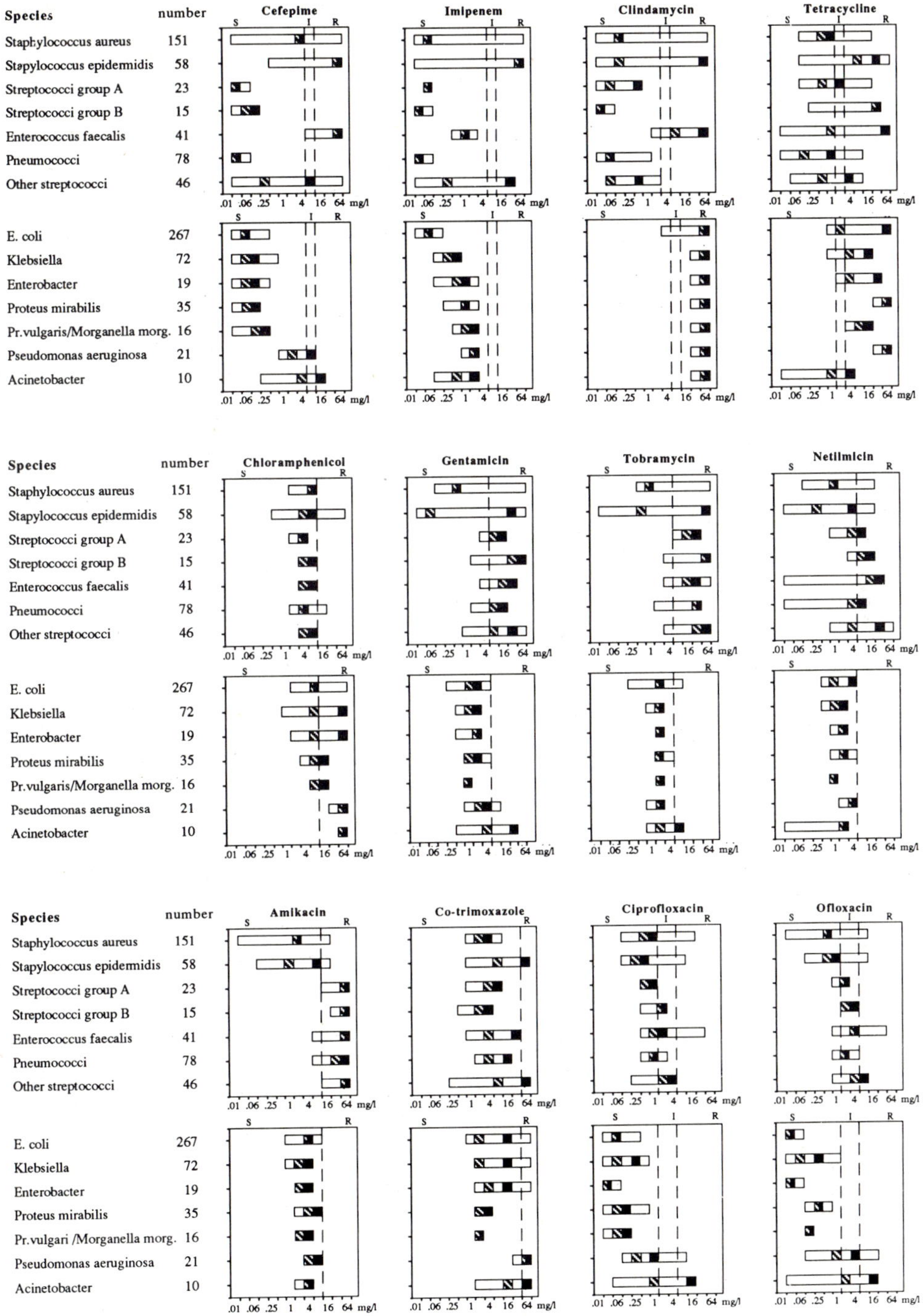

Fig. 1. Antibiotic susceptibility of 852 blood culture isolates to 14 betalactam antibiotics and to 10 other antibiotics. SIR breakpoints according to MIC values (mg/l) used in Sweden (Table I). All betalactamase-producing staphylococci were given an MIC value of 64 mg/l for benzylpenicillin, ampicillin and piperacillin, and all methicillin-resistant staphylococci were given an MIC value of 64 mg/l for betalactam antibiotics.

▧ MIC_{50} ■ MIC_{90} □ Range

Almost all streptococci isolated were sensitive to penicillins, except for enterococci which are naturally penicillin-resistant. Two strains of Streptococcus pneumoniae were not fully sensitive to penicillin at ≥ 0.1 mg/l, one of them had MIC 2.0 mg/l.

Cephalosporins and imipenem

Of the new cephalosporins, cefpirom was as active as cefuroxime against staphylococci, whereas the second and third generation cephalosporins cefotaxim and ceftazidim were slightly less active than cefuroxime against Gram-positive cocci, especially S. aureus. All cephalosporins manifested very limited activity against enterococci. Five strains of the 46 Streptococcus species were identified as Enterococcus faecium and were therefore resistant to imipenem. The 2 Listeria isolates were resistant to all cephalosporins.

Aminoglycosides

The only MRSA strain detected among the 151 S. aureus strains was also resistant to aminoglycosides. Of CNS strains, 10% were resistant to netilmicin, and approximately one-third were resistant both to gentamicin and to tobramycin. No highly aminoglycoside-resistant strains of enterococci were observed.

Other antibiotics

Clindamycin was fully active against S. aureus (except the MRSA strain) and all streptococci, but only against two-thirds of CNS strains and none of the Enterococci.

Tetracycline-resistant isolates were detected among all Gram-positive species. Many group A streptococci (55%) were resistant to tetracycline, compared with less than 10% reported for isolates from tonsillitis (12, 13).

Co-trimoxazole manifested quite good activity against Gram-positive isolates, and none of the E. faecalis isolates were resistant to it.

Quinolone (ciprofloxacin and ofloxacin) resistance was infrequent among staphylococci (2–5%) isolated from blood specimens. Streptococci are known to be moderately resistant to quinolones and we found about one-third of the isolates to be quinolone-resistant. However, only 5% of E. faecalis strains were resistant. Ofloxacin and ciprofloxacin were comparable in activity.

B. Gram-negative isolates (Fig. 1)

Penicillins

A large proportion of E. coli isolates from blood specimens were resistant to *ampicillin* (19%).

Piperacillin was active against 85% of E. coli isolates, 85% of Enterobacter species, 100% of P. mirabilis and indole-positive Proteus species, and 90% of P. aeruginosa. In contrast, only 3% of Klebsiella and 5% of Acinetobacter species were sensitive. The addition of tazobactam (a betalactam inhibitor) to piperacillin potentiated its activity against most Gram-negative species, but not against P. aeruginosa or Acinetobacter strains. The combination of ampicillin and mecillinam manifested better activity against Enterobacteriaceae strains (sensitivity 80%), than did ampicillin alone (45%).

Cephalosporins and imipenem

The blood isolates tested were generally more sensitive to all cephalosporins than were urine and wound isolates collected during the same period at our hospital. Cefepime was the most active, followed by cefpirom, ceftazidime, cefotaxime and cefuroxime. All isolates, except the

2 Xanthomonas maltophilia strains, were sensitive to imipenem. No stably depressed mutants of Enterobacter were found (14).

Aminoglycosides
All of the Enterobacteriaceae were fully sensitive to all of the aminoglycosides (Fig. 1). Resistance to aminoglycosides was only seen among Acinetobacter species.

Other antibiotics (Fig. 1)
Sensitivity of Enterobacteriaceae to co-trimoxazole ranged from 92 to 100%. P. aeruginosa and Acinetobacter species were resistant to co-trimoxazole.

Chloramphenicol was effective against most Enterobacteriaceae, but all P. aeruginosa and Acinetobacter were resistant to it.

Tetracycline was not very effective against Gram-negative isolates.

Quinolones
Enterobacteriaceae were fully sensitive both to ciprofloxacin and to ofloxacin, and no strains were highly resistant to quinolones (i.e. MIC $\geq$ 32) (15). Only 1 resistant strain was found among P. aeruginosa, and some Acinetobacter species were also resistant to quinolones, with MIC_{90} values of 4–16 mg/l.

C. Combined activity against Gram-positive and negative bacteria (*n* = *880*, Table II)
The overall percentage of blood isolates inhibited (susceptibility groups S = sensitive + I = intermediate) by the different betalactam-antibiotics in this study was less than that found in our 1981 study (5). This is probably due to the fact that all methicillin-resistant staphylococci (MRS) were assigned an MIC value of 64 mg/l in the present study.

Although piperacillin alone manifested a rather poor effect (84% of strains being inhibited), in combination with the betalactamase inhibitor, tazobactam, it ranked fourth (95% of strains inhibited). In addition to the 30 MRS strains, 16 were resistant to the combination: 5 Acinetobacter species, 2 Klebsiella species, 5 Streptococcus species, and 4 E. faecalis, altogether 46 strains.

Table II. *Antibacterial activity against 880 Gram-positive and negative bacteria from blood cultures (n = number)*

Percentage of strains inhibited (sensitive plus intermediate).

	Total	Exclusion of	
		Methicillin-resistant staphylococci (*n* = 30)	Enterococcus faecalis (*n* = 41)
Ciprofloxacin	98.6	99.3	98.3
Ofloxacin	98.2	98.8	97.9
Imipenem	95.7	99.0	95.5
Piperacillin/tazobactam	95.0	98.4	94.9
Cefpirom	91.6	94.8	94.9
Cefepime	91.1	94.4	95.4
Co-trimoxazole	90.9	93.9	90.3
Cefotaxime	88.3	91.4	91.5
Chloramphenicol	86.6	88.0	87.6
Netilmicin	82.5	82.5	85.6

Of the cephalosporins, cefotaxime was effective against 88% of strains (or 91% if MRS or E. faecalis were excluded). Both cefpirom and cefepime manifested a very good effect against the blood isolates tested, 92% and 91%, respectively, of strains being inhibited (or 95% for both antibiotics if MRS or E. faecalis were excluded).

The third highest level of activity was found for imipenem, 96% of strains being found to be sensitive, and after exclusion of the 30 MRS, 99% of blood isolates were sensitive (almost identical with the figure of 98.7% obtained in the 1981 study). Now only 8 strains were resistant, 2 Xanthomonas maltophilia, 5 streptococcus species identified as E. faecium, 1 Proteus vulgaris. However, the 30 MRS strains had the Mec gene, and therefore could probably not be treated with imipenem (16).

Quinolones were the most effective drugs tested in this study. Ciprofloxacin and ofloxacin inhibited 98.6% and 98.2% of strains, respectively. Only 12 strains were resistant to ciprofloxacin: 1 Acinetobacter species, 1 S. aureus, 8 CNS and 2 E. faecalis; to ofloxacin, another 4 strains of streptococci were resistant.

D. Comparison of MIC results for the 1981, 1989 and 1992 studies

Blood isolates from the 1981 study (5) were retested in the 1989 study to check reproducibility. There was an increase in S. aureus strains producing betalactamase, from 67% in 1981 to 85% in the present study. No other major significant changes either in MIC_{50} or in MIC_{90} ($>$doubling of median MIC) values were recorded for any species except Acinetobacter. Of the latter, the strains from the 1981 study belonged to the sensitive species, A. bowmanni, whereas all of the 1989 strains belonged to the more resistant species. A. lwoffi or A. calcoaceticus (7). Identical MIC_{50} and MIC_{90} values were found when blood isolates from 1989 (period I) and 1992 (period II) were compared.

E. Comparison with the European collaborative study 1987/88

The present findings confirm the low level of antibiotic resistance earlier reported from North European countries in the European collaborative study (17). For betalactam antibiotics and ciprofloxacin, the present findings show lower frequencies of resistance among staphylococci and P. aeruginosa than was reported in the collaborative study. In the present study, however, E. coli isolates manifested slightly higher resistance to ampicillin – but not to piperacillin – than reported for Swedish isolates in the collaborative study (19% vs. 15% and 10% vs. 12%, respectively). All our E. coli isolates were sensitive to cephalosporins except 2 strains resistant to cefuroxime and 12 resistant to cefoxitin. The reason for the higher ampicillin resistance found for E. coli may be overconsumption of ampicillin during several years, as compared with other antibiotics. The low level of antibiotic resistance among blood isolates from Sweden found in the present study is encouraging for those designing the antibiotic policy and establishing the empirical antibiotic therapy for sepsis patients, but there is always a risk of the development of resistance and the import of resistant strains from abroad, justifying new studies in the future.

ACKNOWLEDGEMENT

In honour and remembrance of Björn Ode, deceased 1990, who initiated and designed this study as a follow-up of his earlier work.

REFERENCES

1. Burma RJA, Horrevorts AM, Wagenvoort JHT. Incidence of multi-resistant gram-negative isolates in eight Dutch hospitals. Scand J Infect Dis Suppl 78: 35–44, 1991.
2. Shah PM, Asanger R, Kahan FM. Incidence of multi-resistance in gram-negative aerobes from intensive care units of 10 German hospitals. Scand J Infect Dis Suppl 78: 22–34, 1991.

3. Fredlund H, Björeman M, Kjellander J, Sjöberg L, Bjorne L, Öhlin A-L. A 10-year survey of clinically significant blood culture isolates and antibiotic susceptibilities from adult patients with hematological diseases at a major Swedish hospital. Scand J Infect Dis 22: 381–391, 1990.
4. Scheel O, Iversen G. Resistant strains isolated from bacteremia patients in northern Norway. Scand J Infect Dis 23: 599–605, 1991.
5. Ode B, Forsgren A, Walder M. Sensitivity of 523 blood culture isolates to 33 antibiotics. Scand J Infect Dis 16: 61–71, 1984.
6. Cowan ST, Steel KJ. Manual for the identification of medical bacteria. London: Cambridge University Press, 1970.
7. Tjernberg I. Antimicrobial susceptibility of Acinetobacter strains identified by DNA-DNA hybridization. APMIS 98: 320–326, 1990.
8. Ericsson HM, Sherris JC. Antibiotic sensitivity testing. Report of an international collaborative study. Acta Pathol Microbiol Scand, Suppl 217, 1971.
9. Swedish Reference Group for Antibiotics: A revised system for antibiotic sensitivity testing. Scand J Infect Dis 13: 148, 1981.
10. Örstavik I, Ödegaard K. A simple test for penicillinase production in Staphylococcus aureus. Acta Pathol Microbiol Scand (B) 79: 855, 1971.
11. McDouglas L, Thornsberry C. The role of beta-lactamase in staphylococcal resistance to penicillinase-resistant penicillins and cephalosporins. J Clin Microbiol 23: 832–839, 1986.
12. Jansson L, Kalin M. Comparative in vitro activity of A-56268 against respiratory tract pathogens. Eur J Clin Microbiol 6: 494–496, 1987.
13. Forsgren A, Walder M. Activity of common antibiotics against Branhamella catarrhalis, Haemophilus influenzae, pneumococci, group A streptococci and Staphylococcus aureus in 1983. Acta Otolaryngol Suppl 407: 43–49, 1984.
14. Livermore DM. Mechanisms of resistance to β-lactam antibiotics. Scand J Infect Dis 78: 7–16, 1991.
15. Jonson M, Walder M, Forsgren A. First clinical isolate of highly fluoroquinolone-resistant Escherichia coli in Scandinavia. Eur J Clin Microbiol Infect Dis 9: 851–853, 1990.
16. Hackbart CJ, Chambers HF. Methicillin-resistant staphylococci: genetics and mechanisms of resistance. Antimicrob Agents Chemother 33: 991–994, 1989.
17. Dornbusch K and The European Study Group of Antibiotic Resistance. Resistance to β-lactam antibiotics and ciprofloxacin in gram-negative bacilli and staphylococci isolated from blood: a European collaborative study. J Antimicrob Chemother 26: 269–278, 1990.

Scand J Infect Dis 26: 77–84, 1994

Incidence and Clinical Significance of Positive Blood Cultures in Febrile Episodes of Patients with Hematological Malignancies

ESA RINTALA

From the Departments of Medicine and Medical Microbiology, Turku University, Turku, Finland

The characteristics of 554 febrile episodes in 126 patients with a hematological malignancy over a 6-year period (1985–90) were reviewed in order to study the current incidence and clinical significance of blood culture positivity. An infection was documented microbiologically in 28% and clinically in 30% of the episodes. Blood cultures were positive in 19% of the febrile episodes. The rate of blood culture positivity was unrelated to the type of hematological malignancy, to neutropenia and to the presence of infection foci. 21% (26/126) of the patients died of sepsis-related causes. Sepsis-related death occurred in 23% of the blood culture positive febrile epidoses, with a median survival time of 2 days. Infection prophylaxis did not reduce either the rate of blood culture positivity or the rate of sepsis-related deaths. Thus, the small proportion of febrile episodes whose fever etiology could be established by blood culture represented 'the tip of the iceberg', i.e. rapidly lethal septic infections with a high mortality rate. This fatality could neither be predicted by a search for infection foci nor prevented by infection prophylaxis.

Esa Rintala, MD, Department of Medicine, Turku University Central Hospital, FIN-20520 Turku, Finland

INTRODUCTION

Blood cultures are routinely taken at the admission of a febrile patient suffering from a hematological malignancy (1). Isolation of bacteria by blood culture is an important prognostic finding, because sepsis in hematological patients with impaired host defence mechanisms carries a high mortality (2).

Although the prognosis of patients with hematological malignancies has improved significantly in recent years (1), sepsis is still a significant cause of death among these patients. Fever frequently accompanies neutropenia in hematological malignanices and may be the first and only sign of sepsis (3). The distinction of sepsis from other causes of fever presents a common and challenging clinical problem in the treatment of hematological patients. Therefore, evaluation of the current incidence and clinical significance of blood culture positivity in febrile patients with a hematological malignancy is needed.

In an attempt to identify patients with a high risk of sepsis, a retrospective analysis of acute febrile episodes was performed in patients with a hematological malignancy. The aims of the study were: 1) to establish the current frequency and etiology of positive blood cultures and the sepsis-related mortality in acute febrile episodes, and 2) to identify the factors that are associated with a positive blood culture and sepsis-related death.

PATIENTS AND METHODS

The patients with a diagnosis of acute or chronic leukemia, multiple myeloma, or myelodysplastic syndrome together with a diagnosis of sepsis, bacteremia, septicemia or fever of unknown origin who were treated at the hematological ward of Turku University Central Hospital between January 1, 1985 and December 31, 1990 were included in this study. Patients with a febrile episode were included if the axillary temperature exceeded 38°C on ≥ 2 occasions within a 12-h period or >38.3°C at least once (4). The febrile episodes were regarded as 2 separate instances if the axillary temperature was <37.5°C for >3 days between 2 fever tops as defined above.

The following data were recorded in each patient: the number of febrile episodes during the study period, the bacterial isolates of blood, urine and other infection sites, the use of infection prophylaxis, the appropriateness of prophylactic antimicrobials, the neutrophil count on admission, focal symptoms and signs, the time interval between the onset of cytotoxic treatment and the onset of fever, the occurrence of sepsis-related death and the survival time.

Two blood samples for bacterial culture were taken on admission or, in hospitalized patients, at the onset of fever. Thereafter, blood was cultured for bacteria daily, or every other day if fever >38°C persisted. If indicated by clinical symptoms and signs, a chest radiograph was taken at the onset of fever. A sample for chemical screening and bacterial culture of urine was collected routinely at the onset of fever.

The blood samples for culture were drawn into Isolator™ tubes (DuPont de Nemours & Co Inc., Wilmington, Delaware, USA). After centrifugation, the sediments were cultured on McLeod (aerobic incubation) and menadione–cysteine enriched brucella blood agars (anaerobic incubation). The plates were inspected daily for 7 days.

Susceptibility testing was performed in parallel with the disk diffusion method (Biodisk AB, Solna, Sweden) on PDM-agar (Biodisk) and with an in-house minimal inhibitory concentration (MIC) microtitre dilution method. Cation-supplemented Mueller-Hinton broth (Biodisk) was used in the MIC method.

Infection prophylaxis was defined as the use of an oral antimicrobial agent with an explicit intention to prevent infections (primary prophylaxis) or infection recurrences (secondary prophylaxis) (5). The prophylaxis was regarded as appropriate if the bacterial isolate proved susceptible to the antimicrobial agent that the patient had been receiving. Prophylaxis was classified as incorrect if an antimicrobial was used that was either found to be ineffective by susceptibility testing or not considered to be an acceptable drug according to standard guidelines (6).

The febrile episode was considered neutropenic if the neutrophil count was $<0.5 \times 10^9/l$ (4).

An infection was considered *microbiologically* documented if there were specific signs and symptoms with respect to an infection that was microbiologically proven by culture or antigen detection (7). An infection was considered *clinically* documented if there were definite signs and symptoms of an infection in an identifiable site and if the etiological agent could not be identified by the microbiological techniques mentioned (7). Febrile episodes not classifiable into either of these 2 categories were defined as *fever of unknown origin* (7).

Sepsis was defined as a blood culture positive febrile episode that was accompanied by a systemic response, i.e. tachypnea (>20 breaths/min), tachycardia (>90 beats/min), and hyperthermia or hypothermia (core or rectal temperature >38.3°C or <35.6°C) (8). In patients with a negative blood culture, signs of invasive disseminated bacterial infection at autopsy were required before a diagnosis of sepsis was established.

Death was considered sepsis-related if it occurred within 7 days of the last positive blood culture and if there were no other obvious causes of death (6). Death within 7 days of admission was regarded as sepsis-related, if the autopsy revealed signs of sepsis, even in the face of negative blood cultures. Survival time was defined as the time between the admission and death.

The blood culture isolate was regarded as a contaminant if coagulase-negative staphylococci or Propionibacterium sp. were cultured in a single blood sample (1, 9, 10). A single blood culture positive for Staphylococcus aureus was considered significant (1).

Statistical methods

Frequencies were compared with the χ^2-test or 2-tailed Fisher's exact test. Student's *t*-test was used to compare means. *P*-values <0.05 were regarded as statistically significant.

RESULTS

There were 554 episodes of fever in 126 patients. 67 (53%) of the patients were men, 59 (47%) women, their mean age being 61 ± 14 yrs (±SD, range 24–91 yrs). Table I shows the diagnoses. 68% (376/554) of the febrile eipsodes were neutropenic.

In 153/554 episodes (28%) an infection was documented microbiologically and in 167/554 episodes (30%) clinically. The cause of fever was unknown in 234/554 episodes (42%).

Blood cultures were obtained in 503/554 (91%) febrile episodes, in 93% of these within 1 hour before empiric antimicrobials were started. The blood culture was positive in 104

Table I. *Diagnoses of the 126 study patients and the numbers of blood culture positive febrile episodes and sepsis-related deaths*

$p = 0.332$, the frequency of the blood culture positive episodes in each diagnosis.
$p = 0.329$, the frequency of the sepsis-related deaths in each diagnosis.

Diagnosis	No. (%) of patients	No. (%) of pos. episodes	No. (%) of sepsis related deaths
Multiple myeloma	43 (34)	25 (26)	9 (35)
Acute myeloblastic leukemia	34 (27)	32 (33)	8 (31)
Chronic lymphocytic leukemia	25 (20)	19 (19)	6 (23)
Acute lymphoblastic leukemia	13 (10)	20 (20)	2 (8)
Chronic myelocytic leukemia	7 (6)	2 (2)	0
Myelodysplastic syndrome	2 (2)	0	1 (4)
Hairy cell leukemia	1 (1)	0	0
Undetermined	1 (1)	0	0
Total	126 (100)	98 (100)	26 (100)

febrile episodes, in 6 of which, >1 blood culture isolate was found, making a total of 113 blood culture isolates recovered. Six contaminants in 6 episodes were found. After exclusion of the contaminates, 107 blood culture isolates were detected in 98 febrile episodes (Fig. 1). The frequency of blood culture positive episodes was 19% (98/503).

The number of blood culture positive febrile episodes was 1.4 ± 0.8 (range 1–5)/patient during the study period. Table II shows the pertinent clinical characteristics of the patients who had blood culture positive/negative febrile episodes. The distribution of the frequency of blood cultures was similar in each type of hematological malignancy (Table I). The blood culture was equally often positive in neutropenic and non-neutropenic episodes, in men and women, and in patients of different ages (Table II). The number of preceding febrile episodes was the same regardless of whether the patient had a positive blood culture or not, and the same was true for the interval between the previous cytotoxic treatment course and the onset of fever (Table II).

Table III shows the foci of the infections at initial clinical evaluation. There were focal signs of infection in 45% (249/554) of febrile episodes, pneumonia and urinary tract infections being most common. Infection foci were found equally often in patients given (15%)/not given (27%) infection prophylaxis ($p = 0.171$). Two of the 3 infections of an

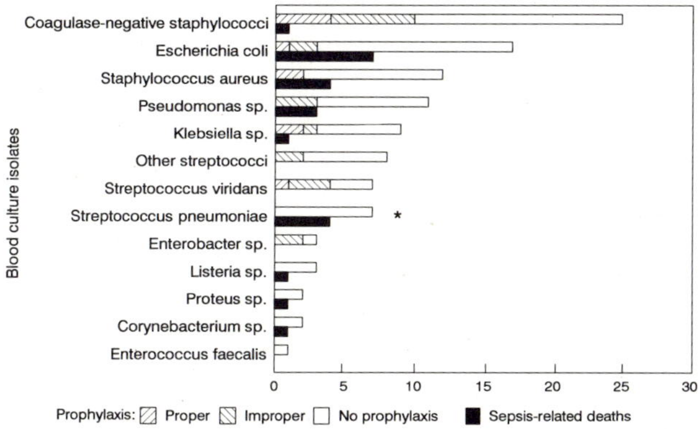

Fig. 1. Blood culture isolates and sepsis-related deaths. The appropriateness of infection prophylaxis according to each isolate is shown. *$p = 0.033$, the rate of sepsis-related death caused by S. pneumoniae.

Table II. *Clinical characteristics of 554 febrile episodes*

Characteristic	Blood culture positive episodes	Blood culture negative episodes	p[a]
No. of episodes	98	405	
Male/female	54/44	236/169	0.582
Age (yrs, mean ± SD, range)	60 ± 16 (24–91)	57 ± 15 (24–91)	0.208
Neutropenia	72	268	0.162
Time from cytotoxic treatment (d)	15 ± 11 (0–52)	16 ± 13 (0–73)	0.737
Survival time (d)	14 ± 22 (0.5–75)	37 ± 26 (1–90)	<0.001
No. of preceding febrile episodes	4 ± 3 (1–14)	5 ± 4 (1–22)	0.306
Infection prophylaxis used	29 (30%)	113 (28%)	0.707

[a] Blood culture positive/negative episodes.

Table III. *Focal infections in blood culture positive and negative febrile episodes*

Infection focus	Blood culture positive (%)	Blood culture negative (%)	p[a]
No focus	60 (61)	245 (60)	0.893
Pneumonia	14 (14)	59 (15)	1.000
Urinary tract infection	7 (7)	21 (5)	0.423
Cellulitis	6 (6)	14 (3)	0.211
Perianal infection	4 (4)	8 (2)	0.208
Stomatitis	3 (3)	17 (4)	0.626
Infection of catheter	2 (2)	1 (0.2)	0.028
Pharyngotonsillitis	1 (1)	15 (4)	0.181
Upper airway infection	1 (1)	19 (5)	0.100
Thrombophlebitis	0	3 (1)	0.397
Gastroenteritis	0	1 (0.2)	0.626
Herpes zoster	0	2 (0.4)	0.490
Total	98 (100)	405 (100)	

[a] Blood culture positive/negative episodes.

indwelling venous catheter were associated with a positive blood culture. No other infection foci predicted blood culture positivity. Infection foci were detected equally often in neutropenic (60%) and in non-neutropenic episodes (56%) ($p = 0.312$).

In 28% (156/554) of febrile episodes in 49% (62/126) of patients, infection prophylaxis was given. Table IV shows the antimicrobials used in infection prophylaxis. The blood culture proved positive in 29 of the febrile episodes in which prophylaxis was given. The use of prophylactic antimicrobials did not affect the rate of blood culture positivity (Table II). Prophylactic antimicrobials were appropriate in 10/29 and incorrect in 18/29 blood culture positive febrile episodes.

The frequency of sepsis-related deaths among episodes with a positive blood culture was 23% (23/98). 18 patients with a negative blood culture died within 7 days of admission; 14 were autopsied. Three of these 14 patients had signs of sepsis. Thus, 21% [(23 + 3)/126] of the patients died of sepsis-related causes and 88% (23/26) of them had a positive blood culture.

Table IV. *Antimicrobials used for infection prophylaxis*

Antimicrobial	No. of febrile episodes
SUT[a]	42
Ciprofloxacin + penicillin + antifungal	19
Ciprofloxacin	19
1st generation cephalosporins	15
Ciprofloxacin + antifungal	13
SUT + antifungal	10
Erythromycin	8
Ciprofloxacin + other antimicrobials	5
Penicillin + other antimicrobials	5
SUT + other antimicrobials	4
1st generation cephalosporins + antifungal	4
Trimethoprim	3
Cefuroxim axetil	2
Ampicillin	1
Other	6
Total	156

[a] SUT = sulfamethoxazole-trimethoprim.

Fig. 1 shows sepsis-related deaths and the blood culture isolates. The deaths caused by Streptococcus pneumoniae sepsis were overrepresented ($p = 0.033$). Of the 7 episodes with blood culture positive for S. pneumoniae, 4 were in multiple myeloma, 2 in chronic lymphocytic leukemia and 1 in acute myeloblastic leukemia. Of these episodes, 57% (4/7) were neutropenic. Of 4 patients who died of pneumococcal sepsis, 2 had multiple myeloma, 1 chronic lymphocytic leukemia and 1 acute myeloblastic leukemia. Of the patients who died of pneumococcal sepsis, 2 were neutropenic and 2 were not.

The frequency of sepsis-related deaths was similar among men and women (15 and 11 patients, respectively, $p = 1.000$). A patient's age at the time of the febrile episode was not predictive of sepsis-related death (63 ± 14 yrs in patients with sepsis-related death and 61 ± 15 yrs without sepsis-related death, $p = 0.613$).

The type of hematological malignancy was not associated with an elevated risk of sepsis-related death (Table I). Febrile episodes with and without a sepsis-related death were equally often neutropenic (18 and 8 episodes, respectively, $p = 0.879$).

The survival time was significantly shorter in episodes with a positive blood culture than with a negative (Table II). The mean survival time in febrile episodes leading to sepsis-related death was 3 days (± 3 d, range 0.5–9 d, median 2 d). Two patients died of sepsis despite infection prophylaxis: 1 had received appropriate antimicrobial, the other did not.

DISCUSSION

Almost half of the febrile episodes in the present study had to be classified as fever of unknown origin despite a thorough search for the etiology. This agrees with earlier studies (7, 11). Only 28% of the febrile episodes were etiologically defined in terms of microbiological findings. In only 19% of the febrile episodes was the blood culture positive, despite the fact that blood samples were cultured in 91% of all episodes and usually very soon after the onset of fever and before the administration of antimicrobials. The etiology of the fever remains obscure in 40–70% of the febrile episodes, even in prospective studies (4, 7, 12). Of the patients who died of sepsis, 88% had a positive blood culture in this study.

Staphylococci and streptococci were frequently detected in blood cultures. Gram-positive bacteria have become increasingly significant pathogens in neutropenic patients, although they are usually associated with a low mortality rate (3, 12, 13).

The rates of blood culture positivity were similar in neutropenic and non-neutropenic episodes and not related to the type of hematological malignancy. These findings suggest that, in general, none of the immunological disturbances characteristic of the various hematological malignancies predispose specifically to a positive blood culture when the patient becomes septic.

Blood culture was positive for S. pneumoniae in 7 febrile episodes in 7 patients, but was significantly overrepresented in the group of sepsis-related deaths. It is noteworthy that none of the patients who died of pneumococcal sepsis received infection prophylaxis. Multiple myeloma and chronic lymphocytic leukemia were well represented in febrile episodes caused by pneumococcal sepsis. Of 4 patients who died of pneumococcal sepsis, 2 had multiple myeloma and 1 chronic lymphocytic leukemia. It is well known that these malignancies are associated with an increased risk of fatal infections caused by encapsulated bacteria (14). Furthermore, most cases of pneumococcal sepsis and half of the episodes of sepsis-related death caused by S. pneumoniae were neutropenic. These findings stress the importance of penicillin as a constituent of prophylactic regimes for neutropenic patients with multiple myeloma and chronic lymphocytic leukemia.

In general, neutropenia did not increase the yield of positive blood cultures, possibly due to the unselected patient population in the present study. More advanced diseases, together with prolonged hospitalization, complicated infections and an increased risk of developing nosocomial sepsis were possibly represented in excess when compared with better selected study populations.

The rate of positive blood cultures was unrelated to the age or sex of the patients. The number of preceding febrile episodes was similar in blood culture positive and negative episodes, indicating that the number of previous infection complications was not associated with a significantly elevated risk of sepsis. The febrile episode usually occurred 2 weeks after the initiation of a cytotoxic treatment course, although at this time point no significantly increased risk of sepsis was found.

The site of an infection, when identifiable, was not related to whether the febrile episode gave a positive blood culture or not (Table III). The only exception was when the infection was caused by an indwelling catheter, but there were only 3 such episodes. In general, the suspicion of sepsis cannot be based on whether there are focal signs or not at the initial clinical evaluation of a febrile patient.

Since the gastrointestinal tract may be the main source of sepsis during neutropenia (15), efforts have been made to suppress the bacterial flora in the gut by administering antimicrobial agents perorally (13). Preliminary studies showed a significant reduction in infections when applying such a policy (16, 17). In the present study, however, infection prophylaxis reduced neither the frequency of focal infections during febrile episodes nor the rate of the blood culture positivity or sepsis-related deaths. The lack of prophylactic effect may have been due to advanced hematological disease, long hospitalization or complicated infections of the patients in the present study. In 62% of the blood cultures taken during infection prophylaxis, the isolate proved resistant to the antimicrobials used for prophylaxis, but this resistance did not raise the mortality rate due to sepsis. It would appear prudent to reassess the policy of infection prophylaxis for patients with a hematological malignancy. The possible benefits of infection prophylaxis in patients with advanced hematological malignancies must be weighed against elevated costs, elevated risk of adverse effects and the risk of creating resistant bacteria. On the other hand, the risk of streptococcal infection, including fatal pneumococcal sepsis, favours the use of penicillin in prophylactic regimes for neutropenic patients with certain hematological malignancies, since such regimens containing quinolones have been found to be associated with an increased frequency of infections caused by Gram-positive bacteria (3, 12).

Sepsis was surprisingly seldom associated with localizing symptoms and findings and it seems that sepsis is not related to focal infection in febrile patients with a hematological malignancy. Focal infections were not specifically associated with blood culture positivity or sepsis-related death. The reason for such pathogenetic disconnection between focal and septic infections is unclear. Further studies are needed to elicit the factors predisposing patients with a hematological malignancy to sepsis rather than to locally restricted infections. Survival time was significantly shorter in the blood culture positive febrile episodes than in the negative (Table II). The median survival time in febrile episodes leading to sepsis-related death was only 2 days. This is important to note, as most blood culture techniques require 2–3 days to complete. Furthermore, the results of early cultures may be difficult to interpret and the results may not always become translated into clinical decisions (18, 19). Rapid and unambiguous techniques for the detection of sepsis in febrile patients with a hematological malignancy are obviously needed.

In conclusion: often no infection could be documented in patients with a hematological malignancy who became suddenly febrile. Blood cultures were positive in only 19% of the febrile episodes. Of these, however, 23% led to sepsis-related death within the succeeding 2–3 days. Thus, the small proportion of febrile episodes in which the etiology of the fever could be established by positive blood culture represented ‘the tip of the iceberg’, i.e. the fraction of infectious complications that had short survival time and high mortality rate. This fatality could neither be predicted by infection foci nor prevented by infection prophylaxis.

Prospective studies are needed to elucidate the mechanisms that predispose patients with a hematological malignancy to the uncontrolled dissemination of bacteria rather than the local restriction of an infection. Early intervention to combat such mechanisms, together with the rapid detection of sepsis, would improve the outcome for septic patients with a hematological malignancy.

ACKNOWLEDGEMENTS

I thank Erkki Eerola, M.D. (Department of Medical Microbiology, Turku University, Turku) for providing the blood culture results and Pentti Huovinen, M.D. (National Institute of Health, Turku) for providing the results of the susceptibility tests.

REFERENCES

1. Meunier F. Infections in patients with acute leukemia and lymphoma. In: Mandell GL, Douglas RG, Bennet JE, eds. Principles and practice of infectious diseases, 3rd edn. New York: Churchill Livingstone, 2265–2275, 1990.
2. Bodey GP, Rodriguez V, Chang H-Y, Narboni G. Fever and infection in leukemic patients. Cancer 41: 1610–1622, 1978.
3. Pizzo PA. Evaluation of fever in the patient with cancer. European Journal of Cancer & Clinical Oncology 25 (Suppl 2): S9–S16, 1989.
4. Hughes WT, Pizzo PA, Wade JC, Armstrong D, Webb CD, Young LS. Evaluation of new anti-infective drugs for the treatment of febrile episodes in neutropenic patients. Clin Infect Dis 15 (Suppl 1): S206–S215, 1992.
5. Froeland SS. Antimicrobial chemoprophylaxis in immunocompromised patients. Scand J Infect Dis Suppl 70: 130–140, 1990.
6. Bryan CS, Reynolds KL, Brenner ER. Analysis of 1186 episodes of gram-negative bacteremia in non-university hospitals: the effects of antimicrobial therapy. Rev Infect Dis 5: 629–638, 1983.

7. Klastersky J, Zinner SH, Calandra T, Gaya H, Glauser MP, Meunier F, Rossi M, Schimpff SC, Tattersall M, Viscoli C, EORTC Antimicrobial Therapy Cooperative Group. Empiric antimicrobial therapy for febrile granulocytopenic cancer patients: lessons from four EORTC trials. European Journal of Cancer & Clinical Oncology 24 (Suppl 1): S35–S45, 1988.
8. Bone RC. Sepsis, the sepsis syndrome, multi-organ failure: a plea for comparable definitions. Ann Intern Med 114: 332–333, 1991.
9. Richet H, Escande MC, Lagrange PH. Lysis centrifugation and slide blood culture systems for diagnosis of bacteremia in immunocompromised patients. Eur J Clin Microbiol Infect Dis 6: 64–67, 1987.
10. Henry NK, Grewell CM, Van Grevenhof PE, Ilstrup DM, Washington II JA. Comparison of lysis-centrifugation with a biphasic blood culture medium for the recovery of aerobic and facultatively anaerobic bacteria. J Clin Microbiol 20: 413–416, 1984.
11. Pizzo PA, Robichaud KJ, Wesley R, Commers JR. Fever in pediatric and young adult patient with cancer. A prospective study of 1001 episodes. Medicine (Baltimore) 61: 153–165, 1982.
12. Pizzo PA. Management of fever in patients with cancer and treatment-induced neutropenia. N Engl J Med 328: 1323–1332, 1993.
13. Klastersky J. Infections in compromised hosts: considerations on prevention. European Journal of Cancer & Clinical Oncology 25 (Suppl 2): S53–S61, 1989.
14. Schimpff SC. Infections in the compromised host – an overview. In: Mandell, Douglas, Bennet, eds. Principles and practice of infectious diseases, 3rd edn. New York: Churchill Livingstone, 2258–2265, 1990.
15. Schimpff SC. Infection prevention during profound granulocytopenia. Ann Intern Med 93: 358–361, 1980.
16. Storring RA, Jameson B, McElwain TJ, Wiltshaw E. Oral non-absorbed antibiotics prevent infection in acute non-lymphoblastic leukaemia. Lancet 2: 837–840, 1977.
17. Enno A, Catovsky D, Darrell J, Goldman JM, Hows J, Galton DAG. Co-trimoxazole for prevention of infection in acute leukaemia. Lancet 2: 395–397, 1978.
18. Campo L, Mylotte JM. Use of microbiology reports by physicians in prescribing antimicrobial agents. Am J Med Sci 296: 392–398, 1988.
19. Rintala E, Kairisto V, Eerola E, Nikoskelainen J, Lehtonen O-P. Antimicrobial therapy of septicemic patients in intensive care units before and after blood culture reporting. Scand J Infect Dis 23: 341–346, 1991.

Scand J Infect Dis 26: 85–93, 1994

Septic Arthritis of the Knee: a 10-Year Review and Long-term Follow-up using a New Scoring System

MARIE STUDAHL[1], BO BERGMAN[2], PETER KÄLEBO[3] and JOHAN LINDBERG[1]

From the Departments of [1]Infectious Diseases, [2]Orthopedic Surgery and [3]Radiology, Östra Hospital, University of Göteborg, Göteborg, Sweden

The case records of 64 patients with 65 episodes of infectious gonarthritis during 1979–88 were reviewed regarding epidemiological, clinical and laboratory data of possible relevance to the course and outcome of the disease. Long-term healing results were evaluated by means of a new scoring system 2–11 years after the acute disease in 46 patients. The infection was acquired by inoculation in 37% and by the hematogenous route in 55%. The major risk factors were trauma to the joint and arthrosis. Staphylococcus aureus was the causative agent in 58% and Streptococci in 15%. Treatment consisted of suction irrigation (86%) or intermittent aspiration (5%) combined with systemic antibiotic treatment. At follow-up, the pain and ache scores of the arthritic joint had decreased by 21% and 16% respectively, compared with the scores of the contralateral control joints. Anatomy and motility were reduced by 9% and 8% respectively. Age <45 was associated with a greater score loss than in older patients. Treatment delayed by >5 days was associated with increased loss of motility. We estimate that 79% of the patients had excellent or good long-term results following treatment of infectious arthritis of the knee. Evaluation of healing after infectious gonarthritis by use of a scoring system is quite feasible and allows comparison of different treatment regimes with improved accuracy.

M. Studahl, MD, Department of Infectious Diseases, Östra Hospital, S-416 85 Göteborg, Sweden

INTRODUCTION

Bacterial infections of the large joints have been reported to occur with an incidence of 2/100,000/year (1). Since the introduction of antibiotics, complete healing can be achieved, but even today severe functional and anatomical sequelae and even death may follow. Host factors as well as exogenous factors influence the outcome and it is difficult to determine the relevant prognostic factors.

One prerequisite for evaluation of the healing result is a method for measuring the condition of the joint. We have applied a scoring system – originally designed to evaluate postoperative healing results – to measure the long-term outcome of septic arthritis in the knee joint, which is the most common target of joint infections (2) and amenable to score evaluation. With this tool we have looked for associations between outcome and prognostic factors.

PATIENTS AND METHODS

All records of patients admitted to the Department of Infectious Diseases, Östra hospital, Göteborg, during 1979–88 with a diagnosis of infectious gonarthritis, were reviewed in 1991. Patients who fulfilled the diagnostic criteria were contacted and re-examined and/or interviewed 2–11 years after the arthritis episode. Patients with infection in a prosthetic joint, or tuberculous infections were not included.

The diagnosis of septic arthritis was based on the following criteria: Clinical signs and symptoms compatible with septic arthritis associated with

1) a positive bacterial culture from synovial fluid (SF) and/or blood, or
2) bacteria demonstrable by microscopy of synovial fluid.

From the patient records, data were collected regarding concomitant and earlier disease, interval between start of symptoms and start of treatment, laboratory data, type and duration of treatment and convalescence.

At follow-up, patients were assessed according to a scoring system which is a modification of that of Larson (3). In our version, 4 categories – anatomy, pain, ache, and motility – are examined and given score-points as shown in Table I. The maximum possible scoring is 50 points. For patients who were evaluated by questionnaire alone, only the pain and ache categories were included.

The arthritic joint (A-joint) scores were compared with those of the contralateral control joint (C-joint) to calculate the loss in score points caused by the disease.

An X-ray examination was made and pictures of the A-joint were compared with the C-joint or with exposures of the A-joint at the time of the acute disease. A standard examination of the knee included a frontal, a lateral and a patellar axial view during weight-bearing. The assessment of arthritic joint damage was focused mainly on the presence of cartilage loss. Joint space narrowing as a sign of damage was graded in 0–4 according to Ahlbäck (4). Associated arthritic findings such as skeletal destruction, erosion, osteophytes and subchondral bone abnormalities were also registered.

Statistical analysis

Continuous variables were analysed by unpaired 2-tailed Student's t-test. Score levels were analysed by either Wilcoxon rank sum test (paired data: A vs C joints) or Mann-Whitney U-test (unpaired data).

Table I. *Modified version of Larson's knee scoring system*

Category	Score points						Max. score points
RANGE OF MOTION	Range	>130°					10 p
		0–45°	Deduct 1 for each 10° of loss	5 p			
		45–90°	Deduct 1 for each 15° of loss	3 p			
		90–130°	Deduct 1 for each 20° of loss	2 p			
ANATOMY	Absence of deformity, no atrophy and no swelling						10 p
	Absence of deformity				*Atrophy* – thigh		
	Angulation	none	2 p		none	2 p	
		present	0 p		1–3 cm	1 p	
					>3 cm	0 p	
	Recurvation	none	1 p				
		present	0 p		*Swelling*		
	Flexionscontracture	none	1 p		none	3 p	
		present	0 p		occasional	1 p	
					persistent	0 p	
	Patelladeformity	none	1 p				
		present	0 p				
PAIN	No pain at motion						15 p
	Slight pain		12.5 p				
	Mild pain		10.0 p				
	Moderate pain		7.5 p				
	Severe pain		2.5 p				
	Disabling pain		0 p				
ACHE	No ache at rest						15 p
	Slight ache		12.5 p				
	Mild ache		10.0 p				
	Moderate ache		7.5 p				
	Severe ache		2.5 p				
	Disabling ache		0 p				
							50 p

RESULTS

Diagnosis

Culture from synovial fluid was performed in 63/65 joints (97%) and bacterial growth was found in 58 cases (92%). The corresponding figures for blood culture were 44/65 (68%) cases cultured whereof 11 (25%) cases grew bacteria.

In all, the diagnosis was based on positive bacteriological culture in synovial fluid and/or blood, in 61/65 cases. For 4 patients the diagnosis was based on the presence of bacteria in synovial fluid demonstrable by microscopy of a Gram-stained slide.

Patients' characteristics

There were 65 infected joints in 64 patients, 1 patient having 2 episodes of arthritis. The age and sex distribution for the 43 males and 22 females is shown in Fig. 1. The mean age of the females was significantly higher (60 ± 20) than that of males (49 ± 20; $p < 0.03$). The age range for all patients was 18–87 years. The patients were evenly distributed over time during the period with 6–11 cases diagnosed each year. All patients were infected in 1 joint only.

Concomitant disease and risk factors

Table II shows earlier and present diseases, as well as risk factors of possible relevance for the course of the arthritis. Operation or trauma immediately preceding the arthritis was the major background factor, being present in 31 patients. Eight operations were elective and 9

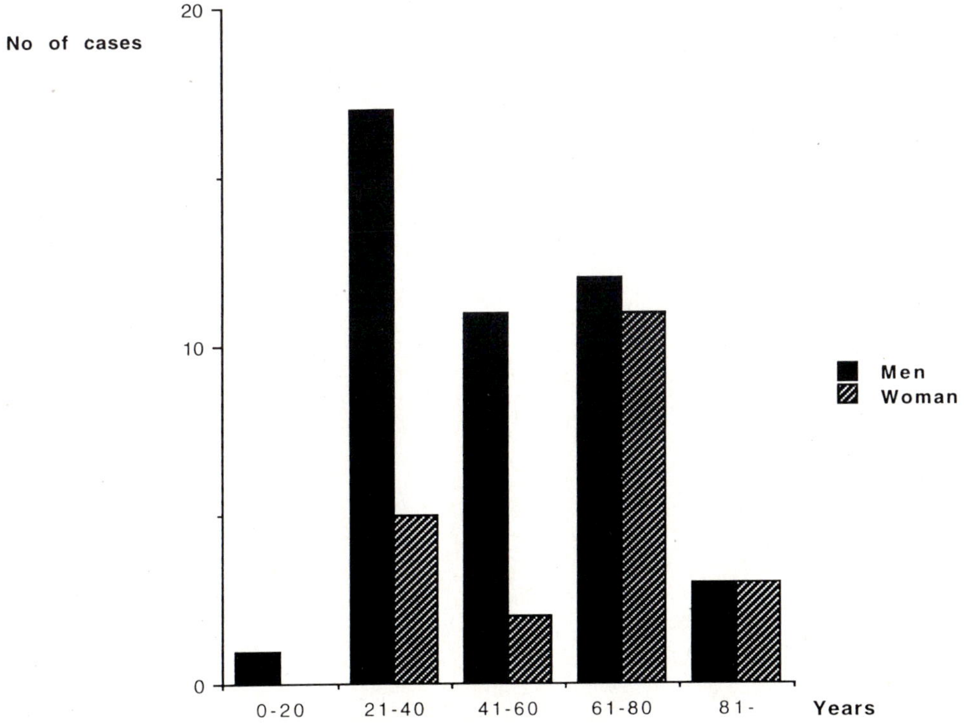

Fig. 1. Age distribution in 64 patients with septic arthritis, 1979–88.

were acute. Previous trauma and/or previous fracture of the arthritic joint was the second most prevalent risk factor, followed by osteoarthritis. There was a low prevalence of background factors unrelated to the joints. Altogether, 52 cases (80%) exhibited at least 1 possible risk factor for septic arthritis.

Route of infection

For 24 patients (37%, 17 males) the infection was acquired by inoculation. For 36 patients (55%, 24 males) without a history of inoculation the infection was regarded as hematogenous. Patients belonging to the latter group were significantly older (58.8 ± 19.4) than patients infected by inoculation (42.2 ± 16.8; $p < 0.001$). Inoculation took place either by operation ($n = 17$), or by a penetrating trauma ($n = 3$), or by corticosteriod injection ($n = 5$). One patient had undergone a minor operation (arthroscopy) and also received an intra-articular corticosteriod injection. In 8 cases, the operation was a major one, and included cruciate ligament operations, osteosynthesis of fractures, and reconstruction of collateral ligaments. Minor surgery in the remaining 9 cases included resection of patella tripartita, resection of a patellar cystic process, meniscal operations, excision of a focus of chondromalacia, lateral release, and open reduction of a fracture. In 5 cases the route of transmission could not be defined because of lack of information.

Bacterial findings

From 61 patients (94%) a positive bacterial culture was obtained (shown in Table III). Staphylococcus aureus was found in 58% and Streptococcus pyogenes in 15%. From 2 patients, 2 species were cultured from the synovial fluid, Enterobacter and other Gram-negative rods in 1 case and E. coli and Enterococci in the other case. Four patients had bacteria demonstrable only in the Gram-stained slide of the synovial fluid; 2 with Gram-positive cocci and 2 with Gram-negative diplococci. One of the latter had an acute epididymitis, while the other 1 had Gonococci cultured from urethra, suggesting a gonococcal etiology of the arthritis.

Laboratory data

Synovial fluid (SF) in 26 analysed cases contained on average 80.8×10^9 WBC/l. 10 patients (31%) had a cell count $< 50 \times 10^9$/l in S.F.; 9 of them yielded bacteria at cultivation (5 were

Table II. *Concomitant disease and risk factors in 65 cases of bacterial gonarthritis*

	No. (%) with risk factor
Trauma associated with the arthritis	25 (35.4)
Fracture and/or operation associated with the arthritis	18 (27.7)
Previous trauma and/or previous fracture of the arthritic joint	17 (26.2)
Osteoarthritis	15 (23.1)
Previous operation on the joint	11 (16.9)
Alcohol abuse	10 (15.4)
Rheumatoid arthritis	6 (9.2)
Systemic corticosteroid treatment	3 (4.6)
Diabetes mellitus	3 (4.6)
Drug abuse	3 (4.6)
Malignant disease	1 (1.5)

Table III. *Bacterial findings of 65 cases of septic gonarthritis*

	No. (%) with bacteria indicated
Staphylococcus aureus	38 (58.4)
Streptococcus pyogenes	10 (15.4)
Pseudomonas spp.	2 (3.1)
E. coli	2 (3.1)
Growth of two species	2 (3.1)
CNS[a]	2 (3.1)
Bacteroides fragilis	1 (1.5)
Enterobacter spp.	1 (1.5)
Haemophilus influenzae	1 (1.5)
Streptococcus pneumoniae	1 (1.5)
Neisseria gonorrhoeae	1 (1.5)

[a]Coagulasnegative staphylococci.

S. aureus). The glucose level was on average 2.4 (0–7.1) mmol/l and the mean protein content 46 (25–63) g/l. The mean ESR was 78 (13–136) mm. 5/65 patients had an ESR <30 mm. The mean value of C-reactive protein was 96 (39–494) mg/l in 31 patients investigated. Only 2 patients had a CRP <50 mg/l.

Treatment

The median and mean intervals from the onset of symptoms until the commencement of adequate antibiotic treatment, called the 'treatment delay', were 1 and 3.5 (0–19) days respectively. All patients were initially given antibiotic intravenously for 10.7 ± 6 days and then orally. The total period of antibiotic treatment was median 80 (mean 123) days. All cases except 6 were treated with suction irrigation (56 cases, 86%) or multiple arthrocentesis (3 cases, 5%). Synovectomy was not performed in any case. The patients were treated in hospital for on average 25.7 days (5–95). This means a cost of about SEK 76,000 (US$ 10,500)/patient with regard to the cost level in 1992. Patients were monitored until clinical resolution for 8.7 months (0–84). One patient died while undergoing treatment, due to abdominal cancer.

Follow-up

35 patients were followed-up by examination and questionnaire and 11 patients by questionnaire only. 18 patients were not followed up: 9 had died and 9 did not respond or were unwilling to participate.

Scoring

35 patients were evaluable in all 4 categories, while 11 patients who were followed up by questionnaire alone were evaluated only regarding the pain and ache categories.

The A-joints received significantly lower mean scores than the C-joints for all 4 categories. However, in 2 patients the A-joint scored higher than the C-joint. For the pain category the mean reduction in scoring points was 21% of the mean score level of the C-joints (14.1 vs 11.3). The ache category was reduced by 16% (14.7 vs 12.4), while the reduction in both anatomy and motility scores was 9% (Table IV). Patients ≤ 45 years old ($n = 21$) had larger

Table IV. *Mean score levels (± SD) in the arthritic joint (A-joint) compared with the control joint (C-joint) regarding anatomy, ache, pain and motility*

Category	C-joint	A-joint	p-value (Wilcoxon)
Ache $n = 46$	14.7 ± 1.5	12.4 ± 3.9	0.0008
Pain $n = 46$	14.1 ± 3.0	11.3 ± 4.4	0.0001
Anatomy $n = 35$	9.7 ± 0.6	8.8 ± 1.3	0.0001
Motility $n = 35$	9.7 ± 0.9	8.8 ± 1.7	0.0004

score loss for pain and ache than older patients ($n = 26$): 33% vs 17.1% ($p = 0.05$) and 26.4% vs 11.5% ($p = 0.05$) respectively. For motility and anatomy there was no difference between the age groups (not shown). At follow-up, 21/35 patients exhibited an anatomical deformity, 10/35 reduced motility, 17/46 increased ache and 20/46 increased pain in the A-joint compared with the C-joint.

Impact of risk factors on the course and outcome

The influence of 6 risk factors on the score loss of the arthritic joint is shown in Table V. Age ≤45 was associated with a greater score loss for ache and pain ($p < 0.05$). Infection by

Table V. *Score loss of the arthritic knee compared with the control knee, related to age, route of infection, treatment delay, earlier trauma, concomitant joint disease and systemic disease*

Risk factor	No.	Ache score loss	Pain score loss	No.	Anatomy score loss	Motility score loss
Age ≤45 yrs	20	4.0 ± 4.2[a]	4.8 ± 4.1[a]	15	0.5 ± 1.1	0.9 ± 1.3
>45 yrs	26	1.7 ± 3.7[a]	2.1 ± 3.8[a]	20	0.5 ± 1.1	1.0 ± 1.5
Route of infection:						
by inoculation	17	3.5 ± 3.9	4.4 ± 4.3	14	0.6 ± 1.2	1.1 ± 1.6
hematogenous	25	2.2 ± 4.1	2.4 ± 3.9	19	1.3 ± 1.2	0.7 ± 1.3
Treatment delay:						
≤5 days	33	2.7 ± 4.0	3.3 ± 4.1	28	1.8 ± 1.3	0.7 ± 1.2[a]
>5 days	10	1.7 ± 3.1	1.7 ± 3.3	5	1.2 ± 0.8	2.2 ± 1.8[a]
Earlier trauma:						
present	9	4.4 ± 4.6	5.6 ± 3.9[a]	7	1.4 ± 0.8	1.4 ± 1.9
absent	36	2.4 ± 3.9	2.9 ± 4.0[a]	28	0.9 ± 1.3	0.8 ± 1.2
Concomitant joint						
disease[b]: present	22	2.7 ± 4.3	3.4 ± 4.2	19	1.3 ± 1.4	0.8 ± 1.2
absent	24	2.7 ± 3.9	3.1 ± 4.1	16	0.6 ± 0.9	1.1 ± 1.6
Systemic disease[c]:						
present	12	2.9 ± 4.5	3.8 ± 4.8	9	0.8 ± 1.1	1.1 ± 1.5
absent	34	2.7 ± 3.9	3.1 ± 3.9	26	1.0 ± 1.3	0.9 ± 1.4

[a] $p < 0.05$ (Mann-Whitney U-test).

[b] Osteoarthritis and/or rheumatoid arthritis.

[c] Alcohol abuse, drug abuse, diabetes, malignant disease, systemic corticosteroid treatment.

Table VI. *Age and sex distribution and mean score levels (±SD) in patients, distributed according to the presence of X-ray sequelae at follow-up*

	Patients with X-ray sequelae	Patients without X-ray sequelae	*p*-value (Mann-Whitney)
No. of patients	9	17[a]	
Males	5	10	
Age	51.8 ± 20.3	50.8 ± 17.6	0.96
Ache score	11.7 ± 3.5	11.2 ± 4.9	1.0
Pain score	11.1 ± 4.2	10.0 ± 5.0	0.6
Anatomy score	8.3 ± 1.0	8.8 ± 1.4	0.14
Motility score	7.7 ± 1.9	9.2 ± 1.4	0.02

[a] Anatomy and motility evaluated in 15 patients.

inoculation was associated with increased score loss for all categories except anatomy, compared with hematogenous infection but the differences were not statistically significant.

Motility score loss was significantly greater in patients with a treatment delay exceeding 5 days than in patients with shorter delay ($p < 0.05$). A history of earlier trauma correlated with increased score loss for pain ($p < 0.05$). There was no significant difference in outcome between patients with vs without systemic or concomitant disease.

X-ray follow-up

For 26 patients X-ray films were available for comparison of A- and C-joints at follow-up or of the A-joint exposed at the time of acute disease and at follow-up. Nine patients (35%) had radiological changes in the A-joint attributable to the arthritis.

A comparison of 9 followed-up patients with sequelae at X-ray with 17 followed-up patients without sequelae is shown in Table VI. Patients with X-ray sequelae had lower mean scores only for motility ($p = 0.02$) compared with patients without sequelae. Age and sex distribution did not differ between the groups with or without sequelae.

DISCUSSION

The present study was performed as a cooperative project between the Departments of Orthopaedics and Infectious Diseases, with the anti-infective therapy centralized to the latter Clinic. This may explain the high proportion of postoperative and post-traumatic joint infections. Children are treated at the Department of Pediatrics and were therefore not included. The higher mean age for women may be due to the predominance in younger ages of post-traumatic and postoperative arthritis – types of joint damage more frequently seen in males than females.

As in many other studies (1, 2, 5–13) S. aureus was the predominant etiological agent, being found in more than half the cases. 15% of the patients had Streptococci, while there were few with Gram-negative organisms. Since no children were included, the paucity of infections with Haemophilus influenzae is not surprising. We found only 1 verified and 2 possible cases of Neisseria gonorrhoeae, which may be due to the declining frequency of gonorrhoea in Sweden during the period.

The treatment delay (mean 3.5 days) was short compared to what has been reported in other studies (5, 8–10). Since the vast majority of patients were treated with suction irrigation for the first 3–5 days it was not possible to make a comparison between this treatment and treatment with multiple arthrocentesis.

An evaluation of the outcome of infectious arthritis has to our knowledge not been made before by use of a scoring system. Instead, knee score investigations presented in the literature compare pre- and postoperative conditions of one joint. We compared the A- and C-joints of each individual on one occasion. The paired examination increases the sensitivity of the assay. However, the 2 patients whose C-joints scored lower than the A-joints illustrate a weak point of the method.

Since the system measures both objective and subjective categories, assessed by the examiner and the patient respectively, it allows an estimation of the multifactorial background of impaired joint function. The categories showing the greatest loss in scoring points were those assessed by the patient. Thus a 21% loss was found for the pain category and 16% for the ache category, while the loss in both motility and anatomy was below 10% (Table IV).

In 80% of the patients we demonstrated the presence of factors that might affect the course and outcome of the disease. Operation or trauma of the joint were the most frequent factors. Only 6 patients had rheumatoid arthritis (3 with corticosteroid therapy), which in some materials is considered as the most common predisposing factor (13). This low figure may be explained by the fact that the patients with septic arthritis and rheumatoid arthritis are often hospitalized at the Department of Rheumatology. Prosthetic joint infections, commonly seen in rheumatological patients, were also excluded from this study. Corticosteroid injection in joints preceded the infection in 5 cases and is a well known cause of septic arthritis (6, 14, 15). However, the complication rate has been estimated to be low (16).

An association was demonstrated between outcome and certain risk factors. A reduced motility score was associated with delayed treatment. This negative impact of delayed treatment on the healing result has been demonstrated by other authors (5, 6, 9, 10). Persisting ache and pain was associated with age ≤ 45 years. The finding that younger patients had a larger score loss than older patients may be explained by the better general condition of the C-joints in younger patients. It may also be due to the predominance of postoperative or post-traumatic infections in the younger patients (16/24), which makes the end result dependent on both the traumatic-operative and the infectious damage. There is probably also a greater demand for perfect healing in younger patients resulting in an experience of more pain than would be the case for an older, less physically active patient. It would therefore seem that younger patients with postoperative/post-traumatic arthritis have less satisfactory healing results from arthritis and that the predominant handicaps are caused by persisting pain and ache for many years (2–11) after the disease.

X-ray changes attributable to the arthritis were found in 9/26 (35%) evaluable patients. The lack of association between X-ray sequelae and the majority of clinical sequelae at follow-up emphasizes the complexity in evaluating the quality of healing.

A comparison of our results with those of other studies on outcome after septic arthritis is difficult, since the translation of a scoring system into other assaying methods will of necessity be arbitrary. Lysholm (17) in his work on knee stabilizing surgery used a modified Larson score. In its latest version (18, 19) 'excellent' corresponds to 50–45 points, 'good' to 44–34, 'fair' to 33–26 and 'poor' corresponds to 25 points and less. Applying these levels to our material indicates that 49% had an excellent result, 30% good, 17% fair and 4% a poor healing result.

These results seem to be good when compared with healing results after infectious arthritis published recently (7, 10, 13, 20). However, these reports include arthritis localized to different joints and are difficult to evaluate regarding the knee infection specifically. Furthermore, a more exact comparison cannot be made because of the different methods used. We find the application of a scoring system for the evaluation of long-term healing results of infectious gonarthritis rational. By such a method, a comparison of results obtained at different centres and by different treatment schedules will be facilitated.

REFERENCES

1. Lidgren L, Lindberg L. Twenty-nine cases of bacterial arthritis. Acta Orthop Scand 44: 263–269, 1973.
2. Esterhai J, Gelb I. Adult septic arthritis. In: Orthpedic Infection 26. Esterhai J, ed. Orthopedic Clinics of North America 503–514, 1991.
3. Smillie. Diseases of the knee joint. Edinburgh and London: Churchill Livingstone, 27–31, 1974.
4. Ahlbäck S. Osteoarthritis of the knee. A radiographic investigation. Acta Radiol Suppl 277, 1968.
5. Cooper C, Cawley MID. Bacterial arthritis in an English health district: a ten year review. Ann Rheum Dis 45: 458–463, 1973.
6. Goldenberg DL, Reed JI. Bacterial arthritis. N Engl J Med 312: 764–769, 1985.
7. Mistelli M, Conen D. Therapie und Prognose der bakteriellen Arthritis: eine retrospektive Analyse. Schweiz Med Wochenschr 121: 932–937, 1991.
8. Lane JG, Falahee MH, Wojtys EM, Hankin FM, Kaaufer H. Pyarthrosis of the knee. Clin Orthop 252: 198–204, 1990.
9. Rosenthal J, Bole GG, Robinson WD. Acute nongonococcal infectious arthritis. Arthritis Rheum 23: 889–897, 1980.
10. Schlapbach P, Ambord C, Blöchlinger AM, Gerber NJ. Bakterielle Arthritis – eine retrospektive Analyse. Schweiz Med Wochenschr 119: 521–526, 1989.
11. Kelly PJ. Bacterial arthritis in the adult. Orthop Clin North Am 6: 973–982, 1975.
12. McCutchan HJ, Fischer RC. Synovial leukocytosis in infectious arthritis. Clin Orthop 257: 226–230, 1990.
13. Meijers KAE, Dijkonans BAC, Hermans J, van den Broek PJ, Cat SA. Nongonococcal infectious arthritis: a retrospective study. J Infect 14: 13–20, 1987.
14. Blackburn WD, Dunn TL, Alarcon GS. Infection versus disease activity in rheumatoid arthritis. Eight years' experience. South Med J 10: 1238–1241, 1986.
15. Montgomery SC, Campbell J. J Bone Joint Surg 71: 540, 1989.
16. Yoshikawa TT. Geriatric infectious diseases: an emerging problem. J Am Geriatr Soc 31: 234–238, 1983.
17. Lysholm J. Arthroscopy in surgery of the knee. Thesis. Linköping University Medical Dissertations, No 106. Linköping, 1981.
18. Ylverton-Tegnér. Cruciate ligament injuries in the knee. Thesis. Linköping University Medical Dissertations, No 203. Linköping, 1985.
19. Andersson AC. Acute anterior cruciate ligament injuries. Evaluation of surgical and non-surgical treatment. Linköping University Medical Dissertations, No 333. Linköping, 1991.
20. Smith MJ. Arthroscopic treatment of the septic knee. Arthroscopy 2: 30–34, 1986.

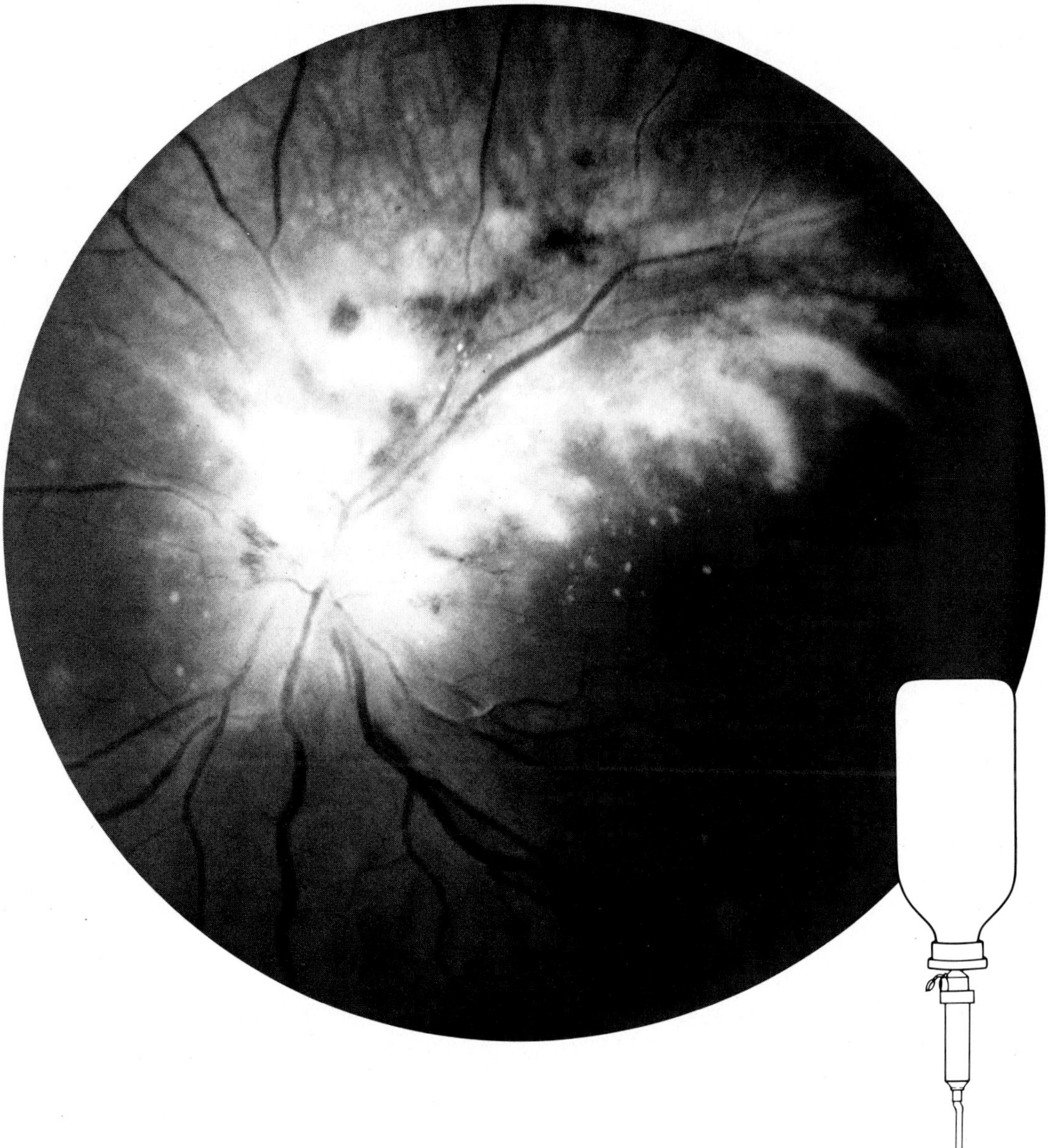

Scand J Infect Dis 26: 95–102, 1994

Klebsiella pneumoniae Meningitis: Prognostic Factors

LOK-MING TANG and SIEN-TSONG CHEN

From the Department of Neurology, Chang Gung Memorial Hospital and Medical College, Taipei, Taiwan

All 42 cases of Klebsiella pneumoniae meningitis diagnosed between 1981 and 1991 were evaluated. These accounted for 13% of patients with blood and/or cerebrospinal fluid culture-proven bacterial meningitis. There was an increased incidence of K. pneumoniae meningitis from the first 6 years of study (7%) to the last 5 years (16%). K. pneumoniae became increasingly important not only in community-acquired meningitis but also in nosocomial meningitis. 12/13 nosocomial cases were patients who had undergone neurosurgical procedures. The overall mortality rate was 43%. The mortality rate in patients with spontaneous meningitis was higher than that in patients with post-traumatic or postoperative meningitis. Factors that adversely affected mortality were age over 60, diabetes mellitus, and severe neurological deficits on admission. The use of third-generation cephalosporins did not reduce the mortality rate.

L.-M. Tang, MD, MSc, Department of Neurology, Chang Gung Memorial Hospital, 199 Tung Hwa North Rd., Taipei, Taiwan

INTRODUCTION

K. pneumoniae meningitis has been considered to be an uncommon infection. In 1948, only 7 cases of K. pneumoniae meningitis were found in a review of 3,377 cases of meningitis (1). In 1957, a study showed that Klebsiella comprised only 1.5% of all cases of meningitis (2). Recently, K. pneumoniae was found to be the causative agent for Gram-negative bacillary meningitis in 14/38 (37%) patients in a study from Taiwan (3).

The treatment of K. pneumoniae meningitis has remained unsatisfactory regarding both mortality and morbidity. In 1975 and 1981, 2 reports of collected series of K. pneumoniae meningitis showed that the mortality rates were 38% and 91% respectively (4, 5). Recently, there have been reports of successful treatment of the infection with third-generation cephalosporins (6–12).

The purpose of this study was to review cases of K. pneumoniae meningitis diagnosed at our institution in order to ascertain the incidence of the disease in acute bacterial meningitis, to delineate the clinical features that are important for the prognosis of the patients and to assess the therapeutic effect of third-generation cephalosporins on the mortality.

MATERIALS AND METHODS

Patients

We reviewed the microbiologic records of cerebrospinal fluid (CSF) and blood cultures and the medical records of patients with bacterial meningitis admitted to Chang Gung Memorial Hospital between 1981 and 1991. Criteria for inclusion were (i) demonstration of K. pneumoniae in CSF culture and history of acute disease and presence of clinical findings of meningeal inflammation, and (ii) demonstration of K. pneumoniae in blood culture, history of acute disease, presence of clinical findings such as headache, fever and nuchal rigidity, and typical CSF features including decreased glucose level, increased protein concentration and pleocytosis with predominant polymorphonuclear cells.

Data on duration of illness, clinical manifestations, associated diseases, head injury or neurosurgical procedure, laboratory findings, use of antibiotics, and outcome were recorded and comparison made between non-fatal and fatal cases. The clinical severity of the illness on admission was classified into 2 stages: **Stage I**: patients with mildly or non-altered consciousness and/or focal neurological signs such as hemiparesis; and **Stage II**: patients in a state of delirium or coma. Only results of the first CSF sample were used. Initial antibiotic therapy was considered appropriate when (*a*) both the antibiotic administered on the day of admission or diagnosis was demonstrated to be effective against K. pneumoniae by

 ISSN 0036-5548

sensitivity testing and (*b*) the antibiotic used was capable of reaching the central nervous system (CNS) in an adequate amount.

Statistical analysis

The mean values of CSF lactate, protein, glucose and leukocyte counts in patient groups were compared by means of Student's *t*-test. Comparison of the risk factors in patient groups was made by means of Fisher's exact test.

RESULTS

There were 42 patients with K. pneumoniae meningitis (31 males and 11 females) aged between 1 month and 78 years (mean, 40 years). 36 patients (85%) were over 20 years of age. One patient was an infant (Fig. 1). Of the 42 patients, only 8 cases were diagnosed between 1981 and 1986, 7% of 114 cases with CSF and/or blood culture-proved bacterial meningitis. In the subsequent years (1987–1991), 34 cases of K. pneumoniae meningitis were diagnosed and accounted for 16.7% of 203 bacteriologically proven cases (Fig. 2).

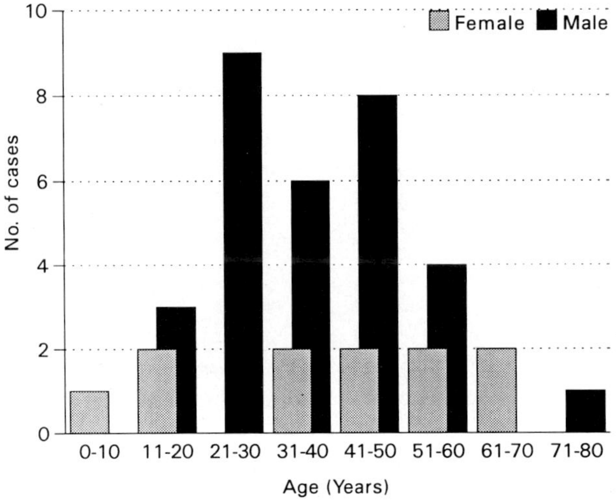

Fig. 1. Distribution by age and sex among 42 patients with Klebsiella pneumoniae meningitis, over 11 years.

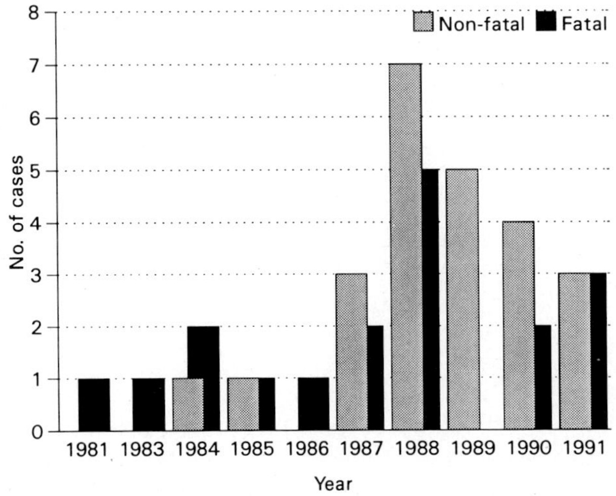

Fig. 2. Number of fatal and non-fatal cases of Klebsiella pneumoniae meningitis, distributed over 11 years, 1981–1991.

The frequencies of underlying conditions in the 42 patients are summarized in Table I. An underlying condition was present in all but 3 patients. The major underlying conditions were head injury, neurosurgical procedure, diabetes mellitus (DM) and CSF leakage. 29 cases were non-hospital acquired. Of the 13 nosocomial cases, 12 were neurosurgical patients. There were 5 patients who had had neurosurgical procedures for head injury, 4 for tumour involving the CNS, 2 for hydrocephalus in haemorrhagic stroke and 1 for spinal stenosis. One of the 13 nosocomial cases was a patient who had received a blood transfusion because of acute blood loss 48 h before presence of clinical findings of meningitis. Of the 13 nosocomial episodes, only 1 occurred during the first 6 years of the study, vis-à-vis 12 during the last 5 years.

The duration of symptoms in patients before antibiotic therapy was initiated ranged from 12 h to 10 days, with a mean of 4.7 days. It was 5.3 days for the patients with head injury and/or neurosurgical procedures and 4 days for those without. On admission, 20 patients had a history of headaches. Fever was present in 37; neck stiffness in 29; and disturbance of consciousness in 35 patients.

A lumbar puncture was performed on all patients. The CSF findings were incomplete in some cases. 13 patients had a leukocyte count $<1000 \times 10^6$/l; 6 survived and 7 died. All 31 patients had an elevated protein level >1 g/l. 23 patients had a CSF glucose level <0.72 mmol/l; 13 survived and 10 died. Only 4 patients did not have a reduced glucose concentration; 3 died and 1 survived. The lactate level was elevated in all 25 patients studied. The differences in CSF protein, glucose and leukocyte count levels between patients who survived and those who died were not significant (Table II). A difference was observed in the mean values of lactate between those who survived and those who died ($t = 2.37$, DF $= 23$, $P < 0.05$). Fig. 3 shows the individual lactate levels of the 25 patients.

Table I. *Underlying conditions in 42 patients with K. pneumoniae meningitis*

Underlying condition	No. of cases (%)[a]	
Head injury		
past	3	(7)
present	13	(31)
Neurosurgical procedure		
past	2	(5)
present	12	(28)
Cerebrospinal fluid leakage	9	(21)
Diabetes mellitus	11	(26)
Malignancy		
nasopharyngeal carcinoma	1	
pulmonary carcinoma	1	
central nervous system	4	(9)
Alcoholism	5	(12)
Liver disease		
cirrhosis	4	(9)
abscess	1	
Pneumonia	3	(7)
Hemorrhagic stroke	2	
Spinal stenosis	1	
Chronic otitis media	1	
Diarrhea	1	

[a] Some patients had more than 1 underlying condition.

Table II. *Mean values ± SD of CSF protein, glucose, lactate and leukocyte count in 42 patients with K. pneumoniae meningitis*

n = no. of patients

Group	No. of patients[a]	Lactate, mmol/l (range)	Protein, g/l (range)	Glucose, mmol/l (range)	Leukocyte, $\times 10^6$/l (range)
Non-fatal	24	13.3 ± 4.3[b] (8.0–21.2) $n = 14$	6.0 ± 5.6 (1.1–21.4) $n = 16$	1.1 ± 2.2 (0.1–9.3) $n = 17$	10146 ± 18771 (35–67680) $n = 19$
Fatal	18	19.0 ± 7.6[b] (4.2–32.0) $n = 11$	6.9 ± 5.2 (1.0–20.6) $n = 15$	1.4 ± 2.3 (0–7.3) $n = 16$	9273 ± 15785 (84–54300) $n = 16$

[a] Not all patients had every test.
[b] $p < 0.05$, Student's t-test.

Positive CSF cultures for K. pneumoniae were obtained in 38 patients. Three had mixed bacterial meningitis; in addition to K. pneumoniae, Enterobacter aerogenes, E. cloacae and Escherichia coli were isolated respectively. Of the 4 patients with negative CSF cultures, all had K. pneumoniae in blood cultures and typical clinical findings of meningeal inflammation. Positive blood cultures were obtained in 23 cases.

Initial antibiotic therapy was considered appropriate in 36 patients. 12 patients received chloramphenicol alone or in combination with gentamicin; 6 (50%) survived and 6 (50%) died. Of the 24 patients treated with cefotaxime, moxalactam or ceftriaxone, 15 (62%) survived and 9 (38%) died. Six patients had inappropriate initial therapy and 3 died despite subsequent use of appropriate therapy. Inappropriate therapy included use of chloramphenicol in 2 patients when K. pneumoniae was subsequently shown to be resistant to the drug, and use of only intravenous gentamicin and penicillin in 4 patients.

Outcome

Of the 42 patients with K. pneumoniae meningitis, 18 died. The overall mortality rate was 43%. Six of the 8 patients (75%) treated in the first 6 years of the study died; all 6 had

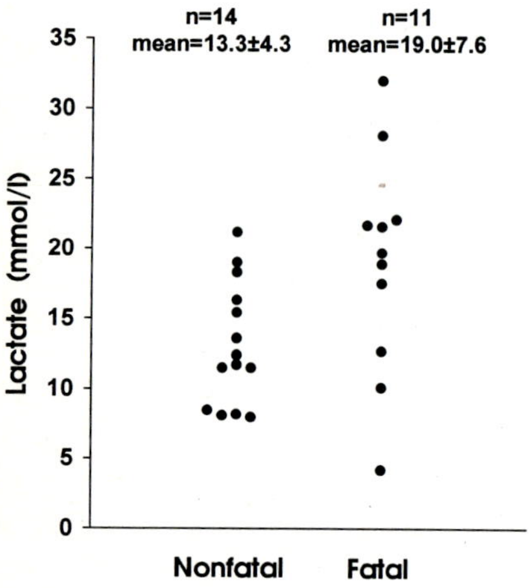

Fig. 3. Cerebrospinal fluid lactate levels in 25 patients with Klebsiella pneumoniae meningitis depicted according to outcome.

spontaneous meningitis, whereas the 2 survivors had post-traumatic meningitis. 12 of the 34 patients (35%) treated in the last 5 years of the study died (6/21 patients with post-traumatic and/or post-neurosurgical meningitis and 6/13 with spontaneous meningitis). The mortality rate in patients with post-traumatic or post-operative meningitis was lower than that in patients with spontaneous meningitis (case fatality rates, 6/23 vs. 12/19, $P < 0.05$, Fisher's exact test, 2-tailed). Prognostic factors were age ($P < 0.02$), Diabetes mellitus ($P < 0.05$) and neurological status on admission ($P < 0.02$) (Table III). The mortality trend was higher in patients with a positive blood culture than in those without (56% vs. 26%), although the difference was not significant ($P > 0.05$).

Table III. *Potential prognostic factors for mortality in patients with K. pneumoniae meningitis*

Factor	Total no. of patients	Patients who died	
		No.	%
Years in which meningitis occurred			
1981–1986	8	6	75
1987–1991	34	12	35
Age (yr)			
0–60	37	13	35[a]
61–80	5	5	100[a]
Sex			
Male	31	13	42
Female	11	5	45
Head injury			
Yes	16	3	18
No	26	15	58
Neurosurgical procedure			
Yes	10	4	40
No	32	14	43
Diabetes mellitus			
Yes	11	8	72[b]
No	31	10	32[b]
Bacteremia			
Yes	23	13	56
No	19	5	26
Cerebrospinal fluid leakage			
Yes	9	1	11
No	33	17	51
Alcoholism			
Yes	4	2	50
No	38	16	42
Duration of symptoms before admission			
<4 days	23	11	47
>4 days	19	7	37
Neurological status on admission			
Stage I	12	0	0[c]
Stage II	30	18	60[c]

[a] $p < 0.02$, Fisher's exact test.
[b] $p < 0.05$, Fisher's exact test.
[c] $p < 0.02$, Fisher's exact test.

All patients in Stage I survived, although 4 of them had symptoms more than 4 days after admission. Of the 30 patients in Stage II, 15 had symptoms for more than 4 days; 8 survived and 7 died. Of the other 15 patients in Stage II who had symptoms for less than 4 days, 4 survived and 11 died.

Follow-up neurological examination was done on 16 of the 23 survivors. The median follow-up period was 11 months (range, 1–36 months). 11 patients resumed a normal life, though there were minor neurological deficits in 4; 3 were disabled but relatively independent; 1 was conscious but severely disabled; and 1 was in a persistent vegetative state.

DISCUSSION

K. pneumoniae is an important cause of nosocomial and community-acquired infections. It accounts for a significant proportion of urinary tract, blood stream, lung, and surgical wound infections (13). The microorganism, however, has been recognized as an uncommon pathogen causing bacterial meningitis. In 1948 Jacob et al. reviewed 3,377 cases of meningitis and found only 7 caused by K. pneumoniae (1). A further study in 1957 found that Klebsiella constituted only 1.5% of all cases of meningitis (2). In our study, K. pneumoniae meningitis accounted for 13% of the 317 patients with culture-proven bacterial meningitis. Furthermore, there was an increasing incidence of K. pneumoniae meningitis from the first 6 years of study (7%) to the last 5 years (16%). The cause of this increase is not known, though the increase in absolute numbers of cases of K. pneumoniae meningitis during the last 5 years may be partly due to the increased number of beds in our hospital. There has been no change in the referral practice of patients sent to us. However, it seems likely that K. pneumoniae meningitis has become more common not only in our hospital, but also in another hospital in Taiwan (3).

K. pneumoniae meningitis usually affects infants and adults but is uncommon between the ages of 2 and 20 years (2). In a review of 32 patients, 6 were less than 1 year of age and 26 (80%) were adults over 20 years old (5). In our study, 36 (85%) of 42 patients were over 20 years of age. However, there were 5 patients (12%) in the age range 11 to 20 years and only 1 infant. The mortality was 100% for the 5 patients over 60 years of age. The poorer prognosis of bacterial meningitis in the elderly has also been observed by others (14, 15). K. pneumoniae meningitis has been shown to be more common in males (2), as also in our study, where males outnumbered females by a ratio of 3 : 1.

K. pneumoniae has become important not only in community-acquired meningitis but also in nosocomial meningitis. In our patients, only 1/8 episodes of meningitis during the first 6 years of study was nosocomial, whereas this was the case in 12/34 patients during the last 5 years. The increased number of nosocomial meningitis cases was due entirely to an increased number of Klebsiella cases in neurosurgical patients. This is consistent with the previous study which showed that Klebsiella is the commonest microorganism isolated from neurosurgical patients with meningitis (4).

The lactate concentration in the CSF has been evaluated in various types of meningitis (16–19). Previous studies emphasized the significance of elevated CSF lactate for differentiation between aseptic and bacterial meningitis (15, 16). That a high CSF lactate may indicate a poor outcome has been noted in conditions such as cerebral malaria (19), cerebral infarction (20) and head injury (21). Nevertheless, the lactate concentration in the first CSF sample from patients with bacterial meningitis was reported to have no prognostic value (22). In our patients with K. pneumoniae meningitis, CSF lactate level was elevated in all 25 patients studied. Patients who had a fatal course had higher CSF lactate levels than those who survived. However, there was a wide distribution of the lactate levels, with a large overlap between the fatal and non-fatal patient groups. Thus, lactate measurement is not useful for predicting outcome. In studies of bacterial meningitis, a CSF leukocyte count $<1000 \times 10^6$/l and a CSF glucose level <0.72 mmol/l were associated with a poor prognosis (23, 24). In our K. pneumoniae meningitis cases, neither of these was an important factor.

Before the era of antibiotic therapy, mortality of the K. pneumoniae meningitis was nearly 100%. In the era of antibiotic therapy with sulfonamides, streptomycin, chlortetracycline and chloramphenicol, the overall mortality was about 50% (25). Before the introduction of third-generation cephalosporins, the main therapeutic approaches for the infection were chloramphenicol, alone or in combination with other antibiotics (4, 5). In 2 studies of K. pneumoniae meningitis treated with chloramphenicol alone or in combination with other antibiotics, the mortality rates were 38% and 91% respectively (4, 5). Third-generation cephalosporins are now the drug of choice for Gram-negative bacillary meningitis (26). In K. pneumoniae meningitis, treatment with third-generation cephalosporins such as cefotaxime or moxalactam has proved successful in some patients (7–9). However, the mortality rate remains high in our patients despite the use of third-generation cephalosporins. Thus of 24 patients with appropriate treatment with cefotaxime, moxalactam or ceftriaxone, 9 (38%) died. It therefore seems that the use of more highly bactericidal antibiotics has not reduced much of the mortality rate in patients with K. pneumoniae meningitis. Perhaps adjunctive therapeutic regimens to lessen subarachnoid space inflammation could improve the prognosis (27).

Previous studies, as well as our own, have shown that the incidence of Diabetes mellitus in patients with K. pneumoniae meningitis is higher than in the general population (28, 29); 11 (26%) of our patients had Diabetes mellitus. We and others (30) have shown that there is an increased mortality of K. pneumoniae meningitis in patients with Diabetes mellitus.

The overall mortality of klebsiella bacteremia has been reported to be some 37% (31). It has been suggested that in K. pneumoniae meningitis, a positive blood culture indicates a poor prognosis (1). In our study, the mortality was not significantly higher in patients with a positive blood culture than in those without.

In Gram-negative bacillary meningitis, the mortality rate in patients with post-traumatic or postoperative meningitis was lower than that in patients with spontaneous meningitis (32). This could be due to a less fulminant course in the former patients. In 1 study of 15 patients with post-traumatic or/and post-neurosurgical K. pneumoniae meningitis and 17 patients with spontaneous K. pneumoniae meningitis, the overall mortality was 91% (5). However, the mortality was much lower (38%) in a study of 13 patients with post-neurosurgical K. pneumoniae meningitis and 2 patients with spontaneous K. pneumoniae meningitis (4). In our study, the overall mortality was 43%, whereas that in patients with post-traumatic or postoperative meningitis was lower than in patients with spontaneous meningitis. This suggests that spontaneous K. pneumoniae meningitis shows a relatively fulminant course.

The neurological status at the beginning of therapy has a significant prognostic implication. The patients in Stage I all survived whereas only 12/30 of those in Stage II (who were in delirium or coma) survived, usually with sequelae. Duration of symptoms prior to treatment of more or less than 4 days is not a prognostic factor. Therefore, failure of treatment is more closely related to the severity of the neurological findings than to the duration of symptoms prior to treatment.

REFERENCES

1. Jacob SS, Top FH. Friedlander bacillus meningitis: report of seven cases with two recoveries. Ann Intern Med 28: 1003–1009, 1948.
2. Spivack AP, Eisenberg GM, Weiss W, Flippin HF. Klebsiella meningitis. Am J Med 22: 865–871, 1957.
3. Jang TN, Wang FD, Wang LS, Yu KW, Liu CY. Gram-negative bacillary meningitis in adults: a recent six-year experience. Journal of the Formosan Medical Association 92: 540–546, 1993.

4. Mangi RJ, Quintiliani R, Andriole VT. Gram-negative bacillary meningitis. Am J Med 59: 829–836, 1975.
5. Cherubin CE, Marr JS, Sierra MF, Becker S. Listeria and gram-negative bacillary meningitis in New York City, 1972–1979: frequent causes of meningitis in adults. Am J Med 71: 199–209, 1981.
6. Ellis-Pegler RB, Lang SDR. Cefoperazone in Klebsiella meningitis: a case report. Drugs 22 (Suppl 1): 69–71, 1981.
7. Landesman SH, Corrado ML, Shah PM, Armenguard M, Barza M, Cherubin CE. Past and current roles for cephalosporin antibiotics in treatment of meningitis: emphasis on use in gram-negative bacillary meningitis. Am J Med 71: 693–703, 1981.
8. Olson DA, Hoeprich PD, Nolan SM, Goldstein E. Successful treatment of gram-negative bacillary meningitis with moxalactam. Ann Intern Med 95: 302–305, 1981.
9. Cherubin CE, Corrado ML, Nair SR, Gombert ME, Landesman S, Humbert G. Treatment of gram-negative bacillary meningitis: role of the new cephalosporin antibiotics. Rev Infect Dis 4: S453–464, 1982.
10. Sandyk R, Brennan MJW. Unusual presentation of primary Klebsiella meningitis: successful treatment with cefotaxime. Postgrad Med J 59: 256–257, 1983.
11. LeFrock JL, Molavi A, Smith B, et al. Effectiveness of cefotaxime in gram-negative meningitis. Neurosurgery 15: 679–682, 1984.
12. Jacobs RF. Cefotaxamine treatment of gram-negative enteric meningitis in infants and children. Drugs 35 (Suppl 2): 185–189, 1988.
13. Farmer JJ III, Kelly MT. Enterobacteriaceae. In: Balows A, Hausler WJ, Herrmann KL, Isenberg HD, Shadomy HJ, eds. Manual of clinical microbiology, 5th edn. Washington DC: American Society for Microbiology, 360–383, 1991.
14. Finland M, Barnes MW. Acute bacterial meningitis at Boston City Hospital during 12 selected years, 1935–1972. J Infect Dis 136: 400–415, 1977.
15. Gorse GJ, Thrupp LD, Nudleman KL, Wyle FA, Hawkins B, Cesario TC. Bacterial meningitis in the elderly. Arch Intern Med 144: 1603–1607, 1984.
16. Brook I, Bricknell KS, Overturf GD, Finegold SM. Measurement of lactic acid in cerebrospinal fluid of patients with infections of the central nervous system. J Infect Dis 137: 384–390, 1978.
17. Komorowski RA, Farmer SG, Hanson GA, Hause LL. Cerebrospinal fluid lactic acid in diagnosis of meningitis. J Clin Microbiol 8: 89–92, 1978.
18. Tang LM. Serial lactate determinations in tuberculous meningitis. Scand J Infect Dis 20: 81–83, 1988.
19. White NJ, Warrel DA, Looareesuwan S, Chanthavanich P, Phillips RE, Pongpaew P. Pathophysiological and prognostic significance of cerebrospinal fluid lactate in cerebral malaria. Lancet 1: 776–778, 1985.
20. Busse O, Hoffmann O. CSF lactate and CT findings in middle cerebral artery infarction: a comparative study. Stroke 14: 960–963, 1983.
21. DeSalles AAF, Kontos HA, Becker DP, Yang MS, et al. Prognostic significance of ventricular CSF lactic acidosis in severe head injury. J Neurosurg 65: 615–624, 1986.
22. Genton B, Berger JP. Cerebrospinal fluid lactate in 78 cases of adult meningitis. Intensive Care Med 16: 196–200, 1990.
23. Tugwell P, Greenwood BM, Warrell DA. Pneumococcal meningitis: a clinical and laboratory study. Q J Med 45: 583–601, 1976.
24. Herson VC, Todd JK. Prediction of morbidity in Hemophilus influenzae meningitis. Pediatrics 59: 35–39, 1977.
25. Bell ALL. Treatment of meningitis due to Friedlander's bacillus. New Engl J Med 252: 1026–1029, 1955.
26. Braun M, Cherubin CE. Gram-negative bacillary meningitis. In: Lambert HP, ed. Infections of the central nervous system. Philadelphia: BC Decker, 150–160, 1991.
27. Tunkel AR, Wispelwey B, Scheld M. Bacterial meningitis: recent advances in pathophysiology and treatment. Ann Intern Med 112: 610–623, 1990.
28. Ayvazian LF. Friedlander Bacillus meningitis successfully treated with streptomycin. Am J Med 5: 470–477, 1948.
29. Thompson AJ, Williams EB, Williams ED, Anderson JM. Klebsiella pneumoniae meningitis. Arch Intern Med 89: 405–420, 1952.
30. Soscia JL, Dibenedetto R, Crocco J. Klebsiella pneumoniae meningitis. Arch Intern Med 113: 569–572, 1964.
31. Montgomerie JZ, Ota JK. Klebsiella bacteremia. Arch Intern Med 140: 525–527, 1980.
32. Berk SL, McCabe WR. Meningitis caused by gram-negative bacilli. Ann Intern Med 93: 253–260, 1980.

Scand J Infect Dis 26: 103–104, 1994

CASE REPORT

Salmonella typhi Meningitis

HENRIQUE LECOUR[1], LURDES SANTOS[1], MARGARIDA OLIVEIRA[1], ALVES PEREIRA[1] and JOANA SIMÕES[2]

From the [1]Department of Infectious Diseases and [2]Microbiology Laboratory School of Medicine, Hospital S. João, Porto, Portugal

Whereas typhoid fever is still an endemic disease in some parts of the world, meningeal involvement in this disease is a rare occurrence. We report a case of Salmonella typhi meningitis in a 70-year-old woman. The patient was treated with ampicillin and the only sequela was right-sided deafness.

H. Lecour, MD, PhD, Department of Infectious Diseases, School of Medicine, Hospital S. João, 4200 Porto, Portugal

INTRODUCTION

Typhoid fever is a less common disease in industrialized countries, where most cases result from infections acquired during travel to endemic areas. In Portugal, however, the disease, as other enteric infections, is still prevalent as a consequence of deficient water supply and sanitation. The incidence in 1991 was 3.26/100,000 inhabitants (1). The most frequent presentation of this salmonellosis is prolonged fever with systemic and intestinal manifestations. When treatment is instituted early, typhoid fever usually runs a benign course. Complications, as well as focal manifestations, are rare. A case of Salmonella typhi meningitis in an adult is presented in this report.

CASE REPORT

Two weeks before admission to the hospital a 70-year-old woman became ill with fever, malaise, headache, anorexia and constipation. One week later, ampicillin, 0.5 g every 6 h, was prescribed, and after 6 days, doxycline was added. During these 2 weeks the patient lost 4 kg. On the day before admission, she became confused and lethargic, and complained of right-sided hypoacusia.

A previous history of diabetes mellitus and arterial hypertension was on record. No other underlying disease was evident. The patient usually drank water from a well, and there was no sanitation at home. No other cases were reported in her family.

On admission the patient was acutely ill, emaciated and febrile (39°C), the mucous membranes were normal and no rash was observed. Her heart rate was 80 beats/min and blood pressure 130/80 mmHg. She was in deep coma (Glasgow score, 5) with severe neck rigidity and Kernig's sign was positive; no focal neurological abnormalities were registered.

A lumbar puncture revealed turbid cerebrospinal fluid under tension, with a cell count of 4,630 cells $\times 10^6$/l, almost all neutrophils, protein 4.07 g/l and glucose 0.06 g/l. The simultaneous blood glucose was 1.55 g/l. Gram-staining of the CSF was negative, but Salmonella typhi sensitive to chloramphenicol, ampicillin and cotrimoxazole was isolated. The results of the cultures from blood, faeces and urine made 2 weeks after onset of the disease, were negative. The standard agglutination test (Widal reaction) done in the third week, was positive for S. typhi, with a titre of 400 for the O antibody and 200 for the H antibody. Two weeks later, the titres were unchanged. The Widal reaction was negative in CSF. The white cell count was 11.4 $\times 10^9$/l, with 90% neutrophils. Results of blood urea and urine analyses were normal.

A brain CAT scan was normal and right-sided hearing loss was confirmed by audiometry. Treatment with intravenous ampicillin, 12 g daily for 3 weeks and dexamethasone, 0.6 mg/kg during the first 3 days was instituted. 24 h after being admitted, the patient recovered from the coma and became afebrile on the following day. A lumbar puncture, done on the second day, showed sterile CSF, with protein 0.92 g/l and glucose 0.73 g/l. Three weeks later, biochemical and cytologic parameters in CSF were normal.

 ISSN 0036-5548

When the patient was discharged the only sequela was the right-sided deafness which persisted 6 months later.

DISCUSSION

With the availability of antibiotic treatment, the clinical course of typhoid fever is nowadays very different from the classic pattern – a serious and prolonged disease frequently with pronounced toxaemia and neurological involvement. Severe headache, sometimes associated with meningismus, but no abnormalities of the CSF, and neuropsychiatric manifestations, including lethargy, confusion, delirium and acute psychotic behaviour, characterized this involvement (2, 3).

Nevertheless, the occurrence of purulent meningitis due to the penetration of S. typhi into the subarachnoid space was a rare event even in the pre-antibiotic era. Only 8 cases of adult meningitis caused by S. typhi were reported before 1940, and since then, 3 more cases have been described (4, 5).

The progressive course of the disease, despite treatment with ampicillin instituted 1 week after onset, can be explained by the low dosage used, as meningitis requires a higher dose.

In contrast to the rare incidence of S. typhi meningitis, other species of the Salmonellae constitute a more common cause of meningitis in children under 2 years of age (6, 7). In our clinical experience, non-typhi Salmonellae spp. were responsible for 14/187 (7.5%) cases of childhood bacterial meningitis, but only observed in neonates and infants where they were the most frequent enteric Gram-negative bacillary cause of meningitis. Species isolated were S. enteritidis, S. wien, S. typhimurium and S. remo (8).

The recent emergence of multiresistant strains of S. typhi in many areas of the world, mainly in Southeast Asia, India and Mexico, can contribute to the occurrence of more serious forms of the disease, since classic treatment is inadequate. Ciprofloxacin or ceftriaxone are effective alternatives to these multiresistant strains. As both drugs also have an adequate penetration into the CSF, possible meningeal involvement can be avoided.

REFERENCES

1. Direcção dos Serviços de Informação de Saúde. Doenças de Declaração Obrigatória 1987–91. Direcção-General de Cuidados de Saúde Primária. Lisboa, 1991.
2. Christie AB. Typhoid and paratyphoid fevers. In: Christie AB, ed. Infectious Diseases – Epidemiology and Clinical Practice. Edinburgh, London and New York: Churchill Livingstone, 55–130, 1974.
3. Hook EW. Salmonella species (including typhoid fever). In: Mandell GL, Douglas Jr RG, Bennett JE, eds. Principles and Practice of Infectious Diseases. New York, Edinburgh, London, Melbourne: Churchill Livingstone, 1700–1716, 1990.
4. Chanmugam D, Machado V, Mihindukulasuriya J. Primary Salmonella typhi meningitis in an adult. BMJ 1: 152, 1978.
5. Hardy C, Bansal A, Lower JA, George CF. Salmonella meningitis following treatment of enteritis with neomycin. Postgrad Med J 60: 284–286, 1984.
6. Denis F, Badiane S, Chiron J, Sow A, Diop Mar I. Salmonella meningitis in infants. Lancet 1: 910, 1977.
7. Appelbaum P, Scragg J. Salmonella meningitis in infants. Lancet 1: 1052–1053, 1977.
8. Lecour H, Seara A, Cordeiro J, Miranda M. Treatment of childhood bacterial meningitis. Infection 17: 343–346, 1989.

Scand J Infect Dis 26: 105–106, 1994

CASE REPORT

AIDS Presenting as Septic Shock Caused by Mycobacterium tuberculosis

MIQUEL VADILLO, XAVIER CORBELLA and JORDI CARRATALA

From the Department of Infectious Diseases, Bellvitge Hospital, University of Barcelona, Barcelona, Spain

Concurrent with the AIDS epidemic, an increasing incidence of tuberculosis has been noted. In HIV-infected patients with immunodeficiency, atypical forms of tuberculosis are seen. A case of disseminated tuberculosis with septic shock in an elderly patient with previously unknown HIV infection is reported.

X. Corbella, MD, Department of Infectious Diseases, Bellvitge Hospital, University of Barcelona, Feixa Llarga s/n, E-08907 L'Hospitalet de Llobregat, Barcelona, Spain

INTRODUCTION

Septic shock is commonly caused by Gram-negative bacteria, whereas Gram-positive cocci are less frequently involved. We report a case in which miliary tuberculosis with septic shock was the initial manifestation of AIDS in an elderly patient with previously unknown HIV infection.

CASE REPORT

A 63-year-old man was brought to the emergency department because of fever and malaise. The patient was awake but listless. His blood pressure was 60/– mmHg, temperature 39°C, respiratory rate 26/min, and pulse rate 120/min. Physical examination showed a lethargic patient with both scleral and cutaneous jaundice. The liver edge descended 6 cm below the right costal margin. Laboratory data were as follows: red-cell count 2.9×10^{12}/l; hematocrit 0.26; hemoglobin 83 g/l; white-cell count 0.7×10^9/l, with 30% lymphocytes, 48% neutrophils and 18% band forms; platelet count, 85×10^9/l; prothrombin time, 47.5%; partial thromboplastin time, 65 s (normal, 35 s); fibrinogen, 3.1 g/l (normal, 1.5–3.5 g/l); and an ethanol gelation test proved negative. Arterial blood gas levels on an inspired oxygen fraction of 0.5 were pH 7.33; $PaCO_2$, 3.46 kPa; PaO_2, 8.4 kPa; bicarbonate, 15 mmol/l. Right ventricular catheterization revealed a central venous pressure of 0 mmHg. The results of urine analysis, chest X-ray and electrocardiography were all normal.

The patient was treated with intravenous fluids and dopamine infusion was started at a dose of 5 µg/kg/min. Blood cultures were obtained, and ceftazidime and amikacin were administered intravenously. 12 h after admission, a dobutamine infusion was started due to persistent hypotension. The patient's respiratory function worsened progressively and mechanical ventilation was instituted 24 h after hospitalization.

On day 2, a preceding one-month history of fever, malaise, weight loss, and jaundice could be elicited. Bronchial and bone marrow specimens were taken, and by Ziehl-Neelsen staining a large number of acid-fast bacilli were demonstrated. Rifampicin 600 mg i.v., isoniazid 300 mg i.v., and ethambutol 1.2 g i.v., qd were started. A test for the presence of HIV antibodies (enzyme-linked immunosorbent assay, ELISA) was performed. A new coagulation study was compatible with disseminated intravascular coagulation: the platelet count fell subsequently, reaching a nadir of 26×10^9/l, the fibrinogen was 1.6 g/l, prothrombin time 50%, the partial thromboplastin time became prolonged (72 s), and the ethanol gelation test became positive. Cultures from blood and urine were negative. The ELISA test for HIV was positive, confirmed by Western blot. Finally, on day 3, the patient died.

At autopsy, multiple caseating granuloma containing numerous acid-fast bacilli in the lungs, mediastinal lymph nodes, liver, spleen, thyroid, stomach, small bowel and pancreas were found. Cultures of bronchial and bone marrow specimens yielded Mycobacterium tuberculosis susceptible to rifampicin, isoniazid, and ethambutol.

DISCUSSION

Fulminant infections associated with hematogenous dissemination of M. tuberculosis are extremely rare, and often result in death before miliary tubercles have time to form (1). This condition, known as "sepsis tuberculosa acutissima", specifically affects severely immunocompromized hosts and can progress to septic shock. To date, only 3 well-documented cases of septic shock have been reported in AIDS patients (2). In addition, Ahuja et al. (3) has described another case, of an intravenous drug addict with esophageal candidiasis and probable AIDS, although testing for HIV had not been performed.

When a local cellular reaction or granuloma is found, M. tuberculosis infection is classified as a different category of disseminated tuberculosis known as acute miliary tuberculosis (1). The presence of granulomatous lesions in HIV-infected patients suggests that M. tuberculosis can cause disease at an earlier stage of immunosuppression (4). In contrast to "sepsis tuberculosa acutissima", the presence of a more adequate inflammatory response converts the disease to the miliary form, which infers a better prognosis.

In our patient, despite widespread multiple caseating granuloma found at autospy, miliary tuberculosis rapidly progressed to a fatal septic shock. In this case, AIDS in a patient with advanced age, and a high mycobacterial load seemed to be the major contributing causes of the fulminant course. No other probable cause of the shock could be identified. Lipoarabinomannan from M. tuberculosis can stimulate, in vitro, the release of tumour necrosis factor from human blood monocytes (5). However, in vivo, it is difficult to surmise whether these or other mycobacterial products could be responsible for the hemodynamic alterations of septic shock.

We conclude that M. tuberculosis should be considered as a possible cause of septic shock in HIV-infected patients, in whom both "sepsis tuberculosa acutissima" and miliary tuberculosis can progress rapidly to a fulminant septic shock. Furthermore, testing for HIV should be recommended in all patients with unusual manifestations of tuberculosis, including even those who are considered to be at low risk for HIV infection.

REFERENCES

1. Clark RA, Blakley SL, Greer D, Smith MHD, Brandon W, Wisniewski TL. Hematogenous dissemination of Mycobacterium tuberculosis in patients with AIDS. Rev Infect Dis 13: 1089–1092, 1991.
2. Gachot B, Wolff M, Clair B, Régnier B. Severe tuberculosis in patients with human immunodeficiency virus infection. Intensive Care Med 16: 491–493, 1990.
3. Ahuja SS, Ahuja SK, Phelps KR, Thelmo W, Hill AR. Hemodynamic confirmation of septic shock in disseminated tuberculosis. Crit Care Med 20: 901–903, 1992.
4. Pitchenik AE, Fertel D, Bloch AB. Mycobacterial disease: epidemiology, diagnosis, treatment, and prevention. Clin Chest Med 9: 425–441, 1988.
5. Moreno C, Taverne J, Mehlert A, Bate CA, Brealey RJ, Meager A, Rook GA, Playfair JH. Lipoarabinomannan from Mycobacterium tuberculosis induces the production of tumor necrosis factor from human and murine macrophages. Clin Exp Immunol 76: 240–245, 1989.

Scand J Infect Dis 26: 107–108, 1994

CASE REPORT

A Case of Fulminant Ecthyma Gangrenosum Associated with Pseudomonas aeruginosa Infection in a Patient with Methylmalonic Acidemia

MOTOHIKO OKANO[1], KAZUNORI KISHIYAMA[2], NORIKO SATAKE[1], SHUJI KUBO[1] and NOBUYOSHI ISHIKAWA[1]

From the [1]Department of Pediatrics and the [2]Department of Dermatology, Kitami Red Cross Hospital, Kitami, Japan

A 6-month-old boy with methylmalonic acidemia died of ecthyma gangrenosum caused by systemic Pseudomonas aeruginosa infection. Subtle malnutrition accompanied by the occasional protein restriction treatment may have underlain the development of serious infection in this case.

M. Okano, MD, Department of Pediatrics, Hokkaido University School of Medicine, North 15 West 7, Kita-ku, Sapporo 060, Japan

INTRODUCTION

Ecthyma gangrenosum is a rare, but distinctive cutaneous disease caused by Pseudomonas aeruginosa (1). P. aeruginosa, commonly present in the hospital environment, appears to have a predilection for causing active infection in the setting of immunodeficiency. In this article, we describe a patient with disseminated and multiple ecthyma gangrenosum associated with methylmalonic acidemia. Subtle malnutrition was suspected to be the major contributory factor causing the disease in this patient.

CASE REPORT

The patient, a Japanese boy, born by caesarean section in breech presentation at 38 weeks' gestation, weighed 2625 g at birth. He had 2 siblings. His 5-year-old elder brother was healthy. However, an older sister had died at 17 days of age due to massive pulmonary hemorrhage of unknown cause. He was admitted to the Department of Pediatrics, Kitami Red Cross Hospital at the age of 2 months, with a diagnosis of acute bronchitis and again at 3 months of age with acute enteritis. Following these episodes, he gradually developed poor suckling and recurrent vomiting with fever, and was again admitted. He was diagnosed as having methylmalonic acidemia on the basis of analyses for various urinary and serum metabolite levels. He was treated with vitamin B_{12}, carnitine and occasional protein restriction.

Despite a couple of acidemic crises, his condition was satisfactorily controlled until 6 months of age, when impetiginous skin lesions appeared periorally and erythematous lesions on his buttocks. Subsequently, the latter lesions spread rapidly, resulting in necrosis and induration (Fig. 1). Multiple indurated hemorrhagic subcutaneous nodules developed on his trunk and extremities. He showed severe pancytopenia, with white blood cell counts of 1.39×10^9/l, hemoglobin levels of 60 g/l, and platelet counts of 43×10^9/l and moderate metabolic acidosis (blood pH; 7.214, base excess of -16.1). His total serum protein levels were 42 g/l; cholesterol, 2.64 mmol/l; copper, 700 μg/l; and zinc, 600 μg/l, respectively. Serum C-reactive protein was markedly increased at 0.24 g/l. Blood cultures proved negative. However, P. aeruginosa and Staphylococcus aureus were both cultured from his throat, ear, skin lesions and stool. He was treated intravenously with ampicillin (150 mg/kg/day) and gentamicin (5 mg/kg/day). However, he deteriorated rapidly, and expired due to massive pulmonary hemorrhage.

At autopsy, extreme hemorrhage in dermal and subcutaneous tissues was seen, together with pronounced necrosis in epidermal and dermal areas and at vascular walls. Hemorrhage was also found in the lungs. Gram-negative rod bacterial colonies were demonstrated in alveolar areas and in systemic perivascular areas of subcutaneous tissues, suggesting septicemia. Additionally, P. aeruginosa was cultured from the affected tissues. Fatty degeneration of the liver was also evident.

 ISSN 0036-5548

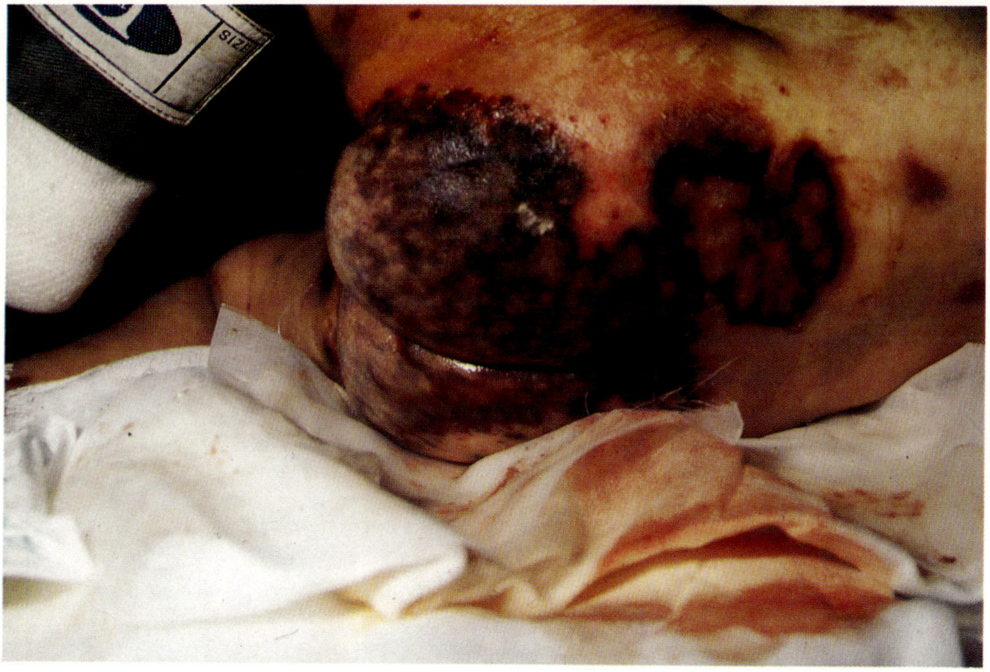

Fig. 1. Extensive necrotic lesion in region of buttocks.

DISCUSSION

Ecthyma gangrenosum is a rare condition, but often occurs in immunologically compromised patients (1). Malnutrition is also considered to be a causative factor. The occasional but long-term protein restriction, which this patient had experienced might have led to subtle nutritional deficiencies. In fact, remarkable fatty change in the liver was evident at autopsy. Although the most common etiologic agent of ecthyma gangrenosum is P. aeruginosa, similar lesions have been described in various infections caused by Aeromonas hydrophilia, S. aureus, Serratia marcescens, Escherichia coli, Klebsiella organisms and fungi (2). Both P. aeruginosa and S. aureus were cultured from multiple lesions in our case. Histopathologically, however, only P. aeruginosa contributed to the lesions, indicating that this organism was the causative agent of ecthyma gangrenosum in this case. Blood cultures proved negative for P. aeruginosa. Nevertheless, septicemia caused by this organism was conceivable, based on the histopathological evaluation and the results of cultures from the lesions at autopsy. P. aeruginosa and S. aureus, cultured from several organs, are both highly sensitive to the antibiotics (ampicillin and gentamicin) used in this patient, yet this regimen proved ineffective. Physicians should therefore remain alert to the possibility of the development of pseudomonas-induced skin lesions during protein prescribed restriction treatment for various metabolic diseases.

ACKNOWLEDGEMENT

The authors would like to thank Dr M. Tateno for his histopathological evaluation, the nursing staff of the Department of Pediatrics, and the laboratory personnel, Kitami Red Cross Hospital.

REFERENCES

1. Boisseau AM, Sarlangue J, Perel Y, Hehunstre JP, Taieb A, Maleville J. Perineal ecthyma gangrenosum in infancy and childhood: septicemic and nonsepticemic forms. J Am Acad Dermatol 27: 415–418, 1992.
2. Wolf JE, Liu HH, Rabinowitz LG. Ecthyma gangrenosum in the absence of Pseudomonas bacteremia in a bone marrow transplant recipient. Am J Med 87: 595–597, 1989.

Scand J Infect Dis 26: 109–110, 1994

CASE REPORT

Reversible Severe Neutropenia after Ceftriaxone

TERAPONG TANTAWICHIEN, KRIANG TUNGSANGA and DARATANA SWASDIKUL

From the Department of Medicine, Chulalongkorn University Hospital, Bangkok, Thailand

A 57-year-old woman developed severe neutropenia during treatment of an upper urinary tract infection with intravenous ceftriaxone. The dosage was 1 g/day for 18 days. There was a return to normal granulopoiesis after the drug was discontinued.

T. Tantawichien, MD, Department of Medicine, Chulalongkorn University Hospital, Bangkok 10330, Thailand

INTRODUCTION

Cephalosporins generally cause few side effects, but adverse hematologic reactions have been reported and included leukopenia, neutropenia, thrombocytopenia, eosinophilia and hypoprothrombinemia (1, 2). Severe neutropenia after cephalosporin therapy is rare, however (1, 3). We report a patient who developed reversible severe neutropenia after ceftriaxone administration.

CASE REPORT

A 57-year-old Thai woman was admitted to Chulalongkorn University Hospital because of drowsiness, fever and vomiting. She was moderately dehydrated and obtunded. Her total white cell count was 18.0×10^9/l with 90% neutrophils and a platelet count of 339.0×10^9/l. Plasma glucose was 30.16 mmol/l and plasma creatinine 97.24 μmol/l. The plasma was positive for ketones. A urine culture grew E. coli with a colony count $>10^5$ colonies/ml. An ultrasonogram of the abdomen revealed a large right renal staghorn calculus and right-sided hydronephosis. She was treated with insulin, oral metoclopramide (30 mg/day for 1 week) and intravenous ceftriaxone (1 g/day). The total leukocyte and neutrophil counts on day 12 of ceftriaxone administration were 4.2×10^9/l and 2.7×10^9/l, respectively. Three days later, a right nephrectomy was performed because of uncontrolled urinary tract infection and technical problems during lithotomy. On the 18th day of hospitalization, leukocyte, neutrophil and platelet counts fell to 3.0×10^9/l, 1.44×10^9/l and 140.0×10^9/l, respectively. Ceftriaxone was discontinued and the patient received parenteral ciprofloxacin and amikacin. Neutrophils decreased further to reach a nadir of 0.17×10^9/l on day 25 of hospitalization (Fig. 1). A bone marrow examination revealed numerous

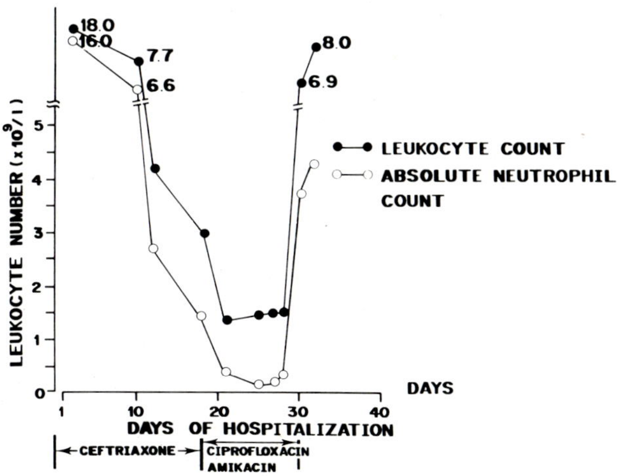

Fig. 1. The course of the leukocyte and neutrophil counts in a case of neutropenia following Ceftriaxone therapy.

granulocytic cells at the promyelocyte/myelocyte stages, lack of mature granulocytes, but normal erythocytic and megakaryocytic cells. Five days later, leukocyte, neutrophil and platelet counts showed a rapid increase to normal levels and defeverescence was noted. A second bone marrow examination was done which showed normal cellularity and granulopoietic maturation.

DISCUSSION

We do not think that sepsis was a likely cause of the severe neutropenia, since infection had been effectively controlled before the granulocyte count reached its nadir on day 25. Metoclopramide can occasionally induce severe neutropenia (4), though it was unlikely to have been the cause of the present severe neutropenia as the dosage was lower and the duration of treatment was shorter than in the reported case (4). Moreover, metoclopramide had been discontinued in our case 2 weeks before leukopenia was observed. The reversible process of severe neutropenia after discontinuation of ceftriaxone in this patient suggests ceftriaxone-induced severe neutropenia.

Severe neutropenia due to ceftriaxone has rarely been described in the English literature (5–7). The total dose (18 g) and the duration of ceftriaxone exposure (18 days) in our case were lower than those reported in previous cases (5–7). They are however in the same range as in patients having ceftriaxone-induced neutropenia [a total dose of 51 ± 29 g (MEAN $\pm$ SD) and a mean duration of treatment 21 days (range 8–25 days)] (3).

Two mechanisms of ceftriaxone-induced neutropenia have been proposed: direct toxicity of ceftriaxone or its metabolites upon the granulocytic progenitor cells in bone marrow (2, 5), and an immunologic process affecting circulating leukocytes or marrow granulopoietic stem cells (8). However, the mechanism of the ceftriaxone-inuced severe neutropenia in our case remains unknown.

The consequences of severe neutropenia include life-threatening bacterial infections (9). It is therefore mandatory to monitor blood counts serially in patients who receive a high daily dose, a high total dose, or are treated with ceftriaxone for a long time.

ACKNOWLEDGEMENT

We thank Professor Henry Wilde for reviewing our manuscript.

REFERENCES

1. Norrby SR. Side effects of cephalosporins. Drugs 34 (Suppl 2): 105–120, 1987.
2. Bang NU, Kammer RB. Hematologic complications associated with β-lactam antibiotics. Rev Infect Dis 5: S380–393, 1983.
3. Naftel KA, Hauser SP, Muller MR. Inhibition of granulopoiesis in vivo and in vitro by β-lactam antibiotics. J Infect Dis 152: 90–98, 1985.
4. Harvey RL, Luzar MJ. Metoclopramide-induced agranulocytosis. Ann Intern Med 108: 214–215, 1988.
5. Rey D, Martin T, Albert A, Pasquali JL. Ceftriaxone-induced granulopenia related to a peculiar mechanism of granulopoiesis inhibition. Am J Med 87: 591–592, 1989.
6. Baciewicz AM, Skiest DJ, Weinshel EL. Ceftriaxone-associated neutropenia (letter). Drug Intell Clin Pharm 22: 826–827, 1988.
7. Nadelman RB, Arlin Z, Wormser GP. Life-threatening complication of empiric ceftriaxone therapy for seronegative Lyme disease. South Med J 84: 1263–1264, 1991.
8. Murphy MF, Metcalfe P, Grint CA, Green AR, Knowles S, Amess JA, Waters AH. Cephalosporin-induced immune neutropenia. Br J Haematol 59: 9–14, 1985.
9. Hughes WT, Armstrong D, Bodey GP, Feld R, Mandell GL, Meyers JD, Pizzo PA, Schimpff NC, Shenep JL, Wade JC, Young LS, Yow MD. Guidelines for the use of antimicrobial agents in neutropenic patients with unexplained fever. J Infect Dis 161: 381–396, 1990.

Scand J Infect Dis 26: 111–115, 1994

CASE REPORT

Delayed Treatment of Pulmonary Blastomycosis Causing Vertebral Osteomyelitis, Paraspinal Abscess, and Spinal Cord Compression

L. MARTIN LAGGING[1], CLYNIECE M. BRELAND[2], DONALD J. KENNEDY[1], THOMAS W. MILLIGAN[2], MARCIA L. SOKOL-ANDERSON[1] and T. ULF WESTBLOM[1]

From [1]The Division of Infectious Diseases and Immunology and [2]the Department of Pathology, Saint Louis University School of Medicine, St. Louis, Missouri, USA

A 36-year-old woman with gallbladder disease had an incidental finding of asymptomatic cavitary lung infection with Blastomyces dermatitidis. No treatment was given initially, and 2 months later she presented with vertebral osteomyelitis, paraspinal abscess, and spinal cord compression due to dissemination of the fungus. The patient recovered following surgical debridement and treatment with 1 g of amphotericin B, followed by itraconazole 400 mg QD for 6 months. In spite of previous reports of the self limiting nature of primary pulmonary blastomycosis in the normal host, antifungal therapy may be needed in cases that do not resolve spontaneously within a short period of time, or if transient immunosuppression may be anticipated as may occur following surgery or after acquisition of other infections.

L. M. Lagging, MD, Division of Infectious Diseases, St. Louis University School of Medicine, 3635 Vista Avenue, FDT-8N, St. Louis, MO 63104, USA

INTRODUCTION

Blastomyces dermatitidis is a dimorphic fungus which is endemic in the south central and midwestern United States (1, 2). Human blastomycosis is acquired by inhalation of aerosolized conidia from the environment leading to a primary pulmonary infection (3). Symptoms, if present, are often nonspecific and can include fever, chills, myalgia, arthralgia, malaise, fatigue, and weight loss (4). The most common clinical finding in those who seek medical attention is pulmonary infection with infiltrates (4) that may clear spontaneously over several weeks (5). If dissemination beyond the lungs occurs, the patient may develop skin lesions, osteomyelitis, genitourinary tract disease, or central nervous system involvement (4, 6–9). Traditionally, amphotericin B has been the drug of choice in treating disseminated blastomycosis (4, 10), but ketoconazole and itraconazole have been used for less severe cases (10, 11). In immunocompetent patients with isolated pulmonary disease, it has been argued that therapy may be unnecessary (5, 12, 13). We report a case of pulmonary blastomycosis where delay in therapy was associated with dissemination of disease with vertebral involvement, abscess formation, and spinal cord compression.

CASE REPORT

A 36-year-old woman was initially hospitalized because of right upper quadrant abdominal pain. Her past medical history had been unremarkable except for a positive PPD skin test on a routine examination 3 years earlier for which she received isoniazid for 1 year. Current workup disclosed iron deficiency anemia, and an incidental 1.5 × 1.5 cm cavitary lung lesion in the posterior left upper lobe (Fig. 1). Bronchoscopy was performed, and cultures showed mixed oral flora with Staphylococcus aureus. Fungal and acid fast

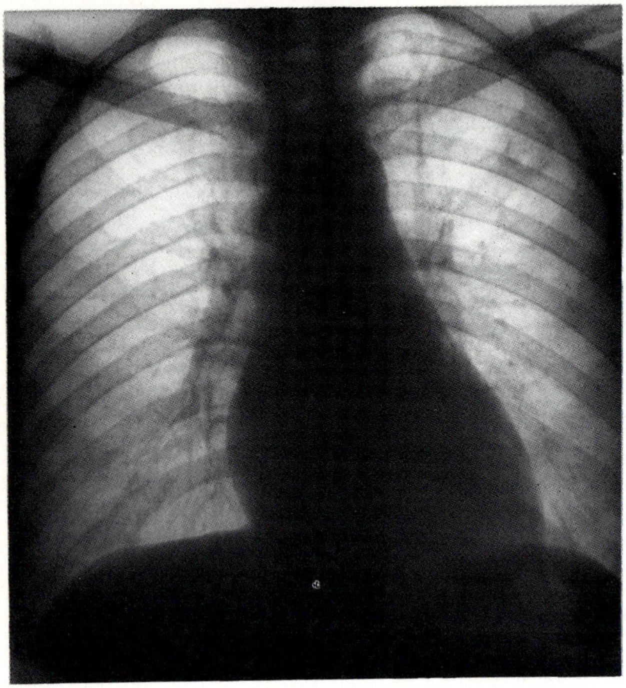

Fig. 1. Initial chest X-ray showing left upper lobe cavitary lesion.

stains were reported as negative. The patient was treated with oral ofloxacin 400 mg BID for 10 days. Two weeks later, cultures at a reference laboratory grew a mold, but this information was not immediately communicated to the treating physician. One month after her first visit, the patient experienced worsening of her right upper quadrant abdominal pain. Alkaline phosphatase was elevated at the time, and a hepatobiliary radioisotope scan was consistent with acute cholecystitis. Cholecystectomy was performed, and histopathology of the gallbladder demonstrated acute and chronic inflammation; fungal stains were negative. The abdominal pain subsequently resolved. A repeat chest X-ray during the hospitalization showed the left upper lobe cavity to have decreased to 1 × 1 cm. Four weeks later she was readmitted with a 3 to 4 week history of night sweats, decreasing appetite, fever of 39°C, and new onset of mid-thoracic back pain that radiated to the left costal margin. The patient denied any cough, shortness of breath, or hemoptysis, but chest X-ray showed persistence of her 1 × 1 cm left upper lobe cavity. Magnetic resonance imaging (MRI) of the spine showed destruction of the Th8 vertebra with spinal cord compression at the same level and a 3 × 4 × 7 cm paraspinal mass (Fig. 2).

Because of the spinal cord involvement, the patient was transferred to St. Louis University Hospital. Upon admission, a 5 × 5 cm round, fluctuant soft tissue mass was noted over vertebra Th8. Babinski reflexes were upgoing bilaterally; the remainder of the neurologic exam was intact. Laboratory examination showed a white cell count of 12.9×10^9/L with normal differential, hemoglobin 82 g/L, ESR 98 mm, and alkaline phosphatase 205 U/L (normal range 33–133). CSF was unremarkable with normal chemistries and normal cell counts. HIV serology was negative, and blastomycosis complement fixation in serum was negative with a titer of <8.

A computer tomography (CT) guided needle aspiration of the spinal mass was performed. Calcofluor white stain on the aspiration material showed multiple 8–10 μm budding yeast. After 5 days, fungal cultures showed growth of a mold, and subsequent culture characteristics were consistent with B. dermatitidis. The same day the aspiration was performed, therapy with amphotericin B was initiated. Three days after initiation of therapy, the mold from the original bronchoscopy 8 weeks prior was found to be DNA probe positive for B. dermatitidis (Accuprobe, Gen-Probe Incorporated) (14, 15). The patient subsequently underwent surgical debridement of the infected area. The inferior portion of vertebra Th7, the entire vertebra Th8, and the superior portion of vertebra Th9 were found to be necrotic. Anterior vertebrectomy with costal bone grafting was performed. At the time of surgery a nodule in the right lower lobe previously undetected on chest X-ray was also excised. Histopathological stains from both the lung and the vertebrectomy specimens showed broad based budding yeasts morphologically identical to those in the previous needle aspirate, and cultures grew B. dermatitidis. The patient was treated with a total dose

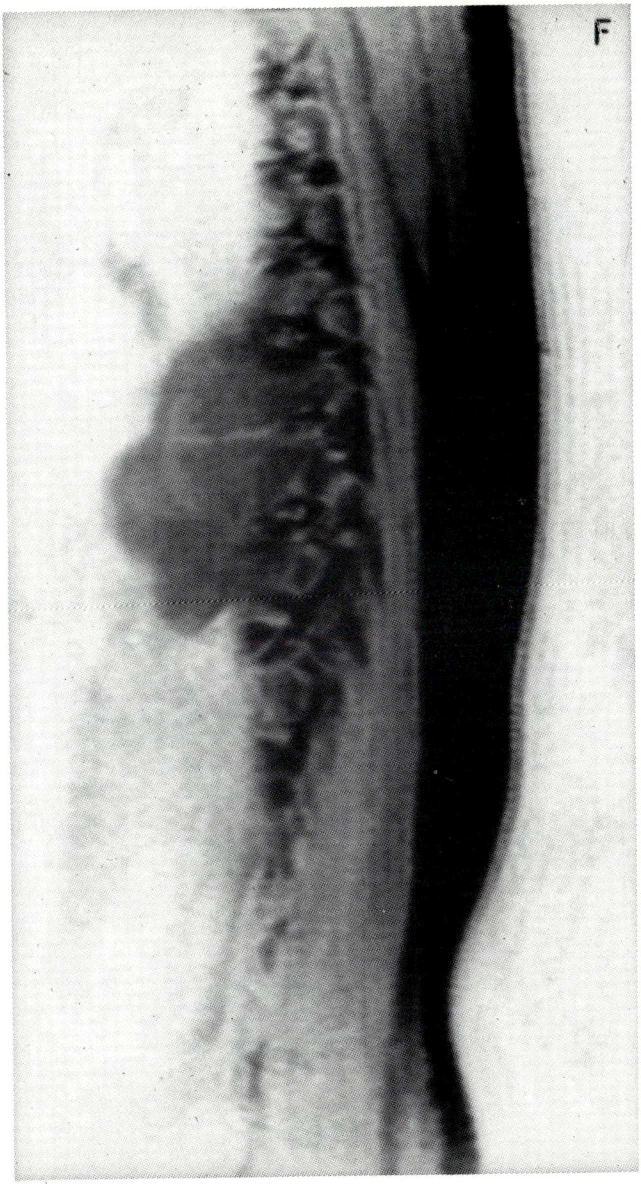

Fig. 2. MRI of spine showing paraspinal abscess extending from vertebra Th7 to Th9.

of 1 gram of amphotericin B, followed by oral itraconazole 400 mg QD for 6 months. She has had a complete recovery. At 6 month follow up, she was asymptomatic, and her chest X-ray had normalized.

During the hospitalization, no immunodeficiency or other underlying infection was identified. Specifically, all cultures and smears for mycobacteria and other pathogenic bacteria were negative, and HIV serology was negative. The exact source of the patient's exposure could not be established; however, 2 months prior to her initial presentation, she had bought soil from a local nursery, and had done extensive replanting of her indoor plants.

DISCUSSION

The need to treat disseminated blastomycosis is well founded. Prior to the advent of effective chemotherapy, disseminated blastomycosis carried a 78% mortality rate (16). Amphotericin B has reduced this fatality rate remarkably, so that a 1 gram course is curative in 87%, and 2 grams curative in 97% of infected patients (4). In recent years, to minimize toxicity, this dosage has been reduced to 500 mg in many patients, followed by extended therapy with ketoconazole or itraconazole (4). In light of the spinal cord compression and proximity to the central nervous system, we opted to treat our patient with a total of 1 gram of amphotericin B, followed by itraconazole for 6 months.

In contrast with disseminated blastomycosis, the most appropriate approach to the patient with acute blastomycosis confined to the lungs has yet to be defined. In one epidemic, B. dermatitidis was recovered from the sputum in 5 of 8 adults after a canoeing trip in northwestern Wisconsin, USA (5). Seven of 8 had abnormal chest X-rays, 6 of which improved spontaneously within 10 weeks. None of the 8 adults were treated with antifungal therapy, and all were in excellent health 5 years later.

In another epidemic in Big Fork, Minnesota, USA, 18 adults and children had blastomycosis diagnosed by culture or skin test (12). 12 of the 18 had an abnormal chest X-ray. None of the patients received antifungal therapy and all were doing well after 1 year.

Based on these 2 epidemics, and a report by Recht et al. (13), it has been suggested that most cases of pulmonary blastomycosis in immunocompetent patients do not require treatment (5, 12, 13), particularly if symptoms are minimal. These recommendations, however, were made when therapy with amphotericin B was the only available option. With the introduction of less toxic oral antifungal drugs such as ketoconazole and itraconazole, the threshold for treating asymptomatic pulmonary blastomycosis should probably be lowered. This is especially true if patients become transiently immunosuppressed as may occur following surgery or after acquisition of other infections.

Dissemination of primary pulmonary blastomycosis may occur in immunocompetent people (7–9). Our patient had an incidental finding of asymptomatic primary pulmonary blastomycosis discovered during workup of gallbladder disease. Aside from possible postoperative immunosuppression, no underlying immunodeficiency was identified during her hospitalization. Because of the delay in making a definitive diagnosis, she initially received no antifungal therapy. We have no way of knowing whether or not earlier therapy would have altered the clinical course in our patient. However, considering the severity of her complications and the availability of oral antifungal drugs with good safety profile (10, 11), it is tempting to conclude that she should have received antifungal therapy for the pulmonary lesion alone when she first presented.

REFERENCES

1. Furcolow ML, Chick EW, Busey JF, Menges RW. Prevalence and incidence studies of human and canine blastomycosis, cases in the United States, 1885–1968. Am Rev Respir Dis 102: 60–67, 1970.
2. Furcolow ML, Busey JF, Menges RW, Chick EW. Prevalence and incidence studies of human and canine blastomycosis. Am J Epidemiol 92: 121–131, 1970.
3. Klein BS, Vergeront JM, Weeks RJ, Kumar UN, Mathai G, Varkey B, Kaufman L, Bradsher RW, Stoebig JF, Davis JP. Isolation of blastomyces dermatitidis in soil associated with a large outbreak of blastomycosis in Wisconsin. N Engl J Med 314: 529–534, 1986.
4. Bradsher RW. Blastomycosis. Clin Infect Dis 14 (Suppl 1): S82–S90, 1992.
5. Cockerill FR, Roberts GD, Rosenblatt JE, Utz JP, Utz DC. Epidemic of pulmonary blastomycosis (Namekagon fever) in Wisconsin canoeists. Chest 86: 688–692, 1984.
6. Witorsch P, Utz JP. North American blastomycosis: a study of 40 patients. Medicine 47: 169–200, 1968.
7. MacDonald PB, Black GB, MacKenzie R. Orthopaedic manifestations of blastomycosis. J Bone Joint Surg [Am] 72: 860–864, 1990.
8. Eickenberg HU, Amin M, Lich R. Blastomycosis of the genitourinary tract. J Urol 113: 650–652, 1975.

9. Goynyea EF. The spectrum of primary blastomycotic meningitis: a review of central nervous system blastomycosis. Ann Neurol 3: 26–39, 1978.
10. Bradsher RW, Rice DC, Abernathy RS. Ketoconazole therapy for endemic blastomycosis. Ann Intern Med 103: 872–879, 1985.
11. Dismukes WE, Bradsher RW, Cloud GC, Chapman SW, George RB, Stevens DA, Girard WM, Saag MS, Bowles-Patton C. Itraconazole therapy for blastomycosis and histoplasmosis. Am J Med 93: 489–497, 1992.
12. Sarosi GA, Hammerman KJ, Tosh FE, Kronenberg RS. Clinical features of acute pulmonary blastomycosis. N Engl J Med 290: 540–543, 1974.
13. Recht LD, Philips JR, Eckman MR, Sarosi GA. Self-limited blastomycosis: a report of thirteen cases. Am Rev Respir Dis 120: 1109–1112, 1979.
14. Kwon-Chung KJ, Bennett JE. Medical mycology. Philadelphia: Lea and Febiger, 58–59, 1992.
15. Stockman L, Roberts GD, Clark KM. Evaluation of a commercially prepared chemiluminescent probe for the culture identification of Blastomyces dermatitidis, Coccidioides immitis, and Cryptococcus neoformans. Abstracts of the 91st General Meeting of the American Society for Microbiology, Abstract F-73, 1991.
16. Martin DS, Smith DT. Blastomycosis: I. A review of the literature. Am Rev Tuber 39: 275–304, 1939.

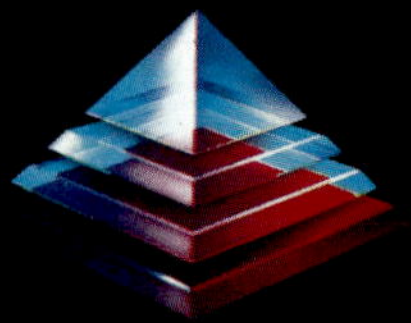

Scand J Infect Dis 26: 117–118, 1994

CASE REPORT

Microscopic Examination of Sperm as the Diagnostic Clue in a Case of Schistosoma haematobium Infection

NIELS OBEL and FINN TRUNK BLACK

From the Department of Medicine and Infectious Diseases, Marselisborg Hospital, University of Aarhus, Denmark

Early diagnosis and treatment of Schistosoma haematobium infections is imperative to prevent chronic manifestations of the disease. Microscopical examination of urine and faeces, and rectal biopsy are widely used standard methods for the rapid diagnosis of schistosomiasis. We report a case in whom numerous Schistosoma haematobium eggs were demonstrated in sperm, even though repeated examination of urine and rectal biopsies had been futile. It is concluded that the case presented demonstrates the importance of using sperm as an alternative sample material when schistosoma eggs are not found in conventional sample materials from male patients suspected of being infected with Schistosoma haematobium.

N. Obel, MD, Department of Medicine and Infectious Diseases, Marselisborg Hospital, University of Aarhus, DK-8000 Aarhus C, Denmark

INTRODUCTION

An estimated 200 million people worldwide are infected with schistosomes. Schistosoma mansoni, Schistosoma japanicum and, less commonly, Schistosoma mekongi and Schistosoma intercalatam inhabit the mesenterial plexus of the infected host. Schistosoma haematobium, in contrast, infects the venules of the urinary bladder. Chronic manifestations of the disease result mainly from irreversible fibrosing lesions developing in response to the schistosoma eggs. Early diagnosis and treatment are therefore imperative. Although sensitive serologic tests for schistosomiasis have been developed, demonstration of parasite eggs is the decisive diagnostic measure in schistosomiasis. We report a case in whom numerous Schistosoma haematobium eggs were demonstrated in sperm even though repeated urinary examinations had been futile.

CASE REPORT

A 35-year-old man consulted the Department of Infectious Diseases after a 3-year stay in Zambia, Namibia, Tanzania and Malawi. Prior to the visit he was vaccinated against yellow fever, cholera and typhoid fever. Chloroquine and paludrine were taken as malarial prophylaxis. Apart from a brief attack of fever of unknown origin, he had felt well during his stay in Africa. The patient had been in frequent contact with fresh water. After his return, he developed tenderness in the left inguinal region and thin, clotting sperm.

Laboratory data: Haemoglobin, 142 g/l; sedimentation rate, 8 mm/h; eosinophil granulocytes, 1.88 x 10^9/l (0.05–0.40 x 10^9/1); leukocytes, 6.6 x 10^9/1; aspartate aminotransferase, 18 U/l (<40 U/l); no protein in urine. Three rectal samples and 6 examinations of urine proved negative for schistosoma eggs. Nevertheless, the patient was found positive by immunofluorescence, using gut-associated schistosoma antigen.

Due to the patient's travel history, eosinophilia, serology and anamnestic information, a sperm sample was obtained in which numerous Schistosoma haematobium eggs were demonstrated microscopically. The number of eggs in the sample material increased considerably when the pellet from centrifugated material was used for microscopy.

The patient was treated with praziquantel, 40 mg/kg body weight. At a 4-month follow-up the subjective complaints had subsided, the eosinophilia disappeared, and Schistosoma haematobium eggs (including calcified eggs) could no longer be demonstrated in semen.

DISCUSSION

Microscopical examination of urine, faeces and of rectal biopsy material is widely used as a standard method for rapid diagnosis of schistosomiasis. The sample material is chosen according to the known location of the parasites – in the venules of the intestines and urinary bladder of the human host. The association of bladder cancer with schistosomiasis is well established (1). Simultaneous presence of schistosoma eggs in prostate biopsies and advanced prostatic cancer has also been reported (2). Furthermore, it has been suggested that schistosoma infection of male genital organs causes infertility (3). Early and precise diagnosis of schistosomiasis is essential in order to avoid the hazards inflicted on the host by this parasite. The case presented is to our knowledge the first report in the literature to demonstrate the importance of using sperm as an alternative sample when schistosoma eggs are not found in conventional sample materials from male patients suspected of harbouring Schistosoma haematobium.

REFERENCES

1. Malik MO, Veress B, Daoud EH, El Hassan AM. Pattern of bladder cancer in the Sudan and its relation to schistosomiasis: a study of 225 vesical carcinomas. J Trop Med Hyg 78: 219–226, 1975.
2. Godec CJ, Grunberger I, Carr GA. Simultaneous presence of schistosomiasis and advanced cancer in prostate. Urology 39: 547–549, 1992.
3. Ogunbanjo BO, Osoba AO, Ochei J. Infective factors of male infertility among Nigerians. Afr J Med Med Sci 18: 35–38, 1989.

Scand J Infect Dis 26: 119–120, 1994

LETTERS TO THE EDITORS

Abdominal Lymphonodal Enlargement in HIV Patients Detected by Ultrasonography

We have read the article by Cassani et al. entitled "Abdominal Lymphoadenopathy Detected by Ultrasonography in HIV-1 Infection: Prevalence and Significance" in Scand J Infect Dis 25: 221–225, 1993 with interest and we would like to make some observations.

Our studies aim to define the meaning of abdominal lymphadenopathy noticed by using Ultrasonography in HIV-1 positive patients.

We have tested 183 patients in various stages of HIV induced disease and have noticed the increased lymph nodes in 80 cases: group I comprised of 72 patients with lymphadenopathy in hepatoduodenal ligament only; group II (8 patients) had enlarged lymph nodes also in other abdominal stations.

All patients, except 2, in group I and all the patients in group II demonstrated evidence of chronic hepatitis (1) or previous hepatitis B, C or D virus infection (2). Four patients from group I also had Non Hodgkin Lymphoma (3).

Patients from group II had systemic CMV infection (4 pts), disseminated mycobacterium avium complex infection (2 pts) (4), disseminated Histoplasmosis (1 pt) (5), diseases which can cause lymphadenopathy also outside the hepatoduodenal ligament. Our results show that the most frequent cause of lymphadenopathy in the hepatoduodenal ligament in HIV patients is chronic hepatitis even if other diseases might cause lymphadenopathy (particularly lymphomas and opportunistic infections). Only in 2 patients with enlarged lymph nodes, who are followed up clinically, no other reasons for the lymphadenopathy besides HIV has been found.

In conclusion, we believe that the finding of abdominal lymphonodal enlargement is not enough to include asymptomatic carriers (Class II, CDC) (6) in group PGL (Class III) unless previous contacts with hepatitis virus or other infectious agents or diseases able to cause such a change can be excluded.

REFERENCES

1. Gore RM, Vogelzang RL, Nemcek AA. Lymphoadenopathy in chronic active hepatitis: CT observations. AJR Am J Roentgenol 151: 75–80, 1988.
2. Messina F, Del Bravo P, Luchi S, Parenti M, Paladini A, Scasso A. Rilievo ecografico di linfonodi nel legamento epatoduodenale e patologia infettiva epatica. Giorn Mal Inf Parass [in press].
3. Nyberg DA, Brooke Jeffrey RB, Federle MP, Bottles K, Abrams DI. AIDS-related lymphomas: evaluation by abdominal CT. Radiology 159: 56–63, 1986.
4. Hulnick DH, Megibow AJ, Naidich DP, Hilton S, Cho KC, Balthazar EJ. Abdominal tuberculosis: CT evaluation. Radiology 157: 199–204, 1985.
5. Randall Radin D. Disseminated hystoplasmosis: abdominal CT findings in 16 patients. AJR Am J Roentgenol 157: 955–958, 1991.
6. Center for Disease Control. Classification system for human T-lymphotropic virus type III/lymphoadenopathy-associated virus infections. Ann Intern Med 105: 234–237, 1986.

Francesco Messina, Paola Del Bravo, Sauro Luchi, Donatella Aquilini and **Antonio Scasso.** Division of Infectious Diseases, Cisanello Hospital, Pisa, Italy

Address for correspondence: F. Messina, MD, Divisione di Malattie Infettive, Ospedale di Cisanello, via Paradisa 2, I-56100 Pisa, Italy

REPLY

Dear Sir,

Dr. Messina and coworkers suggest that the enlargement of deep abdominal lymph nodes detected by ultrasound in HIV positive patients is actually caused by a concomitant chronic hepatitis rather than by the HIV infection. I agree that this hypothesis, already stated in my paper, is particularly pertinent for asymptomatic HIV carriers (CDC – group II) exhibiting lymphadenopathy within the hepatoduodenal ligament. To provide evidence of it, however, a selective association between ultrasonographic findings and liver disease must be obtained; further studies are thus needed, which should obviously take into consideration the prevalence of chronic hepatitis not only in HIV positive patients with deep nodes, as reported by Dr. Messina, but also in non-HIV infected patients.

It is pertinent to recall that in our HIV positive series abdominal lymphadenopathy turned out to be associated with significantly higher serum levels of gammaglobulins and IgG. The same figure was also observed for superficial lymphadenopathy, which are known to represent an element intrinsic to the clinical picture of HIV infection, relevant for a correct classification of the condition and so far clearly unrelated to any hepatic disorder. In HIV positive patients, therefore, deep and superficial nodes appear to have the same significance: both reflect a state of polyclonal B cell activation. If confirmed, these observations suggest that HIV is somehow directly involved in the development of abdominal lymphadenopathy. Likewise, the detection by ultrasound of the above lesions should be properly considered in the HIV infection staging.

Fabio Cassani, Paolo Costigliola, Marco Zoli, Laura Baffoni, Nicola Dentale, Ennio Ricchi, Francesco Chiodo, Germano Pilati, Francesco B. Bianchi and **Emilio Pisi**

Address for correspondence: F. Cassini, MD, Istituto di Clinica Medica Generale e Terapia Medica, Cattedra di Semeiotica Medica II, Policlinico S. Orsola, via Massarenti 9, I-40138 Bologna, Italy

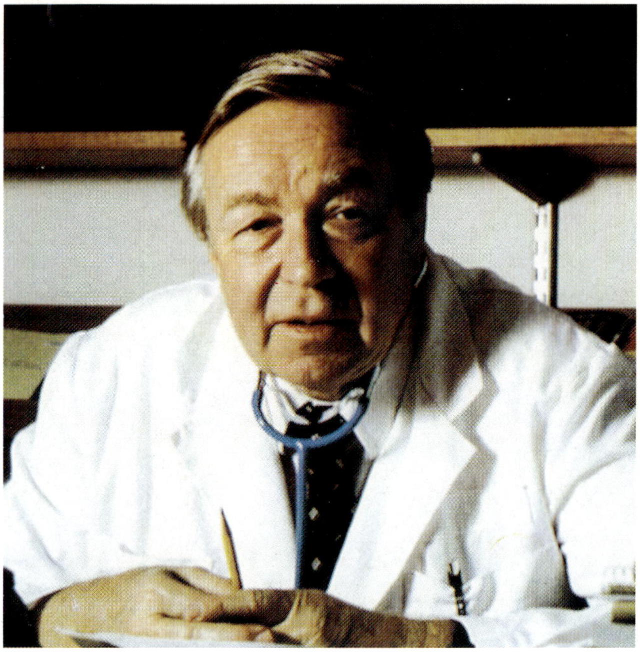

IN MEMORY OF FOLKE NORDBRING

Folke Nordbring died unexpectedly in March 1994. He was born in 1921, received his M.D. at the Karolinska Institute in Stockholm and his clinical training at the University of Uppsala where he became a Ph.D. in microbiology and immunology and a specialist in both paediatrics and infectious diseases. In 1975 he was appointed head of the Department of Infectious Diseases at Uppsala Academic Hospital and in 1980 he moved to Lund to become professor and head of the Department of Infectious Diseases at the University Hospital, a position he held until his retirement in 1987. Folke Nordbring published a large number of scientific articles and monographs in the field of infectious diseases, especially antimicrobial chemotherapy. He was an outstanding teacher, both for the medical students and for his postgraduate students and younger colleagues.

In 1969 Folke Nordbring and a group of infectious disease physicians and microbiologists from the Nordic countries founded the Scandinavian Journal of Infectious Diseases and he became its first editor, a position he held for 24 years. He made this journal a leading international forum for original research in infectious diseases and clinical microbiology, always with an emphasis on the clinical aspects. He was the ideal editor for a scientific journal: fair in the assessments of the submissions, creative and positive in his suggestions for improvements and uncompromising when it came to the scientific quality of articles accepted for publication.

We have lost a good friend and colleague but we are convinced that this journal will continue along Folke Nordbring's lines as one of the main sources of information about new and important research in the field of infectious diseases.

S. Ragnar Norrby — Claus Ola Solberg

Scand J Infect Dis 26: 129–132, 1994

HTLV-II Among Injecting Drug Users in Stockholm

AUD KROOK[1] and JONAS BLOMBERG[2]

From the [1]Department of Immunology, Microbiology, Pathology and Infectious Diseases, Section for Infectious Diseases, Karolinska Institute, Huddinge University Hospital, Stockholm, and the [2]Department of Microbiology, Section for Virology, University of Lund, Lund, Sweden

134 injecting drug users (IDUs) treated at the Department of Infectious Diseases of Roslagstull Hospital, Stockholm, were tested for antibodies to human T-lymphotropic virus, types I and II, by means of 2 HTLV-I/-II peptide-based enzyme immunoassays (EIAs), followed by a whole-virus EIA. Positive EIA reactions were checked and typed by electrophoretic immunoblotting with native HTLV-I and recombinant HTLV-I and -II proteins. 10 IDUs were diagnosed as HTLV-II seropositive. All 10 were of Scandinavian descent. Thus, like HIV-1, HTLV-II infection has entered the injecting drug user population in Stockholm.

J. Blomberg, MD, Department of Medical Microbiology, Section for Virology, Sölvegatan 23, S-223 62 Lund, Sweden

INTRODUCTION

Human T cell lymphotropic virus (HTLV), types I and II, are widespread, with endemic foci in southern Japan and the Caribbean (for a review, see ref. 1). In North America, a relatively high percentage of injecting drug users (IDUs) are HTLV-II seropositive (2). In Europe, HTLV is rare in the general population (3), but HTLV-II does occur in some drug user populations (4). Although the frequency of HTLV infection in Scandinavia seems to be low (5, 6), a surprisingly high prevalence of HTLV-II infection among IDUs (24.5%) was recently reported from Oslo, Norway (7). Additionally 2 cases of HTLV-I and one of HTLV-II infection were observed among IDUs in Malmö, Sweden (6). The prevalence of HTLV infection among IDUs treated at the specialized ward for IDUs with infectious diseases at Roslagstull Hospital, Stockholm, was therefore studied.

MATERIALS AND METHODS

Patients and sera

An extra serum sample was collected prospectively from all the IDUs hospitalized on ward 9 (a specialized ward for IDUs) at Roslagstull Hospital from the date when the ward was opened on October 1st, 1990 until it was moved to Huddinge Hospital on March 3rd, 1992. Serum samples were obtained from 134 patients, out of altogether 157 IDUs. Patient data were coded and test results could not be ascribed to any individual patient. 89 of the 134 patients were men (50% born in 1956 or earlier, range 1941–67) and of the 45 women, 50% were born in 1957 or earlier (range 1943–72). 55 (41%) were HIV-1 positive and all except 3 were of Scandinavian descent. Heroin was the main drug for 71 (53%), and amphetamine for 63 (47%). A positive serology for hepatitis A was seen in 78 (58%), for hepatitis B in 110 (82%) and for hepatitis C in 121 (90%). Only 4 patients were negative in all 3 hepatitis serologies. Three of them were also HIV antibody negative.

Immunoassays and serotyping

All sera were first screened by 2 EIAs for HTLV-I and -II antibodies, 1 proprietary and 1 commercial. In the proprietary test a mixture of the peptides HTLV-I *gag* 102–129, HTLV-I *env* 178–212 and HTLV-II *env* 174–208 adsorbed to microtitre wells, was used. The peptides and their antigenicity were recently described (8). The test was validated against a panel of known HTLV-I and -II positive sera (data not shown). The commercial peptide based HTLV-I and -II antibody test was from Biochrom AG, Berlin, Germany. It also contains peptides from p19 and gp46 of HTLV-I and -II. Reactive sera were further tested in an HTLV whole-virus lysate antibody test (HTLV-I EIA, Abbott, Chicago, IL, USA) according to the instructions of the manufacturer. However, the cut-off level was set to half of that prescribed by the manufacturer. This was because in earlier studies (6, and unpublished results of JB) it was found that the virus lysate EIA could miss a few weakly reactive HTLV-II antibody positive sera. Sera reactive in either of the HTLV peptide antibody tests were subjected to an HTLV-I electrophoretic immunoblot (also called Western blot) (EIB; version 2.3, Diagnostic Biotechnologies, Singapore). Sera which reacted with p19, p24, recombinant gp21 and recombinant gp46 (from either type I or type II) in EIB were considered HTLV-I or -II positive.

RESULTS

Of 134 sera, 31 reacted in either of the HTLV peptide screening assays (Table I A). 14 of these also proved positive in the virus lysate test, using a low cut-off value. 10 of the 31 proved positive in the EIB, with a characteristic HTLV-II reactivity pattern: weak p19, strong p24, strong recombinant gp21 and recombinant type II (but not type I) gp46 bands (Table I B). However, 2 of the 10 reacted markedly weaker than the rest. Had the original cut-off value been used in the virus lysate test, 1 of these 2 weakly HTLV-II reactive sera would have been missed. Two further sera displayed a shadow of EIB reactivity at the ordinary dilution (1/200), but gave a weak HTLV-II-like reactivity when tested at 1/50. The latter 2 sera were not considered HTLV-II positive. Thus, many shades of HTLV-II antibody reactivity from strong to very weak and doubtful occurred. The 10 sera reacted with both *env* and *gag* HTLV proteins, and thus were HTLV antibody positive also according to the WHO criteria (9). Thus, the HTLV-I EIB pattern, and the reactivity with HTLV-II recombinant gp46 – though not with its HTLV-I counterpart – indicated that 10 of 134 IDUs were HTLV-II seropositive. The remaining 19 sera either did not react at all (10 sera), or reacted only weakly with 1 or 2 HTLV proteins: p19 (1 serum), p24 (2 sera), rgp46 type I (1 serum), p24 and p19 (1 serum), p19 + rgp21 (2 sera), p19 + rgp46 type II (2 sera). Due to the 'blind' nature of the study we could not obtain samples for HTLV-I or -II PCR. None of the sera had an HTLV-I antibody reactivity.

Correlation of HTLV seropositivity with clinical data

The HTLV-positive patients comprised 3 females and 7 males (Table II). Their median birth year was 1951 (range 1946–61). Six were heroinists and 4 amphetaminists. All 10 patients were seropositive for hepatitis A, B and C (none had been vaccinated). Seven were HIV-1 seropositive. The sera tested for HTLV were collected between 1990 and 1992.

Table I. *HTLV serology with 134 sera from IDUs*

Method	No.	Pos.
A. *Peptide HTLV-I-II antibody screening*		
Positive in proprietary test only	134	10
Positive in commercial test (Biochrom) only	134	8
Samples where both peptide tests were positive		13
Samples further analysed by virus lysate EIA and EIB		31
B. *Further analyses in sera where either of the 2 peptide tests was positive*		
Virus lysate EIA (HTLV-I) (Abbott; low cut-off[a])	31	14
Western blot (EIB; HTLV-I + recomb. -II)[b]	31	10[c]

[a] The cut-off value recommended by Abbott was halved.
[b] EIB = Electrophoretic immunoblot.
[c] One of the 10 was missed by the commercial peptide EIA test, all 10 were detected by the virus lysate EIA.

Table II. *The 10 IDUs diagnosed as HTLV-II seropositive*

Pat. no.	Birth year	Sex	Abuse	HIV status	Hepatitis status[a]	Serum collected
1	1950	M	Amphet	–	ABC	1990
2	1950	M	Heroin	+	ABC	1990
3	1952	F	Heroin	+	ABC	1990
4	1952	F	Amphet	+	ABC	1990
5	1946	M	Amphet	–	ABC	1991
6	1950	M	Heroin	+	ABC	1991
7	1948	M	Amphet	+	ABC	1991
8	1953	M	Heroin	–	ABC	1991
9	1961	M	Heroin	+	ABC	1992
10	1956	F	Heroin	+	ABC	1992

[a] ABC = hepatitis A, B and C.

DISCUSSION

The diagnosis of an HTLV infection is of clinical consequence. Apart from the well-known HTLV-related diseases adult T cell leukemia and tropical spastic paraparesis, the HTLVs have been reported to hasten the progression of HIV infection in simultaneously HIV-1 and HTLV-I infected persons (10, 11). Hitherto, only sporadic cases of HTLV infection have been observed in Sweden (5, 6, 12). In a study of IDUs from southern Sweden, Denmark and Stockholm, comprising 693 sera from 1987 to 1993, only 3 HTLV antibody-positive cases were observed, all from 1993 in Malmö, Sweden (6). In an unpublished survey of 100 sera from HIV-1-positive persons, including 39 IDUs, collected between 1986 and 1987 in Stockholm, none was HTLV seropositive (personal communication from Dr Anders Sönnerborg). Our observation that at least 10 of 134 IDUs from Roslagstull Hospital in Stockholm were HTLV-II seropositive defines the largest cluster of HTLV infection hitherto known in Sweden. The finding of HTLV seropositive persons of Scandinavian descent, living in Stockholm, indicates that HTLV-II is now established in parts of the native Swedish IDU population, among both heroinists and amphetaminists. Due to the 'blind' nature of the study, the exact neurological status of the patients was not known (13). However, no overt neurological disease was noted among the 10 HTLV-II seropositive patients. Unsuccessful attempts to detect HTLV among Swedish IDUs during the 1980s (6, A. Sönnerborg, personal communication), and the emergence of HTLV seropositive persons during the 1990s (this study, and 6) indicate that the transmission of HTLVs among Swedish IDUs is primarily a phenomenon of the early 1990s. The HTLV seropositive patients were hepatitis A, B and C seropositive and somewhat older than the rest, having had opportunities for HTLV exposure far back in time. As in Norway (7), Italy (4), and North America (2), HTLV-II predominated over HTLV-I in this IDU population. The consistent pattern of association between HTLV-II, rather than HTLV-I, and intravenous drug abuse in such diverse geographical regions, leads to the supposition that HTLV-II may be more transmissible via the intravenous route than HTLV-I is. If there is indeed such a difference between the HTLV types, the mechanism behind it is difficult to envisage.

The finding of 2 sera which react very weakly but with the same pattern as the fully reactive HTLV-II positive sera emphasizes that the confirmation of HTLV-II infection requires very sensitive and specific tests, including PCR, which could not be performed in this study.

An open, prospective study with informed consent in the same patient group is now being set up. This will allow a more detailed clinical investigation, and PCR confirmation of the HTLV-II infection. We also hope to be able to time the HTLV-II infection by testing earlier sera. Knowing that HTLV infection has entered into the IDU population of Stockholm and Malmö, it is now necessary to reappraise whether and how blood donors should be tested for HTLV antibodies in Sweden.

ACKNOWLEDGEMENTS

We are indebted to Elzbieta Vincic for skillful technical assistance, and to Dr Rüdiger Pipkorn for supplying the synthetic peptides. This work was supported by the Department of Environmental Health and Infectious Diseases Control, Karolinska Hospital, Stockholm and the Swedish Medical Research Council, grant no. B09933–03A.

REFERENCES

1. Cann AJ, Chen ISY. Human T-cell leukemia virus types I and II. In: Fields BN, Knipe DM, Chanock RM, Hirsch MS, Melnick JL, Monath TP, Roizman B, eds. Virology, 2nd edn. New York: Raven Press, 1501–1527, 1990.
2. Robert-Guroff M, Weiss SH, Giron JA, Jennings AM, Ginzburg HM, Margolis IB, Blattner WA, Gallo RC. Prevalence of antibodies to HTLV-I, -II and -III in intravenous drug abusers from an AIDS endemic region. JAMA 255: 3133–3137, 1986.
3. Mayer V, Ebbesen P. HTLV-I virus in Europeans: the continuous spread. A meta-analysis. Acta Virol 35: 472–495, 1991.
4. Zanetti AR, Zehender G, Tanzi E, Galli C, Rezza G, Cargnel A, Boschini A, Mari D, Pizzocolo G, Mazzotta F. HTLV-II among Italian intravenous drug users and hemophiliacs. Eur J Epidemiol 8: 702–707, 1992.
5. Blomberg J, Fäldt R. Antibodies to human adult T cell leukemia virus type I associated antigens in Swedish leukaemia patients and blood donors. Br J Haematol 60: 555–557, 1985.
6. Blomberg J, Moestrup T, Frimand J, Hansson BG, Krogsgaard K, Grillner L, Nordenfelt E. HTLV-I and -II in intravenous drug users from Sweden and Denmark. Scand J Infect Dis 26: 23–26, 1994.
7. Holm-Samdahl H, Haukenes G, Kalland KH. HTLV-infeksjon i Norge [HTLV infection in Norway]. MSIS rapport 21: 1, 1993.
8. Blomberg J, Robert-Guroff M, Blattner WA, Pipkorn R. Type- and group-specific continuous antigenic determinants of HTLV. Use of synthetic peptides for serotyping of HTLV-I and -II infection. J Acquir Immune Defic Syndr 5: 294–302, 1992.
9. World Health Organization: proposed WHO criteria for interpreting results from Western Blot assays for HIV-1, HIV-2 and HTLV-I/HTLV-II. Wkly Epidemiol Rec 65: 281–288, 1990.
10. Page JB, Lai SH, Chitwood DD, Klimas NG, Smith PC, Fletcher MA. HTLV-I/II seropositivity and death from AIDS among HIV-1 seropositive intravenous drug users. Lancet 16: 1439–1441, 1990.
11. Pierik LT, Murphy EL. The clinical significance of HTLV-I and HIV-1 in the AIDS epidemic. AIDS Clin Rev 1991: 39–57, 1991.
12. Ryberg B, Blomberg J, Klasse PJ. Tropical spastic paraparesis associated with human T lymphotropic virus type I in an East African naturalised in Sweden. BMJ 295: 1380–1381, 1987.
13. Harrington WJ Jr, Sheremata W, Hjelle B, Dube DK, Bradshaw P, Foung SK, Snodgrass S, Toedter G, Cabral L, Poiesz B. Spastic ataxia associated with human T-cell lymphotropic virus type II infection. Ann Neurol 33: 411–414, 1993.

Scand J Infect Dis 26: 133–136, 1994

Falling Incidence and Prevalence of Hepatitis A in Northern Spain

EMILIO PEREZ-TRALLERO, GUSTAVO CILLA, MERCEDES URBIETA, MIREN DORRONSORO, FERNANDO OTERO and JOSE M. MARIMON

From the Microbiology Service and Infectious Epidemiology Unit Hospital NS Aránzazu, San Sebastián, Spain

The prevalence of hepatitis A virus antibodies was studied using a commercial ELISA method. 2,214 subjects were included, 1,211 in 1992 and 1,003 during 1986–87. In 1992 the seroprevalence rates among subjects 1–9, 10–19, 20–29 and 30–39 years old were 2.4%, 21%, 57.6% and 87.5% respectively, as compared with 7.7%, 37.9%, 80.6% and 98.1% respectively, in a similar group of subjects studied 5 years earlier ($p \leq 0.001$). The reported number of viral hepatitis cases declined from 35.0 per 100,000 people in 1984 to 8.9 per 100,000 in 1992. Concurrently, the age when contracting the disease rose. The mean age for patients acquiring hepatitis A was 15.5 in 1986–88 and 20.1 in 1991–92. The decline in incidence and prevalence of HAV infection indicates a progressive and continuous decrease in HAV circulation in this geographical area.

E. Perez-Trallero, Servicio de Microbiología, Hospital NS Aránzazu, Aptdo 477, E-20080 San Sebastián, Spain

INTRODUCTION

Hepatitis A is a benign disease with a mortality rate of less than 1%. However, because of its high incidence it is a public health problem world-wide that causes large economic losses (1, 2). The age when most infections are acquired varies among countries, socioeconomic strata, and living conditions. In the industrialized countries of Europe, North America and Australia, the incidence and prevalence of hepatitis A has decreased significantly in recent decades. Our study assessed the evolution of hepatitis A in our region in recent years.

MATERIALS AND METHODS

Seroprevalence study

The Guipuzcoa province is located in the northeastern region of the Basque Country and is fronted by the Cantabrian Sea (Atlantic Ocean) and bordered by France to the north. Its 1,997 square kilometers of territory is inhabited by 671,774 people. The population sample for our seroprevalence study consisted of 1,211 subjects enrolled in 1992 and 1,003 enrolled during 1986–87, the latter in another study of subjects with similar socioeconomic status as earlier reported (3). The 1992 sample was divided into 2 groups. The first comprised 603 children and adolescents 1–17 years old who received outpatient care for mild disorders unrelated to liver disease (injuries, minor surgical procedures, etc). The second group comprised 608 women 18–40 years old, randomly selected from those admitted to the maternity ward of Nuestra Señora de Aránzazu Hospital in 1992, which admitted 65% of all women who gave birth in the province (according to the Basque Institute of Statistics). None of the subjects had acute liver disease. The groups included persons of both urban and rural origin who were roughly representative of the middle class. The sample size for each age group was based on the size of the corresponding census population in the province at large and on the prevalence of hepatitis A virus (HAV) antibodies in an earlier study (3) with an acceptable result of $\pm 5\%$ and a confidence level of 95%.

Incidence

Data on the annual incidence of viral hepatitis and hepatitis A in the area were obtained from mandatory infectious disease reports to the EDO (Enfermedades de Declaración Obligatoria) System. Reporting of 'viral hepatitis' has been compulsory in Spain since 1982; cases of hepatitis A, hepatitis B, and unspecified hepatitis are included under this heading. Hepatitis A is an optional subgroup that is not always identified. The age when the hepatitis A infection was acquired was estimated from confirmed cases (presence of IgM anti-HAV) in patients of known age.

Serologic studies

A serum sample obtained from each subject was stored at −40°C until processed. The seroprevalence of hepatitis A was studied by determining total anti-HAV in 1/100 diluted serum using a commercial ELISA method (Hepanostika anti-HAV antibodies, Organon Teknika, Boxtel, The Netherlands). Acute hepatitis A was confirmed by the detection of IgM anti-HAV using commercial ELISA kits (HAVAB M and IMX HAVAB M, Abbott, North Chicago, IL, USA). All tests were carried out according to manufacturer's instructions.

Data analysis

The χ^2-test was used to compare prevalences. Variance analysis (ANOVA, Statcalc Program, Epiinfo 1990, CDC, Atlanta) was used to compare the ages of patients who had the diagnosis hepatitis A.

RESULTS

Prevalence of anti-HAV in the study population

The proportion of immune subjects was smaller in every age group of the 1992 sample than in the 1986–87 sample (Table I). The prevalence of anti-HAV in the 1992 sample was 2.4% (8/334) among children below 10 years of age and increased gradually with age. In 1992 and 1986–87, the 20–29-year-old group had a prevalence of anti-HAV of 57.6% (148/257) and 80.6% (170/211), respectively, and the 30–39-year-old group 87.5% (238/272) and 98.1% (153/156), respectively.

Reported 'viral hepatitis' cases

The number of declared cases of 'viral hepatitis' in the province of Guipuzcoa decreased from 747 in 1984 to 184 in 1991. Likewise, the number of hepatitis A cases diminished from 239 in 1985 to 65 in 1992 (Table II). Information on the incidence of the disease came from 55% of the local general practitioners and pediatricians.

Age when the hepatitis A infection was acquired

During the study period our laboratory acted as a provincial Reference Centre for serologic confirmation of hepatitis A cases. From 1986 to 1992, 621 cases of acute hepatitis A (presence of IgM anti-HAV) were confirmed and 541 (87%) of these patients had a known date of birth. Table III shows the distribution of hepatitis A cases by decades of life. Almost three-fourths of the cases occurred in subjects 10–35 years old. Of cases occurring in subjects below 10 years of age, 84% (117/139) occurred in children 5–9 years old. The mean age of patients with hepatitis A rose during the study period from 15.5 (SD ±9.3) years in 1986–88 to 17.2 (SD ±9.3) in 1989–90 and 20.1 (SD ±10.2) in 1991–92 (ANOVA $F = 9.6$; $p = 0.0002$).

Table I. *Distribution of antibodies to hepatitis A virus (anti-HAV) according to age in Guipuzcoa (Basque Country, Spain) in 1986–87 and 1992*

Age (years)	1986–87 Subjects *n*	(mean age)	Anti-HAV *n*	(%)	1992 Subjects *n*	(mean age)	Anti-HAV *n*	(%)	χ^2	*p*-value
1–9	417	(5.1)	32	(7.7)	334	(5.2)	8	(2.4)	10.3	0.001
10–19	219	(14.7)	83	(37.9)	348	(14.2)	73	(21.0)	19.3	<0.001
20–29	211	(24.8)	170	(80.6)	257	(24.9)	148	(57.6)	28.1	<0.001
30–39	156	(33.3)	153	(98.1)	272	(33.6)	238	(87.5)	14.0	<0.001

Table II. *Incidence of 'viral hepatitis' and 'hepatitis type A' in Guipuzcoa according to weekly reports (general practitioners and pediatricians)*

Year	Cases of viral hepatitis reported	Rate per 100,000	Cases of hepatitis A reported	Rate per 100,000
1984	747	35.0	–	–
1985	455	21.4	239	11.2
1986	427	20.0	237	11.1
1987	440	20.6	271	12.7
1988	424	20.0	276	12.9
1989	290	13.6	159	7.5
1990	365	17.0	150	7.0
1991	270	12.6	135	6.3
1992	184	8.9	65	3.0

Table III. *Age of serologically confirmed (IgM-positive) hepatitis A cases*

Age group (years)	1986–88		1989–90		1991–92	
	n	(%)	*n*	(%)	*n*	(%)
0–9	75	(32.9)	37	(20.9)	27	(19.9)
10–19	79	(34.6)	75	(42.4)	40	(29.4)
20–29	54	(23.7)	47	(26.6)	52	(38.2)
30–39	18	(7.9)	16	(9.1)	15	(11.0)
≥40	2	(0.9)	2	(1.1)	2	(1.5)
Total	228		177		136	
Mean age	15.5	(SD ±9.3)	17.2	(SD ±9.3)	20.1	(SD ±10.2)[a]

[a] ANOVA, $p < 0.001$.

DISCUSSION

Hepatitis A virus is transmitted by the fecal-oral route. Chronic infection does not occur. Hepatitis A virus transmission is promoted by poor hygienic conditions and inadequate water supply. In developing countries, infection in the first decade of life is common (4); in Guipuzcoa and other developed regions, infection occurs later in life. The prevalence of anti-HAV was low in subjects below 10 years of age in the population groups studied in 1986–87 and in 1992.

Of the cases confirmed at our laboratory, about three-fourths occurred in subjects 10–35 years of age. Over a period of time as short as 5 years, we observed a decrease in the prevalence of anti-HAV in all age groups studied. This suggests that the susceptibility of the population of Guipuzcoa to hepatitis A is rapidly increasing. Other studies made in Spain tend to confirm a change in the epidemiological pattern of hepatitis A (5–7). A decrease in the prevalence of anti-HAV among the general population of other Mediterranean countries of Europe has recently been observed. In southern Italy, the prevalence of anti-HAV among children 6–10 years old had fallen to 6.3% in 1988, from 28% in a similar group of subjects 10 years earlier (8). In France, in a study of persons enrolled in a health insurance scheme, the seroprevalence was less than 5% in the 6–15-year-olds, increasing to 39% and 57%, respectively, in the 26–30-year-olds and 31–35-year-olds (9). In Athens, Greece, in 1990 the prevalences of anti-HAV were 2.5%, 6% and 17.5% in subjects 5–9, 10–18 and 19–22 years old, respectively. These figures were substantially lower than those observed 13 years earlier: viz. 30%, 63.2% and 69% respectively (10).

More than a decade ago, the incidence of hepatitis A in the Scandinavian countries was lower than the present-day incidence in the Mediterranean countries. In Sweden, the prevalence of anti-HAV in 1978 was 6.6% in persons below 40 years of age and 1% in those below 20 (11). For Swedish travellers visiting Mediterranean areas of Europe, the risk of acquiring hepatitis A has diminished significantly in recent years (12). The decrease in hepatitis A virus circulation experienced in recent years in most countries of southern Europe will probably allow travellers from non-endemic areas to consider them as non-risk areas.

The outcome of a HAV infection depends on the age at which it occurs. Hepatitis A transmitted during infancy or early childhood usually leads to either asymptomatic infection or only mild, non-specific symptoms without jaundice. However, when young adults become infected they develop more severe icteric disease (4). Although the total number of cases of hepatitis A in Guipuzcoa appears to have diminished, the age at which the disease is acquired is rising. It is thus foreseeable that there will be an increase in symptomatic hepatitis cases among adults in the future. Vaccines have been developed to combat hepatitis A virus to gain control over the infection (2, 13–15). The use of these vaccines will prevent occasional cases of severe disease and also make significant savings in the costs entailed by the disease among the adult population (2, 16).

ACKNOWLEDGEMENTS

This study was supported in part by a research grant from the Department of Health and Consumption of the Basque Government (Convocatory 1992).

REFERENCES

1. World Health Organization. Progress in the control of viral hepatitis: Memorandum of a WHO Meeting. Bull 66: 443–455, 1988.
2. Jilg W. Adult use of hepatitis A vaccine in developed countries. Vaccine 11 (Suppl): S6–S8, 1993.
3. Pérez-Trallero E, Cilla G, Urbieta M, García Bengoechea M. Prevalence of hepatitis A virus infection in Spain. Scand J Infect Dis 20: 113–114, 1988.
4. Gust ID. Epidemiological patterns of hepatitis A in different parts of the world. Vaccine 10 (Suppl): S56–S58, 1992.
5. Salleras L, Brugera M, Vidal J, Taberner JL, Plans P, Jiménez de Anta MT, Rodés J. Cambio del patrón epidemiológico de la hepatitis A en España. Med Clin (Barc) 99: 87–89, 1992.
6. Gil A, González A, Dal-Ré R, Aguilar L, Rey Calero J. Seroprotección frente a hepatitis A, sarampión, rubéola y parotiditis en una población escolar urbana. Med Clin (Barc) 96: 681–684, 1991.
7. Dal-Ré R, Aguilar L, Coronel P. Current prevalence of hepatitis B, A and C in a healthy Spanish population. A seroepidemiological study. Infection 19: 409–413, 1991.
8. Stroffolini T, De Crescenzo L, Giammanco A, Intonazzo V, la Rosa G, Cascio A, Sarzana A, Chiarini A, Dardanoni N. Changing patterns of hepatitis A virus infection in children in Palermo, Italy. Eur J Epidemiol 6: 84–87, 1990.
9. Dubois F, Thevenas C, Caces E, Vol S, Doctoriarena A, Ecault JL, Goudeau A, Tichet J. Seroepidemiologie de l'hepatite A dans six departements du Centre-Ouest de la France en 1991. Gastroenterol Clin Biol 16: 674–679, 1992.
10. Papaevangelou G. Epidemiology of hepatitis A in Mediterranean countries. Vaccine 10 (Suppl): S63–S66, 1992.
11. Iwarson F, Frösner G, Lindholm A, Norkrans G. The changed epidemiology of hepatitis A infection in Scandinavia. Scand J Infect Dis 10: 155–156, 1978.
12. Nordenfelt E. Hepatitis A in Swedish travellers. Vaccine 10 (Suppl): S73–S74, 1992.
13. World Health Organization. Inactivated hepatitis A vaccine. Wkly Epidemiol Rec 67: 261–264, 1992.
14. Anonymous. Hepatitis A: a vaccine at last. Lancet 339: 1198–1199, 1992.
15. Anonymous. Hepatitis A vaccines considered for licensing. JAMA 267: 2007–2008, 1992.
16. Steffen R. Hepatitis A and hepatitis B: risks compared with other vaccine preventable diseases and immunization recommendations. Vaccine 11: 518–520, 1993.

Scand J Infect Dis 26: 137–139, 1994

Three Cases of Acute Hepatitis E Virus Infection Imported into Norway

KJELL SKAUG[1], IVAR JO HAGEN[2] and BENT VON DER LIPPE[2]

From the Departments of [1]Microbiology, [2]Institute of Infectious Disease, Ullevål University Hospital, Oslo, Norway

We report 3 cases of acute hepatitis E virus (HEV) infection imported from Asia. All 3 patients had fever and upper abdominal discomfort preceding jaundice which lasted 2–3 weeks with maximum bilirubin levels of 141–254 mmol/l. The ALT values peaked between 1,347 and 3,690 U/l. Both values normalized within 1–2 months. During the acute phase of the disease, all patients had high levels of IgG and IgM antibodies against HEV (anti-HEV) recombinant and synthetic peptides. The duration of the anti-HEV IgM was about 1–2 months.

K. Skaug, PhD, National Institute of Public Health, Geitmyrsvn. 75, N-0462 Oslo, Norway

INTRODUCTION

Hepatitis E is a self-limiting, acute viral hepatitis that occurs mostly in large outbreaks, particularly in developing countries (1). Sporadic hepatitis E virus (HEV) infections have also been found in industrialized countries, apparently "imported" by immigrants and travellers (2–4).

Currently the diagnosis of an acute HEV infection is made by serological exclusion of acute hepatitis A, B, C and D infection complemented by supportive epidemiological circumstances. More recently, recombinant HEV proteins derived from the cloned virus isolates have been used in anti-HEV immunoassays, such as enzyme immunoassays and immunoblot tests (5).

We here report on 3 cases of acute NANBH caused by HEV.

MATERIALS AND METHODS

Serum specimens were collected from the 3 patients during both acute and convalescent phases of the disease and tested for antibodies to HEV (anti-HEV). From 1 of the patients (case 1), 1 specimen was also drawn approximately 2 months before onset of the hepatitis.

Anti-HEV tests: Recombinant HEV proteins, SG-3 and 8-5, expressed from HEV genomic sequences of the open reading frame 2 (ORF2) and ORF3, of the Burmese strain of HEV, were used in the Abbott HEV EIA to detect anti-HEV IgG. A sample was deemed positive if it also proved positive in a synthetic anti-HEV peptide assay (Abbott). The synthetic HEV peptides spB3-2 and spB4-2 corresponded to contiguous amino acids of the recombinant SG-3 and 8-5 respectively (5).

A sample was deemed positive for anti-HEV IgM if that sample proved positive in an anti-HEV IgM ELISA (Abbott).

CASE REPORTS

Case 1: 30 days after arriving in Norway, a 31-year-old male refugee from Burma was taken ill with fever, nausea and upper abdominal discomfort. The jaundice started shortly afterwards and lasted for approximately 2 weeks. He fully recovered completely within 2 months.

Case 2: A 28-year-old Norwegian male returned to Norway from Nepal after a 5-month long travel through various Asian countries. 60 days after his return, and 7 months after a standard immunoglobulin injection, he was taken ill with fever, slight pain in the upper abdomen, diarrhea and jaundice. Four weeks later he felt completely well.

Case 3: A 31-year-old man from Sri Lanka, now living in Norway, returned from a 5-month visit to India and Bangladesh. 30 days later, he felt sick, had fever, was vomiting, had a slight abdominal pain and jaundice persisting for about 3 weeks. Five weeks later he had recovered completely.

Table I. *Biochemical and serological results on sera from 3 patients with an acute hepatitis E virus infection*

Case no.	Days after symptoms	ALT[a] (U/l)	BIL[b] (mmol/l)	Anti-HEV test results, S/CO[c] HEV EIA[d]	HEV IgM	spB3-2[e]	spB4-2[e]
1	−55	ND[f]	ND	0.9	0.4	0.9	0.9
	5	3,690	141	>7	9.1	3.9	13.7
	19	76	27	>7	4.2	2.3	13.9
	76	ND	ND	5.4	0.8	1.6	5.6
	109	ND	ND	4.8	0.8	1.8	4.6
	274	ND	ND	4.0	ND	ND	ND
	444	ND	ND	3.8	ND	ND	ND
2	7	3,656	ND	>7	7.0	5.6	13.2
	14	1,347	ND	>7	5.5	5.4	13.8
	28	79	ND	6.9	2.2	5.6	12.6
	187	ND	ND	2.8	0.3	2.2	10.1
3	7	1,674	186	>7	2.5	13.3	10.1
	9	1,890	254	>7	3.0	13.3	10.1
	14	1,162	131	>7	1.5	13.3	10.1
	44	56	ND	>7	0.5	13.3	10.1

[a] ALT reference value, male ≤50 U/l.
[b] Bilirubin reference value ≤25 mmol/l.
[c] Sample-/cut-off value ≥1 positive result.
[d] HEV-IgG.
[e] Synthetic peptide.
[f] Not done.

None of the patients had any sign of recent infection with hepatitis A, B, or C virus, cytomegalovirus or Epstein-Barr virus.

The biochemical and serological test results for the 3 cases are presented in Table I. Serum specimens from all 3 patients, collected during the acute phase of the disease, showed strong reactivity against the recombinant antigens and the synthetic peptides. All 3 had detectable anti-HEV IgM which lasted for about 1–2 months. A serum specimen from patient no. 1, collected before the onset of the disease, had no detectable anti-HEV antibodies. During convalescence, sera from patients 1 and 2 showed reduced activity in the anti-HEV EIA test.

DISCUSSION

These 3 cases are as far as we know the first diagnosed acute HEV infections in Norway. All 3 patients had biochemical markers of liver inflammation, and the ALT and bilirubin values peaked between 1,347 and 3,690 U/l and 141–254 mmol/l, respectively. The jaundice lasted for about 2–3 weeks and the bilirubin and ALT levels normalized within 2 months, in accordance with what others have found (6).

HEV outbreaks have been characterized by high attack rates in adults between 15 and 40 years of age. The 3 reported patients were all in the middle-aged adult group. Like hepatitis A, hepatitis E often causes subclinical infection in children (7, 8).

The incubation period for HEV is about 40 days, i.e. generally slightly longer than for hepatitis A virus. Based on the interval between the onset of symptoms and the date of departure from the endemic area, 2 of our patients had a minimum incubation period of 60 days. Similar incubation periods have been described by others (6).

Patient no. 2 had an immunoglobulin (Ig) injection 7 months before developing clinical HEV infection. Thus, in this case, the Ig gave no protection against HEV at the time of infection, approximately 5 months after the injection.

High levels of anti-HEV IgM and IgG were found in the serum specimens taken during the acute phase of the disease, whereafter the IgM disappeared in the early convalescent phase. In 2 patients a decrease in the anti-HEV EIA test results during the convalescent phase was also seen. Similar results have been described by others (9). This may indicate that the anti-HEV EIA test reacts specifically with acute and convalescent sera from recently HEV infected patients only.

REFERENCES

1. Bradley BW. Hepatitis E: epidemiology, aetiology and molecular biology. Med Virol 2: 19–28, 1992.
2. De Cock KM, Bradley DW, Sandford NL, Govindarajan S, Maynard JE, Redeker AG. Epidemic non-A, non-B hepatitis in patients from Pakistan. Ann Intern Med 106: 227–230, 1987.
3. Zaaijer HL, Kok M, Lelie PN, Timmerman RJ, Chau K, van der Pal J. Hepatitis E in The Netherlands: imported and endemic. Lancet 341: 826, 1993.
4. Jardi R, Buti M, Rodriguez-Frias F, Esteban R. Hepatitis E infection in acute sporadic hepatitis in Spain. Lancet 341: 1355–1356, 1993.
5. Dawson GJ, Chau KH, Cabal CM, Yarbough PO, Reyes GR, Mushahwar IK. Solid-phase enzyme-linked immunosorbent assay for hepatitis E virus IgG and IgM antibodies utilizing recombinant antigens and synthetic peptides. J Virol Methods 38: 175–186, 1992.
6. Favorov MO, Fields HA, Purdy MA, Yashina TL, Aleksandrov AG, Alter MJ, Yarasheva DM, Bradley DW, Margolis HS. Serologic identification of hepatitis E virus infections in epidemics and endemic settings. J Med Virol 36: 246–250, 1992.
7. Viswanathan R. Certain epidemiological features of infectious hepatitis during the Delhi epidemic, 1955–1956. In: Hartman FW, LoGrippo GA, Matffer JG, Barron J, eds. Hepatitis Frontiers. Boston: Little, Brown; 207–210, 1957.
8. Hyams KC, Purdy MA, Kaur M, McCarthy MC, Hussain MAM, El-Tigani A, Krawczynski K, Bradley DW, Carl M. Acute sporadic hepatitis E in Sudanese children: analysis based on a new western blot assay. J Infect Dis 165: 1001–1005, 1992.
9. Goldsmith R, Yarboug PO, Reyes GR, Fry KE, Gabor KA, Kamel M, Zakaria S, Amer S, Gaffar Y. Enzyme-linked immunosorbent assay for diagnosis of acute sporadic hepatitis E in Egyptian children. Lancet 339: 328–331, 1992.

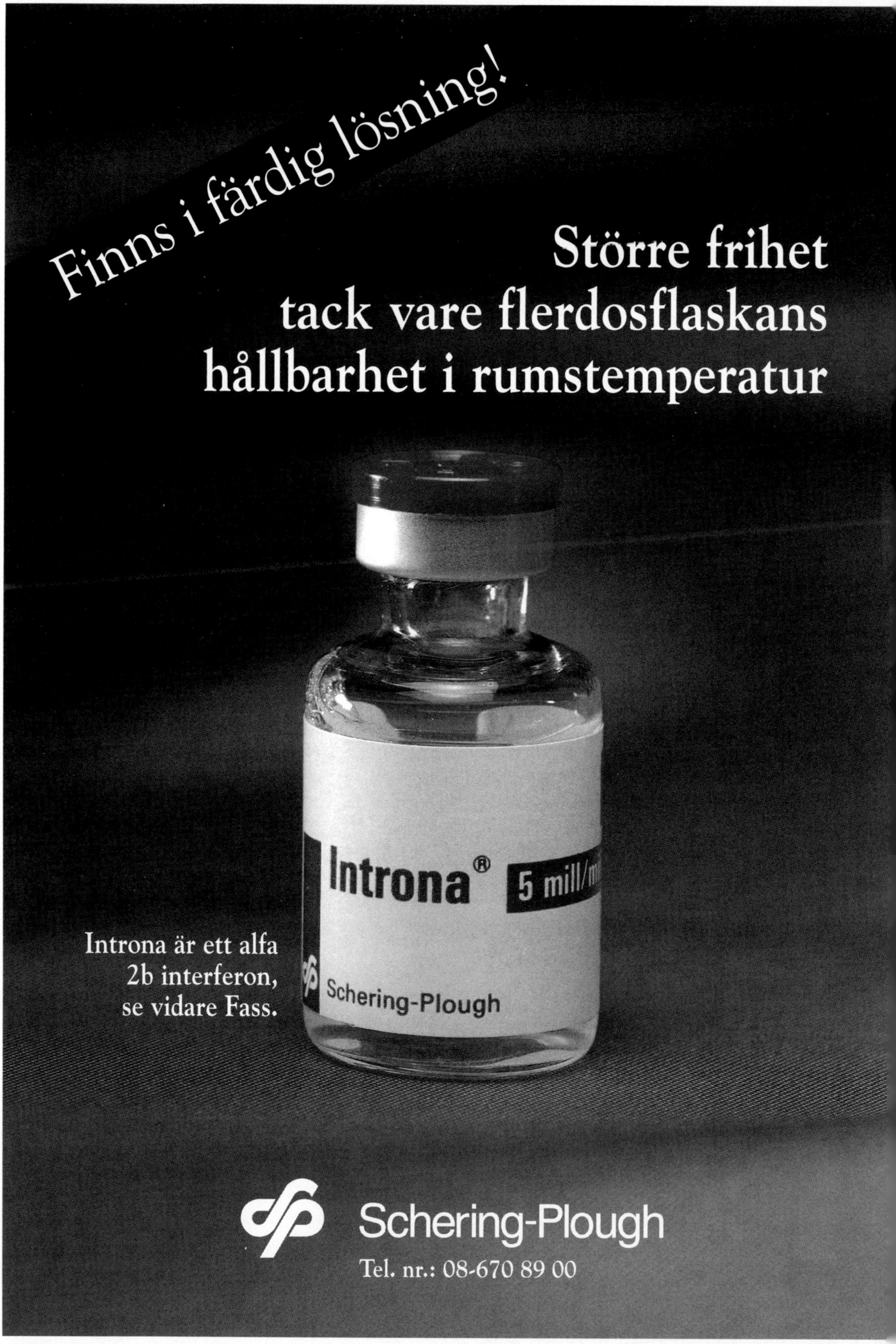
Finns i färdig lösning!
Större frihet
tack vare flerdosflaskans
hållbarhet i rumstemperatur
Introna®
Schering-Plough
Introna är ett alfa
2b interferon,
se vidare Fass.
Schering-Plough
Tel. nr.: 08-670 89 00

Scand J Infect Dis 26: 141–147, 1994

Interferon-γ in Cerebrospinal Fluid from Patients with Viral and Bacterial Meningitis

MARTIN GLIMÅKER[1,2], PER OLCÉN[3] and BIRGER ANDERSSON[4]

From the Departments of [1]Infectious Diseases and [3]Clinical Microbiology and Immunology, Örebro Medical Center Hospital, the [2]Department of Virology, Central Microbiological Laboratory, Stockholm County Council, and the [4]Department of Immunology, National Bacteriological Laboratory, Stockholm, Sweden

Interferon (IFN)-γ was analysed immunologically in cerebrospinal fluid (CSF) sampled in the acute phase from 27 patients (15–66 years) with viral meningitis and from 18 patients (0.5–90 years) with bacterial meningitis. Increased CSF concentrations were observed in 19/27 viral and in 13/18 bacterial cases. CSF-IFN-γ did not distinguish between viral and bacterial meningitis. Five of 8 patients with meningitis due to herpes simplex virus type 2 (HSV-2) had CSF-IFN-γ levels above the highest found in enteroviral meningitis. Thus, a markedly increased CSF-IFN-γ value in patients with suspected viral meningitis ought to indicate HSV-2 etiology. The patients with Streptococcus pneumoniae meningitis (6 adults and 1 child) had significantly higher levels than the 7 children with Haemophilus influenzae meningitis. This may indicate that S. pneumoniae induces more IFN-γ secretion than H. influenzae, and/or that during meningitis, adults are more apt to react with IFN-γ production, than are children.

M. Glimåker, MD, Department of Infectious Diseases, Karolinska Institute, Danderyd Hospital, S-182 88 Danderyd, Sweden

INTRODUCTION

Interferon (IFN)-γ is produced by type 1 T-helper cells and cytotoxic T lymphocytes following antigenic stimulus as well as interleukin (IL)-2 exposure. In addition to its antiviral capacity and effects on the activity of macrophages against intracellular microbes, IFN-γ potentiates the function of polymorphonuclear leukocytes and monocytes against bacteria and fungi (1). Natural killer and B-cells, and expression of HLA antigens, classes I and II, are also stimulated by IFN-γ (1). In meningitis it is of importance that IFN-γ induces or enhances the expression of class II histocompatibility antigens in astrocytes and endothelial cells (2, 3).

Several studies have emphasized the existence of elevated levels of unclassified IFN and of specific IFN-α and IFN-β in CSF during the acute phase in the majority of patients with viral meningitis, whereas undetectable or low CSF levels have been found in most cases of purulent bacterial meningitis (4–13). Local production of specific IFN-γ in cerebrospinal fluid (CSF) has been observed in experimental viral meningitis in mice (14), and in humans with mumps meningitis (15). Elevated IFN-γ levels in CSF were also observed in the majority of cases of herpes simplex encephalitis (16, 17). A few investigations have found elevated levels of CSF-IFN-γ in 50–83% of humans with acute meningitis due to mumps virus and enterovirus and in 19–45% of patients with bacterial meningitis (13, 18, 19). These studies comprised mainly children, while the levels of IFN-γ in CSF from adults with meningitis caused by various organisms have not yet been fully elucidated. This study was conducted primarily in order to assess the potential of measuring IFN-γ in CSF to distinguish acute bacterial from viral meningitis, chiefly in adults, and secondly to elucidate the cellular immune response in CSF during meningitis.

MATERIALS AND METHODS

Inclusion criteria were symptoms indicative of meningitis (fever, headache and neck stiffness) and pleocytosis ($>5 \times 10^6$ leukocytes/l) in CSF. All patients were treated at the Departments of either

Table I. *Characterization of the patient material and results of analysis of the interferon (IFN)-γ levels in cerebrospinal fluid (CSF)*

NA = not applicable

Diagnosis	No. of patients	Median age in years (range)	Females/ Males	Median days (range) from onset of symptoms to sampling of CSF	IFN-γ concentration in CSF: Median IU/ml	Range IU/ml	Proportion elevated >0.94 IU/ml (%)
Viral meningitis							
Enterovirus	15	27 (15–47)	7/8	3 (1–11)	0.9	<0.25–10	7/15 (47)
Herpes simplex type 2	8	25 (20–46)	3/5	1 (0–11)	15.3	2.8–95	8/8
Varicella-zoster	3	25 (21–66)	2/1	4 (2–10)	22.0	3.5–23	3/3
Tick-borne encephalitis	1	38 NA	1/0	6 NA	2.0	NA	1/1
Subtotal	27	27 (15–66)	13/14	2 (0–11)	2.0	<0.25–95	19/27 (70)
Bacterial meningitis							
H. influenzae	7	1 (0.5–2)	4/3	2 (0–8)	0.9	0.4–3.2	3/7 (43)
S. pneumoniae	7	60 (1–90)	2/5	1 (0–2)	14.0	0.95–30	7/7
L. monocytogenes	2	35 (12–48)	1/1	2 (2–2)	30.0	29–31	2/2
N. meningitidis	1	81 NA	0/1	2 NA	0.3	NA	1/1
E. coli	1	0.5 NA	1/0	1 NA	2.0	NA	1/1
Subtotal	18	12 (0.5–90)	8/10	2 (0–8)	2.0	0.3–30	13/18 (72)

Infectious Diseases or Pediatrics at Örebro Medical Center Hospital during the period 1985–90. The patients with viral meningitis formed part of a material of 164 consecutive cases of aseptic meningitis that has been presented elsewhere (20). Those with a bacterial etiology were studied retrospectively. The selection of patients was made according to the availability of CSF specimens and of a viral or bacterial diagnosis. CSF specimens sampled on admission to hospital were available in 27 cases of viral meningitis and 18 of bacterial meningitis. The characterization of the patients and the period from onset of meningeal symptoms to sampling of the acute-phase CSF are presented in Table I. Sera sampled on admission were also available for analysis in the cases of viral meningitis. CSF and sera obtained in the convalescent phase, 2–6 weeks later (median 28 days after onset of symptoms), were available for 16 patients with viral infections according to the protocol used in the previously presented study of aseptic meningitis (20). In none of these cases was the repeat lumbar puncture performed on clinical grounds. CSF samples taken in the convalescent phase were not available in the cases of bacterial meningitis, as these were studied retrospectively.

Viral diagnosis

The enterovirus diagnoses were based on virus isolation from CSF and/or stool samples and/or a significant titre rise in broad-reacting enterovirus serological assays such as the complement fixation test (CTF) and enzyme immunoassay (EIA) for enterovirus. Altogether 15 patients were found to be suffering from meningitis due to 8 different serotypes of enterovirus. Herpes simplex virus type 2 (HSV-2) was deemed to be the etiological agent, on the basis of seroconversion in an EIA using a HSV-2 antigen and/or clinical signs of genital HSV infection in combination with seroconversion in CFT and/or EIA using a HSV type-common antigen. Varicella-zoster virus (VZV) infection was diagnosed clinically (typical zoster blisters) and/or serologically with significant titre-rise in CFT for VZV. Tick-borne encephalitis (TBE) virus was deemed to be the etiological agent in 1 case of TBE-specific IgM and significant titre-rise in TBE-specific IgG-antibodies measured with EIA. Bacterial and fungal cultures from CSF and blood as well as microscopy of Gram-stained CSF proved negative in all 27 patients. CSF antigen detection tests for Haemophilus influenzae, Streptococcus pneumoniae and Neisseria meningitidis were performed, with negative results in 22 of these 27 patients.

Bacterial diagnosis

Microscopy of Gram-stained smears of CSF as well as routinely used aerobic and anaerobic bacterial cultures, including enrichment, were performed on CSF and blood from all patients. The bacterial isolates were identified and typed by routinely used methods. CSF antigen detection tests for H.

influenzae, S. pneumoniae and N. meningitidis were performed in 17 patients. All bacterial diagnoses were based on positive bacterial culture from CSF.

Control group

CSF was sampled, before administration of spinal anesthesia, from the 20 youngest individuals without CNS symptoms who were undergoing surgery outside the CNS and spinal room during 1990. The median age of these individuals (8 females and 12 males) was 62 (range 51–69) years.

Determination of IFN-γ

All specimens were stored at −20°C until analysed. An enzyme-amplified sensitivity immunoassay (EASIA; Medgenix, Brussels, Belgium) was used. Incubations with serum standards and conjugate were done according to the manufacturer's instructions except that the substrate activation by horseradish peroxidase was measured by chemoluminescence (Lumiscan; Labsystems, Tyresö, Sweden) as described elsewhere (20). The results were expressed in international units per ml (IU/ml) after comparison with the standards for IFN-γ included in the assay. The range of reliable measurements was 0.25–95 IU/ml.

Statistical analyses

The Mann-Whitney U-test was used to compare the IFN-γ concentrations in the different etiological groups, as these values were not normally distributed. The χ^2-test was used when compring proportions of elevated levels. Spearman's rank correlation test was performed to ascertain if correlations existed between IFN-γ and the various CSF parameters.

Ethics

The study was approved by the Medical Ethics Committee of Örebro Medical Center Hospital and informed consent was obtained from all patients included in the study according to the Helsinki Declaration.

RESULTS

The upper limit for normal IFN-γ concentrations in CSF was found to be 0.94 IU/ml; i.e. mean + 2SD in the control CSF specimens. The concentrations of IFN-γ in CSF from the patients are given in Fig. 1 and Table I.

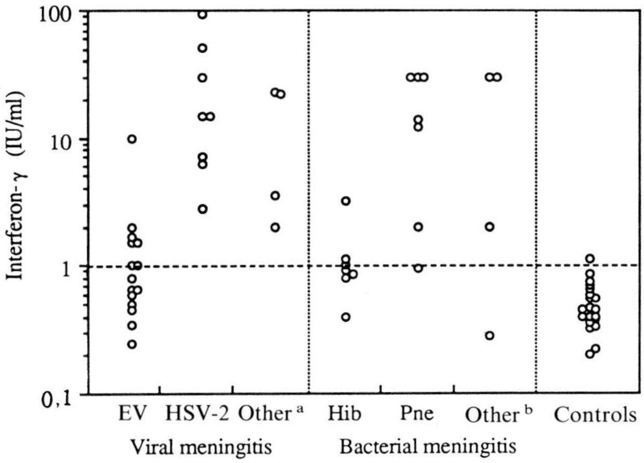

Fig. 1. Concentrations of interferon (IFN)-γ in cerebrospinal fluid from 45 patients with meningitis of different etiologies and from 20 control subjects. EV = enterovirus; HSV-2 = herpes simplex virus type 2; Hib = Haemophilus influenzae type b; Pne = Streptococcus pneumoniae. The interrupted line marks the upper limit of normal values, i.e. mean + 2 SD in the controls. [a] 3 varicella-zoster and 1 tick-borne encephalitis virus. [b] 2 Listeria monocytogenes, 1 Neisseria meningitidis and 1 Escherichia coli.

Viral meningitis cases

Elevated levels of IFN-γ in CSF were observed in 19/27 (70%) cases of viral meningitis, resulting in significantly increased concentrations compared with the control group ($p < 0.001$). All 8 patients with HSV-2 meningitis had elevated levels, which were significantly higher than those in the group with enterovirus infections ($p < 0.001$). All 3 patients with VZV meningitis had clearly elevated levels and a slightly elevated value was observed in the TBE case.

IFN-γ was not detectable (<0.25 IU/ml) in serum sampled in the acute phase in 23/27 patients. Low concentrations were observed in the remaining 4 cases; 2 with HSV-2 meningitis (0.3 and 1.25 IU/ml) and 1 each with enterovirus (1.65 IU/ml) and VZV infection (1.25 IU/ml).

Normal CSF concentrations (<0.94 IU/ml) of IFN-γ were observed in all 16 patients who were tested in the convalescent phase.

Bacterial meningitis cases

Increased levels of IFN-γ were observed in CSF in 13/18 (72%) patients with bacterial meningitis, resulting in significantly higher concentrations than in the control group ($p < 0.001$) but no significant difference when compared with the 27 cases of viral meningitis. The 7 patients (6 adults and 1 child) with meningitis due to S. pneumoniae had significantly higher CSF-IFN-γ levels than the 7 children with H. influenzae meningitis ($p < 0.01$). Both patients with Listeria monocytogenes meningitis had markedly elevated levels, whereas the 81-year-old man with N. meningitidis diagnosis had normal CSF-IFN-γ and the child with E. coli meningitis had only a slightly increased level. Eight of the 9 patients older than 12 years had elevated concentrations of IFN-γ in CSF (median 14, range 0.3–30 IU/ml) whereas only 5/9 children, 2 years old or younger, were found to have elevated levels (median 1.0, range 0.4–30 IU/ml). This difference was not statistically significant ($p = 0.07$).

Correlations to routinely used inflammatory parameters

In the 27 patients with viral meningitis there was a correlation between the IFN-γ concentrations and the numbers of mononuclear leukocytes and the protein levels in CSF ($p < 0.05$ for both correlations). In the group of patients with bacterial diagnoses, CSF-IFN-γ correlated with the number of polymorphonuclear leukocytes in CSF ($p < 0.05$) but not with the protein content in CSF. CSF-IFN-γ did not correlate with the total cell count in CSF in either of these 2 etiological groups.

There was no correlation between the CSF-IFN-γ and the leukocyte count or level of C-reactive protein in peripheral blood, or the body temperature observed when the CSF was sampled.

DISCUSSION

Previous studies have evaluated the levels of IFN-γ in CSF during bacterial and viral (mainly enteroviral) meningitis, predominantly in children (13, 18, 19), whereas our study particularly addressed IFN-γ production in adults with acute meningitis caused by different organisms, including HSV-2. The concentrations of IFN-γ in CSF in the present study were significantly increased in both viral and bacterial meningitis cases, which is consistent with earlier reports (5, 6, 12, 18). Contrary to earlier reported studies (5, 12, 13, 18) we found that the CSF-IFN-γ levels were equally increased in about 70% of both the viral and the bacterial cases; thus no significant difference was observed. This discrepancy could possibly be explained by the difference in the age of patients between this study and the earlier reports.

This hypothesis is supported by the finding in the present study that the adults with bacterial meningitis had higher CSF-IFN-γ levels than did the small children. Thus, it is possible that during bacterial meningitis, adults are more apt to react with IFN-γ production in CSF than are small children.

Another explanation would be that S. pneumoniae more effectively stimulates IFN-γ production than H. influenzae does. This is supported by the findings in the present study that the single child with S. pneumoniae meningitis had a very high CSF concentration of IFN-γ (30 IU/ml) and that significantly higher levels were found in S. pneumoniae meningitis than in H. influenzae meningitis. However, in the earlier studies (12, 13), similar proportions of patients with increased CSF-IFN-γ levels were found in meningitis due to these 2 bacteria. Previous studies have shown that production of unclassified IFN in CSF was induced by S. pneumoniae in 36%, H. influenzae in 25% and by N. meningitidis in 18% of patients with meningitis (5, 6, 12). These results are relatively consistent with our findings regarding H. influenzae, but not regarding S. pneumoniae. This discrepancy may be explained by the fact that we analysed IFN-γ specifically, whereas unspecified IFN (α, -β, and -γ) were measured in the previous studies. An immunoassay, which detects the total amounts of active and inactive forms of IFN-γ, was used in the present study, whereas bioassays, which measure only active forms of the substance, were used in the previous investigations. This difference could also explain the discrepancies.

Just as previous studies have suggested for children (12, 18), our findings indicate that measurement of IFN-γ in CSF cannot be used to distinguish between viral and bacterial meningitis in adults. We found that all patients with HSV-2 meningitis had elevated levels of IFN-γ in CSF, resulting in significantly higher concentrations than in the cases of enteroviral meningitis. Clearly elevated CSF levels of IFN-γ were observed in 2/3 patients with VZV meningitis, whereas the TBE case had a less elevated level. The highest level observed in a patient with enteroviral meningitis was 10.0 IU/ml. Higher levels than this were found in 5/8 HSV-2 patients and in 2/3 VZV cases. This indicates that HSV-2 and possibly also VZV usually are more potent inducers of IFN-γ than are enteroviruses. A markedly increased CSF concentration (>10 IU/ml) of IFN-γ in a patient with presumed viral meningitis ought to indicate a HSV-2 diagnosis, which is a treatable disease. The CSF levels of IFN-γ have previously not been studied in HSV-2 meningitis, but elevated CSF concentrations have been found in HSV encephalitis (16, 17).

The CSF concentration of IFN-γ was completely normalized in the convalescent phase in all viral cases that were tested, which is consistent with earlier findings in children (19). This indicates that CSF-IFN-γ is correlated to disease activity and could be used as an acute phase inflammatory parameter.

It should be kept in mind that, in the present study, the controls were significantly older than the patients, which may have influenced the results regarding proportions of cases with elevated levels.

Since undetectable or very low levels of IFN-γ were observed in acute phase sera from the patients with viral meningitis, the substance seemed to be produced intrathecally in viral meningitis, which is in line with earlier reports (14–16). We again found, as previously observed (19), a correlation between CSF-IFN-γ and the mononuclear cell count in CSF in viral meningitis. This is not surprising, since T lymphocytes are the main source of IFN-γ production (1) and it has been shown that cytotoxic T lymphocytes from CSF secrete IFN-γ in mumps meningitis in humans (15). The correlation between CSF-IFN-γ and the CSF-protein level in viral meningitis, found in the present study, may be due to the fact that both substances reflect the degree of inflammatory activity in CSF. The same covariance, and possibly the fact that IFN-γ enhances the function of polymorhonuclear leukocytes (1), may explain the correlation found between CSF-IFN-γ and the polymorphonuclear cell count in CSF in bacterial meningitis.

The molecular mechanisms that culminate in the generation of mitogen- or antigen-stimulated IFN-γ production are complex and at best only partly defined. Human T helper and suppressor cells – and natural killer cells – can be induced to secrete IFN-γ as a direct response to non-specific mitogens and antigens, or indirectly via IL-2 production (1, 2). IFN-γ can feed back directly to enhance accessory cell function by inducing the expression of class II major histocompatibility complex, stimulating IL-1 production and by augmenting antigen presentation (1). Astrocytes function as antigen-presenting cells in CNS after stimulation by IFN-γ (2). Viruses and other intracellular organisms are known to be potent inducers of IFN-γ production and this substance is the most active antiviral cytokine. Thus, as IFN-γ seems to play an important role for host defence in the CSF during viral meningitis, it is not surprising that we found elevated levels in cases of viral meningitis.

The rationale for IFN-γ production during bacterial meningitis is somewhat more difficult to understand. Other cytokines such as IL-1, -2 and -6, and tumour necrosis factor-α are frequently increased in CSF during bacterial meningitis. IL-2, alone and together with IL-1, and possibly other cytokines as well, may stimulate the T cells to produce IFN-γ (1, 2). Thus, different cytokines seem to act in synergy, which may result in elevated concentrations of IFN-γ in bacterial meningitis. IFN-γ can probably be of value for the host defence against bacterial meningitis by enhancing the function of polymorphonuclear leukocytes and participating in the complex cytokine cascade.

Earlier studies have indicated that the peak IFN-γ levels are usually found some 48 to 72 h after the inception of antigen or mitogen stimulation (21). In the present study, the acute-phase CSF specimens were sampled at different time intervals, 0 to 11 days, after the onset of symptoms. These facts may to some extent explain the relatively wide range of IFN-γ levels that we found within the different etiological groups.

In conclusion, the present study emphasizes that the concentrations of IFN-γ are usually increased in both viral and bacterial meningitis in adults. A markedly elevated CSF-IFN-γ level in a patient with aseptic meningitis indicates meningitis due to HSV-2 rather than enterovirus. The substance cannot be used, however, to distinguish between bacterial and viral meningitis.

ACKNOWLEDGEMENTS

Mrs Katarina Karlén is thanked for expert technical assistance and the Örebro County Council Research Unit is acknowledged for financial support.

REFERENCES

1. Murray HW. Interferon-gamma, the activated macrophage, and host defense against microbial challenge. Ann Intern Med 108: 595–608, 1988.
2. Fontana A, Fierz W. The endothelium-astrocyte immune control system of the brain. In: Miescher PA, Muller-Eberhard H, eds. Seminars in immunopathology. Berlin: Springer, 1985.
3. Fierz W, Endler B, Reske K, Wekerle H, Fontana A. Astrocytes as antigen presenting cells: I. Induction of Ia antigen expression on astrocytes by T cells via immune interferon and its effect on antigen presentation. J Immunol 134: 3785–3793, 1985.
4. Gresser I, Naficy K. Recovery of an interferon-like substance from cerebrospinal fluid. Proc Soc Exp Biol Med 117: 285–289, 1964.
5. Larke RPB. Interferon in the cerebrospinal fluid of children with central nervous system disorders. Can Med Assoc J 96: 21–32, 1967.
6. Haahr S. The occurrence of interferon in the cerebrospinal fluid in patients with bacterial meningitis. Acta Pathol Microbiol Scand 73: 264–274, 1968.

7. Flowers D, Scott GM. How useful are serum and CSF interferon levels as a rapid diagnostic aid in virus infections? J Med Virol 15: 35–47, 1985.
8. Miyazu M, Morishima T, Hanada N, Isomura S, Suzuki S. Types of interferons detected in cerebrospinal fluid from patients with viral infections of the central nervous system. J Infect Dis 152: 1098–1099, 1985.
9. Ichimura H, Shimase K, Tamura I, Kaneto E, Kurimura O, Arimatsu Y, Kurimura T. Neutralizing antibody and interferon-α in cerebrospinal fluid and sera of acute aseptic meningitis. J Med Virol 15: 231–237, 1985.
10. Ho-Yen DO, Carrington D. Alpha-interferon responses in cerebrospinal fluid of patients with suspected meningitis. J Clin Pathol 40: 83–86, 1987.
11. Gustavson-Moringlane IL, Einhorn S, Jarstrand C. Interferon induction and granulocyte function in patients with viral meningitis. J Clin Lab Immunol 26: 85–88, 1988.
12. Chonmaitree T, Baron S. Bacteria and viruses induce production of interferon in the cerebrospinal fluid of children with acute meningitis: a study of 57 cases and review. J Infect Dis 13: 1061–1065, 1991.
13. Raymond J, Benichou C, de Boissieu D, Mensah K, Bergeret M, Lebon P. Absence of intrathecal synthesis of some interferon-α subtypes in bacterial meningitis. J Infect Dis 166: 657–659, 1992.
14. Frei K, Leist TP, Meager A, Gallo P, Leppert D, Zinkernagel RM, Fontana A. Production of B cell stimulatory factor-2 and interferon-γ in the central nervous system during viral meningitis and encephalitis. J Exp Med 168: 149–153, 1988.
15. Martin R, Vallbract A, Kreth HW. Interferon-γ secretion by in vivo activated cytotoxic T lymphocytes from the blood and cerebrospinal fluid during mumps meningitis. J Neuroimmunol 33: 191–198, 1991.
16. Lebon P, Boutin B, Dulac O, Ponsot G, Arthuis M. Interferon γ in acute and subacute encephalitis. BMJ 296: 9–11, 1988.
17. Aurelius E, Andersson B, Forsgren M, Sköldenberg B, Strannegård Ö. Cytokines and other markers of the intrathecal immune response in patients with herpes simplex encephalitis. J Infect Dis (in press).
18. Abbott RJ, Bolderson I, Gruer PJK, Peatfield RC. Immunoreactive IFN-γ in CSF in neurological disorders. J Neurol Neurosurg Psych 50: 882–885, 1987.
19. Minamishima I, Ohga S, Ishii E, Miyazaki C, Hamada K, Akazawa K, Ueda K. Aseptic meningitis in children: correlation between fever and interferon-gamma level. Eur J Pediatr 150: 722–725, 1991.
20. Linde A, Andersson B, Svenson SB, Ahrne H, Carlsson M, Forsberg P, Hugo H, Karstorp A, Lenkei R, Lindwall A, Loftenius A, Säll C, Andersson J. Serum levels of lymphokines and soluble cellular receptors in primary Epstein-Barr virus infection and in patients with chronic fatigue syndrome. J Infect Dis 165: 994–1000, 1992.
21. Kelly CD, Welte K, Murray HW. Antigen-induced human interferon-γ production: differential dependence on interleukin 2 and its receptor. J Immunol 139: 2325–2328, 1987.

Scand J Infect Dis 26: 149–155, 1994

Lyme Borreliosis in Lithuania

LEONAS MOTIEJUNAS[1], JONAS BUNIKIS[1,4], ALAN G. BARBOUR[2,3] and ARIADNA SADZIENE[1,2]

From the [1]Faculty of Medicine, Vilnius University, Vilnius, Lithuania, the Departments of [2]Microbiology, and [3]Medicine, University of Texas Health Science Center, San Antonio, Texas, USA, and the [4]Department of Microbiology, University of Umeå, Umeå, Sweden

The first cases of Lyme borreliosis in Lithuania were diagnosed in 1987, since when the number of reported cases has varied between 50 and 300 per year. In 1988, 354 cases were found through active surveillance. During 1988–91, 3,820 Ixodes ricinus ticks were collected in Lithuania; 11% of adult and 1% of nymphal ticks were infected with borrelia as determined by dark-field microscopy. Infected ticks were found in 27/31 (87%) of the regions investigated. Two isolates of Borrelia were obtained by in vitro cultivation and were shown to be Borrelia burgdorferi according to their reactions with species-specific monoclonal antibodies. From a survey of 6,187 people we estimated that 2,811/100,000 of the Lithuanian population are bitten by ticks every year. The prevalence of antibodies to B. burgdorferi measured by indirect IFA in healthy people varied between 4% and 32%, depending upon occupation and exposure to ticks.

L. Motiejunas, MD, PhD, Faculty of Medicine, Vilnius University, Laboratory of Zoonoses, Gelezinio Vilko 29, Vilnius 2060, Lithuania

INTRODUCTION

Lyme borreliosis (LB) is a common infectious disorder in regions where Ixodes spp. ticks are heavily infested by the spirochaete Borrelia burgdorferi (1). Some manifestations of B. burgdorferi infection in humans, such as erythema chronicum migrans, acrodermatitis chronica atrophicans and Bannwarth's syndrome, have been known in northeastern Europe for many years (2). In Europe, the principal vector for transmission of B. burgdorferi to humans and animals is the sheep tick Ixodes ricinus (3). These ticks are widely distributed in Lithuania and have long been known to be the vector of tick-borne encephalitis virus (4). Three cases of laboratory-confirmed Lyme disease in Lithuania were diagnosed in 1987. These clinical cases prompted clinical and epidemiological investigations of this disease in 1988 with the intention of determining the geographical distribution of Lyme disease and to define ecological, epidemiological and demographic characteristics of LB in Lithuania.

MATERIALS AND METHODS

Tick collection and evaluation

Ixodes ricinus ticks were collected by flagging in forested areas of Lithuania during May through June, in 1988–91. Ticks were collected in 31/44 administrative regions of Lithuania (Fig. 1). The abundance of ticks was measured by flag hour, i.e., the number of ticks attached to a 0.6-m^2 piece of corduroy cloth during a 60-min. survey by dragging. Special attention was paid to recreational areas, such as camping sites and resorts. A total of 51 such locations were evaluated. Wet-mount smears of suspensions of tick intestines in phosphate-buffered saline (pH 7.6) were examined by darkfield microscopy at a magnification of 600 ×. Ticks infected by Borrelia were assessed semi-quantitatively using the following grading system based on numbers of motile spirochaetes with irregular, large coils per 40 fields: 1+, 1–10 organisms; 2+, 10–20 organisms; and 3+, >20 organisms. Two pools of tissue suspensions from microscopically positive ticks were cultured in modified BSK II medium (5). Borrelia spirochaetes were identified by indirect immunofluorescence assay (IFA), according to Barbour et al. (5), using monoclonal antibodies H5332 or H3TS (5) as the primary antibody, and fluorescein-conjugated sheep anti-mouse IgG (obtained from the Gamaleya Institute, Moscow, Russia), as the second antibody.

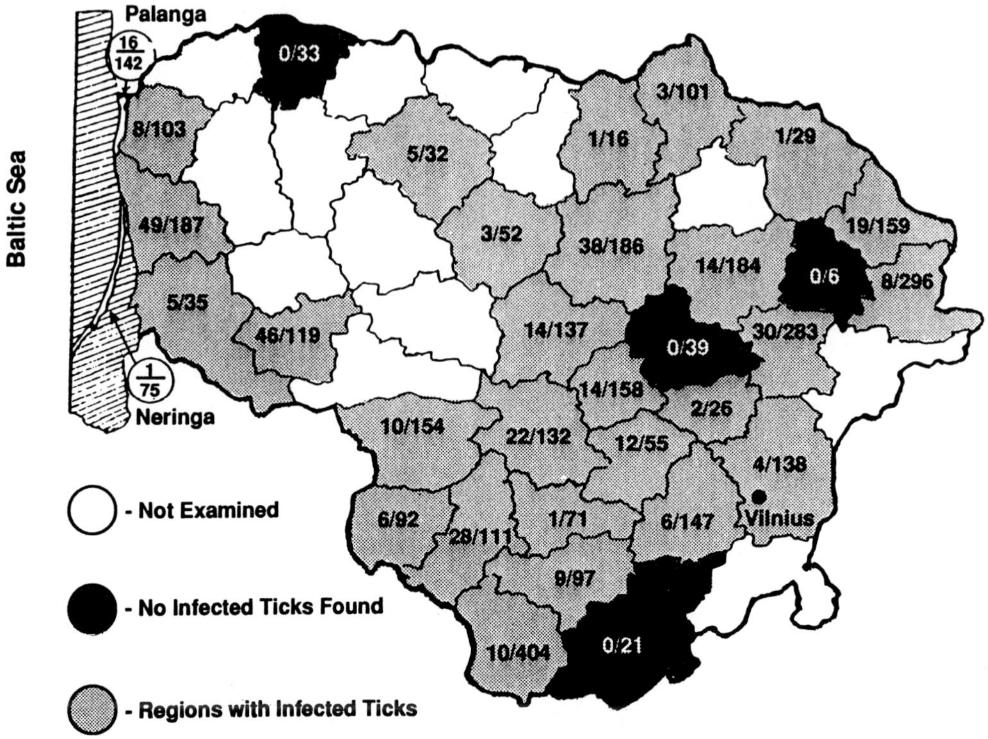

Fig. 1. Geographical distribution of I. ricinus ticks infected with B. burgdorferi in Lithuania (based on 3,820 ticks collected in 31/44 Lithuanian regions during 1988–91). The positions of the most popular resorts in Lithuania, Palanga and Neringa are marked by arrows.

Epidemiological data collection

To determine the frequency of human contact with ticks, we questioned 6,187 people in 10 different administrative regions of Lithuania. Regions were chosen on the basis of ecological differences throughout the republic (6). Subjects were selected randomly among the different age groups, occupations and preferences regarding outdoor activities. The questionnaire, when administered to children <10 years of age, was answered with the assistance of parents or teachers. Information regarding location of the home, living conditions, occupation of the individuals, types of outdoor activities preferred and the amount of time devoted to them, was asked for in the questionnaire. Individuals were also questioned with regard to tick contact during the year of 1989, specifically whether and how many ticks were observed on the body and if they had been embedded.

The prevalence of elevated serum antibody titres to B. burgdorferi within the working population of Lithuania was studied in 3 occupational groups: foresters ($n = 268$), outside field workers ($n = 115$), and veterinarians ($n = 68$). A group of 163 urban industrial workers with little or no occupational tick exposure served as a control group.

Serological methods

Sera were evaluated by IFA. B. burgdorferi sensu lato strain Ip21, isolated in the Baltic region of Russia was used as antigen (7). Fluorescein-conjugated polyvalent sheep anti-human immunoglobulin (Gamaleya Institute, Moscow) was used as the second antibody. Reciprocal Ig antibody titres ≥ 512 were considered indicative of past or present infection with a LB borrelia. Only 1.2% of healthy controls had titres ≥ 512 in a pilot study.

Statistical methods

Epidemiological data from the different regions were analysed by the χ^2 test; p-values <0.001 were considered statistically significant.

RESULTS

Tick collection and evaluation

During 1988–91 we collected 3,820 unengorged nymphal and adult I. ricinus ticks and examined them for the presence of B. burgdorferi (Fig. 1). Ticks were collected in 31 regions and 8 city suburbs of Lithuania (Table I). Infected ticks were found in 27/31 regions and in 6/8 suburbs investigated. In the 4 regions and 2 suburbs where no infected ticks were found, only 6–37 ticks were collected; the average number of ticks collected in the other regions was 124 per region. Overall, 11% of adult ticks and 1% of nymphal ticks were found to be infected. Of the infected ticks, 58% had 1+ infection, 33% a 2+ infection, and 8% a 3+ infection (Table I). The frequency of infected ticks varied widely between the areas surveyed. Whereas in some areas only 2% of the ticks were infected, in other areas as many as 50% were infected. The abundance of ticks also differed widely between different sites in Lithuania, ranging from between 0 and 3 ticks per flag hour on grassy areas, to 30–40 ticks/hour in woods and scrub. This difference in tick density accounted for the different numbers of ticks collected in the various regions (Fig. 1).

Over a 3-year period we collected 1,008 ticks from 51 recreational areas. Ticks from 17 (33%) of these areas were infected with B. burgdorferi. The average rate of tick infection was 3%, and the highest tick infection rate at any one site being 19%. Infected ticks were found in Palanga and Neringa, the most popular Lithuanian resorts, and even in the large city park in the centre of Vilnius (Fig. 1).

Borrelia isolates

From ticks collected from 2 different Lithuanian regions we successfully cultured spirochaete isolates. Cultures were examined by indirect IFA with 2 monoclonal antibodies H5332 and H3TS, which were directed against the OspA protein of a North American strain of B. burgdorferi (5). Monoclonal antibody H5332 became bound to the Lithuanian isolates, whereas monoclonal antibody H3TS did not.

Table I. *Prevalence of B. burgdorferi in Ixodes ricinus ticks collected in Lithuania during 1988–91*

	Infected ticks/examined ticks			Grading of the tick infection[a]			
	Nymphs	Adults					
		Females	Males	1+ infection	2+ infection	3+ infection	No infection
Regions[b]	1/229 (0.5%)	206/1689 (12%)	150/1517 (10%)	211	120	26	3078
City suburbs[c]	2/58 (4%)	15/172 (9%)	11/155	18	7	3	357
Total	3/287 (1%)	221/1861 (12%)	161/1672 (10%)	229 (6%)	127 (3%)	29 (1%)	3435 (90%)

[a] The infectivity of ticks was evaluated by counting the number of motile borrelia-like organisms per 40 fields, as explained in the Materials and Methods section.

[b] Infected ticks were found in 27 of 31 geographical regions examined.

[c] Infected ticks were found in 6 of 8 city suburbs examined.

Epidemiology

Epidemiological data regarding tick exposure for the year 1989 were analysed in 6,187 people (67% male and 32% female) from 10 administrative regions. Those surveyed included people at occupational risk of tick exposure (36%), such as forestry workers, veterinarians, farmers and field workers, people whose work was not associated with outside activities (57%), and people not gainfully employed (7%) such as housewives, retired individuals and children. The number of people questioned in each region varied between 239 and 897 (mean 619). Between April and October 1989, 754 (12%) of these subjects had not been in forested areas, 3,243 (52%) had visited forested areas occasionally (1–5 visits), and 2,190 (36%) frequently (>5 times).

559 (9%) of those questioned had come into contact with a tick, whereof 60% had been bitten by a tick. Many people noticed tick bites several times during the same year; the mean was 1.7 tick bites per person per year. People making regular occupational visits to the forested areas or fields had tick bites 2.5 times more often than those without occupational exposure [324/2,253 (14%) versus 235/3,934 (6%), $p < 0.001$], as noted in the questionnaire. Among 324 people with occupational risk for tick exposure, 173 (53%) had had tick contact during working hours. Among 235 people with no occupational risk of tick exposure, 173 (74%) were bitten during their leisure time. 220/3,243 (7%) people who seldom visited forested areas noticed ticks on their bodies as did 337/2,190 (15%) people who frequently visited forested areas ($p < 0.001$). Only 2 of 754 (0.3%) people who stated that they had never visited a forested area had tick bites. Ticks were 1.7 times more frequently reported in the population above 30 years of age (480/4,926, 10%) than by those less than 30 (79/1,261, 6%) ($p < 0.001$). Tick bites were reported between mid-April and mid-October; 281/559 (50%) bites occurred between the second half of July and the first half of August.

Antibodies to B. burgdorferi were formed in 32% of veterinarians, 22% of field workers, and 14% of foresters. In contrast, only 4% of the urban industry workers had B. burgdorferi antibodies.

DISCUSSION

The data presented in this paper suggest that the major part of the Lithuanian territory is endemic for LB. We thus demonstrated the presence of B. burgdorferi in I. ricinus ticks from 27 regions and 6 city suburbs in which the average tick infection rate was 10%. In only 4 regions and 2 suburbs, were no infected ticks found, but here comparatively few ticks were collected; it is possible that infected ticks would have been detected with a larger sample size also here. If data from the epidemiological survey are extrapolated to the entire population of 3.5 million, we estimated that 2,811/100,000 of the Lithuanian population were bitten by ticks in 1989. Since 10% of these ticks were infected with B. burgdorferi and 1% of the ticks were heavily infected, there is abundant opportunity for B. burgdorferi transmission in Lithuania. A projected number of approximately 1000 cases of LB/year agrees quite well with the number of 354 actual LB cases found in 1988 through active surveillance.

When Lithuanian spirochaete isolates were examined by IFA, they were recognized by monoclonal antibody H5332, but not by H3TS. This finding places the isolates in a group of European B. burgdorferi sensu lato isolates (5), including Ip21 from the Baltic region of Russia (7).

The rate of infection of I. ricinus ticks, the most frequently encountered species of ixodid ticks in Europe, with B. burgdorferi, has been studied in many European countries, including Austria, Czechoslovakia, Germany, Russia, Sweden and Switzerland. The frequency of infected adult ticks varied between countries: 8% in Czechoslovakia (8), 17–30% in Russia

(2), 20% in Austria (3, 9), 11–29% in Germany (3, 10), 15–30% in Sweden (11–13), and 21–36% in Switzerland (3, 14). Most of these studies evaluated ticks for the presence of spirochaetes by immunofluorescence assay or by culturing tick contents (9–12, 14), rather than by using dark-field microscopy or staining with azure-eosin and crystal violet, as in our study and those of others (2, 8). Some authors suggest that the latter techniques are less sensitive for determining rate of infected ticks (13, 15). If this is the case, then the frequency of infected ticks may be underestimated in our study.

The I. ricinus tick is common in all Lithuanian forest areas, and our results suggest that the majority of all I. ricinus populations in the country harbour B. burgdorferi. A similar situation was reported from the Swiss Plateau (14), wooded areas of West Berlin (10), and several areas in Austria (9) and Czechoslovakia (8). In contrast, the distribution of tick-borne encephalitis (TBE) virus is much more focal (2, 4, 16, 17). This could be a reason for the low rates of simultaneous infections with B. burgdorferi and TBE virus, and the low risk for humans to acquire both infections together (17).

The positive Lyme serology among different occupational groups ranged from 4% to 32%, depending on outdoor exposure. The field study results indicate a widespread distribution of Lyme disease spirochaetes in Lithuania, which is consistent with these immunological data. In addition, the high frequency of seropositivity in the generally healthy human groups at risk, such as veterinarians, field workers and rangers, suggests that inapparent B. burgdorferi infections are common in Lithuania, in agreement with reports from Switzerland (18), Austria (3, 19), Germany (20), Sweden (17) and Russia (21).

This study was not designed to evaluate the landscape ecology of Lyme disease in Lithuania, or to determine which specific types of landscapes are most frequently associated with I. ricinus ticks. Nevertheless, the correlation of tick abundance with the peculiarity of landscape (woods and bushes versus grassy areas) suggested that some landscape features may be indicative of the abundance of ticks that are capable of transferring B. burgdorferi spirochaetes. Consequently, these features could be taken into consideration when planning recreation areas, as well as when applying preventive measures to reduce the risk of exposure to Lyme disease vectors. The extent to which tick infections determine the incidence of LB depends on the frequency of person–tick contact. The high rate (up to 50%) of infected ticks in some examined areas and the presence of infected ticks (up to 19%) in recreational areas indicate that it may be helpful to use selected ecologic parameters to identify areas at highest risk for Lyme disease transmission (22). Our study also revealed that outdoor workers ran a 2.5-fold greater risk of tick exposure than indoor workers and those individuals who were not gainfully occupied, although in 74% of the latter 2 populations, contact with ticks had occurred during their leisure activities. The proportion of tick exposure reported by the population over 30 years of age was almost twice that of people below 30 years of age, an observation which suggests that younger people may not have been so careful in examining themselves after being outdoors. All these findings suggest that the performance of preventive measures at different levels, such as ecological, chemical and biological tick control, public health education and self-protection, especially in areas of high risk, would reduce the incidence of LB.

There is still a need for further field studies with regard to natural vertebrate reservoirs of B. burgdorferi in Lithuania, as well as a more detailed comparison of the rates of infection in larvae, nymphal and adult I. ricinus ticks. The present data were in agreement with other studies that have noted a greater prevalence of B. burgdorferi infection in adult I. ricinus, as compared with nymphs (2, 9–12, 14, 23). This probably results from the greater number of potentially infectious blood meals that the adults have ingested in comparison with previous stages (23). It has been pointed out that, despite the greater prevalence of infection in adult

I. ricinus, the nymphal stage of this vector is the most important one for transmission of Lyme disease spirochaetes to humans (23).

Until 1990, the awareness of professional and lay people concerning, as well as the serodiagnostics of Lyme disease were limited. Nevertheless, every year we were informed of about 50–300 new cases of this disease. To complement our epidemiological study, as well as to collect data regarding clinical symptoms and treatment of Lyme disease in Lithuania, we evaluated data from patients with early LB infection. During the 4-year period, active surveillance for LB patients was conducted by contacting doctors of different specialties as well as by directly informing lay people about LB epidemiology and symptoms through the local newspapers and radio. Our study of clinical cases of LB was not designed to evaluate in detail this disease in Lithuania, but rather to show the Lithuanian medical community that LB is a clinical problem in Lithuania and to suggest the main diagnostic and treatment criteria. We observed that the basic clinical symptoms of early LB were similar to those found in studies in other northern and central European countries (11, 24, 25). Thus, our clinical observations indicated that diagnosis of early Lyme disease in Lithuania should be based on: (1) history of tick exposure in an endemic area, (2) characteristic clinical manifestations, and, in some cases (3) positive serology (1, 8).

The results of our investigation clearly show that Lyme disease is a public health and clinical problem in Lithuania. Knowledge of the epidemiology of the disease in this Baltic country enables us to apply the most appropriate control methods. Further acquaintance and familiarity with the disease itself leads to more accurate diagnosis and effective treatment of this emerging infectious disease in Lithuania.

ACKNOWLEDGEMENTS

We thank S. Daujotas and R. Jociene at the laboratory of Zoonoses, Vilnius University, Lithuania, and E. I. Korenberg and his group at Gamaleya Institute, Moscow, Russia for contributions to this study. We thank S. Bergström for valuable suggestions regarding the manuscript.

REFERENCES

1. Steere AC. Lyme disease. N Engl J Med 321: 586–596, 1989.
2. Korenberg EI, Kovalevsky YV, Kuznetsova RI, Fonarev AA, Churilova AA, Antykova LP, Kalinin MI, Kryuchechnikov VN, Mebel BD, Scerbakov SV, Kovtunenko SS. Identification and primary results of treatment for the Lyme disease in North-West of the USSR. Med Parasit and Parasit Dis 5: 75–77, 1988 [in Russian].
3. Stanek G, Pletschette M, Flamm H, Hirschl AM, Aberer E, Kristoferitsch W, Schmutzhard E. European Lyme Borreliosis. In: Lyme disease and related disorders. Ann NY Acad Sci 539: 274–282, 1988.
4. Motiejunas L. Vector-borne infections in Lithuania. Moscow: doctoral thesis, 1–38, 1974 [in Russian].
5. Barbour AG, Heiland RA, Howe TR. Heterogeneity of major proteins in Lyme disease borreliae: a molecular analysis of North American and European isolates. J Infect Dis 152: 478–484, 1985.
6. Piletskis S. Ecologic and vector-associated meaning of different geographical regions of Lithuanian republic. Vilnius: doctoral thesis, 1–48, 1969 [in Lithuanian].
7. Korenberg EI, Kryuchechnikov VN, Kovalevsky YV. Advances in investigations of Lyme borreliosis in the territory of the former USSR. Eur J Epidemiol 9: 86–91, 1993.
8. Kmety E, Renácek J, Vyrosteková V. Investigations of ticks for the presence of Borrelia in Czechoslovakia. Zentralbl Bakteriol Mikrobiol Hyg (A) 263: 460–470, 1986.
9. Radda AC, Burger I, Stanek G, Wewalka G. Austrian hard ticks as vectors of Borrelia burgdorferi; an overview. Zentralbl Bakteriol Mikrobiol Hyg (A) 263: 79–82, 1986.
10. Kahl O, Schmidt K, Schönberg A, Laukamm-Josten U, Knülle W, Bienzle U. Prevalence of Borrelia burgdorferi in Ixodes ricinus ticks in Berlin (West). Zbl Bakt Hyg A 270: 434–440, 1989.
11. Stiernstedt G. Tick-borne Borrelia infection in Sweden. Scand J Infect Dis Suppl 45: 1–70, 1985.

12. Bergström S, Olsén B, Burman V, Gothefors L, Jaenson TGT, Jonsson M, Mejlon HA. Molecular characterization of Borrelia burgdorferi isolated from Ixodes ricinus in Northern Sweden. Scand J Infect Dis 24: 181–188, 1992.
13. Gustafson R, Garduf A, Svenungsson B. Comparison of culture, indirect immunofluorescence, and dark field microscopy for detection of spirochetes from Ixoxes ricinus ticks. Eur J Clin Microbiol Infect Dis 8: 570–572, 1989.
14. Aeschlimann A, Chamot E, Gigon F, Jeanneret J-P, Kesseler D, Walter CH. B. burgdorferi in Switzerland. Zentralbl Bakteriol Mikrobiol Hyg (A) 263: 450–458, 1986.
15. Kovalevsky YV, Kryuchechnikov VN, Korenberg EI. Comparative assessment of two methods of borrelia detection in tick-vector of Lyme disease. Med Parasit and Parasit Dis 1: 45–48, 1988 [in Russian].
16. Wahlberg P, Saikku P, Brummer-Korvenkontio M. Tick-borne encephalitis in Finland. The clinical features of Kumlinge disease during 1959–1987. J Intern Med 225: 173–177, 1989.
17. Gustafson R, Svenungsson B, Gardulf A, Stiernstedt G, Forsgren M. Prevalence of tick-borne encephalitis and Lyme borreliosis in a defined Swedish population. Scand J Infect Dis 22: 297–306, 1990.
18. Fahrer H, van der Linden SM, Sauvain M-J, Zhioua E, Aeschlimann A. The prevalence and incidence of clinical and asymptomatic Lyme borreliosis in population at risk. J Infect Dis 163: 305–310, 1991.
19. Paul H, Gerth H-J, Ackermann R. Infectiousness for humans of Ixodes ricinus containing Borrelia burgdorferi. Zentralbl Bakteriol Mikrobiol Hyg (A) 263: 473–476, 1986.
20. Münchhoff P, Wilske B, Preac-Mursic V, Schierz G. Antibodies against Borrelia burgdorferi in Bavarian forest workers. Zentralbl Bakteriol Mikrobiol Hyg (A) 263: 412–419, 1986.
21. Ananyeva LP, Korenberg EI, Skripnikova IA, Soldatkina LM, Nasonova VA. Clinical and serological study of Lyme disease in the North-Western parts of the USSR. Med Parasit and Parasit Dis 6: 28–31, 1990 [in Russian].
22. Schulze TL, Taylor RCh, Taylor GC, Bosler EM. Lyme disease: a proposed ecological index to assess areas of risk in the Northeastern United States. Am J Public Health 81: 714–718, 1991.
23. Jaenson TGT. The epidemiology of Lyme borreliosis. Parasitology Today 7: 39–45, 1991.
24. Åsbrink E, Olsson I, Hovmark A. Erythema chronicum migrans Afzelius in Sweden. A study on 231 patients. Zbl Bakt Hyg A 263: 229–236, 1986.
25. Weber K, Neubert U. Clinical features of early erythema migrans disease and related disorders. Zbl Bakt Hyg A 263: 209–228, 1986.

Scand J Infect Dis 26: 157–162, 1994

Changing Etiology of Bacteremia in Patients with Hematological Malignancies in Denmark

MAGNUS ARPI[1], M. ALAN VICTOR[2], JENS K. MØLLER[3], VIGGO JØNSSON[2], MOGENS MØRK HANSEN[2], NIELS ANKER PETERSLUND[4] and BRITA BRUUN[1]

From the Departments of [1]Clinical Microbiology and [2]Hematology, Rigshospitalet, Copenhagen, and the Departments of [3]Bacteriology and [4]Hematology, Århus University Hospital, Århus, Denmark

To ascertain whether the microbiological etiology of bacteremia among patients with hematological malignancies has changed in Denmark, the species distribution of clinically relevant blood culture isolates from the Hematological Department at Rigshospitalet, Copenhagen in 1990 was compared with 2 previous studies (1970–72; 1981–85). In addition, time trends of the etiology of bacteremia among hematological patients in Copenhagen (eastern Denmark) and in Århus (western Denmark) were compared. In contrast to many other studies, a significant increase in the proportion of Gram-negative aerobes was observed in Copenhagen (from 43% in 1981–85 to 55% in 1990; $p < 0.05$), whereas in Århus the proportion of Gram-positive aerobes increased steadily during the 1980s (from 34% to 51%; $p < 0.05$). In Copenhagen, non-hemolytic streptococci and Xanthomonas maltophilia increased significantly and accounted for 10% ($p < 0.01$) and 5% ($p < 0.05$) respectively, of all isolates in 1990, whereas Staphylococcus aureus during the 2 decades studied decreased from 25% to 8% ($p < 0.001$). In both regions, a decrease was observed in the proportion of Pseudomonas aeruginosa which accounted for only about 5% of all isolates in 1990. No changes were observed in the rates of anaerobes and yeasts. Several factors may contribute to the reported differences in the etiology of bacteremia among hematological patients, e.g. criteria used to assign the clinical significance of the isolate, blood culture system used, practice of using indwelling intravenous catheters, different policies with respect to antimicrobial treatment, and the degree of immunosuppression. A local surveillance of blood culture isolates is mandatory if changes in etiology and resistance development are to be detected.

M. Arpi, MD, Department of Clinical Microbiology, Frederiksberg Hospital, Ndr. Fasanvej 57, DK-2000 Frederiksberg, Denmark

INTRODUCTION

During recent decades, several investigators have reported changes in the spectrum of microorganisms causing bacteremia in patients with serious immunocompromising diseases, especially among patients with hematological malignancies. Gram-negative bacteria have previously dominated as the most frequent cause of bacteremia (1), but during the last decade there has been a general trend towards a larger proportion of Gram-positive bacteria as causative agents in these patients (1–7). In particular, an increasing incidence of coagulase-negative staphylococcal bacteremia has been reported (1–5). Increasing proportions of non-hemolytic streptococci (1) and multiresistant Corynebacterium spp. (8) have also been observed. Some previously rather uncommon Gram-negative species have also shown an increase, e.g. Enterobacter spp. (9), Pseudomonas spp. other than P. aeruginosa, and X. maltophilia (3, 10). In 2 earlier Danish studies of bacteremia involving patients with hematological malignancies from the same region (1970–72 (11); 1981–85 (12)), Gram-positive and Gram-negative bacteria contributed almost equally as causative agents.

The aim of this study was to elucidate time trends in the etiology of bacteremia in hematological patients admitted from the same region to the Finsen Institute/Rigshospitalet during 2 decades; furthermore, to compare the etiology of bacteremia among hematological patients during the 1980s between eastern and western Denmark.

 ISSN 0036-5548

MATERIALS AND METHODS

The etiology of bacteremia (for the sake of convenience this designation also includes candidemia in this study) among hematological patients admitted to the Hematological Department at Rigshospitalet, Copenhagen, in 1990, was compared with the results from 2 previous Danish studies involving hematological patients from the same region (1970–72 (11); 1981–85 (12)). There were no significant differences in the hematological diagnoses among the patients with bacteremia in the 3 periods investigated. Acute leukemia accounted for 42% (11), 46% (12) and 50%, respectively, while chronic malignant hematological diseases (including lymphomas) accounted for 58% (11), 54% (12) and 50%, respectively.

The distribution of microorganisms from blood cultures from the Hematological Department at Århus University Hospital for 3 selected years (1982, 1986, and 1990) was included to demonstrate time trends in this region, and to be able to compare the etiology of bacteremia among hematological patients from 2 different regions of Denmark. Among the Århus patients, acute leukemia accounted for 32%, 48% and 51% in the years 1982, 1986 and 1990, respectively. The corresponding percentages for chronic malignant hematological diseases were 68%, 52% and 49%.

Selective decontamination of the digestive tract was not used at either of the hematological departments.

Conventional, visually read blood culture systems were used in the 2 previous studies in Denmark (12, 13) and at Rigshospitalet in 1990 (14). At Århus, a conventional blood culture system was employed in 1982 and in 1986 (13), while the automated Bactec NR 660^R was used in 1990.

All blood culture isolates were identified according to conventional laboratory methods (15). The finding of a positive blood culture was not *per se* regarded as proof of bacteremia. Coagulase-negative staphylococci, Corynebacterium spp., Bacillus spp., Propionibacterium spp., and Pseudomonas spp. (except for P. aeruginosa) were regarded as contaminants unless they were isolated from at least 2 separate specimens (12).

If several microbial species were isolated within an interval of 7 days without intervening clinical remission, they were considered as belonging to the same episode and subsequently classified as polymicrobial.

Statistical methods

Fisher's Exact Test was used for paired comparisons. p-values of <0.05 were considered significant.

RESULTS

The etiology of bacteremia among hematological patients admitted to Rigshospitalet in 1990, and in 2 previous Danish studies at the same hematological department, is presented in Table I. In the early 1970s and in the first half of the 1980s, aerobic Gram-positive and Gram-negative bacteria contributed almost equally to bacteremia among these patients. In 1990, a markedly larger proportion of aerobic Gram-negative bacteria contributed to bacteremia among hematological patients as compared with aerobic Gram-positive bacteria, 55% vs. 35% ($p < 0.001$).

The decreasing proportion of Gram-positive aerobes was especially due to a marked decrease in S. aureus and β-hemolytic streptococci. In the period 1970–72, S. aureus was the most common cause of bacteremia, whereas it only ranked as the fifth most common cause in 1990. The rate of coagulase-negative staphylococci fluctuated, being on average 11% during the 2 decades. Of Gram-positive aerobes, only non-hemolytic streptococci increased; the proportion in 1990, 10%, was 10-fold higher than in the 2 previous studies.

Enterobacteriaceae, especially Enterobacter spp., but also Klebsiella spp. and Citrobacter spp. contributed to the increase in Gram-negative aerobic bacteria. E. coli was the most frequent cause of Gram-negative bacteremia during the 2 decades, accounting for about one-fifth of all bacteremia cases. The proportion of X. maltophilia bacteremia increased significantly, whereas a steady decrease of P. aeruginosa was observed. No significant changes in the rates of anaerobes and yeasts were observed.

Table I. *Etiology of bacteremia among hematological patients at the Finsen Institute/Rigshospitalet (eastern Denmark) in 3 selected periods during the time span 1970–1990*

Microorganism	1970–1972 (11) No.	1970–1972 (11) (%)	1981–1985 (12) No.	1981–1985 (12) (%)	1990 No.	1990 (%)	*p*-value
Gram-positive aerobes	48	(48)	87	(44)	55	(35)	NS[a]
S. aureus	25	(25)	24	(12)	12	(8)	<0.001
Coagulase-negative staphylococci	7	(7)	26	(13)	16	(10)	NS
Subtotal staphylococci	32	(32)	50	(25)	28	(18)	<0.05
β-hemolytic streptococci	5	(5)	4	(2)	0	–	<0.05
S. pneumoniae	4	(4)	8	(4)	3	(2)	NS
E. faecalis	2	(2)	12	(6)	3	(2)	NS
Non-hemolytic streptococci	1	(1)	2	(1)	16	(10)	<0.01
Subtotal streptococci	12	(12)	26	(13)	22	(14)	NS
L. monocytogenes	3	(3)	2	(1)	2	(1)	NS
Other	1	(1)	9	(5)	3	(2)	NS
Gram-negative aerobes	46	(46)	85	(43)	85	(55)	<0.05
E. coli	17	(17)	38	(19)	28	(18)	NS
Klebsiella spp.	6	(6)	14	(7)	14	(9)	NS
Enterobacter spp.	4	(4)	9	(5)	14	(9)	NS
Other Enterobacteriaceae	3	(3)	6	(5)	4	(3)	NS
Subtotal Enterobacteriaceae	30	(30)	67	(34)	60	(39)	NS
P. aeruginosa	16	(16)	16	(8)	11	(7)	<0.05
X. maltophilia	0	–	2	(1)	8	(5)	<0.05
Other	0	–	0	–	6[b]	(4)	<0.05[c]
Anaerobes	2	(2)	12	(6)	10	(6)	NS
Bacteroides spp.	2	(2)	4	(2)	1	(0.5)	NS
Clostridium spp.	0	–	7	(4)	7	(5)	NS
Other	0	–	1	(0.5)	2	(1)	NS
Yeasts	3	(3)	16	(8)	5	(3)	NS
Total	99		200		155		

[a] Not significant.
[b] H. influenzae 2, Moraxella sp. 1, B. catarrhalis 1, Pseudomonas sp. 1, Acinetobacter sp. 1.
[c] Comparing 1981–1985 and 1990.

The frequency of polymicrobial bacteremia increased markedly from 5% in 1970–72 to 13% and 14% in 1981–85 and 1990, respectively ($p < 0.05$).

Table II presents the etiology of bacteremia among hematological patients at Århus in 3 selected years during the time span 1982–90. In contrast to the trend in Copenhagen, the proportion of Gram-positive aerobes as the cause of bacteremia increased steadily during the 1980s (especially coagulase-negative staphylococci and enterococci). During the latter part of the 1980s, the proportion of Enterobacteriaceae decreased, especially E. coli. As in Copenhagen, the proportion of P. aeruginosa decreased markedly, and no significant changes were observed for anaerobic bacteria or yeasts. No case of X. maltophilia bacteremia occurred in Århus.

Table II. *Etiology of bacteremia among hematological patients at Århus University Hospital (western Denmark) in 3 selected years during the time span 1982–1990*

Microorganism	1982 No.	1982 (%)	1986 No.	1986 (%)	1990 No.	1990 (%)	p-value
Gram-positive aerobes	22	(34)	37	(38)	84	(51)	<0.05
S. aureus	8	(12)	3	(3)	28	(17)	<0.001[a]
Coagulase-negative staphylococci	5	(8)	8	(8)	24	(14)	NS[b]
Subtotal staphylococci	13	(20)	11	(11)	52	(32)	<0.01[a]
β-hemolytic streptococci	2	(3)	2	(2)	2	(1)	NS
S. pneumoniae	4	(6)	9	(9)	10	(6)	NS
Enterococcus spp.	0	–	1	(1)	7	(4)	NS
Non-hemolytic streptococci	0	–	12	(12)	6	(4)	NS
Subtotal streptococci	6	(9)	24	(25)	25	(15)	NS
L. monocytogenes	1	(1)	0		1	(0.6)	NS
Other	2	(3)	2	(2)	6	(4)	
Gram-negative aerobes	39	(60)	58	(60)	74	(45)	<0.05[a]
E. coli	19	(29)	36	(37)	30	(18)	<0.01[a]
Klebsiella spp.	0	–	7	(7)	16	(10)	<0.01
Enterobacter spp.	2	(3)	2	(2)	9	(5)	NS
Other Enterobacteriaceae	0	–	3	(3)	6	(4)	NS
Subtotal Enterobacteriaceae	21	(32)	48	(49)	61	(37)	NS
P. aeruginosa	18	(28)	10	(10)	8	(5)	<0.001
Other	0	–	0	–	5[c]	(3)	NS
Anaerobes	4	(6)	0	–	5	(3)	NS
Bacteroides spp.	0	–	0	–	5	(3)	NS
Clostridium spp.	4	(6)	0	–	0	–	NS
Other	0	–	1	(1)	0	–	NS
Yeasts	0	–	2	(2)	1	(0.6)	NS
Total	65		97		164		

[a] Comparing 1986 and 1990.
[b] Not significant.
[c] H. influenzae 1, Campylobacter spp. 4.

DISCUSSION

Contrary to many studies (1–7), we could not find an increase of Gram-positive bacteremia cases in hematological patients in eastern Denmark. We found a considerably larger proportion of bacteremia caused by Gram-negative aerobes in 1990 (55%), as compared with the periods 1970–72 (46%) and 1981–85 (43%). However, comparison of the results from hematological patients in 1981–85 (12) and in 1990 with 2 studies on bacteremia in unselected patient populations from 1977–78 (13) and 1983–84 (16) from the same region, revealed a larger proportion of Gram-positive aerobes, especially coagulase-negative staphylococci, among the hematological patients than among patients in the unselected population. The hematological patients also presented with more episodes due to P. aeruginosa, X.

maltophilia and yeasts than did the unselected patient populations. On the other hand, Enterobacteriaceae occurred more often in the unselected material.

Comparison of the etiology of bacteremia among hematological patients from 2 different regions in Denmark, Zeeland (east) and Jutland (west), showed clear differences. Whereas the proportion of Gram-negative aerobes increased in eastern Denmark, Gram-positive aerobes increased in western Denmark. The latter trend resembles the experiences gained at other centres for treatment of hematological diseases (1–7). In patients from eastern Denmark the proportion of non-hemolytic streptococci and X. maltophilia increased significantly, and there was a trend towards a higher rate of Enterobacter bacteremia, which is in agreement with several previous reports (1, 3, 4, 9). A decrease in P. aeruginosa bacteremia was observed in both eastern and western Denmark, which has also been reported by others (1, 6). In eastern Denmark, the rate of S. aureus bacteremia declined markedly, as found by Fredlund et al. in Sweden (4). In the majority of the studies on hematological patients, a clear increase in bacteremia caused by coagulase-negative staphylococci has been reported (1, 3–6). We could not confirm these findings. The proportion of coagulase-negative staphylococci fluctuated in eastern Denmark, while in western Denmark there was a tendency, but not significant, towards a larger proportion at the end of the investigated period. We found no changes in the rates of anaerobic bacteria and yeasts in Denmark, which is in agreement with other studies (3, 4).

It is evident that the etiology of bacteremia among patients with hematological malignancies changes with time, and that the relative proportions of species/groups causing bacteremia differ from hospital to hospital. Several factors probably contribute to these differences.

The criteria used to assign clinical significance of a blood culture isolate, especially regarding coagulase-negative staphylococci, is an important factor. Various criteria are used which of necessity must influence the reported proportions of bacteremia caused by coagulase-negative staphylococci (17). The criterion used in the present study, isolation from >1 blood culture set, is widely used, but may result in an underestimation of the importance of these microorganisms.

Another factor is the blood culture system used. This is known to influence the total yield of microorganisms and the relative proportion of species/groups detected in blood cultures (16, 17).

Differences in the procedures related to use of indwelling intravenous catheters, and especially if blood for culture is drawn from the catheter, are important factors. Several species are known to be catheter-related, e.g. staphylococci, Corynebacterium spp., Enterobacter spp., and X. maltophilia (5, 10, 18).

Different policies with respect to antimicrobial treatment, including the use of prophylaxis, may also affect the etiology of bacteremia. Streptococcal bacteremia has been reported in patients receiving prophylactic therapy with quinolones (7) and X. maltophilia bacteremia has emerged after treatment with imipenem (19). It is noteworthy that an empirical treatment regimen consisting of piperacillin and netilmicin was chosen at Århus University Hospital (20), whereas cefotaxime has mainly been used as initial empirical therapy at Rigshospitalet, followed by imipenem (10). It is quite possible that the use of this treatment regimen was the cause of the difference in incidence of X. maltophilia bacteremia at the 2 hematological departments.

The degree of immunosuppression and the severity of the underlying hematological disease are also of importance.

Several of the species that are seen to have increased their proportion in bacteremia among hematological patients are multiresistant, e.g. X. maltophilia and Corynebacterium jeikeium (5, 10). The rising proportion of X. maltophilia bacteremia in eastern Denmark has caused concern. This species has not, to the best of our knowledge, been reported to be a problem among hematological patients in Scandinavia before. For that reason a thorough elucidation of the epidemiological, microbiological and clinical aspects of these patients has been carried out (10).

This study has demonstrated that it is important to perform a local surveillance of blood culture isolates from hematological patients. Knowledge of the most common causative microorganisms together with knowledge of the outcome of bacteremic episodes, are of the utmost importance in the selection of initial empirical antibiotic regimens. Prompt treatment is essential, and must be instituted even before the causative microorganism has been identified.

REFERENCES

1. Klastersky J. Febrile neutropenia. Focus on antibacterial therapy. Consultant Series in Infectious Disease (3) No. 1: 13, 1992.
2. Pizzo PA, Hathorn JW, Hiemenz J, Browne M, Commers J, Cotton D, Gress J, Longo D, Marshall D, McKnight, Rubin M, Skelton J, Thaler M, Wesley R. A randomized trial comparing ceftazidime alone with combination antibiotic therapy in cancer patients with fever and neutropenia. N Engl J Med 315: 552–558, 1986.
3. Kiehn TE. Bacteremia and fungemia in the immunocompromised patient. Eur J Clin Microbiol Infect Dis 8: 832–837, 1989.
4. Fredlund H, Björeman M, Kjellander J, Sjöberg L, Bjorne L, Öhlin A-L. A 10-year survey of clinically significant blood culture isolates and antibiotic susceptibilities from adult patients with hematological diseases at a major Swedish hospital. Scand J Infect Dis 22: 381–391, 1990.
5. Kiehn TE, Armstrong D. Changes in the spectrum of organisms causing bacteremia and fungemia in immunocompromised patients due to venous access devices. Eur J Clin Microbiol Infect Dis 9: 869–872, 1990.
6. Johansson PJH, Sternby E, Ursing B. Septicemia in granulocytopenic patients: A shift in bacterial etiology. Scand J Infect Dis 24: 357–360, 1992.
7. Pizzo PA. Management of fever in patients with cancer and treatment induced neutropenia. N Engl J Med 328: 1323–1332, 1993.
8. Young VM, Meyers WF, Moody MR, Schimpff SC. The emergence of coryneform bacteria as a cause of nosocomial infections in compromised hosts. Am J Med 70: 646–650, 1981.
9. Bodey GP, Elting LS, Rodriguez S. Bacteremia caused by Enterobacter: 15 years' experience in a cancer hospital. Rev Infect Dis 13: 550–558, 1991.
10. Victor MA, Arpi M, Bruun B, Jønsson V, Mørk Hansen M. Xanthomonas maltophilia bacteremia in immunocompromised hematological patients. Scand J Infect Dis 26: 163–170, 1994.
11. Mortensen N, Mortensen BT, Nissen N. Bacteraemia in patients with leukaemia and allied neoplastic diseases. Scand J Infect Dis 8: 145–149, 1976.
12. Bruun B, Bangsborg J, Hovgaard D, Skinhøj P. Bacteremia and candidemia in hematological malignancies: Microbiological findings and antibiotic susceptibilities. Scand J Infect Dis 20: 503–509, 1988.
13. Bruun B, Sloth K, Bentzon MW, Frederiksen W. A study of bacteremias in Denmark from 1977–1978. Acta Pathol Microbiol Immunol Scand Sect B 90: 309–317, 1982.
14. Arpi M, Larsen SO. Comparison of detection speed and yield in agitated and non-agitated aerobic blood culture bottles. APMIS 100: 1061–1065, 1992.
15. Lennette EH, Balows A, Hausler WJ, Shadomy HJ. Manual of clinical microbiology. American Society for Microbiology. Washington D.C., 1985.
16. Arpi M, Lester A, Frederiksen W. A comparison of a conventional and a radiometric examination of clinical blood cultures with respect to recovery rate and detection time of microorganisms. Acta Pathol Microbiol Immunol Scand Sect B 93: 263–271, 1985.
17. Washington JA and the International Collaborative Blood Culture Study Group. Eur J Clin Microbiol Infect Dis 11: 1115–1128, 1992.
18. Weischer M, Kolmos HJ. Retrospective 6-year study of enterobacter bacteraemia in a Danish university hospital. J Hosp Hyg 20: 15–24, 1992.
19. Elting LS, Khardori N, Bodey GP, Fainstein V. Nosocomial infection caused by Xanthomonas maltophilia: A case-control study of predisposing factors. Infect Control Hosp Epidemiol 11: 134–138, 1990.
20. Møller JK, Bülow P, Bergmann OJ, Ellegaard J. Accumulated microbiological data. Surveillance of infections/antibiotic policy. Ugeskr Læger 151: 1934–1937, 1989.

Scand J Infect Dis 26: 163–170, 1994

Xanthomonas maltophilia Bacteremia in Immunocompromised Hematological Patients

M. ALAN VICTOR[1], MAGNUS ARPI[2], BRITA BRUUN[2], VIGGO JØNSSON[1] and MOGENS MØRK HANSEN[1]

From the Departments of [1]Hematology and [2]Clinical Microbiology, Rigshospitalet, Copenhagen, Denmark

Epidemiological, microbiological and clinical characteristics of 14 episodes of Xanthomonas maltophilia bacteremia in 12 seriously immunocompromised hematological patients, admitted to Rigshospitalet in Copenhagen over the 3-year period 1989–91, were evaluated. The results were compared with a randomly selected control group of 25 patients with Escherichia coli bacteremia. Hospital acquired bacteremia was more common among the patients with X. maltophilia bacteremia ($p < 0.01$). Treatment with broad-spectrum antibiotics before the bacteremic episode was markedly more common among the patients with X. maltophilia bacteremia ($p < 0.001$). The presence of a central venous catheter and previous treatment with corticosteroids were more frequent in patients with X. maltophilia bacteremia ($p < 0.05$). The X. maltophilia blood culture isolates were generally resistant to aminoglycosides and most β-lactams. The mortality rates related to bacteremia caused by X. maltophilia and E. coli were 14% and 20%, respectively.

M. A. Victor, MD, Department of Clinical Microbiology, Copenhagen County Hospital Herlev, Herlev Ringvej, DK-2730, Herlev, Denmark

INTRODUCTION

Xanthomonas maltophilia (Pseudomonas maltophilia) was first described by Hugh and Ryschenkow in 1961 (1). It is a free-living, ubiquitous, motile, Gram-negative, strictly aerobic bacterium that has been isolated from water, soil, animal sources, plant materials, foods, pharmaceuticals, and hospital equipment (2). X. maltophilia is usually a commensal or a contaminant and is part of the transient flora of hospitalized patients (2). It has been reported to be associated with a wide variety of clinical infections, including bacteremia, endocarditis, pericarditis, meningitis, respiratory tract infections, urinary tract infections, and wound infections (2–8). The clinical significance of X. maltophilia isolates is difficult to interpret (3, 8). The vast majority of the reported cases have been of nosocomial origin, and the route of infection has often been unknown (9–11).

Recently, several studies have reported an increasing incidence of X. maltophilia infections in immunocompromised patients, especially among patients with hematological malignancies (8, 10–16). During the last decade, the occurrence of X. maltophilia bacteremia has increased in hematological patients in eastern Denmark (15, 16).

The aim of this study was to describe the epidemiological, microbiological and clinical characteristics of 12 immunocompromised hematological Danish patients with 14 episodes of X. maltophilia bacteremia. In order to identify specific risk factors which characterized these patients, a control group of 25 hematological patients with E. coli bacteremia, at the same department and during the same period, were included in the study.

MATERIALS AND METHODS

In the 3-year period 1989–91, X. maltophilia was isolated from 50 blood culture sets from 15 bacteremic episodes in 13 immunocompromised hematological patients admitted to the Hematological Department, Rigshospitalet, Copenhagen. From the same period, 26/70 hematological patients with E. coli bacteremia were evaluated in order to provide a reference group (first patient from each month was selected). One patient with a polymicrobial bacteremia with X. maltophilia and E. coli was excluded from the study, resulting in 14 episodes of X. maltophilia bacteremia and 25 episodes of E. coli bacteremia.

Definitions

Bacteremia vs. contamination: Each blood culture was evaluated to determine whether the isolate represented a clinically significant bacteremia or a contamination. The decision was based on several factors, including sampling procedure (direct or catheter-sampled specimen), number of positive bottles in each blood culture set, culture results from other body sites, physical and laboratory examination, underlying disease, and instrumentation (17).

Prognostic group: The patients were divided into 3 prognostic groups based upon diagnosis, the actual state of the malignant disease (excluding the bacteremic episode), and possibility of obtaining remission:
Group I: Patients with estimated survival of 'years',
Group II: Patients with estimated survival of 'months', and
Group III: Patients with estimated survival of 'weeks' (18).

Hospital vs. community acquired bacteremia: The designation hospital acquired bacteremia was used for all patients from whom the first positive blood culture was obtained on or after the third day in hospital or following instrumentation or surgery, regardless of the length of hospitalization (19).

Polymicrobial bacteremia: More than 1 clinically significant organism isolated from a single blood culture or from separate blood cultures within a week (15).

Treatment with broad-spectrum antibiotics and corticosteroids: All treatments given within a month before the first positive blood culture was obtained were included.

Mortality: Any death within a week after the first positive blood culture was regarded as a bacteremia-related death, regardless of whether competitive causes of death were present or not (18).

Blood culture method: A 3-bottle system (2 aerobic and 1 anaerobic bottle) designed for bedside inoculation of 10 ml blood, was used (Media Department, Statens Seruminstitut, Copenhagen (15)). All isolates from blood and other body sites were identified according to conventional laboratory methods (2).

Antibiotic susceptibility testing: A tablet diffusion method was used (Neo-Sensitabs^{R}, Rosco Diagnostica, Tåstrup, Denmark (20)) on Danish blood agar (Media Department, Statens Seruminstitut).

Statistical analysis

Fisher's Exact Test was used for paired comparisons. p-values <0.05 were considered significant.

RESULTS

Table I compares epidemiological characteristics for patients with mono- and polymicrobial X. maltophilia and E. coli bacteremias. On average, 4 positive blood cultures were obtained per episode of X. maltophilia bacteremia (range: 1–10). In 11 of the 14 episodes, ≥2 blood cultures were found positive. In these severely immunocompromised patients, we were unable to designate any of the actual blood culture isolates as contaminants. All positive blood cultures with X. maltophilia were obtained from a central venous catheter (CVC). In only 2 episodes was a peripheral blood culture obtained, and in both instances growth of X. maltophilia. In 12 of the E. coli episodes, the blood cultures were only obtained from a CVC, 10 only from a peripheral vein, and in 3 episodes obtained from both a CVC and a peripheral vein.

The 2 groups were roughly comparable with respect to sex distribution and underlying hematological diseases (Table I). Acute myelogenous leukemia dominated in both groups, followed by malignant lymphoma. The average time lag between diagnosis of the hematological disease and the actual bacteremia was roughly the same in both groups, about 2 years. There was a tendency toward a short estimated survival (weeks) among patients with

Table I. *Comparison of epidemiological characteristics among hematological patients with mono- and polymicrobial X. maltophilia and E. coli bacteremias*

	X. maltophilia			E. coli			
	Total (14)[a]	Mono-microbial (8)	Poly-microbial (6)	Total (25)	Mono-microbial (18)	Poly-microbial (7)	*p*-value
Sex (males/females)	6/8	2/6	4/2	8/17	4/14	4/3	
Age (yr.)							
mean	34	32	37	50	49	55	
range	7–68	7–47	18–68	19–73	19–72	29–73	
Hematological diagnoses							NS[b]
acute myelogenous leukemia	7	2	5	11	9	2	
myelodysplasia	1	1		3	3		
acute lymphatic leukemia	1	1		1		1	
chronic lymphatic leukemia				1	1		
malignant lymphoma	4	3	1	7	3	4	
Mb. Waldenström				1	1		
severe aplastic anemia	1	1		1	1		
Prognostic group (estimated survival)							NS
I: 'years'	2	2		7	5	2	
II: 'months'	8	2	6	17	12	5	
III: 'weeks'	4	4		1	1		
Hospital acquired bacteremia	12	8	4	7	5	2	<0.01
Days hospitalized[c]							
mean	23	32	13	7	6	8	
range	0–73	7–73	0–38	0–66	0–66	0–44	

[a] Number of episodes in parentheses.
[b] Not significant.
[c] Length of stay during the actual admission until the first positive blood culture was obtained.

monomicrobial bacteremia caused by X. maltophilia, 50% vs. 6% among patients with monomicrobial E. coli bacteremia ($p = 0.2$).

Patients with X. maltophilia bacteremia were generally younger than patients with E. coli bacteremia. Markedly more patients with X. maltophilia bacteremia were <40 years of age as compared with patients with E. coli bacteremia, especially when comparing patients with monomicrobial bacteremia, 75% vs. 28% ($p < 0.05$).

Hospital acquired bacteremia was significantly more common among patients with X. maltophilia bacteremia, totally and also among patients with monomicrobial bacteremia ($p < 0.01$) (Table I). The majority (64%) of patients with X. maltophilia bacteremia had been hospitalized >2 weeks when the first positive blood culture was obtained, compared with only 16% of those with E. coli bacteremia ($p < 0.01$).

There was a tendency (not significant) for polymicrobial bacteremia to be more common among patients with X. maltophilia bacteremia, 43% (E. cloacae 3, Citrobacter sp. 1, coagulase-negative staphylococci 3, non-hemolytic streptococci 1, Corynebacterium jeikeium 1), than among patients with E. coli bacteremia, 28% (K. pneumoniae 3, E. cloacae 1,

Aeromonas sp. 1, coagulase-negative staphylococcus 1, non-hemolytic streptococci 3, C. perfringens 1).

Body temperature in patients with monomicrobial X. maltophilia bacteremia was on average lower than among patients with monomicrobial E. coli bacteremia (39.1°C (range 38.1–40.5°C) vs. 39.9°C (range 38.1–41.5°C)). Septic shock was observed in 2 patients, 1 with X. maltophilia and 1 with E. coli bacteremia.

In 11 episodes of X. maltophilia bacteremia (79%) the strain was also isolated from local sites. In 6 of the episodes there was clinical suspicion of 1 or several local infections (CVC infection 4, pleural empyema 1, dental abscess 1, anal ulceration 1, labial ulceration 1). Seven clinically suspected foci were culture verified in patients with E. coli bacteremia (urinary tract infection 2, anal abscess 2, pneumonia 2, pharyngitis 1).

Table II compares 4 predisposing factors for the 2 patient groups. The number of patients with neutropenia and the degree and duration of neutropenia was the same in both groups. The presence of a CVC and treatment with broad-spectrum antibiotics a month before the bacteremic episode was markedly more common among patients with X. maltophilia bacteremia (also with regard to monomicrobial bacteremias ($p < 0.05$)). All patients with X. maltophilia bacteremia had a CVC. In 4 cases the CVC was removed during the bacteremic episode. In 12 episodes of X. maltophilia bacteremia, ≥2 broad-spectrum antibiotics had been given prior to the bacteremia, most often a combination of a β-lactam and netilmicin (83%). The most commonly used antibiotics were cefotaxime (92%), netilmicin (83%; always in combination with another antibiotic), imipenem (50%), ciprofloxacin (42%), and vancomycin (42%). Only 24% of patients with E. coli bacteremia had been treated with broad-spectrum antibiotics within a month before the bacteremic episode, mainly with cefotaxime and netilmicin.

Previous treatment with corticosteroids also occurred more frequently among patients with X. maltophilia bacteremia. In all monomicrobial episodes with X. maltophilia bacteremia,

Table II. *Predisposing factors in hematological patients with mono- and polymicrobial X. maltophilia and E. coli bacteremias*

	X. maltophilia			E. coli			
	Total (14)	Mono-microbial (8)	Poly-microbial (6)	Total (25)	Mono-microbial (18)	Poly-microbial (7)	*p*-value
Neutropenia ($<0.5 \times 10^9$/l)	12	8	4	20	15	5	NS[a]
Days of neutropenia							
mean	14	10	19	14	12	19	
range	2–38	2–21	2–38	2–42	2–41	4–42	
Central venous catheter	14	8	6	15	11	4	<0.05[b]
Treatment with broad-spectrum antibiotics	12	8	4	6	3	3	<0.001[b]
Treatment with corticosteroids	11	6	5	9	5	4	<0.05[c]

[a] Not significant.
[b] Comparing monomicrobial bacteremias.
[c] Comparing total numbers.

the patients had 3 or all of the 4 risk factors, whereas only 3 patients with monomicrobial E. coli bacteremia (12%) has so many risk factors ($p < 0.001$).

Once the bacteriological diagnosis was established, all the monomicrobial episodes of X. maltophilia bacteremia were treated with antibiotics, depending on the results of in-vitro susceptibility tests. Ceftazidime (63%), ciprofloxacin (63%) and tobramycin (50%; always in combination with another antibiotic) were the most commonly used antibiotics. 17 (94%) of the monomicrobial episodes with E. coli were treated with antibiotics, cefotaxime (65%) and netilmicin (59%) being the antibiotics most often used. 64% of the patients with X. maltophilia bacteremia and 80% of the patients with E. coli bacteremia improved during the antibiotic treatment (defervescence of fever and clinical improvement).

A fatal outcome (within 1 week) related to bacteremia was observed in 2 episodes (14%) of X. maltophilia bacteremia (2 monomicrobial bacteremias) and in 5 episodes (20%) of E. coli bacteremia (2 monomicrobial, 3 polymicrobial bacteremias). However, at the time of writing, 11/12 patients (92%) with X. maltophilia bacteremia had died, on average 4 months (range 0–15) after the first positive blood culture was obtained. In comparison, 17/25 patients (68%) with E. coli bacteremia had died, on average 3 months (range 1–14) after the first positive blood culture.

The X. maltophilia isolates were generally resistant to aminoglycosides and most β-lactams. The most active agents were sulphonamide and chloramphenicol, followed by ciprofloaxacin and tetracycline. The most active β-lactam was ceftazidime (50% of strains susceptible). All isolates were resistant to ampicillin, cefuroxime, imipenem, and trimethoprim.

DISCUSSION

The clinical significance of X. maltophilia isolates is difficult to interpret (8, 10–16). However, Khardori et al. regarded all their 7 blood culture isolates as representing bloodstream infections (8). Accordingly we were not able to designate any of the blood culture isolates in the present study as contaminants.

To identify specific risk factors in patients with X. maltophilia bacteremia, a control group of episodes of E. coli bacteremia was included in this study, as E. coli is still the most common Gram-negative species isolated from blood cultures from hematological patients in Denmark (16). Without a reference group it would be more difficult to determine whether the results reflected characteristics of X. maltophilia bacteremia as such, or rather characteristics of the patient population studied.

We found a high frequency (43%) of polymicrobial X. maltophilia bacteremias in our study, as has also been reported by others (6, 11). The proportion of polymicrobial E. coli bacteremias (28%) was also higher in the present study than in unselected patient populations, where the rate of polymicrobial bacteremia is about 10% (21). The immunocompromised status of our patients and the large number of predisposing factors, especially the large number of CVC drawn blood cultures, probably explain the high proportion of polymicrobial bacteremias.

In the present study, the vast majority of X. maltophilia bacteremias were hospital acquired, thus agreeing with the results reported by Morrison et al. (6). The proportion of hospital acquired E. coli bacteremias in our control group was significantly lower. Most of the patients with X. maltophilia bacteremia in our study had also been hospitalized >3 weeks before the onset of bacteremia, i.e. 3 times as long as the patients in the E. coli control group. Long hospitalization before onset of bacteremia was also found by others (8, 11).

In the present study, septic shock was experienced in only 1 episode of X. maltophilia bacteremia, which was a significantly lower rate than the 43% reported by Elting et al. (11).

Most of the patients with X. maltophilia bacteremia in our study were neutropenic, i.e. $<0.5 \times 10^9$/l. This figure agrees with Khardori et al. who found that all their patients with cancer had neutropenia, defined as $\leq 1.0 \times 10^9$/l (8), though in another study of X. maltophilia bacteremia in cancer patients, of whom half had hematological malignancies, only 42% had neutropenia ($<1.0 \times 10^9$/l) (11).

The presence of a CVC was the most common predisposing factor among patients with X. maltophilia bacteremia in the present and in previous studies (8, 11).

We found that treatment with broad-spectrum antibiotics within a month of the bacteremic episode was significantly more common among patients with X. maltophilia bacteremia than among those in the E. coli control group. This also tallied with the study by Khardori et al., whose X. maltophilia bacteremia patients had all received imipenem (8). In our study, imipenem had been given before the onset of bacteremia in 6 of the bacteremic episodes with X. maltophilia. In a case-control study of factors predisposing to clinically significant nosocomial infection with X. maltophilia, Elting et al. found that imipenem treatment was >10 times more frequent among cases than among controls (22). We also found that previous treatment with corticosteroids was more frequent among patients with X. maltophilia bacteremia.

In the present study, a clinically suspected portal of entry was culture, verified in 6 episodes of X. maltophilia bacteremia, mainly from CVC insertion site or CVC tip. This was consistent with a previous study where the portal of entry was identified in about half of the patients, mainly from a CVC (11). The reservoir of X. maltophilia and the route of transmission of X. maltophilia remain largely unknown (8). Some studies report isolation of X. maltophilia from the respiratory tract (6, 8), while others suggest the gastrointestinal tract as a likely reservoir (11). In contrast, Rosenthal claimed that systemic infection with X. maltophilia was more likely to derive from the environment than from an endogenous source (23). Newer diagnostic tools, e.g. serology (24) and ribotyping (25) could possibly be used to elucidate the epidemiological characteristics of X. maltophilia.

About 2/3 of the patients with X. maltophilia bacteremia in our study responded to treatment (antibiotics and in 4 cases removal of the CVC), which accords with results reported by others (8, 11). In the study by Elting et al., it was shown that administration of appropriate antibiotics was an important prognostic factor, although not as significant as removal of the CVC which had a response rate of 100%, irrespective of the appropriateness of antibiotic therapy (11).

Mortality related to X. maltophilia bacteremia was low in the present study. Morrison et al. found a crude mortality rate in nosocomial X. maltophilia bacteremia of 33%, and cancer patients had an average mortality rate of 52% due to various X. maltophilia infections (6). Among other things, different definitions of bacteremia-related death could probably explain the observed differences in the mortality rate. In our study, there was a trend (not significant) towards a higher overall mortality among patients with X. maltophilia bacteremia as compared with the E. coli bacteremia patients. Perhaps X. maltophilia signifies poor prognosis rather than being the cause of death.

The X. maltophilia blood culture isolates in the present study were generally resistant to aminoglycosides and most β-lactams, which is in agreement with several previous studies (6, 8, 10, 26). The most active agents in our study were sulphonamide, chloramphenicol, ciprofloxacin and tetracycline, a finding also made by several other investigators (3, 6, 8). A very high susceptibility (98–100%) to trimethoprim-sulfamethoxazole was reported in several studies (6, 8), but lower susceptibility rates to ciprofloxacin (8, 24), chloramphenicol (8), and tetracycline (3) have also been reported. Like others, we found all isolates to be resistant to imipenem (8, 24). As the number of strains investigated in the present study was small, a more extensive study involving 100 recently isolated clinical strains is now in progress.

REFERENCES

1. Hugh R, Ryschenkow E. Pseudomonas maltophilia, an Alcaligenes-like species. J Gen Microbiol 26: 123–132, 1961.
2. Lennette EH, Balows A, Hausler WJ, Shadomy HJ. Manual of clinical microbiology. Washington DC: American Society for Microbiology, 1985.
3. Gilardi GL. Infrequently encountered Pseudomonas species causing infection in humans. Ann Intern Med 77: 211–215, 1972.
4. Holmes B, Lapage SP, Easterling BG. Distribution in clinical material and identification of Pseudomonas maltophilia. J Clin Pathol 32: 66–72, 1979.
5. Zuraleff JJ, Yu VL. Infections caused by Pseudomonas maltophilia with emphasis on bacteremia: case reports and a review of the literature. Rev Infect Dis 4: 1236–1246, 1982.
6. Morrison AJ, Hoffmann KK, Wenzel RP. Associated mortality and clinical characteristics of nosocomial Pseudomonas maltophilia in a university hospital. J Clin Microbiol 24: 52–55, 1986.
7. Muder RR, Yu VL, Dummer JS, Vinson C, Lumish RM. Infections caused by Pseudomonas maltophilia. Expanding clinical spectrum. Arch Intern Med 147: 1672–1674, 1987.
8. Khardori N, Elting L, Wong E, Schable B, Bodey GP. Nosocomial infections due to Xanthomonas maltophilia (Pseudomonas maltophilia) in patients with cancer. Rev Infect Dis 12: 997–1003, 1990.
9. Gardner P, Griffin WB, Swartz MN, Kunz LJ. Non-fermentative gram-negative bacilli of nosocomial interest. Am J Med 48: 735–749, 1970.
10. Marshall WF, Keating MR, Anhalt JP, Steckelberg JM. Xanthomonas maltophilia: An emerging nosocomial pathogen. Mayo Clin Proc 64: 1097–1104, 1989.
11. Elting LS, Bodey GP. Septicemia due to Xanthomonas species and non-aeruginosa Pseudomonas species: increasing incidence of catheter-related infections. Medicine 69: 296–306, 1990.
12. Kiehn TE. Bacteremia and fungemia in the immunocompromised patient. Eur J Clin Microbiol Infect Dis 8: 832–837, 1989.
13. Kiehn TE, Armstrong D. Changes in the spectrum of organisms causing bacteremia and fungemia in immunocompromised patients due to venous access devices. Eur J Clin Microbiol Infect Dis 9: 869–872, 1990.
14. Kerr KG, Corps CM, Hawkey PM. Infections due to Xanthomonas maltophilia in patients with hematological malignancy. Rev Infect Dis 13: 762, 1991.
15. Bruun B, Bangsborg J, Hovgaard D, Skinhøj P. Bacteremia and candidemia in hematological malignancies: microbiological findings and antibiotic susceptibilities. Scand J Infect Dis 20: 503–509, 1988.
16. Arpi M, Victor MA, Møller JK, Jønsson V, Mørk Hansen M, Peterslund NA, Bruun B. Changing etiology of bacteremia in patients with hematological malignancies in Denmark. Scand J Infect Dis 26: 157–162, 1994.
17. Weinstein MP, Reller LB, Murphy JB, Lichtenstein KA. The clinical significance of positive blood cultures: a comprehensive analysis of 500 episodes of bacteremia and fungemia in adults. I. Laboratory and epidemiologic observations. Rev Infect Dis 5: 35–53, 1983.
18. Hovgaard D, Skinhøj P, Bangsborg J, Bruun B, Mørk Hansen M, Nissen NI. Bacteremia and candidemia in hematological malignancies: clinical findings. Scand J Infect Dis 20: 495–501, 1988.
19. Garner JS, Jarvis WR, Emori TG, Horan TC, Hughes JM. CDC definitions for nosocomial infections. Am J Infect Control 16: 128–140, 1988.
20. Casals JB, Pringler N. Antimicrobial testing using Neo-Sensitabs, 9th ed., Rosco-Diagnostica, 1991.
21. Eykyn SJ, Gransden WR, Phillips I. The causative organisms of septicemia and their epidemiology. J Antimicrob Chemother 25 (Suppl C): 41–58, 1990.
22. Elting LS, Khardori N, Bodey GP, Fainstein V. Nosocomial infection caused by Xanthomonas malthophilia: a case-control study of predisposing factors. Infect Control Hosp Epidemiol 11: 134–138, 1990.
23. Rosenthal SL. Sources of pseudomonas and acinetobacter species found in human culture materials. Am J Clin Pathol 62: 807–811, 1974.

24. Schable B, Rhoden DL, Hugh R, Weaver RE, Khardori N, Smith PB, Bodey GP, Anderson RL. Serological classification of Xanthomonas maltophilia (Pseudomonas maltophilia) based on heat-stable O antigens. J Clin Microbiol 27: 1011–1014, 1989.
25. Bingen EH, Denamur E, Lambert-Zechovsky NY, Bourdois A, Mariani-Kurkdjian P, Cezard J-P, Navorro J, Elion J. DNA restriction fragment length polymorphism differentiates crossed from independent infections in nosocomial Xanthomonas maltophilia bacteremia. J Clin Microbiol 29: 1348–1350, 1991.
26. Garcia-Rodriguez JA, Garcia Sanchez JE, Garcia-Garcia MI, Garcia Sanchez E, Munoz Bellido JL. Antibiotic susceptibility profile of Xanthomonas maltophilia. In vitro activity of β-lactam/β-lactamase inhibitor combinations. Diagn Microbiol Infect Dis 14: 239–243, 1991.

Scand J Infect Dis 26: 171–178, 1994

Risk Factors for Listeriosis in Denmark, 1989–1990

ANNETTE JENSEN, WILHELM FREDERIKSEN and PETER GERNER-SMIDT

From the Department of Clinical Microbiology, Statens Seruminstitut, Copenhagen S, Denmark

Dietary risk factors for listeriosis were examined, and the risk levels of listeriosis according to specific underlying diseases were evaluated, in order to study the basis for prevention. Questionnaires from 50 listeriosis patients and 40 matching control persons were analysed. Unpasteurized milk was a risk food for sporadic listeriosis, and an outbreak of a European epidemic strain of Listeria monocytogenes was obviously linked to a blue-mould cheese or a hard cheese. Leukaemia, AIDS and renal transplantation were found to be associated with >1000-fold risk of acquiring listeriosis, compared with healthy persons. As a part of prevention, persons running a high risk of contracting listeriosis should be individually informed about food hygiene and risk foods.

A. Jensen, MD, Bøgeløvsvej 4, DK-2830 Virum, Denmark

INTRODUCTION

Listeriosis, caused by the bacterium Listeria monocytogenes, is a serious, foodborne disease (1, 2). Active tracing of disease sources by questionnaire studies has helped identify the origin of outbreaks and sporadic disease. Such sources have been: contaminated, ready-to-eat or raw foods consumed without further preparation, e.g. milk, cheese, paté, turkey sausages, sea foods, and vegetables, mushrooms and coleslaw [see (2) and (3)]. The ultimate evidence of the sources was produced by microbiological examination of food.

Among an increasing number of cases of listeriosis, the Danish laboratory surveillance recorded a self-limited outbreak with unknown source from 1985 to 1987 (4). To actively forestall new outbreaks and also to identify risk foods in sporadic listeriosis, we developed the Danish case-control questionnaire study described here.

Many conditions, such as AIDS, auto-immune disease, cancer, diabetes mellitus, dialysis, immunosuppressive treatment, liver disease, organ transplantation, pregnancy and T-cell immunodeficiencies (2, 5, 6), predispose to listeriosis, but the relative risk of contracting listeriosis can only be estimated when prevalence data are accessible. We found it important to evaluate the risk level for certain predisposing conditions, and to identify which conditions needed specific attention by preventive efforts.

MATERIALS AND METHODS

Between January 1989 and May 1991, all laboratory-reported Danish cases and matching control persons were asked to attend a consecutive, open questionnaire study. A case was defined as an ill person, or a mother and her unborn or newborn infant, from whom L. monocytogenes was demonstrated. Species identification and serotyping were performed at Statens Seruminstitut, Copenhagen. Phage typing was performed by J. Rocourt, Institute Pasteur, Paris.

On the reporting day, the nurse attending the listeriosis patient was asked to hand a questionnaire to the patient (or to a person who could answer for the patient) and one to a control person who was hospitalized at the same department on the same date as the patient. The control person was matched with respect to questionnaire period, geographical area of hospital admission, age, and gender. The questionnaire dealt with more than 50 food items consumed during 1 month preceding the date of the L. monocytogenes positive specimen.

Questionnaire data were subjected to univariate analysis by the SAS statistical program (Andreas Habicht, IMSOR, The Technical University of Denmark, DK-2800 Lyngby). The χ^2-test and Fisher's exact test were used (2-tailed; significance level 0.05).

The risk of acquiring listeriosis for persons with underlying conditions was evaluated by correlating information from the listeriosis patients' hospital records to contemporary Danish prevalence data concerning health, disease, and drug sales.

RESULTS

Epidemiology

Listeriosis in Denmark since 1981 is described quarterly in Fig. 1. During recent years the incidence rate has been 6–7 cases/10^6 inhabitants/year. From March 1989 to December 1990, one-third, 26 cases, became ill with a strain of serogroup 4, phagovar 2389/2425/3274/2671/47/108/340, hence referred to as the EPI strain. The remaining strains were with few exceptions of unrelated phagovars, non-epi strains. Thus, this study describes both an outbreak and sporadic listeriosis.

EPI cases, like non-epi cases, were found in most parts of Denmark, but were more frequent in the suburbs of the second largest town, Aarhus. Adult EPI patients differed from adult non-epi patients by more frequently having meningitis (65% vs. 40%); and by a lower mortality during hospitalization (26% vs. 47%). The rate of materno-fetal cases (12% vs. 17%) and the average age of adult cases (59 years vs. 60 years) were similar in EPI cases and non-epi cases.

The EPI strain was clearly community acquired, i.e. not nosocomial; all EPI patients were hospitalized because of listeriosis and all positive specimens were collected within 3 days after admission (Table I). In contrast, 11/32 of the non-epi type specimens were collected after more than 3 days in hospital; 10 of these 11 patients had septicaemia, only 1 had meningitis, and all but 1 had predisposing conditions. The ratio meningitis/septicaemia in cases of listeriosis detected within 3 days of hospitalization was the same for EPI cases, 15/7, as for non-epi cases, 14/7.

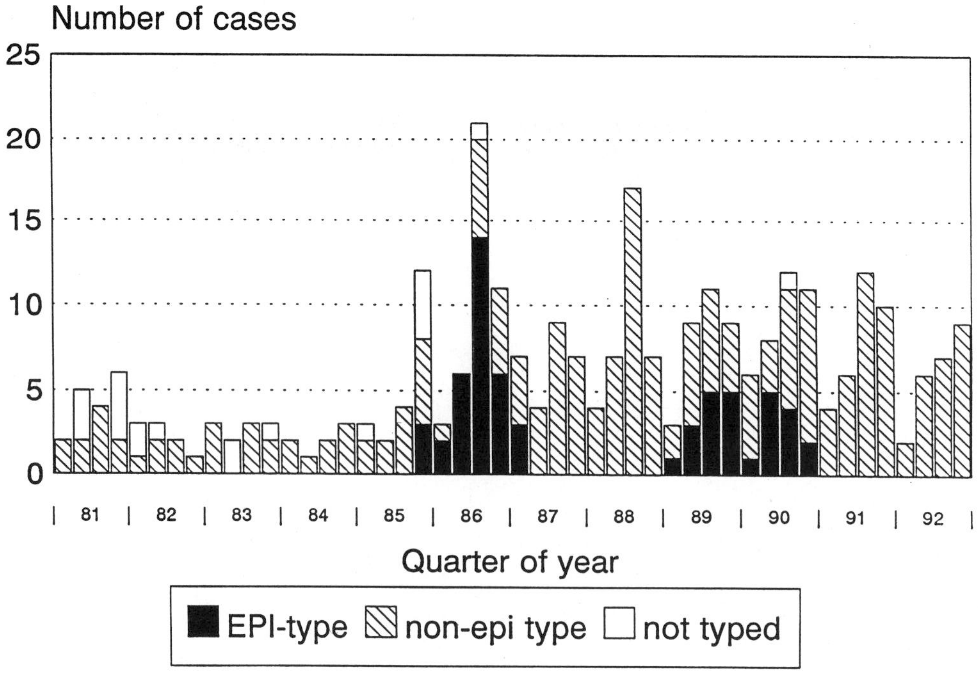

Fig. 1. Listeriosis in Denmark, 1989–90.

Table I. *Clinical presentation of the 59 adult cases of listeriosis 1989–1990 in relation to the period in hospital before collection of the listeria-positive specimen*

Listeria type	Clinical presentation	Underlying condition	0–1 day	2–3 days	4–6 days	1 week–5 months	Unknown
EPI	Meningitis	–	7	–	–	–	–
		+	8	–	–	–	–
EPI	Septicaemia	–	1	1	–	–	1
		+	5	–	–	–	–
Non-epi	Meningitis	–	8	1	–	–	–
		+	5	–	1	–	–
Non-epi	Septicaemia	–	1	1	1	–	1
		+	1	4	1	8	2
Unknown	Septicaemia	+	–	–	–	1	–

Table II. *Case-control questionnaire analysis results described by Odds Ratios; only results with Odds Ratio >2 are shown*

	All[a]	Sporadic[b]	Outbreak[c]	Outbreak[d]
Paté	8.1(*)[e]	–	–	2.2[e]
Unpasteurized milk	2.4[e]	8.6(*)[e]	–	–
Pasteurized milk	2.4	–	–	–
Fruit and vegetables	–	–	9.2*	9.9*
Blue mould cheese (all five brands)	–	–	2.8	2.9
Brand X of blue mould cheese	–	–	3.0	4.6*
Nature medicine	2.9	–	–	–
Medicine (excl. steroid/chemother.)	2.4(*)	–	–	–
Steroid	20.7**[e]	18.3**[e]	25.0**[e]	2.5
Chemotherapy	16.3**[e]	16.1**[e]	16.7**[e]	–
Steroids and/or chemotherapy	30.5***[e]	30.7***[e]	30.0***[e]	–

[a] All listeriosis cases compared with control persons.
[b] Listeriosis cases with non-epi phagovars compared with control persons.
[c] Listeriosis cases with the EPI-phagovar compared with control persons.
[d] Listeriosis cases with the EPI-phagovar compared with non-epi cases plus control persons.
[e] The Odds Ratio value is unknown higher, because zero-consumption between control persons was calculated by replacing zero with the value 0.5. Significance levels: (*) $p < 0.1$; * $p < 0.05$; ** $p < 0.01$; *** $p < 0.001$.

Questionnaire

90 questionnaires were answered, 50 from listeriosis patients and 40 from control persons. Most of the questionnaires unanswered by listeriosis patients concerned patients who had died. Not all participants answered all questions. An analysis of the questionnaire results is shown in Table II. For clarity, only results with statistical significance and Odds Ratio (OR) >2 are shown.

Unpasteurized milk and paté were only consumed by listeriosis patients, but not by 33 and 34 controls, respectively. Unpasteurized milk was consumed by 9% patients (OR undefined >8.6; CI 0.6–117; $p < 0.08$) and paté was consumed by 11% patients (OR undefined >8.1; CI 0.6–101; $p < 0.07$).

Steroid- and/or chemotherapy were more frequent among listeriosis patients (25/66) than among controls (0/25) (OR undefined >30.5; CI 4.3–217; $p < 0.0001$), and the significance values were similar for EPI patients and non-epi patients. Other drugs, i.e. apart from steroid and chemotherapy, were taken by 32/50 listeriosis patients, but by only 17/40 controls (OR 2.4; CI 0.9–6.2; $p = 0.07$), but no specific drug was dominant. Antacids and non-steroid anti-inflammatoric drugs were equally frequently taken by listeriosis patients and control persons (20%).

EPI patients more often consumed blue-mould cheeses and fruit-and-vegetables, compared with non-epi patients and controls. Fruit-and-vegetables answers were far too disparate to allow of calculations. However, 5 different Danish blue-mould cheeses were reported by name, and 1 of these, Brand X, was consumed by significantly more EPI patients (6/16), than by non-epi patients and controls (6/46) (OR 4.6; CI 1.0–21; $p = 0.03$).

Food investigations

The EPI strain was grown from food items submitted by 2 EPI patients, in smoked cod roe and in boiled chicken, respectively. Cross-contamination from other foods could not be excluded. The first patient was an otherwise healthy renal transplanted woman who had also eaten the Brand X blue-mould cheese at the same meal, 2 days before her symptoms of septicaemia started. One plastic bag with 3 opened packages of foods from the meal (Brand X blue-mould cheese, smoked cod roe and onion sausage) was received by the Veterinary Control for examination, but the EPI type was isolated only from the cod roe after enrichment of 25 g of each food. L. monocytogenes, but not the EPI type, was isolated in the factory from cod roe. Blue-mould cheese and onion sausage were not studied further. The second patient was an elderly woman living alone who died before information was collected; the origin of the chicken was unknown.

The EPI strain was found at routine dairy checks in 3 Mid-Jutland cheese dairies, never in 1988, but during 1989 in 7 different brand specimens of a popular hard cheese type, during 1990 in 1 hard cheese specimen, and during 1991 in 1 dairy milieu specimen. Moreover, the EPI strain was demonstrated in one French imported hard cheese in 1990. The implicated Danish hard cheese type is so popular that it was consumed by more than 90% of both the listeriosis patients and the control persons. We have no information about routine dairy checks of blue-mould cheese.

Though lots of other Danish industrial foods, mayonnaise salads, fish, meat products and some cheese shop utensils were examined and found positive for listeria, the EPI type was never found among hundreds of these strains.

Underlying conditions

Underlying conditions for listeriosis are reported in Table III. Each case is mentioned only once according to the most relevant diagnosis. For example, steroid treatment in leukaemia is mentioned under leukaemia, and splenectomy was a fact in 2 patients, one of whom also had leukaemia while the other underwent renal transplantation. The 23 remaining patients include 12 with various health weaknesses, such as age >80 years ($n = 4$), non-insulin-dependent diabetes mellitus ($n = 2$), drug abuse ($n = 1$), heart disease ($n = 1$), chronic bronchitis with cor pulmonale ($n = 1$), apoplexia ($n = 1$), aortic aneurysm ($n = 1$), and aneurysm of a cerebral artery ($n = 1$). It is remarkable that all 3 study patients with renal transplants were ill with the EPI type. All were women, and were transplanted at the same centre, but years apart. They lived more than 100 km apart, and they were admitted for listeriosis to different hospitals at different times, 1 and 8 months after the first case, respectively.

Risk levels

The risk levels for listeriosis in relation to various underlying conditions were calculated (Table IV).

Table III. *Underlying conditions in all Danish cases with listeriosis, 1989 and 1990*

Underlying condition	EPI cases *N*	(%)	Non-epi cases *N*	(%)	Total *N*	(%)
None	10	(43)	13	(37)	23	(39)
Leukaemia and lymphoma	4	(17)	9	(26)	14[a]	(24)
Intra-abdominal cancer	2	(9)	5	(14)	7	(12)
AIDS	1	(4)	2	(6)	3	(5)
Chronic alcoholism	1	(4)	1	(3)	2	(3)
Steroid treatment	1	(4)	2	(6)	3	(5)
Renal transplant	3	(13)	–		3	(5)
Systemic lupus erythematosus	–		2	(6)	2	(3)
Insulin-dependent diabetes	1	(4)	1	(3)	2	(3)
Total, adult cases	23	(98)	35	(101)	59	(99)
Materno-fetal cases	3	(12)	7	(17)	10	(15)

[a] One patient with unknown phagovar.

Table IV. *Listeriosis risk levels per year in Denmark, 1989–90, related to predisposing conditions*

Reference[d]	Predisposing condition	Listeriosis[a] 1989 + 1990	Prevalence[b] 1/1 1990	Risk[c]/10^6 disposed/year
(A)	Acute leukaemia ALL + AML	5	250	10,000
(B)	AIDS in Denmark per 31.12.89	3	223	6,726
(C)	Myelomatosis	2	450	2,222
(D)	Chronic lymphatic leukaemia CLL	3	700	2,143
(E)	Chronic myeloid leukaemia CML	1	260	1,900
(F)	Renal transplant	3	1,350	1,111
(G)	Systemic lupus erythematosus	2	1,750	571
(H)	Systemic steroid therapy	19	50,000	190
(I)	Intra-abdominal cancer	7	26,839	130
(J)	Materno-fetal = liveborn	10	60,000	83
(K)	Antacid therapy	13	100,000	65
(L)	Insulin-dependent diabetes	2	20,000	50
(M)	Non-insulin-dependent diabetes	3	80,000	19
(N)	Chronic alcoholism	2	60,000	17
(P)	Age ≥ 60 years	34	1.0×10^6	17.0
(P)	Age 25–59 years[e]	21	2.4×10^6	4.4
(P)	Age 1–24 years[e]	4	1.6×10^6	1.3
(P)	Danish inhabitant	69	5×10^6	6.9
(Q)	Outbreak of EPI-type	26	5×10^6	2.6
(Q)	Healthy[ef]	11	5×10^6	1.1

[a] Number of listeriosis cases during the years 1989 and 1990.
[b] Prevalence, or the condition incidence/year multiplied by the average life time after diagnosis.
[c] $(a/2) \times (1{,}000{,}000/b)$.
[d] The reference list in Danish can be provided by the author.
[e] Materno-fetal cases excluded.
[f] Patients with health weaknesses excluded (see text, page 174).

Malignant haematological and lymphatic tissue diseases, AIDS included, represented the highest risk levels, >1000-fold the risk in healthy persons. (Jurado (7) estimated a similar incidence, $1150/10^6$ AIDS patients.) All of our 3 AIDS patients were males, with the disease in a quiet phase. One surviving 44-year-old with previously unknown HIV status went down with EPI-type meningitis, and soon after had pneumocystis pneumonia. He was also found to have Kaposi sarcoma, like the 2 other AIDS patients who were ill with non-epi types. One was a 71-year-old man who died the third day of meningitis, and the other a 55-year-old prednisolone-treated man who died 38 days after septicaemia.

Abdominal cancer preceding listeriosis included cancer of the stomach, colon, rectum (2 cases), ovary, prostate and liver. Listeriosis patients did not have any of the other common cancers of the lung, skin, breast or urinary bladder.

The 2 alcoholic listeriosis patients needed injections of vitamin B during hospitalization. They had no signs of alcohol-related diseases.

The pregnancy-associated risk level was 83 cases/10^6 newborns (25 EPI/million and 58 non-epi/million live births, respectively). This contrasts with the risk level during the Danish outbreak in 1986, of 253/10^6 live births (8). In the USA, an active surveillance project found a relative risk of 120 sporadic cases/10^6 births (1).

The risk levels of listeriosis during treatment with the specific drugs, steroids and antacids, were estimated by comparing the listeriosis patients' use with the registered drug sales in Denmark in daily defined doses.

DISCUSSION

Our study identified certain risk foods, also found by others: unpasteurized milk (2, 9–11) and paté (2, 12, 13). Some 10% of Danish sporadic cases might be prevented by abandoning consumption of unpasteurized milk. However, these foods could only explain a minor proportion of the sporadic cases. Therefore more knowledge about risk foods is necessary. In a multistate case-control study on sporadic listeriosis in the USA, 32% of sporadic cases could be attributed to eating soft cheeses or food purchased from grocery delicatessen counters, while eating undercooked chicken increased the risk among immunosuppressed patients (3).

The EPI strain implicated in this Danish outbreak was contracted domestically; no patient had been abroad. The strain is of international epidemiological interest, since 2 other large European outbreaks have been caused by exactly the same phagovar, but the sources were obviously at least 3 different foods: in the Swiss outbreak of 1983–87, contaminated soft cheese caused 122 cases (14), and the French outbreak in 1992 involved 279 cases caused by pork tongue in aspic (15). There are indications that the Danish source was a cheese product, either the Brand X blue-mould cheese, as significantly indicated by the questionnaire, or the hard cheese as indicated by the dairy control cultures.

The EPI outbreak in Denmark of 1989–90 differed epidemiologically from the Danish outbreak which ended 2 years earlier (4); the materno-fetal rate was lower (12% vs. 43%), the mean age of non-materno-fetal cases was higher (59 years vs. 47 years), and the geographical distribution was different (more cases near Aarhus vs. in Greater Copenhagen). The explanation for the differences between the 2 outbreaks might be that they were caused by 2 different food sources.

Our questionnaire data collecting method differed from other studies by reacting immediately after reporting of the listeria finding, and in using a written form. In that way we avoided delay and time-consuming interviews at inconvenient times. Some possible infection risk situations eluded the questionnaire, but were mentioned by 3 patients with non-epi strains. One younger man had meningitis symptoms in the aeroplane home from a tour to Paris, where 2 days earlier he had tasted cheeses in a street market. One mother gave birth prematurely, a few days after home slaughtering of a steer. Another mother became ill while her husband was cleaning out a sheep stable; he alone drank raw cowmilk; both had a short febrile spell and diarrhea 1 week before the wife gave birth prematurely. The last-mentioned case indicates that information on household members' health and their diet should be considered important. Also early examination for excretion of listeria in faeces from household members could be a help in identifying sources (16–18).

In planning the study we chose a questionnaire period of 1 month, like most other authors; few used as long as 3 months (19). Later, others have used 3 weeks (12). Since all people have a short memory regarding food consumption, it is essential that the questionnaire period is as short as possible respecting the incubation period. The incubation period for listeriosis is undetermined, but suggested to be from 1 up to several weeks (1). However, according to recent reports where sources are confirmed by typing and the time of exposure is known, the incubation period seems to be 1–4 days (20–23), as in experimental animal studies with oral administration of listeria (24). Therefore, in surveillance studies a questionnaire period of ≤2 weeks preceding the listeria-positive specimen seems reasonable.

Questions about foods should be general, but for commonly consumed foods, detailed information may be needed (batch name, durability, factory name, food store). If questions are too broad, specific brand names are forgotten. Therefore a detailed, up-to-date brand list should be put as a reminder to the patient.

Prevention of large outbreaks of foodborne diseases is a matter of concern for industrial food production hygiene. However, the food industry is so huge that absolute surveillance is impossible. HACCP (Hazard Analysis of Critical Control Points) principles are now applied to an increasing extent in food production in order to ensure microbiologically safe foods (25). However, L. monocytogenes is a widely distributed environmental pathogen and may not be eradicated from all food items. Therefore consumers should generally be informed about the constant risk connected with eating potentially contaminated foods, about hygiene and cross-contamination, and that refrigerator temperature can only delay growth of L. monocytogenes. The immense importance of predisposing immunodeficiencies was confirmed by our calculations of risk levels for different conditions. Therefore persons with a high risk of listeriosis should be individually informed about food hygiene and risk foods.

It was indicated that one-third of sporadic listeriosis cases in Denmark were nosocomial (defined as isolation of listeria >3 days after admission). In Barcelona, as many as 42% of listeriosis cases were nosocomial (defined as isolation of listeria 10–51 days after admission) (26). Nosocomial sources may be difficult to identify, because it can be assumed that a low grade of contamination is enough to make weakened patients ill. Therefore hospital kitchens preparing food for immunocompromised persons should be highly aware of safe cooking and hygiene – and not only for the sake of the rare listeria-disease, but also because of other pathogenic food-borne microorganisms.

REFERENCES

1. WHO Working Group. Foodborne listeriosis. Bull World Health Organ 66: 421–428, 1988.
2. Farber JM, Peterkin PI. Listeria monocytogenes, a food-borne pathogen. Microbiol Rev 9: 476–511, 1991.
3. Schuchat A, Deaver KA, Wenger JD, Plikaytis BD, Mascola L, Pinner RW, Reingold AL, Broome CV, and the Listeria Study Group. Role of foods in sporadic listeriosis. JAMA 267: 2041–2045, 1992.
4. Samuelsson S, Rothgardt NP, Carvajal A, Frederiksen W. Human listeriosis in Denmark 1981–1987 including an outbreak November 1985–March 1987. J Infect 20: 251–259, 1990.
5. Rocourt J, Jacquet C. Listeria – listeriosis. 1989–1990 List of references. WHO Collaborating Centre for Foodborne Listeriosis, 1–78, September 1991.
6. Carvajal A, Samuelsson S, Rothgardt NP, Frederiksen W. The treatment of Listeria monocytogenes infections in the central nervous system. Acta Microbiol Hung 36: 159–163, 1989.
7. Jurado RL, Farley MM, Pereira E, Harvey RC, Schuchat A, Wenger JD, Stephens DS. Increased risk of meningitis and bacteremia due to Listeria monocytogenes in patients with human immunodeficiency virus infection. Clin Infect Dis 17: 224–227, 1993.

8. Frederiksen B, Samuelsson S. Feto-maternal listeriosis in Denmark 1981–1988. J Infect 24: 277–287, 1992.
9. Potter ME, Kaufmann AF, Blake PA, Feldman RA. Unpasteurized milk. JAMA 252: 2048–2052, 1984.
10. Fleming DW, Cochi SL, MacDonald KL, Brondum J, Hayes PS, Plikaytis BD, Holmes MB, Audurier A, Broome CV, Reingold AL. Pasteurized milk as a vehicle of infection in an outbreak of listeriosis. N Engl J Med 312: 404–407, 1985.
11. Linnan MJ, Mascola L, Lou XD, Goulet V, May S, Salminen C, Hird DW, Yonekura ML, Hayes P, Weaver R, Audurier A, Plikaytis BD, Fannin SL, Kleks A, Broome CV. Epidemic listeriosis associated with Mexican-style cheese. N Engl J Med 319: 823–828, 1988.
12. McLauchlin J, Hall SM, Velani SK, Gilbert RJ. Human listeriosis and paté: a possible association. BMJ 303: 773–775, 1991.
13. Kittson E. A case cluster of listeriosis in Western Australia with links to paté consumption. Eleventh International Symposium on Problems of Listeriosis. 11–14 May, 1992: Abstr. 18.
14. Bille J. Epidemiology of human listeriosis in Europe, with special reference to the Swiss outbreak. In: Miller AJ, Smith JL, Somkuti GA, eds. Foodborne listeriosis. Society for Industrial Microbiology, 71–74, 1990.
15. Goulet V, Lepoutre A, Rocourt J, Courtieu AL, Dehaumont P, Veit P. Épidémie de listériose en France. Bull Epidemiol Hebd 4: 13–14, 1993.
16. Mascola L, Sorvillo F, Goulet V, Hall B, Weaver R, Linnan M. Fecal carriage of Listeria monocytogenes – Observations during a community-wide, common-source outbreak. Clin Infect Dis 15: 557–558, 1992.
17. Jensen A. Excretion of Listeria monocytogenes in faeces after listeriosis: rate, quantity and duration. Med Microbiol Lett 2: 176–182, 1993.
18. Schuchat A, Deaver K, Hayes PS, Graves L, Mascola L, Wenger JD. Gastrointestinal carriage of Listeria monocytogenes in household contacts of patients with listeriosis. J Infect Dis 167: 1261–1262, 1993.
19. Schlech WF, Lavigne PM, Bortolussi RA, Allen AC, Haldane EV, Worth AJ, Hightower AW, Johnson SE, King HS, Nicholls ES, Broome CV. Epidemic listeriosis – evidence for transmission by food. N Engl J Med 308: 203–206, 1983.
20. Kerr KG, Dealler SF, Lacey RW. Materno-fetal listeriosis from cook-chill and refrigerated food. Lancet ii: 1133, 1988.
21. Junttila J, Brander M. Listeria monocytogenes septicemia associated with consumption of salted mushrooms. Scand J Infect Dis 21: 339–342, 1989.
22. Facinelli B, Varaldo PE. Ignorance about listeria. BMJ 299: 738, 1989.
23. Azadian BS, Finnerty GT. Cheese-borne listeria meningitis in immunocompetent patient. Lancet i: 322–323, 1989.
24. Farber JM, Daley E, Coates F, Beausoleil N, Fournier J. Feeding trials of Listeria monocytogenes with a non-human primate model. J Clin Microbiol 29: 2606–2608, 1991.
25. Anonymous. Listeria monocytogenes. Recommendations by The National Advisory Committee on Microbiological Criteria for Foods. Int J Food Microbiol 14: 185–246, 1991.
26. Nolla-Salas J, Antó JM, Almela M, Coll P, Gasser I, Plasencia A, and the Collaboratory Study Group of Listeriosis of Barcelona. Eur J Clin Microbiol Infect Dis 12: 157–161, 1993.

Scand J Infect Dis 26: 179–187, 1994

Chlamydia Pneumoniae (TWAR): a common agent in acute bronchitis

GÖRAN FALCK[1], LENA HEYMAN[2], JUDY GNARPE[3] and HÅKAN GNARPE[3]

From the [1]Department of Family Medicine, University Hospital, Uppsala, the [2]Community Health Centre Solsidan, Ludvika and the [3]Department of Clinical Microbiology, Gävle Central Hospital, Gävle, Sweden

Patients seeking medical attention for respiratory infections were investigated with serology and culture for Chlamydia pneumoniae to investigate the prevalence of C. pneumoniae in a specific geographical area and its association with respiratory disease. Evidence for C. pneumoniae infection was found in approximately 25% of cases. 71% of patients with C. pneumoniae had symptoms from the lower respiratory tract as compared to 29% of the others. We conclude that C. pneumoniae can be a major cause of acute bronchitis.

G. Falck, MD, Apoteksgårdens Vårdcentrum, S-714 22 Kopparberg, Sweden

INTRODUCTION

In Sweden, acute bronchitis is generally regarded to be a result of viral infection. There is no consensus about antibiotic treatment (1), however, symptomatic treatment is recommended (2). Despite this recommendation, antibiotic treatment was given to 63% of patients with bronchitis in Sweden during 1991 (3).

Antibiotics are usually prescribed before the etiologic agent is known. The choice of drug has therefore to be based on epidemiological data of the prevalences of different etiological agents in acute bronchitis. These data are most often based on empirical studies of the etiology of community acquired pneumonia. It is therefore important to have accurate information on the prevalence of different infectious agents. Interest has earlier been focused on Mycoplasma pneumoniae because of its periodical appearance (4). In the past year, increased attention has been focused on Chlamydia pneumoniae (TWAR) as a common cause of acute bronchitis (5).

In the summer of 1992, the possible association of C. pneumoniae with unexpected sudden death among elite orienteers was reported (6). This has not yet been proven. Seven of the last 8 orienteers who died were found to have geographical connections with an area in the mid part of Sweden. In addition to this, the sudden death of a 16-year-old girl while jogging in November 1992 focused interest on the geographical area in which we based our investigation.

The objective of the study was to investigate the prevalence of infections associated with C. pneumoniae in a clinical material from this same geographical area during the fall of 1992.

MATERIALS AND METHODS

Patient population

Inclusion criteria were: consecutive patients older than 10 years seeking medical attention for respiratory infections with symptoms of at least 1 week's duration at 2 community health centres during October through December 1992. The investigation was extended to an additional 3 health centres during a couple of weeks in late November/early December 1992. During this period 96 patients were included. A total of 158 patients were initially enrolled, but 30 did not meet the inclusion criteria (no ongoing infection, seeking medical attention because of general anxiety) and another 14 did not appear for reexamination.

 ISSN 0036-5548

114 patients examined on 2 occasions remained, 53 men and 61 women. The mean and median ages were 31.5 and 36, and 26 and 34 years for men and women, respectively, ranges were 12–65 and 14–82 years.

Clinical investigation

A thorough history was obtained at inclusion. Patients with presumed bacterial infections were given antibiotic treatment.

A specimen for culture of C. pneumoniae was taken with ENT swab from the tonsil area and from tonsillar crypts, if present, from 101 of the patients (88.6%). The swab was immersed in 2SP medium and kept at +4°C, then sent to the Department of Clinical Microbiology at the Gävle Central Hospital (a distance of 150 km). The time interval between collection of specimens and their arrival at the laboratory varied between 18–28 h. All specimens were frozen at −70°C on arrival at the laboratory. Cultures for M. pneumoniae were not done.

A serum specimen was taken for serological investigations of C. pneumoniae and M. pneumoniae antibodies at inclusion. A second specimen was obtained after 4–16 (usually 8–12, mean 9) weeks. At the same time a second specimen for culture was taken from 84 of the patients (73.7%), this time from the back of the throat.

Microbiology

All specimens for culture were cultured in HL (human lung) cells for 72 h according to an earlier described procedure (7, 8) and stained with monoclonal antibodies to chlamydial lipopolysaccharide (Pathfinder, Kallestad) and with monoclonal antibodies specific for C. pneumoniae, kindly donated by Dr Kenneth Persson, Malmö, Sweden.

Chlamydia serology

All sera were investigated for presence of IgG, IgM and IgA antibodies to Chlamydia species using egg-cultured elementary bodies from C. trachomatis, serovars D-K, C. psittaci and C. pneumoniae, strain IOL 207, as antigens. All sera initially positive in a screening test for IgM were retitrated after absorption with Protein A Sepharose (CL-4B, Pharmacia, Uppsala, Sweden). All sera were incubated with antigen overnight at 4°C and then incubated with antihuman antibody to IgG, IgM or IgA (Dakopatts A/S, Denmark) for 30 min. The microimmunofluorescence determinations were read in a Zeiss UV microscope at ×400 with oil immersion by 2 experienced microbiologists.

Isolated IgM titers of ≥16, IgG titers of ≥1024, or a 4-fold change in titer of IgG, IgM or IgA were considered to be indicators of recent infection with C. pneumoniae.

Mycoplasma pneumoniae serology

All sera were tested for antibodies to M. pneumoniae by use of a latex agglutination test, Serodia Myco II[9] (Fujibio Diagnostics). A 4-fold change in titer or titers of ≥1024 were considered as indication of recent infection. Serologic investigations regarding a possible viral etiology were not done due to economic considerations.

RESULTS

A majority of the 114 included patients had an acute onset of disease but several had persisting symptoms for 1–12 weeks before inclusion. Four of the patients (no. 1, 4, 28, 81) had earlier visited the clinic for the same symptoms and were regarded as relapses at the time of inclusion.

70 patients (61%) had specific IgG titers of ≥64 to C. pneumoniae indicating earlier exposure. 72% (38/53) of men and 52% of women had IgG (Fig. 1). 48 (42%) of the patients had specific IgA titers of ≥16 to C. pneumoniae (males 45%, females 39%) (Fig. 2).

IgG antibodies were both more prevalent and found in higher titers in men, especially in younger age groups (Fig. 1). IgA antibodies were also found more often in men than in women (Fig. 2). Men had higher geometric mean titers (GMT) than women, which was most notable under the age of 20 (Fig. 3).

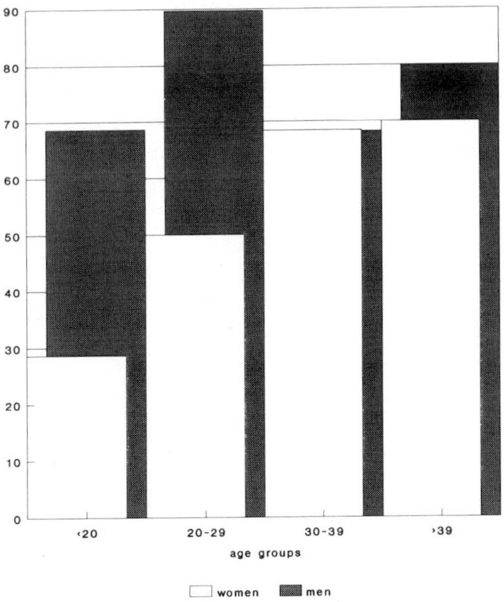

Fig. 1. Percentage of patients with specific IgG antibodies (≥ 64) to C. pneumoniae related to age and sex.

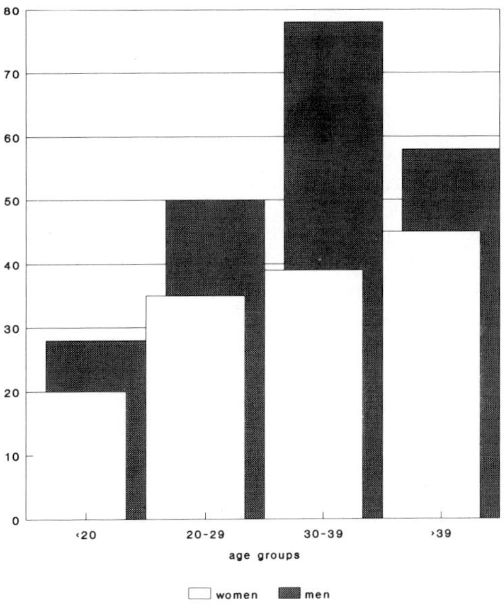

Fig. 2. Percentage patients with specific IgA antibodies (≥ 16) to C. pneumoniae related to age and sex.

11 patients (10%) had a 4-fold change in antibody titers to C. pneumoniae; 7 (7%) for IgG antibodies and 4 (4%) for IgA. Isolated IgM antibodies were found in 8 patients (7%), 6 of whom were women, and IgG titers of ≥ 1024 were found in 9 patients (8%) (Table I). A number of additional patients were found to have IgG titers of 512 and were most likely infected with C. pneumoniae according to their clinical histories and serologically verified infections in other family members.

Serological indications of M. pneumoniae infection were found in 2 patients, neither of whom had antibodies to C. pneumoniae.

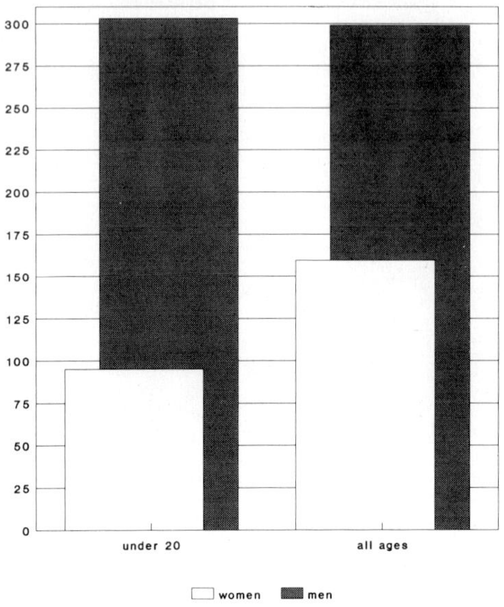

Fig. 3. Geometric mean titers of specific IgG antibodies in men and women to C. pneumoniae related to sex.

Table I. *Clinical and serological findings in patients with C. pneumoniae infection*
NS = no symptoms

Patient no.	Sex/age	Time interval[a]	Diagnosis[b]	Chlamydia pneumoniae inverted titer (MIF) IgG	IgM	IgA	Treatment given
Confirmed C. pneumoniae infection; 4-fold IgG rise or IgM ≥ 16							
1	F/71	2	pneumonia	1024	64	128	doxycycline clarithromycin
		12	NS	2048	0	128	
9	M/50	8	pharyngitis	512	16	0	doxycycline
		17	NS	512	0	16	
11	M/64	8	bronchitis+	0	0	64	doxycycline
		17	cor incomp.	64	0	16	
28	F/47	9	bronchitis	16384	16	128	doxycycline clarithromycin
		19	NS	2048	0	32	
29	F/41	8	sinusitis	512	16	32	doxycycline
		17	NS	1024	0	16	
37	M/18	3	bronchitis	512	0	16	erythromycin
		13	NS	128	0	0	
52	F/40	4	bronchitis	512	16	0	none
		10	NS	256	0	0	
58	F/69	4	bronchitis	0	0	0	doxycycline
		13	dyspnoa	64	0	0	
63	F/17	4	bronchitis	0	32	0	erythromycin
		8	NS	0	0	0	
82	F/76	48	bronchitis	512	64	64	doxycycline clarithromycin
		60	NS	512	0	32	

Table I (continued)

Patient no.	Sex/age	Time interval[a]	Diagnosis[b]	Chlamydia pneumoniae inverted titer (MIF) IgG	IgM	IgA	Treatment given
Confirmed C. pneumoniae infection; 4-fold IgG rise or IgM ≥ 16							
90	M/20	3	bronchitis	32	0	0	none
		13	NS	128	0	0	
100	F/32	3	sinusitis	32	0	0	doxycycline
		10	NS	1024	0	0	
101	F/16	1	pharyngitis	64	0	16	none
		12	NS	256	0	16	
106	M/25	2	pharyngitis	0	0	0	erythromycin
		15	NS	64	0	16	
154	M/64	2	bronchitis	1024	0	128	erythromycin
		10	NS	1024	32	64	
Probable C. pneumoniae infection; 4-fold IgA titer change							
4	F/58	24	bronchitis	1024	0	64	doxycycline clarithromycin
		37	NS	2048	0	256	
15	M/32	8	bronchitis	256	0	64	doxycycline
		11	NS	128	0	16	
19	F/54	4	bronchitis	512	0	64	doxycycline
		16	NS	512	0	16	
69	F/21	6	bronchitis	512	0	32	doxycycline
		16	NS	512	0	0	
Probable C. pneumoniae infection; IgG ≥ 1024 and simultaneous IgA ≥ 16							
3	F/34	4	pharyngitis	512	0	128	doxycycline
		11	NS	1024	0	64	
10	F/16	8	bronchitis	1024	0	64	doxycycline
		19	NS	1024	0	32	
61	M/20	4	bronchitis	512	0	128	erythromycin
		18	NS	1024	0	128	
71	M/26	12	bronchitis	1024	0	0	none
		23	NS	1024	0	16	
118	M/11	3	bronchitis	2048	0	16	erythromycin
		8	NS	2048	0	16	
132	F/33	4	rhinitis	1024	0	32	none
		13	NS	1024	0	32	
140	F/27	3	pharyngitis	1024	0	16	doxycycline
		8	rhinitis	1024	0	0	
150	M/17	3	bronchitis	1024	0	128	doxycycline
		10	NS	1024	0	64	
161	F/37	4	bronchitis	1024	0	16	doxycycline
		12	NS	1024	0	16	

[a] Time interval in weeks after onset.

[b] Dominating symptom/complaint at time of examination.

One patient was positive in culture at inclusion (1.0%), and 3 (3.6%) at the second examination. Two of these 4 had a clinical relapse a couple of weeks before the second culture was obtained. One additional patient (patient 79) was culture positive on reexamination. He is presented as a representative case although he did not meet the inclusion criteria (Table II).

Three patients with serological evidence of C. pneumoniae infection (patients no. 1, 4, 11) required hospitalization. None of the other patients were hospitalized during the observation period. No specific symptom signifying infection with C. pneumoniae could be defined, however, 71% of the patients with serologic evidence of C. pneumoniae infection had symptoms from the lower respiratory tract as compared to 29% of the other patients.

86% of the patients with serologic evidence of C. pneumoniae infection (24 patients) had been given antibiotics: 18 had been given doxycycline, 4 of them clarithromycin, and 6 erythromycin. Four of the patients (14%) received no antibiotic treatment.

62% of the remaining patients had been treated with antibiotics, 10 with phenoxymethyl penicillin, 26 with doxycycline, 13 with erythromycin and 1 each tetracycline and clarithromycin. 31 patients did not receive antibiotics. In 4 patients there was no information about antibiotic prescriptions.

Three individual cases are presented below. One (case 28) is described because of a long persistence of symptoms in spite of repeated antibiotic treatments; another (case 79) because of relatively mild symptoms with positive culture, and a third (case 132) with influenza following a C. pneumoniae infection.

Table II. *Patients with positive culture for C. pneumoniae. Clinical and serological data*

NS = no symptoms

Patient no.	Sex/age	Time interval[a]	Diagnosis[b]	Result of culture	Chlamydia pneumoniae IgG	IgM	IgA	Treatment given
23	F/26	4	pharyngitis	–	0	0	0	doxycycline
		10	NS	+	0	0	0	none
		14	NS	–	0	0	0	none
40	M/25	1	pharyngitis increased transaminases	+	64	0	0	erythromycin
		4	NS	–	128	0	0	none
		10	NS	–	128	0	0	none
79	M/17	6	conjunctivitis	–	128	0	0	none
		16	rhinitis	+	256	0	0	none
		22	NS	–	64	0	0	none
83	F/31	1	rhinitis	–	64	0	0	none
		11	bronchitis	+	64	0	0	none
		15	NS	–	128	0	16	none
132	F/33	4	rhinitis	–	1024	0	32	none
		13	Influenza	+	1024	0	32	doxycycline
		17	NS	–	1024	0	32	none

[a] Time interval in weeks after onset.

[b] Dominating symptom/complaint at time of examination.

CASE REPORTS

Case 28

A 47-year-old woman, a smoker with a history of repeated respiratory infections, came to the outpatient clinic in the midst of October 1992 with a recent history of increasing hoarseness and coughing for 5 weeks. She had pharyngitis and some ronchi at examination. She was given doxycycline 100 mg × 1 for 14 days. She returned in early November. After an initial improvement during treatment, symptoms had reappeared with increased signs of obstruction and productive coughing. Pharyngitis and basal ronchi on both sides were found on examination. Peak Expiratory Flow (PEF) was 350 l/min, the leukocyte count was 4.9×10^9/l and the ESR was 8 mm/h. Chest X-ray was normal. The patient was given doxycycline 100 mg × 2 for another 10 days. After an initial improvement at the beginning of the treatment she experienced increasing hoarseness. The findings at examination were unchanged: swollen vocal cords on examination. Serological examination showed an IgG titer of 16,384, IgM of 16 and IgA of 128, to C. pneumoniae. The patient was again treated with doxycycline, 100 mg × 2 for 3 weeks along with inhalation steroids.

10 days after the end of this antibiotic treatment the patient had a clinical relapse with symptoms of bronchitis. She was then given clarithromycin, 250 mg × 2 for 14 days. At reexamination in the beginning of February, there were no signs of infection, however there were remaining signs of obstruction, and the PEF was 380 l/min. The patient was advised to continue with inhalation steroids. Serological investigation of the second serum specimen showed IgG titer of 2048, IgM < 16 and IgA of 32.

Case 79

A 17-year-old man, member of a team of bandy players, which had an increased number of respiratory infections during the fall of 1992, fell ill with ear ache and a sore throat in mid-October. Several of the other players had had temporary periods of chest pains and 1 had been hospitalized for suspected myocarditis. Specimens for C. pneumoniae culture and blood for serology were taken when the whole team was examined in the end of November. At this time the patient had mild conjunctivitis of the left eye but was otherwise without symptoms or signs of disease. He became ill 1 week before reexamination in early February with rhinitis and a sore throat of 4 days duration. No further symptoms developed and he was not given antibiotic treatment. Serological examinations showed an IgG titer of 128 increasing to 256 before finally falling to 64. Culture for C. pneumoniae was positive at the second examination (Table II).

Case 132

A 33-year-old male who was an active orienteer, had purulent rhinitis and pharyngitis, and frontal headache 1 month before the first examination in the beginning of December. The pharynx had a granular appearance at examination, otherwise there were no abnormal findings. Antibiotics were not given. The patient was reexamined in the beginning of February and was at that time healthy. He became ill again in mid February with symptoms of fever, headache and coughing with signs of obstruction. He was treated with doxycycline 100 mg × 2 for 2 weeks and was subjectively free of symptoms and signs at reexamination 1 month later. Antibody titrations showed on all 3 occasions IgG titer of 1024, IgM < 16 and IgA of 32. Culture for C. pneumoniae was positive on the second occasion. Serological examination revealed that the last infection was caused by influenzae B virus.

DISCUSSION

The high prevalence of patients with specific antibodies to C. pneumoniae suggests that C. pneumoniae may be endemic in the area (10). This is supported by similar findings in an adjacent county (11). We have earlier found a difference in teenage males and females (12) as well as in healthy blood donors (11). The findings of this investigation are in agreement as males, particularly young males, had antibodies of both IgG and IgA classes in higher titers than females. 75% of the patients with IgM antibodies were females. This may suggest that the females with IgM had their first infection with the organism whilst most males were reinfected.

Saikku and coworkers (13) have interpreted IgA antibodies as a sign of persistent or chronic infection. We found that IgA antibodies disappeared along with the clinical improvement seen after antibiotic treatment at a more rapid rate than IgG antibodies in this patient material. These patients are being followed for 1 year.

In an area with a high prevalence of C. pneumoniae a large number of persons have antibodies due to earlier exposures, and there may also be a number of subjectively healthy carriers (8). IgG antibodies may remain elevated for a considerable time. It is therefore difficult to conclude anything regarding recent exposure using IgG antibody levels as an indicator. The choice of a cut off value as an indication of recent infection has to be arbitrary and dependent on the epidemiological situation as well as the technique used for determination. Grayston and coworkers have suggested ≥ 512 (5). We have seen a number of patients with a persisting IgG titer of 512 for more than 1 year without signs and symptoms of disease. We therefore decided to use 1024 as the breakpoint to indicate recent infection. This was supported by the fact that all 9 patients with high IgG also had IgA antibodies and 1 of them was positive in culture (case 132). These findings agree with those of Chirgwin et al. in a study from Brooklyn (14). The low number of positive cultures in our investigation may be due to losses in viability during transportation and to the fact that the initial specimens for culture were taken from the tonsils. Like Chirgwin, we found a patient (case 23) with positive culture and clinical signs who did not develop an antibody response. One possible explanation may be asymptomatic carriage of C. pneumoniae (11, 15) and that the symptoms were due to other etiologic agents or that the immunologic stimulation was too small to stimulate an antibody response (16), although this seems less likely. It is also possible that the antibiotic treatment given may have suppressed the antibody response (17).

The prevalences of M. pneumoniae and C. pneumoniae vary in different studies depending on the epidemiological situation and the laboratory techniques used. The results of this investigation suggest that C. pneumoniae was a likely cause of infection in approximately 20% of cases if patients with relapses were excluded whilst M. pneumoniae may have been associated with the disease in at most 2% of cases. This is an agreement with our earlier finding that C. pneumoniae is one of the most common causes of community acquired pneumonia in our area (18). Our findings here suggest that C. pneumoniae is important as an etiologic agent in respiratory tract infections other than pneumonia.

This investigation was not designed as a study of treatment efficacy, however, some observations were made. There was most likely a temporary shift in the prescription pattern of antibiotics during the time of this investigation. This was caused by the suspected association between C. pneumoniae and sudden death in young individuals. Four patients regarded as experiencing a relapse of C. pneumoniae infection were only temporarily improved by doxycycline in spite of extended treatment periods (e.g. case 28). This is in agreement with the observations of Hammerschlag et al. (17).

Our findings demonstrate the need of a continuous surveillance of the spectrum of causative agents in lower respiratory tract infections as a base for choice of antibiotic preparation for treatment.

ACKNOWLEDGEMENTS

This investigation was supported by grants from Dalarna Research Institute, Gävleborgs läns Research and Developmental Fund and by a special grant from the Swedish Government.

REFERENCES

1. Howie JGR, Richardson IM, Gill G, Durno D. Respiratory illness and antibiotic use in general practice. J R Coll Gen Pract 21: 657–663, 1971.
2. Strandberg K, Veerman B, Lönnerholm G, eds. Pharmacotherapy in lower respiratory tract infections. Uppsala: Medical Products Agency, 2: 119–131, 1991.

3. Nordenstam I, Wennberg M, Kristoferson K. Swedish statistics on medicines 1991 (Svensk Läkemedelsstatistik). Stockholm: Apoteksbolaget, 1992.
4. Mycoplasma pneumoniae (Editorial). Lancet 337: 651–652, 1991.
5. Grayston JT, Campbell LA, Kuo CC, Mordhorst CH, Saikku P, Thom DH, Wang SP. A new respiratory tract pathogen: Chlamydia pneumoniae strain TWAR. J Infect Dis 161: 618–625, 1990.
6. Wesslén L, Påhlson C, Friman G, Fohlman J, Lindquist O, Johansson C. Myocarditis caused by Chlamydia pneumoniae (TWAR) and sudden unexpected death in a Swedish elite orienteer. Lancet 340: 427–428, 1992.
7. Cles LD, Stamm WE. Use of HL cells for improved isolation and passage of Chlamydia pneumoniae. J Clin Microbiol 28: 938–940, 1990.
8. Gnarpe J, Gnarpe H, Sundelöf B. Endemic prevalence of Chlamydia pneumoniae in subjectively healthy persons. Scand J Infect Dis 23: 387–388, 1991.
9. Gnarpe J, Lundbäck A, Sundelöf B, Gnarpe H. Prevalence of Mycoplasma pneumoniae in subjectively healthy individuals. Scand J Infect Dis 24: 161–164, 1992.
10. Saikku P. The epidemiology and significance of Chlamydia pneumoniae. J Infect Suppl 1: 27–34, 1992.
11. Gnarpe H, Gnarpe J. Increasing prevalence of specific antibodies to Chlamydia pneumoniae in Sweden. Lancet 341: 381, 1993.
12. Gnarpe H, Gnarpe J, Unge P, Sundelöf B. Chlamydia pneumoniae in acute myocardial infarction in Sweden 1989. In: Mårdh PA, Saikku P, eds. Chlamydial Infections of the Genital and Respiratory Tracts and Allied Conditions. Uppsala: Centre for STD Research, 84–90, 1991.
13. Saikku P, Leinonen M, Tenkanen L, Linnanmäki E, Ekman MR, Manninen V, Mänttäri M, Frick MH, Huttunen JK. Chronic Chlamydia pneumoniae infection as a risk factor for coronary heart disease in the Helsinki heart study. Ann Intern Med 116: 273–278, 1992.
14. Chirgwin K, Roblin PM, Gelling M, Hammerschlag MR, Schachter J. Infection with Chlamydia pneumoniae in Brooklyn. J Infect Dis 163: 757–761, 1991.
15. Hyman CL, Augenbraun MH, Roblin PM, Schachter J, Hammerschlag MR. Asymptomatic respiratory tract infection with Chlamydia pneumoniae TWAR. J Clin Microbiol 29: 2082–2083, 1991.
16. Berdal BP, Scheel O, Ögaard AR, Hoel T, Gutteberg TJ, Ånestad G. Spread of subclinical Chlamydia pneumoniae infection in a closed community. Scand J Infect Dis 24: 431–436, 1992.
17. Hammerschlag MR, Chirgwin K, Roblin PM, Dumornay W, Mandel L, Smith P, Schachter J. Persistent infection with Chlamydia pneumoniae following acute respiratory illness. Clin Infect Dis 14: 178–182, 1992.
18. Sundelöf, B, Gnarpe J, Gnarpe H, Darougar S. Chlamydia pneumoniae pneumonia in Sweden. In: Bowie WR, Caldwell HD, Jones RP, Mårdh PA, Ridgway GL, Schachter J, Stamm WE, Ward ME, eds. Chlamydial infections. Cambridge University Press, 426–428, 1990.

Scand J Infect Dis 26: 191–197, 1994

Effect of Loracarbef and Amoxicillin on the Oropharyngeal and Intestinal Microflora of Patients with Bronchitis

MARIANNE FLOOR[1,2], FRANK VAN AKKEREN[3], MAJA ROZENBERG-ARSKA[1], MAARTEN VISSER[1], AD KOLSTERS[1,2], HENRIËTTE BEUMER[1,2] and JAN VERHOEF[1]

From the [1]Eykman-Winkler Institute, University Hospital Utrecht, [2]U-Gene Research, Utrecht, and [3]General Practice, Amsterdam, The Netherlands

The effect on the oropharyngeal and intestinal microflora and the efficacy and tolerance of loracarbef (200 mg b.i.d. for 7 days) versus amoxicillin (500 mg t.i.d. for 7 days) were compared in 80 patients with bronchitis. The oropharyngeal samples of 18% of patients in the amoxicillin group and 5% of patients in the loracarbef group revealed a new Gram-negative species around days 8–10. The presence of other aerobic bacteria than found at baseline in the faeces occurred in 38% of patients treated with amoxicillin compared with 31% in the loracarbef group on days 8–10. After treatment, no loracarbef- or amoxicillin-resistant aerobic Gram-negative bacteria were found in faecal samples in the loracarbef group, while amoxicillin- or loracarbef-resistant (E. coli) strains appeared in 35% of patients receiving amoxicillin ($p < 0.001$). Treatment success occurred by days 8–10 in all 40 patients receiving loracarbef, compared with 90% in the amoxicillin group, on days 21–28, in 93% and 90% respectively. The results of this study indicate that the use of loracarbef leads to minor changes in the normal oropharyngeal and intestinal microflora compared with amoxicillin, while almost no resistant Gram-negative bacteria emerge after treatment with loracarbef.

M. Floor, MD, U-Gene Research, Bolognalaan 40, 3584 CJ Utrecht, The Netherlands

INTRODUCTION

Respiratory tract infections are the most common infections encountered in general medical practice. Antibiotics are commonly prescribed for such conditions. A negative effect of the administration of antibiotics can be changes in the endogenous oropharyngeal and intestinal flora. When the number of microorganisms diminishes as a result of antimicrobial therapy, overgrowth of bacteria already present and colonization with potentially pathogenic microorganisms can occur. The use of antibiotics can also promote the development of antimicrobial resistance and spread of these resistant bacteria into the environment.

Treatment with antibiotics is a frequent cause of diarrhea, reported in up to 25% of patients taking antibiotics (1). C. difficile – and/or its toxins – is found in about half of all hospitalized patients with antibiotic-associated diarrhea (2); the incidence in outpatients is uncertain.

Loracarbef, an agent of the carbacephem class of β-lactam antibiotics, is highly effective against the common respiratory tract pathogens and has a good safety profile. The results of clinical studies indicate that loracarbef is effective and safe in the treatment of acute bronchitis or exacerbations of chronic bronchitis (3, 4). Approximately 90% of loracarbef is absorbed from the gastrointestinal tract after oral administration and the kidney is the major route of elimination. In healthy volunteers, loracarbef caused minor changes in both the oropharyngeal and the intestinal microflora (5).

The purpose of the present study was to investigate in patients with bronchitis the effect on the oropharyngeal and intestinal microflora of loracarbef, as well as of amoxicillin, a commonly prescribed drug in general practice. In addition the efficacy and tolerance of both drugs was studied.

PATIENTS AND METHODS

Patients and drug administration

80 outpatients >18 years with either acute bronchitis or an acute exacerbation of chronic bronchitis and the presence of purulent sputum were enrolled in this study. Chronic bronchitis was defined according to the American Thoracic Society statement as being a chronic or recurrent productive cough present on most days for a minimum of 3 months a year and for at least 2 successive years. An acute exacerbation was defined in terms of symptoms and levels of severity (type 1 the most severe level) described by Anthonisen et al. (6). Patients were recruited from 9 general practitioners in The Netherlands.

In this double-blind study, patients were randomized to receive either loracarbef at a dosage of 200 mg twice daily for 7 days or amoxicillin at a dosage of 500 mg (two 250 mg capsules) 3 times daily for 7 days. Each patient received 6 capsules/day (2 loracarbef capsules plus 4 capsules of placebo or 6 amoxicillin capsules). The randomization was done by Eli Lilly Company in blocks of 4 patients.

Patients with the following conditions were excluded from the study: pregnancy or lactation; hypersensitivity to cephalosporins or penicillins; any condition, including significant underlying or concomitant disease, that, in the opinion of the investigator, could preclude evaluation of response; treatment with any experimental drug during, or within 28 days prior to this study; concurrent antimicrobial therapy or antimicrobial therapy within 4 weeks preceding the pre-therapy evaluations; inability of patients to return for follow-up examinations; earlier inclusion in the present study; known impaired liver- or renal function as determined by elevation in any liver function test more than 3× the upper limit of normal or serum creatinine >220 μmol/l; diarrhea (≥3 watery stools/24 h) within 14 days prior to this study; concomitant therapy with anti-secretory drugs (e.g. H2-antagonists) and/or antacids. The study protocol was approved by the Medical Ethics Committee of the University Hospital, Utrecht. Informed consent was obtained from all patients.

Procedures

Each patient was clinically examined 3 times: before treatment, between days 8 and 10 and days 21 to 28. At the same time oropharyngeal and faecal samples were collected. A sputum sample was collected at the first visit and at the 2 post-treatment visits if the patient was able to produce sputum. The second and third visit included monitoring of possible side effects of the used drug. The patient received a diary in which to record any stool characteristics and side effects.

Microbiological procedures

Oropharyngeal cultures were obtained by gargling 10 ml of 0.9% NaCl solution in the mouth for 10 sec and collecting this rinsing fluid in a sterile, calibrated tube. The tube was stored at 4°C for a maximum of 24 h. Counting of bacteria was done using CLED/MacConkey dipslides (Orion Diagnostica, Espoo, Finland). Pathogens were identified using standard laboratory procedures. Faecal specimens (±1 g) were collected in a transport medium containing cysteine peptone and yeast extract and stored at 4°C for a maximum of 24 h. After homogenization, 20-fold serial dilutions were made in cysteine peptone broth. Samples of selected dilutions were plated on different media for aerobic and anaerobic culture. For the isolation and counting of anaerobic bacteria, Reinforced Clostridial Agar (Oxoid, Basingstoke, Hants, England) and Clostridium Difficile Agar (Oxoid) were used. All stool specimens were tested for the presence of C. difficile toxin in a cytotoxin assay with monkey kidney cells (Vero cells). For the isolation and counting of aerobic bacteria the dilutions were subcultured on MacConkey agar (Oxoid), selective for Gram-negative rods, blood agar for staphylococci, Bile Esculine and Salt Tolerance agar (Difco, Detroit, MI, USA) for enterococci and Sabouraud and dextrose agar (Merck, Darmstadt, Germany) selective for yeasts. Identification of Enterobacteriaceae was done using Enterotube II (Hoffmann-La Roche, Basle, Switzerland) and of non-fermenters using Oxifermtube (Hoffmann-La Roche). S. aureus was determined by DNase and coagulase assays and enterococci by growth on Bile Esculine agar and tolerance to salt. The lowest detectable number of bacteria with the methods used was 2.0 $\log_{10}$ cfu/g of faeces.

A Gram stain from each sputum sample was examined to determine the number of leukocytes and epithelial cells. A sputum sample was considered reliable for culture if it contained <10 epithelial cells and ≥25 polymorphonuclear leukocytes/low-power microscopic field. Microorganisms were isolated and identified according to standard bacteriological methods. The antibiotic susceptibility for loracarbef and amoxicillin was determined for all pathogens isolated from the sputum samples and for the aerobic Gram-negative rods isolated from the oropharyngeal and faecal specimens. The susceptibility was determined by agar diffusion by standard methods (7), using loracarbef (30 μg) and amoxicillin (10 μg) discs (Oxoid). Bacterial isolates were regarded as sensitive to loracarbef if the inhibition zone was

≥ 18 mm. Isolates were considered sensitive to amoxicillin if the inhibition zone was ≥ 29 mm for staphylococci and non-enterococcal streptococci, ≥ 20 mm for H. influenzae and M. catarrhalis and ≥ 14 mm for enteric Gram-negative bacteria.

Evaluation

The second oropharyngeal samples were evaluated for the colonization by other aerobic species than found in the baseline samples and the emergence of resistant Gram-negative rods. The faecal samples were evaluated for changes in the total numbers of aerobic and anaerobic bacteria in the follow-up samples, compared with the baseline samples, for the emergence of resistant Gram-negative rods, for the isolation of increased numbers of enterococci and yeasts and for the emergence of C. difficile and/or C. difficile toxin in the follow-up samples.

Diarrhea was defined as the occurrence of ≥ 3 watery stools/24 h. The occurrence of 1–2 watery stools/24 h or ≥ 3 loose stools/24 h was called 'loose stools'.

Clinical response to therapy was assessed at the 2 post-treatment visits and defined as follows: cure was defined as the elimination of signs and symptoms of infection with no recurrence in the post-therapy period; improvement was defined as the significant but incomplete resolution of signs and symptoms of infection; failure was defined as signs and symptoms not subsiding or improving during therapy.

All data was analysed with SPSS/PC+ Version 4.0.1 (SPSS Inc., Chicago, IL, USA) using the paired t-test for comparison of numbers of bacteria isolated in the quantitative faecal cultures and the χ^2-test. Statistical significance was assumed at $p < 0.05$.

RESULTS

All 80 patients enrolled in the study were evaluable for the assessment of the effect of the study drugs on the oropharyngeal and intestinal microflora and regarding their clinical efficacy. The 2 treatment groups were comparable with respect to age, male/female ratio and kind of bronchitis (Table I). A pathogen was cultured from the sputum of 10 patients (12.5%). In the amoxicillin group, 14 patients experienced a type 1 exacerbation compared with 7 patients in the loracarbef group.

Effect on the oropharyngeal microflora

Initial oropharyngeal cultures revealed the presence of H. influenzae and Acinetobacter spp in 2 patients treated with amoxicillin and the presence of M. catarrhalis in 3 patients in the loracarbef group. In none of these 5 patients were Gram-negative bacteria cultured from the follow-up samples.

In 7 patients treated with amoxicillin (18%), a new pathogen was cultured in the second oropharyngeal sample. Five samples contained Enterobacter spp (3 strains were resistant to amoxicillin, 2 were resistant to both study drugs), while 2 samples contained M. catarrhalis, sensitive to both study drugs.

The oropharyngeal samples of 2 patients treated with loracarbef (5%) contained a pathogen in the second oropharyngeal sample. In one sample, Acinetobacter spp (resistant

Table I. *Patient characteristics*

Characteristics	Loracarbef	Amoxicillin
Total no. of patients	40	40
Mean age (yr) (SD)	57 (18)	59 (17)
Male/female ratio	18/22	22/18
No. of patients with:		
Acute bronchitis	28	23
Type 1 exacerbation	7	14
Type 2 exacerbation	3	3
Type 3 exacerbation	2	0

to both study drugs) was cultured; in the other, M. catarrhalis sensitive to loracarbef and amoxicillin was found. The oropharyngeal samples obtained at day 21–28 did not show any of the pathogens isolated previously.

Effect on the intestinal microflora

The effect of both drugs on numbers of bacteria is shown in Tables II and III. The total number of anaerobic bacteria remained unchanged both during and after therapy with loracarbef and amoxicillin. Total numbers of aerobic Gram-negative bacteria were significantly higher on days 8–10 than at baseline in patients treated with amoxicillin, whereas in patients treated with loracarbef, no increase was found in the numbers of these bacteria. Enterococci were cultured on days 8–10 in (not significantly) higher numbers than at baseline in 8 patients treated with loracarbef. Enterococci were cultured in one (days 8–10) sample in the amoxicillin group. The numbers of yeasts tended to increase insignificantly in both groups during therapy, but returned to baseline numbers on days 21–28.

The presence of other aerobic bacteria than found at baseline occurred in a slightly higher percentage of patients in the amoxicillin group (15/40 patients, 38%) than in the loracarbef group (12/39 patients, 31%) on days 8–10 (Table IV). 39 patients in the loracarbef group were evaluable for this aspect, as the culture of 1 patient had been lost. 13/15 new acquired bacteria in the amoxicillin group were Klebsiella spp, while 6 different strains appeared in the loracarbef group.

No loracarbef or amoxicillin-resistant aerobic Gram-negative bacteria were found in faecal samples of patients treated with loracarbef, compared with 14 amoxicillin or loracarbef resistant strains (35%) in patients receiving amoxicillin ($p < 0.001$) (Table IV). In all these patients, E. coli strains were found, 10 of which were resistant to amoxicillin, 1 strain

Table II. *Mean numbers of bacteria in faeces of 40 patients treated with loracarbef*

	Mean log number/g faeces ± SD		
	Baseline	Days 8–10	Days 21–28
Anaerobic bacteria	9.4 ± 1.5	9.4 ± 1.6	9.3 ± 1.9
Aerobic Gram-negative bacteria	6.0 ± 2.6	6.3 ± 2.4	6.2 ± 2.6
Enterococcus faecalis	2.3 ± 1.2	2.8 ± 2.1	2.3 ± 1.2
Yeasts	2.6 ± 1.1	3.0 ± 1.7	2.6 ± 1.3

Table III. *Mean numbers of bacteria in faeces of 40 patients treated with amoxicillin*

	Mean log number/g faeces ± SD		
	Baseline	Days 8–10	Days 21–28
Anaerobic bacteria	9.0 ± 2.2	9.2 ± 1.9	9.2 ± 2.3
Aerobic Gram-negative bacteria	7.3 ± 2.1	8.1[a] ± 1.9	7.1[b] ± 2.8
Enterococcus faecalis	2.2 ± 1.0	2.1 ± 0.6	2.2 ± 1.0
Yeasts	2.5 ± 0.8	2.9 ± 1.3	2.6 ± 1.1

[a] Significant compared with baseline ($p = 0.03$; paired t-test).
[b] Significant compared with days 8–10 ($p = 0.03$; paired t-test).

Table IV. *Gram-negative bacteria in the faecal samples at days 8–10 (culture 2) and/or days 21–28 (culture 3), compared with baseline*

	Loracarbef ($n = 39$)	Amoxicillin ($n = 40$)
Presence of other Gram-negative bacteria	12 (31%)	15 (38%)
In: culture 2	7	9
cultures 2 & 3	2	5
undetermined[a]	3	1
Emergence of resistant Gram-negative bacteria	0 (0%)	14 (35%)
In: culture 2	0	7
cultures 2 & 3	0	4
undetermined[a]	0	3

[a] No culture at days 21–28.

(resistant to amoxicillin at baseline) developed resistance to loracarbef too, and 3 strains became resistant to both study drugs.

Other aerobic bacteria than found in the baseline samples or resistant Gram-negative bacteria, that emerged in the intestinal flora on days 8–10, were still present on days 21–28 in about 1/3 of patients treated with amoxicillin, compared with 1/6 of patients treated with loracarbef (Table IV). Neither C. difficile nor C. difficile toxin was detected in any stool specimen.

Adverse events

18 patients treated with loracarbef and 15 treated with amoxicillin experienced an adverse event. In this study, particular attention was paid to the occurrence of diarrhea or loose stools during therapy with the study drugs. In the loracarbef group, 8 patients registered in their diaries the occurrence of diarrhea and 5 reported loose stools. One of these patients experienced diarrhea 1 week after termination of treatment with loracarbef; another patient had loose stools during treatment with loracarbef and then diarrhea 3 days after completion of treatment. The faecal cultures on days 8–10 of the loracarbef patients with diarrhea revealed Citrobacter spp., Klebsiella spp., and E. coli in 2 cases, while in the 4 other samples, no other aerobic bacteria than found at baseline were cultured. Six amoxicillin-treated patients had diarrhea during therapy and 6 patients had loose stools. In 4 of these patients experiencing diarrhea, Klebsiella spp. was cultured from their faecal sample, 1 patient had both E. coli resistant to amoxicillin and Klebsiella spp. cultured, while the sixth patient had no changes in faecal flora compared with baseline.

Other adverse events probably or possibly related to the study drugs were headache, vaginitis, vaginal fluor, nausea and decreased appetite in the loracarbef group and dry mouth, exanthema, tingling fingers and headache in the amoxicillin group. The adverse events were of mild to moderate severity and therapy did not have to be interrupted due to these events.

Clinical efficacy

Treatment success (cure or improvement) occurred by days 8–10 in all 40 (100%) patients receiving loracarbef, compared with 36 (90%) in the amoxicillin group, and on days 21–28 in 37 (93%) and 36 (90%) patients respectively (differences were not statistically significant). By days 8–10, there were 4 failures in the amoxicillin group, while failure after initial improvement occurred by days 21–28 in 1 patient in each group. In 2 patients treated with loracarbef and 3 patients treated with amoxicillin, the clinical response could not be determined on days 21–28.

DISCUSSION

Broad-spectrum antibiotics are commonly used for the treatment of upper and lower respiratory tract infections. Since none of these antibiotics differ greatly with respect to clinical efficacy, as confirmed in this study, other aspects must determine which drug will be chosen for therapy. One of these aspects is the influence of the drug on the oropharyngeal and intestinal microflora. Many studies investigating the effect of new drugs on the oropharyngeal and intestinal microflora are performed in healthy volunteers. It is also of interest to study this effect in patients.

The normal flora of the digestive tract provides a so-called colonization resistance to the establishment of potential pathogens (8). Antibiotic treatment may diminish this colonization resistance, leading to overgrowth of already present bacteria or promoting the invasion of new microorganisms. In this study, treatment with amoxicillin – and to a lesser extent with loracarbef – resulted in colonization of the oropharynx and intestines with new, potentially pathogenic Gram-negative bacteria. Amoxicillin is known to affect the anaerobic bacteria (9), while treatment with loracarbef resulted in a decrease of bifidobacteria and eubacteria in healthy volunteers (5). In the present study the total numbers of anaerobic bacteria remained unchanged both during and after therapy with the study drugs. However, we have not accounted for the various strains of anaerobic bacteria.

C. difficile is one of the microorganisms that might profit from the decrease in colonization resistance. In hospitalized patients, C. difficile and/or its toxins are found in about half of all patients with antibiotic-associated diarrhea (2). Moreover, in healthy volunteers taking oral cephalosporins, C. difficile has been detected in up to 92% of volunteers (10). In the present study neither C. difficile nor its toxin was detected.

Although amoxicillin had in this study a significantly greater effect on the faecal flora than had loracarbef, diarrhea and loose stools were reported in almost equal numbers in both treatment groups. These numbers were higher than reported previously (11), but one must take into account that the occurrence of diarrhea or loose stools was registered by the patients in their diaries and not by the general practitioner. Not all patients reporting diarrhea had a change in their faecal flora. The latter will be partly due to the fact that faecal samples were collected at fixed time points and not at the moment the patient had diarrhea.

Antibiotic therapy can also promote the development of antimicrobial resistance and the spread of these resistant bacteria to other individuals (12). In the present study, colonization of the oropharynx with Acinetobacter spp. resistant to loracarbef occurred in only 1 patient, compared with 5 patients in the amoxicillin group, whose oropharyngeal sample of days 8–10 revealed a new Gram-negative species resistant to amoxicillin. No loracarbef- or amoxicillin-resistant Gram-negative bacteria were detected in the faecal samples of the loracarbef patients. Treatment with amoxicillin on the other hand resulted in the emergence of resistant strains in the faecal samples of 35% of the patients.

The results of this study indicate that loracarbef is efficacious in the treatment of bronchitis. Moreover, the use of loracarbef, compared with amoxicillin, led to minor changes in the normal oropharyngeal and intestinal microflora and almost no emergence of resistant Gram-negative bacteria occurred during or after treatment with loracarbef.

ACKNOWLEDGEMENTS

This study was supported by a grant from Eli Lilly Nederland B.V. We thank the participating general practitioners for their help: R. P. H. Beijaert, A. M. E. Drost, N. P. van Duijn, R. C. van Leeuwen, C. van der Smagt, L. Smit, A. M. Steenhuisen and J. van Zwieten.

REFERENCES

1. Bartlett JG. Antibiotic-associated diarrhea. Clin Infect Dis 15: 573–581, 1992.
2. George WL, Rolfe RD, Finegold SM. C. difficile and its cytotoxin in feces of patients with antimicrobial agent associated diarrhea and miscellaneous conditions. J Clin Microbiol 15: 1049–1053, 1982.
3. Dere WH. Acute bronchitis: results of U.S. and European trials of antibiotic therapy. Am J Med 92 (Suppl 6A): 53S–57S, 1992.
4. Zeckel ML. Loracarbef (LY163892) in the treatment of acute exacerbations of chronic bronchitis: results of U.S. and European comparative clinical trials. Am J Med 92; Suppl 6A: 58S–64S, 1992.
5. Nord CE, Grahnen A, Eckernäs SA. Effect of loracarbef on the normal oropharyngeal and intestinal microflora. Scand J Infect Dis 23: 255–260, 1991.
6. Anthonisen NR, Manfreda JR, Warren CPW, Hershfield ES, Harding GKM, Nelson NA. Antibiotic therapy in exacerbations of chronic obstructive pulmonary disease. Ann Intern Med 106: 196–204, 1987.
7. National Committee for Clinical Laboratory Standards. Performance standards for antimicrobial disc susceptibility tests. Approved standard M2-A4. National Committee for Clinical Laboratory Standards. Villenova, Pa, 1990.
8. Van der Waaij D. The colonization resistance of the digestive tract in experimental animals and its consequences for infection prevention, acquisition of new bacteria and the prevention of spread of bacteria between cage mates. In: Van der Waaij D, Verhoef J, eds. New criteria for antimicrobial therapy. Amsterdam, Oxford: Excerpta Medica, 43–52, 1979.
9. Vollaard EJ, Clasener HAL, Saene HKF van, Muller NF. Effect on colonization resistance: an important criterion in selecting antibiotics. DICP 24: 60–66, 1990.
10. Chachaty E, Depitre C, Mario N, Bourneix C, Saulnier P, Corthier G, Andremont A. Presence of Clostridium difficile and antibiotic and β-lactamase activities in feces of volunteers treated with oral cefixime, oral cefpodoxime proxetil, or placebo. Antimicrob Agents Chemother 36: 2009–2013, 1992.
11. Therasse DG. The safety profile of loracarbef: clinical trials in respiratory, skin and urinary tract infections. Am J Med 92 (Suppl 6A): 20S–25S, 1992.
12. Nord CE, Kager L, Heimdahl A. Impact of antimicrobial agents on the gastrointestinal microflora and the risk of infections. Am J Med 76: 99–106, 1984.

Scand J Infect Dis 26: 199–207, 1994

Intestinal Parasites in Refugees and Asylum Seekers Entering the Stockholm Area, 1987–88: Evaluation of Routine Stool Screening

ANNA PERSSON and LARS ROMBO

From the Department of Immunology, Microbiology, Pathology and Infectious Diseases, Division of Infectious Diseases, Karolinska Institut, Huddinge Hospital, Stockholm, Sweden

In order to evaluate the results of routine screening for intestinal parasites, the medical records of 4592 refugees and asylum seekers arriving in the Stockholm area from January 1987 to December 1988 were reviewed. 3938/4592 (86%) delivered stool specimens for examination and intestinal parasites were demonstrated in 651/3938 (17%). Protozoa, mainly Giardia intestinalis, were found in 403/3938 (10%) and helminths, mainly nematodes, in 277/3938 (7%). Intestinal parasites were most frequently recovered in subjects coming from the Indian subcontinent/South-east Asia and Africa (infection rates 39% and 25%, respectively). Extensive variations in the prevalence of intestinal parasite infection in various ethnic groups (range 4%–39%) were largely attributable to variations in prevalence of helminthic infections (range 2%–34%). Origin from the tropics or subtropics as well as low age, male sex, rural region of domicile before/during exile and short length of stay in Sweden were related to intestinal parasitic infection. Lack of data on morbidity in untreated asymptomatic carriers, limited risks for transmission of the recovered parasites in Sweden as well as the expenses for screening indicate a need for reconsideration of the present praxis of mass screening in favour of a selective screening of high-risk groups based on country of origin and age.

A. Persson, MD, Department of Immunology, Microbiology, Pathology and Infectious Diseases, Karolinska Institute, Huddinge Hospital, S-141 86 Huddinge, Sweden

INTRODUCTION

Intestinal parasites belong to the most common infective agents of mankind and affect billions of the world population, predominantly in the tropical and subtropical areas. The recent large reflux of refugees and asylum seekers from highly endemic areas into low or non-endemic industrialized countries therefore lead to an increased import of intestinal parasites prompting decisions on screening routines.

Health policies for migrant population differ between various receiving countries. In Sweden, a health screening at the expense of the government has been offered to all refugees and asylum seekers since the middle of the 1980's. According to current guidelines from The Swedish National Board of Health, routine stool examination for ova and parasites has only been recommended for persons coming from non-European countries (1), but is in reality offered to anybody, regardless of country of origin.

Apart from regular tabulations of notifications of Giardia intestinalis and Entamoeba histolytica to the National Bacteriological Laboratory, only scarce information has been published on the occurrence of intestinal parasites in the refugee population entering Sweden since the screening was started (2–5). Little attention has been paid to the cost of mass screening policy and to the impact of screening on personal and/or public health.

In this study we report on the prevalence of intestinal parasites in different groups of refugees and asylum seekers detected by routine stool screening and the cost for this screening. We have also studied factors associated with increased risk for intestinal parasitic infection and discuss the possible implications of the presented data on current screening policy.

SUBJECTS AND METHODS

Between January 1987 and December 1988, 5125 persons were seen at a center which provided a screening program to assess the state of health of refugees and asylum seekers arriving in the Stockholm area. Medical records for 4592 (97%) of these subjects were available.

3938/4592 (86%) of the subjects delivered stool samples for examination and were included in this study. The median duration of stay in Sweden at the time for examination was 120 days (range 2 days to 4 years). No substantial differences in distribution with regard to age, sex, time spent in Sweden, years of schooling, ethnic origin and region of domicile were found between subjects who delivered a stool specimen and those who did not.

Demographic characteristics

Age, sex, region of domicile prior to entry to Sweden, level of education and ethnic distribution of the studied population are presented in Table I.

The largest groups consisted of subjects from Latin America (the majority from Chile) and Asia, followed by minor groups from Africa (the majority from Ethiopia) and from Eastern Europe. The heterogeneity of the Asian population with regard to socioeconomic background and ethnic origin necessitated division in minor subgroups from Iran, the Middle East/Turkey and the Indian subcontinent/South East Asia.

The mean age was 25 years and nearly one third (31%) of subjects were aged 15 years and younger. 50% (1375/2729) of persons aged 16 years and older were males.

The group coming from the Indian subcontinent consisted to a greater extent of large families as compared to other groups (data not shown).

Screening procedure

All screening procedures were voluntary and interpreters were always available. Both children and adults were examined in a standardized way. The evaluation included medical history recorded by specially trained nurses, physical examination and following laboratory investigations: complete blood count with erythrocythe indexes, liver function test (s-ALAT), hepatitis B virus serology (HBsAg), syphilis serology (VDRL), dipstick urinanalysis, Mantoux 2 TU, chest X-ray and examination of a single fecal sample for ova and parasites. Furthermore, HIV-serology, schistosoma serology and thick blood films were performed if the examined persons came from a country highly endemic for HIV-infection, schistosomiasis and/or malaria.

Oral and written explanation of the stool collection procedure was given to each person. Stool specimens were collected in containers with formaldehyde preservative and returned to the laboratory by mail usually within 2 weeks. Stool was examined with the formol-ether concentration method using iodine for staining. Non-pathogenic intestinal protozoa were reported by the laboratory but not recorded in this study.

Table I. *Demographic characteristics of the refugees and asylum seekers screened 1987–88 at the Health Center in the Stockholm County*

Ethnic origin	Number examined (%)	Male sex (%)	Children <16 yrs (%)	Urban region of domicile (%)[a]	Yrs of schooling Means[b]
Africa	385 (10)	191 (50)	139 (36)	283 (74)	9
Eastern Europe	316 (8)	139 (44)	84 (27)	288 (91)	11
Indian Subc./S.E. Asia	143 (4)	91 (64)	39 (27)	97 (68)	11
Iran	731 (18)	362 (50)	213 (29)	678 (93)	11
Latin America	1627 (41)	841 (52)	484 (30)	1455 (90)	10
Middle East/Turkey	736 (19)	398 (54)	250 (34)	554 (75)	7
Total	3938 (100)	2020 (51)	1209 (31)	3365 (85)	10

[a] 308/3938 persons have incomplete data on region of domicile.
[b] Only persons aged 19 yrs included.

Statistical methods

Statistical analyses were performed using the Statistical Analysis System (SAS) and Statistical Package BMDP on personal computer. The χ^2 method was used for comparison of proportions. The influence of different factors on the prevalence of intestinal parasitic infections was analyzed in a stepwise multiple logistic regression model. The factors considered were ethnic origin, age, region of domicile, sex, education (years of schooling) and duration of stay in Sweden.

RESULTS

Stool specimens were obtained from 3938 subjects and parasites were detected in 651 (17%). Multiple findings were observed in 68/3938 (2%).

403/3938 (10%) were infected with potentially pathogenic protozoa, G. intestinalis more than twice as frequent (298/403) as E. histolytica (118/403).

277/3938 (7%) were infected with helminths, infections with nematodes being most common (202/277). Trichuris trichiura was the most frequently found worm, followed by Ascaris lumbricoides, while hookworm was more scarcely represented (Table II).

Factors associated with presence of intestinal parasitic infections

140/3938 subjects are not included because of incomplete data. Fewer parasites were detected in stools after longer time spent in Sweden and found in 19% of those who were examined within 4 months after arrival ($n = 1920$), as compared to 14% in those examined after 4 months ($n = 1878$), $p < 0.001$. Lower frequency of infection was observed both for protozoa (12% versus 8%, $p < 0.001$) and helminths (8% versus 6%, $p < 0.05$). No substantial differences in ethnic origin, socioeconomic background or age distribution were observed in groups examined within 4 months after arrival compared with groups examined after residence exceeding 4 months (data not shown).

Table II. *Prevalence of intestinal parasites in the refugees and asylum seekers screened 1987–88 at the Health Center in the Stockholm County*

	Tropical/subtropical origin (%)[a]		Other origin		Total (%)
	Adults	Children[b]	Adults	Children[b]	
Number examined	350	178	2379	1031	3938 (100)
Number positive stools	71 (20)	81 (46)	323 (14)	176 (17)	651 (17)
Protozoa	18 (5)	21 (12)	233 (9)	141 (14)	403 (10)
E. histolytica	7 (2)	5 (3)	83 (3)	23 (2)	118 (3)
G. intestinalis	11 (3)	17 (10)	148 (6)	122 (12)	298 (8)
Helminths	58 (17)	66 (37)	108 (5)	45 (4)	277 (7)
A. lumbricoides	15 (4)	20 (11)	50 (2)	14 (1)	99 (3)
E. vermicularis	0	0	3 (<1)	3 (<1)	6 (<1)
Hookworm	8 (2)	13 (7)	4 (<1)	0	25 (<1)
S. stercoralis	2 (<1)	0	3 (<1)	0	5 (<1)
T. trichiura	32 (9)	28 (16)	25 (1)	17 (2)	102 (3)
Taenia	4 (1)	2 (1)	7 (<1)	0	13 (<1)
H. nana	6 (2)	16 (9)	17 (<1)	15 (1)	54 (1)
S. mansonii	3 (<1)	5 (3)	0	0	8 (<1)
D. dendriticum	1 (<1)	0	3 (<1)	2 (<1)	6 (<1)

[a] Africa and the Indian subcontinent/South East Asia.
[b] Individuals aged 15 years and below.

Country of origin

The country of origin was the strongest predictor over all covariates and highly indicative of the presence of parasitic infection after correction for age, sex, region of domicile, years of schooling and length of stay in Sweden.

With prevalence of parasitic infection in Eastern Europe at the baseline, highest odds ratios were found for subjects coming from the tropics: 16 (95% confidence interval 8–33) for persons from the Indian subcontinent/South East Asia and 8 (95% confidence interval 4–15) for Africans. Odds ratio for the Middle East/Turkey was 6 (95% confidence interval 3–12) and 4 and 4 (95% confidence interval 2–8) for Latin America and Iran, respectively.

Infection rates in ethnic groups are presented in Table III. The uneven distribution of parasitic infection with regard to ethnic origin ($p < 0.001$) was mostly due to variations in prevalence of helminthic infections.

The highest rates of helminthic infections were found in subjects from the Indian subcontinent/South East Asia and in Africans, 34% and 20%, respectively. Rates in remaining groups of refugees from the Middle East/Turkey, Iran, Latin America and Eastern Europe were consistently lower and ranged from 12% to 2%.

Protozoan infections were more uniformly distributed through various ethnic groups and the frequency of parasitic recovery in the stools was generally lower (range 12% to 3%).

Region of domicile

308/3938 subjects are not included because of incomplete data. Overall frequency of intestinal infection was higher in subjects coming from rural areas (72/265, 27%) than in subjects coming from urban areas (515/3365, 15%). The difference ($p < 0.001$) was due to the increased prevalence of helminthic infections in persons from rural areas (17%) as compared to the prevalence in persons from urban areas (6%), whereas the prevalence of protozoan infections was almost the same in both groups, 11% versus 10%.

Age

The overall prevalence of parasitic infection varied with age ($p < 0.001$) (Table IV). Children were more often infected than adults both with respect to pathogenic protozoa (13% versus 9%, $p < 0.001$) and helminths (9% versus 6%, $p < 0.001$). The highest frequency of parasitic infection (23%) was found in school children and reflected higher prevalence of helminthic infection in this group (12%), twice the prevalence in both preschool children (6%) and adults (6%).

Table III. *Prevalence and cost/detection of intestinal parasites in the refugees screened 1987–88 at the Health Center in the Stockholm County, by country of origin*

Ethnic origin	Number examined A	Helminths (%)	Protozoa (%)	Parasites (%) C	Cost/detected parasite $D = A \times B^a/C$
Africa	385	76 (20)	26 (8)	96 (25)	$140
Indian Subc./S.E. Asia	143	48 (34)	13 (9)	56 (39)	$89
Eastern Europe	316	2 (<1)	10 (3)	12 (4)	$922
Iran	731	29 (4)	74 (10)	101 (14)	$253
Latin America	1627	39 (2)	199 (12)	234 (14)	$243
Middle East/Turkey	736	83 (11)	81 (11)	152 (21)	$169
Total	3938	277 (7)	403 (10)	651 (17)	$212

[a] B = cost/stool examination $35.

Table IV. *Prevalence of intestinal parasites in the refugees and asylum seekers screened 1987–88 at the Health Center in the Stockholm County, by age group*

Age group	Number examined	Protozoa (%)	Helminths (%)	Parasites (%)
Children	1209	162 (13)	111 (9)	257 (21)
Preschool 0–6 years	514	69 (13)	30 (6)	92 (18)
School 7–15 years	695	93 (13)	81 (12)	165 (24)
Adults >15 years	2729	241 (9)	166 (6)	394 (14)
Total	3938	403 (10)	277 (7)	651 (17)

No corresponding difference in the overall frequency of protozoan infections was seen between preschool and school children. However, parasite-specific prevalences showed that rates of infection with G. intestinalis were decreasing with age, from 13% in preschool children to 10% in school children and 6% in adults ($p < 0.001$) as opposed to rates of infection with E. histolytica.

Sex

Men were more frequently infected than women, 18% ($n = 1988$) and 15% ($n = 1890$) respectively, $p < 0.05$.

Years of schooling

The frequency of parasitic infection did not vary significantly by the level of education (years of schooling).

Cost for stool screening

The center's cost for a stool examination was 35 USD at the time for the screening. The total cost for the initial stool screening (only the costs for diagnostic procedure taken into account) was thus calculated to 137 830 USD for 3938 stool examinations. This corresponds to 212 USD per stool finding.

Since the cost per detected case is inversely proportional to the prevalence there was considerable variation in cost/detected parasite in the ethnic groups. Thus, the cost ranged from 89 USD per parasitic infection in refugees from the Indian subcontinent/South East Asia (prevalence of parasitic infection 39%) to 922 USD in population from Eastern Europe (prevalence 4%) (Table III).

If the screening had been restricted to groups with high frequency of parasitic infections, i.e. children regardless of country of origin and adults with origin from a country in the tropics and subtropics (Indian subcontinent/S.E. Asia and Africa) 50% (328/651) of the stool findings would be caught for the cost of 166 USD/stool finding. The cost for each intestinal parasite recovered outside this group was 258 USD.

DISCUSSION

Socioeconomic background, state of health and nutrition of the migrant population entering industrialized countries often differ favourably from the average in their countries of origin, as was also seen in this study. The screened population was heterogenous, but nearly all subjects were in apparent good state of health and nutrition.

The extensive variations in prevalence of intestinal parasitic infections encountered in various ethnic groups do not necessarily correspond to the true epidemiology in countries of origin. They merely reflect specific living and socioeconomic conditions in the particular community from which refugees or asylum seekers arrive. Still, country of origin was shown to be the strongest predictor of parasitic infection, which is in agreement with what has been found in a study of refugees and refugee claimants entering Canada (6).

Two groups with high rates of helminthic infections were identified, Africans and Asians from the Indian subcontinent and South East Asia, i.e. refugees and asylum seekers coming from the tropics and subtropics.

In the Asian group, intrafamilial aggregation of parasitic infections may also have contributed to the particularly high infection rate in this subgroup.

Parasite burden in these groups was also potentially more pathogenic as multiple infections, particularly with A. lumbricoides, T. trichiura and hookworm were more common (data not shown) and parasites such as Schistosoma mansoni and Strongyloides stercoralis were recovered.

Asymptomatic infections are by far most common in migrant populations and as expected gastrointestinal symptoms did not correlate with presence of intestinal parasites in the present study.

It is generally agreed that intestinal parasites rarely cause subsequent disease in the presently healthy carriers and a vast majority of carriers remain asymptomatic, but few solid data on morbidity of most intestinal parasitic infections are available (7, 8).

E. histolytica, S. stercoralis, A. lumbricoides and hookworm have been considered to merit detection and treatment, even in the absence of symptoms, because of latency and/or potential risk for serious life-threatening disease. Still, there is no documented increase in use of health care due to complications following undetected intestinal parasitic infections in countries where mass screening is not applied (6, 9, 17, 18).

Health risks also diminish with time. Lower infection rates in refugees examined after longer stay in Sweden could be ascribed to spontaneous loss of parasites over time, reflecting the natural history of parasitic infection in the absence of reinfection. In Central American immigrants with overall prevalence of intestinal parasites exceeding 50% no helminths were found in individuals who had been in the United States for more than 3 years (10).

Prevention of transmission has been a major objective for screening of migrants and it is often argued in support for screening that elimination of infections reduces risk of stigmatization of a migrant population.

In reality, most intestinal parasites are not easily transmitted in Sweden and the preventive effect of screening is marginal. High sanitary standards and high level of hygiene create a sufficient barrier for spread of soil-transmitted helminths. Lack of specific intermediate hosts interrupts life cycles of other parasites as oriental flukes or schistosomas, and makes their transmission virtually impossible.

Infections with G. intestinalis and E. histolytica deserve special concern because of their potential for person-to-person spread.

The average level of protozoan infection in the screened population was 10% and predominantly due to the presence of G. intestinalis, which was particularly common in preschool children. Similar age distribution for G. intestinalis and low frequency of infection with E. histolytica were also reported in other migrant populations (5, 6, 10). The occurrence of these protozoa is assumed to be generally low in industrialized countries. Overall prevalence estimates reported for general Canadian or American population did not generally exceed 10% (6, 7, 10–12). As only older prevalence studies are available (13–16) little is known about the present reservoir of these protozoa in Sweden and other Nordic countries.

However, they are invariably present, G. intestinalis being associated with diarrhoeal outbreaks in children day-care centers (17–19), institutions and hospital wards (20) and both parasites with accidental breakdowns in sewage systems (21, 22). Sexual transmission is also documented in homosexual men (23).

Apart from children adopted from abroad, refugees and asylum seekers are the only groups screened for intestinal parasites on routine basis, whereas a considerable number of persons with the same background, i.e. relatives to persons already granted asylum, resettled refugees and immigrants visiting their home countries are not examined.

Moreover, refugees and immigrants are certainly not the only ones accounting for a potential indigenous transmission. A large and increasing part of the indigenous Swedish population travels abroad and a considerable number stay for long periods in areas with poor sanitation and contaminated water supplies with an obvious risk for being infected by intestinal parasites (24, 25). These travellers are not screened, but rates of infections with intestinal protozoa comparable with those observed in certain groups examined in this study were found in Swedish personnel working in developing countries for the Swedish International Development Authority and their families on medical evaluation after return to Sweden (26).

Expected spontaneous recovery from infection also emphasizes the importance of the evaluation of screening activities on prevalence of infection, particularly as poor impact of screening programs on rates of some parasitic infections is reported (9, 10, 27, 28). Many factors, such as limited reliability of a single stool examination, poor compliance, ineffective treatment, possible reinfection within groups, or new infections acquired during visits in native countries, can affect elimination and at the same time contribute to persistence of infection within a refugee population despite intervention.

To date, no comprehensive cost-effectiveness or cost-benefit studies have been performed on the overall contribution of screening programs to personal and public health. Lack of data on morbidity in untreated asymptomatic carriers as well as on secondary infection rates restricts the economic evaluation of screening strategies (29, 30).

However, even strictly economic considerations based on calculation of the costs of stool examination could be helpful in making rational decisions, highlighting the relation of prevalence to cost/detected parasite. In the present screening, differences in cost per detected parasite were nearly tenfold between groups with high and low prevalence.

Facing the situation where the benefits of screening on personal and public health can be questioned on grounds as least as valid as those used in support for intervention we suggest a reconsideration of the present praxis of mass screening in favor of the screening of selected refugee groups as follows:

A selective screening based on country of origin of refugees coming from the tropics and subtropics should reduce costs but still detect infections with parasites of more prominent pathogenic potential and individuals with high parasite burden.

A continued screening of children, irrespective of country of origin is appropriate because of increased risk for person-to-person transmission and vulnerability during growth.

Similarly, screening should be considered for other vulnerable subgroups as those disabled by disease or malnutrition, candidates for institutional care for candidates for immunosuppressive therapy.

ACKNOWLEDGEMENT

We are grateful to all personnel working at the Health Center during the period of the study for their devoted and skilled work.

REFERENCES

1. The Swedish National Board of Health. Health care for refugees and asylum seekers. General guidelines. Stockholm Allmänna förlag 1988. Allmänna råd från Socialstyrelsen 1988: 8 [in Swedish].
2. Castor B. Health screening of immigrants. Lövens litteratur information 20: 129–137, 1988 [in Swedish].
3. Blixth G, Mjönes S, Jepsson A. Medical care for refugees in a rural community. Clinical examination during the period November 19, 1985–December 31, 1986. Allmännmedicin 9: 171–173, 1988 [in Swedish].
4. Berglund G, Brune L, Finizia M. What health care measures are needed by refugee children? Läkartidningen 89: 4494–4497, 1992 [in Swedish].
5. Gustavson-Moringlane IL, Gustafsson E. Results of health control of 1000 refugees. Important with early examination. Läkartidningen 82: 3052–3054, 1985 [in Swedish].
6. Godue CB, Gyorkos TW. Intestinal parasites in refugee claimants: A case study for selective screening? Can J Public Health 81: 191–195, 1990.
7. WHO Expert Committee. Public health significance of intestinal parasitic infections. Bull World Health Organ 65: 575–588, 1987.
8. Cook GC. The clinical significance of gastrointestinal helminths – a review. Trans R Soc Trop Med Hyg 80: 675–685, 1986.
9. Gyorkos WT, Mac Lean JD, Viens P, Chheang Ch, Koskin-Nelson E. Intestinal parasite infection in the Kampuchean Refugee population 6 years after resettlement in Canada. J Infect Dis 166: 413–417, 1992.
10. Salas SD, Heifetz R, Barret-Connor E. Intestinal parasites in central American Immigrants in the United States. Arch Intern Med 50: 1514–1516, 1990.
11. Kappus KK, Juranek DD, Roberts JM. Results of testing for intestinal parasites by state diagnostic laboratories, United States, 1987. MMWR CDC Surveill Summ 40: 25–45, 1991.
12. Gyorkos T, Meerovitch E, Prichard R. Estimates of intestinal parasite prevalence in 1984: Report of a 5-year follow-up survey of provincial laboratories. Can J Public Health 78: 185–187, 1987.
13. Engbaek K, Olesen Larsen S. The incidence and significance of Giardia lamblia and other intestinal parasites in children in day-institutions. Ugeskr Laeger 140: 14–17, 1978 [in Danish].
14. Engbaek K, Olesen Larsen S. Intestinal parasites in schoolchildren. Correlation between incidence and some social parameters. Ugeskr Laeger 140: 9–13, 1978 [in Danish].
15. Böe J. Occurence of human intestinal protozoa in Norway. Acta Med Scand 113: 321–328, 1943.
16. Svensson R. Studies on human intestinal protozoa. Acta Med Scand Suppl 70, 1935.
17. Christensson B, Jacobson B, Ryd G. Giardiasis among children in day care centers in 2 northern communities in Stockholm. Läkartidningen 89: 763–764, 1992 [in Swedish].
18. Tjernström K, Alvin A, Christensson B, Ryd G. An outbreak of giardiasis among children in family day nurseries. Läkartidningen 89: 764–765, 1992 [in Swedish].
19. Bergman G, Dahl IL. Giardiasis at child care centres in Sweden. Läkartidningen 76: 4263–4264, 1979 [in Swedish].
20. Castor B. Giardiasis in three Swedish institutions. Läkartidningen 78: 950–951, 1981 [in Swedish].
21. Anderson Y, De Jong B. An outbreak of giardiasis at a ski resort in Sweden. Water Science and Technology 21: 143–146, 1989.
22. Neringer R, Andersson Y, Eitrem R. A waterborne outbreak of giardiasis in Sweden. Scand J Infect Dis 19: 85–90, 1987.
23. Emtestam L, Lindberg B, Pehrsson PO, Ringertz O, Sandström E. Sexually transmitted intestinal pathogens among homosexual men in Stockholm. Läkartidningen 80: 2747–2748, 1983 [in Swedish].
24. Sterner G, Lantorp K, Lidman K. Giardiasis – a problem of present interest in Sweden. Nord Med 86: 1343–1346, 1971 [in Swedish].
25. Pehrsson PO. Amoebiasis in non-endemic country. Epidemiology, presenting symptoms and diagnostic methods. Scand J Infect Dis 15: 207–214, 1983.
26. Stenbeck JL, Sjöblom N-G. Diseases among Swedish International Development Authority employees – 5 years' data. Health risks during work in developing countries. Läkartidningen 80: 4433–4436, 1983 [in Swedish].

27. Gyorkos TW, Frappier-Davignon L, Mac Lean JD, Viens P. Effect of screening and treatment on imported intestinal parasites infections: results from a randomized, controlled trial. Am J Epidemiol 129: 763–761, 1989.
28. Molina CD, Molina MM, Molina JM. Intestinal parasites in Southeast Asian refugees two years after immigration. West J Med 149: 422–425, 1988.
29. Anderson JP, Moser RJ. Parasite screening and treatment among Indochinese refugees. JAMA 253: 2229–2235, 1985.
30. Barret-Connor E. Direct dollar costs and savings of screening stool examination for eggs and parasites in adult Southeast Asian Refugees. Am J Trop Med Hyg 31: 466–468, 1982.

Scand J Infect Dis 26: 209–214, 1994

CASE REPORT

Stomatococcus mucilaginosus Septicemia in Two Bone Marrow Transplanted Patients

EVA ANDSTRÖM[1,2], SOLGUN BYGDEMAN[3], SIV AHLÉN[3], ANDERS HEIMDAL[4] and BERTIL NYSTRÖM[3]

From the [1]Department of Transplantation Surgery, [2,3]Division of Infectious Diseases, and [4]Department of Oral Surgery, Huddinge Hospital, Stockholm, Sweden

A 44-year-old man with chronic myeloid leukemia and a 10-year-old boy with adrenoleukodystrophy, both admitted for bone marrow transplantation in December 1992, developed clinical signs of septicemia within 2 weeks after transplantation. Three strains of Stomatococcus mucilaginosus were isolated from blood cultures. These were among the first cases of S. mucilaginosus infection diagnosed at our Laboratory and the first reported from Scandinavia. S. mucilaginosus is part of the endogenous oral flora. Both patients had signs of oral mucositis. All 3 strains were isolated earlier with the Laboratory's present blood culture system, compared with the one in use before spring 1992.

E. Andström, MD, Department of Immunology, Microbiology, Pathology and Infectious Diseases, Division of Infectious Diseases, Karolinska Institut, Huddinge Hospital, S-141 86 Huddinge, Sweden

INTRODUCTION

Stomatococcus mucilaginosus belongs to the family Micrococcaceae. It is part of the normal flora of the human upper respiratory tract (1). It was first described as a human pathogen in 1978 (2). Between 1985 and 1992, 41 additional cases of infection due to S. mucilaginosus have been reported (3, 4). S. mucilaginosus has been isolated from patients with septicemia, endocarditis and catheter-associated infections, most often in immunosuppressed patients or patients with intravenous drug abuse, cardiac valve disease, or indwelling vascular catheters.

This report describes 2 of the first cases to be published in Scandinavia, both observed in December 1992 at the Department of Transplantation Surgery, Huddinge Hospital, Stockholm, Sweden.

CASE REPORT

Case 1 (Fig. 1)

A 44-year-old male (UPN 373) with chronic myeloid leukaemia in a second chronic phase was admitted for bone marrow transplantation (BMT). On admission he was sero-positive for cytomegalovirus (CMV), varicella-zoster virus (VZV) and herpes simplex virus (HSV). Conditioning started 5 days before BMT according to the routine of the Department (5). Prophylaxis against graft-versus-host disease (GVHD) was given (cyclosporin and methotrexate) (6). Gut decontamination included ciprofloxacin and amphotericin B.

On day 6 after BMT, after being aplastic for 2 days, the patient became subfebrile. The following day, co-trimoxazole and amikacin medication was instituted. During the ensuing 24 h he developed clinical signs of septicemia. Simultaneously he developed an oral mucositis. The antibiotic regimen was changed to vancomycin and imipenem-cilastin.

S. mucilaginosus was isolated in blood cultures from days 6 and 7 after BMT in the aerobic (but not in the anaerobic) bottle in 4 blood cultures. Further blood cultures on days 13, 14, 17 and 19 were all negative. No other microbiological findings during this period could explain the patient's septicemia.

Case 2 (Fig. 2)

A 10-year-old boy (UPN 375) with adrenoleukodystrophy for 1 year, was admitted for bone marrow transplantation. Conditioning consisted of busulphan and cyclophosphamide. Prophylaxis against

Fig. 1. Case 1.

Blood cultures:	Day		
	−8	+	
	−7	+	
	−6	+	
	−5	+	←start of conditioning
	−4	+	
	−3	+	
	−2	+	
	−1	+	
	0	+	←bone marrow transplantation
	1	+	
	2	+	
	3	+	
	4	+	←aplastic phase
	5	+	
S. mucilaginosus→	6	+	←subfebrility
S. mucilaginosus→	7	+	←co-trimoxazole and amikacin
	8	+	←clinical septicemia, antibiotics changed to vancomycin, imipenem-cilastin
	9	+	
	10	+	
	11	+	←granulocyte colony stimulating factor, granulocyte transfusions
	12	+	
negative→	13	+	
negative→	14	+	
	15	+	←afebrile
	16	+	
negative→	17	+	
	18	+	←evidence of engraftment (WBC $> 0.2 \times 10^9/l$)
negative→	19	+	
	20	+	

GVHD and treatment was the same as in case 1. During conditioning, he developed difficulty in taking the drugs orally even though he had no visible oral ulcers. Two days after BMT he became subfebrile and on the fifth day post-BMT his temperature increased to 39°C. Treatment with co-trimoxazole and amikacin was initiated following routine cultures and pulmonary X-ray. A slight oral mucositis was noted, which progressed during the following day. Staphylococcus aureus, sensitive to both antibiotics used, was isolated in blood cultures. On day 8 after BMT a small localized pulmonary infiltrate in the right lingular lobe was noted on chest radiography. Antibiotic therapy was changed to vancomycin and imipenem-cilastin. As the pulmonary infiltrates continued to increase, diagnostic bronchoscopy with bronchoalveolar lavage (BAL) was performed on day 13 after BMT. CMV antigen was demonstrated in cell culture from BAL. Ganciclovir was instituted. The patient was seronegative for CMV prior to transplantation and the donor was seropositive. The pulmonary X-ray findings were interpreted as a septic reaction.

In a blood culture on day 10 after BMT, S. mucilaginosus was isolated from the aerobic (but not from the anaerobic) bottle. No other microbiological findings were made which could explain the patient's septic and deteriorating state despite 5 days of antibiotic treatment for a S. aureus septicemia of a sensitive strain.

Engraftment was observed on day 14 after BMT. Simultaneously his fever was reduced to subfebrility, which persisted for another 6 weeks and was interpreted as sign of a primary CMV infection.

Laboratory findings

From all 4 positive blood cultures from the first patient (UPN 373) 2 strains of S. mucilaginosus were isolated (BO 9209996 I and II). From 1 blood culture from patient UPN 375, 1 strain was isolated (BO 9210539). All 3 strains grew in the Bactec 860[R] blood culture

Fig. 2. Case 2.

		Day		
		−8	+	←start of conditioning
		−7	+	
		−6	+	
		−5	+	
		−4	+	
		−3	+	
		−2	+	
		−1	+	
		0	+	←bone marrow transplantation
		1	+	
		2	+	←subfebrility
		3	+	
		4	+	
Blood cultures:	S. aureus →	5	+	←pulmonary X-ray negative
	negative →	6	+	←co-trimoxazole and amikacin
	negative →	7	+	
	negative →	8	+	←infiltrate right lingular lobe
		9	+	antibiotics changed to vancomycin + imipenem-cilastin
	S. mucilaginosus →	10	+	Liposomal amphotericin B added
		11	+	
		12	+	
		13	+	←bronchoalveolar lavage
		14	+	←evidence of engraftment
		15	+	
	negative →	16	+	←ganciclovir (CMV antigen in BAL)
		17	+	granulocyte colony stimulating factor due to leukopenia (CMV?)
		18	+	
		19	+	
		20	+	

system (Becton Dickinson Diagnostic Instrument Systems, USA) within 72 h. Their most prominent features were: greyish-white, smooth, mucoid, non-haemolytic colonies with an unusually strong adherence to the agar surface, a microscopic morphology resembling that of micrococci, catalase negativity and growth only in the aerobic bottle. The colonies were extremely difficult to emulsify in broth.

On the first subculture the strains grew well on haematin agar in 5% CO_2 atmosphere but not on horse blood agar, except for a satellite phenomenon close to the S. aureus streak. The results of the biochemical tests (Table I) verified the preliminary diagnosis of S. mucilaginosus. Both strains from case 1 were ciprofloxacin resistant, also co-trimoxazole resistant. The strain from case 2 was co-trimoxazole resistant, but sensitive to ciprofloxacin.

In order to check the sensitivity of our present (Bactec 860^R) and former (Signal^R Oxoid Ltd, England) blood culture systems for S. mucilaginosus, bottles were inoculated with 10 ml each of dilutions in human blood with 100, 10 and 1 colony-forming unit (cfu)/ml of the 3 S. mucilaginosus strains BO 9209996 I and II and BO 9210539. Fig. 3 illustrates when growth was first observed with the 2 blood culture systems of the 3 different patient strains in the 3 dilutions.

All 3 strains had been subcultured several times after their primary isolation before this experiment.

Table I. *Biochemical tests of our 3 isolates of Stomatococcus mucilaginosus*

	Stomatococcus mucilaginosus		
Test/substrate	BO9209996 I	BO9209996 II	BO9210539
Arginine dihydrolase	−	−	−
Arabinose	−	−	−
Beta-galactosidase	+	+	+
Catalase	−	−	−
Citrate	−	−	−
Deoxyribonuclease	−	−	−
Esculin	+	+	+
Gelatin hydrolysis[a]	+	+	+
Glucose oxidation	+	+	+
Glucose fermentation	+	+	+
Growth in 6.5% NaCl	−	−	−
Growth on hematin agar			
in 5% CO_2	+	+	+
in air	−	−	+
Growth on horse-blood agar			
in 5% CO_2	+/−	+/−	+/−
in air without satellite	−	−	−
in air, only satellite growth	+	+	+
Hemolysis	−	−	−
H_2S	−	−	−
Indole	−	−	−
Lactose	−	−	−
Leucine arylamidase	+	+	+
Mannitol	−	−	−
Melibiose	−	−	−
Nitrate reduction	+	+	+
ONPG	−	−	−
Oxidase	−	−	−
Pyrolidone arylamidase	+	+	+
Raffinose	−	−	−
Sodium hippurate	+	−	+
Sorbitol	−	−	−
Sucrose	+	+	+
Trehalose[a]	+	+	+
Urea	−	−	−
Voges-Proskauer	+	+	+

[a] After 4 days incubation.

DISCUSSION

The 2 cases of S. mucilaginosus infection described here are among the first to be reported from Scandinavia. Both occurred in bone marrow transplant patients within 2 weeks after transplantation. Bone marrow transplantations have been performed at Huddinge Hospital for more than a decade, and nearly 400 patients have been treated (5). Why have cases of S. mucilaginosus infection not been observed earlier?

The Bactec 860[R] system detected growth of S. mucilaginosus earlier than the Signal[R] system. It could be that cases have escaped detection with the Signal[R] system earlier used at our Laboratory.

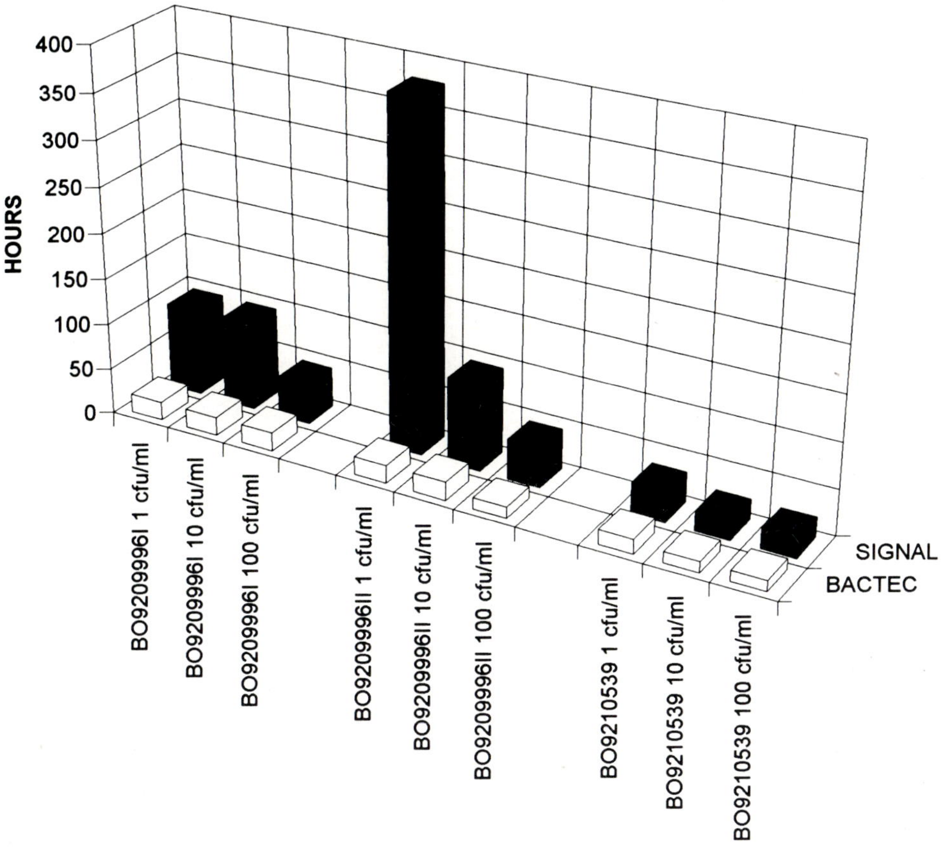

Fig. 3. Number of hours required for growth of 3 different strains of S. mucilaginosus in 2 different blood culture systems.

S. mucilaginosus may conceivably be mistaken for diphtheroids, micrococci, or coagulase-negative staphylococci. S. mucilaginosus belongs to the endogenous oral microflora and may thus be translocated from the oral cavity to the bloodstream if oral mucosal lesions are present, as in these 2 patients (7). Oral application of non-absorbable antimicrobial agents is a common prophylactic measure to reduce colonization of the oral cavity with non-endogenous microorganisms, but is usually not directed against endogenous oral micro-organisms (8). Since April 1992, oral prophylaxis in BMT patients at Huddinge Hospital has been reduced to tooth-brushing with a soft brush and saline. The gut decontamination regimen includes ciprofloxacin, but 2 of the 3 S. mucilaginosus strains in these patients were ciprofloxacin resistant. As a number of reports from different parts of the world during the past few years have described this species as a cause of severe infection in immunocompromised patients, we may expect further cases. Factors contributing to this are the more aggressive chemotherapy used, which causes breakdown of mucous membranes in the oral cavity (9), and the use of prophylactic antimicrobial regimes with a poor effect on Gram-positive microorganisms. Furthermore, improved blood culture systems will probably facilitate the isolation of fastidious microorganisms like S. mucilaginosus, as indicated by our present observations.

REFERENCES

1. Bergan T, Kocur M. Stomatococcus mucilaginosus gen. nov., sp. nov., ep. rev., a member of the family Micrococcaceae. Int J Syst Bacteriol 32: 374–377, 1982.
2. Rubin SJ, Lyers RW, Murcia AJ. Endocarditis associated with cardiac catheterization due to a Gram-positive coccus designated Micrococcus mucilaginosus incertae sedis. J Clin Microbiol 7: 546–549, 1978.
3. Kaufhold A, Reinert RR, Kern W. Bacteremia caused by Stomatococcus mucilaginosus: Report of seven cases and review of the literature. Infection 20: 213–220, 1992.
4. Langbaum M, Eyal FG. Stomatococcus mucilaginosus septicemia and meningitis in a premature infant. Pediatr Infect Dis J 11: 334–335, 1992.
5. Ringdén O, Aschan J, Boström L, Dahllöf G, Tollemar J, Paulin T, Gahrton G, Groth CG, Klaesson S, Lindquist R, Ljungman P, Lönnquist B, Persson U, Shanwell A, Winiarski J. Allogenic bone marrow transplantation at Huddinge Hospital and strategies to improve survival. In: Terasaki PI, ed. Clinical Transplants 1990. California: UCLA Tissue Typing Laboratory.
6. Ringdén O, Pihlstedt P, Markling L, Aschan J, Båryd I, Ljungman P, Lönnqvist B, Tollemar J, Janossy G, Sundberg B. Prevention of graft-versus-host disease with T cell depletion or cyclosporin and methotrexate. A randomized trial in adult leukemic marrow recipients. Bone Marrow Transplant 7, 221–226, 1991.
7. Heimdahl A, Mattsson T, Dahllöf G, Lönnquist B, Ringdén O. The oral cavity as a port of entry for early infections in patients treated with bone marrow transplantation. Oral Surg Oral Med Oral Pathol 68: 711–716, 1989.
8. Heimdahl A, Gahrton G, Groth CG, Lundgren G, Lönnquist B, Ringdén O, Nord CE. Selective decontamination of alimentary tract microbial flora in patients treated with bone marrow transplantation. A microbiological study. Scand J Infect Dis 16: 51–60, 1984.
9. Mattsson T, Heimdahl A, Dahllöf G, Nilsson B, Lönnquist B, Ringdén O. Variables predicting oral mucosal lesions in allogenic bone marrow recipients. Head Neck 13: 224–229, 1991.

Scand J Infect Dis 26: 215–217, 1994

CASE REPORT

A Highly Unusual Combination of Pulmonary Pathogens in an HIV Infected Patient

KARINE GILLET-JUVIN[1], MARC STERN[2], DOMINIQUE ISRAËL-BIET[3], DOMINIQUE PENAUD[2], and FRANÇOISE CARNOT[3]

From the Departments of [1]Pulmonary Diseases, and [2]Pathology, Laennec Hospital, Paris, and the [3]Department of Pulmonary Diseases, Foch Hospital, Suresnes, France

We report on a case with an unusual combination of pulmonary pathogens including Pneumocystis carinii, Rhodococcus equi and Toxoplasma gondii in an HIV infected patient. The multiple microbiological procedures required to ascertain the etiological diagnoses of pneumonitis in HIV-seropositive subjects are discussed.

K. Gillet-Juvin, MD, Service du Pr Even, Hopital Laennec, 42 rue de Sèvres, F-750 07 Paris, France

INTRODUCTION

The combination of 3 different pathogens as the cause for infectious pneumonitis is exceptional. This case report illustrates the diagnostic problems encountered in HIV-seropositive patients and the requirement of multiple microbiological procedures to ascertain the etiologies.

CASE REPORT

A 30-year-old HIV infected caucasian male presented with a productive cough, minor hemoptysis, night sweats and 4 weeks fever. He had been an IV drug user, treated with AZT and monthly aerosolized pentamidine (AP) for 2 years. His clinical status had so far been CDC class IV A. On admission, the patient's general and respiratory condition was serious. PaO_2 at room air was 79 mmHg and $PaCO_2$ 35 mmHg. Chest X-ray disclosed bilateral upper lobe infiltrates, with a clear excavation of the left apical lobe. The WBC count was 3.4×10^9/l with 80% neutrophils, ESR 128 mm and CD4 cell count was 10×10^6/l with negative p24 antigenemia. A first fiberoptic bronchoscopy with bronchoalveolar lavage (BAL) and a protected brush sampling performed 2 weeks earlier had been negative; a second fiberoptic bronchoscopy was therefore performed with BAL in the right middle lobe, multiple transbronchial biopsies (TBB) in the right upper lobe, bronchial washings and a protected brush in the left upper lobe. The BAL cellularity was normal (0.391×10^9 cells/l, 82% macrophages, 12% lymphocytes and 6% PMN); BAL remained negative for parasites, fungi, bacteria and mycobacteria. In contrast, a Gomori-Grocott staining of the TBB specimens disclosed the presence of Pneumocystis carinii (PC) cysts. Surprisingly, numerous Toxoplasma gondii were also found on hematoxylin and eosin staining. Moreover, the protected brush and the bronchial washings grew a Gram-positive organism, subsequently identified as Rhodococcus equi. The patient denied any contact with horses or farm animals during the months before admission. Blood cultures remained negative, as well as toxoplasmosis antigenemia, and a CT of the brain was normal. Toxoplasma serology, known as positive for 2 years, was unmodified. Because of a previous allergy to sulfonamides, the treatment was started with pyrimethamin, clindamycin, dapsone against both toxoplasmosis and Pneumocystis carinii pneumonia (PCP) and erythromycin plus rifampicin against the Rhodococcus equi according to the in vitro sensitivity pattern.

The patient's condition initially improved with a diminishing size of the cavitation and a decrease of the infiltrates. The PC and the T. gondii were no longer present on TBB specimens obtained 6 weeks later, while the Rhodococcus equi still grew in the bronchial washings. The patient died 3 months later with widespread Rhodococcus pneumonitis.

DISCUSSION

This case not only illustrates the combination of multiple opportunistic agents causing pulmonary infections during HIV disease, but also highlights atypical presentation of pulmonary toxoplasmosis, and underscores the role of a complete fiberoptic evaluation, including bronchial washings, BAL and TBB to ensure correct diagnoses. The toxoplasmosis pneumonitis was initially very unlikely for several reasons: Its most common chest X-ray presentation is a diffuse interstitial pattern (1, 2) and the upper lobe infiltrates in patients under preventive AP rather argue for an atypical presentation of PCP (3, 4). Moreover, pulmonary involvement is observed almost exclusively in the presence of central nervous system disease (5). A suspected diagnosis of toxoplasmosis pneumonitis, has been diagnosed by bronchial biopsies until recently when Oksenhendler et al. (1) obtained a positive diagnosis by BAL in 10 of 11 cases. The combination of PC and T. gondii, unusual in their clinical and radiological presentation, was further complicated by the discovery of a third organism, Rhodococcus equi, in the protected brush samples. It is an aerobic, Gram-positive organism, occasionally responsible for pulmonary cavitation in AIDS patients. The clinical features and the chest X-ray of our patient are similar to the few cases previously reported (6, 7). The diagnosis of a Rhodococcus equi infection is not problematic. It needs prolonged antibiotic treatment and frequent reassessment due to evolution of resistance to antibiotics (8). If not treated this organism will expose the patient for the risk of developing a destructive pneumonitis. The etiologic relationship of each pathogen remains debatable. That of R. equii is strongly argued for by the cavitary pneumonia and its repeated isolation by culture. PC is also a very likely pathogen in this classical form of PCP during AP treatment. The toxoplasma infection remains doubtful in this localized form without a disseminated disease. No reports of this form of presentation has been published until now. All 3 pathogens found were obtained with multiple procedures performed during fiberoptic bronchoscopy, including TBB. The fact that BAL remained negative was probably due to that it was performed in an unaffected lobe. However, also if performed in an affected lung segment increasing the chance of a diagnosis of PC (9), it is likely that T. gondii would have remained undiagnosed. Transbronchial biopsies markedly increases the diagnostic sensitivity of the fiberoptic procedure and must be proposed if a first BAL remains negative for the diagnosis of localized pneumonitis particularly in severely immunosuppressed patients (10).

REFERENCES

1. Oksenhendler E, Cadranel J, Sarfati C, Katlama C, Datry A, Marche C, Wolf M, Roux P, Derouin F, Clauvel JP. Toxoplasma gondii pneumonia in Patients with the acquired immunodeficiency syndrome. Am J Med 88: 5-18N–5-21N, 1990.
2. Goodman PC, Schnapp LM. Pulmonary toxoplasmosis in AIDS. Radiology 184: 791–793, 1992.
3. Jules-Elysee KM, Stover DE, Zaman MB, Bernard EM, White DA. Aerosolized pentamidine: effect on diagnosis and presentation of Pneumocystis carinii pneumonia. Ann Int Med 112: 750–757, 1990.
4. Edelstein H, McCabe RE. Atypical presentations of pneumocystis carinii pneumonia in patients receiving inhaled pentamidine prophylaxis. Chest 98: 1366–1369, 1990.
5. Schnapp LM, Geaghan SM, Campagna A, Fahy J, Steiger D, Ng V, Hadley K, Hopewell PC, Stansell JD. Toxoplasma gondii pneumonitis in patients infected with the human immunodeficiency virus. Arch Intern Med 152: 1073–1077, 1992.
6. Emmons W, Reichwein B, Winslow DL. Rhodococcus equi infection in the patients with AIDS: literature review and report of an unusual case. Rev Infect Dis 13: 91–96, 1991.
7. Drancourt M, Bonnet E, Gallais H, Peloux Y, Raoult D. Rhodococcus equi infection in patients with AIDS. J Infect 24: 123–131, 1992.

8. Nordmann P, Chavanet P, Caillon J, Duez JM, Portier H. Recurrent pneumonia due to rifampicin-resistant Rhodococcus equi in a patient infected with HIV. J Infect 24: 104–108, 1992.
9. Baughman RP, Dohn MN, Shipley R, Buchsbaum JA, Frame PT. Increased pneumocystis carinii recovery from the upper lobes in pneumocystis pneumonia. The effect of aerosol pentamidine prophylaxis. Chest 103: 426–432, 1993.
10. Gillet-Juvin K, Cadranel J, Isarël-Biet D, Antoine M, Carnot F, Akoun G, Mayaud C. Interest of concurrent transbronchial biopsy and bronchoalveolar lavage for the diagnosis of localized pneumonitis in HIV infected patients. (Abst 3180), VIII International Conference on AIDS, Amsterdam, 1992.

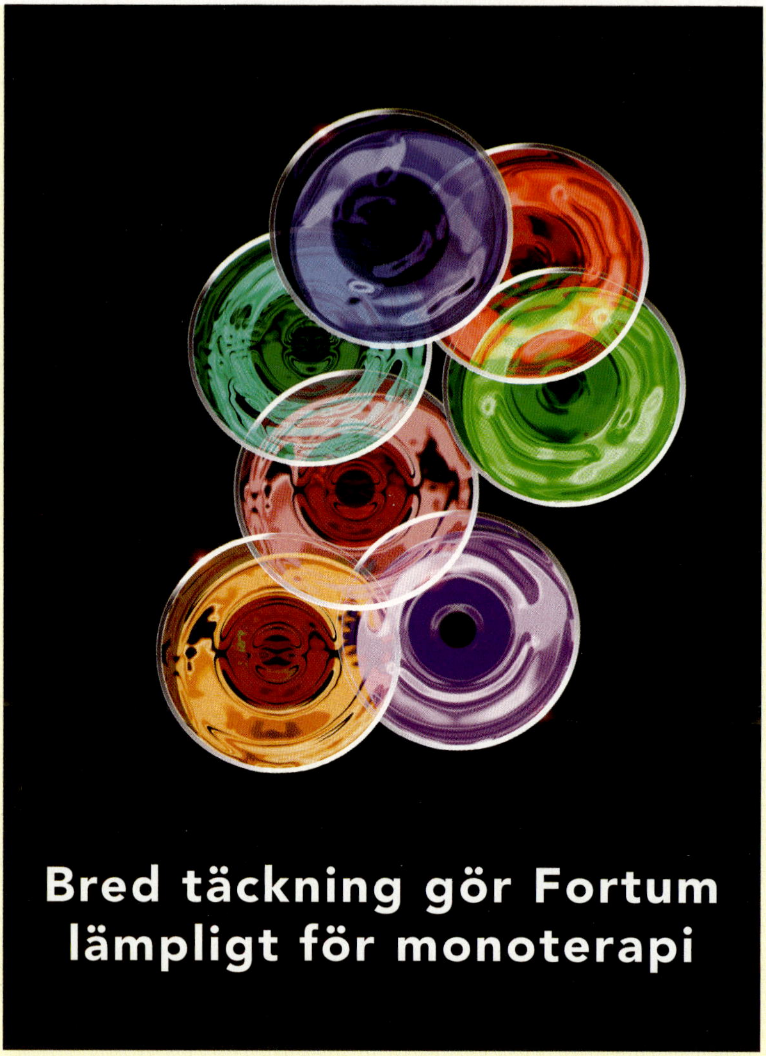
Bred täckning gör Fortum
lämpligt för monoterapi

Scand J Infect Dis 26: 219–221, 1994

CASE REPORT

Left Vocal Cord Palsy: An Unusual Presentation of a Mycotic Aneurysm of the Aorta Caused by Salmonella cholerasuis

PAUL CHAN[1,2], JENG JONG HUANG[3] and YU JEN YANG[3]

From the [1]Institute of Clinical Medicine of National Yang Ming Medical College, [2]Medical Department of Taipei Municipal Chung Hsiao Hospital, [3]National Cheng Kung University Hospital at Tainan, Taiwan

A 67-year-old man was admitted to hospital because of fever, productive cough and a concomitant hoarseness. A para-aortic lesion was found on chest X-ray, and bronchoscopy revealed a left vocal cord palsy. Due to rapid enlargement of the lesion, angiography was performed, which revealed a pseudoaneurysm at the descending aorta. Operation disclosed an infected aneurysm with rupture, and tissue culture yielded Salmonella cholerasuis. The findings of a mycotic aneurysm and hoarseness due to compression of the left recurrent laryngeal nerve is a rare and serious combination caused by salmonella, previously unreported in the medical literature.

P. Chan, MD, No. 87, Tung Teh Road, NanKang, Taipei, Taiwan 11532, R.O.C.

INTRODUCTION

Hoarseness associated with heart disease was first described by Ortner (1) in 1889, in patients with mitral stenosis. It was later proved that the hoarseness was caused by compression of the left recurrent laryngeal nerve by cardiovascular structures (2, 3), such as a large aortic aneurysm (3, 4). Mycotic aneurysms are also uncommon, with sporadic cases reported only occasionally in the medical literature (5–10). Here we report on an unusual case of mycotic aneurysm of the descending aorta caused by Salmonella cholerasuis, with associated hoarseness due to compression of the left recurrent laryngeal nerve by the large aneurysm.

CASE REPORT

A 67-year-old man had suffered from fever and productive cough for about 2 months. He had visited a local hospital where pneumonia was diagnosed. Concomitantly, the patient experienced haemoptysis, chest pain and hoarseness. Bronchoscopy revealed left vocal cord palsy without intrapulmonary lesions. Because a malignancy was suspected, radiotherapy was considered. However, the patient was referred to another hospital because of rapid expansion of the peri-aortic lesion, as revealed by a chest X-ray. Physical examination revealed an ill-looking man, with normal body temperature, blood pressure 110/70 mmHg, pulse 72/min and respiratory rate of 19/min. The white blood cell count was 11.7×10^9/l, while haemoglobin and platelet counts were normal. The erythrocyte sedimentation rate was 85 mm/h and C-reactive protein >30 mg/l. Blood sugar and creatinine values were normal. Because of suspicion of a mycotic aneurysm of the aorta, angiography, computer-assisted tomography and magnetic resonance imaging were performed (Fig. 1). Angiography revealed a pseudoaneurysm arising from the origin of the descending aorta.

Intravenous antimicrobial therapy was initiated with cefatriaxone sodium 1 g twice daily and amikacin 500 mg twice daily. An emergency operation was performed, and a large pseudoaneurysm (10×10 cm) was found at the descending aorta, with invasion of lung tissue and rupture. It was located just distal to the subclavian artery, with compression of the aortopulmonary window. In situ graft replacement was performed, with total debridement of necrotic tissues, from which S. cholerasuis was grown, although blood culture proved negative. The pathologist reported necrotising aortitis with thrombus formation. The patient was treated with antibiotics for another 4 weeks after the operation, followed by oral ofloxacin 200 mg twice daily for 6 months after being discharged with normal phonation. His condition was unremarkable 2 years after discharge.

 ISSN 0036-5548

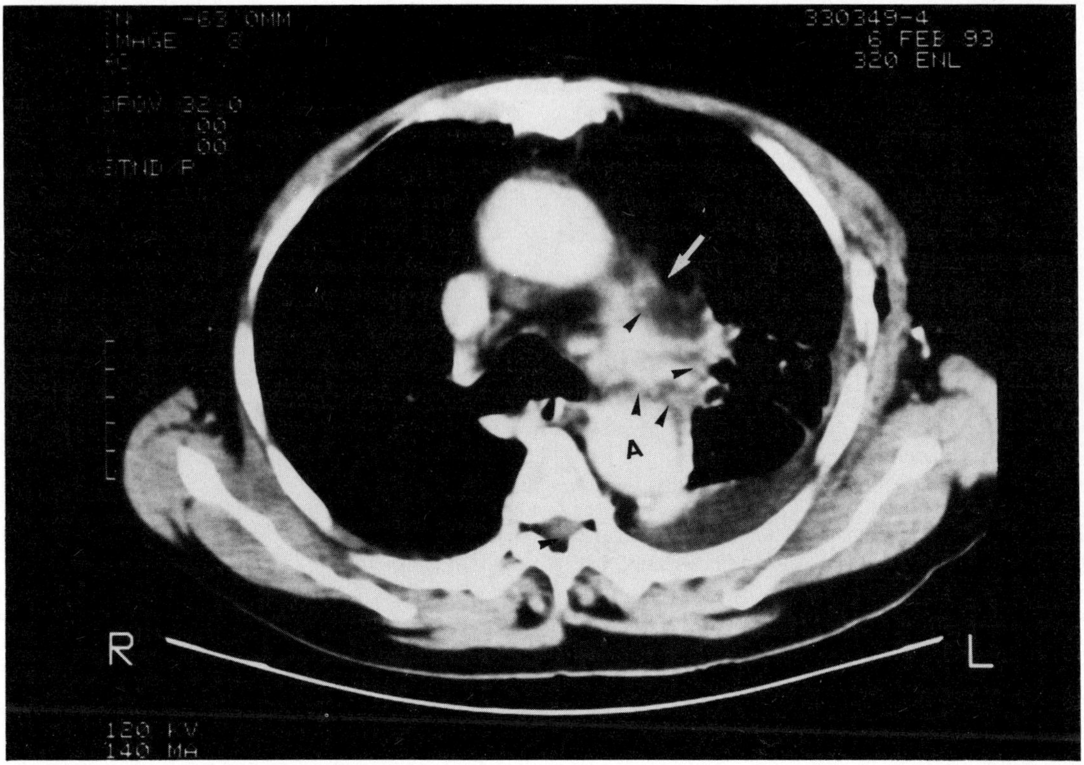

Fig. 1. Contrast-enhanced CT revealing a pseudoaneurysm arising from the ventral aspect of proximal descending aorta (*A*), located at the aortopulmonary window (*white arrow*) with inflammation and leakage (*arrowheads*).

DISCUSSION

Mycotic aneurysms constitute 0.8% to 2.8% of all aortic aneurysms (8, 11). The diagnosis of mycotic aneurysm is based on a high degree of suspicion, plus a clinical presentation of fever, leukocytosis and abdominal or back pain, in addition to a pulsatile abdominal mass if the aneurysm is located in the abdomen, especially in older patients (11). Patients who have an increased risk of endothelial damage because of diabetes mellitus, hypertension or smoking are at particular risk (11, 12). The prognosis in patients with mycotic aneurysms is usually poor, because of technical difficulty in completely eradicating the infectious focus, plus the insidious onset which often results in rupture before effective treatment can be initiated (8, 11, 13).

Conservative treatment is incapable of preventing the almost 100% mortality (11). However, recent reports have shown that a combination of surgical treatment and intensive antimicrobial therapy dramatically improves survival prospects (6, 8).

Hoarseness from left recurrent laryngeal nerve palsy associated with cardiovascular diseases (Cardiovocal or Ortner syndrome) is an unusual entity which has been reported to occur in 0.5% of patients with mitral stenosis (2); it is even rarer in other heart diseases (3). The left recurrent laryngeal nerve branches from the left vagus nerve at the anterolateral border of the aortic arch in a space between the main pulmonary artery and aortic arch (aortic window), just behind the ligamentum arteriosum. Therefore compression of the nerve can be caused by a dilated pulmonary artery, a persistent ductus arteriosus, or lesions of the aortic arch such as aneurysms (syphilitic, atherosclerotic or mycotic). The hoarseness associated with cardiovocal syndrome is usually reversible following successful interventional treatment (3).

Retrospective analysis of this patient's clinical course revealed that initially he had had an infected aortic aneurysm of the descending aorta which continued to expand because of the progressive inflammatory processes and subsequent destruction of the aortic wall, resulting in rapid expansion of the aneurysm to a large size. Compression of the recurrent laryngeal nerve resulted in hoarseness several days subsequent to fever and cough. The operative findings revealed a mycotic aneurysm 10 cm in diameter which caused the compression of the aortopulmonary window. Whereas aneurysms of the thoracic aorta are not uncommon, aneurysms leading to a cardiovocal syndrome are rare, probably depending on the size and the direction of the expansion. This case illustrates 2 rare clinical entities of which clinicians should be aware in order to make possible a timely diagnosis whereby appropriate therapy can be given.

REFERENCES

1. Ortner NI. Recurrenslahmung bei mitral Stenose. Wien Klin Wochenschr 10: 753–755, 1897.
2. Camishion RC, Gibbon JH, Pierucci L, Kida J. Paralysis of left recurrent laryngeal nerve secondary to mitral valve disease: report of two cases and literature review. Ann Surg 163: 818–827, 1960.
3. Chan P, Lee CP, Ko JT, Hung JS. Cardiovocal (Ortner's) syndrome: Left recurrent laryngeal nerve palsy associated with cardiovascular disease. Eur J Med 1: 492–495, 1992.
4. Zelman S, Nice GW. Recurrent left laryngeal nerve paralysis in atherosclerotic heart disease. JAMA 149: 1292–1292, 1952.
5. Cull DL, Winter RP, Wheeler JR, Gregory RT, Snyder SO, Galye RG, Parent NF III. Mycotic aneurysm of the suprarenal abdominal aorta. J Cardiovasc Surg 33: 181–184, 1992.
6. Pasic M, Carrel T, Vogt M, Segesser L, Turina M. Treatment of mycotic aneurysm of the aorta and its branches: the location determines the operative technique. Eur J Vasc Surg 6: 419–423, 1992.
7. Mehmet CO, McNicholas KW, Serra JS, Spagna PM, Lemole GM. Review of Salmonella mycotic aneurysms of the thoracic aorta. J Cardiovasc Surg 30: 99–103, 1989.
8. Chan FY, Crawford ES, Coselli JS, Safi HJ, Williams TW. In situ prosthetic graft replacement of mycotic aneurysm of the aorta. Ann Thorac Surg 47: 193–203, 1989.
9. Trairatvorakul P, Sriphojanart S, Sathapatayavongs B. Abdominal aortic aneurysms infected with Salmonella: problems of treatment. J Vasc Surg 12: 16–19, 1990.
10. Chan P, Lan CK, Wan YL. Salmonella cholerasuis bacteremia and mycotic aneurysm of abdominal aorta – report of 5 cases. Chang Gung Med J 12: 115–120, 1989.
11. Parkhurst GF, Decker JP. Bacterial aortitis and mycotic aneurysm of aorta: report of 12 cases. Am J Pathol 31: 821–835, 1955.
12. Cohen PS, O'Brien TF, Schoenbaum SC, Medeiros AA. The risk of endothelial infection in adults with salmonella bacteremia. Ann Intern Med 89: 931–932, 1978.
13. Bennett DE. Primary mycotic aneurysms of the aorta. Arch Surg 94: 758–765, 1967.

Scand J Infect Dis 26: 223–224, 1994

CASE REPORT

Abscess of the Submandibular Gland Caused by Salmonella typhimurium Biotype 10

AINA MØLLER HEILESEN and PER-HENRIK CHRISTENSEN

From the Department of Clinical Microbiology, Central Hospital, and the Department of Otorhinolaryngology, Sct. Josef Hospital, Esbjerg, Denmark

From an abscess of the submandibular gland, Salmonella typhimurium biotype 10 was isolated in pure culture. The patient had no history of gastroenteritis, and Salmonella could not be isolated from faeces.

A. Heilesen, MD, Department of Clinical Microbiology, Central Hospital, DK-6700 Esbjerg, Denmark

INTRODUCTION

The cause of Salmonella infection and abscess development is mostly supposed to be haematogenous spread from a primary infection of the gastrointestinal tract (1). Although abscesses are described in almost any organ (2), we have been unable to find any published report of abscess of the submandibular gland due to Salmonella typhimurium.

CASE REPORT

A 52-year-old previously healthy male whose occupation is transporting pigs from farms to the slaughterhouse, felt a swelling of the left submandibular region 10 days before hospitalization. Two days later he developed fever, severe pain and trismus. Upon physical examination at the Department of Otorhinolaryngology, there was no swelling of the pharynx and no stone in the submandibular duct. The submandibular gland was firm and enlarged, without fluctuation. The skin was normal, as was the physical examination in other respects.

Antibiotic treatment was initiated with gentamicin and ampicillin. Next day the temperature was normal, but the patient had developed redness and fluctuation of the submandibular region. The abscess was incised and a $5 \times 4 \times 3$ cm cavity was left open. Gentamicin was discontinued, and on day 4 ampicillin was replaced by oral pivampicillin. Five days after the incision, Salmonella typhimurium, biotype 10 was isolated in pure culture from the sample. The strain proved sensitive to all antibiotics tested. Oral ciprofloxacin replaced pivampicillin, and was continued for 10 days. 13 days after hospitalization the patient was transferred to the outpatient clinic. During hospitalization, an insulin-demanding diabetes mellitus was detected, for which the patient commenced treatment. Other laboratory values were normal.

DISCUSSION

The incidence of Salmonella infections has increased worldwide (3–7). Undercooked eggs and egg-containing foods are found to be very important vehicles for Salmonella enteritidis and S. typhimurium (8, 9). Our patient had no history of travelling abroad and no one in the family or close contacts had had any sign of Salmonella infection. However, diabetes mellitus is described as being 1 of the underlying predisposing diseases in salmonellosis in humans (5, 10).

The present patient had transported Salmonella-infected pigs, but had no history of skin lesion or abscess as described by Blasco et al. (11). Mandal and Brennand have described fever in only 54% in a 15-year retrospective study of bacteriaemia in salmonellosis (1), and gastroenteritis is seen in about half of the patients (5).

Since the numbers of cases of non-typhoid salmonellosis is increasing, and as secondary infections may develop weeks, months or years after the initial bacteremia (12), probably because Salmonella is a facultative intracellular organism with the ability to survive and grow in phagocytes (13), we consider it important that clinicians be aware of the different clinical pictures that salmonellosis may present.

REFERENCES

1. Mandal BK, Brennand J. Bacteraemia in salmonellosis: a 15 year retrospective study from a regional infectious diseases unit. BMJ 297: 1242–1243, 1988.
2. Cohen JI, Bartlett JA, Corey GR. Extra-intestinal manifestations of salmonella infections. Medicine 66: 349–388, 1987.
3. Maguire HCF, Codd AA, Mackay VE, Rowe R, Mitchell E. A large outbreak of human salmonellosis traced to a local pig farm. Epidemiol Infect 110: 239–246, 1993.
4. Chalker RB, Blaser MJ. A review of human salmonellosis. Rev Infect Dis 10: 111–122, 1988.
5. Lester A, Eriksen NHR, Nielsen H, Nielsen PB, Friis-Møller A, Bruun B, Scheibel J, Gaarslev K, Kolmos JH. Non-typhoid salmonella bacteraemia in greater Copenhagen 1984 to 1988. Eur J Clin Microbiol Infect Dis 1991: 486–490, 1991.
6. Salmonella surveillance summary for 1986. CDC, 1988.
7. Rodrigue DC, Tauxe RV. International increase in salmonella enteritidis: a new pandemic? Epidemiol Infect 105: 21–27, 1990.
8. St. Louis ME, Morse DL, Potter ME, DeMelfi TM, Guezewich JJ, Tauxe RV, Blake PA. The emergence of grade A eggs as a major source of salmonella enteritidis infections. JAMA 259: 2103–2107, 1988.
9. Hedberg CW, David MJ, White KE, MacDonald KL, Osterholm MT. Role of egg consumption in sporadic salmonella enteritidis and salmonella typhimurium infection in Minnesota. J Infect Dis 167: 107–111, 1993.
10. Bello EF, Pien FD. Salmonella dublin neck abscess. Arch Otolaryngol 111: 476–477, 1985.
11. Blasco AC, Valdivieso FB, Ayala IA, Munoz AY, Jimenez AA. Infecciones focales por salmonella no typhi: revision de mestra casuistica y comparacion con otras series. Rev Clin Esp 191: 71–75, 1992.
12. Koshi G. Uncommon manifestations of salmonella infections. Indian J Med Res 64: 314–321, 1976.
13. Conlan JW, North RJ. Early pathogenesis of infection in the liver with the facultative intracellular bacteria listeria monocytogenes, francisella tularensis, and salmonella typhimurium involves lysis of infected hepatocytes by leucocytes. Infect Immun 60: 5164–5171, 1992.

Scand J Infect Dis 26: 225–228, 1994

CASE REPORT

Successful Combined Surgical and Medical Treatment of Fusarium Infection after Bone Marrow Transplantation

MICHAEL E. ELLIS[1], HUGH CLINK[2], DEREK YOUNGE[3] and BO HAINAU[4]

From the Departments of [1]Medicine, [2]Oncology, [3]Orthopedic Surgery and [4]Pathology and Laboratory Medicine, King Faisal Specialist Hospital and Research Center, Riyadh, Kingdom of Saudi Arabia

The usual management of opportunistic fusarium infection in the immunocompromized patient is with systemic antifungals, despite which little impact is made on the mortality which approaches 100%. We describe a case of fusarium infection of the foot in a bone marrow transplant recipient which was successfully managed with local wide excisional surgery and intravenous liposomal amphotericin B.

M. E. Ellis, MD, Department of Medicine, King Faisal Specialist Hospital and Research Centre, P.O. Box 3354, Riyadh 11211, Kingdom of Saudi Arabia

CASE REPORT

A 29-year-old Sudanese male with centroblastic lymphoma had received conditioning with carmustine, etoposide, cytarabine, and melphalan prior to autologous bone marrow transplantation. Prophylactic antimicrobials included acyclovir and oral fluconazole 200 mg daily from the 1st day of neutropenia (2nd post-transplant day white cell count 0.1×10^9/l). Nine days after transplant, he complained of local tenderness on the plantar aspect of the left foot. Examination revealed an area of local tenderness over the flexor digitorum profundus muscle. He was febrile, at 38.5°C. Five days later, a 1 cm round, raised reddened area with central necrosis appeared (Fig. 1). Biopsy showed marked infiltration by septated hyphae with parallel borders, branching at acute angles consistent with either aspergillus or fusarium (Fig. 2). Treatment was commenced with intravenous amphotericin B, 0.5 mg/kg, increasing over 3 days to 1 mg/kg, together with rifampicin 600 mg orally daily. He remained profoundly neutropenic and febrile with a daily intermittent peak of up to 38.6°C. Granulocyte–monocyte colony stimulating factor (GMCSF) (300 μg subcutaneously daily) was given to aid neutrophil recovery and function, in a potentially life threatening situation.

Fusarium spp was identified on culture of the skin biopsy and treatment was changed to liposomal amphotericin B (3 mg/kg daily) on the 16th post-transplant day. After a further 14 days (29th transplant day) of antifungal therapy – a total of 2.5 g of amphotericin B – he was apyrexial, the white cell count had risen to 1.4 (58% polymorphs) but the lesion had increased in size to approximately 1.3 cm diameter. Over this period, he had remained well systemically – notably he had no cough or dyspnea, no facial pain, headache or nasal discharge. Plain radiology and CT scan of the chest, sinuses and abdomen were normal.

At this time, he underwent surgical excision of the lesion. The surgeon removed an eclipse of skin and soft tissue (2.5×4.0 cm). Pathological examination revealed a half inch embedded broken hypodermic needle (the patient recalled subsequently having had an episode of sharp pain in his sole on walking barefoot in another hospital several weeks prior to his transplantation). Histologically, the resection lines showed that the margins of the resected tissue were free of fungal infection. The white cell response to GMCSF continued and this was discontinued 3 days after the operation (32nd transplant day), on which the white cell count was 6.1×10^9/l (66% neutrophils). Ambisome was continued for 13 days after the operation (42nd transplant day). At this time, the wound had healed normally and the peripheral white cell count and differential remained normal. At follow-up, 6 months later, he remained well and had no evidence of local or systemic fungus infection.

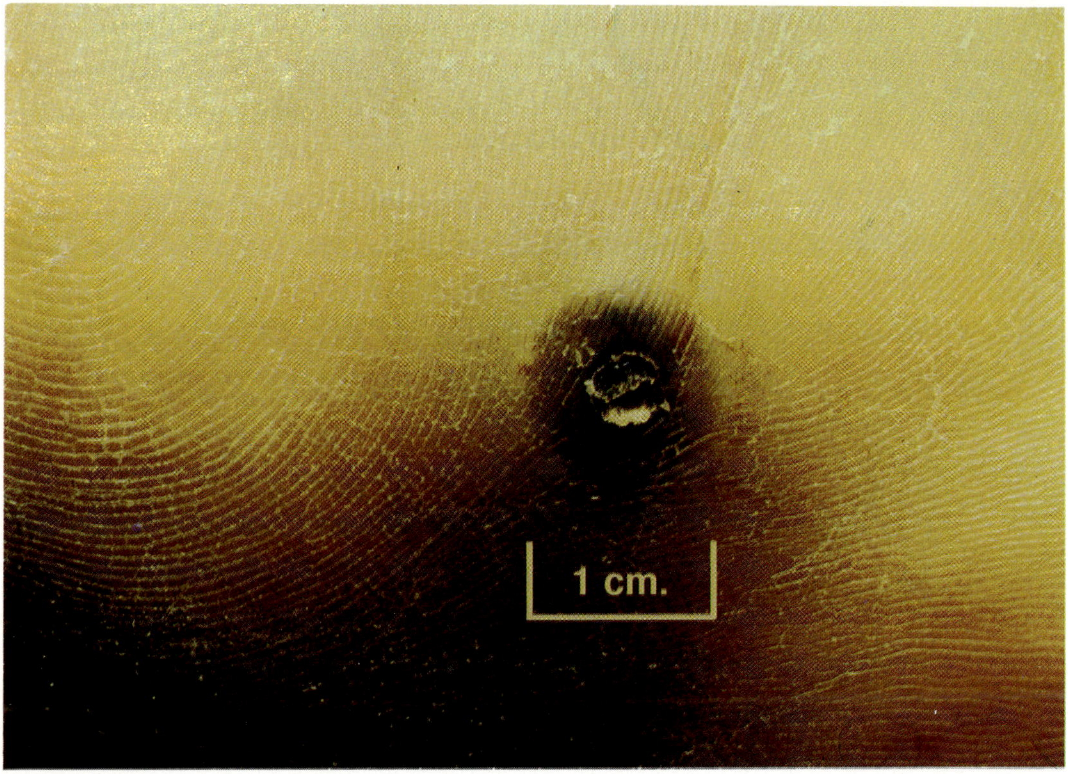

Fig. 1. Photograph of foot lesion.

DISCUSSION

Fusarium spp is an emerging pathogen in patients with hematological malignancy, a major risk factor being severe and prolonged neutropenia. Differentiation from aspergillus is possible only by culture, but is crucial since fusarium is usually resistant to the azoles and to amphotericin B, and liposomal encapsulated amphotericin B has been used successfully in a few cases (1). It was of some concern that, despite the prophylactic use of fluconazole, this infection had developed. The portal of entry for most cases of disseminated fusarium infection is usually the upper respiratory tract, sinuses, or lungs. Localized fusarium infection is, however, well described secondary to localized trauma, but occurring mainly in immunocompetent patients (2, 3). Our patient had no pulmonary or systemic features, and with the recent history of trauma suggested that the skin lesion was a manifestation of a primary inoculation source rather than a feature of hematogenous dissemination. There is nothing in the literature to suggest that local subcutaneous foci of fusarium pose any lesser risk for dissemination, compared with patients who acquire it via a pulmonary focus. On the contrary, there is evidence that other fungal infections, which are acquired via a primary cutaneous/inoculation route in immunocompromized patients, act as a focus for dissemination. This has been demonstrated with aspergillosis (4, 5).

In view of the risk of opportunistic fungi disseminating from such a cutaneous source, it is reasonable to remove the focus in its entirety. The decision to adopt this approach in our patient was further strengthened by the known poor response of established fungal infection to antifungal treatment (6). Although administration of systemic antifungal antimicrobials is

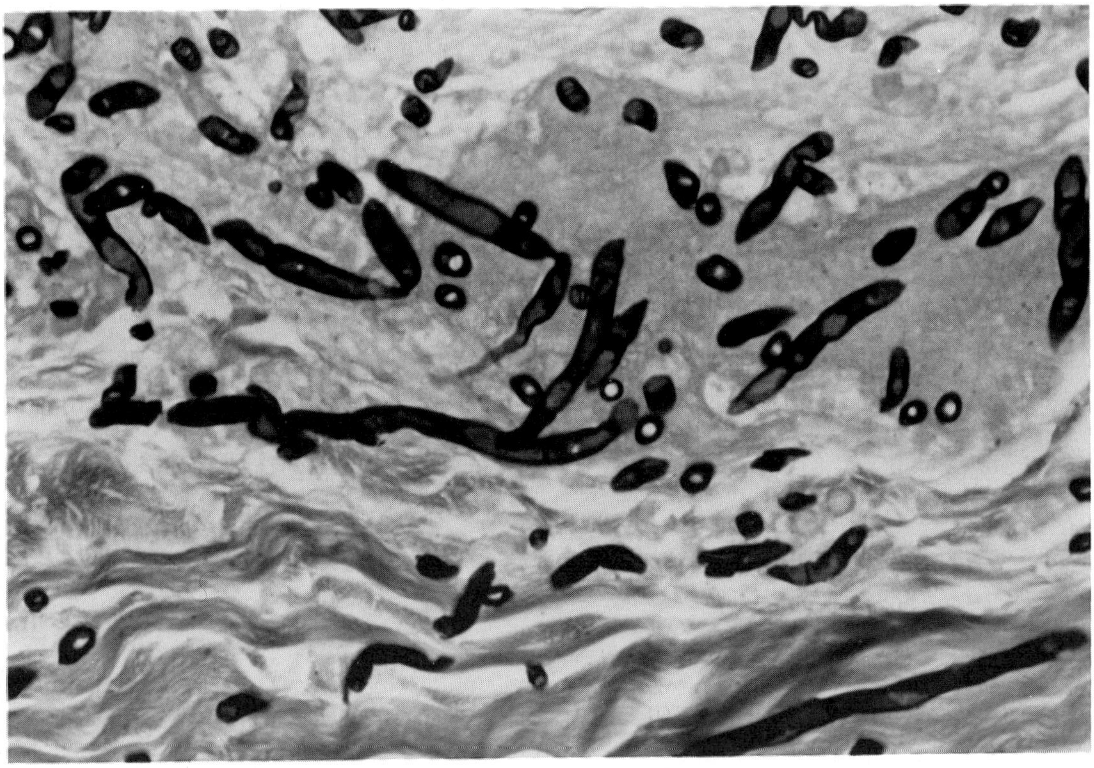

Fig. 2. Micrograph of the biopsy, showing dichotomic branching septate hyphae. The morphology is consistent with either aspergillus or fusarium. Grocott-methenamine-silver stain. Magnification ×800.

the standard approach, surgical removal of pulmonary opportunistic fungal infections in the immunocompromized host, with the primary aim of reducing dissemination, has been described in a few cases in the literature, but it is not clear what effect this had on recurrence of disseminated fungal disease or patient outcome (7, 8). To our knowledge, a surgical approach has not previously been described for primary skin fusarial infection in bone marrow transplant patients. A key factor in the response to fungal infection is recovery of neutrophils – undoubtedly this would have played a major role in this case. Nevertheless, better results compared with historical controls are claimed in some patients who undergo surgical resection of their fungal foci (7, 9). In our patient, however, despite a rising white count, the lesion was noted to grow in size. Moreover, despite excellent surgical access, we dared not leave open the possibility of dissemination, or indeed of recurrence during any subsequent graft failure.

Since such fungi produce angioinvasion, we could not rule out the possibility that distant hematogenous spread might have occurred at a subclinical level, though it was hoped that this would have been prevented by the relatively early surgical intervention undertaken. Indeed, this is unlikely, as after 2 months' follow-up, the patient remains clinically well. Skin healing was normal in our patient, probably aided by the granulocyte response to GMCSF.

We recommend in immunocompromized patients that early local excision of anatomically accessible opportunistic fungal foci be undertaken in situations where the site clearly represents the portal of entry, provided such sites are surgically accessible and the patient's general condition permits surgical intervention.

REFERENCES

1. Viviani MA, Tortorano AM, Malaspina C, Grancini A, Crofrancesco E. Efficacy of Ambisome in the treatment of Fusarium infection in a leukemic patient. XI Congress of the International Society of Human and Animal Mycology 1991 (Abstract).
2. Page JC, Friedlander G, Dockery OL. Postoperative fusarium osteomyelitis. J Foot Surg 21: 174–176, 1982.
3. Hiemenz JW, Kennedy B, Kwon-Chung KJ. Invasive fusarioses associated with an injury by a stingray barb. J Med Vet Mycol 28: 209–213, 1990.
4. Langlois RP, Flegel EF, Meakins JL, Morehouse DD, Robson HG, Guttman RD. Cutaneous aspergillosis with fatal dissemination in a renal transplant recipient. Can Med Assoc J 120: 673–675, 1980.
5. Allo MD, Miller J, Townsend T, Tan C. Primary cutaneous aspergillosis associated with Hickman intravenous catheters. N Engl J Med 317: 1105–1108, 1987.
6. Anaissie E. Opportunistic mycoses in the immunocompromised host: experience at a cancer center and review. Clin Infect Dis 14 (Suppl 1): S43–53, 1992.
7. Lupinetti FM, Behrendt DM, Giller RH, Trigg ME, de Alarcon P. Pulmonary resection for fungal infection in children undergoing bone marrow transplantation. J Thorac Cardiovasc Surg 104: 684–687, 1992.
8. Lupinetti FM, Giller RH, Trigg ME. Operative treatment of fusarium fungal infection of the lung. Ann Thorac Surg 49: 991–992, 1990.
9. Berger LA. CT scanning for invasive fungal disease. In: "Trends in Invasive Fungal Infections II" Conference. Manchester, 1993.

Scand J Infect Dis 26: 233–238, 1994

HISTORICAL REVIEW

Effect of Introduction of Sulphonamides on the Incidence of and Mortality from Puerperal Sepsis in a Swedish County Hospital

ULF HÖGBERG

From the Department of Obstetrics and Gynaecology, Umeå University Hospital, Umeå, Sweden

The effect of sulphonamides on the incidence of and mortality from puerperal sepsis in a county hospital between 1931 and 1950 was evaluated in a retrospective cohort study. The impact of antibiotics was evaluated by epidemiological methods. The incidence of puerperal sepsis decreased following the introduction of sulphonamides. The risk of contracting puerperal sepsis was reduced 80%. Whereas the fatality rate remained unaffected, patients treated with antibiotics had a significantly shorter duration of fever.

U. Högberg, MD, Department of Obstetrics and Gynaecology, University Hospital, S-901 87 Umeå, Sweden

INTRODUCTION

Before the age of antisepsis, puerperal sepsis was the major complication in early obstetrical practice. That it was caused by an infectious agent was suspected in the 18th century when Denman (1768), in England, suggested that the disease was carried by physicians and midwives from one mother to another. In 1772, White said that the discharges of septic puerperal women were contagious and Gordon (1795) stated "... this disease seized women only as were visited or delivered by a practitioner or taken care of by a nurse who had previously attended patients affected with the disease. In short, I have evident proofs of its infectious nature."

The epidemiology of puerperal sepsis was well described by contemporary Swedish obstetricians, who reported that it affected impoverished unmarried women suffering from malnutrition. Outbreaks then occurred concomitant with outbreaks of erysipelas and scarlet fever. Anaemia probably also contributed to the high fatality rate of puerperal sepsis. Almost 50% of women who contracted the disease died. At its worst, 20% of mothers died from puerperal sepsis. Some years, no women died in Swedish lying-in hospitals. Evidently the women's high susceptibility to the streptococcus at that time, together with a contracted pelvis and anaemia, produced difficult obstetric situations with a high mortality (1).

Oliver Wendell Holmes (1843) and Ignaz Semmelweiss (1844) both described the mode of transmission of puerperal sepsis and suggested means to prevent it (2). Once these were accepted, the effect was dramatic. Antisepsis was estimated to reduce septic maternal mortality 96% in lying-in hospitals and 63% in rural home deliveries in Sweden during the late 19th century (1). The spread of this new technology to all mothers took time. It was not until 1931–35 that the national mortality figures for puerperal sepsis reached the level that the lying-in hospitals achieved in 1881–1900 (3). Mortality from puerperal sepsis continued to decline in Europe from the beginning of the 20th century. This was probably due to further improvements in antiseptic measures, improvements in surgical techniques, and possibly better nutritional standards with less anaemia in pregnant women. Some decrease in the incidence of puerperal sepsis may also have been a result of the introduction of new technology developed during the 1930s. This included the typing of streptococci, charting their source and mode of spread, with the identification and treatment of carriers, isolation of infected cases, use of masks, etc. (2).

The earliest sulphonamides (prontosil and sulphanilamide) were effective against the streptococcus (4, 5). Sulphonamides were introduced into obstetric practice in 1935 (6) and that they were responsible for the decline of puerperal sepsis seems indisputable (7).

In Sweden, a sharp reduction in the mortality rate from puerperal sepsis was reported during the 1940s that was associated with the introduction of antibiotics (8, 9). However, this relationship, which appeared obvious to clinicians, has been questioned. Antibiotics have been suggested not to have had any certain effect on the decline in national mortality rates from puerperal sepsis in Sweden between 1930–38 and 1939–51 (10).

The aim of this study was therefore to further evaluate the effect of antibiotics on the incidence and mortality of puerperal sepsis in a retrospective cohort study.

METHODS

Sundsvall is the central region of the timber and paper industry in Sweden. There were 27,124 registered births between 1931 and 1950 at the county hospital's obstetric department. The archives of Sundsvall's hospital's obstetric unit's files and the records for this period have been examined. However, complete files were not available for 1932, 1933, and 1939 and these years were excluded. All cases in the files with a diagnosis of endometritis and puerperal sepsis, fever, salpingitis, haemorrhage, thrombosis, urinary infection, or gonorrhoea were registered; as were interventions including caesarean section, forceps delivery, perforation of membranes, internal version and extraction, manual removal of placenta and curettage. The following data were included for each case: maternal age and parity, intercurrent diseases such as heart disease, pregnancy and delivery complications, operations performed, medicines, haemoglobin (%), time span of labour, time span from rupture of the membranes to delivery, time span from third stage, birth weight, neonatal complications, duration of fever (days) and puerperal care, birth weight, and neonatal outcome. The data were registered and computerized using the Quest program.

Annual reports of Sundsvall's hospital and national statistics from Statistics Sweden, have also been used.

The following definitions are used in the study. Parity is defined as the number of previous pregnancies ending in registered births or stillbirths. Fatality rate is defined as the number of deaths/number of diagnosed cases. Cause-specific mortality is defined as the number of deaths/100,000 population at risk. Incidence rate refers to the number of cases/1,000 population at risk.

Measures of potential impact refer to the effect of a change in certain risk factor distribution. The impact of antibiotics is presumed to be 'preventive' regarding the incidence. To estimate the potential impact, both the relative risk that can be ascribed to a certain protective factor, and the incidence/prevalence of the same factor in the population are required. The prevented fraction is defined as the quotient between the cases that would have occurred in the absence of the projective factor minus the cases that did occur (prevented cases), and the cases that did occur (11, 13).

Unpaired *t*-test was used to compare the periods before and after the introduction of antibiotics.

RESULTS

The incidence of endometritis/puerperal sepsis at the obstetric unit in Sundsvall during the 1930s was high, 23.0–56.0/1,000 deliveries, with no sign of a decline during that decade. An abrupt reduction was seen in 1940–41/1942–43. For comparison, other indicators of obstetric outcome, such as perinatal mortality and the incidence of low birth weight (<2,500 g) declined between 1931 and 1950, but at slower rate, with reductions of 47.5% and 35.5%, respectively. Further, the slope of the decline is quite different (Fig. 1).

Sulphonamides were introduced in Sundsvall during 1941. In that year, there were 87 cases of endometritis/puerperal sepsis on the maternity ward, 26 of them treated with sulphonamides. Only 2 cases of puerperal infection were registered in 1942, both treated with sulphonamides. Newly delivered mothers who had had complicated deliveries requiring the use of forceps, caesarean section, or in whom perforation of membranes, internal version, extraction

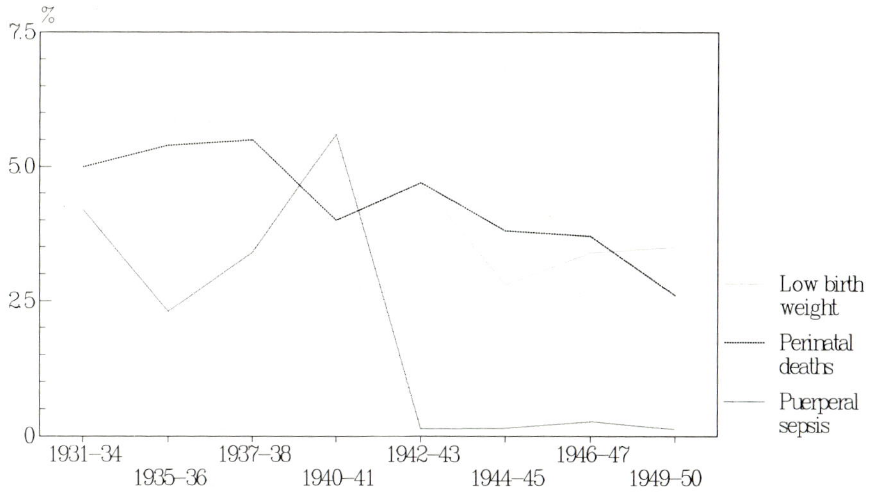

Fig. 1. Number of cases of puerperal sepsis, low birth weight and perinatal deaths per 100 births, Maternity of Sundsvall 1931–50.

of the placenta and curettage had been undertaken also received sulphonamides. Penicillin was introduced in 1945 and the indications for its use were the same as for sulphonamides. However, in Sundsvall's obstetric unit, sulphonamides were still preferred for the treatment of endometritis/puerperal sepsis even after the introduction of penicillin (Table I).

The patients who were diagnosed as having endometritis/puerperal sepsis were compared by unpaired *t*-test for the two periods 1931–40/1942–50. No differences regarding maternal age, parity, birth weight, or delivery time were observed. A slightly increased haemoglobin level was noted. The only significant change was the duration of fever, which decreased from 7.1 to 4.9 days after the introduction of antibiotics, indicating a less severe course of puerperal infection (Table II).

The risk of contracting puerperal sepsis was reduced by 95% (RR = 0.05) after the introduction of antibiotics (Table III).

Although the incidence of puerperal infection was considerably reduced and the disease became less severe, the fatality rate was unaffected after the introduction of antibiotics. The estimated case-fatality rate of puerperal sepsis/endometritis remained unchanged between 1946 and 1950 when compared with 1936 to 1940, despite antibiotics having been available during the former period (Table IV). The estimated case fatality rate is uncertain as there were only 14 cases, and only 6 received sulphonamides and none received penicillin during 1946 to 1950.

Table I. *No. of parturients/puerperas treated with sulphonamide or penicillin during the years 1941–50. Only sulphonamides were used on the indication of puerperal sepsis, Maternity of Sundsvall*

	1941	1942	1943	1944	1945	1946	1947	1948
No. of patients treated with sulphonamides (all)	52	42	24	32	17	37	3	7
– diagnosis puerperal sepsis	26	2	1	1	3	7	0	0
No. of patients treated with penicillin	–	–	–	–	2	3	5	10

Table II. *Comparison of certain maternal variables by means during the years 1931–41/1942–50 when antibiotics were available during the latter period, Maternity of Sundsvall*

	1931–41 No.	Mean	1942–50 No.	Mean	*p*-value
Maternal age	266	25.5	23	26.9	0.34
Parity	266	1.5	16	1.4	0.75
Hb (%)	174	67%	22	73%	0.02
Labour (h)	257	22.3	15	18.5	0.53
Birth weight (g)	264	3439	15	3342	0.48
Days with fever	266	7.0	22	4.8	0.001
Days of care	266	11.8	23	9.4	0.02
Third stage (min)	263	13.1	13	13.5	–

Table III. *Puerperal sepsis/endometritis per 1,000 live births, Maternity of Sundsvall, before and after the introduction of antibiotics*

Period	No. of births	No. of puerperal sepsis	Rate (%)	RR[a]	Cases prevented	PF[b]
1931–40	7,496	266	3.55	1	–	–
1942–50	13,407	23	0.17	0.05	476-23 = 453	95%

[a] relative risk.
[b] prevented fraction.

Table IV. *Incidence of puerperal sepsis/endometritis/1,000 live births, Maternity of Sundsvall 1936–40 (except 1939), and 1946–50; cause-specific mortality of puerperal sepsis/100,000 live births in Sweden 1936–40/1946–50 and case fatality rate/100 diagnosed cases of puerperal sepsis/endometritis*

	1936–40	1946–50
Incidence	32.9	1.9
Mortality	62	3.5
Case fatality rate	1.9	1.8

DISCUSSION

Evaluation of medical technology is biased when using historical controls, often over-emphasising the influence of new treatments (13). The question of the effect of antibiotics on the mortality decline of infectious diseases cannot be definitely resolved retrospectively, but the results from this study suggest the presence of a causal relationship. The study questioning this relationship did not take into account the sulphonamides were not fully introduced in Sweden obstetrics until 1941–42 (10). Further, no other cause of maternal death declined during the 1940s to the same extent as did puerperal sepsis. Moreover, the age shift in the parturient population during the 1940s had a negligible effect on the mortality from sepsis, but not other causes of maternal death (3).

The abrupt decline in the incidence of puerperal sepsis coincided with the introduction of sulphonamides, suggesting a relationship. Other outcome measurements, such as low birth weight and perinatal mortality should be better related to socio-economic factors and antenatal and delivery performance, thus declining at a slower rate and supporting the results of this study. Further, the practice of using sulphonamides, as well as penicillin, for other indications then puerperal sepsis, for example prophylactically in patients undergoing instrumental delivery, should have had a major impact on the prevention of outbreaks of puerperal sepsis (Table I).

Thus, there seems to be evidence supporting a causal relationship between the declining incidence of puerperal infections and the introduction of antibiotics. The assumed impact on the incidence of puerperal infection is within the same range as was noticed when antiseptic technique was introduced in the lying-in hospitals during the 19th century, when puerperal septic mortality declined by 95% (1, 14).

This study showed that antibiotics shorten the course of puerperal infection. A reduction in case-fatality rate could not be found, probably because of the small number of women with puerperal infection receiving antibiotics. However, the introductory trials of the drug in Britain in 1936 and 1937 did show a case fatality reduction, from 25% to 4.7%, and 13.5% to 1.4% respectively (15, 16).

That fatal puerperal sepsis is a multifactorial condition is evident in obstetrics in developing countries. Even today, the use of antibiotics will not solve the problems of patients' delay, contracted pelvis, anaemia and exhaustion. An indirect indication of better reproductive health in Swedish mothers during the 1940s was their improved haemoglobin level. This may have been related to improved nutrition, as well as to antenatal care which reached more than 60% of the pregnant population in Sweden between 1946 and 1950 (3, 14).

The dramatically lower incidence of puerperal sepsis could be due to the prophylactic use of antibiotics in patients with complicated deliveries with prolonged labour, premature rupture of the membranes, complicated forceps delivery, abdominal delivery, internal version, perforation, or extraction of placenta. This practice successfully prevented new cases of puerperal infection in otherwise anaemic and exhausted mothers in poor physical condition, resulting in an overall declining incidence of puerperal sepsis and ensuing deaths (17). Antibiotic prophylaxis is still given and is of value, for example in prolonged labour and abdominal delivery (18).

Clinicians accept the therapeutic efficacy of antibiotics in puerperal sepsis. Thus antibiotics appear to be effective in reducing the death rate from puerperal sepsis. Although declining streptococcal virulence may also have played a part in the decline in mortality from puerperal fever, its role was minor compared with that of antibiotics (19). The war against puerperal sepsis took 100 years, and was won by two achievements, antiseptic techniques and the introduction of antibiotics.

REFERENCES

1. Högberg U, Wall S, Broström G. The potential impact of medical technology on maternal mortality in 19th century. Int J Gynaecol Obstet 23: 489–497, 1985.
2. Baird D. The evolution of modern obstetrics. Lancet 2: 557–661, 1960.
3. Högberg U, Joelsson I. The decline of maternal mortality in Sweden, 1931–1980. Acta Obstet Gynecol Scand 64: 583–592, 1985.
4. Domagk G. Ein Beitrag zur Chemotherapie der bakteriellen Infektionen. Dtsch Med Wochenschr 61: 250–253, 1935.
5. Foerster R. Sepsis im Anschluss an ausgedehnte Periporitis. Heilung durch Streptozon. Z Haut- und Geschlechtskrankheiten 45: 549–550, 1933.
6. Anselm E. Unsere Erfahrungen mit Prontosil bei Puerperalfieber. Dtsch Med Wochenschr 61: 264, 1935.
7. McKeown T, Record RG, Turner RD. An interpretation of the decline of mortality in England and Wales during the twentieth century. Popul Stud 29: 391–422, 1975.

8. Furstenberg N. Maternal mortality – a statistical analysis of earlier and present prognosis in childbirth. Acta Obstet Gynecol Scand 28: 103–109, 1949.
9. Klintskog E. Maternal mortality in Sweden – an investigation based on official Swedish statistics. Acta Obstet Gynecol Scand 50: 361–377, 1950.
10. Hemmminki E, Paakulainen Y. The effect of antibiotics on mortality of infectious diseases. Am J Publ Health 66: 1180–1184, 1976.
11. Kleinbaum DG, Kupper LL, Morgenstern H. Epidemiologic Research, Principles and Quantitative Methods. London: Lifetime Learning Publications, 1982.
12. Walter S. Calculation of attributable risks from epidemiological data. Int J Epidemiol 7: 175–182, 1978.
13. Chalmers I, Enkin M, Keirse M. Effective Care in Pregnancy and Childbirth: Oxford, Oxford University Press, 1989.
14. Högberg U. Maternal Mortality in Sweden. Umeå University Medical Dissertation, New Series 156, 1985.
15. Colebrook L. Kenny M. Treatment with Prontosil of puerperal infections due to haemolytic streptococci. Lancet 2: 1319–1322, 1936.
16. Foulis MA, Barr JB. Prontosil album in puerperal sepsis. BMJ 445–446, 1937.
17. Klein M, Clahr J. Factors in the decline of maternal mortality. JAMA 168: 237–242, 1958.
18. Smaill F. Prophylactic antibiotics in caesarean section (all trials). In: Enkin MW, Keirse MJNC, Renfrew MJ, Neilson JP eds. Pregnancy and Childbirth Module. 'Cochrane Database of Systematic Reviews': Review No 03690 18 December 1992. Oxford: Update Software, Spring 1993.
19. Loudon I. Death in Childbirth – An International Study of Maternal Care and Maternal Mortality 1800–1950. Oxford: Oxford University Press, 1992.

Submitted November 25, 1993; accepted March 10, 1994

Scand J Infect Dis 26: 239–247, 1994

Cytomegalovirus Infection Rate among Heart Transplant Patients in Relation to Anti-thymocyte Immunoglobulin Induction Therapy

KIM KROGSGAARD[1], SØREN BOESGAARD[2], JAN ALDERSHVILE[2], HENRIK ARENDRUP[2], SVEND AAGE MORTENSEN[2], GÖSTA PETTERSON[3], and THE COPENHAGEN HEART TRANSPLANT GROUP

From the Departments of [1]Infectious Diseases M, [2]Medical Department B and [3]Thoracic Surgery RT, Rigshospitalet, University of Copenhagen, Copenhagen, Denmark

During a 2-year period, 49 patients underwent heart transplantation at Rigshospitalet, Copenhagen. Nine (18%) were females and the mean age for all patients was 44 years (range 14–56 years). Immunosuppressive therapy included cyclosporin, azathioprine and steroids in all patients. 43 patients received in addition short-term (approx. 4 days) induction treatment with anti-thymocyte immunoglobulin (ATG). 17 patients received ATG Fresenius®, 2.5 mg/kg/day or ATGAM®, 12.5 mg/kg/day, whereas the remaining 26 patients received ATG Merieux®, 2.5 mg/kg/day. Prophylactic antimicrobial chemotherapy included ceftriaxone, acyclovir (1 g daily), nystatin, and pyrimethamine in toxoplasmosis mismatch patients. Serological assays for cytomegalovirus (CMV), Epstein-Barr virus, varicella-zoster virus, herpes simplex virus, legionella and toxoplasmosis as well as CMV and bacterial culturing were carried out before transplantation, at regular intervals and when clinically indicated. Five patients developed septicaemia. Nine had pulmonary bacterial infections, including 2 cases of legionella pneumonia. Two had Clostridium difficile diarrhoea. Three patients had Pneumocystis carinii pneumonitis. 24 patients (49%) had evidence of CMV infection/reactivation. Seven out of 10 CMV mismatch (pos donor/neg recipient) patients and 3 out of 12 CMV match (pos donor/pos recipient) patients developed clinical CMV disease. The rate of CMV infection/reactivation was significantly higher among patients who had CMV-positive donors ($p < 0.01$) and among patients receiving ATG Merieux® induction treatment ($p < 0.0001$). Logistic regression analysis showed that both positive CMV donor status and ATG Merieux® induction treatment were significant independent predictors of CMV infection. Six patients (12%) died. Two out of 4 infection related deaths could be ascribed to CMV disease.

K. Krogsgaard, MD, PhD, Department of Medicine, Division of Infectious Diseases, College of Physicians and Surgeons of Columbia University, 630 West 168th Street, New York, NY 10032, USA

INTRODUCTION

Infection is an important factor contributing to morbidity and mortality in heart transplant patients (1, 2). In most series, infections seem to be a contributory factor in about half of all fatal cases (1, 2). The heart transplant patient is a compromised host, the degree of immune suppression being the result of underlying cardiac disease, surgical trauma, immobilization and necessary immunosuppressive medications. Most centres use a triple drug regimen including steroids, azathioprine and cyclosporin (3). In addition, cytolytic treatment with anti-thymocyte globulin (ATG) or OKT3 is an effective tool not only for the treatment of rejection, but also as induction therapy to delay the first rejection and probably also prevent early severe rejections (4). As yet, there is no consensus about the advantage of induction therapy when all possible adverse effects are taken into account. Information on the relative potency, antibody specificity, and adverse effects of the various immunoglobulin preparations is very limited.

Of the various pathogens implicated in post-heart transplantation infections, cytomegalovirus (CMV) is probably the most important (5–7). CMV may give rise to an influenza-like mild illness with low-grade fever, as well as a severe disease with organ manifestations such as pneumonitis, hepatitis, colitis and carditis (8, 9). In addition, CMV has in some retrospective reports been implicated as a triggering and contributory factor in acute and chronic allograft rejection and vasculopathy (10, 11). Although CMV disease is more frequent and severe among CMV mismatch patients (CMV-positive donor to CMV-negative recipient), CMV may also be a problem in CMV-positive recipients (6, 8). Various prophylactic regimens are available but the cost-effectiveness profile remains unclear. The low-dose acyclovir used to prevent herpes simplex has little effect on CMV and is most probably insufficient as CMV prophylaxis (12, 13). Ganciclovir may diminish CMV morbidity among CMV-positive patients (14). However, ganciclovir causes bone marrow suppression and is therefore not an attractive drug to combine with other immunosuppressive drugs.

In the present survey on infections after heart transplantation we report clinical and microbiological findings during the first 6 months following heart transplantation in the first 49 patients from Copenhagen. In the program 3 different preparations of ATG were used to induce immune suppression; no specific CMV prophylaxis was given, and CMV disease was left untreated unless severe organ involvement was present.

MATERIALS AND METHODS

Patients

Heart transplantation started in Denmark in October 1990 and in the following 2-year period 49 patients underwent transplantation at Rigshospitalet, Copenhagen. 40 patients (82%) were males and the mean age for all patients was 44 years (range: 14–56 years). The underlying cardiac disease among males was: dilated cardiomyopathy, 18 (45%); ischaemic heart disease, 21 (52.5%); and congenital heart disease, 1 (2.5%). Among females 6 (67%) had dilated cardiomyopathy and 3 (33%) ischaemic heart disease. The survey was restricted to the first 6 months after transplantation.

Immune suppression protocols

The regimen included steroids, azathioprine and cyclosporine. Three different preparations of ATG were used: ATGAM® (horse anti-human thymocyte globulin), ATG Fresenius® (rabbit anti-human thymocyte globulin), ATG Merieux® (rabbit anti-human thymocyte globulin). According to the manufacturers, equipotent immunosuppressive doses most probably are: ATG Merieux®, 2.5 mg/kg, approximately equal to ATG Fresenius® 4 mg/kg and ATGAM® 25 mg/kg. Early in the program ATG induction (ATGAM® or Fresenius®) was given only to patients with reduced renal function (Cr^{51}-EDTA clearance < 60 ml/min) while from patient no. 24 onward, all received induction with ATG Merieux®.

Among the first 23 patients, 6 received horse ATG (ATGAM®; 12.5 mg/kg/day; mean 3.7 days, range 3–4 days), 11 had rabbit ATG (ATG Fresenius®; 2.5 mg/kg/day; mean 4.4 days, range 3–7 days), and 6 did not receive any ATG induction. The remaining 26 patients had rabbit ATG Merieux® (2.5 mg/kg/day; 3.8 days, range 3–5 days). ATG induction was continued until the whole-blood-specific cyclosporin level exceeded 240 ng/ml.

Moderate and persistent mild rejections were treated with methylprednisolone 0.5–1.0 g daily for 3 days. Myocardial biopsies were taken weekly for 6 weeks, every second week for 6 weeks, monthly for 3 months, and thereafter every third month and degree of rejection classified according to ISHLT criteria (15).

Prophylactic antimicrobial chemotherapy

Prophylactic antimicrobiol chemotherapy included two 3 g doses of ceftriaxone, acyclovir 1 g/day for 3 months, nystatin 6 MU/day for 4–6 weeks, and if mismatch for toxoplasmosis, pyrimethamine 25 mg/day for 6–8 weeks.

Microbiological examinations

On a routine basis, all patients were examined as follows: Bacterial cultures from nose, pharynx, urine and blood were raised from all patients before transplantation and on days 2, 4, 7. Titres of IgG and IgM CMV antibodies were determined using enzyme immune assays (State Serum Institute, Copenhagen) before transplantation and at weeks 1, 2, 4, 6, 8 and 3 and 6 months after transplantation. CMV cultures from urine, saliva and blood were obtained at weeks 1, 2, 4, 6, 8, and 12. Culturing was done at the State Serum Institute, Copenhagen.

Herpes simplex titres (HSV), Epstein Barr virus (EBV), varicella-zoster virus (VZV), legionella titres, and toxoplasmosis titres were assayed before transplantation and at weeks 1, 6, 8, and 3 and 6 months after transplantation. All analyses were performed using routine diagnostic tests. The toxoplasmosis analysis included IFAT as well as ELISA IgG and IgM (State Serum Institute, Copenhagen). In addition, both CMV and bacterial cultures as well as other microbiological examinations were performed when clinically indicated.

Definition of CMV infection/reactivation/disease

Primary CMV infection was diagnosed based upon IgG anti-CMV seroconversion, detection of IgM anti-CMV, CMV culturing, or histological demonstration of CMV inclusion bodies. CMV reactivation/reinfection was diagnosed based upon the finding of a fourfold increase in IgG anti-CMV titre, detection of IgM anti-CMV, CMV culturing, or histological demonstration of CMV inclusion bodies.

Early seroconversions (i.e. within the first 2 weeks) were considered passive transfusion transfer of CMV antibodies and not true seroconversions if titres declined rapidly or antibodies disappeared.

CMV disease was diagnosed if CMV infection/reactivation/reinfection was associated with 1) fever ($\geq 38°C$), 2) an influenza-like illness with or without pneumonitis, colitis, hepatitis, or carditis, and 3) absence of any other probable explanation for the symptoms (infection or rejection).

Statistics

Analysis of difference in proportions was carried out using Fisher's exact test. Multivariate analysis was carried out using logistic regression analysis. The level of type 1 error was fixed at 5%.

RESULTS

A survey of the clinically overt infections is given in Table I.

Bacterial infections

Septicaemia developed in 5 (10%) patients and the etiologies among 3 recovering patients were Staphylococcus epidermidis (2) and Listeria monocytogenes (1). Fatal Klebsiella oxytoca septicaemia developed in 1 patient who had been treated repeatedly for rejections. Another patient with protein-losing enteropathy died from septic shock with several microorganisms isolated from the blood (Staphylococcus aureus, Staphylococcus epidermidis and non-haemolytic streptococci) as well as positive blood tests for Candida albicans antigen (Cantec). In addition, Serratia marsescens was cultured from the blood of a patient who had sudden onset of febrile illness and prompt response to antibiotic treatment. Due to the clinical condition the event was not registered as septicaemia.

Nine patients (18%) had pneumonia. The aetiology was Legionella pneumophila in 2 cases and Pseudomonas maltophilia, Streptococcus pneumoniae, Haemophilus parainfluenzae and

Table I. *Clinically significant infections in Danish heart transplant patients in relation to transplantation (Tx)*

	No. of patients	Weeks after Tx median (range)
Septicemia	5	4 (2–11)
Pneumonia	9	3 (2–21)
Pneumocystis carinii pneumonitis	3	16 (11–26)
Clostridium difficile diarrhea	2	5, 18
CMV disease	10	6 (3 – 8)

Staphylococcus epidermidis in 1 case each. The diagnosis of legionellosis was established in both patients by immune fluorescence (IF) on bronchial lavage (BAL) fluid and the type was determined by significant increases in titres. The last patient had secondary Pseudomonas maltophilia pneumonia due to pulmonary embolism with abscess formation. The aetiology remained undetermined in a further 2 patients.

Two patients had severe diarrhoea, and in both Clostridium difficile was isolated and treated with oral vancomycin.

Symptomatic urinary tract infection was registered in 1 patient (faecal streptococci). One patient had an abscess after a recent tooth extraction.

Parasitic infections

18 (37%) patients were negative for toxoplasmosis antibodies and 13 of these had a toxoplasmosis-negative donor. The remaining 5 (10%) had a positive donor and received pyrimethamine prophylaxis. 31 (63%) patients were toxoplasmosis-positive, of whom 9 had a toxoplasmosis-positive donor. No patient developed clinical or serological evidence of de novo toxoplasmosis acquisition or reactivation.

The diagnosis Pneumocystis carinii pneumonitis was verified by microscopical examination of BAL fluid in 3 patients. All patients were treated with intravenous high dosage of sulfamethoxazole with trimethoprim for 3 weeks.

CMV infection and other viral infections

Of the 49 patients, 19 were CMV-negative, of whom 10 (53%) had a positive donor (CMV mismatch). Among the 10 CMV mismatch patients, 9 (90%) developed CMV infection (Table II). Seven of the 10 (70%) developed clinical CMV disease, of whom 1 with pneumonitis received treatment (see below) with ganciclovir, while the remaining 6 patients had clinically self-limiting disease which did not require treatment. Table II summarises the serological findings in relation to clinical CMV disease. Two (20%) CMV mismatch patients died. One developed a febrile illness with influenza-like symptoms and a slight decrease in leukocyte and platelet counts on day 40. The symptoms subsided 10 days later without treatment. On day 60 this patient suddenly and unexpectedly died at home. Postmortem examination showed CMV inclusion bodies in liver, kidney, lungs and heart. The other patient developed CMV pneumonitis on day 34. The diagnosis was established clinically and confirmed by culturing CMV from BAL. Subsequently ganciclovir 5 mg/kg body weight twice daily was started on day 36. After 4 weeks the dose was decreased to 5 mg/kg body weight once daily for 2 weeks further. On day 77 the patient was transferred to his home town hospital where he later had a relapse of CMV pneumonitis complicated with pulmonary and cerebral aspergillosis from which he died 6 months after transplantation.

Of the 49 patients, 30 were CMV-positive, of whom 12 (40%) had a positive donor. Seven of these 12 (58%) developed CMV reactivation/reinfection and 3 (25%) had clinical CMV disease which was mild, self-limiting in all cases and not treated.

In the group of 18 CMV-positive and 9 CMV-negative recipients with negative donors, no CMV disease was seen (a summary of the serological and clinical findings in relation to CMV is depicted in Table II).

Table III summarises some demographic variables, morbidity and mortality in relation to ATG induction regimen. Overall morbidity and mortality did not differ in the 2 groups and there was no difference regarding rejection rate in the 2 groups (timing, duration, severity, treatment and effect on heart function not analysed).

The rate of CMV infection/reactivation was significantly higher among patients who had a CMV-positive donor ($p < 0.01$) and among patients receiving ATG Merieux® induction

Table II. *Serological and CMV culture findings in 49 Danish heart transplant patients in relation to recipient and donor CMV status and transplantation (Tx)*

	No. of patients, ( ) indicates treatment with ganciclovir	Weeks after Tx median and range
Recipient negative, donor positive (CMV mismatch)	10	
CMV infection	9	
4-fold IgG anti-CMV increase	4	8(2–26)
IgM anti-CMV positive	8	7(6–10)
CMV culture positive	5[a]	6(5–10)
CMV disease	7(1)	6(6–8)
Recipient and donor positive (CMV match)	12	
CMV infection/reactivation	7	
4-fold IgG anti-CMV increase	5	8(6–26)
IgM anti-CMV positive	3	8(8–24)
CMV culture positive	7	7(3–13)
CMV disease	3(0)	7(3–8)
Recipient positive, donor negative (CMV match)	18	
CMV infection/reactivation	8	
4-fold IgG anti-CMV increase	6	7(6–13)
IgM anti-CMV positive	3	8(4–13)
CMV culture positive	4	6(1–7)
CMV disease	–	
Recipient negative, donor negative (CMV match)	9	
CMV infection	0	

[a] In 1 patient, CMV was detected histologically.

treatment ($p < 0.0001$). There was also a trend towards a higher rate of clinical CMV disease in the latter group but the difference did not reach statistical significance ($p = 0.06$). Positive CMV recipient status was not associated with a higher CMV infection/reactivation rate. In a logistic regression analysis, both positive CMV donor status and ATG Merieux® induction treatment were found to be significant independent predictors of CMV infection.

The 2 patients who died from or in relation to CMV disease received ATG (1 Fresenius® and 1 Merieux®). The 2 deaths not related to infection could be ascribed to early acute rejection in a patient who did not receive ATG and in the other to subclavian venous thrombosis with massive pulmonary embolism occurring after retransplantation for poor primary donor organ function unrelated to rejection.

EBV, VZV and HSV antibodies were detected before transplantation in the majority (95%) of the patients. No patient had serological findings suggestive of either primary infection or reactivation. However, 1 patient developed monodermatomal herpes zoster.

DISCUSSION

The present study confirms previous findings that infections are an important factor contributing to morbidity and mortality within the first 6 months in heart transplant patients (1, 2). During the period covered by this survey, 6 deaths (12%) occurred, of which 4 were related to infection. Two deaths related to bacterial infections were in patients who had had

Table III. *Demographic variables, donor CMV status, infections, rejections, and mortality in relation to anti-thymocyte immunoglobulin (ATG) induction treatment in 49 consecutive Danish heart transplant patients. All patients received standard triple-drug immune suppression in addition to induction (see materials and methods). Detailed information on ATG dosage is included in "Patients"*

PCP: pneumocystis carinii pneumonitis, CMV: cytomegalovirus, * $p < 0.0001$ (Fisher's exact test), ** $p = 0.06$ (Fisher's exact test).

	A No ATG	B ATGAM®	C ATG Fresenius®	A + B + C	ATG Merieux®
No. of patients	6	6	11	23	26
Females/males	1/5	2/4	1/10	4/19	5/21
Mean age (years)	40	48	44	44	44
CMV-positive	2	4	6	12	18
CMV-positive donor	1	4	3	8	14
Pulmonary infections	–	1	3	4(17%)	5(19%)
Septicaemia	–	2	2	4(17%)	1(4%)
Clostridium difficile diarrhea	–	–	–	–	2
PCP	–	–	–	–	3
CMV infection/ reactivation	–	2	2	4(17%)*	20(77%)*
CMV disease	–	1	1	2(9%)**	8(31%)**
Patients with rejections	3[a]	4	4[b]	11(48%)	13(50%)
Absolute no. of rejections	7	10	8	25	31
Rejection rate	1.16	1.67	0.73	1.09	1.19
Deaths related to infection	–	–	2	2	2
Deaths unrelated to infection	1	–	1	2	–
Mortality rate				17%	8%

[a] Including 1 early fatal rejection.
[b] Including 1 with recurrent rejections and fatal septicaemia.

a complicated postoperative course with surgical and cardiac problems resulting in multi-organ failure. In 1 patient the main problem had been recurrent rejections. In such patients the infection should be looked upon as a factor contributing to rather than the cause of the fatal outcome. In contrast 2 deaths were most likely directly attributable to CMV infection. One patient died suddenly and unexpectedly, having recovered from a mild and apparently self-limiting CMV disease. In light of the postmortem findings of CMV infection in many organs including the myocardium it seems likely that the patient died from an arrhythmia caused by CMV-induced cardiac inflammation. The other patient died from relapsing primary CMV pneumonitis eventually (according to the postmortem findings) complicated by disseminated aspergillosis. The fact that CMV infection/reactivation was seen in half of the patients, that approx. 20% had CMV disease and that CMV was associated with fatal outcome in 2 cases emphasizes that CMV is the most important single pathogen in terms of both mortality and morbidity. Several studies have shown that CMV infection occurs most frequently among CMV mismatch patients with a risk of more frequent and severe clinical CMV disease. However, CMV infection and disease may also be a problem in a substantial number of CMV-positive patients who reactivate their latent CMV or who become reinfected with a different CMV strain from a CMV-positive graft. Thus, CMV problems may be anticipated in the majority of heart transplant patients.

In order to minimize CMV problems one could either embark upon early CMV diagnosis, or give CMV prophylaxis to all patients at risk. The present findings show that the available diagnostic methods are of limited value (Table II). In CMV mismatch patients, IgM anti-CMV developed in 6 out of 7 patients with CMV disease but the positive test coincided with rather than preceded the clinical symptoms (Table II). Both IgG seroconversion and culturing proved to be of limited sensitivity. Among the CMV-positive patients with positive donors 3 out of 12 developed CMV disease which could not be predicted by using IgG antibody or CMV culture. It is evident that the development of a test which can predict clinical CMV disease should be given high priority. Meanwhile the only options are treatment and prophylaxis. Hitherto our policy has been to treat only severe CMV disease. One may speculate whether treatment, and earlier treatment respectively would have saved our 2 patients. The sudden death might be unrelated to CMV. The present study further supports that acyclovir in a dose 1 g/day is of limited value for preventing CMV disease. High-dose acyclovir, i.e. 4 g/day, may be of some value (16, 17) and has recently been included in our protocol for CMV mismatch recipients. Newer prodrugs to acyclovir are being introduced into the market. In a recent paper it was shown that ganciclovir reduced CMV morbidity in CMV-positive heart transplant patients, whereas the authors were unable to show a beneficial effect in the high-risk CMV mismatch patients (14). Considering the fact that ganciclovir may only be administered parenterally and has a pronounced tendency to cause bone marrow suppression, this agent does not seem to be the ideal prophylactic CMV drug. Specific CMV hyperimmune globulins seem to be effective for both prophylaxis and treatment but are too expensive for routine use (18).

ATG's are potent immunosuppressive preparations which may be employed both in the treatment of severe or recurrent rejections and for induction in combination with the usual triple regimen to minimize the risk of early rejection and to reduce cyclosporin toxicity. In the present series the first 23 patients received no ATG, or ATG ATGAM®, or ATG Fresenius®, as compared with the last 26 patients who all received ATG Merieux® as induction treatment. The important finding is that there was a significantly higher CMV infection/reactivation rate and a pronounced trend towards a higher CMV disease rate in the patients who received ATG Merieux®. The rationale of ATG induction therapy is to clear the early postoperative course from the rejection problem and in this respect it is very effective but the long-term impact of this treatment remains to be further studied.

By univariate analysis the CMV infection/reactivation rate was found to be significantly higher among patients who had CMV-positive donors, whereas a positive CMV recipient status was not associated with a higher CMV infection/reactivation rate. Multivariate analysis showed that positive CMV donor status and ATG Merieux® induction treatment were both significant independent predictors of CMV infection/reactivation.

The increased rate of CMV infection/reactivation is on its own not surprising, as ATG is a known potent reactivator of latent viruses (19). It was unexpected, however, that the use of ATG Merieux® which is presumed to be the most potent ATG preparation, would have such an impressive effect when given as induction therapy for a period of only 3–4 days. The information about relative potency and equipotent doses of different ATG preparations provided by the manufacturers seems very uncertain and information about antibody specificity is also limited. It is also interesting to note that the 3 cases of PCP occurred among patients treated with ATG Merieux®. The present findings extend previous findings in renal transplant recipients showing that ATG induction treatment increases the incidence of CMV infection (20). Comparing the ATG preparations is difficult, however. They vary in many aspects, of which potency and specificity are only two. The question about the importance of antibody specificity is interesting. Costanzo-Nordin et al. recently showed that the monoclonal specific anti CD3 OKT3 induction treatment was a predictor of CMV infection among patients receiving either OKT3 for 14 days or low-dose horse ATG for 9 days (5).

In conclusion, CMV is the single most important pathogen known in infections seen during the first 6 months after heart transplantation. Furthermore, our findings suggest that even a short course of heavy immunosuppression has a significant impact on CMV infection/reactivation rate.

REFERENCES

1. Kriett JM, Kaye MP. The Registry of the International Society for Heart Transplantation: seventh official report, 1990. J Heart Transplant 9: 323–330, 1990.
2. Grossi P, De Maria R, Caroli A, Zaina MS, Minoli L. The Italian Study Group on Infections in Heart Transplantation. Infections in heart transplant recipients: the experience of the Italian heart transplant program. J Heart Lung Transplant 11: 847–866, 1992.
3. Renlund D, O'Connell JB, Bristow MR. Strategies of immunosuppression in cardiac transplantation. Semin Thorac Cardiovasc Surg 2: 181–188, 1990.
4. Laske A, Gallino A, Schneider J, Baur EP, Carrel T, Pasic M, von Segesser LK, Turina MI. Prophylactic therapy in heart transplantation: monoclonal versus polyclonal antibody therapy. J Heart Lung Transplant 11: 557–563, 1992.
5. Costanzo-Nordin MR, Swinnen LJ, Fisher SG, O'Sullivan EJ, Piforre R, Hereaux AI, Mullen GM, Johnson MR. Cytomegalovirus infections in heart transplant recipients: relationship to immunosuppression. J Heart Lung Transplant 11: 837–846, 1992.
6. Andersson R, Sandberg T, Berglin E, Jeansson S. Cytomegalovirus infections and toxoplasmosis in heart transplant recipients in Sweden. Scand J Infect Dis 24: 411–417, 1992.
7. Gorensek MJ, Stewart RW, Keys TF, McHenry MC, Goormestic M. A multivariate analysis of the risk of cytomegalovirus infection in heart transplant recipients. J Infect Dis 157: 515–522, 1988.
8. Smyth RL, Scott JP, Borysiewicz, Sharploes LD, Stewart S, Wreghitt TG, Gray JJ, Higenbottom TW, Wallwork J. Cytomegalovirus infection in heart-lung transplant recipients: risk factors, clinical associations and response to treatment. J Infect Dis 164: 1045–1050, 1991.
9. Augustine SM, Yeo CJ, Buchman TG, Achuff SC, Baumgartner WA. Gastrointestinal complications in heart and in heart-lung transplant patients. Transplantation 10: 547–555, 1991.
10. Loebe M, Schuler S, Zais O, Warnecke H, Fleck E, Hetzer R. Role of cytomegalovirus infection in the development of coronary artery disease in the transplanted heart. J Heart Transplant 9: 707–711, 1990.
11. Sharples LD, Caine N, Mullins P, Scott JP, Solis E, English TAH, Large SR, Schofield PM, Wallwork J. Risk factor analysis for the major hazards following heart transplantation – rejection, infection, and coronary occlusive disease. Transplantation 52: 244–252, 1991.
12. Goodrich JM, Mori M, Gleaves CA, DuMond C, Cays M, Ebeling DF, Buhles WC, DeArmond B, Meyers JD. Early treatment with ganciclovir to prevent cytomegalovirus disease after allogenic bone marrow transplantation. N Engl J Med 325: 1601–1607, 1991.
13. Dunn DL, Mayoral JL, Gillingham KJ, Loeffler CM, Brayman KL, Kramer MA, Erice A, Balfour HH, Fletcher CV, Bolman RM, Matas AJ, Payne WD, Sutherland DER, Najarian JS. Treatment of invasive cytomegalovirus disease in solid organ transplant patients with ganciclovir. Transplantation 51: 98–106, 1991.
14. Merigan TH, Renlund DG, Keay S, Bristow MR, Starnes V, O'Connell JB, Resta S, Dunn D, Gamberg P, Ratkovec RM, Richenbacher WE, Millar RC, DuMond C, DeAmond B, Sullivan V, Cheney T, Buhles W, Stinson EB. A controlled trial of ganciclovir to prevent cytomegalovirus disease after heart transplantation. N Engl J Med 326: 1182–1186, 1992.
15. Billingham ME, Cary NR, Hammond ME, Kemnitz J, Marboe C, Callister HA, Snovar DC, Winters GL, Zerbe A. A working formulation for the standardization of nomenclature in the diagnosis of heart and lung rejection: Heart rejection study group. J Heart Transplant 9: 587–593, 1990.
16. Meyers JD, Reed EC, Shepp DH, Thornquist M, Dandliker PS, Vicary CA, Flournoy N, Kirk LE, Kersey JH, Thomas ED. Acyclovir for prevention of cytomegalovirus infection and disease after allogenic marrow transplantation. N Engl J Med 318: 70–75, 1988.

17. Balfour HH, Chace BA, Stapleton JT, Simmons RL, Fryd DS. A randomized, placebo-controlled trial of oral acyclovir for the prevention of cytomegalovirus disease in recipients of renal allografts. N Engl J Med 320: 1381–1387, 1989.
18. Havel M, Teufelsbauer H, Laczkovics A, Kurz R, Wolner E. Cytomegalovirus hyperimmunoglobulin prophylaxis in the prevention of cytomegalovirus infection in immunosuppressed heart transplant patients. Transplant Proc 22: 1805–1806, 1990.
19. Rubin RH. Impact of cytomegalovirus infection on organ transplant recipients. Rev Infect Dis Suppl 7: S754–S762, 1990.
20. Boyce NW, Hayes K, Gee D, Holdsworth SR, Thomson NM, Scott D, Atkins RC. Cytomegalovirus infection complicating renal transplantation and its relationship to acute transplant glomerulopathy. Transplantation 45: 706–709, 1988.

Submitted October 6, 1993; accepted January 10, 1994

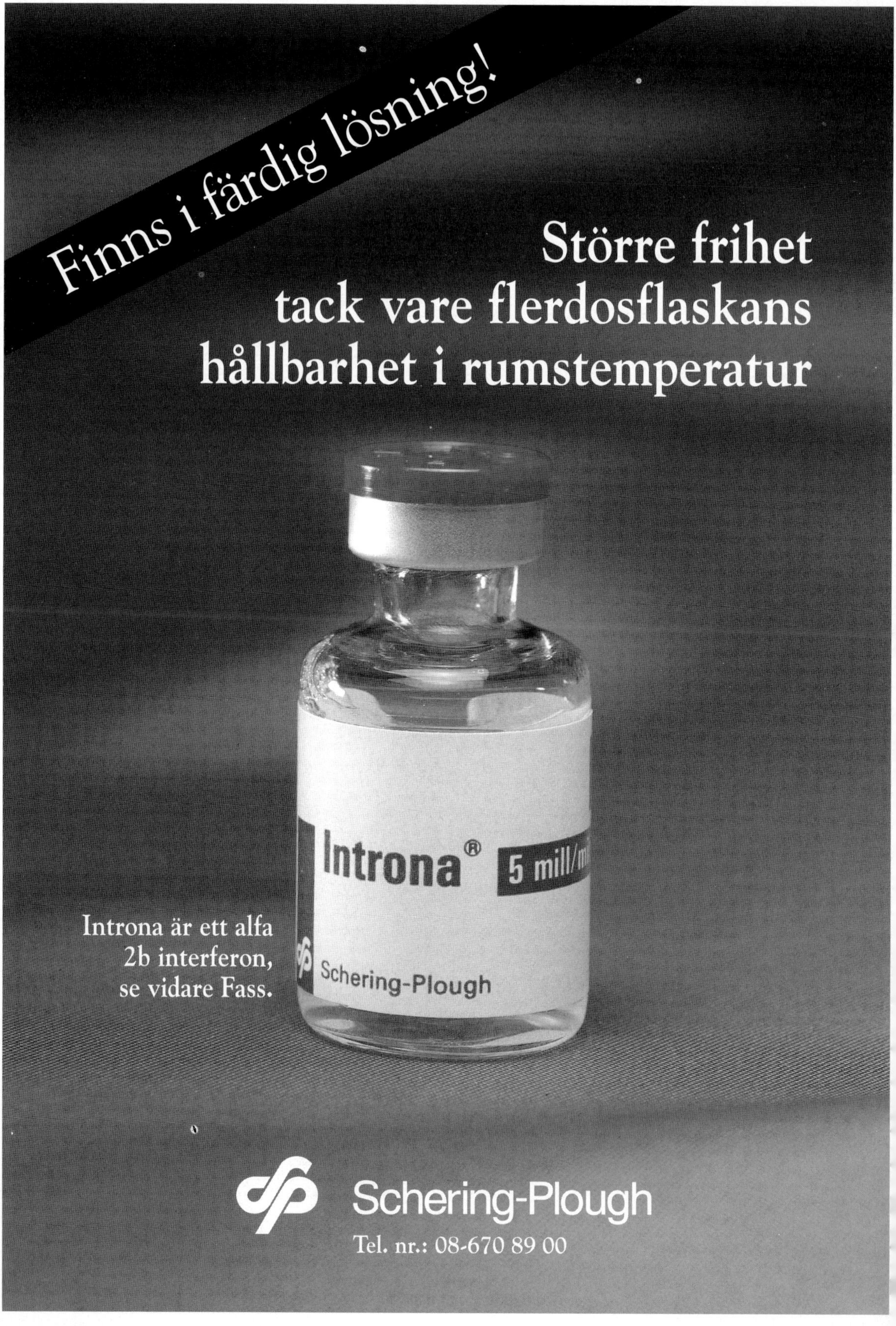
Finns i färdig lösning!
Större frihet
tack vare flerdosflaskans
hållbarhet i rumstemperatur
Introna® 5 mill/m
Schering-Plough
Introna är ett alfa
2b interferon,
se vidare Fass.
Schering-Plough
Tel. nr.: 08-670 89 00

Scand J Infect Dis 26: 249–254, 1994

PCR for the Diagnosis of Enteroviral Meningitis

ANDERS THORÉN[1,2] and ANDERS WIDELL[2]

From the Departments of [1]Infectious Diseases and [2]Medical Microbiology, Section of Clinical Virology, University of Lund, Malmö General Hospital, Malmö, Sweden

A 2-step 'semi-nested' enterovirus PCR was developed and applied to CSF and serum specimens from 27 consecutive patients with aseptic meningitis. CSF and sera from 8 patients with non-enteroviral diagnoses were included as negative clinical controls. Enterovirus RNA was detected in CSF by PCR in 15 of the patients with aseptic meningitis, compared with 6 by virus culture. Acute-phase sera proved positive for enterovirus RNA in 11 patients, thus increasing the number of PCR-positive patients to 18. Convalescent-phase sera were all negative by PCR. The correlation of a positive or negative PCR result in CSF and/or serum versus combined conventional virology (serology and isolation from 1–3 sites, i.e. CSF, stool and throat) was 78%. All negative controls were negative by PCR. PCR is a reliable and sensitive diagnostic tool for the detection of enteroviral infections. Both CSF and acute-phase serum should be considered for testing.

A. Thorén, MD, Department of Infectious Diseases, Malmö General Hospital, S-214 01 Malmö, Sweden

INTRODUCTION

Application of the polymerase chain reaction (PCR) to detect enteroviral RNA has been developed for a direct and rapid diagnosis of clinically important enteroviral infections (1–6). In general, the unique sensitivity of the PCR reaction has been used on the samples related to the target organ of infection, such as cerebrospinal fluid (CSF) in meningitis, where conventional virus culture often fails (7).

A viremic stage occurs in systemic enteroviral infections (8) and in a previous retrospective report we have demonstrated enteroviral RNA by PCR in stored sera from patients with enteroviral meningitis (4). Blood samples are readily obtained, compared with CSF or various organ biopsies. The aim of this study was to perform and compare PCR analysis of serum and CSF in a prospectively collected patient material with suspected enteroviral meningitis. By analysing acute and convalescent-phase sera by PCR, signs of prolonged or persistent infections were also sought.

MATERIALS AND METHODS

Patients

Consecutive patients with suspected viral meningitis attending the Department of Infectious Diseases and the Department of Pediatrics, Malmö General Hospital, during 1991–92 were enrolled. Patients with signs of Borrelia infection or Guillain-Barré syndrome were excluded as were also patients with known non-enteroviral aetiology. The duration of prodromal clinical symptoms – if present – were the duration of meningeal symptoms prior to lumbar puncture were recorded, as was age, sex and CSF cell count. CSF, acute and convalescent serum drawn 2–4 weeks later were prospectively collected and kept frozen at −20°C.

Clinical control subjects

Eight patients undergoing lumbar puncture during the course of the study were used as negative controls, since a definite alternative diagnosis had been established. The following diagnoses were represented: embolia cerebri (1), haemorrhagia cerebri (1), bacterial meningitis (1 with Streptococcus pneumoniae and 1 with meningococci), gasteroenteritis (1), influenza A (1), Borrelia meningitis (1), pneumonia (1).

 ISSN 0036-5548

Virus culture and serology

Virus isolation and typing was performed from throat, CSF and stool using green monkey kidney cells and human embryonic fibroblasts as previously described (4). A complement fixation test was performed on paired sera against 2 antigens, coxsackie virus B5 and echovirus 18 (4). To assay the sensitivity of enterovirus PCR, stocks of coxsackie virus B5 and echovirus 18 (used as antigens in the complement fixation tests) and a clinical isolate of coxsackie virus B3 were cultured on Vero cells and the titres were determined by examination of the cytopathic effect from virus dilutions, from which the $TCID_{50}$ was calculated. Tenfold dilutions in phosphate-buffered saline (PBS) or fetal calf serum were made from the virus stock solutions and these dilutions were used to establish the sensitivity of the PCR.

RNA extraction

Samples of 100 µl of serum, CSF or PBS were extracted according to the acid guanidinium thiocyanate-phenol-chloroform method with modifications described by Widell et al. (9). RNA extraction was performed on batches of 10 samples, each including 5 clinical samples, 4 technical negative controls (PBS) and 1 positive control containing 3×10^1 $TCID_{50}$ coxsackie B3 virus diluted in fetal calf serum.

Combined reverse transcription and PCR

Three primers selected from the conserved regions of the 5′ end of the genome were used as described previously (4). The primers E1 (CACCGGATGGCCAATCCA) and R1 (ATTGTCACCATAAGC-AGCCA) served as outer and inner downstream primers respectively and R2 (CCTCCGGCCCCT-GAATGCGGCTAAT) as upstream primer in the 2-step 'seminested' PCR reaction where E1 + R2 were used in the first PCR and R1 + R2 in the second PCR reaction. The concentration of all primers was 0.5 µM in PCR I and II.

The reaction was performed as previously described by Widell et al. concerning hepatitis C virus RNA (9). The reaction volumes of 50 µl contained 9.5 µl of RNA extract plus 40.5 µl reaction mix including primer E1 and R2 (0.5 µM). The reaction was performed at 43°C for 1 h (reverse transcription) followed by denaturation at 94°C for 5 min, annealing at 45°C for 2 min plus denaturation at 94°C for 1 min, 35 cycles, and finally an extension at 72°C for 5 min. All temperatures were tube temperatures (Hybaid Thermal Reactor, Hybaid, Teddington, England).

The second PCR was performed with 5 µl from the first reaction transferred to 45 µl of the PCR mix with R2 + R1 serving as primers. The reaction was started at 94°C for 1 min followed by 45°C for 10 s, 30 cycles (tube temperatures).

The PCR products were visualized by agarose gel electrophoresis whereby the first PCR reaction was expected to give a 196 bp band and the second reaction a 154 bp band.

Precautions against contamination

Precautions adhered to the criteria specified by Kwok and Higuchi (10). The different major steps in the PCR were performed in different rooms completely isolated from each other. Filter tips were used in all stages.

RESULTS

The sensitivity of the PCR assay calculated from extractions of serial dilutions of titrated enterovirus corresponded to 3×10^2 $TCID_{50}$ in the first PCR reaction and 3×10^{-2} $TCID_{50}$ in the second reaction.

Clinical samples were stored for 1 year at maximum. Within that time the distribution of PCR-positive samples did not correlate with the duration of storage.

Clinical findings

27 patients with meningitis were enrolled, 16 female and 11 male. Of the 27 patients 25 appeared during the expected enterovirus season in July through November; only 2 were enrolled in December–June, both negative in all enteroviral diagnostic tests including PCR. There were 21 adults, age ranging 16–44 years and 6 children, 2 weeks to 12 years old. Only 1 child was younger than 1 month; this child had a nosocomial neonatal infection.

The CSF findings were compatible with aseptic meningitis with cells ranging from $10–200 \times 10^6$/l. Two patients, however, presented and were treated as cases of bacterial meningitis. They had 810 polynuclear + 370 mononuclear cells and 660 polynuclear + 307 mononuclear cells × 10^6/l, respectively. Bacterial cultures from CSF were negative. Both these patients had evidence of enteroviral meningitis: PCR positive CSF and culture positive stool.

The PCR result of CSF did not correlate to the number of white or red cells, nor to the protein level in the total material.

Virological results

The results of virus serology and virus isolation from CSF, throat and stool are shown in Table I together with the PCR results in acute-phase sera and CSF. All technical controls (PBS) in the PCR tests were negative as well as CSF and serum from the control subjects with different diagnoses. The PCR results of the convalescent-phase sera, 2–4 weeks after the meningitis episode, were also negative.

Table I. *Age and summary of virological findings and PCR analysis of 27 patients with aseptic meningitis*

+ = positive result. – = negative result. nd = not done.

		Conventional virus assays					PCR	
	Age (yrs)	Serology[a]	Vir. culture CSF	Vir. culture throat	Vir. culture stool	≥ one pos. vir. finding	PCR CSF	PCR acute serum
1	0.05	–	CB2	nd	CB2	yes	+	nd
2	19	nd	–	–	–	no	+	+
3	17	+	E11	nd	E11	yes	+	+
4	32	+	–	nd	E6	yes	+	+
5	29	–	–	–	nd	no	+	+
6	16	nd	–	–	–	no	+	+
7	24	+	E11	nd	nd	yes	+	+
8	37	–	CA9	–	–	yes	+	+
9	7	nd	–	E30	E30	yes	+	+
10	12	–	–	nd	CA	yes	+	–
11	28	+	–	E30	E30	yes	+	–
12	32	+	–	–	nd	yes	+	–
13	23	+	–	E18	E18	yes	+	–
14	3	h[b]	–	CB5	CB5	yes	+	–
15	10	+	–	nd	CA9	yes	+	–
16	32	+	–	nd	nd	yes	–	+
17	7	nd	E11	nd	E11	yes	–	+
18	3	+	–	nd	CB2	yes	–	+
19	23	–	–	–	–	no	–	–
20	29	–	–	nd	–	no	–	–
21	19	–	–	E14	nd	yes	–	–
22	29	–	–	nd	nd	no	–	–
23	23	–	–	–	CB5	yes	–	–
24	24	–	–	–	–	no	–	–
25	40	–	–	–	–	no	–	–
26	44	+	E22	–	–	yes	–	–
27	23	–	–	–	–	no	–	–
No. positive patients/ tested (%)		10/23 (43%)	6/27 (22%)	5/16 (31%)	12/21 (57%)	18/27 (67%)	15/27 (55%)	11/26 (42%)

[a] ≥4-fold elevated titre in paired sera.

[b] High, but equal titres in paired sera.

A prodromal phase, mainly upper respiratory symptoms, was seen in 13/27 patients. When this phase was absent, the duration of 'prodromal' symptoms was considered as equal with the meningeal symptoms prior to lumbar puncture (Fig. 1). When the duration of prodromal and meningeal symptoms prior to lumbar puncture was compared with the PCR findings, a correlation to the duration of prodromal symptoms versus positive PCR test in CSF and/or serum was seen (Fig. 1) and also versus CSF culture and serology (Table I).

In CSF, enterovirus RNA was detected in 15/27 patients whereas only 6 patients were positive with virus isolation. Positive PCR results of CSF and serum were mostly, but not completely, in agreement and by combined results from the 2 PCR analyses, a total of 18 patients were PCR positive.

A correlation of positive or negative PCR results with conventional virology was found in 21/27 (78%) patients. The PCR was positive in both serum and CSF in 3 patients where culture was negative and serology negative or missing (due to lack of convalescent serum). On the other hand, 3 patients were PCR negative but had indications of enteroviral aetiology in conventional tests: one of them was culture positive in CSF for echovirus 22 which is known to be missed in enterovirus PCR due to sequence divergency (1, 11). The remaining 2 had a positive throat and stool virus culture respectively, as the only indication of enteroviral infection (see Table I, patients 21 & 23). Both these patients had a long duration of prodromal symptoms prior to lumbar puncture, 8 and 14 days, respectively.

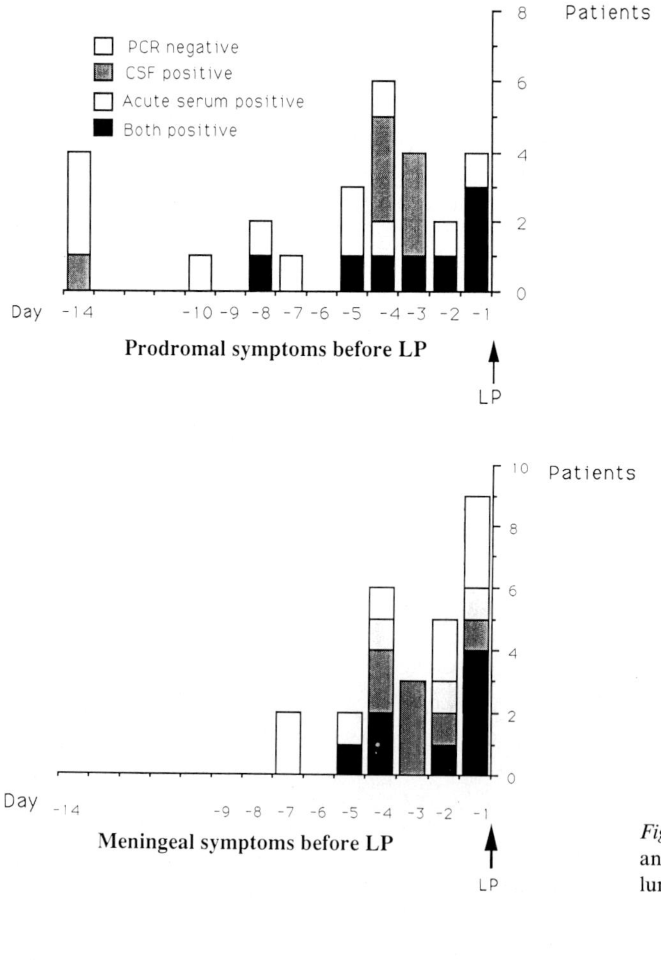

Fig. 1. Duration of prodromal and meningeal symptoms before lumbar puncture (days).

Assuming 100% specificity (no false positives) of all assays, the sensitivity may be calculated as follows (21 patients positive in at least one assay): PCR-CSF: 71%, PCR serum: 52%, PCR for CSF and serum combined: 86% and all conventional methods combined: 86%.

DISCUSSION

The sensitivity was high in this 2-step enterovirus PCR assay, corresponding to a virus titre of 10^{-2} $TCID_{50}$. Such a high sensitivity is needed to detect virus present in CSF or serum as shown by us and others previously (4, 6). As indicated by the results of virus culture, larger amounts of virus are present in stool and a 1-step PCR assay would be quite sufficient to detect enterovirus in stool (5).

The selection of primers for a so-called nested PCR was based on the conserved parts of the enteroviral genomes so far sequenced. According to available data from GenBank there are several closely spaced options for different downstream primers (like E1, R1 etc) but few conserved regions suitable for upstream PCR primers. In our previous report we have shown that a 'seminested' assay with a common upstream primer in the first and second reaction will increase the sensitivity (4). A similar assay was also applied on CSF PCR by Glimåker et al. (6).

A useful enterovirus detecting assay should be specific. There are great similarities between the conserved regions of the enteroviral genomes and those of the rhinoviruses, and some published downstream primers have also been shown to amplify rhinoviral RNA. This should not apply to the primers in our assay due to mismatches in the 3′ end of the E1 primer to rhinoviruses (1).

The high sensitivity of a nested PCR is, however, double-edged: there is a risk of false-positive results unless strict precautions are taken. All results must be validated against contamination controls including a sufficient number of technical negative controls (10). Moreover, even with these precautions taken account of, reports of enteroviral RNA detected by PCR, such as persistent infections in chronc fatigue syndrome and chronic myocardial disease, must be evaluated with great caution (12, 13). The relevance of enteroviral RNA in myocardial samples has been questioned by Weiss et al., who found an equal distribution of enteroviral RNA in myocardial biopsies from patients with suspected enteroviral cardiomyopathy and myocardium from controls (14). This finding underlines the importance of carefully selected patients serving as controls.

All technical controls (PBS) were negative in this study as well as CSF and serum from patients serving as controls. The 23 available convalescent sera were also negative, in agreement with the lack of clinical signs of persistent infection.

Accordance of positive and negative PCR results from CSF and serum versus the combined results from conventional virology was found in 78% of the patients. A definite diagnosis of enteroviral aetiology by demonstration of virus or viral RNA from CSF and or serum could be done by PCR in 86% of the 21 patients where enterovirus was indicated by any method, compared with 26% by virus culture of CSF. Serology gave a positive result in 11 patients (52%) but the delay in time to obtain paired sera hampers its clinical usefulness. The true sensitivity of any enterovirus assay cannot be calculated from this study which represents patients with unknown aetiology.

The PCR assay yielded 3 positive patients who tested negative by combined conventional virology. However, the PCR missed 1 patient with echovirus 22. This has been observed in other studies and depends on the divergent sequence of the viral genome and has led to the suggestion of a reclassification of echovirus 22 from the enterovirus group (11).

The other 2 patients who proved negative by PCR had a positive virus culture from throat or stool, respectively, as the only indication of enteroviral aetiology. If they represent a true enteroviral infection, the negative PCR results might be explained by the relatively long delay between the onset of prodromal symptoms and lumbar puncture, 14 and 8 days respectively. The viraemic stage may then have passed and virus been cleared from blood and CSF by formation of antibodies (Fig. 1).

One of the drawbacks of PCR compared with virus culture is the lack of epidemiological information, since the result will not reveal the enterovirus type. Molecular–biological typing has been tried, but is not yet practical for routine use (3). Virus culture is thus still indicated in epidemic situations and when polio is suspected on clinical grounds, for instance in patients with palsies.

This study has confirmed the results of our previous retrospective study that PCR analysis of serum can reveal an enterovirus meningitis (4) and, when added to the PCR analysis of CSF, will increase the sensitivity of the method.

ACKNOWLEDGEMENTS

The authors wish to thank: Siv Månsson for skilful and pleasant introduction into the RNA-PCR routines of the laboratory. Karin Ahlfors for efficient support in collection of samples and typing of strains. This study was supported by funds from Alfred Österlunds Foundation and the Medical Faculty, University of Lund.

REFERENCES

1. Zoll GJ, Melchers WJG, Kopecka H, Jambroes G, van der Poel HJA, Galama JMD. General primer-mediated polymerase chain reaction for detection of enteroviruses: application for diagnostic routine and persistent infection. J Clin Microbiol 30: 160–165, 1992.
2. Rotbart HA. Enzymatic RNA amplification of the enteroviruses. J Clin Microbiol 28: 438–442, 1990.
3. Chapman NM, Tracy S, Gauntt CJ, Fortmueller U. Molecular detection and identification of enteroviruses using enzymatic amplification and nucleic acid hybridization. J Clin Microbiol 28: 843–850, 1990.
4. Thorén A, Robinson AJ, Maguire T, Jenkins R. Two-step PCR in the retrospective diagnosis of enteroviral viraemia. Scand J Infect Dis 24: 137–141, 1992.
5. Glimåker M, Abebe A, Johansson B, Ehrnst A, Strannegärd Ö. Detection of enteroviral RNA by polymerase chain reaction in faecal samples from patients with aseptic meningitis. J Med Virol 38: 54–61, 1992.
6. Glimåker M, Johansson B, Olcén P, Ehrnst A, Forsgren M. Detection of enteroviral RNA by polymerase chain reaction in cerebrospinal fluid from patients with aseptic meningitis. Scand J Infect Dis 25: 547–557, 1993.
7. Rotbart HA, Kinsella JP, Wasserman RL. Persistent enterovirus infection in culture-negative meningoencephalitis: Demonstration by enzymatic RNA amplification. J Infect Dis 161: 787–791, 1990.
8. Prather SL, Dagan R, Jenista JA, Menegus MA. The isolation of enteroviruses from blood: A comparison of four processing methods. J Med Virol 14: 221–227, 1984.
9. Widell A, Månsson A-S, Sundström G, Hansson BG, Nordenfelt E. Hepatitis C virus RNA in blood donor sera detected by the polymerase chain reaction: Comparison with supplementary hepatitis C antibody assays. J Med Virol 35: 253–258, 1991.
10. Kwok S, Higuchi R. Avoiding false positives with PCR. Nature 339: 237–238, 1989.
11. Coller BG, Chapman NM, Beck MA, Pallansch MA, Gauntt CJ, Tracy SM. Echovirus 22 is an atypical enterovirus. J Virol 64: 2692–2701, 1990.
12. Gow JW, Behan WMH, Clements GB, Woodall C, Riding M, Behan PO. Enteroviral RNA sequences detected by polymerase chain reaction in muscle of patients with postviral fatigue syndrome. BMJ 302: 692–696, 1991.
13. Jin O, Sole MJ, Butany JW, Chia WK, McLaughlin PR, Liu P, Liew CC. Detection of enterovirus RNA in myocardial biopsies from patients with myocarditis and cardiomyopathy using gene amplification by polymerase chain reaction. Circulation 82: 8–16, 1990.
14. Weiss LM, Liu X-F, Chang KL, Billingham ME. Detection of enteroviral RNA in idiopathic dilated cardiomyopathy and other human cardiac tissues. J Clin Invest 90: 156–159, 1992.

Submitted November 29, 1993; accepted January 24, 1994

Scand J Infect Dis 26: 255–261, 1994

Variability of the E2/NS1 Region of Swedish Hepatitis C Virus Strains and Its Correlation to Genotypes

BO JOHANSSON[1], ZHI-BING YUN[1] and ANDERS SÖNNERBORG[1,2]

From the Departments of [1]Virology, Central Microbiological Laboratory, Stockholm County Council and [2]Infectious Diseases, Huddinge Hospital, Karolinska Institute, Stockholm, Sweden

Serum RNA was extracted from 5 Swedish patients infected with hepatitis C virus (HCV). The N-terminal part of the genomic region coding for the gp70 (E2/NS1), including the hypervariable domain of the E2 protein, was reverse transcribed and amplified by the polymerase chain reaction (PCR) using biotinylated primers. The amplicon was immobilized on magnetic polystyrene beads coated with streptavidine. Solid-state sequencing was carried out on the bound single-stranded DNA, after denaturation. The results of phylogenetic sequence analysis and calculated ratios of transition and transversion mutations showed that 4 of the strains clustered together with the USA prototype strains HCV-1 and HCV-H (genotype I), while 1 strain was close to the Japanese isolate HCV-J, and particularly to isolate HCV-BK (genotype II). Possible antigenic epitopes in the Swedish strains were mapped in the HVR region.

B. Johansson, PhD, The Stockholm County Council, Central Microbiological Laboratory, Department of Virology, Box 70470, S-107 26 Stockholm, Sweden

INTRODUCTION

Hepatitis C virus (HCV), a proposed member of the virus family flaviviridae, is responsible for most of the cases of post-transfusion non-A non-B hepatitis, worldwide. The genome of HCV is a positive-stranded RNA molecule, about 9.5 kb long, which encodes a polyprotein of about 3,000 amino acids. Following a 3–400-nucleotides long, 5′-untranslated region, reading frames for core and envelope (E1 and E2/NS1), as well as 4 additional non-structural proteins (NS2–NS5) have been identified (1–3). The E2/NS1 product is a glycoprotein of about 70 kd size (gp70).

The sequence of the HCV genome shows marked diversity due to mutations among virus strains (4), and a region corresponding to 31 amino acids in the N-terminal part of gp70 has been named a 'hypervariable region' (HVR) (5). The mutations can be classified as transitions (Ts) or transversions (Tv). Ts are changes from purine to purine, or pyrimidine to pyrimidine, whereas Tv are changes from purine to pyrimidine, and vice versa. Based on sequence variability among strains from different geographical locations, 6 different genotypes have been proposed (6).

Since escape mutations of the HCV genome have been localized to the HVR (7), neutralizing antibodies induced by different types of the virus may not be cross-reactive. Therefore, future vaccine production may have to be aimed at locally prevalent viral strains. The purpose of this study was to identify antigenic regions in HVR of HCV strains from Sweden.

MATERIALS AND METHODS

Patients

All 5 patients in this study suffered from chronic hepatitis, and were positive for HCV both using a second generation antibody ELISA test (Abbott Laboratories, Chicago, IL) and PCR in the 5′ non-coding region (8). Two of the patients had received infected blood transfusions, and 3 were intravenous drug abusers. All had been infected in Sweden. None of the patients had undergone any treatment. They were randomly selected.

 ISSN 0036-5548

Extraction of RNA and PCR

Extraction of HCV RNA from the serum samples, reverse transcription (RT) and PCR were performed as described elsewhere (8). The PCR primers were flanking the hypervariable region of the HCV genome (Fig. 1), and the downstream primer 145 was used as RT primer for c-DNA synthesis. The PCR reactions were performed in a nested configuration (Fig. 1: PCR 1 and 2A) with primers described by Kato et al. (9). The 144 and 145 primers were used as outer primer (593 bp fragment) and 146 and 147 as inner primers (454 bp fragment). The 146 or 147 primer was biotinylated to make possible the catching of the amplicon on streptavidin-coated magnetic beads (Dynal A/S, Oslo, Norway). In some PCR reactions the second round of amplification (Fig. 1: PCR 1 and 2B or 2C) was designed to separately amplify the 5′ and 3′ parts of the sequence in an overlapping fashion. This was done in order to amplify strains which were impossible to amplify using the previously described primers (454 bp fragment). Thus, biotinylated primer 146 and primer YD1 (Fig. 1) were used as inner primers for the upstream fragment (208 bp), and biotinylated primer 147 and primer YU2 (Fig. 1) for the downstream fragment (297 bp).

Sequencing reaction

Solid-state DNA sequencing of the PCR-amplified inner fragments was performed using M-280 streptavidin Dynabeads essentially according to the manufacturer's instructions (Dynal A/S, Oslo, Norway). When only 1 amplified band could be seen after agarose gel electrophoresis of the PCR product, 40 μl of this was mixed directly with the beads. However, when more bands were present (unspecific products), the correct fragment was purified from a preparative agarose gel (10) and 100–300 ng DNA was mixed with the beads. After NaOH treatment of the beads, to produce single-stranded DNA, and elution of the complementary strand using the MPC magnetic tube rack (Dynal) the biotinylated strand bound to the beads was sequenced with the downstream 3′ PCR primer as sequencing primer. The non-bound complementary DNA strand was also sequenced, using the other PCR primer, after neutralization of the eluate. The sequencing reaction was performed with the Sequenase ver. 2.0 kit (USB, Cleveland, OH, USA), according to the manufacturer's instructions. 6% polyacrylamide gels were used with wedge spacers (0.4–1.2 mm), and they were run for 2–3.5 h at 55°C. Autoradiography was accomplished by using Hyperfilm β MAX X-ray film (Amersham, Buckinghamshire, England). PCR products from individual HCV strains were sequenced in 3–5 independent experiments.

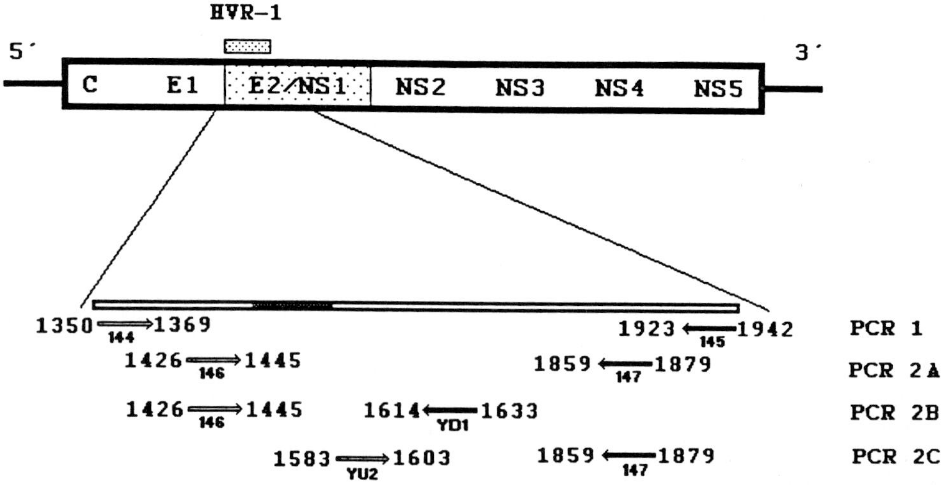

Fig. 1. Map of the HCV genome, and the locations of the PCR primers. The numbers flanking the primer-arrows are the nucleotide positions in the HCV-1 strain. Primer-sequences are: 5′CTGCTCCG-GATCCCACAAGC 3′ (144), 5′GTATCATTTTCACCCCAGCT 3′ (145), 5′TCTCCATGGTGGGGA-ACTGG 3′ (146), 5′GGGCTGGGAGTGAAGCAATA 3′ (147), 5′ACACCAACGGCAGTTGGCAC 3′ (YU2), 5′TCATTGCAGTTCAGGGCCGT 3′ (YD1). Arrows corresponding to sense primers are unfilled, and those corresponding to antisense primers are black.

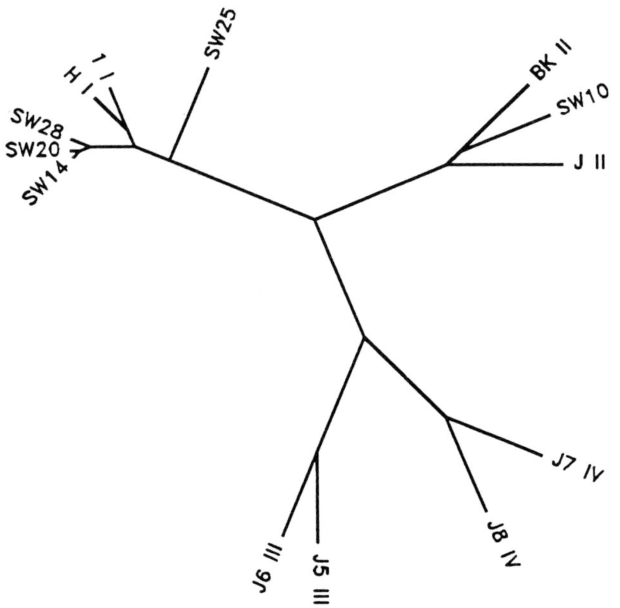

Fig. 2. Phylogenetic analysis of DNA sequence data from the E2/NS1 region. The analysis was performed using the DNADIST program of the Phylip vers. 3.4 package. The distance matrix was converted to an unrooted phylogenetic tree by using the NEIGHBOR and DRAWTREE programs of the same package.

Sequence analysis

The DNA sequence data was stored and converted to protein data using the DNASIS/PROSIS microcomputer program, version 7.0 (Hitachi Software Engineering America Ltd., CA, USA). Predictions of antigenic sites and protein chain flexibility were performed with the ANTIGEN and FLEXPRO modules of the PC/Gene program vers. 6.7 (Intelligenetics Inc., CA, USA). DNA sequences from 2 representatives of the 4 established genotypes were retrieved from GenBank release 73. Alignment of the DNA sequences was performed with the Clustal V program of Higgins et al. (11, 12). Analysis of the aligned data was carried out by using the DNAPARS, and the DNADIST (D option) programs of the Phylip ver. 3.4 package, implemented for IBM compatible microcomputers. The input order of the sequences was randomized (20 jumbles). The distance matrix generated by the latter program was clustered by the programs KITSCH or NEIGHBOR of the Phylip package. The protein sequence data was aligned by using the MACAW program (vers. 1.05) of Schuler et al. (14), and analysed by the PROTPARS program of Phylip.

The DRAWTREE program of the Phylip package was used for production of graphical output from the phylogenetic analysis of the other programs. This program produces unrooted representations of the data, which is the most suitable alternative, when the ancestors of HCV are not known.

Pairwise comparisons of the aligned DNA sequences of most strains were performed by hand, and the mutations counted and classified as transitions (Ts; A ↔ G or C ↔ T) or transversions (Tv; A ↔ C, A ↔ T, G ↔ C or G ↔ T).

RESULTS

DNA sequences

A set of DNA sequence data from 8 different HCV strains HCV-1, H, J, BK, J5, J6, J7 and J8, was recovered from GenBank (R. 73). These strains represent 4 different genotypes of HCV: HCV-1 and H (I), HCV-J and BK (II), HCV-J5 and J6 (III) and HCV-J7 and J8 (IV) (15). These sequences, from genomic positions 1452 to 1856 in HCV-1, were aligned with our sequence data (GenBank accession no. L16889-93) from 5 Swedish HCV infected patients (not shown; alignments can be obtained from the authors). The alignment agreed closely with the previously sequenced HCV strains from the USA and Japan. As expected, the greatest variability was found in the hypervariable domain, corresponding to the region between nucleotides 1491 and 1587 of HCV-1 (not shown).

The aligned sequences were analysed using the phylogeny programs in the Phylip package (vers. 3.4). A representative unrooted dendrogram obtained with NEIGHBOR is shown in Fig. 2. All the previously sequenced HCV strains clustered as expected in the 4 genotypic groups. It is also evident that 4 of the Swedish strains, SW14, 20, 28 and 25, cluster with the USA prototype strains HCV-1 and H in genotype group I. Strain SW10, however, is very clearly associated with the Japanese prototype strain HCV-J in group II, but seems to be slightly more related to the HCV-BK strain in this group.

Analysis of the Ts/Tv ratios (16) for representative HCV strains from the same or different genotype groups (Table I), supports the results from the phylogenetic tree construction. Thus, ratios higher than 1.0 were obtained from this genomic region by members of the same genotype group, and values between 0.4 and 0.8 from members of different groups. The Ts/Tv ratios of the Swedish strains SW10, SW20 and SW25 and strains from the different groups (Table I) were clearly in accordance with the phylogenetic tree analysis. This is illustrated even more clearly by a scatterplot of the frequency of transversions, in percentage of total mutations, against the percentage nucleotide sequence divergence for homologous (intragenotype) and heterologous (intergenotype) comparisons (Fig. 3), as demonstrated by Tanaka et al. (16).

The datapoints for the intragenotype (A in Fig. 3; HCV-strains: 1/H; 1/SW20; J5/J6; J7/J8; BK/SW10; 1/SW25; J/BK; SW20/SW25), and intergenotype (B in Fig. 3; HCV-strains: J6/J7; 1/SW10; J5/SW25; BK/J7; BK/J5; 1/J5 + J8/SW25, superimposed; 1/J + SW10/SW25, superimposed; J8/SW20; 1/J7; BK/SW20; BK/SW25; J8/SW10; SW10/SW20; J5/SW20; J5/SW10) comparisons form distinctly separate clusters when this region of the HCV genome is analysed.

Protein sequences

The protein sequences derived from the DNA sequence data were aligned, and the hypervariable region was clearly discernible at the very N-terminal domain of the E2 protein (not shown; alignments can be obtained from the authors). The phylogenetic analysis performed with PROTPARS, shows the expected clustering of the members of the 4 genotypes (Fig. 4). The 4 Swedish strains (SW14, 20, 25 and 28), which clustered with the genotype I group using DNA data, is apparently less closely associated with this group when protein sequence data are used. The SW10 strain is, however, still related to genotype group II.

A scan of the HVR sequences for antigenic sites and protein chain flexibility, using the ANTIGEN and FLEXPRO programs of the PC/Gene package, points to the second half of

Table I. *Ratios between base transition and transversion (Ts/Tv) mutations in the E2/NS1 region*[a]

	I	II	III	IV	SW10	SW20	SW25
I	**4.1**	0.6	0.6	0.5	0.8	**2.2**	**1.5**
II		**1.3**	0.6	0.6	**1.6**	0.5	0.5
III			**2.2**	0.8	0.4	0.4	0.6
IV				**2.1**	0.5	0.5	0.6
SW10						0.5	0.5
SW20							**1.1**

[a] The HCV isolates compared were: 1/H; 1/J; 1/J5; 1/J7; J/BK; BK/J5; BK/J7; J5/J6; J6/J7; J7/J8; 1/SW10; BK/SW10; J5/SW10; J8/SW10; 1/SW20; BK/SW20; J5/SW20; J8/SW20; 1/SW25; BK/SW25; J5/SW25; J8/SW25; SW10/SW20; SW10/SW25; SW20/SW25.
Values above 1.0 are in bold letters.

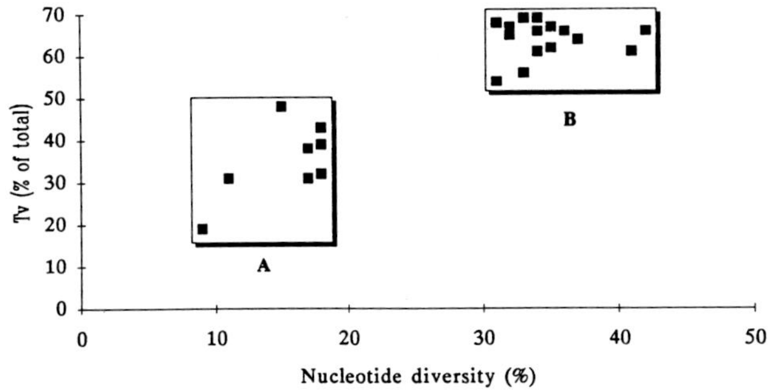

Fig. 3. The rate of base transversions as a function of nucleotide sequence divergence in the E2/NS1 region. The same intra- and intergenotype comparisons of base transversions (Tv) as a percentage of total number of mutations (Tv + Ts) and percentage nucleotide sequence divergence were made as shown in Table I. (*A*) Cluster of all intragenotype comparisons; (*B*) cluster of all intergenotype comparisons. The datapoints in ascending order according to % Tv, and when at the same value, according to % nucleotide diversity, represent comparisons between the HCV strains: 1/H; 1/SW20; J5/J6; J7/J8; BK/SW10; 1/SW25; J/BK; SW20/SW25 (cluster A) and J6/J7; 1/SW10; J5/SW25; BK/J7; BK/J5; 1/J5 + J8/SW25; 1/J + SW10/SW25; J8/SW20; 1/J7; BK/SW20; BK/SW25; J8/SW10; SW10/SW20; J5/SW20; J5/SW10 (cluster B).

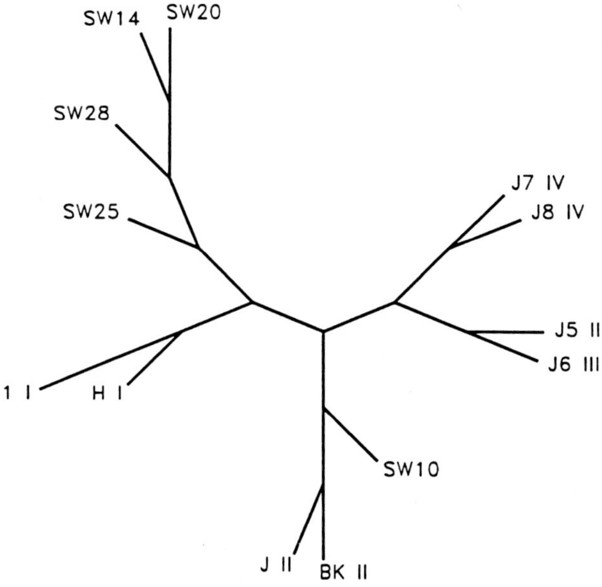

Fig. 4. Phylogenetic analysis of protein sequence data from the E2/NS1 region. The analysis was performed using the PROTPARS program of the Phylip vers. 3.4 package.

this domain (amino acids 21–29 of HVR) as a major antigenic determinant in all the genotypes of HCV analysed in this communication, except for HCV-BK and J8. In HCV-BK, maximal chain flexibility was still in the second half of the HVR domain.

DISCUSSION

It proved difficult to interpret the sequence data from the E2/NS1 region by using direct sequencing from the PCR products, probably because of the 'quasispecies' nature of HCV (17), and the exceptional sequence variability of the hypervariable region. This resulted, in some cases, in a faint background of sequence from minor HCV variants in the sample. However, reliable data could be assembled by repeated sequencing of the same samples, and by using the shorter overlap PCR products as templates.

The phylogenetic analysis of the DNA sequence data in the E2/NS1 region shows clearly a close relationship of 4 Swedish HCV strains (SW14, 20, 25 and 28) with the genotype I group of strains from the USA. The apparently less close association found when using protein sequences is probably not as statistically reliable as the DNA data, because the only algorithm available is based on parsimony. A total of 6 genotypic groups of HCV has been proposed (6). However, no sequence information in the E2/NS1 region for the strains of groups V and VI was available. One Swedish strain, SW10, was clearly most related to the Japanese genotype group II. This strain was obtained from a patient who had received a HCV-infected blood-transfusion in Sweden. The source of the infected blood was not established, however.

As recently shown by Tanaka et al. (16), the ratios of the numbers of transitions and transversions found by pairwise comparison of sequences can be used in order to classify HCV strains into the different genotypic groups. Using whole genomic sequences or sequences from the NS5 region, they obtained ratios of 4.0 to 24 for members of the same group, and 0.6 to 1.1 for those from different groups. The latter values are in good agreement with our results with the N terminal part of the E2/NS1 region. However, the values for members in the same genotype groups were consistently lower than the corresponding data of Tanaka et al. (16), viz. 1.1 to 4.1. This is probably related to the region chosen for the analysis. If the analysis of HCV-1 and HCV-H (group I) sequences is confined to the HVR region only, the Ts/Tv ratio will be 11 to 12 (16).

The conclusions from this mutation analysis agreed closely with the phylogenetic results, i.e. the genotype classification of the Swedish strains was confirmed.

Evidence of immune selection of HCV envelope glycoprotein sequence variants has recently been presented (7). Using 8-residue peptides, corresponding to the hypervariable region, these authors found linear epitopes subjected to immune selection in the 2 HCV strains HCV-18 and Th, which partly overlaps the antigenic sites of the C-terminal part of the region predicted in this communication. One of the Swedish strains (SW25), as well as prototype strain HCV-H, shows the sequence QNIQLI of HCV strain Th (7). This sequence was, however, shifted slightly towards the C-terminal, compared with the predicted epitopes. A peptide of this composition was found to bind antibodies in plasma from patients infected with the HCV Th strain (7). This sequence information for an apparently important epitope in the gp70 protein of the Swedish strains, might be of value for future vaccine development.

ACKNOWLEDGEMENTS

This study was supported by grants from the Martin Rind Foundation and from the Karolinska Institute. The expert technical assistance of Ms. Åsa Staland is gratefully acknowledged.

REFERENCES

1. Kato N, Hijikata M, Ootsuyama Y, Nakagawa M, Ohkoshi S, Sugimura T, Shimotohno K. Molecular cloning of the human hepatitis C virus genome from Japanese patients with non-A non-B hepatitis. Proc Natl Acad Sci USA 87: 9524–9528, 1990.
2. Takamizawa A, Mori C, Fuke I, Manabe S, Murakami S, Fujita J, Onishi E, Andoh T, Yoshida I, Okayama H. Structure and organization of the hepatitis C virus genome isolated from human carriers. J Virol 65: 1105–1113, 1991.
3. Choo QL, Richman KH, Han JH, Berger K, Lee C, Dong C, Gallegos C, Coit D, Medina Selby R, Barr PJ, Weiner AJ, Bradley DW, Kuo G, Houghton M. Genetic organization and diversity of hepatitis C virus. Proc Natl Acad Sci USA 88: 2451–2455, 1991.

4. Houghton M, Weiner AJ, Han JH, Kuo G, Choo QL. Molecular biology of the hepatitis C viruses: implications for diagnosis, development and control of viral disease. Hepatology 14: 381–388, 1991.
5. Weiner AJ, Brauer MJ, Rosenblatt J, Richman KH, Tung K, Crawford K, Bonino F, Saracco G, Choo QL, Houghton M, Han JH. Variable and hypervariable domains are found in the regions of HCV corresponding to the Flavivirus envelope and NS1 proteins and the Pestivirus envelope glycoproteins. Virology 180: 842–848, 1991.
6. Mori S, Kato N, Yagyu A, Tanaka T, Ikeda Y, Petchclai B, Chiewsilp P, Kurimura T, Shimotohno K. A new type of hepatitis C virus in patients in Thailand. Biochem Biophys Res Commun 183: 2451–2455, 1991.
7. Weiner AJ, Geysen HM, Christopherson C, Hall JE, Mason TJ, Saracco G, Bonino F, Crawford K, Marion CD, Crawford KA, Brunetto M, Barr PJ, Miyamura T, McHutchinson J, Houghton M. Evidence for immune selection of hepatitis C virus (HCV) putative envelope glycoprotein variants: potential role in chronic HCV infections. Proc Natl Acad Sci USA 89: 3468–3472, 1992.
8. Yun Z-B, Lindh G, Weiland O, Johansson B, Sönnerborg A. Detection of hepatitis C virus (HCV) antibodies in serum and liver histology in Swedish blood donors. J Med Virol 39: 57–61, 1993.
9. Kato N, Ootsuyama Y, Tanaka T, Nakagawa M, Nakazawa T, Muraiso K, Ohkoshi S, Hijikata M, Shimotohno K. Marked sequence diversity in the putative envelope proteins of hepatitis C viruses. Virus Res 22: 107–123, 1992.
10. Ayehunie S, Johansson B, Sönnerborg A, Zewdie D, Britton S, Strannegård Ö. Sequence analysis of selected regions of the env (V3 loop and gp41) and gag (p7) reading frames of Ethiopian human immunodeficiency virus type 1 strains. Arch Virol 128: 229–239, 1993.
11. Higgins DG, Bleasby, AJ, Fuchs, R. CLUSTAL V: improved software for multiple sequence alignment. Comput Appl Biosci 8: 189–191, 1992.
12. Higgins DG, Sharp PM. Fast and sensitive multiple sequence alignments on a microcomputer. Comput Appl Biosci 5: 151–153, 1989.
13. Felsenstein, J. Phylogenies from molecular sequences: inference and reliability. Annu Rev Genet 22: 521–565, 1988.
14. Schuler GD, Altschul SF, Lipman DJ. A workbench for multiple alignment construction and analysis. Proteins 9: 180–190, 1991.
15. Okamoto H, Kurai K, Okada S-I, Yamamoto K, Lizuka H, Tanaka T, Fukuda S, Tsuda F, Mishiro S. Full-length sequence of a hepatitis C virus genome having poor homology to reported isolates: comparative study of four distinct genotypes. Virology 188: 331–341, 1992.
16. Tanaka T, Kato N, Hijikata M, Shimotohno K. Base transitions and base transversions seen in mutations among various types of the hepatitis C viral genome. FEBS Lett 315: 201–203, 1993.
17. Martell M, Esteban JI, Quer J, Genesca J, Weiner A, Esteban R, Guardia J, Gomez J. Hepatitis C virus (HCV) circulates as a population of different but closely related genomes: quasispecies nature of HCV genome distribution. J Virol 66: 3225–3229, 1992.

Submitted September 30, 1993; accepted January 6, 1994

Scand J Infect Dis 26: 263–270, 1994

Serum Hepatitis C Virus RNA Levels in Chronic Hepatitis C – Importance for outcome of interferon alfa-2b treatment

ZHI BING YUN[1], OLLE REICHARD[2], MARGARET CHEN[1], JOAKIM LUNDEBERG[3], GUNNAR NORKRANS[4], ARIL FRYDEN[5], ANDERS SÖNNERBORG[1,6] and OLA WEILAND[6]

From the Departments of [1]Virology, Central Microbiological Laboratory of the Stockholm County Council, Stockholm, [2]Infectious Diseases, Karolinska Institute, Danderyds Hospital, Danderyd, [3]Biochemistry and Biotechnology, Royal Institute of Technology, Stockholm, [4]Infectious Diseases, East Hospital, University of Gothenburg, Gothenburg, [5]Infectious Diseases, University Hospital of Linköping, Linköping, and [6]Immunology, Microbiology, Pathology and Infectious Diseases, Division of Infectious Diseases, Karolinska Institute, Huddinge Hospital, Huddinge, Sweden

Sera from 39 out of 40 patients with chronic hepatitis C virus (HCV) infection who had been treated for 60 weeks with interferon alfa-2b proved initially HCV RNA positive by reversed transcriptase polymerase chain reaction (PCR). These patients were analysed for genotype and quantitatively for HCV RNA levels prior to treatment by using a competitive PCR method with colorimetric detection of the amplified products. HCV RNA levels were correlated to outcome of treatment, mode of acquisition, histology and HCV genotype. The median pretreatment HCV RNA level in sustained responders ($n = 15$) with eradication of the viremia and normalization of serum ALT levels lasting 24 weeks post treatment was significantly lower than that in the combined group of non-sustained responders ($n = 9$) and non-responders ($n = 15$), 2.52×10^5 vs 8.90×10^5 genome equivalents per ml serum, $p < 0.0125$, respectively. 10 out of 17 patients with HCV RNA levels lower than the median level (5.64×10^5 genome equivalents per ml serum) had a sustained response to interferon treatment versus only 5/22 with levels equal to or higher than the median level, $p = 0.04$. No significant pretreatment differences in median HCV RNA levels according to mode of acquisition, genotype, or liver histology prior to treatment were seen. It is concluded that a low pretreatment HCV RNA level seems to be indicative of a sustained response to interferon alfa-2b treatment, whereas a high level seems to be indicative of a non-sustained or non-response. In the individual patient, however, the levels varied widely irrespective of response category.

O. Weiland, MD, PhD, Department of Infectious Diseases 173, Huddinge Hospital, S-141 86 Huddinge, Sweden

INTRODUCTION

It is now well known that hepatitis C virus (HCV) infection is the major cause of both parenteral and sporadic non-A, non-B hepatitis (1–3), and that it has potentially serious long-term consequences including liver cirrhosis and hepatocellular carcinoma (3–5). Tests to detect antibodies to recombinant antigens are used for a serologic diagnosis of HCV infections (6–8). HCV is a positive-stranded RNA virus (9). HCV RNA can be detected in serum by reversed transcription polymerase chain reaction (RT-PCR) (10, 11), a direct evidence of viremia. Viremia levels have been assessed semiquantitatively by limiting dilution RT-PCR, an expensive and laborious method (12, 13), by competitive RT-PCR assay (14, 15) and recently by a new branched DNA signal amplification method (16). Using this latter method, some authors have found that viremia levels are higher in patients who acquired their infection via transfusion than from health care work or intravenous drug abuse (16), whereas others have not (17). Furthermore, it has been suggested that patients with chronic hepatitis C who have lower viremia levels are more likely to respond to interferon treatment in a sustained fashion than those with higher levels (14–16, 18, 19).

 ISSN 0036-5548

In the present study we used a sensitive recently developed competitive PCR method with colorimetric detection of the amplified product to quantify HCV RNA levels in serum prior to interferon treatment and to correlate these to the ultimate outcome of treatment (20). We also analysed the outcome of treatment according to genotype as determined by Okamoto et al. (21), and correlated genotype, histology prior to treatment, and mode of acquisition to the HCV RNA levels prior to treatment.

MATERIAL AND METHODS

40 patients with chronic HCV infection who had been treated with interferon alfa-2b for 60 weeks at a dosage of 3 MU 3 times a week were chosen as detailed elsewhere (22). The original treatment study was performed in 1990–92 and included 40 patients who completed the treatment, 21 men and 19 women, mean age 46 years (range 18–74). 25 had aquired their HCV infection from blood transfusions, 7 from earlier intravenous drug abuse, 1 from tattooing and the remaining 7 from unknown causes (22). All were positive for anti-HCV by second generation ELISA (Abbott Laboratories, North Chicago, IL, USA) and confirmed by second generation RIBA (4-RIBA, Chiron Corp., Emerville, CA, USA). All but 1 were HCV RNA positive in serum prior to treatment. In a liver biopsy performed within 6 months of treatment, 9, 21 and 10 patients were found to have chronic persistent hepatitis (CPH), chronic active hepatitis (CAH) and CAH with suspected or developed cirrhosis (Ci), respectively, as classified by criteria recommended by an international group, with slight modifications (23, 24).

Patients were defined as: **sustained responders** to treatment if the mean ALT levels during the last 2 months of treatment became normal and stayed normal 6 months past treatment; as **non-sustained responders** if the mean ALT levels after being normal during the last 2 months of treatment rose again during 6 months of follow-up post treatment; and as **non-responders** if the ALT level at treatment cessation was above the upper limit of normal (22). Sera drawn prior to treatment and stored as −25°C from all 40 patients were available for quantification of HCV RNA levels and genotyping.

Extraction of HCV RNA and PCR

Extraction of HCV RNA from the serum samples, reverse transcription (RT) and PCR were performed as described earlier (10, 11). Primers were chosen from the 5′-nontranslated region. In brief, HCV cDNA was synthesized in a total volume of 25 μl RT mixture using 1 μM downstream outer primer, 5 units M-MuLV reverse transcriptase (Boehringer Mannheim, Germany), 10 units RNasin (Boehringer Mannheim) and 10 μl extracted RNA. After double PCR, a 260 bp fragment was produced. The PCR product was assayed by agarose gel electrophoresis.

Quantification of HCV RNA

Quantification of the amount of HCV RNA was performed using a method based on competitive PCR and colorimetric detection of the amplified products, as earlier described (20, 25). After the RT, one-tenth of the resulting cDNA, and the same volume of serially diluted cloned HCV competitor DNA, were co-amplified by nested PCR. The competitor DNA consisted of the amplified regions of the wild-type HCV cDNA with an internal region substituted with the *lac* operator sequence. The PCR products were specifically quantitated by a colorimetric solid-phase assay. This assay reproducibly detects 10 HCV genome equivalents. The intra-assay variation is 10–15%, whereas the inter-assay variation is 15–20%. This assay is more robust than methods which do not include an internal standard (20).

Genotyping of HCV RNA

Genotyping was performed using PCR with type-specific primers, by which altogether 4 genotypes can be identified (21). Extraction of the HCV RNA was followed by RT and first-round amplification in the same tube, which contained two universal primers no. 256 and no. 186, 5 units M-MuLV reverse transcriptase and 1 unit *Taq* polymerase. Firstly, the RT-PCR mixture was incubated at 37°C for 60 min followed by heating at 95°C for 2 min and then HCV cDNA was amplified directly in conjunction with the PCR program described earlier by Okamoto et al. (21). After nested PCR, genotypes I, II, III and IV can be obtained by using a universal upstream primer no. 104 together with 4 specific downstream primers no. 132, no. 133, no. 134 and no. 135, respectively. 20 μl of nested PCR product was subjected to electrophoresis on a 3% Nusieve agarose gel.

Statistical methods

Statistical methods were performed with Fishers' exact test and the Mann-Whitney U-test on a Macintosh computer using the Statview II program.

RESULTS

15 patients were classified as sustained responders, all of whom became HCV RNA negative with normal ALT levels, 9 as non-sustained responders, 1 of whom became HCV RNA negative, and 16 as non-responders, 1 of whom became HCV RNA negative 6 months post treatment. One patient was negative already prior to treatment, as detailed elsewhere (22).

HCV RNA levels prior to treatment

HCV RNA levels prior to treatment ranged between 3.20×10^3 and 7.96×10^6 genome equivalents/ml serum, median 5.64×10^5.

The HCV RNA levels according to response category to treatment are shown in Fig. 1. For the patients with sustained response, non-sustained response and non-response the median levels were 2.52×10^5, 1.90×10^6 and 8.00×10^5 genome equivalents/ml serum, respectively. Patients with sustained response had a significantly lower median pretreatment HCV RNA level than the combined group of patients with non-sustained and non-response ($p < 0.0125$). Sustained responders also had a significantly lower median pretreatment HCV RNA level than non-sustained responders ($p < 0.009$) whereas the difference from patients with non-response did not reach statistical significance ($p < 0.07$). 10/17 patients with HCV RNA levels below the median level (5.64×10^5 genome equivalents/ml serum) had a sustained response, versus only 5/22 with levels equal to or higher than the median level ($p = 0.04$).

In the individual patients in the respective treatment outcome category the levels differed widely. Levels thus ranged from 3.20×10^3 to 5.12×10^6, 5.04×10^5 to 7.96×10^6 and 3.40×10^4 to 7.60×10^6 genome equivalents/ml serum among sustained, non-sustained, and non-responders, respectively.

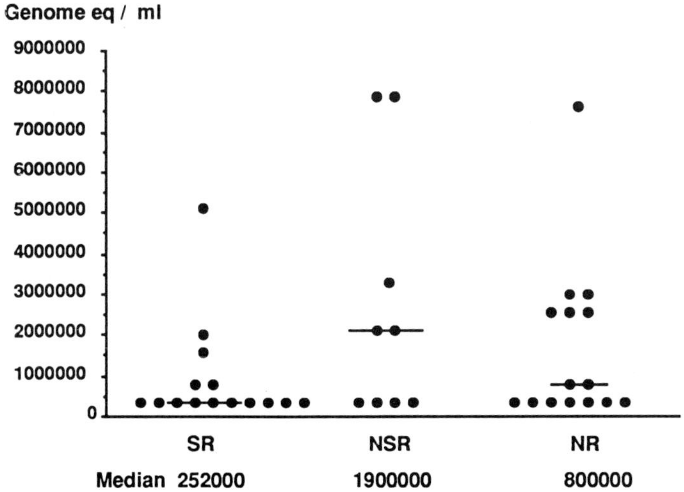

Fig. 1. Pretreatment HCV RNA titres in serum according to response category presented as genome equivalents/ml serum. Bar shows median titre in each response category. SR = sustained response ($n = 15$), NSR = not sustained response ($n = 9$) and NR = non-response ($n = 15$). For details, see Material and Methods.

Genotyping

Genotyping according to Okamoto et al. (21) was possible in 36/39 (92%) HCV RNA positive patients (as amplified with primers from the 5′NT regions of the genome), whereas 3 were untypable with the core-derived primers used for genotyping. 16, 8 and 9 patients had genotype I, II or IV, respectively. Three had mixed types, whereof 2 genotypes I and II and 1 genotypes I and IV.

HCV RNA levels in different genotypes

The median HCV RNA level found in patients with genotypes I, II and IV was 6.38×10^5, 3.29×10^5 and 8.00×10^5 genome equivalents/ml serum, respectively, as depicted in Fig. 2. The median levels did not differ significantly between patients with different genotypes. Patients with genotype II tended to have a lower median HCV RNA level than patients with genotype IV, but not significantly so ($p = 0.06$, Mann-Whitney U-test).

Treatment outcome according to genotype

When the different genotypes were analysed according to outcome of treatment 9/16 (56%), 2/8 (25%) and 3/9 (33%) patients with genotype I, II and IV, respectively, responded in a sustained fashion. These differences did not reach statistical significance.

HCV RNA levels according to mode of acquisition and histology

HCV RNA levels were also analysed according to mode of acquisition but again no significant differences were found. The median level for patients with acquisition from transfusion, prior intravenous drug abuse (including 1 patient who acquired his disease from tattooing) or sporadic cause shown in Fig. 3 were 7.14×10^5, 5.64×10^5 and 8.00×10^4 genome equivalents/ml serum, respectively, differences which were not significant. Age and mode of acquisition were related, however, since significantly more patients aged ≥ 40 had acquired their infection via blood transfusion than those <40 (18/23 vs 7/17, $p < 0.05$). However, no significant difference in the median HCV RNA levels before treatment was seen

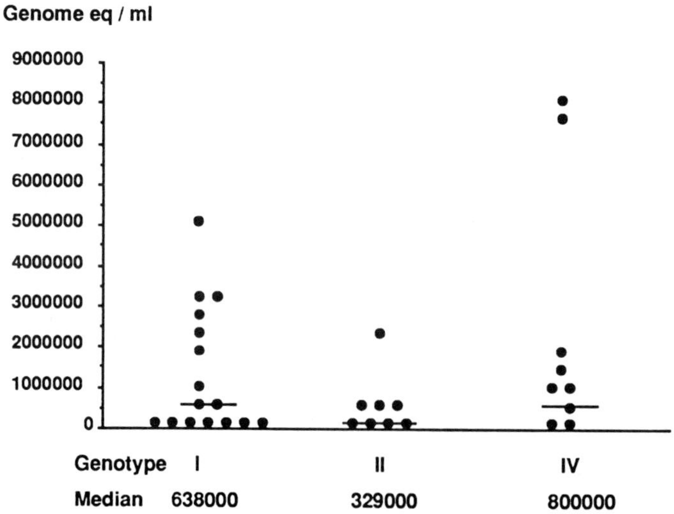

Fig. 2. Pretreatment HCV RNA titres in serum according to genotype according to Okamoto et al. (21) presented as genome equivalents/ml serum. Bar shows median titre for each genotype. Genotype I ($n = 16$), genotype II ($n = 8$) and genotype IV ($n = 9$).

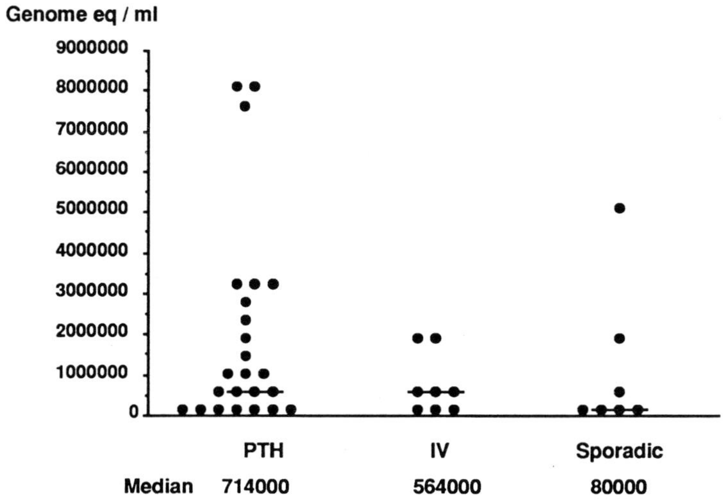

Fig. 3. Pretreatment HCV RNA titre in serum according to mode of acquisition of the hepatitis C virus infection presented as genome equivalents/ml serum. Bar shows median titre in each category. PTH = transfusion/s ($n = 24$), IV = intravenous drug use ($n = 8$ including one patient who got his infection from tattooing), and Sporadic = sporadic cause ($n = 7$).

according to age above vs. below 40. We also analysed the levels according to histological findings prior to treatment as shown in Fig. 4. The median levels among patients with CPH, CAH and CAH with suspected or developed cirrhosis were 4.80×10^5, 7.96×10^5 and 4.58×10^5 genome equivalents/ml serum, respectively, differences that were not significant. As earlier analysed, no difference in treatment outcome was found according to pretreatment histological findings (22).

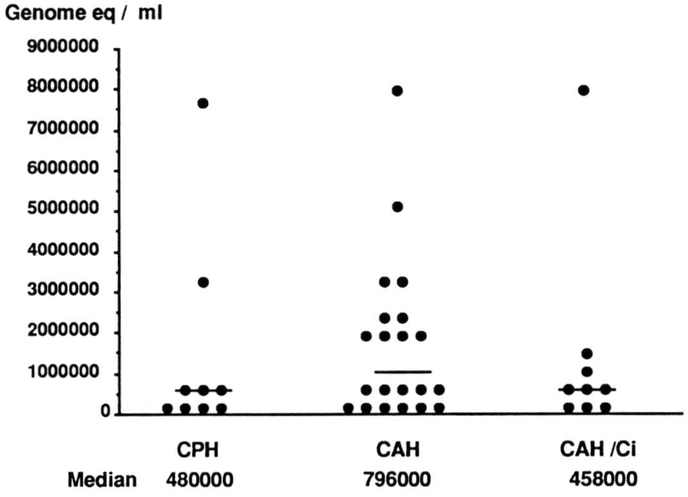

Fig. 4. Pretreatment HCV RNA titres in serum according to histology prior to treatment presented as genome equivalents/ml serum. Bar shows median titre in each category. CPH = chronic persistent hepatitis ($n = 9$), CAH = chronic active hepatitis ($n = 21$), and CAH/Ci = CAH with suspected or developed cirrhosis ($n = 9$).

DISCUSSION

The most important finding in this study was that patients with sustained response to interferon alpha-2b treatment, meaning eradication of the viremia and normalization of the aminotransferase levels lasting 6 months post treatment (22), had the lowest median pretreatment HCV RNA levels, thus confirming the findings of others (14–16, 18, 19). Sustained responders thus had a significantly lower median pretreatment level than the combined group of patients with a non-response or a non-sustained response. In contrast to the findings by Lau et al. (16) but in agreement with the findings of Kodali et al. (17) we could not find a significant difference in the viremia level among groups with different modes of acquisition of their hepatitis C virus infection. Thus patients with acquisition via blood transfusion/s did not have a median HCV RNA level in serum significantly different from those who had acquired the infection via remote earlier intravenous drug abuse (7.14×10^5 vs 5.64×10^5 genome equivalents/ml serum). Our results may be due to the fact that we used a very sensitive quantification method, with which it was possible to quantify all HCV RNA positive patients, as opposed to the bDNA method, which does not detect HCV RNA levels below a detection limit of 350,000 genome equivalents/ml (16).

The amount of circulating HCV RNA in our patients before treatment vaired roughly between 10^3/ml and 10^7/ml, which is in line with what others have found (15, 16, 26), levels lower than those usually found among patients with replicating chronic hepatitis B virus infection. It has been reported that HCV RNA levels in serum increase with advancing liver disease seen histologically, which parallels an increasing resistance to interferon treatment (27). In contrast to this we could not find any correlation between the pre-treatment histological findings and the outcome of treatment. In fact, patients with CAH with suspected or developed cirrhosis responded just as well as patients with less pronounced histological disease (28). Furthermore, in agreement with the findings of Lau et al. (16) we could not find any correlation with the histological grading and the viremia levels prior to treatment.

In the study by Lau et al., genotypes were not determined, but the question was raised whether genotypes were correlated to the outcome of treatment and to the levels of viremia before treatment. When using the genotyping system as proposed by Okamoto et al. (21) we could not find any significant differences in response rates or median pretreatment viremia levels between patients with different genotypes, in accordance with the findings of Kobayashi et al. (19). Genotype III, however, which seems to be associated with a high response rate, was not represented in our patient material (15). Differences between genotypes could have been missed, however, since the number of patients studied was relatively small and the more recently described genotype V (29) was not detected using this system. A non-significant trend was found towards a higher median HCV RNA pre-treatment serum level in patients with genotype IV vs genotype II. In a recent European study from France, patients with genotype II were found to respond less well to interferon treatment and to have more advanced liver disease than patients with other genotypes (30). Others have also found that patients with genotype II seem to respond less well to interferon treatment (15). We could not find any difference in response rate according to genotype, although patients with genotype I tended to respond in a sustained fashion more often than those with genotype II or IV (9/16 vs 5/17), a difference which was not significant. The most common genotype noted among our patients was genotype IV, in contrast to findings in France and Italy, where genotype II seems to be most prevalent (30).

To conclude, we found that a low median pre-treatment HCV RNA level, as determined by a competitive PCR method with colorimetric detection of the amplified product, seems to be indicative of a sustained response to interferon alfa-2b treatment, whereas a high median pre-treatment titre seems to be indicative of a non-sustained or non-response. In the individual patient, however, the pre-treatment titres varied widely, in agreement with the findings of others (14), thus making a prediction of the response based on the HCV RNA pre-treatment titre difficult.

ACKNOWLEDGEMENT

This investigation was supported by grants from the Karolinska Institute Stockholm, and from Schering-Plough AB, Sweden.

REFERENCES

1. Alter M, Margolis H, Krawczynski K, Judson F, Mares A, Alexander J, Hu P, Miller J, Gerber M, Samplinger R, Meeks E, Beach M, for the Sentinental Counties chronic non-A and non-B hepatitis study. The natural history of community-acquired hepatitis C in the United States. N Engl J Med 327: 1899–1905, 1992.
2. Farci P, Alter H, Wong D, Miller R, Shih J, Jett B, Purcell R. A long-term study of hepatitis C virus replication in non-A, non-B hepatitis. N Engl J Med 325: 98–104, 1991.
3. Mattsson L, Sönnerborg A, Weiland O. Outcome of acute symptomatic non-A, non-B hepatitis: a 13-year follow-up study of hepatitis C virus markers. Liver 13: 274–278, 1993.
4. Tremolada F, Casarin C, Alberti A, Drago C, Tagger A, Ribero M, Realdi G. Long-term follow-up of non-A, non-B (type C) posttransfusion-hepatitis. J Hepatol 16: 273–281, 1992.
5. Kiyosawa K, Sodeyama T, Tanaka E, Gibo Y, Yoshisawa K, Nakano Y, Furuta S, Akahane Y, Nishioka K, Purcell R, Alter H. Interrelationship of blood transfusion, non-A, non-B hepatitis and hepatocellular carcinoma: Analysis by detection of antibody to hepatitis C virus. Hepatology 12: 671–675, 1990.
6. Kuo G, Choo Q, Alter HJ, Gitmik GL, Redeker AG, Purcell RH, Miyamura T, Dienstag JL, Alter MJ, Stevens CE, Tegtmeier GE, Bonino F, Colombo M, Lee WS, Kuo C, Berger K, Shuster JR, Overby LR, Bradley DW, Houghton M. An assay for circulating antibodies to a major etiologic virus of human non-A, non-B hepatitis. Science 244: 362–364, 1989.
7. Van Der Poel C, Cuypers H, Reesink H, Weiner A, Quan S, Di Nello R, Van Boven J, Winkel I, Mulder-Folkerts D, Exel-Ohlers P, Schaasberg W, Leentvaar-Kuypers A, Polito A, Houghton M, Lelie P. Confirmation of hepatitis C virus infection by new four-antigen recombinant immunoblot assay. Lancet 337: 317–319, 1991.
8. Mattsson L, Gutierrez R, Dawson G, Lesniewski R, Mushahwar I, Weiland O. Antibodies to recombinant and synthetic peptides derived from the hepatitis C virus genome in long-term-studied patients with posttransfusion hepatitis C. Scand J Gastroenterol 26: 1257–1262, 1991.
9. Houghton M, Weiner A, Han J, Kuo G, Choo Q-L. Molecular biology of the hepatitis C viruses: implications for diagnosis, development and control of viral disease. Hepatology 14: 381–388, 1991.
10. Brillanti S, Garson J, Tuke P, Ring C, Briggs M, Masci C, Miglioli M, Barbara L, Tedder R. Effect of alfa-interferon therapy on hepatitis C viraemia in community-acquired chronic non-A, non-B hepatitis: a quantitative polymerase chain reaction study. J Med Virol 34: 136–41, 1991.
11. Yun Z, Lindh G, Weiland O, Johansson B, Sönnerberg A. Detection of hepatitis C virus (HCV) RNA by PCR related to HCV antibodies in serum and liver histology in Swedish blood donors. J Med Virol 39: 57–61, 1993.
12. Shindo M, Di Bisceglie A, Cheung L, Shih W-K, Cristiano K, Feinstone S, Hoofnagle J. Decrease in serum hepatitis C viral RNA during alpha-interferon therapy for chronic hepatitis C. Ann Intern Med 115: 700–704, 1991.
13. Weiland O, Zhang Y-Y, Widell A. Serum HCV RNA levels in patients with chronic hepatitis C given a second course of interferon alpha-2b treatment after relapse following initial treatment. Scand J Infect Dis 25: 25–30, 1993.
14. Hagiwara H, Hayashi N, Mita E, Takehara T, Kasahara A, Fusamoto H, Kamada T. Quantitative analysis of hepatitis virus RNA in serum during interferon alfa therapy. Gastroenterology 104: 877–883, 1993.
15. Yoshioka K, Kakumu S, Wakita T, Wakita T, Ishikawa T, Itoh Y, Takayanagi M, Higashi Y, Shibata M, Morishima T. Detection of hepatitis C virus by polymerase chain reaction and response to interferon-alpha therapy: relationship to genotype virus. J Hepatol 16: 293–299, 1992.

16. Lau J, Davis G, Kniffen J, Qian K-P, Urdea M, Chan C, Mizokami M, Neuwald P, Wilber J. Significance of serum hepatitis C virus RNA levels in chronic hepatitis C. Lancet 341: 1501–1504, 1993.
17. Kodali V, Gordon S, Silverman A, Urdea M, Chan C, Wilber J. Levels of hepatitis C virus (HCV) RNA correlate with liver histology but not with mode of transmission. Hepatology 18: Abstract 97 AASLD, 1993.
18. Martinot-Peignoux M, Marcellin P, Poteau M, Erlinger S, Benhamou J. HCV-RNA quantification and response to interferon treatment in patients with chronic hepatitis C. Hepatology 18: Abstract 747 AASLD, 1993.
19. Kobayashi Y, Watanabe S, Konishi M, Yokoi M, Kakehashi R, Kaito M, Kondo M, Hayashi Y, Jomori T, Suzuki S. Quantification and typing of serum hepatitis C virus RNA in patients with chronic hepatitis C treated with interferon-beta. Hepatology 18: 1319–1325, 1993.
20. Yun Z, Lundeberg J, Johansson B, Hedrum A, Weiland O, Uhlén M, Sönnerborg A. Colorimetric detection of competetive PCR products for quantification of hepatitis C viremia. J Virol Methods 47: 1–14, 1994.
21. Okamoto H, Sugiyama Y, Okada S, Kurai K, Akahane Y, Sugai Y, Tanaka T, Sato K, Tsuda F, Miyakawa Y, Mayumi M. Typing hepatitis C virus by polymerase chain reaction with type-specific primers: application to clinical surveys and tracing infectious sources. J Gen Virol 73: 673–679, 1992.
22. Reichard O, Foberg U, Frydén A, Mattsson L, Norkrans G, Sönnerborg A, Wejstål R, Yun Z-B, Weiland O. High sustained response rate and clearence of viraemia in chronic hepatitis C following treatment with interferon alfa-2b for 60 weeks. Hepatology 19: 280–285, 1994.
23. International Group. Acute and chronic hepatitis revisited. Lancet 2: 914–919, 1977.
24. Schvarcz, R, Glaumann H, Weiland O, Norkrans G, Wejstål R, Frydén A. Histological outcome in interferon alpha-2b treated patients with chronic posttransfusion non-A, non-B hepatitis. Liver 11: 30–38, 1991.
25. Lundeberg J, Wahlberg J, Uhlen M. Rapid colorimetric quantification of PCR-amplified DNA. Biotechniques 10: 68–75, 1991.
26. Hagiwara H, Hayashi N, Mita E, Naito M, Kasahara A, Fusamoto H, Kamada T. Quantitation of hepatitis C virus RNA in serum of asymptomatic blood donors and patients with type C chronic liver disease. Hepatology 17: 545–550, 1993.
27. Gretch D, Han J, Wilson R, Carithers R, Bush M, Sayers M, Corey L. High titre hepatitis C virus infection is associated with advanced disease stage and resistance to interferon. Hepatology 18: Abstract 125 AASLD, 1993.
28. Reichard O, Glaumann H, Norkrans G, Wejstål R, Frydén A, Schvarcz R, Weiland O. Histological outcome in patients with chronic hepatitis C given a 60 weeks interferon alfa-2b treatment course. Liver 14: in press, 1994.
29. Okamoto H, Tokita H, Sakamoto M, Horikita M, Kojima M, Iizuka H, Mishiro S. Characterization of the genomic sequence of type V (or 3a) hepatitis C virus isolates and PCR primers for specific detection. J Gen Virol 74: 2385–2390, 1993.
30. Nosbaum J, Pol S, Gigou M, Okamoto H, Féray C, Poussin K, Paterlini P, Berthelot P, Mishiro S, Bréchot C. HCV genotype II is associated to liver cirrhosis, cancer and low response to interferon alpha in European patients. Hepatology 18: Abstract 127 AASLD, 1993.

Submitted January 31, 1994; accepted March 21, 1994

Scand J Infect Dis 26: 275–282, 1994

Microtiter Assay for Colorimetric Detection of in vitro Amplified Chlamydia trachomatis Sequences

JOAKIM LUNDEBERG[1], LENA BONDESSON[2], ANDERS HEDRUM[2], LENA GRILLNER[3], MALIN STARK[1], GEO VON KROGH[2] and MATHIAS UHLÉN[1]

From the [1]Department of Biochemistry and Biotechnology, Royal Institute of Technology, the Departments of [2]Dermatology and Venereology, and [3]Clinical Microbiology, Section of Virology, Karolinska Hospital, Stockholm, Sweden

An integrated diagnostic method for colorimetric detection of polymerase chain reaction (PCR) products in a microtitre format is described. The amplified material is labelled by using modified PCR primers introducing a biotin molecule and a *lac* operator handle. Positive samples are identified, after immobilization onto streptavidin-coated microtitre wells, using a reporter fusion protein consisting of the Escherichia coli *lac* repressor and β-galactosidase. The analysis of the PCR products is thus, from a practical point of view, identical with the enzyme-linked immunosorbent assay (ELISA) using the enzymatic activity of β-galactosidase. Here, we show that the assay can be used for rapid and simple detection of Chlamydia trachomatis in an automated format. The reported analysis of 90 urethral patient samples, using this microtitre assay, indicates that this technique is more sensitive and more specific than culture technique.

M. Uhlén, Department of Biochemistry and Biotechnology, Royal Institute of Technology, S-100 44 Stockholm, Sweden

INTRODUCTION

Chlamydia trachomatis, an obligate intracellular pathogen, is one of the major causes of genital tract infections. Many chlamydial infections are asymptomatic and the conventional culture techniques have a sensitivity of only 80–85% (1). This represents a clinical dilemma, since undiagnosed infections may cause sequelae, in particular severe pelvic inflammatory disease (2, 3). Accordingly, simple laboratory methods with improved specificity and sensitivity that are applicable for mass screening purposes are needed. The polymerase chain reaction (PCR) (4) makes possible – in theory – the detection of a single molecule and offers new possibilities for chlamydia detection (5, 6). The PCR – but also recent immunological techniques – have been shown to reduce the time between sample collection and diagnosis.

We have earlier described a DNA detection system, i.e. DIANA (detection of immobilized amplified nucleic acids), for colorimetric detection of amplified material (7, 8) based on solid-phase technology. Different solid supports have been investigated. Lundeberg et al. used Sepharose beads as solid support which required centrifugation for sedimentation and had generally poor kinetics (7). Wahlberg et al. used magnetic beads as solid support, enabling rapid and easy handling with good kinetics (8). Furthermore, the magnetic bead also enabled direct sequencing of the amplified material for investigation of the selected target region.

Here, we show that a simple and cost-effective microtitre plate format can be used, making the procedure more suitable as a large-scale diagnostical method. No instrumentation is needed except for standard plate washers and plate readers, present in most clinical laboratories. A clinical study of 90 urethral patient samples, obtained from a venereal disease clinic, was carried out using this microtitre-based DNA assay. A comparison of the described method with a standard cell culture assay and an immunological ELISA method for urine samples was performed.

MATERIALS AND METHODS

Patients

Altogether 90 men attending a venereal disease clinic at Karolinska Hospital were enrolled after giving informed consent. Approval had been given by the Medical Ethics Committee. The patients included had urethral discharge and/or dysuria or were sexual partners of verified chlamydia positive patients.

Clinical specimens

Initially a smear was prepared from the urethra to count the number of polymorphonuclear leukocytes and to search for presence of intracellular diplococci. Hereafter specimens were taken from the distal 3–4 cm of the male urethra with 2 cotton-tipped swabs (ENT, Swedish Hospital Supply, Mölndal, Sweden). A specimen for culture was taken with the first swab and placed immediately in a transport buffer (20 mM phosphate buffer (pH 7.0)/6.48 g/l sucrose/10 mg/l gentamicin/2.5 mg/l amphotericin B/100 mg/l vancomycin/10% fetal calf serum). The second swab was placed into a sterile tube containing 200 µl 1 × PCR buffer (10 mM Tris-HCl (pH 8.3)/1.5 mM $MgCl_2$/50 mM KCl/0.1% Tween 20) for PCR analysis. If not tested within 24 h, specimens for culture were stored at −70°C until they were tested. All specimens used for PCR analysis were stored at −70°C until tested. A total of 90 samples were collected and analysed with both culture and PCR analysis. On 53 occasions, urine was collected for ELISA analysis. The urine was provided after the swabs had been taken. Finally a specimen was taken for cultivation of gonococci.

Chlamydia trachomatis culture

The culture of Chlamydiae in McCoy cell monolayer was performed as described by Ripa and Mårdh (1). The cultures were fixed in ethanol after incubation in 5% CO_2 at 37°C for 48 h and stained with a FITC-conjugated monoclonal antibody, MicroTrak Chlamydia trachomatis Confirmation test (Syva Co, Palo Alto, CA, USA) and examined for inclusions in an inverted fluorescence microscope. Of the 90 samples analysed, 16 were culture positive (Table I).

Antigen detection

53 urine samples were tested in parallel with ELISA. Urine samples (10 ml) were collected as first catch in the morning or after 4 h incubation in the bladder. The urine was centrifuged at 2500 × *g* for 10 min and the pellet was dissolved in 1 ml IDEIA Chlamydia Test transport medium (Celltech Diagnostic Ltd, Cambridge, England). Specimens were stored at +4°C if analysed within 4 days; otherwise they were frozen at −70°C until tested. The enzyme immunoassay used was the IDEIA Chlamydia Test and was performed according to the instructions by the manufacturer. Positive results by IDEIA were confirmed by immunofluorescence after centrifugation of the specimen in the transport media at 2500 × *g* for 10 min. 25 µl of the cell pellet was spotted on a glass slide, dried and fixed in acetone for 5 min and

Table I. *Detection of Chlamydia trachomatis*

			PCR product analysed by[a]	
Group	Specimen	Culture	Gel electro-phoresis	DIANA
A	15, 27, 32, 34, 40, 43, 47[b], 52[b], 55[b], 59, 62[b], 69[b], 78, 82, 86[b]	Pos	Pos	Pos
B	3, 38, 46, 48[b], 50, 84[b]	Neg	Pos	Pos
C	87[b]	Pos	Neg	Neg
D	68 samples	Neg	Neg	Neg

[a] The result of 2 independent in vitro amplifications using 2 different detection methods are presented. No divergent results were found among the duplicates.

[b] Indicates ELISA-positive samples.

stained with monoclonal antibody, MicroTrak Direct Test (Syva Co, Palo Alto, CA, USA). The finding of 2 or more elementary bodies was considered confirmation of a positive result. Of the 53 samples analysed, 9 were ELISA-positive (Table I).

DNA amplification

The PCR was performed, in duplicate, in a nested procedure as described elsewhere (8) with some minor changes. Briefly, the clinical swabs were introduced directly into the PCR tube containing reagents for the outer amplification in a total volume of 50 µl and rubbed against the wall of the tube. The outer amplification with primers RIT23 and RIT24 (Table II) was carried out for 35 cycles and the subsequent inner amplification (20 cycles) with primers RIT25 and RIT26 (Table II) used 5 µl of the resulting outer amplification as template. Both PCR runs were performed in a 50 µl volume containing: 10 mM Tris-HCl (pH 8.3)/1.5 mM $MgCl_2$/50 mM KCl/0.1% Tween 20/0.2 mM dNTPs/0.2 µM primer/1.5 U of AmpliTaq polymerase (Perkin Elmer, Norwalk, CT, USA). The amplification was performed on a Perkin-Elmer 9600 (Perkin Elmer, Norwalk), and temperature profile was 96°C for 0.5 min/60°C for 0.5 min and 72°C for 1 min. The first cycle of the outer PCR was preceeded by 5 min at 94°C to lyse the target cells. As a positive control in the DNA amplifications, C. trachomatis serovar L2, kindly supplied by Dr Håkan Gnarpe (Gävle Hospital, Gävle, Sweden), was used. In addition to negative patient samples, water was used as negative control in every PCR experiment. To minimize cross-contamination in the amplification procedure, 3 separate rooms were used, 1 for mixing PCR reagents, 1 for the transfer of specimens and 1 for PCR and DIANA analysis. In addition, positive displacement pipettes (Gilson, Rainin, MA) were used for transfer of material between outer and inner PCR run. Of the 90 analysed specimens, 21 were found positive by agarose gel-electrophoresis (Table I).

Colorimetric microtitre analysis

The microtitre plates for coating, E.I.A./R.I.A. plate (Costar, Cambridge, MA, USA), were prepared by mixing 100 µl PBS (10 mM phosphate buffer (pH 7.4)/150 mM NaCl), 100 µl coating buffer (0.05 M carbonate buffer, pH 9.7) and 0.6 µl streptavidin (1 mg/ml, Boehringer Mannheim, Germany) and incubated overnight at +4°C. The plates were rinsed 3 times with 0.2% Tween 20 in PBS and blocked with 2% BSA (bovine serum albumin) in PBS at 37°C for 1 h and finally rinsed 4 times with 0.2% Tween 20 in PBS before use. PCR mixture (20 µl) and 80 µl DIANA buffer (0.1 M Tris-HCl (pH 7.5)/0.15 M NaCl/0.1% Tween/1.0 mM $MgCl_2$/10 mM β-mercaptoethanol) were added to the streptavidin-coated plates and incubated for 20 min at room temperature. The microtitre plates were then washed once with DIANA buffer. The solid support with immobilized DNA was mixed with 50 µl of fusion protein, LacI-β-Galactosidase (Dynal AS, Oslo, Norway), and incubated for 20 min. The solid support was washed 4 times with DIANA buffer before adding 100 µl chromogenic substrate, *o*-nitrophenyl-β-*D*-galactoside (ONPG, 1.25 mg/ml). Absorbance was determined after 30 min at 405 nm by an ELISA spectrophotometer (EAR 340AT, SLT Instruments, Austria). Of the 90 analysed specimens, 21 proved positive by DIANA (Table I and Fig. 3).

Cloning of the CrP target region

The CrP region of C. trachomatis serovar L2 was amplified with the outer primers RIT23 and RIT24 (Table II) using the conditions described above. The resulting amplified product was directly cloned into the PCRII vector using the TA cloning system from Invitrogen (San Diego, CA, USA). A clone containing the target region was identified and verified by solid-phase DNA sequencing (9). The

Table II. *Oligonucleotides*

Name	Sequence	Region[a]
RIT23	5′-GCAATGGTTTCTTACTGTGGA-3′	1013–1033
RIT25	5′-BIOTIN-GGACATAAAAATACAGCAAGC-3′	1034–1054
RIT26[b]	5′-*AATTGTTATCCGCTCACAATT*-TTCTTTCACAGTCCAAACTAC-3′	1256–1276
RIT24	5′-AGGAGTTTGTGCTCTTACTAG-3′	1310–1330

[a] Nucleotide position according to Clark et al. (16).
[b] Nucleotides in italics correspond to the lac operator sequence.

concentration and purity of prepared plasmid DNA was determined by absorbance according to Maniatis et al. (10). The plasmids were subsequently serially diluted (1 : 10) in 10 mM Tris-HCl (pH 8.3) and 10 ng/μl yeast tRNA (Boehringer-Mannheim, Germany). These were amplified by PCR, as described above, and 3 μl of the PCR product was loaded and analysed on a 2% agarose gel and stained with ethidium bromide.

RESULTS

General principle

The general principle for the colorimetric detection of PCR-amplified material in a 96-well format is depicted in Fig. 1. The target DNA is amplified using the PCR in a nested procedure, with a general set of an outer primer pair and an inner primer pair with 1 biotinylated primer and 1 primer containing the E. coli *lac*-operator DNA sequence. The amplified material is bound to streptavidin-coated microtitre plate walls, taking advantage of the strong and specific interactions between biotin and streptavidin. The solid phase allows the isolation and subsequent handling of target DNA in a highly specific manner. The E. coli *lac* operator incorporated during the 'inner' PCR run, is detected by the interaction of a recombinant fusion protein consisting of the E. coli *lac* repressor and β-galactosidase which allows for colorimetric analysis after addition of chromogenic substrate. The results can be measured in standard ELISA plate readers at 405 nm.

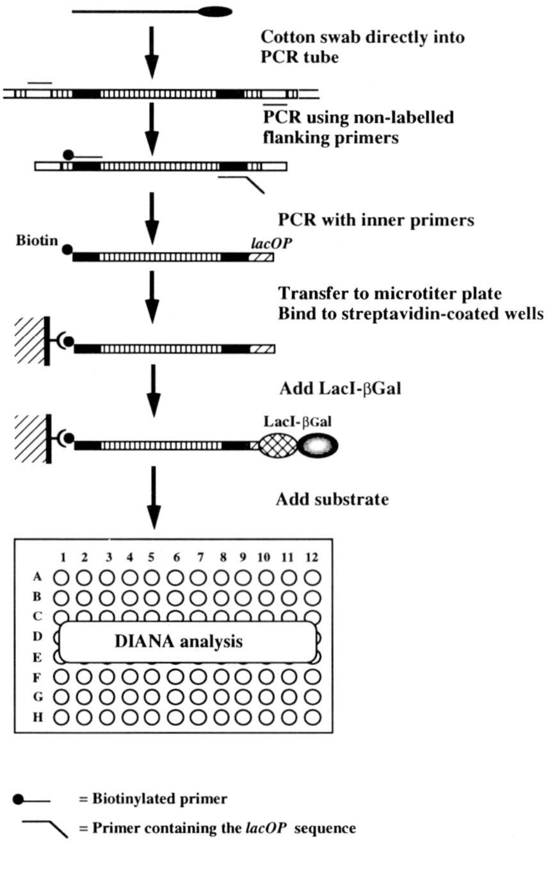

Fig. 1. Schematic outline of sample preparation, PCR and colorimetric DIANA assay for the detection of immobilized amplified nucleic acids using streptavidin-coated microtitre wells.

Sensitivity of the specific primers for the CrP region

The sensitivity of the in vitro amplification was investigated by PCR detection of a serially diluted plasmid construct comprising the CrP region. Known amounts of plasmid were diluted down to theoretical single copy level and amplified using the described approach with the CrP specific primers in a nested configuration. The resulting amplified material was analysed by agarose gel-electrophoresis and ethidium bromide staining (Fig. 2). The results show a specific fragment of 264 bp through the dilution series. The last dilution step that is successfully amplified corresponds to 2 plasmid molecules. Note the constant intensity of the amplified fragments in each lane down to the lane corresponding to 2 plasmid copies. This shows that the PCR-plateau has been reached for all samples in the dilution series and suggests that the nested CrP primers have a high sensitivity and can detect single molecules. In addition, to analyse the variation of the colorimetric DIANA step, 7 parallel amplifications of a dilution step corresponding to 100 CrP plasmids were performed and subsequently detected using the DIANA assay. The resulting average absorbance value of the 7 samples was 0.927 with a standard deviation of 0.067. The same 7 amplified samples analysed 12 days later had an average absorbance of 0.965 with a standard deviation of 0.077. This shows a low intra- and interassay variation of the colorimetric detection with the same amplified material. However, the interassay variation increases when the variation of the PCR is taken into account. Yun et al. (11) have recently shown that the complete analysis including both the PCR step and DIANA analysis have an interassay variation up to 21%.

Detection of Chlamydia trachomatis

90 clinical specimens of urogenital origin were used to evaluate the DIANA using a standard cell culture assay as the 'golden standard'. 53 urine specimens were also analysed by ELISA, carried out in parallel. A C. trachomatis serovar L2 strain was used as a positive control in the DIANA assay.

The gene encoding the outer membrane Cys-rich protein (CrP) found in C. trachomatis, was chosen as target region for amplification as it has earlier been shown to accurately detect chlamydia in clinical samples (8). (However, other genes can also be used, such as the major outer membrane protein (MOMP) gene or ribosomal genes (12–14)). The amplification of the CrP region yielded an outer fragment of 318 bp (35 cycles) and an inner fragment of 264 bp (20 cycles) (8). This shorter biotinylated (264 bp) fragment obtained after the second PCR step is efficiently immobilized to the streptavidin-coated microtitre wells for the subsequent analysis (data not shown).

The results of the assay are presented in Table I. Group A consisted of 15 samples which were positive by culture analysis, agarose gel-electrophoresis, and by DIANA. Group B consisted of 6 specimens which were all culture-negative but positive using PCR and

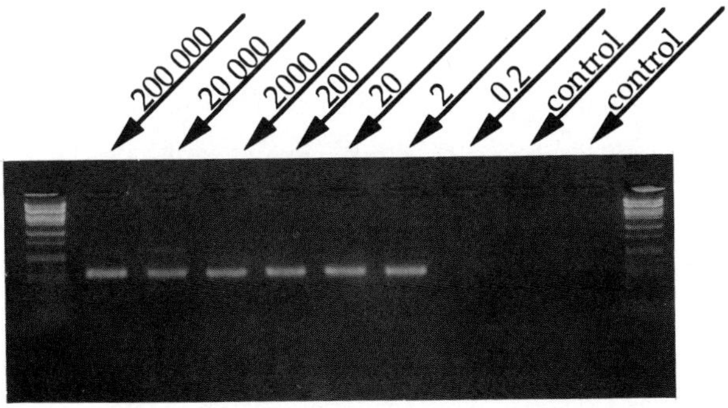

Fig. 2. The result after nested PCR using the CrP primers on a 1:10 dilution series of a plasmid containing the CrP target region. Three microlitres of the PCR product was loaded onto a 2% agarose gel and stained with ethidium bromide for subsequent detection.

DIANA. Noteworthy in this group were 2 specimens (48 and 84) which proved to be ELISA-positive, thus corroborating the PCR analysis result of the same specimens. Among the other 4 PCR-positive, culture-negative specimens that were collected, 2 came from patients with urethritis and 2 from patients with sexual partners who had verified chlamydial infection, the latter also supporting the PCR results. In group C, 1 specimen was positive in both culture and urine analysis, but negative when using PCR/DIANA. The largest group, (D), consisted of 68 samples which were all negative whether using either cultivation, PCR, or DIANA. Five samples were taken on a Friday and therefore frozen at $-70°C$ before cultivation. No divergent results were obtained with these samples, compared with the other assays.

The comparison of the ELISA analysis of the urine samples (53 patients) with the other assays showed that a majority of specimens (39 cases) were negative in all of the alternative assays and in 6 cases positive in all tests (Table I). The remaining 8 cases showed divergent results: in 3/8 cases the urine samples were negative but positive by culture, PCR, or DIANA. Two of 8 cases were found negative by both ELISA and culture yet positive with PCR and DIANA. One of 8 cases was positive by both ELISA and culture but negative by PCR and DIANA. In 2 cases ELISA, PCR and DIANA were positive whereas culture was negative (Table I).

The samples that proved positive in the colorimetric DIANA analysis are shown in Fig. 3. The absorbance at 405 nm of the 2 parallel PCR amplifications after 30 min were analysed, but showed little variation (data not shown). Their average absorbance value is presented for the different patients. The parallel samples of 2 patients (55 and 78) exhibit lower absorbance values, but they are easily distinguished from the background signal. However, this suggests the presence of a potent PCR inhibitor in these 2 sample, indicating that nested PCR is vital

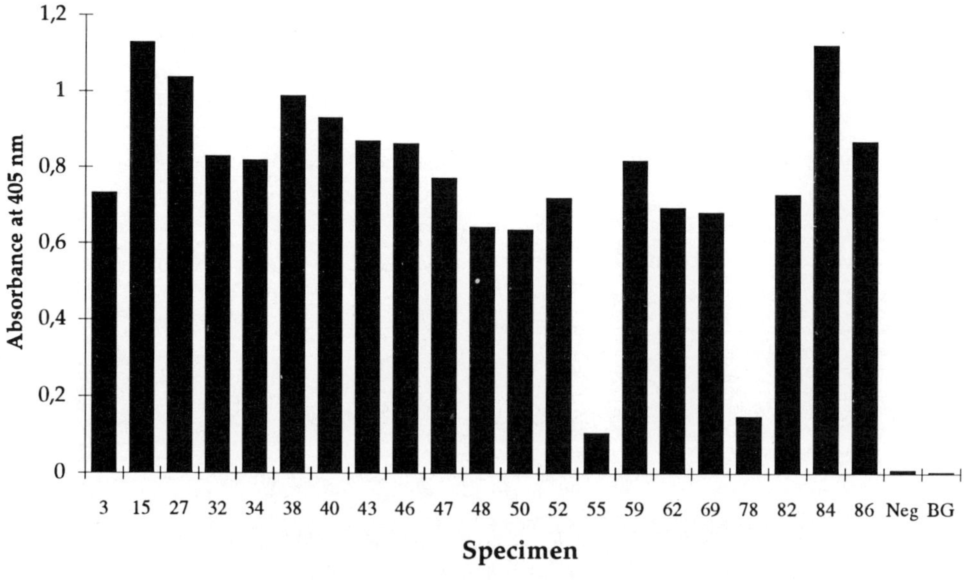

Fig. 3. Comparison between DIANA positive samples. The change in absorbance (405 nm) at room temperature was analysed with an ELISA spectrophotometer (EAR 340AT, SLT Instruments, Austria) after 30 min. A sample was considered positive when its mean value exceeded that of a negative control plus 3 standard deviations. The negative specimens have an average absorbance of 0.010 in with a standard deviation of 0.008. Background signal (BG) has an average absorbance of 0.005.

for reliable C. trachomatis detection. A single PCR amplification step would in these 2 cases probably not be sufficient for PCR detection of the target bacteria. The negative samples have an average absorbance (at 405 nm) of 0.010 (s.d. = 0.008), while the average background have 0.005. These results show very low background signals with minor variations after the nested PCR.

DISCUSSION

Cell culture isolation of Chlamydia trachomatis, has so far been considered the most sensitive and specific method for identifying C. trachomatis. This method, which is relatively cumbersome and time-consuming, also demonstrates a suboptimal sensitivity in the range of 80–85% (1). PCR for detection of chlamydia offers advantages like rapidity and improved sensitivity (12–14). However, one factor limiting the use of PCR for screening purposes has been the lack of an automatable and non-radioisotopic detection system for the amplified material; the available techniques rely on hybridizations and/or gel electrophoresis and are not well suited for reproducible large-scale screening.

An assay system combining a nested in vitro amplification of a selected target DNA sequence to make possible 'single-molecule detection' and a colorimetric analysis in an ELISA format has been developed for chlamydia. The system has a number of advantages, including *(i)* an easy template preparation step (patient swabs are put directly into PCR tubes), *(ii)* a quick and efficient capturing (20 min) and colorimetric detection (20 min) after a nested PCR procedure, *(iii)* a convenient ELISA format, *(iv)* its generality enabling easy adaptation of other pathogens. Thus, a complete analysis of a patient specimen with improved sensitivity can be performed in less than 1 working day, including amplification and analysis.

The results indicate improvements in sensitivity, using PCR and DIANA, compared with both tissue culture and urine analysis by ELISA. Six additional specimens were diagnosed as positive (group B). Two of these proved positive by ELISA in urine, thus verifying the PCR results. One culture and ELISA positive sample proved negative using PCR. This could have been due to differences in sample collection technique, since different specimens were used for culture and PCR. The first of the 2 cotton swabs taken from the patients was always transferred to the tube to be used for cultivation in order to ensure that this reference method would have the highest possible positivity rate. Obviously, PCR has the potential of being more sensitive than culture analysis, since it identifies DNA from the organism and does not require viable bacteria. In these experiments we have simply placed a patient swab directly in the PCR tube for amplification, thus avoiding time-consuming extractions and preparations of DNA. For this approach we have replaced the transport medium, which normally contains fetal calf serum, a potential PCR inhibitor, with a simple PCR buffer. No statistical analysis has been made on the included material due to the limited number of samples. However, the results indicate that a higher degree of sensitivity is achieved with the described approach. The high sensitivity of the PCR system is also demonstrated by the successful PCR detection of a sample containing 2 plasmid copies (encoding the CrP target region) in an end-dilution experiment.

The coated microtitre plates make the handling of the PCR products identical with the ELISA procedures, which has obvious advantages. No centrifugation, filtration or precipitation is needed and the instruments for microtitre plates used here are already available at most clinical and research laboratories (i.e., plate washers and readers). A further improvement to make possible large-scale screening of urine samples would be to combine the DIANA microtitre analysis with immunomagnetic purification of elementary bodies directly in urine (15) which effectively eliminates PCR inhibitors and therefore can yield a more even colorimetric signal for all samples. The development of a 1-tube nested procedure (Stark, Uhlén and Lundeberg, unpublished data) enhances the approach still further, making possible an integrated approach for DNA detection of Chlamydia trachomatis.

ACKNOWLEDGEMENTS

We are grateful to Drs S. Ståhl and P-Å. Nygren for useful discussions. This work was supported by the Swedish Board for Technical Development and the Nordic Industrial fund.

REFERENCES

1. Ripa KT, Mårdh PA. Cultivation of Chlamydia trachomatis in cycloheximide-treated McCoy cells. J Clin Microbiol 6: 328–331, 1977.
2. Paavonen J. Pelvic inflammatory disease. Semin Dermatol 9: 126–132, 1990.
3. Weström LV. Chlamydia trachomatis – clinical significance and strategies of intervention. Semin Dermatol 9: 117–125, 1990.
4. Mullis KB, Faloona FA. Specific synthesis of DNA in vitro via a polymerase-catalyzed chain reaction. Methods Enzymol 155: 335–350, 1987.
5. Bobo L, Coutlee F, Yolken RH, Quinn T, Viscidi RP. Diagnosis of Chlamydia trachomatis cervical infection by detection of amplified DNA with an enzyme immunoassay. J Clin Microbiol 28: 1968–1973, 1990.
6. Claas HCJ, Wagenvoort JHT, Niesters HGM, Tio TT, van Rijsoort-Vos JH, Quint WGV. Diagnostic value of the polymerase chain for Chlamydia detection as determined in a follow up study. J Clin Microbiol 29: 42–45, 1991.
7. Lundeberg J, Wahlberg J, Holmberg M, Pettersson U, Uhlén M. Rapid colorimetric detection of in vitro amplified DNA sequences. DNA Cell Biol 9: 287–292, 1990.
8. Wahlberg J, Lundeberg J, Hultman T, Uhlén M. General colorimetric method for DNA diagnostics allowing direct solid-phase genomic sequencing of the positive samples. Proc Natl Acad Sci USA 87: 6569–6573, 1990.
9. Hultman T, Ståhl S, Hornes E, Uhlén M. Direct solid phase sequencing of genomic and plasmid DNA using magnetic beads as solid support. Nucleic Acids Res 17: 4937–4946, 1989.
10. Maniatis T, Fritsch EF, Sambrook J. Molecular Cloning: a Laboratory Manual, Cold Spring Harbor: Cold Spring Harbor Laboratory University Press, 1982.
11. Yun Z, Lundeberg J, Johansson B, Hedrum A, Weiland O, Uhlén M, Sönnerborg A. Colorimetric detection of competitive PCR products for quantification of hepatitis C virus. J Virol Methods [in press 1994].
12. Dutilh B, Bébéar C, Rodriguez P, Vekris A, Bonnet J, Garret M. Specific amplification of a DNA sequence common to all Chlamydia trachomatis serovars using the polymerase chain reaction. Res Microbiol 140: 7–16, 1989.
13. Griffais R, Thibon M. Detection of Chlamydia trachomatis by the polymerase chain reaction. Res Microbiol 140: 139–141, 1989.
14. Pollard DR, Tyler SD, Ng C-W, Rozee KR. A polymerase chain reaction (PCR) protocol for the specific detection of Chlamydia spp. Mol Cell Probes 3: 383–389, 1989.
15. Hedrum A, Lundeberg J, Paulson C, Uhlén M. Colorimetric detection of in vitro amplified Chlamydia trachomatis in urogenital samples using immunomagnetic separation. PCR Methods and applications 2: 167–171, 1992.
16. Clark IA, Ward EW, Lambden PR. Molecular cloning and sequence analysis of a developmentally regulated cysteine-rich outer membrane protein from Chlamydia trachomatis. Gene 71: 307–314, 1988.

Submitted June 28, 1993; accepted February 6, 1994

Scand J Infect Dis 26: 283–287, 1994

Arcanobacterium haemolyticum and Streptococcal Pharyngitis

PETTERI CARLSON[1], OLLI-VEIKKO RENKONEN[2] and SIRKKA KONTIAINEN[1,2]

From the [1]Department of Medical Microbiology, Aurora Hospital, and the [2]Department of Bacteriology and Immunology, University of Helsinki, Helsinki, Finland

Arcanobacterium haemolyticum was recovered from 0.5% of throat cultures of 3,922 patients seeking medical attention because of sore throat. Most of the patients positive for A. haemolyticum were 15–25 years old, and had fever (80%), lymphadenopathy (67%), pharyngeal exudate (69%) or skin rash (23%). In this age group, 2% of the throat cultures proved positive for A. haemolyticum. All A. haemolyticum strains were susceptible to penicillin, erythromycin, cephalexin and clindamycin, but resistant to trimethoprim/sulphamethoxazole. In half of the patients with A. haemolyticum it was the only bacterial pathogen isolated, while in the remainder, beta-haemolytic streptococci were also detected. As expected, beta-haemolytic streptococci were much more frequent than A. haemolyticum in the throat cultures.

S. Kontiainen, MD, Department of Medical Microbiology, Aurora Hospital, Nordenskiöldinkatu 20, FIN-00250 Helsinki, Finland

INTRODUCTION

Acute pharyngitis is a frequent reason for seeking medical attention, especially in the younger age groups (1). In addition to group A beta-haemolytic streptococci, groups G and C have been implicated in streptococcal sore throat (2–5). Arcanobacterium haemolyticum (previously Corynebacterium haemolyticum; 6) has also been reported to cause pharyngitis, especially in adolescents and young adults (7–12). Pharyngitis caused by A. haemolyticum clinically resembles that caused by streptococci (7, 9), and may be accompanied by a skin rash resembling scarlatina. A. haemolyticum in pharyngitis has been reported from Sweden (7, 11) but not from the other Nordic countries. We tested throat culture samples from patients with pharyngitis for A. haemolyticum and beta-haemolytic streptococci during a 14-month period. We now report the results of our study.

MATERIALS AND METHODS

Samples

All throat culture samples ($n = 3{,}922$) sent to the Division of Bacteriology, Department of Medical Microbiology, Aurora Hospital, Helsinki, Finland, during a 14-month period (Nov. 1991–Dec. 1992) were studied. Samples were from patients with acute pharyngitis who were visiting the primary health care centres in the City of Helsinki area (500,000 inhabitants). The samples were transported to the laboratory either in modified Stuart transport tubes (Transpocult^R, Orion Diagnostica, Espoo, Finland; $n = 1{,}788$) or on Streptocult^R (Orion Diagnostica) culture slides ($n = 2{,}134$). Some of the Streptocult^R cultures ($n = 957$) were screened by laboratory technicians at the primary health care centres and only those with beta-haemolytic colonies suspected of being streptococci were sent for serogrouping. A clinical history was obtained from patients culture positive for A. haemolyticum.

Cultures

Swab specimens and growth from Streptocult^R were streaked on A. haemolyticum selective plates and on sheep blood agar plates. The selective medium used for isolating A. haemolyticum was a modification of that described by Brenwald et al. (13) and contained 2% Trypticase Soy Agar (BBL, Cockeysville, MD, USA), 1.1% Mueller Hinton Broth (BBL), 0.85% agar (BBL), 5.0% defibrinated horse blood, 8.8 mg/l colistin (Sigma Chemical Co., St. Louis, MO, USA), 5 mg/l oxolinic acid (Sigma) and 8 mg/l

 ISSN 0036-5548

mupirocin (provided by SmithKline, Beecham, UK). After 48 h incubation at 35°C in a humidified atmosphere of 5% CO_2 in air, colonies suspected of being A. haemolyticum or beta-haemolytic streptococci were further cultured on sheep blood agar plates.

Identification of A. haemolyticum

A. haemolyticum was identified by typical colony morphology, beta-haemolysis, Gram strain, negative catalase test (3% H_2O_2), positive DNase test (Bacto DNase Test Agar, Difco, Detroit, USA), positive lipase test on egg yolk agar (14), positive reverse CAMP test (15) and a typical APICoryne (Bio Merieux, Marcy-l'Etoile, France) profile. A. haemolyticum ATCC 9345 was used as reference strain.

Serogrouping of beta-haemolytic streptococci

Latex agglutination (Streptex^R, Wellcome Diagnostics, Dartford, Kent, England) was used for serogrouping the beta-haemolytic streptococci. Only Voges-Proskauer negative (by Voges-Proskauer diagnostic tablets, Rosco Diagnostica, Taastrup, Denmark) haemolytic strains which agglutinated with anti-group C antibody were considered group C beta-haemolytic streptococci.

Susceptibility to antimicrobial agents

The minimum inhibitory concentrations (MIC) for phenoxymethylpenicillin, erythromycin, clindamycin, tetracycline, cephalotin and trimethoprim/sulphamethoxazole of the A. haemolyticum strains were determined with the E-test^R (Biodisk, Solna, Sweden). For MIC testing, Mueller-Hinton II Agar (BBL) supplemented with 5% defibrinated sheep blood and inoculated according to NCCLS (16) was used. S. aureus ATCC 29213, E. faecalis ATCC 29212 and A. haemolyticum ATCC 9345 were used as quality control strains.

RESULTS

Patients

The majority of samples, 86%, were from patients <40 years of age. The age groups most frequently sampled were 1–6, 14–18 and 22–27 years old, and 21%, 6% and 11% of the samples, respectively, were from these age groups. In the youngest age groups the sex ratio was about equal, but in the older groups the majority were females. For example, 70% of the 22–27-year age group were females.

Frequency of A. haemolyticum

A. haemolyticum was isolated from 19 patients (0.5%, Table I). 10 of the isolates were from samples sent in Stuart transport tubes and 9 from Streptocult^R culture slides. Eight of the 9 isolates from Streptocult^R were from culture slides prescreened for beta-haemolytic streptococci. Patients with A. haemolyticum were older than patients with group A streptococci ($p < 0.001$), but younger than those with group G streptococci ($p < 0.001$). The mean ages of female and male patients with A. haemolyticum were similar (p = NS). In the age group 15–25 years, 2% of the patients were culture-positive for A. haemolyticum.

Frequency of beta-haemolytic streptococci

Beta-haemolytic streptococci were isolated from 1,047 samples (27%): 61% were of group A, 23% of group G, 9% of group C and 7% of group B (Table I). Throat cultures of females more often proved positive for beta-haemolytic streptococci than did those of males. Patients with group A streptococci were younger than those harbouring group G ($p < 0.001$) or other streptococci (Table I). The age group most often affected by group A streptococci were the 3–11-year-olds, while group C and G were most often detected in age groups 14–30 and 20–30 years, respectively. Male patients with group A, C or G streptococci were younger ($p < 0.001$) than female patients with these streptococci.

Isolates of beta-haemolytic streptococci greatly outnumbered those of A. haemolyticum in the throat cultures, and 11/19 patients with A. haemolyticum also had beta-haemolytic

Table I. *Characteristics of pharyngitis patients yielding A. haemolyticum and beta-haemolytic streptococci in culture*

Bacterium	No. of patients (F/M ratio)	Mean age (SD)	Mean age (SD)	Highest incidence in age group, years
Arcanobacterium haemolyticum	19 (0.7)	20.4 (5.5)[a]	20.5 (4.3)[b] 20.4 (6.5)	15–25
Streptococci group A	634 (1.2)	17.7 (13.2)	20.7 (13.9) 14.1 (11.2)	3–11
group B	74 (2.7)	25.8 (15.4)	25.3 (14.1) 27.1 (18.8)	17–28
group C	95 (1.6)	21.3 (11.6)	23.5 (12.2) 17.8 (9.9)	14–30
group G	244 (1.9)	25.1 (15.6)	26.5 (15.4) 22.7 (15.7)	20–30

[a] p-values by Student's t-test A. haemolyticum vs. group A streptococci, $p < 0.001$; vs. group B streptococci, $p < 0.001$; vs. group C, p = NS; and vs. group G streptococci, $p < 0.001$; and group A vs. group B, $p < 0.001$; vs. group C, $p < 0.001$; vs. group G, $p < 0.001$; group C vs. group G, $p < 0.001$ and vs. B, $p < 0.001$.

[b] Mean age of female patients first, then that of male patients. p-values females vs. males, A. haemolyticum p = NS; group A $p < 0.001$; group B p = NS; group C $p < 0.001$; and group G $p < 0.001$.

streptococci in the throat: 4 patients had group A beta-haemolytic streptococci, 2 group G, 4 group C and 1 group B. Group A and G beta-haemolytic streptococci were most often isolated in February–April and in October–December, while the frequency with which group B and C streptococci were isolated was similar throughout the year. A. haemolyticum was isolated in spring and autumn.

Susceptibility to antimicrobial agents

All A. haemolyticum strains were susceptible to phenoxymethylpenicillin (MIC ≤ 0.064 μg/ml), erythromycin (MIC ≤ 0.023 μg/ml), clindamycin (MIC ≤ 0.094 μg/ml) and cephalotin (MIC ≤ 0.047 μg/ml), but resistant to trimethoprim/sulphamethoxazole (MIC > 32/608 μg/ml). Two of the isolates were resistant to tetracycline (MIC 24 μg/ml), while the rest were sensitive (MIC ≤ 0.25 μg/ml).

Clinical symptoms

Tonsillar exudate was detected in 11/16 patients (69%) with A. haemolyticum, fever in 12/15 (80%), and cervical lymphadenopathy in 8/12 (67%). Rhinitis or cough was reported by 3/8 patients (38%). Three patients out of 13 (23%) had a scarlatiniform rash. Most of the patients (14/19) with A. haemolyticum were successfully treated with phenoxymethyl penicillin (0.6 g 3 times a day for 10 days). One patient with A. haemolyticum had tonsillitis requiring hospitalization. Beta-haemolytic streptococci were not detected in her throat culture, she had no heterophilic antibodies (Monospot^R-test), had a fever of 40°C, swallowing difficulties, a white blood cell count of 23.0×10^9/l and the C-reactive protein level in serum was 189 mg/l. She was treated with parenteral cefuroxime followed by oral cefuroxime axetil, and recovered uneventfully.

DISCUSSION

Arcanobacterium haemolyticum was detected in 2% of the throat cultures from 15–25 year old patients with pharyngitis. This is similar to the frequency described in Sweden (7, 11) and Belgium (12). In 8/19 patients (42%) A. haemolyticum was the only bacterial pathogen isolated, while in 11 patients, beta-haemolytic streptococci were also found. The frequency with which A. haemolyticum was isolated without accompanying beta-haemolytic streptococci is lower than that reported from Sweden (7, 11), Belgium (12), USA (8) and Great Britain (10), but similar to that reported from Greece (9). The reason why we detected A. haemolyticum as the only pathogen less often than in most previous reports may be due to the fact that a quarter of the samples we studied had been prescreened for beta-haemolytic streptococci.

We could not repeat the throat cultures after the treatment and do not know whether the patients might have harboured A. haemolyticum after full clinical recovery. Others, however, have shown that A. haemolyticum could not be detected after treatment (8, 10), and that throat carriers of A. haemolyticum are rare (7, 17).

The disease associated with the growth of A. haemolyticum in throat cultures in the patients described here resembled that described previously. Typical rash was detected in one-fifth of the patients. This is similar to that previously reported in Scandinavia (11), but less than in some other reports (7–9).

All strains of A. haemolyticum were sensitive to all the antimicrobial agents recommended for the treatment of tonsillitis, phenoxymethylpenicillin, oral cephalosporins, erythromycin and clindamycin. Thus in spite of reports of penicillin tolerance of A. haemolyticum strains (18), clinical symptoms disappeared in all the patients during penicillin treatment.

There are a few published reports of seasonality in the isolation rates of A. haemolyticum. In Belgium, however, no seasonality was found in the isolation rate of A. haemolyticum (12). Although the numbers of A. haemolyticum isolated in this study were small, the seasonality in its isolation rate was similar to that of group A streptococci.

A. haemolyticum and group A beta-haemolytic streptococci were isolated from males and females equally often, and the majority of patients with group G, B and C streptococci were females. The mean ages of female and male patients with A. haemolyticum were similar, while males with group A, G and C streptococcal isolates were significantly younger than females. Patients with group A streptococci were generally younger than patients with group G. This is in agreement with a previous study of children with pharyngitis (4).

A. haemolyticum may thus be isolated from throat culture specimens of patients with pharyngitis with or without lymphadenopathy and may sometimes be accompanied by scarlatiniform rash. The isolation of A. haemolyticum may follow a seasonal pattern; it affects young adults and can be found as the sole bacterial pathogen in the throat cultures. Treatment aimed at streptococcal tonsillitis is likely to eradicate A. haemolyticum. Cultures for A. haemolyticum are indicated to recover a potential pathogen in young patients with pharyngitis.

ACKNOWLEDGEMENTS

We thank SmithKline Beecham for the kind gift of mupirocin and Leena Saraste for help in preparing the manuscript.

REFERENCES

1. Norrby R. Clinical aspects on bacterial infections in the upper respiratory tract. Scand J Infect Dis Suppl 39: 14–18, 1983.
2. Cimolai N, Elford RW, Bryan L, Anand C, Berger P. Do the beta-hemolytic non-group A streptococci cause pharyngitis? Rev Infect Dis 10: 587–601, 1988.

3. Turner JC, Hayden GF, Kiselica D, Lohr J, Fishburne CF, Murren D. Association of group C beta-hemolytic streptococci with endemic pharyngitis among college students. JAMA 264: 2644–2647, 1990.
4. Gerber MA, Randolph MF, Martin NJ, Rizkallah MF, Cleary PP, Kaplan EL, Ayoub EM. Community-wide outbreak of group G streptococcal pharyngitis. Pediatrics 87: 598–603, 1991.
5. Turner JC, Fox A, Fox K, Addy C, Garrison CZ, Herron B, Brunson C, Betcher G. Role of group C beta-hemolytic streptococci in pharyngitis: epidemiologic study of clinical features associated with isolation of group C streptococci. J Clin Microbiol 31: 808–811, 1993.
6. Collins MD, Jones D, Schofield GM. Reclassification of "Corynebacterium haemolyticum" (McLean, Liebow & Rosenberg) in the genus Arcanobacterium gen. nov. as Arcanobacterium haemolyticum nom. rev., comb. nov. J Gen Microbiol 128: 1279–1281, 1982.
7. Banck G, Nyman M. Tonsillitis and rash associated with Corynebacterium haemolyticum. J Infect Dis 154: 1037–1040, 1986.
8. Miller RA, Brancato F, Holmes KK. Corynebacterium haemolyticum as a cause of pharyngitis and scarlatiniform rash in young adults. Ann Intern Med 105: 867–872, 1986.
9. Karpathios T, Drakonaki S, Zervoudaki A, Coupari G, Fretzayas A, Kremastinos J, Thomaidis T. Arcanobacterium haemolyticum in children with presumed streptococcal pharyngotonsillitis or scarlet fever. J Pediatr 121: 735–737, 1992.
10. Fell HWK, Nagington J, Naylor GRE. Corynebacterium haemolyticum infections in Cambridgeshire. J Hyg 79: 269–274, 1977.
11. Selander B, Ljungh Å. Corynebacterium haemolyticum as a cause of nonstreptococcal pharyngitis. J Infect Dis 154: 1041, 1986.
12. Cambier M, Janssens M, Wauters G. Isolation of Arcanobacterium haemolyticum from patients with pharyngitis in Belgium. Acta Clin Belg 47: 303–307, 1992.
13. Brenwald NP, Teare EL, Mountfort LK, Tettmar RE. Selective medium for isolating Arcanobacterium haemolyticum. J Clin Pathol 43: 610, 1990.
14. Sutter VL, Citron DM, Edelstein MAC, Finegold SM. Wadsworth Anaerobic Bacteriology Manual. Belmont, CA: Star Publishing Company, 111–112, 1985.
15. Clarridge JE. The recognition and significance of Arcanobacterium haemolyticum. Clin Microbiol Newsl 11: 41–48, 1989.
16. National Committee for Clinical Laboratory Standards. Performance standards for antimicrobial disk susceptibility test, 4th ed., vol. 10, no. 7. Approved standard M2-A4. Villanova, Pa: National Committee for Clinical Laboratory Standards, 1990.
17. Fell HWK, Nagington J, Naylor GRE, Olds RJ. Infections in man with Corynebacterium haemolyticum. J Med Microbiol 6: vii, 1973.
18. Nyman M, Banck G, Thore M. Penicillin tolerance in Arcanobacterium haemolyticum. J Infect Dis 161: 261–265, 1990.

Submitted October 18, 1993; accepted January 6, 1994

Scand J Infect Dis 26: 289–296, 1994

Community-acquired Pyelonephritis in Adults: Characteristics of E. coli Isolates in Bacteremic and Non-bacteremic Patients

RISTO IKÄHEIMO[1], ANJA SIITONEN[3], ULLA KÄRKKÄINEN[2], JUHA MUSTONEN[1], TARJA HEISKANEN[3] and P. HELENA MÄKELÄ[3]

From the Departments of [1]Medicine and [2]Clinical Microbiology, Kuopio University Hospital, Kuopio, and [3]National Public Health Institute, Helsinki, Finland

Escherichia coli strains isolated from the urine in 49 consecutive episodes of community-acquired pyelonephritis in adult women were characterized for adhesins and hemolysin production. The mean age of the patients was 56 years and 47% had at least 1 compromising condition. P fimbriae was found in 67% and hemolysin production in 35% of the strains; these figures were significantly ($p < 0.001$) higher than the corresponding figures (11% for each) among 287 strains isolated from stool of healthy adults (Siitonen A. J Infect Dis 1992; 166: 1058–1065). The prevalence of Non-P mannose-resistant adhesins and type 1C fimbriae was low (4 and 8%, respectively) and did not differ significantly from the corresponding prevalences (1 and 7%) in healthy adults. 74% fo the pyelonephritic (but only 22% of the stool) isolates had at least 1 of these 4 virulence factors ($p < 0.001$) and 37% and 7%, respectively, had at least 2 ($p < 0.001$). Nevertheless, the strains represented a wide variety of O:K serotypes without any indication of specially virulent clones. Of the 49 patients 15 had concomitant bacteremia, and in all except 2 compromised elderly patients the urinary and blood isolates were identical.

R. Ikäheimo, MD, Department of Medicine, Kuopio University Hospital, FIN-70211 Kuopio, Finland

INTRODUCTION

The role of a number of bacterial characteristics in the pathogenesis of pyelonephritis caused by Escherichia coli has been the subject of many epidemiological and experimental studies, as recently reviewed by Johnson (1). The ability of the bacteria to attach to the epithelial cells of the urinary tract has been established as the most important single determinant in establishing acute pyelonephritis. This attachment is mediated by adhesins, of which P fimbriae are the most important; these fimbriae have been found to play a decisive role in the pathogenesis of acute pyelonephritis both in children (2–6) and in adults (7–11). In acute cystitis, Non-P mannose-resistant (MR) adhesins (previously called X adhesins) have also been shown to play a role (4, 12–15). Most E. coli strains also express type 1 fimbriae, which are probably not involved in urinary tract infection (UTI) (1). The pathogenetic role of type 1C fimbriae, a fourth type of adhesin, has also remained obscure, although their prevalence has been higher among strains associated with UTI than among fecal control strains (13, 16–18). Hemolysin production has been found to be associated with E. coli strains causing clinically more severe forms of UTI (1). Virulent clones characterized by their O:K:H serotype have been identified among strains isolated from pyelonephritis episodes (4, 19, 20). Nevertheless, there are still only a few published prospective epidemiological studies on urinary isolates from adults. Many studies have also been flawed by a lack of adequate control material. We therefore initiated prospective studies on UTI in adults. 178 consecutive cases of lower community-acquired UTI and 148 cases of nosocomial UTI have been described in recent publications (13, 17). A large control material of E. coli strains isolated from stool from healthy adults has been described recently (21). The present study is an analysis of E. coli isolated from the urine or blood of 49 consecutive women with

 ISSN 0036-5548

community-acquired acute pyelonephritis and shows that these strains differ in characteristic ways both from strains causing cystitis and from strains in stool of healthy adults.

MATERIALS AND METHODS

Patients

49 women with community-acquired acute pyelonephritis caused by E. coli were treated at Kuopio University Hospital in Eastern Finland between June 1989 and September 1990. Their mean age was 56 years (range 20–89 years). The patients had been referred from community health centres in the area because of fever and a suspicion of acute pyelonephritis. All patients were initially examined by the clinician on duty and later by the clinician responsible for the study (R.I.). The case history was obtained, physical examination done and laboratory parameters (erythrocyte sedimentation rate (ESR), total white blood cell count (WBC), C-reactive protein (CRP), serum creatinine, urinary sediment, urine and blood cultures) were determined. Most of the patients underwent ultrascanning of the kidneys to exclude urinary tract obstruction. 45 patients were examined by intravenous pyelography.

The diagnosis of acute pyelonephritis was based on the presence of significant bacteriuria ($\geq 10^5$ bacteria/ml urine), increased CRP (≥ 30 mg/l), pyuria, fever ≥ 38°C, and clinical signs and symptoms of acute pyelonephritis including costovertebral angle tenderness, without concurrent symptoms of any other infection. The patients with bacteremia fulfilled the above criteria and their blood cultures proved positive for E. coli.

The patients were also stratified into groups according to the presence of underlying predisposing conditions as follows:

(1) Non-compromised patients ($n = 26$), i.e. no conditions predisposing to UTI.
(2) Compromised patients ($n = 23$), with either diabetes (4 patients), corticosteroid (immunosuppressive) treatment (5 patients), or urological abnormality (1 patient with mild pelvic-ureteral stenosis, 1 with nephrolithiasis, 2 with cortical scars/parenchymal reduction, 2 with hydronephrosis, 1 with ureter and pelvis duplex, and 1 patient with rotated kidney. Eight patients had only one predisposing condition and 6 had more than one of these conditions.

Laboratory findings

Blood samples obtained before institution of antimicrobial treatment were analysed by conventional methods for ESR, CRP and WBC.

Bacteria

E. coli strains were identified by standard methods (22), and stored at −70°C in skim milk until further analysed. They were then subcultured on non-selective cystine-lactose agar and subsequently twice on colonization factor antigen agar to enhance the expression of adhesins (23).

Fimbrial analysis

MR hemagglutination was detected by agglutination of human group O erythrocytes in the presence of 0.1 M methyl-a-D-mannoside (M-6882, Sigma Chemical Co, St. Louis, MO) on glass slides kept over crushed ice (3).

The strains were tested for P fimbriae with the P-specific agglutination test (PF test, Orion Diagnostica, Espoo, Finland) as earlier described (24).

Strains showing MR hemagglutination without having P fimbriae were defined as possessing Non-P MR adhesins (21).

The identification of type 1C fimbriae was based on bacterial agglutination with specific polyclonal and monoclonal antibodies (received from A. Pere, Orion Diagnostica, Espoo, Finland) followed by indirect immunofluorescence assay (16, 25).

Hemolysin production

The production of hemolysin was tested on sheep blood agar plates. Strains producing a clear halo after overnight culture at 35°C were defined as hemolysin-positive.

Serotyping

O grouping and capsular identification of the strains were performed as described (21).

Ribotyping

Restriction fragment length polymorphism of ribosomal RNA genes (ribotyping) was used to compare the genotypes of the blood and urinary isolates of the bacteremic patients (26, 27).

Chromosomal DNA of the strains was isolated with a DNA extractor (Applied Biosystems, Foster City, CA) and digested with Hind III (Boehringer Mannheim Biochemica, Mannheim, Germany) restriction endonuclease according to manufacturer's instructions. After Southern blotting onto a Hybond™-N+ (Amersham International plc, Amersham, Bucks, England) nylon membrane, the plasmid pKK3535 carrying the 5S, 16S and 23S rRNA genes (28) was used as a probe. A commercial kit (DIG, Boehringer Mannheim) was used for labelling the probe, hybridization and detection of the hybrids (29).

Statistics

The χ^2-test and Student's unpaired *t*-test were used to compare the significance of differences.

RESULTS

Host characteristics and response to infection

Of the 49 patients with acute pyelonephritis, 15 had concomitant bacteremia (Table I). Patients with bacteremia were older ($p < 0.05$) and more often had compromising conditions than the patients without bacteremia. CRP ($p < 0.001$) and WBC ($p < 0.05$) values were higher in bacteremic patients than in patients without bacteremia. There were no statistically significant differences in clinical laboratory parameters between non-compromised and compromised patients, but the latter were older.

Adhesins and hemolysin production

67% of the 49 urinary strains were positive for P fimbriae (Table I). P fimbriation was somewhat more frequent among strains isolated from non-compromised patients (77%) than from compromised patients (57%). In the non-compromised patients with bacteremia, 83% (5/6) and in patients without bacteremia, 75% (15/20) of the strains expressed P fimbriae. The corresponding figures in the compromised patients were 56% and 57%. The differences

Table I. *Host and virulence-associated characteristics and response to infection in non-compromised and compromised patients with acute pyelonephritis (PN) with or without bacteremia*

Non-P = Non-PMR adhesins, Type 1C = Type 1C fimbriae, % comprom = percentage of compromised patients.

	Total	Non-compr. patients	Comprom. patients	PN without bacteremia	PN with bacteremia
No. of pats.	49	26	23	34	15
(% comprom)	(23)	(0)	(100)	(41)	(60)
Mean age (years)	56	48[a]	66[a]	51[b]	68[b]
ESR (mm/h)	50(±22)	46(±18)	55(±26)	47(±20)	57(±26)
CRP (mg/l)	131(±70)	135(±70)	126(±60)	114(±60)[c]	168(±53)[c]
WBC ($\times 10^9$/l)	12(±4)	12(±4)	13(±4)	11(±4)[d]	14(±4)[d]
P fimbriae (%)	65	73	57	68	60
Non-P (%)	4	4	4	3	7
Type 1C (%)	8	8	9	6	13
Hemolysin (%)	35	31	39	32	40

[a] $p < 0.01$ (Student's *t*-test).
[b] $p < 0.05$ (Student's *t*-test).
[c] $p < 0.001$ (Student's *t*-test).
[d] $p < 0.05$ (Student's *t*-test).

in the frequencies between the groups were not statistically significant. The frequency of P fimbriation was the same both in patients <60 years of age and in patients >60 years old (66.7% vs. 68%).

Only 4% of the isolates expressed Non-P MR adhesins, 8% type 1C fimbriae and 35% hemolysin. Strains of patients with bacteremia did not differ significantly from those of patients without bacteremia in any of these parameters.

K antigens and their association with adhesins

78% (38/49) of the strains were capsulated, with K1 in 27%, K5 in 12%, K2 in 10%, K13 in 4% and K7 in 2%. 22% had other, unidentified capsular antigens. Capsulated strains were somewhat more often (74%) P-fimbriated than strains without capsule (46% P-fimbriated, $p > 0.05$). No other characteristics showed an association with the presence or absence of a capsule or with any specific capsular type.

O antigens and their association with adhesins and hemolysin production

Altogether 47% of the strains were O-groupable with the sera used and fell into 10 O serogroups with 1 to 4 strains each. O18 was the most common O group (8.2%), followed by O2 and O6 (both 6.1%).

78% of the O-groupable, but only 58% of the non-typable (NT) and Rough strains wee P-fimbriated. All O1, O2, O6, O7, O16, O25 and O86 strains were P-fimbriated. Hemolysin production (altogether 35%) was associated with O4, O6, O16, O18 and O86 strains. There was a wide spectrum of various O:K combinations and we could not identify any penetrating O:K serotype to suggest a pyelonephritic clone.

Correlation of strains isolated from urine and blood

Of the 49 patients, 15 had concomitant bacteremia. 11 of these had the same E. coli strain in the urine as in the blood, judging by the phenotype (Table II), but in 4 patients the isolate from the blood differed from the corresponding urinary strain in 1 or more of the phenotypic characteristics. When the 15 strain pairs were further analysed by ribotyping, 17 different

Table II. *Comparison of E. coli strains from the urine and blood of 15 patients with bacteremia*

Patient no.	Phenotype: Urine	Phenotype: Blood	Ribotyping[a]
1.	O2:K7:1C+:P+	O2:K7:1C+:P+	Identical
2.	O4:K2:Hly+:Non-P+	O4:K2:Hly+:Non-P+	Identical
3.	O6:K5:Hly+:1C+:P+	O6:K5:Hly+:1C:P+	Identical
4.	O16:K1:Hly+:P+	O16:K1:Hly+:P+	Identical
5.	O18:K1	O18:K1	Identical
6.	O18:K1	O18:K1	Identical
7.	**O18:K5:Hly+:P+**	**ONT:K+**	**Different**
8.	O25:K+:P+	O25:K+:P+	Identical
9.	O25:K+:Hly+:P+	O25:K+:Hly+:P+	Identical
10.	OR:K1:Hly+:P+	OR:K1:Hly+:P+	Identical
11.	**OR:K−:P+**	**OR:K+:P+**	**Identical**
12.	ONT:K5	ONT:K5	Identical
13.	ONT:K+:P+	ONT:K+:P+	Identical
14.	**ONT:K−:P+**	**ONT:K+:P+**	**Identical**
15.	**ONT:K−**	**ONT:K1:P+**	**Different**

[a] 17 different ribotypes were identified among the 30 strains.

ribotypes were identified and 13 of the 15 pairs of the strains appeared to be identical (Table II). These included the 11 pairs found identical by phenotyping, but also 2 of the strain pairs (patients 11 and 4) that had shown differences in phenotype. In both these cases the urinary isolate had been non-capsulated (K−), and the blood isolate capsulated (K+), a difference that could indicate selection for encapsulation in the circulation. We believe therefore, that these pairs are identical. Two further strain pairs (from patients 7 and 15) that had shown larger differences in phenotype also differed by ribotyping.

DISCUSSION

The main purpose of this prospective study was to obtain a more detailed picture of the characteristics of E. coli strains causing community-acquired pyelonephritis in adult women. To evaluate the significance of the findings, the data obtained were compared with those found in other clinically relevant materials by ours (Fig. 1). Such E. coli materials were available to us as collected at the same time from patients with either community-acquired cystitis or nosocomial UTI in the same Kuopio area, and from stool from healthy persons and examined by the same methods (13, 17, 21). Furthermore, these results are compared with those from the previous available studies in adult pyelonephritis.

The present study confirms the prominent role of P-fimbriated E. coli as the main cause of acute pyelonephritis also in adults. In this respect the pyelonephritis isolates (67% P-fimbriated) differed from isolates both from community-acquired (25% P-fimbriated) and nosocomial UTI (12% P-fimbriated) and from normal stool (11% P-fimbriated) (Fig. 1). P-fimbriated strains were even more frequent (77%) in pyelonephritis of non-compromised patients; in this group, 5/6 (83%) strains from bacteremic patients were P-fimbriated. However, there were no statistically significant differences in the frequency of P fimbriation between the urinary and blood isolates (Table I). Instead, the compromised patients and patients with bacteremia were significantly older than the non-compromised patients without bacteremia. This is presumably speaking for a role for host conditions predisposing to E. coli bacteremia spreading from the urinary tract.

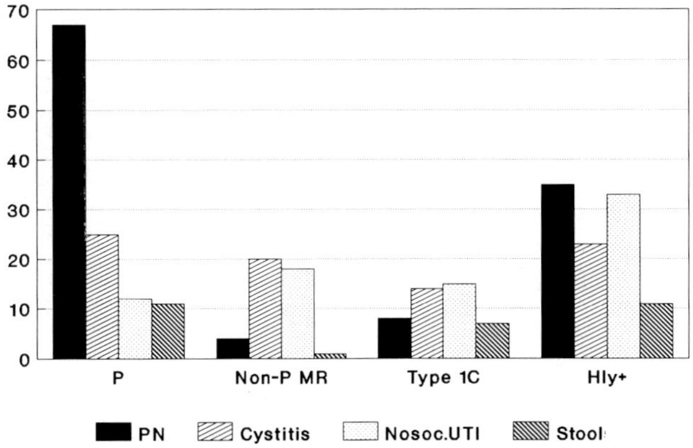

Fig. 1. Prevalence (percent) of virulence-associated factors of 49 strains from pyelonephritis (PN), of 178 strains from cystitis (Ref. 8), of 148 strains from nosocomial UTI (Ref. 4) and of 287 strains in stool from healthy adults (Ref. 11). P = P fimbriae, Non-PMR = Non-P MR adhesins, Type 1C = Type 1C fimbriae, Hly+ = Hemolysin production. Statistically significant differences: PN vs Cystitis: P fimbriae: $p < 0.001$ (χ^2), Non-P MR adhesins: $p = 0.02$ (χ^2); PN vs Nosoc. UTI: P fimbriae: $p < 0.001$ (χ^2), Non-P MR adhesins: $p = 0.035$ (χ^2); PN vs Stool: P fimbriae: $p < 0.001$ (χ^2), Hemolysin: $p < 0.001$ (χ^2).

In the previous studies made in adults, Jacobson et al. found 27 of the 30 E. coli strains (90%) expressing P fimbriae (9); in Sandberg's study, 80% of the pyelonephritic strains were P-fimbriated (7). In bacteremic patients with acute pyelonephritis the prevalence of P fimbriation was 92% (23/25 strains from women) in Brauner's study (8) and 62% in Johnson's study (10). However, all E. coli strains from bacteremic non-compromised patients were P-fimbriated in the latter study. The same was true in a recent study by Otto et al. (11) who found all 18 strains in healthy patients with bacteremia, but only 71% of strains from non-bacteremic patients, expressing P fimbriae. The patients with bacteremia were older than those without bacteremia also in this study, but the older patients did not have more complicating factors than the younger ones.

The role of Non-P MR adhesins has long been unclear in the pathogenesis of UTI, although some studies have suggested a role for these adhesins in acute cystitis (1). Our recent studies in patients with lower UTI (13, 17) have shown a strong and independent role of Non-P MR adhesins in the virulence of E. coli causing cystitis found in nearly 20% of the strains. In the present study only 4% of the strains from women with acute pyelonephritis expressed these adhesins, which is even fever than described in earlier studies (14–15); the use of several different human or sheep blood cells in these earlier studies may at least partly explain the difference. Fig. 1 clearly indicates an association of these adhesins with lower- but not with upper-UTI.

The prevalence of type 1C fimbriae has been reported in only a few studies (13, 16, 17, 25). Their higher frequency in UTI than in stool from healthy persons has suggested that type 1C fimbriae may have a role in the pathogenesis of human UTI. Fig. 1 shows that type 1C fimbriae were more prevalent among strains causing cystitis or nosocomial UTI, and of low prevalence in strains causing pyelonephritis and in stool from healthy persons. However, the frequent association of type 1C fimbriation with other virulence characteristics prompted us to perform a multivariate analysis of all these materials; it indicated that type 1C fimbriae do not play an independent role in the establishment of UTI (18).

Hemolysin production has in many studies been associated with severe UTI (1). The present study shows that this epidemiological association also applies to E. coli from adult pyelonephritis. But also hemolysin is usually found in strains with other virulence-associated characteristics, and had a negligible, independent role in the multivariate analysis (18).

Altogether 71% of the pyelonephritis isolates, but only 22% of the strains in stool from healthy adults had at least 1 virulence-associated factor (either P fimbriae or Non-P MR adhesin, type 1C fimbriae or hemolytic activity) ($p < 0.001$). The corresponding figures were 54% in community-acquired cystitis and 45% in nosocomial UTI. 37% of the pyelonephritis isolates, but only 7% of fecal controls had 2 or more of these factors ($p < 0.001$). These figures are in harmony with reports from other materials and confirm the significance of virulence factors in the severe forms of UTI also in adults.

A wide range of O antigens and O:K serotypes were identified among the pyelonephritis strains and there was no indication of a clone or clones characteristic of pyelonephritis. Several virulent clones or virulence-associated traits of E. coli have been described in pyelonephritis of basically healthy children (4, 19, 20) suggesting that in a healthy population only especially virulent bacteria can cause ascending infection, leading to the selection of these rare clones. Also studies in adults (7, 11) have reported, that certain serotypes (O1:K1:H7, O4:K12:H1, O7:K1:H−, O16:K1:H6, O16:K1:H− and O75:K5:H−) were dominant among urinary isolates. A large proportion of the patients in the present study were elderly and many of them had medical conditions predisposing to pyelonephritis. This adult population thus clearly differs from pediatric pyelonephritis, but not extensively from the above-mentioned adult materials. We conclude, however, that in the adults also host factors are important in the establishment of the disease. Thus the selection pressure for rare, exceptionally virulent clones could be less in the adults (with age and other predisposing factors) than in basically healthy children.

The 15 patients who had concomitant E. coli bacteremia, were older and had more often a compromising condition than the patients with pyelonephritis without bacteremia. At the same time, the E. coli strains causing bacteremia did not differ from those causing pyelonephritis without bacteremia, suggesting that host factors rather than bacterial virulence were decisive in determining whether or not the bacteria would invade the circulation, causing 'urosepsis'. 11 pairs of strains from blood and urine were identical in respect of all the phenotypic characteristics studied and also in genomic ribotyping. In 2 patients, there were minor differences in the O:K serotype, but ribotyping indicated that also these strains were identical. Interestingly, in both of these pairs, the blood isolates were encapsulated, whereas the corresponding urinary isolates were non-capsulated. In 2 further patients, the blood and urinary isolates were clearly not identical. These 2 patients were elderly women with diabetes and minor urinary tract abnormality, i.e. severely compromised patients. It seems possible that in these patients there was more than one E. coli strain causing UTI, and the one conserved for analysis was not the one that had invaded the blood. An alternative explanation would be an extra-urinary focus as the source of the bacteremia, but it seems less probable; all these patients had clinical and laboratory findings typical of pyelonephritis without other infectious foci.

The present study confirms the strong association of P fimbriae and, to a lesser extent, of hemolysin, with acute pyelonephritis also in adult women. Instead, the prevalence of Non-P MR adhesins was very low compared with that in lower UTI. There was no indication of a pyelonephritic clone suggesting that host factors play a prominent role in the establishment of pyelonephritis in adults, whereas especially virulent bacteria represented by rare clones are necessary to cause pyelonephritis in children. Those 15 patients who had bacteremia associated with the pyelonephritis were older and more often had compromising conditions than the non-bacteremic patients, whereas the E. coli strains of these 2 patient groups did not differ from each other, likewise speaking for the role of host factors.

ACKNOWLEDGEMENTS

This study was supported by the Emil Aaltonen foundation. We thank Dr A. Pere (Orion Diagnostica) for the antisera against type 1C fimbriae. We thank also Dr Eveliina Tarkka for giving good advice in evaluating the results of ribotyping and Liisa Immonen and Kaisa Jousimies for excellent technical assistance.

REFERENCES

1. Johnson JR. Virulence factors in Escherichia coli urinary tract infection. Clin Microbiol Rev 4: 80–128, 1991.
2. Källenius G, Möllby R, Svenson SB, Helin I, Hultberg H, Cedergen B, Winberg J. Occurrence of P-fimbriated Escherichia coli in urinary tract infections. Lancet 2: 1369–1372, 1981.
3. Väisänen V, Elo J, Tallgren LG, Siitonen A, Mäkelä PH, Svanborg-Eden C, Källenius G, Svenson SB, Hultberg H, Korhonen T. Mannose-resistant haemagglutination and P antigen recognition are characteristic of Escherichia coli causing primary pyelonephritis. Lancet 2: 1366–1369, 1981.
4. Väisänen-Rhen V, Elo J, Väisänen E, Siitonen A, Orskov I, Orskov F, Svenson SB, Mäkelä PH, Korhonen TK. P-fimbriated clones among uropathogenic Escherichia coli strains. Infect Immun 43: 149–155, 1984.
5. Westerlund B, Siitonen A, Elo J, Williams PH, Korhonen TK, Mäkelä PH. Properties of Escherichia coli isolates from urinary tract infections in boys. J Infect Dis 158: 996–1002, 1988.
6. de Man P, Cläeson I, Johanson I, Jodal U, Svanborg-Eden C. Bacterial attachment as a predictor of renal abnormalities in boys with urinary tract infection. J Pediatr 115: 915–922, 1989.
7. Sandberg T, Kaijser B, Lidin-Janson G, Lincoln K, Orskov F, Orskov I, Stokland E, Svanborg-Eden C. Virulence of Escherichia coli in relation to host factors in women with symptomatic urinary tract infection. J Clin Microbiol 26: 1471–1476, 1988.

8. Brauner A, Leissner M, Wretlind B, Julander I, Svenson SB, Källenius G. Occurrence of P-fimbriated Escherichia coli in patients with bacteremia. Eur J Clin Microbiol 4: 566–569, 1985.
9. Jacobson SH, Lins L-E, Svenson SB, Källenius G. P fimbriated Escherichia coli in adults with acute pyelonephritis. J Infect Dis 152: 426–427, 1985.
10. Johnson JR, Roberts PL, Stamm WE. P fimbriae and other virulence factors in Escherichia coli urosepsis: association with patient's characteristics. J Infect Dis 156: 225–229, 1987.
11. Otto G, Sandberg T, Marklund B-I, Ulleryd P, Svanborg C. Virulence factors and pap genotype in Escherichia coli isolates from women with acute pyelonephritis, with or without bacteremia. Clin Infect Dis 17: 448–456, 1993.
12. O'Hanley P, Low D, Romero I, Lark D, Vosti K, Falkow S, Schoolnik G. Gal-Gal binding and hemolysin phenotypes and genotypes associated with uropathogenic Escherichia coli. N Engl J Med 313: 414–420, 1985.
13. Ikäheimo R, Siitonen A, Kärkkäinen U, Mäkelä PH. Virulence characteristics of Escherichia coli in nosocomial urinary tract infection. Clin Infect Dis 16: 785–791, 1993.
14. Novicki B, Svanborg-Eden C, Hull R, Hull S. Molecular analysis and epidemiology of the Dr. hemagglutinin of uropathogenic Escherichia coli. Infect Immun 57: 446–451, 1989.
15. Arthur M, Johnson CE, Rubin RH, Arbeit RD, Campanelli C, Kim C, Steinbach S, Agarwal M, Wilkinson R, Goldstein R. Molecular epidemiology of adhesin and hemolysin virulence factors among uropathogenic Escherichia coli. Infect Immun 57: 303–313, 1989.
16. Pere A, Leinonen M, Väisänen-Rhen V, Rhen M, Korhonen TK. Occurrence of type-1C fimbriae on Escherichia coli strains from human extraintestinal infections. J Gen Microbiol 131: 1705–1711, 1985.
17. Ikäheimo R, Siitonen A, Kärkkäinen U, Kuosmanen P, Mäkelä PH. Characteristics of Escherichia coli in acute community-acquired cystitis of adult women. Scand J Infect Dis 25: 705–712, 1993.
18. Siitonen A, Martikainen R, Ikäheimo R, Palmgren J, Mäkelä PH. Virulence associated characteristics of Escherichia coli in urinary tract infection: a statistical analysis with special attention to type 1C fimbriation. J Microbiol Pathog 15: 65–75, 1993.
19. Lomberg H, Hellström M, Jodal U, Leffler H, Lincoln K, Svanborg-Eden C. Virulence-associated traits in Escherichia coli causing first and recurrent episodes of urinary tract infection in children with or without vesicoureteral reflux. J Infect Dis 150: 561–569, 1984.
20. Orskov F, Orskov I. Summary of a workshop on the clone concept in the epidemiology, taxonomy, and evolution of the Enterobacteriaceae and other bacteria. J Infect Dis 148–157, 1983.
21. Siitonen A. Escherichia coli in fecal flora of healthy adults: Serotypes, P and type 1C fimbriae, Non-P MR adhesins and hemolytic activity. J Infect Dis 166: 1058–1065, 1992.
22. Farmer III JJ, Kelly MT. Enterobacteriaceae. In: Balows A, Hausler Jr WJ, Herrman KL, Isenberg HD, Shadomy HJ, eds. Manual of Clinical Microbiology. Washington DC: American Society for Microbiology, 360–383, 1991.
23. Evans DG, Evans DJ Jr, Tjoa W. Hemmagglutination of human group A erythrocytes by enterotoxigenic Escherichia coli isolated from adults with diarrhea: correlation with colonizing factor. Infect Immun 18: 330–337, 1977.
24. Kärkkäinen U, Ikäheimo R, Katila M-L, Mäntyjärvi R. P fimbriation of Escherichia coli strains from patients with urosepsis demonstrated by a commercial agglutination test (PF TEST). J Clin Microbiol 29: 221–224, 1991.
25. Pere A, Novicki B, Saxen H, Siitonen A, Korhonen TK. Expression of P, type-1, and type-1C fimbriae of Escherichia coli in the urine of patients with acute urinary tract infection. J Infect Dis 156: 567–574, 1987.
26. Grimont F, Grimont PAD. Ribosomal nucleic acid gene restriction patterns as potential taxonomic tools. Ann Microbiol (Paris) 137B: 165–175, 1986.
27. Bingen EH, Denamur E, Picard B, Goullet P, Lambert-Zechovsky NY, Brahimi N, Mercier J-C, Beaufils F, Elion J. Molecular epidemiology unravels the complexity of neonatal Escherichia coli acquisition in twins. J Clin Microbiol 30: 1896–1898, 1992.
28. Brosius J, Ullrich A, Raker MA, Gray A, Dull TJ, Gutell RR, et al. Construction and fine mapping of recombinant plasmids containing the rrnB ribosomal RNA operon of E. coli. Plasmid 6: 112–118, 1981.
29. Tarkka E, Åhman H, Siitonen A. Ribotyping as an epidemiologic tool for Escherichia coli. Epidemiol Infect [in press 1994].

Submitted September 29, 1993; accepted January 16, 1994

Scand J Infect Dis 26: 297–300, 1994

Acute Suppurative Thyroiditis: A Ten-year Review in a Taiwanese Hospital

LONG-BIN BENJAMIN JENG[1], JEN-DER LIN[2] and MIIN-FU CHEN[1]

From the Departments of [1]Surgery and [2]Internal Medicine, Chang Gung Medical College, Chang Gung Memorial Hospital, Taipei, Taiwan, R.O.C.

12 patients with acute suppurative thyroiditis were treated over a 10-year period. Their ages ranged from 2–81 years. Eight of them had a pre-existing thyroid mass. A piriform sinus fistula was demonstrated in one of the 2 patients with a history of recurrent infections. Cultures of the pus taken from the infected glands grew Gram-positive streptococci in 4 patients, Gram-negative bacteria in 4, and anaerobic bacteria in 1; the other 3 were sterile. Both patients who grew Klebsiella pneumonia were diabetic. Most of the patients received drainage in addition to systemic antibiotics. Only 2 patients had recurrence during the follow-up period. We present a review of our experience with this uncommon infection.

L.-B. B. Jeng, MD, Department of Surgery, Chang Gung Memorial Hospital, 5, Fu-Hsing Street, Kwei-Shan Shiang, Tao-Yuan, Taiwan, R.O.C.

INTRODUCTION

The thyroid gland is rarely the victim of an acute bacterial infection because of its anatomical position (1), capsule (2), rich system of blood and lymphatic supply (1–3), and its high iodine content (1). There are several possible routes of infection in acute suppurative thyroiditis (AST) according to Hazard (4), though in most cases the origin is usually not obvious. Recently, Miyauchi et al. (1, 5) reported the existence of a piriform sinus fistula as the route of infection. In most cases, an esophagogram revealed the fistula.

We treated 12 patients with AST over a 10-year period. Only 1 was found to have a piriform sinus fistula. Two diabetic patients presented with unusual Klebsiella pneumonia ASTs secondary to bacteremia. We review here our experience with this uncommon infection.

MATERIALS AND METHODS

Patients

12 patients with AST were treated at Chang Gung Memorial Hospital during the 10-year period from 1982 to 1991. The clinical characteristics of these 12 patients are summarized in Table I. There were 8 female and 4 male patients. Their ages ranged from 2 to 81 years (mean 38 years). Eight of them had a pre-existing thyroid mass either on one side or bilaterally. The diagnoses of the masses included nodular goitre in 6 patients and chronic thyroiditis and anaplastic cancer, in 1 patient each. Fever, neck pain and swelling were the most common symptoms and signs. Nine patients had peripheral white blood cell counts exceeding 10×10^9/l. Two of the 3 patients without leukocytosis were diabetic. The thyroid function tests showed that all patients were in a euthyroid state.

Diagnostic procedures

Sonographic examinations were performed in most cases to exclude an extrathyroid infection and to perform an aspiration for cytological study under echoguidance. Esophagography was carried out in 2 patients with a history of recurrent AST, whereof 1 demonstrated a piriform sinus fistula.

RESULTS

Bacteriology

The pus taken from the infected thyroid glands was cultured and grew Gram-positive streptococci in 4 patients, Gram-negative bacteria in 4 and anaerobic bacteria in 1; the other 3 were sterile. Of the Gram-negative bacteria identified 2 proved to be Klebsiella pneumoniae and the others E. coli and pseudomonas. Both patients who grew Klebsiella pneumonia were

 ISSN 0036-5548

Table I. *Clinical characteristics of 12 patients with acute suppurative thyroiditis*

Str. = streptococcus, Anaerobic: Bacteroid distasonis, Bacteroid melaninegenicus, Fusobacterium nucleatum. Drainage +: incision and drainage, −: not drained. Antibiotics: PcG: benzyl penicillin, GM: gentamicin, AM: amikacin.

Case no.	Age (y) /sex	Pre-existing neck mass	WBC count ($\times 10^9$/l)	Diabetes	Bacteria cultured	Anti-biotics	Duration	Drainage	Recurrence
1	28/F	Left side	13	No	Str. GrD	PcG + GM	14 d	+	No
2	2/F	No	12.8	No	Sterile	PcG	7 d	+	Yes
3	6/F	No	14	No	Str.	PcG	7 d	−	No
4	81/F	Bilateral	15.2	No	Sterile	PcG	7 d	+	No
5	51/F	No	6.6	Yes	K. pneumonia	PcG + GM	4 d	+	No
						Keflin + GM	2 d		
						Mandole + AM	15 d		
6	58/F	Bilateral	11.7	No	E. coli	PcG + GM	3 d	+	No
						Keflin + AM	15 d		
7	54/F	Right side	15.7	No	Pseudomonas	PcG + GM	14 d	−	No
8	55/M	Left side	6.9	Yes	K. pneumonia	PcG + GM	4 d	−	No
						Keflin + GM	14 d		
9	18/M	No	8.6	No	Str. viridans	PcG + GM	14 d	+	Yes
10	24/F	Left side	14.6	No	Str. GrD	PcG	7 d	+	No
11	50/F	Bilateral	20.7	No	Sterile	PcG + GM	14 d	+	No
12	27/M	Left side	12	No	Anaerobic	PcG + GM	4 d	+	No

diabetic. The pseudomonas infection had resulted from a percutaneous aspiration during an echographic study for a thyroid nodule.

Treatment

All the patients received systemic antibiotics. Usually, benzyl penicillin and gentamicin were administered initially and then changed according to the results of the culture and sensitivity tests. The duration of antibiotic therapy varied from 7 to 21 days, depending on the patient's clinical response (Table I). Three patients had percutaneous aspiration only, while the other 9 patients underwent incision and drainage. In addition to drainage, 2 of these 9 patients underwent thyroidectomy because of the size of the thyroid mass and severity of the infection. Two patients had a fistula excised. Only 1 of them had a piriform sinus fistula demonstrated preoperatively (case 9).

Recurrences

During the follow-up period from 2 to 10 years, there were 2 recurrences (Table I). Both of these patients had a fistula excised during drainage of the abscess. The first patient (case 2) was a 2-year-old child in whom a fistula was found while performing the surgical drainage. The fistula was excised, though we suspect that it was only partially excised, since no preoperative esophagogram was performed. The other patient (case 9), a 28-year-old woman with preoperative esophagographic demonstration of fistula also developed recurrence, although the fistula was excised. The cause of the recurrence remains unknown.

DISCUSSION

Gram-positive bacteria such as streptococci, staphylococci and pneumococci are the most frequent causative organisms in acute suppurative thyroiditis (2). Berger has reviewed 224 patients with thyroid infection reported in the English literature since 1900 (6). Of these, 153 had acute bacterial infection. The bacteriological findings from 85 specimens of pus or thyroid tissue confirmed that Gram-positive cocci were the most common pathogens (62/85). Gram-negative bacilli were found in 12 patients, with Enterobacteriaceae being the most common (7/12). The 5 other rare Gram-negative bacilli included: Haemophilus influenza in 2 patients and Pseudomonas aeruginosa (7), Actinobacillus actinomycetemcomitans and E. coli (8) in one each.

Since 1983, only a few reports have appeared (9–13). A review of these continues to show the incidence of AST caused by Gram-negative bacteria to be rare. In our series, there was a relatively large proportion of Gram-negative bacterial infections (4/12). Three patients had a positive blood culture for the same organism. One was caused iatrogenically by percutaneous aspiration, which was performed to diagnose a thyroid nodule. In certain regions and in selected patients, AST caused by Gram-negative bacteria may not be as rare as suggested in the literature. This makes it important to confirm the diagnosis by culture to ensure the appropriateness of the antibiotic treatments.

With direct inoculation of either staphylococci or streptococci into the carotid artery in dogs, Womack & Cole failed to produce thyroid infections (14). The experiment revealed the inherent resistance to infection of the thyroid gland, ascribed to its rich vascularity, anatomic isolation and high iodine content. If this barrier is breached by an internal fistula, the thyroid may become infected. The piriform sinus fistulae reported by Miyauchi et al. originally in 1981 (5) and more recently in 1990 (1) drew attention to this unusual route of thyroid infection. The characteristic clinical features included (i) onset in infancy and childhood, (ii) left lobe involvement, and (iii) frequent recurrence unless the fistula was extirpated completely. In 38 of 42 patients, examined by barium meal, a fistula was found. 25 patients with complete fistulectomy had no recurrence, whereas of the 16 patients without fistulectomy, 6 had recurrences. We performed a barium study in only 2 patients (cases 1 and 9). One had a fistula; the other patient (case 2) with a history of recurrent infections, had surgical exploration. A fistula was found and resected but there was a recurrence. This suggests that follow-up esophagography is necessary in patients with recurrent infections.

The other route of AST is by hematogenous spread, which was previously believed to be the most common (2). We believe this to be the route in our 2 cases of infection by Klebsiella pneumoniae. Both cases were diabetic with Klebsiella bacteremia, though no definite origin could be determined. The relationship between Klebsiella pneumoniae bacteremia and diabetes has been noted by Cheng et al. (15) in cases of pyogenic liver abscesses with septic metastatic lesions. They suggested that the impairment of chemotaxis, phagocytosis and the bactericidal function of phagocytes in diabetics make these patients more vulnerable to disseminated K. pneumoniae infection. Also, because diabetic patients have intimal layer damage of the vessels, they are predisposed to such a hematogenous spread. Both diabetic patients had normal white blood cell counts in the peripheral blood. We wonder if this is indirect evidence of impaired chemotaxis.

To summarize: Gram-negative bacteria caused one-third of our AST cases. Culture and sensitivity testing of aspirates from the infected thyroid gland is mandatory for the choice of antibiotics. If the cultures reveal K. pneumoniae, diabetes should be suspected and appropriate treatment given. Both the infecting organism and the diabetic state should be controlled in order to get a good clinical response.

ACKNOWLEDGEMENTS

The authors thank Dr Bullard for his help in English correction and Ms. Yang for her expert preparation of this manuscript.

REFERENCES

1. Miyauchi A, Matsuzuka F, Kuma K, Takai S. Piriform sinus fistula: An underlying abnormality common in patients with acute suppurative thyroiditis. World J Surg 14: 400–405, 1990.
2. Hay ID. Thyroiditis: A clinical update. Mayo Clin Proc 60: 836–843, 1985.
3. Lambert MJ III, Johns ME, Mentzer R. Acute suppurative thyroiditis. Am Surg 46: 461–463, 1980.
4. Hazard JB. Thyroiditis: a review. Am J Clin Pathol 25: 289–298, 1955.
5. Miyauchi A, Matsuzuka F, Takai S, Kuma K, Kosak G. Piriform sinus fistula: a route of infection in acute suppurative thyroiditis. Arch Surg 116: 66–69, 1981.
6. Berger SA, Zonszein J, Villamena P, Mittman N. Infectious disease of the thyroid gland. Rev Infect Dis 5: 108–122, 1983.
7. Weissel M, Wolf A, Linkesch W. Acute suppurative thyroiditis caused by pseudomonas aeruginosa (letter). BMJ 2: 580, 1977.
8. Saksouk F, Salti IS. Acute suppurative thyroiditis caused by Escherichia coli. BMJ ii: 23–24, 1977.
9. Svenungsson B, Lindberg AA. Acute suppurative salmonella thyroiditis: clinical course and antibody response. Scand J Infect Dis 13: 303–306, 1981.
10. Miller D, Hill JL, Sun CC, O'Brien DS, Heller JA, Jr. The diagnosis and management of piriform sinus fistula in infants and young children. J Pediatr Surg 18: 377–381, 1983.
11. Hirata A, Saito S, Tsuchida Y, Hazama H, Iwanaka T, Shima K, Hori T. Surgical management of piriform sinus fistula. Am Surg 50: 454–457, 1984.
12. Smeal WE, Schenfeld LA, Caroff RJ. Acute suppurative thyroiditis in a 3-year-old boy. Postgrad Med 80: 100–107, 1986.
13. Evengard B, Julander I. Suppurative staphylococcus aureus thyroiditis. Scand J Infect Dis 18: 483–485, 1986.
14. Womack NA, Cole WH. Normal and pathologic repair in the thyroid gland. Arch Surg 23: 466–476, 1931.
15. Cheng DL, Liu YC, Yen MY, Liu CY, Wang RS. Septic metastatic lesions of pyogenic liver abscess: Their association with Klebsiella pneumoniae bacteremia in diabetic patients. Arch Intern Med 151: 1557–1559, 1991.

Submitted November 15, 1993; accepted January 10, 1994

Scand J Infect Dis 26: 301–305, 1994

Increasing Resistance to Penicillin in Streptococcus pneumoniae in Southern Sweden

KARL EKDAHL[1] and CARL KAMME[2]

From the Departments of [1]Infectious Diseases and [2]Clinical Microbiology, Lund University Hospital, Lund, Sweden

The susceptibility to penicillin of 6 prevalent pneumococcal types isolated from nasopharynx in 1992 was compared with that of corresponding types from 1980–82. The 6 types or groups, 6, 9, 14, 15, 19 and 23, constituted 78% of consecutive isolates. 19/204 isolates in 1992 were intermediately resistant (MIC 0.12–1.0 mg/l) in comparison with 1/194 from 1980–82 ($p < 0.001$). Resistant strains (MIC ≥ 2 mg/l) were not found. Of group 15, no fewer than 10/31 isolates were intermediately resistant, which may support the clonal origin and spread of penicillin-resistant pneumococci. At least 5.0% of nasopharyngeal isolates are now intermediately resistant to penicillin. This figure is substantially higher than the 2% earlier reported in Sweden.

C. Kamme, MD, Department of Clinical Microbiology, Lund University Hospital, Sölvegatan 23, S-223 62 Lund, Sweden

INTRODUCTION

The emergence and spread of penicillin-resistant Streptococcus pneumoniae is the result of the vast oral consumption of antibiotics for more than 4 decades. In the 1970s and 1980s, a worldwide spread of resistant strains occurred (1–3).

In Europe, reported frequencies vary between countries: below 5% in Belgium, Britain and Switzerland, 44% in Spain and 58% in Hungary (1–4). A rapid increase from 2.9% in 1989 to 12% in 1990 occurred in France, while from Iceland a clonal spread of resistant type 6 pneumococcus was recently reported (5, 6).

In Sweden, the preferred antibiotic for upper respiratory tract infections (URTI), including primary acute otitis media, is phenoxymethyl penicillin. In 1987 the pharmacy sales figures for phenoxymethyl penicillin and amoxicillin were 5.6 and 0.67 DDD/1000 inhabitants/day, respectively. Consumption increased to 6.8 DDD for phenoxymethyl penicillin and 1.3 DDD/1000 inhabitants/day for amoxicillin, amoxicillin/clavulanic acid in 1992 (7). In that year 60% of children aged 0–4 years received a course of phenoxymethyl penicillin and 31% a course of amoxicillin, amoxicillin/clavulanic acid. The number of prescriptions of amoxicillin for this age group nearly tripled from 1987 to 1992 (7). (The defined daily dose (DDD) for a drug is established on the basis of the average daily dose on its main indication in adults. Thus, drug consumption, expressed as DDD/1000 inhabitants/day, gives a rough estimate of the number of patients receiving standard treatment with a given drug. DDD for phenoxymethyl penicillin is 2 g and for amoxicillin, 1 g) (7).

In spite of this large consumption the reported frequency of intermediately penicillin-resistant (MIC 0.12–1.0 mg/l) and resistant (MIC ≥ 2 mg/l) pneumococci among clinical isolates has not exceeded 2% until the latest national survey, performed in 1987 (8, 9).

In the present investigation the susceptibility to benzylpenicillin and phenoxymethyl penicillin of the 6 most common groups or types in nasopharyngeal isolates in 1992 (6, 9, 14, 15, 19, and 23) was compared with corresponding types isolated in 1980–82. The aim was to ascertain if any significant increase in the MICs had occurred over the 10-year period, especially any upward shift among the susceptible strains as has been reported by other investigators (10).

MATERIALS AND METHODS

Bacterial strains

The strains from 1980–82 were lyophilized isolates from the nasopharynx in children 1–8 years of age with RTIs. They were collected from October to March and were not consecutive. The strains from 1992 were consecutive isolates from the nasopharynx in out-patients with RTIs, 204 patients 1–8 years old and 23 patients aged 15–65 years. The isolates were collected from September to December and screened for types/groups 6, 9, 14, 15, 19, and 23 until the number of each type/group corresponded to the number of surviving old isolates. Typing was performed by the *quellung* reaction with antisera from Statens Seruminstitut, Copenhagen, Denmark. The typing of group 15 strains was performed by Dr Jørgen Henrichsen, Statens Seruminstitut.

Antibiotics

Benzylpenicillin and phenoxymethyl penicillin were provided as standard powder. The drug solutions, weight compensated for potency, as well as the agar dilution plates, were prepared on the day of use.

Determination of MICs

In order to get a reliable estimate of the density of the inocula, the capsular material was eliminated or reduced by aerobic subculturing before determining the MIC.

Two μl of log-phase cultures in Todd Hewitt broth was inoculated with a multipoint inoculator onto the surface of horse blood agar (as control) and horse blood agar containing 2-fold dilutions of the antibiotics. The size of the inoculum was $5 \times 10^4 - 1 \times 10^5$ CFU/ml. The plates were incubated at +37°C in air for 20 h when the MICs were determined, defined as the lowest concentration of the drug not yielding any visible growth.

In each test, old and freshly isolated strains of the same type were inoculated onto the same plates. Thus, any inter-assay variation could not influence the comparison between old and recent isolates.

Inter-assay variation

Three strains, S. pneumoniae L15532, S. pneumoniae L378 and Micrococcus luteus L56 served as controls and were included in each test. The inter-assay variation of phenoxymethyl penicillin was 1 dilution step for all 3 strains, 1 dilution step of benzylpenicillin for 2 and ±1 dilution step for 1 of the strains.

The E-test® (Biodisk AB, Solna, Sweden) was done according to the instructions of the manufacturer.

Statistics

The χ^2-test with Yates' correction and Fisher's exact, 2-tailed test were used.

RESULTS

Benzyl penicillin

In 1992, 19/204 isolates were intermediately resistant (MIC 0.12–1.0 mg/l) in comparison with 1/194 from 1980–82 ($p = 0.0002$). The difference between old and recent isolates was also significant for group 15 alone ($p = 0.004$) and for the other 5 taken together ($p = 0.011$) (Table I). No resistant strains (MIC $\geq$ 2 mg/l) were found. The intermediately resistant strains were isolated in patients living in different parts of the county, none of them belonging to the same family, day nursery or school.

Among susceptible isolates of groups 6, 9, 19, and 23, there were fewer recent isolates with low MICs (0.008–0.016 mg/l) than among the old strains. Taking these groups together and also including type 14, the difference in this respect was significant; 158/174 from 1992 versus 138/173 from 1980–82 ($p = 0.006$).

Group 15 showed an opposite tendency, with an increased number of MICs of 0.008–0.016 among recent isolates (NS) (Table I).

Of all group 15 isolates, there were significantly more type 15A ($p = 0.007$) among the intermediately resistant than among the susceptible isolates (Table II).

Table I. *Susceptibility to benzylpenicillin of nasopharyngeal strains of Streptococcus pneumoniae isolated in 1980–1982 and 1992*

MIC (mg/l)	Group 6, 30%[a]		Group 9, 7%[a]		Type 14, 9%[a]		Group 15, 6%[a]		Group 19, 12%[a]		Group 23, 14%[a]	
	-80–82	-92	-80–82	-92	-80–82	-92	-80–82	-92	-80–82	-92	-80–82	-92
0.008	2	3	5	5	6	5		1	9	3	3	2
0.016	40	37	14	12	17	19	11	20	27	25	35	27
0.03	3	2		3	5		9		4	5	3	10
0.06		2								4		
0.12		1						2				
0.25						3		7	1	3		
0.5								1		1		
1.0												1
No. of strains	45	45	19	20	28	27	20	31	41	41	41	40
Intermediately resistant	0	1	0	0	0	3	0	10	1	4	0	1

[a] Distribution of types/groups among consecutive isolates.

Table II. *Benzylpenicillin: Distribution of susceptible and intermediately resistant pneumococcal types 15A, B and C*

	Type 15A	Type 15B	Type 15C	Type 15F	Total
Susceptible	1	7	13	0	21
Intermediately resistant	5[a]	3	2	0	10
Total	6	10	15	0	31

[a] The number of type A strains was significantly higher among the intermediately resistant than among the susceptible isolates ($p = 0.007$).

The MICs of the altogether 20 intermediately resistant isolates (0.12–1.0 mg/l) recorded with the plate dilution method were checked with the E-test, which gave the same range (0.094–1.0 mg/l).

Phenoxymethyl penicillin

A few strains had slightly, but insignificantly higher MICs of phenoxymethyl penicillin than of benzylpenicillin.

DISCUSSION

A significant increase in MICs occurred in the 6 prevalent pneumococcal types/groups isolated in 1992, in comparison with these types/groups from 1980–82. A gradual increase in resistance was evident both above and below the breakpoint (0.06 mg/l) as well as a distinct separation of susceptible and intermediately resistant isolates, as seen for group 15.

The reported figure, less than 2%, for intermediately resistant and resistant pneumococci in the national survey in 1987, is obviously no longer valid in Southern Sweden (10), where the figure is now at least 5%, taking the frequency of the types/groups into consideration (Table I).

The gradual increase in MICs in recent isolates may either indicate selection of less susceptible strains in the normal pool of pneumococci or, as suggested, represent small mutational steps possibly leading to increased resistance if such strains are subjected to further ecological pressure (10).

10/31 recent group 15 isolates were distinctly separate from the susceptible ones. This pattern was possibly in agreement with the randomly occurring acquisition of gene fragments from related species in the respiratory tract and seems to support the clonal origin and spread of penicillin-resistant pneumococci (11–14).

The nasopharynx in children is the main reservoir for pneumococci as well as for Haemophilus influenzae and Moraxella catarrhalis. Pneumococci spread easily in crowded settings, in day nurseries for instance. Resistant strains are able to colonize the nasopharynx in children as easily as susceptible strains and without the support of antibiotic pressure (15). However, an antimicrobial agent active against susceptible pneumococci in the nasopharynx may enhance the selection and spread of resistant strains. This has been shown in Spain, where the rate of penicillin-resistant pneumococci increased in proportion to increasing consumption of aminopenicillins (2). In 1983 the prescription of amoxicillin in Spain was 10.34 DDD/1000 inhabitants/day, which was twice that in France, where the frequency of penicillin-resistant pneumococci rose from virtually nil in 1986 to 2.9% in 1989 and to 12% in 1990 (5, 16).

In Sweden, phenoxymethyl penicillin is recommended for URTIs including primary acute otitis media, since amoxicillin does not offer any therapeutic advantage in otitis and also appears to have a less desirable ecological effect in selecting β-lactamase-producing H. influenzae than has phenoxymethyl penicillin (17–20). The amoxicillin/clavulanic acid combination does not differ in any of these respects from amoxicillin alone (21, 22).

The predominant reason for prescribing oral penicillins is URTIs, but there has not been any epidemiological explanation in Sweden for the continuously increasing consumption of these drugs, especially amoxicillin and amoxicillin/clavulanic acid. In 1987, 8% of patients with acute otitis media and 2% of patients with URTIs were given amoxicillin, in contrast to 20% and 6% in 1992, respectively. In children the figures for 1992 were even higher, 29% for otitis media (0–4 years of age) and 12% for URTIs (0–14 years of age) (7).

There is no doubt that the spread of penicillin-resistant respiratory tract pathogens is boosted by the vast and uncritical prescribing of oral penicillins to outpatients. When antibiotic resistance starts to emerge, the frequency of resistant strains is low and slowly increasing but will sooner or later accelerate until the situation gets out of control. A less liberal antibiotic policy is obviously necessary and may possibly retard or prevent the further increase in penicillin resistance in pneumococci in Sweden.

ACKNOWLEDGEMENTS

This investigation was supported by grants from the Faculty of Medicine, University of Lund.

The authors are indebted to: Dr Jørgen Henrichsen, Statens Seruminstitut, Copenhagen, for typing the group 15 strains and for valuable viewpoints on the manuscript; to Dr Anders Ekedahl, Apoteksbolaget, for help with the drug sales statistics; and to Lennart Olbjer for checking our statistical calculations.

REFERENCES

1. Klugman KP. Pneumococcal resistance to antibiotics. Clin Microbiol Rev 3: 171–196, 1990.
2. Baquero F, Martínez-Beltrán J, Loza E. A review of antibiotic resistance patterns of Streptococcus pneumoniae in Europe. J Antimicrob Chemother Suppl C, 28: 31–38, 1991.
3. Applebaum PC. Antimicrobial resistance in Streptococcus pneumoniae: an overview. Clin Infect Dis 15: 77–83, 1992.
4. Marton A, Gulyas M, Munoz R, Tomasz A. Extremely high incidence of antibiotic resistance in clinical isolates of Streptococcus pneumoniae in Hungary. J Infect Dis 163: 542–548, 1991.

5. Geslin P, Buu-Hoi A, Frémaux A, Acar JF. Antimicrobial resistance in Streptococcus pneumoniae: an epidemiological survey in France, 1970–1990. Clin Infect Dis 15: 95–98, 1992.
6. Kristinsson KG, Hjálmarsdóttir MA, Steingrímsson, O. Increasing penicillin resistance in pneumococci in Iceland. Lancet 339: 1606, 1992.
7. Swedish statistics on medicines (Svensk läkemedels-statistik). Stockholm: Apoteksbolaget, 1992.
8. Kallings I, Bengtsson S, Christensen P, Holm SE, Lind L, Kalin M. Antibiotic sensitivity of Haemophilus influenzae, Streptococcus pneumoniae, Streptococcus pyogenes and Branhamella catarrhalis isolated from upper respiratory tract infections in Sweden. Scand J Infect Dis Suppl 39: 100–105, 1983.
9. Kallings I, Christensen P, Olsson-Liljequist B, Danielsson D, Burman LG, Holm S, Bengtsson S, Kaijser B, Kalin, M. Aktuell antibiotikakänslighet hos luftvägspatogener i Sverige. Läkartidningen 84: 2407, 1987 [in Swedish].
10. Handwerger S, Tomasz A. Alterations in penicillin-binding proteins of clinical and laboratory isolates of pathogenic Streptococcus pneumoniae with low levels of penicillin resistance. J Infect Dis 153: 83–89, 1986.
11. Dowson CG, Hutchinson A, Woodford N, Johnson AP, George RC, Spratt BG. Penicillin-resistant viridans streptococci have obtained altered penicillin-binding protein genes from penicillin-resistant strains of Streptococcus pneumoniae. Proc Natl Acad Sci USA 87: 5858–5862, 1990.
12. Dowson CG, Hutchison A, Brannigan JA, George RC, Hansman D, Líñares J, Tomasz A, Smith JM, Spratt BG. Horizontal transfer of penicillin-binding protein genes in penicillin-resistant clinical isolates of Streptococcus pneumoniae. Proc Natl Acad Sci USA 86: 8842–8846, 1989.
13. Chalkley LJ, Koornhof HJ, Intra- and inter-specific transformation of Streptococcus pneumoniae to penicillin resistance. J Antimicrob Chemother 26: 21–28, 1990.
14. Potgieter E, Chalkley LJ. Reciprocal transfer of penicillin resistance genes between Streptococcus pneumoniae, Streptococcus mitior and Streptococcus sangius (letter). J Antimicrob Chemother 28: 463–465, 1991.
15. Radetsky MS, Johansen TL, Lauer BA, Istre GR, Parmelee SW, Wiesenthal AM, Glode MP. Multiply resistant pneumococcus causing meningitis: its epidemiology within a day-care centre. Lancet 2: 771–773, 1981.
16. Col NF, O'Connor RW. Estimating worldwide current antibiotic usage: Report of Task Force 1. Rev Infect Dis 9 (Suppl 3): 232–243, 1987.
17. Puhakka H, Virolainen E, Aantaa E. Treatment of acute otitis media in children-penicillin V or amoxicillin? Acta Otolaryngol Suppl (Stockh) 386: 108–111, 1982.
18. Qvarnberg Y. Acute otitis media. A prospective clinical study of myringotomy and antimicrobial treatment. Acta Otolaryngol Suppl (Stockh) 375: 1–157, 1981.
19. Freijd AA, Rynell-Dagöö B. Isolation of nasopharyngeal beta-lactamase-producing Haemophilus influenzae in relation to antibiotic treatment of acute otitis media in infants. Acta Otolaryngol (Stockh) 95: 351–357, 1983.
20. Scheifele DW, Fussell SJ. Ampicillin-resistant Haemophilus influenzae colonizing ambulatory children. Am J Dis Child 135: 406–409, 1981.
21. Stenström C, Lundgren K, Ingvarsson L, Bertilson SO. Amoxycillin/Clavulanate versus amoxycillin in recurrent otitis media and therapeutic failure in children. Acta Otolaryngol (Stockh) 111: 120–129, 1991.
22. Jonsson L, Eliasson I, Kamme C, Mölstad S. Selektion av β-laktamasproduktion i luftvägsfloran under behandling med amoxicillin resp. amoxicillin/klavulansyra [in Swedish]. Abstract 48 GP. Svenska Läkaresällskapets Riksstämma 1992.

Submitted October 5, 1993; accepted March 3, 1994

Världens bredaste antibiotika-sortiment.

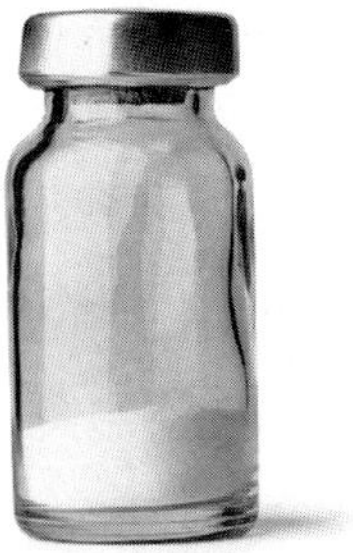

AZACTAM® (AZTREONAM)
MOT BAKTERIER.

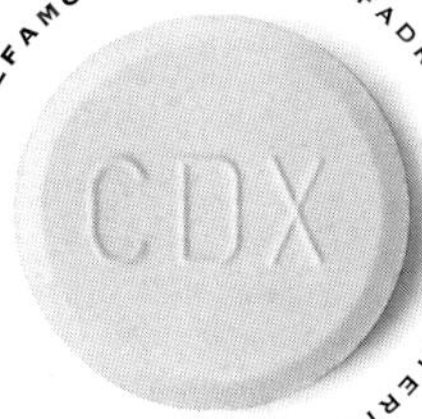

CEFAMOX® LÖSLIG (CEFADROXIL) MOT BAKTERIER.

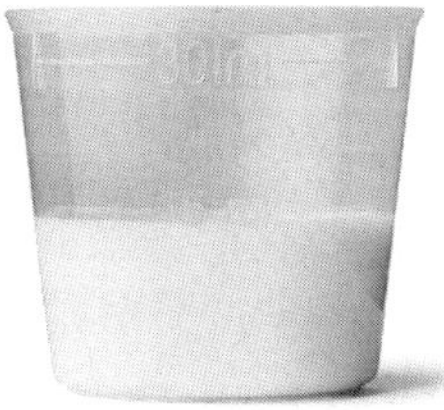

MYCOSTATIN® (NYSTATIN)
SVAMPMEDEL.

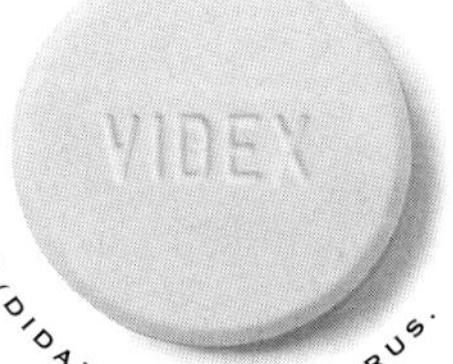

VIDEX® (DIDANOSIN) MOT VIRUS.

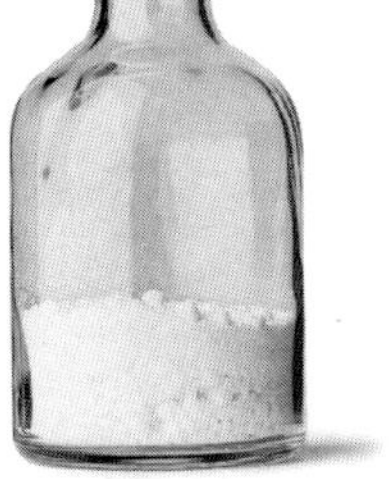

PENTREXYL® (AMPICILLIN)
MOT BAKTERIER

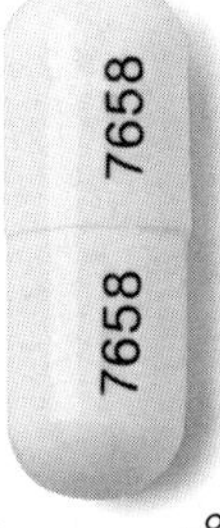

DICLOCIL® (DIKLOXACILLIN) MOT BAKTERIER.

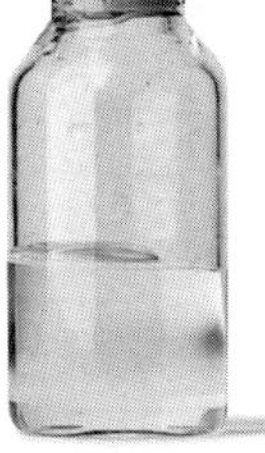

BIKLIN® (AMIKACIN)
MOT BAKTERIER.

AZACTAM (AZTREONAM). ANTIBIOTIKUM AV MONOBACTAM-TYP. INJEKTIONS- OCH INFUSIONSSUBSTANS 1G, 2 G. INDIKATIONER: INFEKTIONER ORSAKADE AV AZTREONAMKÄNSLIGA BAKTERIER, T EX SEPTIKEMI, ÖVRE URINVÄGSINFEKTIONER, KOMPLICERADE NEDRE URINVÄGSINFEKTIONER, NEDRE LUFTVÄGSINFEKTIONER ORSAKADE AV GRAMNEGATIVA BAKTERIER SAMT GONORRÉ. **BIKLIN (AMIKACIN).** BREDSPEKTRUMANTIBIOTIKUM. INJEKTIONSVÄTSKA 250 MG/ML. INDIKATIONER: INFEKTIONER AV ALLVARLIG ELLER LIVSHOTANDE KARAKTÄR SPECIELLT DÅ ETIOLOGIN ÄR OKÄND ELLER GRAMNEGATIV SEPTIKEMI BEFARAS. VID ALLVARLIGA INFEKTIONER AV OKÄND ETIOLOGI BÖR PREPARATET KOMBINERAS MED ETT BETALAKTAMANTIBIOTIKUM I AVVAKTAN PÅ ODLINGS- OCH RESISTENSBESKED. **CEFAMOX (CEFADROXIL).** ANTIBIOTIKUM AV CEFALOSPORINTYP. KAPSLAR 500 MG, TABLETTER 1G, PULVER TILL MIXTUR 100 MG/ML. INDIKATIONER: INFEKTIONER ORSAKADE AV MIKROORGANISMER KÄNSLIGA FÖR CEFADROXIL, EXEMPELVIS NEDRE OCH ÖVRE URINVÄGSINFEKTIONER, HUD- OCH MJUKDELSINFEKTIONER OCH ÄVEN ÖVRE LUFTVÄGSINFEKTIONER SÅSOM STREPTOKOCKTONSILLIT, DÄR PENICILLINBEHANDLING INTE GIVIT ÖNSKAD EFFEKT ELLER ÄR OLÄMPLIG AV ANDRA SKÄL. **DICLOCIL (DIKLOXACILLIN).** PENICILLINASSTABILT PENICILLIN. KAPSLAR 250 MG, 500 MG, PULVER TILL MIXTUR 12,5 MG/ML, INJEKTIONS- OCH INFEKTIONSSUBSTANS 0,5 G, 1 G, 2 G. INDIKATIONER: INFEKTIONER ORSAKADE AV PENICILLINASPRODUCERANDE STAFYLOKOCKER. **FUNGIZONE (AMFOTERICIN B).** ANTIBIOTIKUM MOT GENERALISERAD

Scand J Infect Dis 26: 309–316, 1994

Treatment of Clostridium difficile Associated Diarrhea and Colitis with an Oral Preparation of Teicoplanin; a Dose Finding Study

THE SWEDISH CDAD STUDY GROUP*

92 patients with antibiotic-associated diarrhea were randomized to receive oral teicoplanin 100 mg twice daily for 7 days (BID group); or 50 mg 4 times daily for 3 days, followed by 100 mg twice daily for 4 days (QID group) in a randomized, double-blind, multicentre study. Clostridium difficile was demonstrated by culture and/or cytotoxin test in 49 (53%) patients, of whom 47 (23 male, 24 females, mean age 65 years; 23 in the BID group, 24 in the QID group) were evaluable for clinical efficacy. Prior treatment with cephalosporins was registered in 49%, isoxazolyl-penicillins in 33% and clindamycin in 20% of the C. difficile positive patients. On the last day of treatment, 96% (23 of 24 patients) in the QID group were found cured, compared with 70% (16 of 23 patients) in the BID group ($p = 0.02$). On days 2 and 3 of treatment, QID group patients had significantly fewer loose stools per day ($p < 0.05$) than those of the BID group. Clinical recurrence, within 4 weeks post-treatment, occurred in 35% and 33% of the patients in the BID and QID groups, respectively. The bacteriological elimination rate 4 weeks post-treatment was 55% in the BID group and 59% in the QID group. The study was terminated prematurely due to the unexpectedly high clinical failure and recurrence rate in C. difficile positive patients treated with the BID dosage regimen.

J. Wiström, MD, PhD, Department of Infectious Diseases, University Hospital of Umeå, S-901 85 Umeå, Sweden

INTRODUCTION

The spectrum of Clostridium difficile-associated disease ranges from self-limiting diarrhea to severe and sometimes life-threatening colitis (1–4). Treatment with vancomycin, metronidazole or bacitracin may afford prompt alleviation, but symptomatic and bacteriological relapses are frequent (4–10).

---

* Members of the Swedish CDAD study group: Principal investigator: Johan Wiström, Department of Infectious Diseases and Clinical Bacteriology, University Hospital, Umeå, Sweden; Investigators: Rolf Lundholm, Department of Infectious Diseases and Clinical Bacteriology, University Hospital, Umeå, Sweden; Mårten Prag, Eva Törnkvist, Department of Infectious Diseases and Clinical Microbiology, Örebro Medical Centre Hospital, Örebro, Sweden; Rolf Maller, Steffan Ånsehn, Department of Infectious Diseases and Clinical Bacteriology, University Hospital, Linköping, Sweden; Per-Erik Åbom, Bertil Hoorn; Department of Infectious Diseases and Clinical Bacteriology, Ryhov Hospital, Jönköping, Sweden; Gunnel Nyström, Lars-Olof Mentzing, Department of Infectious Diseases and Clinical Bacteriology, Karlstad Hospital, Karlstad, Sweden; Erling Myhre, Claes Schalén, Independent evaluator: S. Ragnar Norrby, Department of Infectious Diseases and Clinical Microbiology, University Hospital, Lund, Sweden; Claus Holmen, Jörgen Hannover Larsen, Department of Infectious Diseases and Clinical Bacteriology, Boden Hospital, Boden, Sweden; Sven-Åke Hedström, Department of Infectious Diseases, Halmstad Hospital, Halmstad, Sweden; Sverker Eriksson, Department of Infectious Diseases, Norrköping Hospital, Norrköping, Sweden; Anders Strömberg, Bengt Wretlind, Department of Infectious Diseases and Clinical Bacteriology, Danderyds Hospital, Danderyd, Sweden; Göran Bondesson, Astra Arcus AB, Södertälje, Sweden; Ian Harding, Merrel Dow Research Institute, Reading Road, Winnersh, Berkshire RG11 5HQ, England. Present address: Thackelay's Research Consultancy, 8 Corner Cottage, Horton, Devizes, Wiltshire, SN10 3NB, England; Microbiological coordinator: Carl Erik Nord, Department of Oral microbiology, Karolinska Institute, University Hospital, Huddinge, Sweden.

Teicoplanin is a new non-absorbable glycopeptide antibiotic, structurally related to vancomycin (11). Teicoplanin has a high in vitro activity against C. difficile, with minimal inhibitory concentrations ranging from <0.007 to 2.0 mg/l, compared with 0.125 to 4.0 mg/l for vancomycin (11–14). Studies on oral treatment of C. difficile associated diarrhea, using the parenteral formulation of teicoplanin, have given favourable results (14, 15).

As with vancomycin, there is reason to develop a preparation of teicoplanin suitable for oral use. In the present study 2 different dosage regimens of a capsule of teicoplanin were compared for treatment of C. difficile-associated diarrhea and colitis.

PATIENTS AND METHODS

Study design

This was a prospective, coordinated, randomized, double-blind (double-dummy), clinical, multicentre, dose-finding trial to assess the efficacy of 2 different dosage regimens of an oral capsule formulation of teicoplanin for the treatment of C. difficile associated diarrhea. It was performed between September 1989 and March 1991 at 10 Departments of Infectious Diseases in Sweden. The study was approved by the relevant regional research Ethics Committees. All patients gave witnessed verbal informed consent to participate.

The 2 dose regimens were chosen on the basis of available microbiological and clinical data for oral teicoplanin treatment of C. difficile infections (11, 12). In order to detect a 25%-unit difference in cure rate between the 2 different dosage regimens, and assuming a cure rate of 90% for the best treatment, at least 80 patients with C. difficile had to be enrolled in the trial. This was based on a 2-tailed χ^2 test at the 5% level and with a power of 80% to detect the difference.

An interim analysis by the independent evaluator revealed a higher failure and recurrence rate than initially anticipated and the study was therefore terminated prematurely with only 49 C. difficile positive patients included.

Patients

Patients aged ≥18 years with diarrheal disease, either known or on clinical grounds strongly suspected to be due to C. difficile, and who had received antibacterial therapy within the last 6 weeks were eligible for the trial. Exclusion criteria were pregnancy and nursing, hypersensitivity to vancomycin or teicoplanin, treatment with teicoplanin, vancomycin, fusidic acid, bacitracin or imidazole derivatives during the preceding 6 days, known non-infectious diarrhea (inflammatory bowel disease), infectious diarrhea due to micro-organisms other than C. difficile, treatment for C. difficile induced diarrhea during the preceding 6 weeks, HIV and/or hepatitis B infection and previous inclusion in the study. Patients fulfilling inclusion (but not exclusion) criteria, who had a history of diarrhea and ≥4 loose stools or ≥2 loose stools plus any of the following symptoms: fever >38°C rectal temperature or abdominal cramp during the previous 24 h period were eligible for randomization.

Treatment regimen

Patients were randomized to start treatment with either teicoplanin 100 mg twice daily for 7 days (BID group) or teicoplanin 50 mg 4 times daily for 3 days, followed by teicoplanin 100 mg twice daily for 4 days (QID group). Capsules containing 50 mg of teicoplanin sodium and fully identical placebo capsules containing maize starch and talc (manufactured by Marion Merrell Dow Pharmaceuticals Ltd. U.K. and distributed by Astra Arcus, Södertälje, Sweden) were delivered in code numbered blister packs with 8 capsules for each day. Treatment was always initiated with active medication (dose one of day one). All doses were given at least 1 h before a meal.

Patients were hospitalized on enrolment but could be discharged during the study period if there was a marked improvement. Written and verbal instructions about the conduct of the trial were given together with diary cards for daily registration of tablet intake, stool frequency, stool consistency, body temperature, and presence or absence of vomiting and abdominal pain. Concurrent medication including antibiotics (but not vancomycin, metronidazole, fusidic acid or bacitracin), were given at the discretion of the investigator and recorded on the case record form.

A history of possible gastrointestinal symptoms experienced after therapy was obtained on day 5 to 7 after completed treatment (first follow-up). The last follow-up was performed 4 weeks after the end of treatment when the patient was seen by one of the investigators and diary cards were checked.

A serum sample for routine haematology and renal and liver function tests was obtained before the start of treatment, on the last day of treatment in hospitalized patients, in case of relapse and at the follow-up 4 weeks after the end of treatment.

Adverse reactions were registered by asking an open-ended question about unusual symptoms during treatment.

Evaluation of efficacy and safety

All decisions concerning classification and evaluation of efficacy and safety were taken before the patient data were divided into treatment groups and the randomization code was broken. To be included in the efficacy analysis, the patients had to have demonstrable C. difficile cytotoxin or verified presence of C. difficile in the faecal specimen obtained on enrolment. To be included in the safety analysis the patient must have taken at least 1 dose of the study drug.

The course of illness was assessed daily during treatment, with one end-point on the last day of treatment and the main end-point at the last follow-up, 4 weeks post-treatment. Patients were classified as, cured (<1 loose stool/24 h without additional symptoms), improved (2 loose stools/24 h without additional symptoms or 1 loose stool/24 h with accompanying symptoms), or failed. Recurrence was defined as cure followed by return to inclusion criteria during the follow-up period of 4 weeks after treatment. The day when treatment was started was defined as day 1.

Bacteriological efficacy for C. difficile was defined as: elimination (negative culture and cytotoxin assay at follow-up), persistence (identification of C. difficile and/or cytotoxin before and after treatment), relapse (culture positive and/or cytotoxin positive after initial elimination).

Microbiological procedures

Faecal samples for culture on routine selective media for the presence of C. difficile (16), Salmonella spp., Shigella spp., Campylobacter spp., and Yersinia enterocolitica, and for C. difficile cytotoxin assay were obtained on enrolment, the day after completion of treatment in hospitalized patients, in the event of relapse, and at follow-up 4 weeks after treatment. C. difficile cytotoxin B was assayed on cell-lines according to the routine procedures at the local laboratory, an effect which was neutralized by C. difficile antitoxin (SBL, Stockholm, Sweden). Specimens were frozen within 3 h if delay in processing of more than 24 h was anticipated.

Statistical methods

Wilcoxon's 2-sample test was used to compare treatment results at the last follow-up, the time to clinical cure, and the mean number of loose stools per day. Clinical and bacteriological outcome at the last follow-up was assessed as the overall effect for the whole scale of cured/improved/recurrence/failure and elimination/relapse/persistence, respectively. Chi-square tests (or when appropriate Fisher's exact test) were used to compare cure rates and incidence of adverse reactions between treatment groups. A 95% CI is given when appropriate. Statistical analyses was performed using Statview™ (Abascus Inc., Berkeley, CA, USA) and Epi Info™ (USD Inc., Stone Mountain, GA., USA).

RESULTS

Demographic data for the 92 patients randomized for treatment before the study was terminated, the 49 who had demonstrable C. difficile cytotoxin and/or positive culture for C. difficile before start of treatment and the 47 (96% of C. difficile positive) patients evaluable for efficacy are given in Table I. The large proportion of patients yielding positive assays for C. difficile (2), may be explained by the use of relatively strict inclusion criteria with regard to clinical suspicion of this infection. Two C. difficile positive patients (1 culture positive/ toxin negative) who did not fulfil the inclusion criteria with respect to the required number of loose stools per day were excluded from evaluation of efficacy. One patient in the QID group discontinued treatment on day 3 due to nausea, but was included in the clinical evaluation for efficacy. The mean duration of treatment was 6.8 days (range 3–7 days) in both treatment groups.

Table I. *Characteristics of the patient population before randomization to treatment with teicoplanin 100 mg BID for 7 days (BID group) or 50 mg QID for 3 days followed by 100 mg BID for 4 days (QID group)*

Patient characteristics	Dosage regimen	
	BID group	QID group
No. of patients randomized and analysed for safety	43	49
Gender (male/female)	22/21	19/30
Mean age (years; range)	59(21–92)	58(16–88)
No. of patients with concomitant non-infectious disease	25	24
No. of C. difficile positive patients	24	25
No. of patients analysed for clinical efficacy	23	24
Gender (male/female)	13/10	10/14
Mean age (years; range)	65(45–86)	64(26–88)
Mean number of loose stools on inclusion	7.8	7.6
No. of patients with watery stools on inclusion (%)	10(44)	14(55)

Cephalosporins, isoxazolyl-penicillins and clindamycin were the antibiotics most frequently administered to the patients during the 6 weeks preceding enrolment in the study (Table II). Among the 34 patients treated with cephalosporins prior to enrolment administration of an oral cephalosporin was registered on 14 occasions (13 with cefadroxil and 1 with cefaclor) and parenteral cephalosporins on 34 occasions (15 each with cefotaxime or cefuroxime and 4 with ceftazidime). Treatment with a cephalosporin ($p = 0.02$) and clindamycin ($p = 0.1$) was more common in C. difficile positive than in C. difficile negative patients, while the converse was true for beta-lactams other than cephalosporins and isoxazolyl-penicillins ($p = 0.01$) (Table II).

Clinical results

On the last day of treatment the clinical cure rate (% of patients cured) among patients evaluable for efficacy was 70% (16 of 23 patients) in the BID group compared with 96% (23

Table II. *Antibiotic treatment during a period of 6 weeks preceding the inclusion in the study; patients with multiple medication appear several times*

Antibiotic treatment	No. patients (%)	
	Clostridium positive ($n = 49$)	Clostridium negative ($n = 43$)
Single antibiotic	18(37)	24(56)
≥3 antibiotics	16(33)	8(19)
Cephalosporin	24(49)	10(23)*
Isoxazolyl-penicillin	16(33)	12(28)
Clindamycin	10(20)	3(7)
Beta-lactam antibiotics other than cephalosporins and isoxazolyl-penicillins	10(20)	21(49)*
Other antibiotics	20(41)	15(35)

* Denotes statistical significance between C. difficile positive and negative patients, $p < 0.05$.

of 24 patients) in the QID group ($p = 0.02$). At this time 3 BID patients (13%) were classified as improved, whereas 4 patients (17%) were failures. One patient (4%) in the QID group failed treatment. Clinical recurrence occurred within 4 weeks post-treatment in one-third of the patients in both treatment groups (Table III). No difference was found between QID and BID treatment in the overall clinical outcome ($p = 0.08$) at the last follow-up 4 weeks post-treatment (a mean of 27 days after treatment) (Table III).

The clinical outcome for the 5 evaluable patients (3 BID and 2 QID) who had positive C. difficile culture and negative cytotoxin assay in their pre-treatment samples did not differ from that of the cytotoxin-positive subjects, 2 of these patients were classified as cured (1 in each group) and 1 patient each as having improvement (BID group), failure (BID group) or recurrence (QID group).

The mean number of loose stools per day was significantly ($p = <0.05$) lower on day 2 (4.0 vs 7.2) and on day 3 of treatment (2.7 vs 4.4) in patients of the QID group than in those of the BID group. No statistically significant difference was found during treatment between the BID and QID groups with respect to the number of patients who experienced watery diarrhea or in the initial mean time to cure (4.9 days for the BID group compared with 4.4 days for the QID group, $p = >0.6$).

The 2 C. difficile positive patients not included in the efficacy analyses were cured. 14 evaluable patients (9 BID and 5 QID) received concomitant antibiotic treatment (6 subjects a quinolone, 2 each a cephalosporin or ampicillin, and 1 each clindamycin, imipenem, doxycycline and gentamicin) during the time for study medication. Among these patients clinical cure was recorded in 9 (64%), improvement in 1 (7%), recurrence in 3 (22%) and failure in the 1 patient (7%). Patients with recurrence were older than those with cure (mean age 74 vs 61 years). 11 of 24 evaluable women (46%) experienced recurrence, compared with 5 of 23 men (22%) ($p = 0.1$).

The 43 initially C. difficile negative patients were in most cases not evaluated further until the end of treatment (mean of 6 days) or until the time of discharge from hospital. At this point, 39% (7/18) and 78% (18/23) of the assessable cases were classified as cured in the BID group and QID group, respectively ($p = 0.02$), while 22% (4/18) and 4% (1/23) respectively

Table III. *Clinical and bacteriological outcome at last follow-up, 4 weeks post-treatment, in C. difficile positive patients after treatment with teicoplanin 100 mg BID for 7 days (BID group) or 50 mg QID for 3 days followed by 100 mg BID for 4 days (QID group)*

	No. (%) of patients		
Outcome	BID group	QID group	Total
A) *Clinical outcome**	($n = 23$)	($n = 24$)	($n = 47$)
Clinical cure	8(35)	15(63)	23(49)
Clinical improvement	3(13)	0	3(6)
Clinical recurrence	8(35)	8(33)	16(34)
Clinical failure	4(17)	1(4)	5(11)
B) *Bacteriological outcome***	($n = 22$)	($n = 24$)	($n = 46$)
Bacteriological elimination	12(55)	14(59)	26(56)
Bacteriological relapse	3(13)	8(33)	11(24)
Bacteriological persistence	7(32)	2(8)	9(20)

Statistical difference between BID and QID groups, * $p = 0.08$, ** $p = 0.4$.

had improved. The remaining 39% (7/18) of patients in the BID group and 17% (4/23) in the QID group were clinical failures.

Adverse events

Nine adverse advents were reported from 7 of the 92 patients evaluable for safety, 3 of 43 patients (7%) in the BID and 4 of 49 patients (8%) in the QID group (CI, −12.0% to 9.6%; $p = >0.6$), respectively. In the BID group a 61-year-old woman, classified as a clinical failure, died on day 4 due to a combination of lymphoma and pseudomembranous colitis without perforation. Her colitis had improved considerably at that time, from 19 watery loose stools on enrolment to 4 loose stools during the 24 h prior to death. Furthermore 1 patient in the BID group complained of vomiting and nausea, leading to treatment withdrawal on day 3, and one other patient experienced exanthema. In the QID group 1 patient each complained of metallic taste, pruritus, arthralgia and hallucinations and 1 patient with history of alcohol abuse experienced paranoid symptoms. There were no tendencies towards more frequent abnormal laboratory values in either treatment group.

Bacteriological results on inclusion

Of the 49 patients with positive C. difficile culture and/or cytotoxin assay in pre-treatment samples, 33 (68%) were cytotoxin and culture positive, 5 (10%) were cytotoxin positive only, 5 (10%) were cytotoxin positive and had no assessable culture and 6 (12%) were culture positive only. Two campylobacter and 2 salmonella infections were found among the C. difficile negative patients in the pre-treatment samples.

Bacteriological outcome

46 patients were evaluable for bacteriological outcome, 22 in the BID and 24 in the QID group, respectively (Table III). The elimination rate of C. difficile did not differ between the BID and QID groups (55% vs. 59%) (Table III).

Bacteriological elimination was found in 81% (21/26) of patients from both groups with clinical cure or improvement, in 25% (4/16) of patients with clinical recurrence, in 25% (1/4) of assessable patients with clinical failure and in 79% (11/14) of the patients who received concomitant antibiotic treatment.

DISCUSSION

Although terminated prematurely, this is the only study so far to have evaluated oral teicoplanin capsules for empirical treatment of clinically suspected C. difficile associated diarrhea. Among evaluable patients, the QID regimen proved superior to the BID regimen, and gave a significantly higher cure rate and lower mean number of loose stools during the first stage of treatment as well as higher rates of initial bacterial elimination. The clinical curve (70%) rate observed at the end of treatment among patients treated with BID dosage regimen was lower than anticipated and this, together with a high clinical recurrence rate, was the main reason for terminating the study. The clinical results obtained with the QID dosage are on the other hand comparable with those observed in a number of clinical trials with varying dosage regimens of vancomycin or metronidazole (4–9, 15).

Previous studies employing the parenteral formulation of teicoplanin for oral treatment of C. difficile associated colitis have reported excellent results (14, 15). In one study, 100 mg of parenteral teicoplanin twice daily (identical to the daily dose used in this study) for 10 days was compared with vancomycin 500 mg 4 times a day (15). Clinical recurrence occurred in only 2 (8%) and bacteriological relapse/persistence in 5 (19%) of 26 teicoplanin-treated patients, while 4 (20%) of 20 vancomycin-treated patients recurred and in 9 (45%) C. difficile was not eliminated. Differences in the patient population, study design and duration of treatment may have contributed to the discrepancy in results obtained with oral teicoplanin in that study and the present one. However, the pharmacokinetic properties of the oral formulation (capsule) used in the present study may have differed from that of the parenteral formulation previously used (14, 15). Although faecal concentrations of teicoplanin were not monitored in this study it is possible that the concentrations of teicoplanin achieved, especially with the BID dosage, in patients suffering from frequent loose stools in the early stage of their disease, were inadequate to eradicate or even suppress C. difficile.

Endogenous presence of C. difficile despite high levels of antibiotic in the stools, re-establishment of C. difficile by bacterial spores not affected by treatment, and reinfection from exogenous sources, have been suggested as possible explanations of bacterial relapses and clinical recurrence (4, 8, 9, 17–19). Approximately 20–25% of patients treated with vancomycin or metronidazole experience recurrent diarrhea (4–9, 15), which is less than the 33–35% recurrence rate reported here. High rates of bacteriological persistence and relapse, similar to that found in the present study, have also been reported following vancomycin treatment of C. difficile infection (4, 7–9, 14). Elimination of C. difficile is however only partly related to clinical cure (4, 6–9, 15, 18) as illustrated by our result in which asymptomatic persistence or relapse of C. difficile occurred in approximately 20% of patients with clinical cure.

Discontinuation of antibiotic therapy is recommended for initial treatment of C. difficile-associated diarrhea (2, 3). In this study no differences were seen in clinical or bacteriological outcome in patients with or without continued treatment with other antibiotics. The number were too low to allow any firm conclusion to be drawn but it is conceivable that such treatment, if indicated, can be continued using antibiotics with as little selective pressure on the faecal flora as possible.

The specific aetiology of antibiotic-associated diarrhea not caused by C. difficile has not been elucidated, nor is it known whether these patients will benefit from specific antibiotic treatment (2). In the present study, treatment with the QID regimen proved to be significantly more effective than the BID regimen also among this category of patients. This observation might mean that at least certain patients with antibiotic-associated diarrhea in whom present routine tests, despite their high sensitivity (2), fail to detect C. difficile or its toxin could benefit from specific antibiotic treatment.

Our results confirm previous observations that antibiotics which make an appreciable impact on the anaerobic intestinal flora, such as cephalosporins and lincosamides, are the agents most frequently blamed for precipitating C. difficile disease (2, 3, 20).

In conclusion, a high initial cure rate was achieved in the treatment of C. difficile associated diarrhea, by using an oral preparation of teicoplanin in a dosage regimen of 50 mg 4 times daily for 3 days followed by 100 mg twice daily for 4 days. This regimen was superior to a dosage of 100 mg teicoplanin twice daily for 7 days. However, clinical recurrence was noted in one-third of the patients and bacteriological persistence or relapse in nearly half of those treated with both regimens. Further clinical, bacteriological and pharmacokinetic studies, in comparison with other commonly used agents, are warranted in order to establish an appropriate oral formulation of teicoplanin as well as the most effective, convenient and least costly dosage regimen for treatment of C. difficile associated diarrhea.

ACKNOWLEDGMENTS

This study was supported by a grant from the Marion Merrell Dow Research Institute, Winnersh, England and Astra Arcus AB, Södertälje, Sweden.

REFERENCES

1. Aronsson B, Möllby R, Nord CE. Diagnosis and epidemiology of Clostridium difficile enterocolitis in Sweden. J Antimicrob Chemother 14 (Suppl D): 85–95, 1984.
2. Bartlett JG. Antibiotic associated diarrhea. Clin Infect Dis 15: 573–581, 1992.
3. Fekety R, Shah AB. Diagnosis and treatment of Clostridium difficile colitis. JAMA 269: 71–75, 1993.
4. Wilcox MH, Spencer RC. Clostridium difficile infection: responses, relapses and reinfections. J Hosp Infect 22: 85–92, 1992.
5. Keighley MRB, Burdon DW, Arabi Y, Alexander-Williams J, Thompson H, Youngs D, Johnson M, Bentley S, George RH, Mogg GAG. Randomised controlled trial of vancomycin for pseudomembranous colitis and postoperative diarrhoea. BMJ 2: 1667–1669, 1978.
6. Teasley DG, Gerding DN, Olson MM, Peterson LR, Gebhard RL, Schwartz MJ, Lee JT. Prospective randomised trial of metronidazole versus vancomycin for Clostridium-difficile-associated diarrhoea and colitis. Lancet 2: 1043–1046, 1983.
7. Young GP, Ward PB, Bayley N, Gordon D, Higgins G, Trapini JA, McDonald MI, Labrooy J, Hecker R. Antibiotic-associated colitis due to Clostridium difficile: double-blind comparison of vancomycin with bacitracin. Gastroenterology 89: 1038–1045, 1985.
8. Bartlett JG, Tedesco FJ, Shull S, Lowe B, Chang T. Symptomatic relapse after oral vancomycin therapy of antibiotic-associated pseudomembranous colitis. Gastroenterology 78: 431–434, 1980.
9. Walters BAJ, Robert SR, Stafford R, Senevirarne E. Relapse of antibiotic associated colitis: endogenous persistence of Clostridium difficile during vancomycin therapy. Gut 24: 206–212, 1983.
10. Johnson S, Homann SR, Bettin KM, Quick JN, Clabots CR, Peterson LR, Gerding DN. Treatment of asymptomatic Clostridium difficile carriers (fecal excretors) with vancomicin or metronidazole. A randomized, placebo controlled trial. Ann Intern Med 117: 297–302, 1992.
11. Babul N, Pasko M. Teicoplanin: A new glycopeptide antibiotic complex. Drug Intell Clin Pharm 22: 218–226, 1988.
12. Newsom SW, Matthews J, Rampling AM. Susceptibility of Clostridium difficile strains to new antibiotics: quinolones, efrotomycin, teicoplanin and imipenem. J Antimicrob Chemother 15: 648–650, 1985.
13. Bartoloni A, Colao MG, Orsi A, Dei R, Giganti E, Parenti F. In-vitro activity of vancomycin, teicoplanin, daptomycin, ramoplanin, MDL 62873 and other agents against staphylococci, enterocooci and Clostridium difficile. J Antimicrob Chemother 26: 627–633, 1990.
14. de Lalla F, Privitera G, Rinaldi E, Ortisi G, Santoro D, Rizzardini G. Treatment of Clostridium difficile-associated disease with teicoplanin. Antimicrob Agents Chemother 33: 1125–1127, 1989.
15. de Lalla F, Nicolin R, Rinaldi E, Scarpellini P, Rigoli R, Manfrin V, Tramarin A. Prospective study of oral teicoplanin versus oral vancomycin for therapy of pseudomembranous colitis and Clostridium difficile-associated diarrhea. Antimicrob Agents Chemother 36: 2192–2196, 1992.
16. George LW, Sutter LV, Citron D, Finegold SM. Selective and differential medium for isolation of Clostridium difficile. J Clin Microbiol 9: 214–219, 1979.
17. Young GP, Bayley N, Ward P, St John DJB, McDonald MI. Antibiotic-associated colitis caused by Clostridium difficile: relapse and risk factors. Med J Aust 144: 303–306, 1986.
18. Johnson S, Calbots CR, Linn FV, Olson MM, Peterson LR, Gerding DN. Nosocomial Clostridium difficile colonisation and disease. Lancet 336: 97–100, 1990.
19. McFarland LV, Surawicz CM, Stamm WE. Risk factors for Clostridium difficile carriage and C. difficile-associated diarrhea in a cohort of hospitalized patients. J Infect Dis 162: 678–684, 1990.
20. Aronsson B, Möllby R, Nord CE. Antimicrobial agents and Clostridium difficile in acute enteric disease: epidemiological data from Sweden, 1980–1982. J Infect Dis 151: 476–481, 1985.

Submitted December 14, 1993; accepted February 16, 1994

Scand J Infect Dis 26: 317–320, 1994

Resistance to Fluoroquinolones in Pseudomonas aeruginosa and Klebsiella pneumoniae

JOHAN RYDBERG, CHARLOTTE LARSSON and HÅKAN MIÖRNER

From the Department of Medical Microbiology, University Hospital of Lund, Lund, Sweden

The fluoroquinolone sensitivity of Pseudomonas aeruginosa and Klebsiella pneumoniae was studied by determinations of Minimum Inhibitory Concentrations (MICs) of norfloxacin and ciprofloxacin in consecutive clinical isolates. In P. aeruginosa, resistance or reduced susceptibility (MIC ≥ 8 mg/l for norfloxacin and ≥ 2 mg/l for ciprofloxacin) was found in 17% (9/54) of the isolates. Reduced susceptibility (MIC ≥ 2 mg/l for norfloxacin) was found in 12% (10/84) of K. pneumoniae isolates. P. aeruginosa strains isolated in 1991 had reduced susceptibility to both norfloxacin and ciprofloxacin significantly more often than isolates from 1984–85 ($p = 0.02$). 10/84 K. pneumoniae strains from 1991 had reduced susceptibility to norfloxacin, compared with 1/34 from 1984–85. This difference was not statistically significant ($p = 0.11$).

J. Rydberg, MD, Department of Medical Microbiology, Sölvegatan 23, S-223 62 Lund, Sweden

INTRODUCTION

The fluoroquinolones are very effective antibiotics against most Gram-negative aerobic and microaerophilic bacteria. They interact with the bacterial enzyme DNA gyrase and thereby interfere with the DNA-supercoiling in sensitive bacteria (1). Two main modes of resistance have been described: bacteria may become resistant to fluoroquinolones via mutations in the A subunit of the DNA-gyrase, or via permeability changes in the cell membrane (2, 3).

Norfloxacin was introduced in Sweden in 1986 and was soon adopted as an important antibiotic against urinary tract infections. Ciprofloxacin has been used since 1988 for treatment of urinary tract infections, but also against other infections caused by Gram-negative and Gram-positive bacteria. The main advantages of these antibiotics, when compared with other antibacterials, are their activity against P. aeruginosa, also when given orally, and their very low MIC values for Enterobacteriaceae. However, we have recently observed a large number of isolates of P. aeruginosa and K. pneumoniae with diminished susceptibility to fluoroquinolones. This finding prompted a study of the fluoroquinolone sensitivity of consecutive clinical isolates of P. aeruginosa and K. pneumoniae. Isolates from blood cultures obtained in 1984 and 1985 were used as control strains.

MATERIALS AND METHODS

Clinical samples

From clinical urine specimens sent to our laboratory, 92 consecutive isolates of K. pneumoniae from 84 patients, and 61 consecutive isolates of P. aeruginosa from 54 patients were obtained during a 3-month period. Duplicate specimens were excluded from further evaluation.

The urine specimens came from both outpatients and hospitalized patients from several different community care centres, clinics and wards in 3 different towns. In no case did more than 2 of the specimens come from the same community care centre or hospital clinic. The samples were cultured overnight on blood-agar plates and McConkey plates in a semi-quantitative manner, using routine techniques. All isolates were saved on deep agar for further MIC-testing. The initial species identification of all strains with reduced susceptibility was verified with API-20E or API-NE (Bio-Mérieux, Marcy-l'Etoile, France).

Susceptibility testing

MICs of norfloxacin and ciprofloxacin were determined with an agar dilution method on PDM II agar (AB Biodisk, Solna, Sweden). The klebsiella strains were also tested for nalidixic acid. For all isolates

 ISSN 0036-5548

with reduced susceptibility, the MIC was determined in parallel with the E-test (AB Biodisk, Solna, Sweden) (4). The concordance between the E-test and agar dilution MIC was very good. In the few cases with minor discrepancy, the MICs of agar dilution were used in the presentation of results.

Control strains

Strains of P. aeruginosa ($n = 27$) and K. pneumoniae ($n = 34$) isolated from blood cultures in 1984 and 1985, before the introduction in Sweden of fluoroquinolones, were used as controls. The strains had been kept at −80°C in calf serum. They were thawed and subcultured to PDM II agar and their norfloxacin and ciprofloxacin MICs were determined with the E-test.

Statistics

Fisher's exact test was used to calculate statistical correlations.

RESULTS

In this consecutive study of urinary tract isolates, 84 K. pneumoniae strains were tested. 12% of K. pneumoniae isolates (10 of 84 strains) had reduced susceptibility to norfloxacin with MIC ≥ 2 mg/l. Five percent (4 of the original 84 strains) had reduced susceptibility (MIC ≥ 2 mg/l) to ciprofloxacin. All 10 strains with reduced susceptibility to norfloxacin were resistant to nalidixic acid with MIC ≥ 64 mg/l. One of the 34 control strains from 1984–85 had reduced susceptibility to norfloxacin and none to ciprofloxacin (Table I).

Altogether 54 consecutive strains of P. aeruginosa were tested. Nine strains (17%) of P. aeruginosa had MIC ≥ 8 mg/l to norfloxacin and were resistant (Table II). Among these 9 strains, 7 had MIC ≥ 8 mg/l to ciprofloxacin and were resistant to this drug as well. The remaining 2 were of intermediate susceptibility.

None of the 27 control strains were resistant to norfloxacin or ciprofloxacin. This discrepancy in sensitivity between the strains from 1991 and 1984–85 was statistically significant (Table II).

Table I. *Reduced susceptibility to norfloxacin and ciprofloxacin in Klebsiella pneumoniae*

	Klebsiella pneumoniae		
	1991 ($n = 84$)	1984–85 ($n = 34$)	p-value
Norfloxacin (MIC ≥ 2 mg/l)	12% (10)	3% (1)	0.11 ns
Ciprofloxacin (MIC ≥ 2 mg/l)	5% (4)	0% (0)	0.25 ns

Table II. *Resistance to norfloxacin and reduced susceptibility to ciprofloxacin in Pseudomonas aeruginosa*

	Pseudomonas aeruginosa		
	1991 ($n = 54$)	1984–85 ($n = 27$)	p-value
Norfloxacin (MIC ≥ 8 mg/l)	17% (9)	0% (0)	0.02
Ciprofloxacin (MIC ≥ 2 mg/l)	17% (9)	0% (0)	0.02

DISCUSSION

This study has demonstrated the emergence of resistance (MIC $\geq$ 8 mg/l) or decreased susceptibility (MIC $\geq$ 2 mg/l) to the fluoroquinolones norfloxacin and ciprofloxacin in consecutive clinical isolates from 1991 of P. aeruginosa, and a trend in the same direction for K. pneumoniae.

The fluoroquinolones were introduced in Sweden in 1986 with norfloxacin for use against urinary tract infections. One of their advantages was their vigorous activity against P. aeruginosa. Ciprofloxacin is also used against respiratory tract infections, including treatment of infections in patients suffering from cystic fibrosis, where P. aeruginosa is a major pathogen.

In Sweden, norfloxacin has a central role in the treatment of urinary tract infections, both in hospital and in primary health care. The fluoroquinolones have obvious advantages by virtue of their oral use also against difficult-to-treat organisms, high activity against urinary tract pathogens and their high degree of safety. However, during recent years, international reports have documented a decreased susceptibility to fluoroquinolones in P. aeruginosa, e.g. from 98.6% sensitive isolates in 1986 to 86.3% in 1989 (5). Our study confirms that the same development has occurred in Sweden. Furthermore, the P. aeruginosa strains not only had reduced susceptibility but were definitely resistant according to Swedish recommended break-points, with MICs $\geq$ 8 mg/l for both norfloxacin and ciprofloxacin. The occurrence of resistance in P. aeruginosa is perhaps not too surprising, but the number of resistant isolates is so high that susceptibility of P. aeruginosa to fluoroquinolones can no longer be taken for granted.

There have also been reports on increasing resistance to fluoroquinolones in Campylobacter species (6, 7) and in staphylococci (5). The finding in the present consecutive non-selected material, of 12% K. pneumoniae with reduced susceptibility to norfloxacin, is striking as the Enterobacteriaceae have been considered almost invariably sensitive to fluoroquinolones. Rare exceptions have even been published as case reports (8). A highly fluoroquinolone-resistant E. coli strain was reported earlier from Sweden (9) and 3% E. coli strains with reduced susceptibility to norfloxacin and lomefloxacin were found in a study from 3 different counties in southern Sweden. Almost all of these E. coli strains came from one of the 3 counties, indicating that there are regional differences in susceptibility to fluoroquinolones (10). When analysing recent data from our laboratory, the results from 1991 are confirmed by findings in urinary isolates from 1993. Judged by the disc diffusion test, 10% of 125 consecutive K. pneumoniae isolates and 21% of 86 consecutive P. aeruginosa isolates from urine were resistant to norfloxacin. This development must be monitored carefully and may become a challenge to the future usefulness of fluoroquinolones as empirical drugs in complicated urinary tract infections.

REFERENCES

1. Hooper DC, Wolfson JS. Mode of action of the new quinolones: New data. Eur J Clin Microbiol Infect Dis 10: 223–231, 1991.
2. Bryan LE, Bedard J. Impermeability to quinolones in Gram-positive and Gram-negative bacteria. Eur J Clin Microbiol Infect Dis 10: 232–239, 1991.
3. Bryan LE, Bedard J, Chamberland S, Wong S. Quinolone antimicrobial agents: mechanism of action and resistance development. Clin Invest Med 12: 14–19, 1989.
4. Baker CN, Stocker SA, Culver DH, Thornsberry C. Comparison of the E-test to agar dilution, broth microdilution, and agar diffusion susceptibility testing techniques by using a special challenge set of bacteria. J Clin Microbiol 29: 533–538, 1991.
5. George RC, Ball LC, Norbury PB. Susceptibility to ciprofloxacin of nosocomial Gram-negative bacteria and staphylococci isolated in the UK. J Antimicrob Chemother 26 (Suppl F): 145–156, 1990.

6. Endtz HP, Ruijs GJ, van Klingeren B, Jansen WH, van der Reyden T, Mouton RP. Quinolone resistance in campylobacter isolated from man and poultry following the introduction of fluoroquinolones in veterinary medicine. J Antimicrob Chemother 27: 199–208, 1991.
7. Wretlind B, Strömberg A, Östlund L, Sjögren E, Kaijser B. Rapid emergence of quinolone resistance in Campylobacter jejuni in patients treated with norfloxacin. Scand J Infect Dis 24: 685–686, 1992.
8. Lopez-Brea M, Alarcon T. Isolation of fluoroquinolone-resistant Escherichia coli and Klebsiella pneumoniae from an infected Hickman catheter. Eur J Clin Microbiol Infect Dis 9: 345–347, 1990.
9. Jonsson M, Walder M, Forsgren A. First clinical isolate of highly fluoroquinolone-resistant Escherichia coli in Scandinavia. Eur J Clin Microbiol Infect Dis 9: 851–853, 1990.
10. Neringer R, Forsgren A, Hansson C, Ode B and the south Swedish Lolex study group. Lomefloxacin versus norfloxacin in the treatment of uncomplicated urinary tract infections: three-day versus seven-day treatment. Scand J Infect Dis 24: 773–780, 1992.

Submitted October 19, 1993; accepted February 1, 1994

Scand J Infect Dis 26: 321–327, 1994

Impact of Metronidazole Resistance on the Eradication of Helicobacter pylori

LESLIE A. NOACH[1], WIES L. LANGENBERG[2], MAURO A. BERTOLA[3], JAAP DANKERT[2] and GUIDO N. J. TYTGAT[1]

From the Departments of [1]Gastroenterology and Hepatology, and of [2]Microbiology, Academic Medical Centre, Amsterdam, and [3]Brocades Pharma Yamanouchi Group, Leiderdorp, The Netherlands

We investigated how often Helicobacter pylori was resistant to metronidazole before treatment in 283 H. pylori positive patients and whether the in vitro susceptibility to metronidazole could predict the clinical outcome of several drug regimens containing metronidazole. Metronidazole susceptibility was tested using either disc diffusion or plates containing metronidazole. Metronidazole-resistant strains were found in 41% of patients before their first anti-H. pylori treatment course. In patients with metronidazole-susceptible isolates, eradication was achieved in 74% after colloidal bismuth subcitrate (CBS) with metronidazole and in 91% after triple therapies consisting of CBS, metronidazole and amoxicillin or tetracycline. Dual therapies of 1 or 4 weeks' duration and triple therapies lasting 1 week were ineffective in patients with metronidazole-resistant strains. A 4-week course of triple therapy could still eradicate H. pylori in 68% of patients with metronidazole-resistant strains, but at the cost of significant side-effects. It is concluded that metronidazole resistance is common and is generally associated with a poor outcome of anti-H. pylori therapies containing metronidazole. Alternative drug schedules are urgently needed for patients with metronidazole-resistant H. pylori.

L. A. Noach, MD, PhD, Department of Gastroenterology and Hepatology, Academic Medical Center, Meibergdreef 9, 1105 AZ Amsterdam, The Netherlands

INTRODUCTION

Eradication of Helicobacter pylori is associated with healing of gastritis and a markedly reduced relapse rate of both duodenal and gastric ulcers (1–6) but is difficult to achieve. Most single-drug regimens have been incapable of eradicating H. pylori (7–10). Higher success rates have been obtained with combinations of bismuth compounds and 1 or 2 antibiotics (10–12).

In vitro studies have shown that colloidal bismuth subcitrate (CBS) and ampicillin, as well as CBS and metronidazole act synergistically against H. pylori (13). Clinically, there is evidence to show that combinations of bismuth salts and nitroimidazoles (such as metronidazole and tinidazole) are more effective than regimens consisting of bismuth compounds and amoxicillin (8, 10, 12). The beneficial results of combinations of bismuth and metronidazole have been attributed to the fact that metronidazole, in contrast to amoxicillin, is secreted in gastric juice (8, 14, 15).

A major drawback to the use of nitroimidazoles is the occurrence of resistance to these drugs. Many investigators have ascribed failure of therapy to this phenomenon (16–21). It remains unclear whether the addition of a second antibiotic to a bismuth compound and nitroimidazoles, or prolongation of the therapy, can overcome therapy failure due to nitroimidazole resistance (16, 17).

The aim of this study was to determine the effect of metronidazole resistance on the clinical outcome of several drug regimens containing metronidazole, of varying duration.

PATIENTS AND METHODS

Between 1988 and 1992, metronidazole susceptibility tests were performed on isolates of H. pylori from 283 consecutive patients (104 women, 179 men) who were later treated in a series of open studies with either dual therapy (CBS and metronidazole) or triple therapy (CBS, metronidazole and amoxicillin or tetracycline) for 7–28 days. Isolates were obtained from antral biopsies before initiating therapy. Only patients for whom results of culture and histology before therapy as well as at least 4 weeks after cessation of therapy were available, were evaluated for this study. Patients were considered H. pylori negative if both cultures of H. pylori were negative and haematoxylin-eosin staining showed no microorganisms at least 4 weeks after the end of therapy.

Compliance with the prescribed study medications was assessed by interview during the out-patient visit 4 weeks after the end of treatment. Patients who took <75% of the medication were excluded from the study. In addition, patients were asked to report any side-effects during this visit.

Details of the patients treated with the 5 different regimens are shown in Table I.

Susceptibility tests

Metronidazole susceptibility tests were performed on blood-agar either by disc diffusion using commercially available discs containing 5 μg metronidazole (1988–October 1991) or on plates containing metronidazole 8 mg/l (after October 1991) as previously described by others (7, 8, 22).

To ascertain agreement between both tests, both tests were performed in a subgroup of 35 patients and related to the outcome of therapy.

In both tests, the plates were incubated under micro-aerophilic conditions at 37°C, and zone diameters of inhibition were measured after 4–5 days of incubation. Isolates that grew within a zone diameter of <15 mm with the disc diffusion test or on the plate containing metronidazole were considered resistant to metronidazole. Strains with isolated colonies growing inside the inhibition zone were designated resistant, whatever the size of the inhibition zone.

Statistics

Statistical analysis was performed by using the 2-tailed χ^2-test with Yates' correction when appropriate and the Fisher's exact test. A p-value <0.05 was considered significant.

Table I. *Details of patients treated with anti-H. pylori regimens*

	D1[a] CBS 7d MNZ 7d	D2[b] CBS 28d MNZ 10d	T1[c] CBS 28d MNZ 10d AMX 28d	T2[d] CBS 7d MNZ 7d AMX 7d	T3[e] CBS 7d MNZ 7d TET 7d
Male	16	52	40	34	46
Female	13	37	19	11	32
Age (yr)					
20–39	10	25	13	10	17
40–59	13	36	26	27	43
>60	6	28	20	8	18
NWE[f]	25	70	52	31	63
IMM[g]	4	19	7	14	15
FD[h]	20	28	28	20	20
PUD[i]	9	61	31	25	58
Total	29	89	59	45	78

[a] D1 = CBS 120 mg qid + metronidazole (MNZ) 500 mg tid for 7 days.
[b] D2 = CBS 120 mg qid for 28 days + MNZ 500 mg tid during the last 10 days.
[c] T1 = CBS 120 mg qid for 28 days + MNZ 500 mg tid for 10 days + amoxicillin (AMX) 375 mg tid for 28 days.
[d] T2 = CBS 120 mg qid + MNZ 500 mg tid + AMX 375 mg tid for 7 days.
[e] T3 = CBS 120 mg qid + MNZ 500 mg tid + tetracycline (TET) 500 mg qid for 7 days.
[f] NWE = patients originally from north-west European countries.
[g] IMM = immigrants from Mediterranean, African and Latin-American countries.
[h] FD = functional dyspepsia without a history of peptic ulceration.
[i] PUD = current or past evidence of duodenal and/or gastric ulceration.

RESULTS

Susceptibility testing using either disc diffusion or metronidazole plates was performed in 300 pretreatment isolates from 266 patients treated with one of the above-mentioned regimens and from 17 patients treated with 2 regimens after failure of the first treatment.

Comparison of the results of the disc diffusion test and metronidazole plate in 35 patients before the start of regimen D2 revealed that both tests agreed regarding susceptibility and resistance in 19 and 10 isolates respectively. In the disc diffusion test, 6 isolates had colonies inside the inhibition zone or a diameter of growth inhibition <15 mm, whereas the metronidazole plate suggested susceptibility. As both positive and negative predictive values regarding success or failure of therapy with the metronidazole plate were slightly higher (60% and 80% respectively) than with the disc diffusion test (53% and 56% respectively), we chose the former for the determination of metronidazole resistance from October 1991.

Pretreatment susceptibility tests identified 116 (41%) patients with metronidazole-resistant strains.

Metronidazole-resistant strains were found more often in women than in men and more often in immigrants (all from (sub)tropical countries) than in Northwest Europeans, but differences between sexes as well as between populations failed to reach statistically significant levels ($p = 0.065$ and $p = 0.310$ respectively) (Fig. 1). Nor were there any statistically significant differences in the levels of resistance between the different age groups or between patients with current vs. past evidence of duodenal ulceration and patients with functional dyspepsia.

Table II shows that the efficacy of the various treatment schedules was significantly greater in patients with metronidazole-susceptible isolates than in patients with resistant strains. The

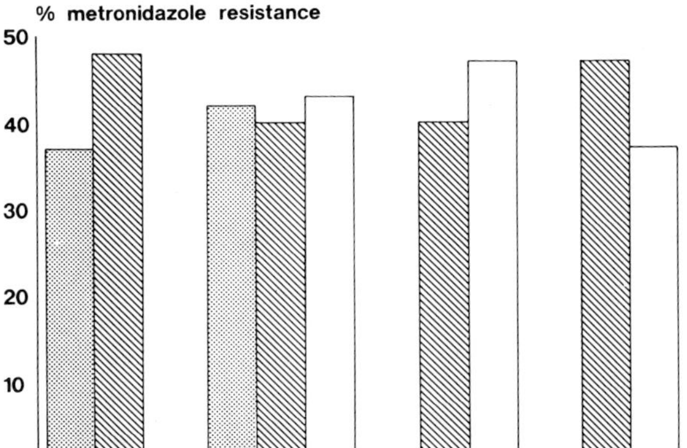

Fig. 1. Metronidazole-resistant H. pylori in different patient groups before treatment.

Table II. *Eradication rates in patients with metronidazole-susceptible (S) and resistant isolates (R) with different therapies*

	D1 CBS 7d MNZ 7d	D2 CBS 28d MNZ 10d	T1 CBS 28d MNZ 10d AMX 28d	T2 CBS 7d MNZ 7d AMX 7d	T3 CBS 7d MNZ 7d TET 7d
S	7/11 (64%)	43/57 (75%)	37/40 (93%)	8/12 (67%)	47/49 (96%)
R	4/18 (22%)	7/32 (22%)	13/19 (68%)	8/33 (24%)	11/29 (38%)

triple therapies (T1 + T2 + T3) appeared to be significantly more effective than both dual regimens in patients with susceptible isolates (D1 + D2) ($p = 0.002$). In patients with pretreatment resistant strains, the eradiction rate with regimen T1 was significantly higher than with dual therapies ($p < 0.001$) and other triple schedules ($p = 0.003$). Significant side-effects, occurring in 48% of patients receiving the 4-week course of triple therapy, gave occasion to interrupt treatment in 3 patients.

DISCUSSION

Nitroimidazoles combined with bismuth compounds can eradicate H. pylori in some 40–80% of patients (2, 11, 12, 17, 18, 22). When amoxicillin or tetracycline is added to such drugs, eradication rates exceeding 90% may be achieved (3, 5, 23, 24). However, the reported success rates vary considerably between investigators. Different results may be attributed to differences in drug formulations, dosage, duration of therapy courses, patient compliance and antibiotic resistance (8, 25, 26).

As appears from the present study, pretreatment metronidazole resistance clearly affects the results of dual and triple therapies. In patients with susceptible isolates, we achieved eradication in 50/68 (74%) of patients with both dual therapies and in 92/101 (91%) patients with the triple therapies. In subjects harbouring metronidazole-resistant H. pylori, treatment often failed. However, the 4-week triple regimen (T1) could still eradicate H. pylori in about two-thirds of patients infected with metronidazole-resistant strains. Although our patient population with resistant isolates treated with the latter regimen was small, this observation supports Burette's hypothesis that triple therapy of longer duration can overcome therapy failure due to metronidazole resistance (17). It remains unclear whether this favourable effect results from prolonged administration of CBS and amoxicillin, or from the intrinsic effects of metronidazole itself. It has been postulated that patients may be infected with multiple strains of H. pylori and that some of these strains are still susceptible to metronidazole. Borody et al. found that 14 days of triple therapy combined with omeprazole resulted in high eradication rates even in a limited number of patients with metronidazole-resistant strains (27). Again, it has not been clarified whether the repeated use of metronidazole, or of CBS and tetracycline, or the addition of omeprazole was responsible for this observation.

Metronidazole resistance has been associated with previous use of metronidazole or tinidazole. High prevalence rates are reported in patients from (sub)tropical countries where these drugs are often administered for the treatment of amoebiasis or other intestinal parasites (8, 28, 29). The more frequent use of nitroimidazoles in women for treatment of various vaginal infections and as perioperative prophylaxis for hysterectomy has also been suggested to contribute to a high rate of resistance (30).

In our study, a relatively high level of pretreatment metronidazole resistance was detected (41%), in comparison with other studies from Holland and neighbouring Northwest European countries (Table III). 19% of our patients were immigrants from Mediterranean, African and Latin-American countries. We found a prevalence rate of metronidazole resistance of 47% in this group, as opposed to 40% in Northwest European natives. This non-significant difference may only partly explain the relatively high rate of resistance detected in our patients. We have not investigated whether previous use of nitroimidazoles in our patients may have contributed to the high rate of resistance found.

It has been postulated that metronidazole resistance develops due to a diminished ability of strains to achieve a sufficiently low redox potential under micro-aerobic conditions for the necessary reduction of metronidazole (32). A mutation in the nitroreductase of the organism is thought to be responsible for this resistance.

Table III. *Reported prevalence rates of metronidazole resistance in various countries*

	Prevalence
Finland (16, 28)	27–36%
Sweden (28)	10%
Great Britain (19, 28, 31)	19–33%
Ireland (11, 28)	7–20%
The Netherlands (28, 30)	6–41%
Belgium (17, 28, 29)	24–29%
France (28)	25%
Spain (28)	6%
Portugal (28)	23%
Italy (28)	23%
Greece (28)	45%
Canada (28)	35%
Australia (18)	17%
Zaire (8)	84%

Currently, no universally accepted standard procedure exists to detect metronidazole susceptibility. Methodological factors may have been responsible for differences observed in the level of resistance. With the disc diffusion test, we detected 17% more resistant isolates than with the metronidazole plate. As the majority of susceptibility tests in this study have been performed by disc diffusion, this may have contributed to our relatively high percentage of resistant strains.

Nitroimidazoles have proved to be effective drugs in the treatment of H. pylori infection when combined with a bismuth compound and a second antibiotic, provided that the patient harbours a metronidazole-susceptible strain. The likelihood that patients with nitroimidazole-resistant strains will respond to metronidazole is too low to recommend its use in this group. Although prolonged treatment with triple regimens may succeed in eradicating H. pylori in a considerable number of patients with the resistant form, side effects of such regimens are not negligible. Moreover, the unrestricted use of nitroimidazoles is likely to increase the incidence of metronidazole resistance (33). Therefore, clinicians should not prescribe nitroimidazoles without prior testing for susceptibility. If a patient appears to be infected with nitroimidazole-resistant organisms, alternative drug schedules such as CBS and clarithromycin, or omeprazole and amoxicillin or clarithromycin, should be the first choice for these patients (34, 35).

REFERENCES

1. Coghlan JG, Humphries H, Dooley C, Keane C, Gilligan D, McKenna D, Sweeney E, O'Morain C. Campylobacter pylori and recurrence of duodenal ulcers: a 12 month follow-up study. Lancet 2: 1109–1111, 1987.
2. Marshall BJ, Goodwin CS, Warren JR, Murray R, Blincow ED, Blackbourn SJ, Philips M, Waters TE, Sanderson CR. Prospective double-blind trial of duodenal ulcer relapse after eradication of Campylobacter pylori. Lancet 2: 1437–1441, 1988.
3. Borody T, Cole P, Noonan, S, Morgan A, Lenne J, Hyland L, Brandl S, Borody EG, George LL. Recurrence of duodenal ulcer and Campylobacter pylori infection after eradication. Med J Aust 151: 431–435, 1989.
4. Rauws EAJ, Tytgat GNJ. Cure of duodenal ulcer associated with eradication of Helicobacter pylori. Lancet 335: 1233–1235, 1990.
5. George LL, Borody TJ, Andrews P, Devine M, Moore-Jones D, Walton M, Brandl S. Cure of duodenal ulcer after eradication of Helicobacter pylori. Med J Aust 153: 145–149, 1990.

6. Graham DY, Lew GM, Klein PD, Evans DG, Evans DJ, Saeed ZA, Malaty HM. Effect of treatment of Helicobacter pylori infection on the long-term recurrence of gastric or duodenal ulcer. A randomized controlled study. Ann Intern Med 116: 705–708, 1992.
7. Bayerdörffer E, Ottenjann R. The role of antibiotics in Campylobacter pylori associated peptic ulcer disease. Scand J Gastroenterol Suppl 142: 93–100, 1988.
8. Glupczynski Y, Burette A. Drug therapy for Helico-bacter pylori infection: problems and pitfalls. Am J Gastroenterol 85: 1545–1551, 1990.
9. Graham DY, Klein PD, Opekun AR, Smith KE, Polasani RR, Evans DJ, Evans DG, Alpert LC, Michaletz PA, Yoshimura HH, Adam E. In vivo susceptibility of Campylobacter pylori. Am J Gastroenterol 84: 233–238, 1989.
10. Rauws EAJ. Therapeutic attempts at eradication of Campylobacter pylori. Eur J Gastroenterol Hepatol 1: 34–41, 1989.
11. O'Riordan T, Mathai E, Tobin E, McKenna D, Keane C, Sweeney E, O'Morain C. Adjuvant antibiotic therapy in duodenal ulcers treated with colloidal bismuth subcitrate. Gut 31: 999–1002, 1990.
12. Bell GD, Weil J, Powell K, Jobson R, Harrison G, Gant PW, Jones PH, Owen RJ, Moreno M, Trowell JE. Helicobacter pylori treated with combinations of tripotassium dicitrato bismuthate and metronidazole: efficacy of different treatment regimens and some observations on the emergence of metronidazole resistance. Eur J Gastroenterol Hepatol 3: 819–822, 1991.
13. Van Caekenberghe DL, Breyssens J. In vitro synergistic activity between bismuth subcitrate and various anti-microbial agents against Campylobacter pyloridis (C. pylori). Antimicrob Agents Chemother 31: 1429–1430, 1987.
14. Veldhuyzen van Zanten SJO, Goldie J, Hollingsworth J, Siletti C, Richardson H, Hunt RH. Secretion of intravenously administered ampicillin, erythromycin and metronidazole in gastric juice. Implications for management of Helicobacter pylori. J Clin Pathol 45: 225–227, 1992.
15. Lamouliatte H, Cayla R, Meyer M, Demotes-Moinard F, Vincon G, Quentin-Nourry C, Vialette G, Mégraud F. Pharmacokinetics of oral and intravenous amoxillin in human gastric mucosa [Abstract]. Gastroenterology 102: A107, 1992.
16. Rautelin H, Seppala K, Renkonen OV, Vainio U, Kosunen TU. Role of metronidazole resistance in therapy of Helicobacter pylori infections. Antimicrob Agents Chemother 36: 163–166, 1992.
17. Burette A, Glupczynski Y, De Prez C. Evaluation of various multi-drug eradication regimens for Helicobacter pylori. Eur J Gastroenterol Hepatol 4: 817–823, 1992.
18. Goodwin CS, Marshall BJ, Blincow ED, Wilson DH, Blackbourn S, Phillips M. Prevention of nitroimidazole resistance in Campylobacter pylori by coadministration of colloidal bismuth subcitrate: clinical and in vitro studies. J Clin Pathol 41: 207–210, 1988.
19. Logan RPH, Gummett PA, Misiewicz JJ, Karim QN, Walker MM, Baron JH. One week eradication regimen for Helico-bacter pylori. Lancet 338: 1249–1252, 1991.
20. De Koster E, Nyst JF, Deprez C, Glupczynski Y, Otero J, Denis P, Van Geel J, Buset M, De Reuck M, Deltenre M. Towards a coherent HP treatment strategy [Abstract]. Ital J Gastroenterol 23 (Suppl 2): 103, 1991.
21. Bell GD, Powell K, Burridge SM, Pallecaros A, Jones PH, Gant PW, Harrison G, Trowell JE. Experience with "triple" anti-Helicobacter pylori eradication therapy: side-effects and the importance of testing the pretreatment bacterial isolate for metronidazole resistance. Aliment Pharmacol Ther 6: 427–435, 1992.
22. Weil J, Bell GD, Morden A, Harrison G, Gant PW, Jones PH, Trowell JE. Helicobacter pylori infection treated with a tripotassium dicitrato bismuthate and metronidazole combination. Aliment Pharmacol Ther 4: 651–657, 1990.
23. McColl KEL, Fullarton GM, Chittajalu R, El Nujumi AM, MacDonald AMI, Dahill SW, Hilditch TE. Plasma gastrin, daytime intragastric pH and nocturnal acid output before and at 1 and 7 months after eradication of Helicobacter pylori in duodenal ulcer subjects. Scand J Gastroenterol 26: 339–346, 1991.
24. Borody TJ, George LL, Brandl S, Andrews P, Lenne J, Moore-Jones D, Devine M, Walton M. Helicobacter pylori eradication with doxycycline-metronidazole bismuth subcitrate tripletherapy. Scand J Gastroenterol 27: 281–284, 1992.
25. McNulty CAM. Bacteriological and pharmacological basis for the treatment of Campylobacter pylori infection. Gastroenterol Clin Bio 13: 96B–100B, 1989.
26. Graham DY, Lew GM, Malaty HM, Evans DG, Evans DJ, Klein PD, Alpert LC, Genta RM. Factors influencing the eradication of Helicobacter pylori with triple therapy. Gastroenterology 102: 493–496, 1992.

27. Borody TJ, Brandl S, Andrews P, Jankiewicz E, Ostapowicz NH. Helicobacter pylori eradication failure (EF) – further treatment possibilities [Abstract]. Gastroenterology 102: A43, 1992.
28. Glupczynski Y. Metronidazole resistance in Helicobacter pylori: results of the second multicenter in vitro study [Abstract]. Ital J Gastroenterol 23 (Suppl 2): 107, 1991.
29. Glupczynski Y, Burette A, De Koster E, Nyst JF, Deltenre M, Cadranel S, Bordeaux L, De Vos D. Metronidazole resistance in Helicobacter pylori [Letter]. Lancet 335: 976–977, 1990.
30. Becx MCJM, Janssen AJHM, Clasener HAL, de Koning RW. Metronidazole resistant Helicobacter pylori [Letter]. Lancet 335: 539–540, 1990.
31. Weil J, Bell GD, Powell K, Jobson R, Trowell JE, Gant P, Jones PH. Helicobacter pylori and metronidazole resistance [Letter]. Lancet 336: 1445, 1990.
32. Cederbrant G, Kahlmeter G, Ljungh Å. Proposed mechanism for metronidazole resistance in Helicobacter pylori. J Antimicrob Chemother 29: 115–120, 1992.
33. Tytgat GNJ, Axon ATR, Dixon MF, Graham DY, Lee A, Marshall BJ. Helicobacter pylori: causal agent in peptic ulcer disease? Working party report from World Congress of Gastroenterology 1990, Sydney. Oxford: Blackwell Scientific Publications, 36–45, 1990.
34. Bayerdörffer E, Mannes GA, Sommer A, Hochter W, Weingart J, Hatz R, Lehn N, Ruckdeschel G, Dirschedl P, Stolte M. High dose omeprazole combined with amoxicillin eradicates Helicobacter pylori. Eur J Gastroenterol Hepatol 4: 697–702, 1992.
35. Logan RPH, Gummett PA, Hegarthy BT, Walker MM, Baron JH, Misiewicz JJ. Clarithromycin and omeprazole for Helicobacter pylori [Letter]. Lancet 340: 239, 1992.

Submitted October 25, 1993; accepted January 12, 1994

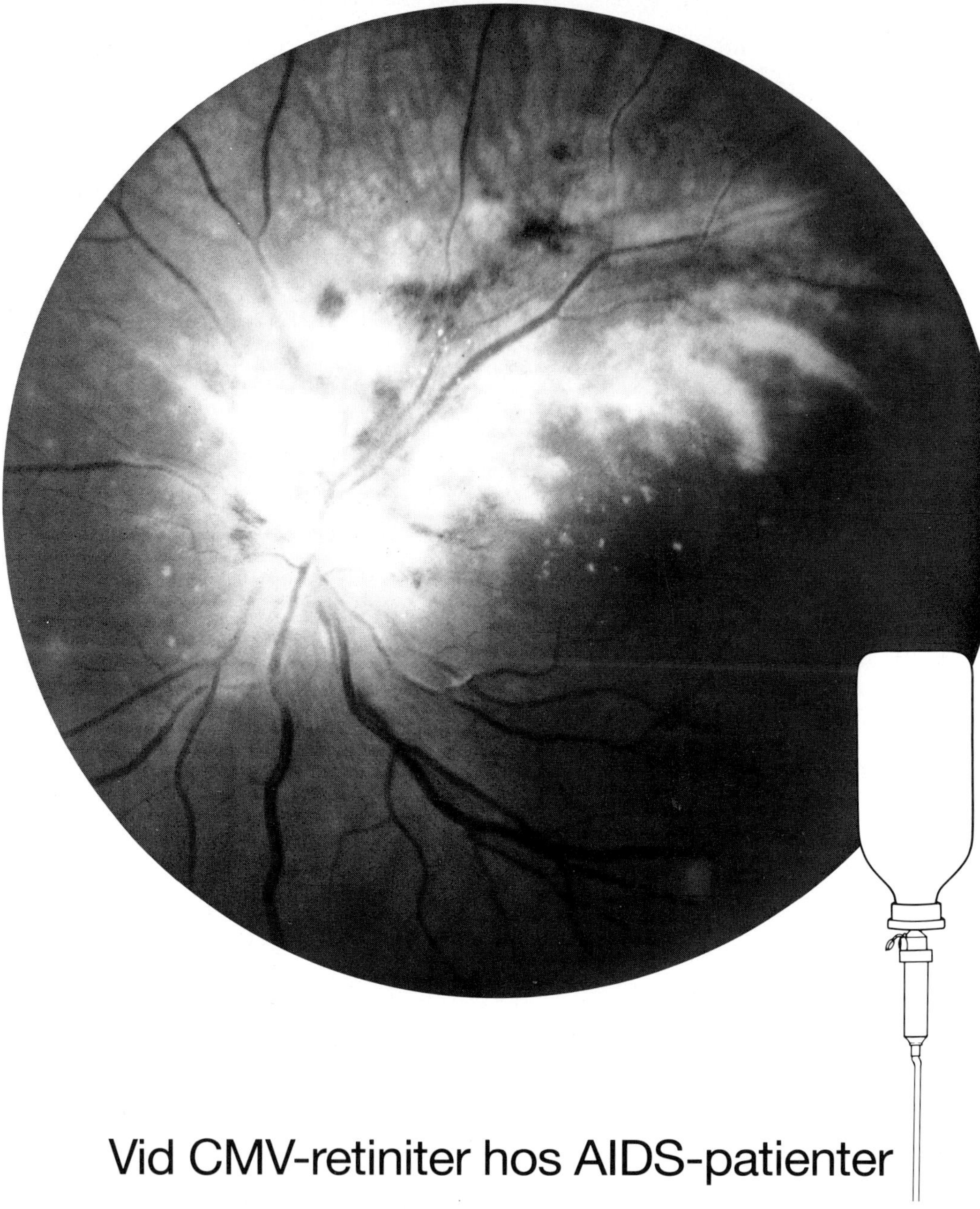

Scand J Infect Dis 26: 329–337, 1994

Serum Antibody Titres to Shigella Lipopolysaccharides and Invasion Plasmid Antigens in Healthy Costa Rican and Swedish Women

ROSARIO ACHÍ[1,2], LEONARDO MATA[2] and ALF A. LINDBERG[1]

From the [1]Department of Clinical Bacteriology, Karolinska Institute, Huddinge Hospital, Huddinge, Sweden, and the [2]Instituto de Investigaciones en Salud (INISA), University of Costa Rica, San José, Costa Rica

Specific serum antibody titres to defined lipopolysaccharides (LPS) of Shigella spp. and Salmonella serogroup B (BO) and Shigella invasion plasmid antigens (Ipa) were determined by enzyme immunoassays in healthy Costa Rican women from low ($n = 34$), middle ($n = 36$) and high ($n = 19$) socioeconomic conditions and from 64 Swedish women. Specific IgG antibody titres were the highest, in particular to the S. flexneri Y LPS, with mean titres of 750 (SD = 360), 690 (380), and 820 (300) for the Low, Middle and High Costa Rican groups respectively. Lower titres were recorded against S. sonnei and S. dysenteriae type 1. Titres against Salmonella LPS were very low (<250). In Swedish women, significantly lower serum anti-LPS titres were found ($p < 0.05$). No statistically significant differences regarding socioeconomic conditions or serum anti-LPS titres were seen in the Costa Rican groups ($p > 0.05$). Mean IgG-titres to the Ipa of 330 (150), 220 (170) and 140 (110) were found for the 3 Costa Rican groups, respectively. The IgG and IgM titres to Ipa in serum from the Low group were significantly higher than those of the High group ($p < 0.05$). The mean serum IgG titre of 70 (90) for the Swedish women was significantly lower than that of the Low and Middle groups ($p < 0.05$), but similar to that of the High group ($p > 0.05$). High IgG anti-Ipa titres were found in 38% from the Low, 19% from the Middle but none in the High group (mean value of the High group +2 SD). The anti-Ipa antibodies in the Costa Rican groups seemed to be a better indicator of Shigella exposure than were anti-LPS antibodies. A good degree of correlation was found between serum and colostrum IgA anti-Ipa titres (0.651, $p < 0.001$), and serum S. flexneri LPS and colostrum IgA anti-S. flexneri LPS antibody titres (0.607, $p < 0.001$).

A. A. Lindberg, MD, Department of Clinical Bacteriology F82, Huddinge Hospital, S-141 86, Huddinge, Sweden

INTRODUCTION

Shigellosis plays a major role for morbidity and mortality in several developing countries (1). Despite the indicators of good health in Costa Rica there are various vulnerable groups, particularly those living in overcrowded conditions with bad sanitation, that are still affected by enteric diseases (2). Previous studies have suggested that Shigella is a minor cause of diarrhea in Costa Rican populations (2, 3). However, the high anti-S. flexneri titres we found in colostrum from Costa Rican mothers with middle and particularly with poor-socioeconomic conditions, contrasting with significantly lower titres in the wealthy women ($p < 0.05$) (4), strongly suggested that Shigella could be quite a prevalent pathogen among these groups. Also, the significantly higher anti-invasion plasmid antigen titres in colostrum from the poor mothers ($p < 0.05$) (5), corroborates the previous observations regarding antibodies to the Shigella LPSs. It should be kept in mind that as shigellosis can be a mild disease, not requiring medical attention, it may therefore go unrecorded in epidemiological studies (6).

Virulence in Shigella requires the expression of both chromosomal and plasmid genes (7–11). Of these, the complete expression of the chromosomally coded lipopolysaccharide (LPS) portion, harbouring the specific O-antigens, is a prerequisite for virulence (9). Other antigens necessary for virulence in shigellae are those coded for by a large extrachromosomal

 ISSN 0036-5548

invasion plasmid, designed as the invasion plasmid antigens (Ipa) (7, 8, 10, 11). These protein antigens are shared by all virulent Shigella spp. and by enteroinvasive Escherichia coli (EIEC) strains. Antibody responses to shigellae are primarily elicited against these 2 main groups of surface antigens (7, 9).

Several studies have evaluated humoral responses to Shigella antigens in serum (12–16), as well as at the mucosal level (16–19). However, only a limited number of them have simultaneously compared responses to both LPSs and Ipa (16, 20, 31).

High serum antibody titres to Shigella were observed in healthy Vietnamese (13, 20). The presence of high titres in healthy individuals from areas where shigellosis is highly prevalent may complicate the observation of significant differences in nutritional status, geographical area and age groups may also complicate the drawing of conclusions during serological studies regarding Shigella exposure (16, 18, 20, 21). The Costa Rican groups studied here comprised healthy women from the same geographical area, were of similar nutritional status and age, but probably differed regarding exposure to enteric pathogens.

The aim of the present study was to determine the titres of class-specific antibodies to the main surface antigens of Shigella, LPS and Ipa, in serum from healthy Costa Rican women from different socioeconomic conditions and to compare them with the titres of Swedish women who are seldom exposed to enteric bacterial pathogens. We also wanted to compare the titres in serum with those found at the secretory level (4, 5) and to determine the degree of correlation between serum and colostrum (4, 5) antibody titres of the same individual, against the Ipa and LPS antigens.

MATERIALS AND METHODS

Study groups

Healthy Costa Rican women enrolled during 1989 in the metropolitan area of San José and with varying socioeconomic status constituted the study groups. Parameters of socioeconomic condition, including household income, place of prenatal care and place of delivery, were used for selection of the groups (4). A total of 34 healthy women, living in overcrowded slums around the city, with a very low family income (<20,000 colones/month; 1 $U.S. = 85 colones), and attending a public hospital (San Juan de Dios Hospital) for delivery, constituted the low socioeconomic condition group (Low). The high socioeconomic standard group (High) comprised 19 women attending private maternity clinics (household income >150,000 colones/month). The middle socioeconomic condition group (Middle) was defined as those women ($n = 36$) living in intermediate conditions (income 30,000–70,000 colones/month) compared with the Low and High groups (4). All mothers had a normal pregnancy, and their nutritional status was assumed to be similar in all three groups. All gave birth to normal babies with an average birth weight of >3,000 g (4). Serum samples from 64 randomly selected pregnant Swedish women, visiting Huddinge Hospital for routine examinations and representing a population with a low degree of exposure to infectious enteric diseases, were also analysed.

Serum samples

Venous blood samples from the Costa Rican women were collected 1 and 30 days after delivery. Specimens were centrifuged and serum separated, aliquoted and frozen at −70°C until transported in dry ice to Sweden for analyses. Serum samples from the Swedish women were analyzed soon after collection.

Lipopolysaccharide antigens (LPS)

Phenol–water-extracted, chemically defined LPSs available from previous investigations: Salmonella typhimurium serogroup BO (23), Shigella dysenteriae type 1 (24), Plesiomonas shigelloides (the same O-antigen as Shigella sonnei) (25) and Shigella flexneri Y (26) were used as antigens in EIAs.

Invasion plasmid antigens (Ipa-s)

Water extracts from both a rough Escherichia coli K12 strain (SP10), carrying the invasion plasmid (pWR110) of a Shigella flexneri 5 isolate, M90T (27, 28) and from a plasmid-free parent strain (J53) were prepared according to Oaks et al. (15), with modifications as previously described (5). After the extraction procedure, a water extract rich in Ipa-s was obtained and the total protein concentration was determined by Lowry's method (29). Extracts were kept frozen at −20°C until use.

Enzyme immunoassays (EIAs)

The EIA for the LPSs was performed as previously described (23). Wells were coated with 100 μl of antigen at concentrations of 5 μg/ml for S. flexneri and 10 μg/ml for the other LPSs, in 50 mM carbonate buffer, pH 9.6. The EIA for Ipa was performed according to Oaks (15). 100 μl of each water extract at a protein (Ipa-s) concentration of 20 μg/ml for both SP10 and J53 strains, diluted in 50 mM phosphate-buffered saline (PBS), pH 7.4, was used to coat the immune plates (Costar, Costar Corporation, Cambridge, Mass.). Unsaturated wells were blocked with 100 μl of 5% fetal calf serum for 1 h at room temperature (5). Serum samples were diluted 1:1,000 in PBS, with 1% fetal calf serum. Alkaline phosphatase conjugated rabbit anti-human IgA (1:2,000), IgG (1:4,000) and IgM (1:2,000) from Dakopatts, Copenhagen, Denmark, were used. The titres of anti-LPS antibodies were expressed as relative titres: the optical density (OD) values (405 nm, 100 min) times the dilution factor (=1,000). The optimal dilution for colostrum samples was also 1:1,000 as previously described (4). In order to increase the specificity of the Ipa assay, samples were tested against extracts from both the SP10 and J53 strains. Optical densities (OD) were recorded after 100 min at 405 nm. The reported optical density value was calculated as OD–SP10 minus OD–J53. Data are reported as relative titres, defined as the OD times the dilution factor of the sample (=1,000). High antibody titres were defined as those titres over the cut-off value (mean value + 2 SD for the High group from Costa Rica).

Total immunoglobulin determinations

Total IgA, IgG and IgM of Costa Rican serum samples were determined by nephelometry (30).

Statistical methods

The non-parametric Kolmogorov–Smirnov test was used to determine differences between socioeconomic groups. Simple Regression Analysis was used to correlate serum and colostrum antibody titres.

RESULTS

Total immunoglobulin determinations

Total mean (SD) serum-IgA concentrations of 3.23 (0.96), 2.95 (0.86) and 2.61 (0.88) g/l; IgG of 13.19 (2.80), 12.44 (3.04) and 10.43 (2.81) g/l; and IgM of 3.74 (1.62), 3.39 (1.56), 3.38 (1.50) g/l, were found in samples 1 day after delivery in the Low, Middle and High groups, respectively. Similar IgA and IgM values were found 30 days later. IgG values of 15.90 (3.36), 15.20 (2.91), and 13.43 (2.93) g/l, for the respective groups, were found on day 30. A tendency to lower IgG mean values was observed in the 3 groups 1 day after delivery as compared with the mean values on day 30. However, no significant differences were found regarding day post delivery or socioeconomic conditions ($p > 0.05$).

Serum antibody titres against the LPS antigens

Mean relative IgA titres of 310 (SD = 140) for Shigella flexneri Y and 120 (50) for Salmonella BO LPS in the Low group were found in sera collected 1 day after delivery (Fig. 1). The IgA titres in sera collected day 30 post partum were very similar (data now shown). Comparable serum titres against the 2 LPS antigens were observed in the Middle and High groups. Relative-IgG titres of 130 (70), 140 (70) and 140 (90) against the Salmonella BO LPS were found in sera from mothers in the three socioeconomic groups at day 1 post-delivery. Against the Shigella flexneri Y LPS, mean titres of 750 (360) in the Low, 690 (380) in the Middle and 820 (410) in the High group were found on day 1 post delivery (Fig. 1). Similar figures were observed 30 days later (not shown). Mean antibody titres against Shigella sonnei and Shigella dysenteriae were intermediate. Mean IgM anti-Shigella flexneri titres of 610 (300), 460 (270) and 550 (260) for the Low, Middle and High groups, respectively were

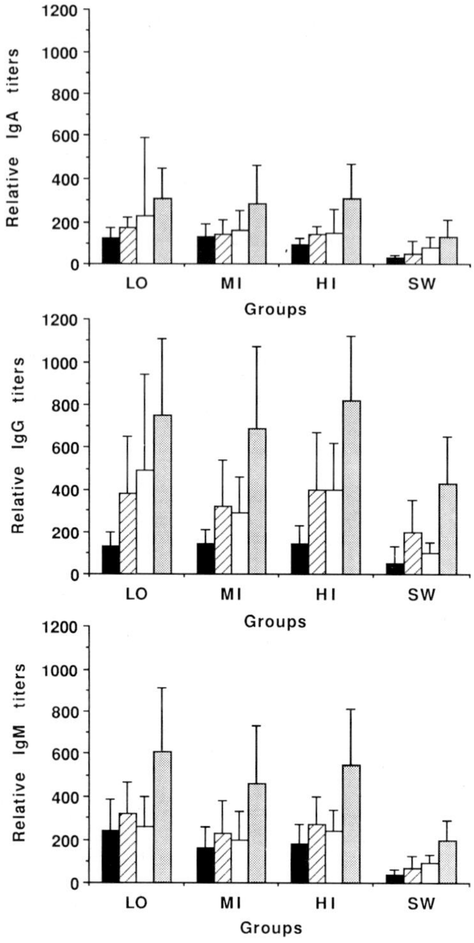

Fig. 1. Relative titres of IgA, IgG and IgM antibodies against the lipopolysaccharide antigens of Salmonella serogroup BO, S. dysenteriae type 1, S. sonnei and S. flexneri found in Costa Rican women with Low (LO), Middle (MI) and High (HI) socioeconomic conditions, and Swedish women (SW). Vertical bars represent the standard deviation.

found 1 day post delivery and remained unchanged 1 month later (Fig. 1). No statistical differences regarding socioeconomic status or day post delivery were found in the Costa Rican groups ($p > 0.05$). In the Swedish samples, only low titres to the LPSs were found (Fig. 1) and they were significantly lower than those of any of the Costa Rican groups ($p < 0.05$).

Serum antibody titres against the Ipa

The mean serum antibody titres to Ipa of shigellae in serum of the Costa Rican women are shown in Fig. 2. The Low group had the highest relative mean values, of 140 (120), 330 (150) and 100 (80) for IgA, IgG and IgM, respectively, in serum samples collected 1 day after delivery. Similar values were observed in samples collected 30 days later (Fig. 2). In the High group, titres of 70 (50), 140 (110) and 30 (20) for IgA, IgG and IgM respectively were found on day 1. The mean serum IgG and IgM titres in the Low group were significantly higher ($p < 0.05$) than those of the High group, while the IgA titres were similar ($p > 0.05$). Significantly lower IgG titres were observed in the Middle compared to the Low group ($p < 0.05$). In the Swedish samples, only very low mean anti-Ipa titres of 20 (20), 70 (90) and 20 (20) for the IgA, IgG and IgM respectively, were observed (Fig. 2). Titres in this group

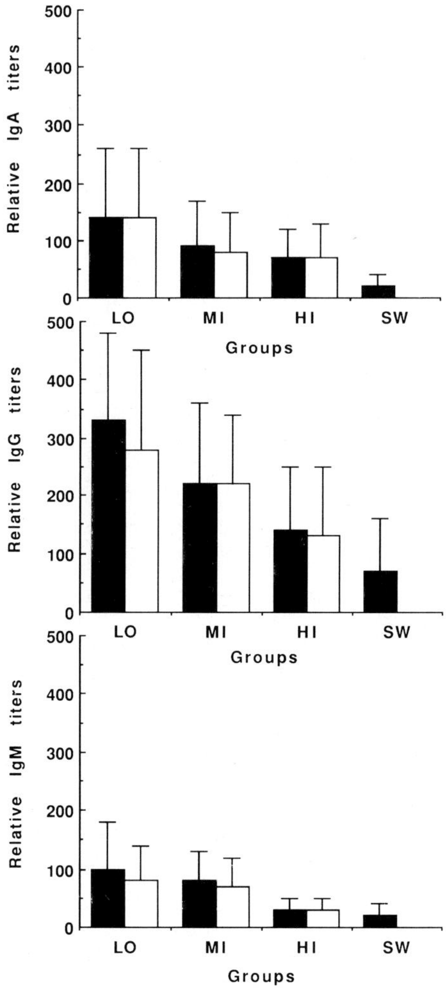

Fig. 2. Relative titres of IgA, IgG and IgM antibodies against the invasion plasmid antigens (Ipa) in Costa Rican sera from women with Low (LO), Middle (MI), and High (HI) socioeconomic conditions, and Swedish women (SW) 1 and 30 days post delivery. Vertical range bars denote standard deviation.

were significantly lower ($p < 0.05$) than those of the Costa Rican Low and Middle groups. Comparable IgG and IgM titres were observed for the Swedish and the High groups ($p > 0.05$), while significantly higher IgA titres ($p < 0.05$) were found in the Costa Rican High group.

High antibody titres against the S. flexneri Y LPS and the Ipa

When titres from the High group of Costa Rica (days 1 and 30) were used to calculate a cut-off value (mean + 2 SD), 5–6% of samples in the different groups showed high serum IgA-titres against Shigella flexneri Y LPS (Table I). Similar figures were found for IgG: 3% in the Low and 6% of samples in the Middle group had high titres. For IgM titres, 15% of the samples in the Low, 3% in the Middle and none of the High group had a high titre (Table I). Similar figures for day 30 were noted (data not shown). This relative comparison showed that 29%, 38% and 47% of samples (day 1) from the Low group had high IgA, IgG and IgM anti-Ipa titres, respectively, as compared with the High group with relatively low titres only (Table I). Similar results were observed in serum samples from day 30 post delivery (data not shown).

Table I. *Number of serum samples with high[a] anti-Shigella flexneri Y LPS and anti-Ipa antibody titres in the Costa Rican (different socioeconomic conditions) and Swedish groups*

Group	Day post delivery	Anti-S. flexneri Y LPS IgA	IgG	IgM	Anti-Ipa IgA	IgG	IgM
Costa Rican							
Low	1	2/34[b] (6%)	1/34 (3%)	5/34 (15%)	10/34 (29%)	13/34 (38%)	16/34 (47%)
Middle	1	2/36 (6%)	2/36 (6%)	1/36 (3%)	3/36 (26%)	7/36 (19%)	15/36 (42%)
High	1	1/19 (5%)	0/19	0/19	1/19 (5%)	0/19	0/19
Swedish		0/64	0/64	0/64	0/64	0/64	0/64

[a] Samples above the cut-off value (mean value + 2 standard deviations for the High group) = IgA = 630, IgG = 1,420 and IgM = 1,070 for anti-LPS and IgA = 180, IgG = 350, IgM = 60 for anti-Ipa antibodies.

[b] Number of positive samples/total number of samples.

Correlations

Comparison of anti-Ipa and anti-Shigella flexneri Y LPS antibody titres in serum of Costa Rican mothers in the Low group. A good degree of correlation was found between serum-antibody titres of the IgA isotype and those of the IgG class against the Shigella flexneri Y LPS ($r = 0.573, p < 0.001$). A slight, non-significant correlation ($r = 0.300, p > 0.05$) was found between serum IgA and IgG antibody titres against Ipa. The correlation between serum IgG antibody titres against the LPS antigens of S. flexneri Y and Ipa was not significant ($r = 0.340, p > 0.05$). No significant correlations were found between the IgA and IgM antibody titres.

Comparison between anti-Ipa and anti-LPS antibody titres in serum and colostrum of Costa Rican mothers in the Low group. A significant correlation ($r = 0.651, p < 0.001$) between serum IgA anti-Ipa titres and the corresponding colostrum-IgA anti-Ipa titres was observed. The comparison of colostrum IgA anti-Ipa antibodies and serum IgG anti-Ipa antibodies also demonstrated a good correlation ($r = 0.500, p < 0.05$). The serum IgA antibody titres against the LPS of Shigella flexneri Y LPS showed a close correlation with the colostrum IgA antibody titres against the same LPS ($r = 0.607, p < 0.001$). The correlation between IgA in colostrum and IgG antibodies in serum was not significant ($r = 0.352, p > 0.05$). Correlations comparing IgM titres were not significant either.

DISCUSSION

The availability of specific and sensitive enzyme immunoassays using defined antigens is a key factor in serological studies. Measurement of specific antibody titres may permit accurate comparisons in sero-epidemiological surveys, individual serodiagnosis of shigellosis and of antibody responses during vaccination trials. Obviously, before such studies can be carried out on a large scale, basic information about populations from diverse geographical areas and of different degrees of exposure should be available. For the Costa Rican groups studied here, the High group could be used as a control of low exposure for the same geographical area. As most of the studies have been based mainly on shigellosis patients in highly endemic areas, the controls had titres that were already high (12–14, 16). This may interfere with the observation of significant differences between cases and control groups. Information from these Costa Rican populations, in addition to that from the 'unprimed' Swedish individuals (13, 20, 31), complemented with observations in previous studies in Vietnam (13, 20) and Bangladesh (32), offers a good background for the antibody responses to LPS and Ipa antigens in healthy groups differently exposed to this enteropathogen.

As expected, serum antibodies of the IgG isotype were the highest, but IgM and IgA titres were also present. They were mainly against the S. flexneri Y LPS, while those against the other shigellae and particularly salmonella were relatively low. The titres to the LPSs in the 3 Costa Rican groups were found to be intermediate as compared with the higher titres ($>1,000$) in serum of healthy Vietnamese populations (13, 20). This suggests that the frequency of exposure is generally lower even for individuals of the Low group. These baseline titres were significantly higher than those of the 'unprimed' Swedish group, which may be interpreted as denoting previous contact with Shigella, but the actual differences in exposure were not reflected here. The similar mean anti-LPS titres in the 3 groups suggest that women living in deprived circumstances have probably experienced only a few Shigella episodes. The results regarding the anti-Ipa titres support these conclusions (Fig. 1). They were approximately half of those seen in healthy Vietnamese populations (710 ± 190 for IgG), determined with the same assay (5). However, here the titres in the Low and Middle groups were significantly higher than those of the Swedish group, while the titres in the High group were similar to those seen in the Swedish women. This indicates that at the serum level, the anti-Ipa antibodies represent a better indicator of the frequency of exposure, at least for the groups studied here.

The IgA anti-Ipa antibodies were significantly more numerous in all Costa Rican groups than in the Swedish women ($p < 0.05$). The IgG and IgM titres in the High group did not differ from the Swedish titres. Even though the titres are relatively low, the IgA anti-Ipa titres seem to be present also in populations with a probable low exposure. This indicates previous contact with shigellae also for individuals in the High group. The fact that some 30–40% of the women in the Low group had high serum IgA and IgG anti-Ipa titres tallies with our finding of high anti-S. flexneri Y LPS and anti-Ipa titres in colostrum (4, 5), suggesting relatively frequent exposure in these groups. Moreover, the good degree of correlation when comparing colostrum and serum Iga titres with the S. flexneri LPS and particularly with the Ipa in the same individual and serum IgG anti-Ipa and colostrum IgA anti-Ipa, indicates that even though elicited by independent mechanisms, rises at both the mucosal and the peripheral level occur following infection. The independent responses of anti-LPS and anti-Ipa antibodies may be due mainly to both the nature of the antigen and the antigenic presentation on the bacterial surface. Proteins (Ipa) are T-cell dependent antigens, whereas saccharide antigens (LPS) can polyclonally stimulate the B cells directly to APC, even when administered in small doses (33).

For individual diagnosis in 'unprimed' – and perhaps also in not too heavily exposed – populations, a notable rise in the anti-Ipa titres during infection is likely to be observed. In an endemic area such as Vietnam, the already high titres in the individual seem to make serodiagnosis based on Ipa a less useful tool (20). Instead, a rise in anti-LPS antibody response occurs after each infection.

Secretory antibodies reflect the maternal gut exposure to microbial antigens (i.e. the intestinal immunity of the mother) (22, 34). They seem to give a better estimate of the actual exposure level, than do serum levels. We are of the opinion that the significantly higher titres in colostrum of the poor Costa Rican women to the LPS antigens, particularly to S. flexneri, represent a more reliable indicator of the higher Shigella exposure in this group. The similar baseline titres of serum indicate that the Costa Rican exposure to shigellae is lower than in highly endemic areas like Vietnam. This also indicates the independence of the mucosal immune system (22). For this reason, immune responses at both the peripheral and the mucosal level should be compared in epidemiological studies and vaccination trials.

Positive correlations between serum and colostrum antibody titres were found in the most exposed groups, as the degree of exposure is probably enough to elicit responses at both secretory and serum levels, even though they seem to be independently stimulated (22).

Even though secretions (including colostrum and breast milk) seem to be more reliable indicators of recent exposure to Shigella, sampling at these levels is not always likely and then relative serum antibody titres, if interpreted and compared correctly, may offer quite useful information during serological studies.

The finding of antibody titres in colostrum and serum against the S. flexneri and S. sonnei LPSs and the Ipa suggested that shigellae are more prevalent in Costa Rica than has been assumed. Therefore, we have initiated a study on the presence of shigellae both in infant patients and in a healthy population from the low socioeconomic conditions, using culture and a combined immunomagnetic polymerase chain reaction (IMS-PCR) based assay, where the shigellae are captured by shigella LPS-specific monoclonal antibodies and PCR products detected by dot-blot using a specific probe conjugated to alkaline phosphatase (35). This study has documented a Shigella frequency of 8% in healthy and up to 26% in diarrheal patients at the hospital (unpublished data), lending credence to our findings that both the Ipa and LPS titres reflect the prevalence of shigellae in Costa Rica.

ACKNOWLEDGEMENTS

This work was supported by the Karolinska International Research Training (KIRT) Programme founded by the Swedish Agency for Research Cooperation with Developing Countries (SAREC) and The Swedish Medical Research Council (grant no. 16X-656).

REFERENCES

1. Bennish ML, Wojtyniak BJ. Mortality due to shigellosis: community and hospital data. Rev Infect Dis 13 (Suppl. 4): S245–251, 1991.
2. Mata L, Rosero L. National health and social development in Costa Rica: a case study of intersectoral action. Pan American Health Organization, technical paper N13, 1988.
3. Achí R, Mata L, Vives M, Pizarro D. Aspectos clínico-epidemiológicos de la criptosporidiosis en Costa Rica. Rev Med Hosp Nal Ninos (Costa Rica) 20: 45–58, 1985.
4. Achí R, Cam PD, Forsum U, Karlsson K, Sáenz P, Mata L, Lindberg AA. Titres of class-specific antibodies against Shigella and Salmonella lipopolysaccharide (LPS) antigens in colostrum and breast milk of Costa Rican, Swedish and Vietnamese mothers. J Infect 25: 89–105, 1992.
5. Cam PD, Achí R, Lindberg AA, Pál T. Antibodies against invasion-plasmid coded antigens of shigellae in human colostrum and milk. Acta Microbiol Hung 39: 263–270, 1992.
6. The prospects of immunizing against Shigella spp. In: Institute of Medicine. New vaccine development: establishing priorities. Vol 2. Disease of importance in developing countries. Washington, DC: National Academy Press, 329–337, 1986.
7. Hale TL, Sansonetti PJ, Schad PA, Austin S, Formal SB. Characterization of virulence plasmid and plasmid-associated outer membrane proteins in Shigella flexneri, Shigella sonnei and Escherichia coli. Infect Immun 40: 340–350, 1983.
8. Hale TL. Genetic basis of virulence in Shigella species. Microbiol Rev 55: 206–224, 1991.
9. Lindberg AA, Kärnell A, Weintraub A. The lipopolysaccharide of Shigella bacteria as a virulence factor. Rev Infect Dis 13 (Suppl. 4): S279–284, 1991.
10. Sansonetti PJ. Genetic and molecular basis of epithelial cell invasion by Shigella species. Rev Infect Dis 13 (Suppl. 4): S285–292, 1991.
11. Yoshikawa M, Sasakawa C. Molecular pathogenesis of shigellosis: a review. Microbiol Immunol 35: 809–824, 1991.
12. Cohen D, Block C, Green MS, Lowell G, Ofek I. Immunoglobulin M, A, and G antibody response to lipopolysaccharide O antigen in symptomatic and asymptomatic Shigella infections. J Clin Microbiol 27: 162–167, 1989.

13. Ekwall E, Cam PD, Trach DD, Taube A, Lindberg AA. Shigella flexneri O-antigen-specific enzyme immunoassay: class-specific antibody titres against lipopolysaccharide antigens in healthy Vietnamese and Swedish populations. Serodiagn Immunother 2: 47–61, 1988.
14. Lindberg AA, Cam PD, Chan N. Shigellosis in Vietnam. Rev Infect Dis 13 (Suppl. 4): S231–237, 1991.
15. Oaks EV, Hale TL, Formal SB. Serum immune response to Shigella protein antigens in Rhesus monkeys and humans infected with Shigella spp. Infect Immun 53: 57–63, 1986.
16. Oberhelman RA, Kopecko DJ, Salazar-Lindo E, Gotuzzo E, Buysse JM, Venkatesan MM, Yi A, Fernández-Prada C, Guzmán M, León-Barúa R, Sack RB. Prospective study of systematic and mucosal immune responses in dysenteric patients to specific Shigella invasion plasmid antigens and lipopolysaccharides. Infect Immun 59: 2341–2350, 1991.
17. Cleary TG, West MS, Ruiz-Palacios G, Winsor DK, Calva JJ, Guerrero ML, Van R. Human mild secretory immunoglobulin A to Shigella virulence plasmid coded antigens. J Pediatr 118: 34–38, 1991.
18. Cruz JR, Carlsson B, Hofvander Y, Holme DT, Hanson LÅ. Studies of human milk: II. Concentration of antibodies against Salmonella and Shigella in milk of women from different populations and the daily intake by their breast-fed infants. Acta Paediatr Scand 74: 338–341, 1985.
19. Schultsz C, Qadri F, Hossain SA, Ahmed, Ciznar I. Shigella-specific IgA in saliva of children with bacillary dysentery. Microbiol Immunol 89: 65–72, 1992.
20. Cam PD, Pál T, Lindberg AA. Immune response against lipopolysaccharide and invasion plasmid coded antigens of shigellae in Vietnamese and Swedish dysenteric patients. J Clin Microbiol 31: 454–457, 1993.
21. Cohen D, Slepon R, Green M. Sociodemographic factors associated with serum anti-Shigella lipopolysaccharide antibodies and shigellosis. Int J Epidemiol 20: 546–550, 1991.
22. Bergmann K-Ch, Waldman RH. Stimulation of secretory antibody following oral administration of antigen. Rev Infect Dis 10: 939–950, 1988.
23. Carlsson HE, Lindberg AA, Hammarström S, Ljunggren Å. Quantitation of Salmonella O-antibodies in human sera by enzyme-linked immunosorbent assay (ELISA). Int Arch Allergy Appl Immunol 48: 485–494, 1975.
24. Lindberg AA, Haeggmann S, Karlsson K, Cam PD, Trach DD. The humoral antibody response to shigella dysenteriae type 1 infections as determined by ELISA. Bull WHO 62: 597–606, 1984.
25. Ekwall E, Haeggmann S, Kalin M, Svenungsson B, Lindberg AA. Antibody response to Shigella sonnei infection determined by an enzyme-linked immunosorbent assay. Eur J Clin Microbiol 2: 200–205, 1983.
26. Lindberg AA, Ekwall E, Carlin N. Shigella flexneri O-antigen specific enzyme immunoassay: lipopolysaccharides and synthetic glycoconjugates as antigens. Serodiagn Immunother Infect Dis 2: 63–78, 1988.
27. Formal SB, Gemski P, Baron LS, LaBrec EH. Genetic transfer of Shigella flexneri antigens to Escherichia coli K-12. Infect Immun 1: 279–287, 1970.
28. Sansonetti PJ, Kopecko DJ, Formal SB. Involvement of a plasmid in the invasive ability of Shigella flexneri. Infect Immun 35: 852–860, 1982.
29. Lowry OH, Rosebrough NJ, Farr AL, Randall RJ. Protein measurement with the Folin phenol reagent. J Biol Chem 193: 267–275, 1951.
30. Fink PC, Römer M, Haeckel R. Measurement of proteins with the Behring Nephelometer. A multicentre evaluation. J Clin Chem Biochem 27: 261–276, 1989.
31. An L, Zhao CR, Ekwall E, Forsum U, Lindberg AA. Serum antibody responses against Shigella lipopolysaccharides and invasion plasmid-coded antigens in Shigella infected Swedish patients. Scand J Infect Dis, 1993.
32. Raqib R, Tzipori S, Islam M, Lindberg AA. Immune responses to Shigella dysenteriae 1 and Shigella flexneri lipopolysaccharide and polysaccharide antigens in Bangladeshi patients with shigellosis. Serodiagn Immunother Infect Disease 1: 37–45, 1993.
33. Jann K, Westphal O. Microbial polysaccharides. In: Sela M, ed. The antigens, vol III. New York: Academic Press, 89–95, 1975.
34. Hanson LÅ. The mammary gland as an immunological organ. Immunol Today 3: 168–172, 1982.
35. Islam D, Lindberg AA. Detection of Shigella dysenteriae type 1 and Shigella flexneri in feces by immunomagnetic isolation and polymerase chain reaction. J Clin Microbiol 30: 2801–2806, 1992.

Submitted September 29, 1993; accepted January 12, 1994

Scand J Infect Dis 26: 339–347, 1994

Serological Follow-up after Treatment of Borrelia Arthritis and Acrodermatitis Chronica Atrophicans

SUSANNE HAMMERS-BERGGREN[1], ANNE-METTE LEBECH[4], MATS KARLSSON[1], ULF ANDERSSON[3], KLAUS HANSEN[4] and GÖRAN STIERNSTEDT[2]

From the Departments of Infectious Diseases, Karolinska Institute, [1]Danderyd Hospital, Danderyd and [2]Huddinge Hospital, Huddinge, and [3]the Department of Pediatrics, Karolinska Institute, Division of Rheumatology, St. Göran's Hospital, Stockholm, Sweden, and [4]the Borrelia Laboratory, Department of Infection Immunology, Division of Biotechnology, Statens Seruminstitut, Copenhagen, Denmark

To study the serological response to Borrelia burgdorferi after treatment of late Lyme borreliosis, consecutive serum samples from 20 patients with Borrelia arthritis and 21 with acrodermatitis chronica atrophicans were analysed with capture IgM ELISA and indirect IgG ELISA, both using B. burgdorferi flagella as antigen. Seven patients had positive IgM OD values, whereas all 41 had positive IgG OD values before therapy. In the majority, highly elevated IgG OD values were seen. All patients improved after antibiotic therapy, 32 recovering completely, while 9 had sequelae. At follow-up after 6 months to 5 years, 4/7 patients became negative in IgM ELISA, whereas 3 still had slightly elevated IgM OD values 6 months, 1 year and 4.5 years, respectively, after therapy. Only one patient became negative in IgG ELISA during follow-up, although a significant decline in IgG OD values was seen in 22 of the remaining 40 initially IgG-positive patients. The serological response after successful treatment of Borrelia arthritis and acrodermatitis chronica atrophicans may persist for several years even with highly elevated IgG OD values in patients who have recovered completely.

S. Hammers-Berggren, MD, Department of Infectious Diseases, Danderyds, Sjukhus, S-182 88 Danderyd, Sweden

INTRODUCTION

Earlier studies on the antibody response to Borrelia burgdorferi have shown a persisting IgG antibody response after spontaneous recovery from neuroborreliosis (1) and Lyme arthritis (2, 3). In epidemiological screening surveys, a large proportion of healthy persons without a previous or present history of Lyme borreliosis have been found to be seropositive to B. burgdorferi (4–6). Sometimes highly elevated IgG titres against B. burgdorferi have been demonstrated even in asymptomatic persons otherwise found in late manifestations of Lyme borreliosis such as neuroborreliosis with encephalomyelitis, Borrelia arthritis (BA) and acrodermatitis chronica atrophicans (ACA) (2, 3, 7–9). As antibiotic therapy was not given to these asymptomatic patients, doubts have been raised as to whether a latent infection might be present (3). It is therefore of interest to study the serological response after adequate antibiotic therapy of late manifestations of Lyme borreliosis.

BA, described by Steere et al. as Lyme arthritis in 1976 (10), and confirmed by a positive antibody response against B. burgdorferi in serum in conjunction with the exclusion of other causes of joint inflammation, is classified as the second or third stage of Lyme borreliosis (11, 12). A large proportion of such patients have highly elevated antibody titres against B. burgdorferi, mainly of IgG class, at diagnosis (2, 3, 8, 13, 14). ACA is usually diagnosed on typical clinical findings in combination with a positive antibody response, mainly of IgG class, against B. burgdorferi (9, 15). ACA is classified as a third-stage manifestation of Lyme borreliosis (11, 15) and in the majority of patients high IgG titres are found at diagnosis (9). Positive IgM OD values against B. burgdorferi are more seldom found in these late manifestations of Lyme borreliosis (2, 3, 8, 9).

The aim of the present study was to investigate the kinetics and duration of the antibody response against B. burgdorferi following antibiotic treatment of late Lyme borreliosis. Consecutive serum samples from patients treated for BA and ACA were analysed with a capture IgM ELISA and an indirect IgG ELISA, both using B. burgdorferi flagella as antigen and the results were correlated to the clinical outcome.

MATERIALS AND METHODS

Patients

Patients with BA and patients with ACA admitted to the Department of Infectious Diseases, Danderyd Hospital or the Department of Pediatrics, Division of Rheumatology, St. Göran's Hospital, Stockholm, between 1986 and 1991 were included in the study.

Borrelia arthritis

The diagnosis of BA was based on a typical clinical picture (10) and positive serology against B. burgdorferi. Other causes of joint inflammation were excluded by culture of the synovial fluid in all patients with monoarthritis, by the measurement of rheumatoid factor, antinuclear antibodies, antistreptolysin O titre, streptococcal anti-DNAse titre, antibodies to Yersinia enterocolitica type 3 and antibodies to Salmonella serotypes BO and DO. 20 patients with BA were included, for whom pretreatment and follow-up characteristics are shown in Table I.

All patients received antibiotic treatment. Benzyl penicillin 3 g q 8 h (in children 100–150 mg/kg/day) for 10–14 days was given intravenously (i.v.) to 12 patients, 4 received doxycycline 200 mg q 24 h orally 2–4 weeks, 3 received benzyl penicillin 3 g q 8 h i.v. for 10–14 days followed by doxycycline 200 mg q 24 h orally for 14 days and 1 patient received cefotaxime 2 g q 12 h i.v. for 14 days followed by doxycycline 200 mg q 24 h orally for 14 days.

Table I. *Clinical data of patients with Borrelia arthritis*

Number of patients	20
Children/adults	11/9
Male/female	10 (6 children)/10 (5 children)
Age	8–69 years, median 14 years
Preceding tick-bite within 3 months	5
Preceding erythema migrans	1
Clinical manifestations	
Clinical picture of joint inflammation	
One/several brief attacks of arthritis	18
Chronic arthritis[a]	2
Number of joints involved	
Monoarthritis	11
Oligoarthritis	8
Polyarthritis	1
Joint involved	
Knee	18
Elbow	3
Wrist	3
Ankle	2
Shoulder	1
Pretreatment symptom duration	2.5 weeks–3 years, median 6.5 months
Follow-up time	6 months–5 years, median 3.5 years
Improvement	20
Complete recovery[b]	19 (including 2 patients with chronic arthritis)
Sequelae	1, effusion of ankle 6 months posttreatment

[a] Chronic arthritis = continual joint inflammation for ≥1 year (11, 12).
[b] Complete recovery = no relapse of arthritis within 6 months' follow-up after last treatment course.

Four of the 20 patients were retreated due to persisting or new symptoms of arthritis. One patient was retreated with cefotaxime i.v. for 14 days followed by doxycycline orally for 14 days, 3 weeks after initial treatment with oral doxycycline. One other patient received ceftriaxone 2 g q 24 h i.v. for 14 days, 2 years after an initial treatment course with benzyl penicillin i.v. Two patients initially treated with penicillin i.v. received repeated antibiotic treatment regimens including oral doxycycline, oral penicillin and i.v. ceftriaxone. One of these 2 patients responded after a course of ceftriaxone 1 g q 24 h i.v. for 14 days, one year after the initial treatment. In the other patient, synovectomy was ultimately performed 15 months after the initial treatment.

Acrodermatitis chronica atrophicans

The diagnosis of ACA was based on a typical clinical picture (15) and positive serology against B. burgdorferi. 21 patients with ACA were included, in whom pretreatment and follow-up characteristics are shown in Table II.

All these patients received antibiotic therapy. Penicillin V 1 g q 8–12 h 3 weeks was given orally to 12 patients, 7 received doxycycline 100–200 mg q 24 h orally for 2–3 weeks and 2 patients received benzyl penicillin 3 g q 8 i.v. for 10 days. Due to persistent symptoms, 3 patients were retreated with oral doxycycline 1.5 and 9 months, respectively, after the initial treatment course with penicillin orally in 2 patients and benzyl penicillin i.v. in the third, 7 months after the initial treatment course.

Serology

Serum samples from all patients were analysed with a capture IgM ELISA and an indirect IgG ELISA, both using B. burgdorferi flagella as antigen. The methods have been described earlier in detail (16, 17). Briefly, in the capture IgM ELISA the solid phase is coated with μ-chain specific rabbit antihuman IgM, binding to human IgM antibodies in sera diluted 1/200. B. burgdorferi-specific IgM antibodies react with the test antigen consisting of a B. burgdorferi flagella biotin-avidin-peroxidase complex. Bound flagella are visualized adding O-phenylenediamine substrate with H_2O_2. In the indirect IgG ELISA, microtitre plates are coated with purified B. burgdorferi flagella. Serum samples diluted 1/200 are added and specific antibodies become bound. The binding is detected by adding peroxidase-conjugated rabbit anti-human IgG antibodies and O-phenylenediamine substrate with H_2O_2. In both assays the optical density (OD) is read spectrophotometrically and cut-off, 0.500 in the IgM ELISA and 0.180 in the IgG ELISA is defined as the 98% percentile of OD values obtained in sera from 200 healthy controls (16, 17). Consecutive serum samples from each patient are analysed simultaneously on the same microtitre plate. A 2-fold decrease or increase in the OD value in consecutive serum samples is considered significant for both the capture IgM ELISA and the indirect IgG ELISA.

Table II. *Clinical data of patients with acrodermatitis chronica atrophicans (ACA)*

Number	21
Male/female	4/17
Age	13–88 years, median 67 years
Preceding erythema migrans (EM) on the same extremity	7
Time to prior EM	6 months–8 years
Clinical manifestations	
ACA	16
ACA + peripheral neuropathy of affected limb	5
ACA + arthropathy	0
Pretreatment symptom duration	3 months–10 years, median 2 years
Follow-up time	10 months–4 years, median 2 years
Improvement	21
Complete recovery	13 (62%)
Sequelae	8 (38%)
Inflammation/atrophy of skin	3
Inflammation/atrophy of skin + underlying neuropathy	3
Neuropathy but no skin affection	2

The first serum sample in each patient was drawn before initiation of antibiotic therapy, except in 2 patients with ACA. In these 2, the first serum sample was drawn 2 and 3 months, respectively, after commencing antibiotic treatment.

RESULTS

Borrelia arthritis

Pretreatment. Four of the 20 patients had positive IgM OD values and all had positive IgG OD values against B. burgdorferi. In the 4 patients with positive IgM OD values, the range was 0.520 – >2.500 (median 1.390) and in the 20 patients with positive IgG OD values the range varied between 0.350 and >2.500 (median 1.020).

Two of the patients with positive IgG OD value only were initially negative in the IgM ELISA but had developed borderline IgM OD values (0.540 and 0.560) after 1 and 2 months of observation, respectively.

Follow-up

IgM OD values

The serum IgM OD value kinetics in the 6 positive patients are shown in Fig. 1A. Of the 4 initially IgM-positive patients, including 1 with borderline OD value and 2 patients with slightly positive IgM ELISA within 2 months of treatment, 3 patients became negative in IgM ELISA during follow-up when tested after 1 month, 9 months and 4 years, respectively. The remaining 3 patients still had positive IgM OD values against B. burgdorferi 6 months, 1 and 4.5 years, respectively, after antibiotic treatment. A significant decline was seen in 2 patients after 3 and 6 months, respectively, while the third had an unchanged borderline OD value during the follow-up time of 1 year.

IgG OD values

The serum IgG OD value kinetics are shown in Fig. 1B. A general decline in the IgG OD values is evident. Of the 20 IgG-positive patients, only 1 turned negative in the IgG ELISA during follow-up when tested after 4 years, while 19 patients still had positive IgG OD values at follow-up after 6 months to 5 years (median 3.5 years). In 13/19 patients a significant decline in the IgG OD value was seen during follow-up for 6 months to 4 years (median one year).

Patients with increasing OD values during follow-up

Two patients (nos. I and II, Fig. 1B) showed 1 and 2 peaks in the IgG OD value, respectively. Both patients had relapses of their arthritides simultaneously with the OD value increase. They had been treated with oral doxycycline and i.v. penicillin G, respectively. Both were negative in the IgM ELISA. Patient no. I was retreated with cefotaxime i.v. followed by doxycycline orally and recovered completely. Patient no. II was retreated orally with repeated antibiotic courses and finally with ceftriaxone i.v. and responded.

Patients with highly elevated IgG antibodies during follow-up

Three patients had declining though highly elevated IgG OD values for years after antibiotic treatment and/or synovectomy (Fig. 1B). All 3 recovered. The first patient was IgM negative. She responded to treatment with penicillin i.v. followed by doxycycline orally and developed no further symptoms of arthritis when followed for 3.5 years.

The second patient had a positive IgM OD value against B. burgdorferi, which declined significantly within 3 months of commencing antibiotic therapy with penicillin i.v. She

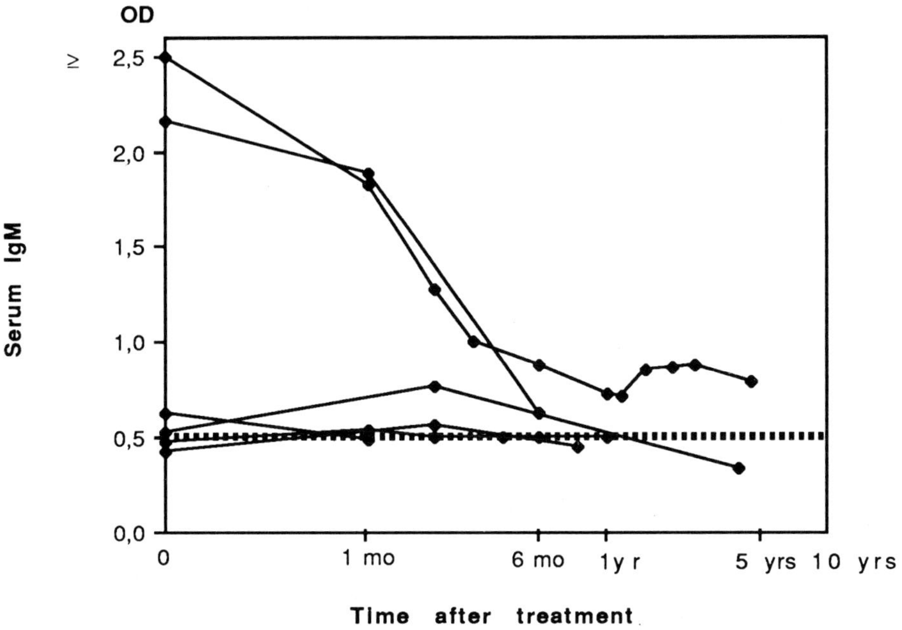

Fig. 1A

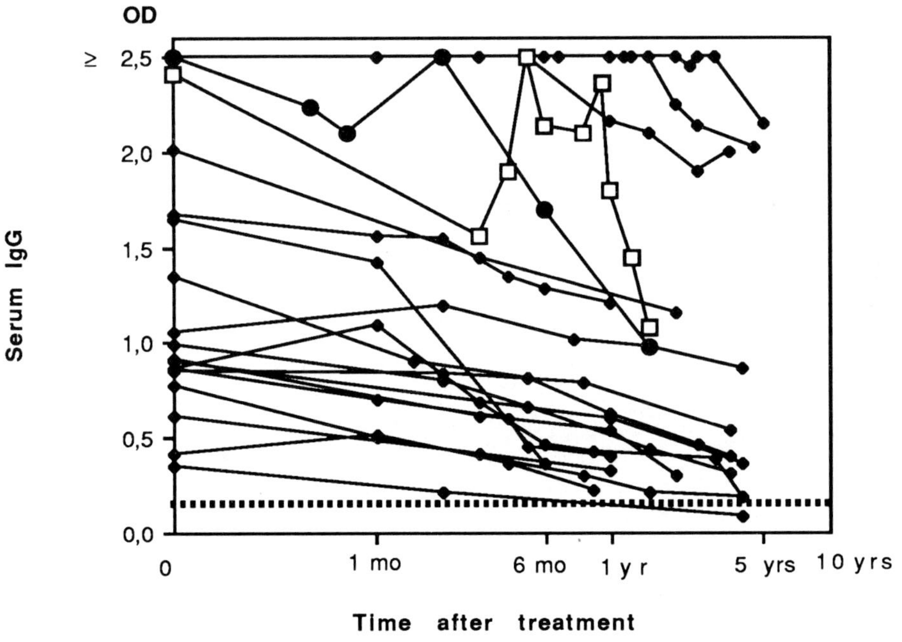

Fig. 1B

Fig. 1 A and B. Serum IgM and serum IgG OD values against Borrelia burgdorferi before treatment and during follow-up in 20 patients with Borrelia arthritis. Horizontal dotted lines mark the cut-off. Mo = months, yrs = years. – ● – = patient no. I. – □ – = patient no. II.

developed chronic gonarthritis and received repeated antibiotic courses. Ultimately she was synovectomized 15 months after the initial antibiotic course and responded.

The third patient was negative in the IgM ELISA. She had chronic arthritis prior to the first antibiotic course with penicillin i.v. She did not respond and was retreated with ceftriaxone i.v. 2 years after the first treatment, whereafter her continuous joint inflammation ceased.

Acrodermatitis chronica atrophicans

Pretreatment

None of the 19 patients who had a serum drawn before treatment had a positive IgM OD value, whereas all 19 had positive IgG OD values (range 0.990– >2.500, median 1.800).

Follow-up

IgM OD values

One patient (no. III, see below) with no pretreatment sample available and whose first serum was drawn 2 months after the onset of antibiotic therapy had a positive IgM OD value against B. burgdorferi (OD value 0.610). The IgM OD value was still positive 3 months later. At follow-up after 1.5 years she was negative in the IgM ELISA.

IgG OD values

The kinetics of serum IgG OD values are shown in Fig. 2. A general decline in the IgG OD values was seen in the 21 IgG-positive patients, although all positive still had IgG OD values when followed for 10 months–4 years (median 2 years). In 9 of the 21 patients a significant

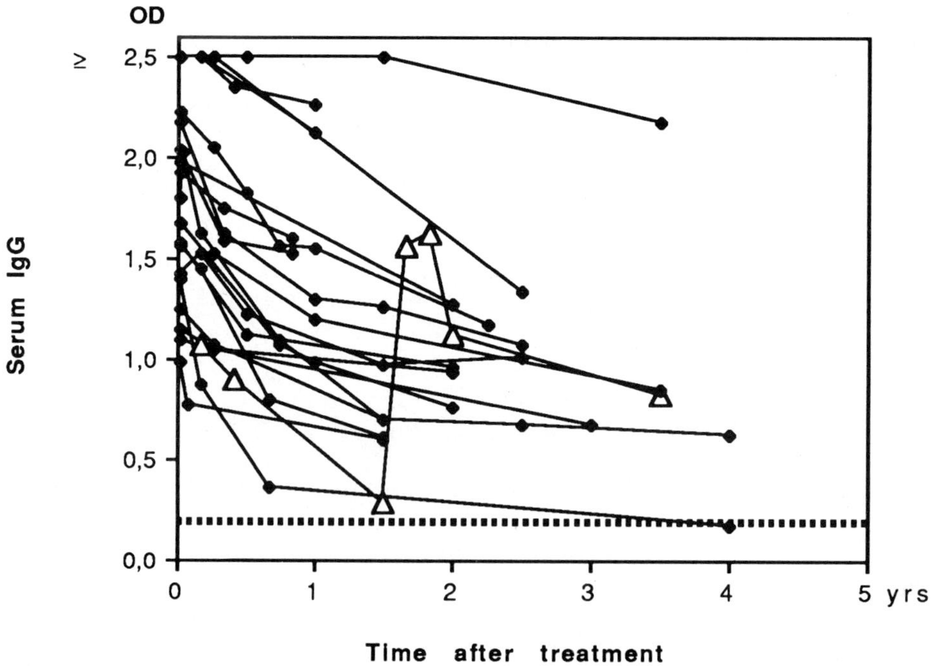

Fig. 2. Serum IgG OD values against Borrelia burgdorferi before treatment and during follow-up in 21 patients with acrodermatitis chronica atrophicans. Horizontal dotted line marks the cut-off. Yrs = years. – △ – = patient no. III.

decline in the IgG OD value was seen during follow-up for 8 months–3.5 years (median 2 years).

Patients with increasing antibody OD values during follow-up

One patient (no. III, Fig. 2) with symptoms of ACA 1.5 years before therapy, made a complete clinical recovery after treatment with oral doxycycline 200 mg q 24 h for 3 weeks. She had a slightly elevated IgM OD value 2 months after therapy but was negative after 1.5 years. At this time her IgG OD value had declined significantly. Two months later, during the summer, she developed facial palsy and headache and was once again admitted to hospital. No lumbar puncture was performed, but a serum analysis showed a significant rise in the IgG OD value against B. burgdorferi. The IgM OD value was negative. She was again treated with doxycycline 200 mg q 24 h orally for 14 days and recovered completely. A second decrease in the IgG OD value was determined 4 months later. A follow-up serum sample drawn 3.5 years after treatment of ACA and 2 years after treatment of the facial palsy, however, still showed an elevated IgG OD value against B. burgdorferi (Fig. 2).

Patients with highly elevated IgG antibodies during follow-up

Three patients with ACA, one of them with simultaneous neuropathy, continued to have highly elevated IgG OD values for 1 year or more after treatment (Fig. 2). Two of the patients recovered completely during follow-up, while 1 patient improved but still had signs of dermatitis and hypo-anesthesia 1 year after antibiotic therapy.

DISCUSSION

Earlier long-term follow-up studies on patients with Lyme arthritis have shown a persistent IgG antibody response to B. burgdorferi during several years of follow-up (2, 3). The patients in these studies were untreated or had only received short-term oral antibiotic therapy for a preceding EM. Another study demonstrated a persistent IgG response to B. burgdorferi for 2 years after antibiotic treatment of Lyme arthritis, but the kinetics were not studied as only 1 post-treatment sample was analysed (18).

The present study demonstrates that the kinetics of the antibody response following antibiotic treatment of late manifestations of Lyme borreliosis, such as BA and ACA with clinical recovery shows a gradual decline, though elevated antibodies, mainly of the IgG class, may persist for several years. However, it is possible that the specific IgG antibody response to B. burgdorferi even after late manifestations of Lyme borreliosis may disappear over time, as half of the 41 patients in the present study showed a significant decline of the IgG OD value during follow-up after therapy.

In epidemiological screening surveys, healthy persons without a previous or present history of Lyme borreliosis are sometimes found to have very high IgG titres against B. burgdorferi (4–6). In the present study, we found some patients with declining but still very high IgG OD values during follow-up for 1 to several years, even though most of them had recovered completely. Patients with BA or ACA may be misdiagnosed or have mild clinical symptoms not calling for a medical examination. While spontaneous recovery from ACA is not known to occur (19), Steere et al. found a spontaneous recovery rate of relapsing B. burgdorferi caused arthritis in 10–20% per year (20). Another possibility of recovery from BA and ACA without a correct diagnosis is that the individuals have received one or several antibiotic treatment courses for other infections, e.g. respiratory tract infections. These theories may explain why even very high IgG titres can occasionally be found without indication of disease activity.

IgM positivity against B. burgdorferi in patients with BA and ACA has earlier been considered insignificant, as a high percentage of positive rheumatoid factor was found in these patients (9, 21). By using the IgM capture ELISA with a directly labelled antigen, the problem with false IgM positivity due to rheumatoid factor is solved (16). Furthermore, one can expect a higher frequency of true IgM positivity against B. burgdorferi in the capture assay, as the disadvantage of the IgG antibody competition in the indirect ELISA is eliminated (16).

Fewer than 20% of the patients with BA and ACA had positive IgM OD values at diagnosis and in 5 of 7 patients only borderline or slightly elevated values were demonstrated. Therefore, the IgM antibody response as a parameter of treatment effect will not be suitable in patients with late Lyme borreliosis. However, as all the patients in the present study improved after therapy, the gradual decline in the IgG OD value in almost all patients during follow-up may have been a laboratory parameter indicating treatment efficacy. Analogously, the rising IgG OD values in 2 patients with relapsing arthritides before retreatment could indicate treatment failure (Fig. 1B).

The possibility of incorrect diagnosis in the 41 patients may be one factor contributing to the persistence of the antibody response after antibiotic therapy. However, as the 20 patients had a typical medical history of BA, other etiologies of arthritis were excluded, and as 21 patients had typical findings of ACA on clinical examination, this suspicion seems unlikely – although it cannot be completely excluded.

One patient with a BA of the knee showed a significant decrease in IgM OD value after the first antibiotic course with i.v. penicillin, despite the development of chronic gonarthritis. This finding, together with the fact that repeated antibiotic courses in this patient did not cure the arthritis, may indicate that not only live spirochetes but also immunological mechanisms are involved in the pathogenesis of BA in some patients. The IgM OD value was still slightly elevated 4.5 years after treatment and more than 3 years after recovery following synovectomy. Consequently, an elevated IgM OD value may not always indicate early or current infection.

The patient with ACA (no. III) and a rapid rise in the serological response after treatment with oral doxycycline for 3 weeks probably had a B. burgdorferi reinfection, causing the headache, facial palsy and the significant increase in the IgG OD value. The initial therapy given for ACA in this case has earlier been demonstrated to be effective for the treatment of neuroborreliosis (22), which is why a latent infection in the nervous system seems to be an unlikely explanation.

In conclusion, the IgG antibody response after treatment of BA and ACA may persist for years even with highly elevated IgG OD values but in the absence of clinical disease activity. Consequently, a single serum sample with IgG antibodies to B. burgdorferi must always be correlated to the clinical picture. The gradual decrease in the IgG OD values against B. burgdorferi in the majority of patients is probably an effect of antibiotic treatment, although the same finding may occur during spontaneous recovery in patients with arthritis. Reinfection may maintain seropositivity.

ACKNOWLEDGEMENT

We thank Dorthe Søeberg Pedersen for excellent technical assistance.

REFERENCES

1. Krüger H, Reuss K, Rohrbach E, Pflughaupt K-W, Martin R, Mertens HG. Meningoradiculitis and encephalomyelitis due to Borrelia burgdorferi: a follow-up study of 72 patients over 27 years. J Neurol 236: 322–328, 1989.

2. Stiernstedt G, Granström M. Ixodes ricinus spirochete infection as the cause of postinfectious arthritis in Sweden. Scand J Rheumatol 14: 336–342, 1985.
3. Craft JE, Grodzicki RL, Steere AC. Antibody response in Lyme disease: evaluation of diagnostic tests. J Infect Dis 140: 789–795, 1984.
4. Steere AC, Taylor E, Wilson ML, Levine JF, Spielman A. Longitudinal assessment of the clinical and epidemiological features of Lyme disease in a defined population. J Infect Dis 154: 295–300, 1986.
5. Gustafson R, Svenungsson B, Gardulf A, Stiernstedt G, Forsgren M. Prevalence of tick-borne encephalitis and Lyme borreliosis in a defined Swedish population. Scand J Infect Dis 22: 297–306, 1990.
6. Berglund J, Eitrem R. Tick-borne borreliosis in the archipelago of southern Sweden. Scand J Infect Dis 25: 67–72, 1993.
7. Stiernstedt G, Granström M, Hederstedt B, Sköldenberg B. Diagnosis of spirochetal meningitis by enzyme-linked immunosorbent assay and indirect immunofluorescence assay in serum and cerebrospinal fluid. J Clin Microbiol 21: 819–825, 1985.
8. Hammers-Berggren S, Andersson U, Stiernstedt G. Borrelia arthritis in Swedish children: clinical manifestations in 10 children. Acta Paediatr 81: 921–924, 1992.
9. Hansen K, Åsbrink E. Serodiagnosis of erythema migrans and acrodermatitis chronica atrophicans by the Borrelia burgdorferi flagellum enzyme-linked immunosorbent assay. J Clin Microbiol 27: 545–551, 1989.
10. Steere AC, Malawista SE, Snydman DR, Shope RE, Andiman WA, Ross MR, Steele FM. Lyme arthritis. An epidemic of oligoarticular arthritis in children and adults in three Connecticut communities. Arthritis Rheum 20: 7–17, 1977.
11. Steere AC. Medical progress: Lyme disease. N Engl J Med 321: 586–596, 1989.
12. Herzer P. Joint manifestations of Lyme borreliosis in Europe. Scand J Infect Dis Suppl 77: 55–63, 1991.
13. Kryger P, Hansen K, Vinterberg H, Pedersen FK. Lyme arthritis among Danish patients with arthritis. Scand J Rheumatol 19: 77–81, 1990.
14. Herzer P, Wilske B. Lyme arthritis in Germany. Zbl Bakteriol Mikrobiol Hyg A 263: 268–274, 1986.
15. Åsbrink E, Hovmark A, Olsson I. Clinical manifestations of acrodermatitis chronica atrophicans in 50 Swedish patients. Zbl Bakteriol Mikrobiol Hyg A 263: 253–261, 1986.
16. Hansen K, Pil K, Lebech A-M. Improved immunoglobulin M serodiagnosis in Lyme borreliosis by using a μ-capture enzyme-linked immunosorbent assay with biotinylated Borrelia burgdorferi flagella. J Clin Microbiol 29: 166–173, 1991.
17. Hansen K, Hindersson P, Strandberg-Pedersen N. Measurement of antibodies to Borrelia burgdorferi flagellum improves serodiagnosis in Lyme disease. J Clin Microbiol 26: 338–346, 1988.
18. Feder HM, Gerber MA, Luger SW, Ryan RW. Persistence of serum antibodies to Borrelia burgdorferi in patients treated for Lyme disease. Clin Infect Dis 11: 894–900, 1992.
19. Åsbrink E. Cutaneous manifestations of Lyme borreliosis. Scand J Infect Dis Suppl 77: 44–50, 1991.
20. Steere AC, Schoen RT, Taylor E. The clinical evolution of Lyme arthritis. Ann Intern Med 107: 725–731, 1987.
21. Kujala GA, Steere AC, Davis JS. IgM rheumatoid factor in Lyme disease: correlation with disease activity, total serum IgM, and IgM antibodies to Borrelia burgdorferi. J Rheumatol 14: 772–776, 1987.
22. Karlsson M, Hammers-Berggren S, Lindqvist L, Stiernstedt G, Svenungsson B. Comparison of intravenous penicillin G and oral doxycycline for treatment of Lyme neuroborreliosis. Neurology [accepted 1994].

Submitted January 4, 1994; accepted March 6, 1994

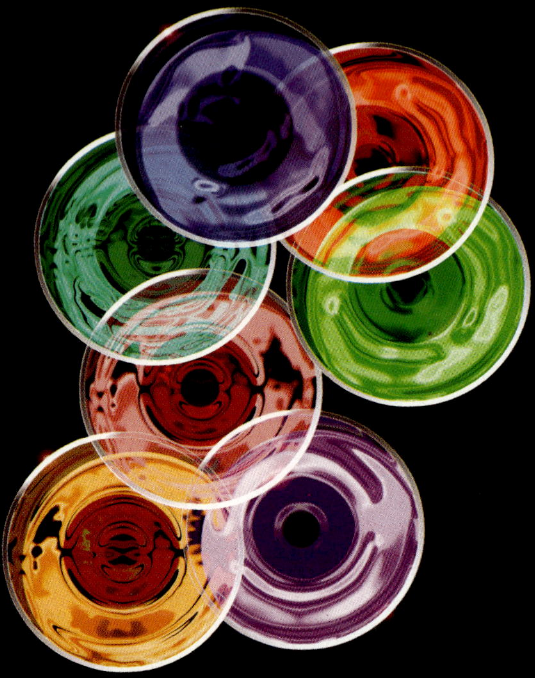

Bred täckning gör Fortum lämpligt för monoterapi

Sedan Fortum (ceftazidim) introducerades har monoterapi vid behandling av febrila patienter med nedsatt infektionsförsvar blivit accepterad.

Tack vare Fortums antibakteriella egenskaper är behandlingen lika effektiv som vid kombinationsterapi. Dessutom är den enklare, vilket sparar såväl tid som pengar.

Fortum kan även ges till patienter med försämrad njurfunktion. Vid behandling av denna patientgrupp se FASS.

FORTUM®

Bred täckning – effektiv behandling

Injektionsflaska 250 mg, 500 mg, 1 g, 2 g. Infusionsflaska 1 g, 2 g.

Glaxo ANTIBIOTIKASEKTIONEN BOX 263 431 23 MÖLNDAL. TELEFON 031-67 09 00

REFERENSER

Pizzo PA, Hathorn JW, Miemenz J et al. N Engl J Med 1986; 315: 552-8.
De Pauw BE, Feld R, Deresinski S et al. 6th International Symposium on infections in the immunocompromised Host. Peebles, Scotland June 3-6, 1990.
Novakova I, Donnelly P, de Pauw B. Scand J Infect Dis 22: 705-71 (1990)
Parr MD, Hansen LA, Rapp RP. Drug Intell Clin Pharm 1988; 22:628-31.
Mondorf AW, Mondorf W, Banzer S. 5th Mediterranean Congress of Chemotherapy, Cairo 1986: Abst. 0196.
Sanders JW, Powe NR, Moore RD. J Infect Dis 1991; 164:907:16.

Scand J Infect Dis 26: 349–355, 1994

Prevalence of Borrelia burgdorferi in Selected Tick Populations in Finland

JUHA JUNTTILA, RAILI TANSKANEN and JAAKKO TUOMI

From the Department of Microbiology and Epizootology, College of Veterinary Medicine, Helsinki, Finland

The purpose of the studies was to determine the prevalence of Borrelia burgdorferi sensu lato in selected populations of Ixodes ricinus in Finland and to secure strains of the spirochete for further characterization. 1,210 Ixodes ricinus ticks (399 females, 419 males and 392 nymphs) were collected during June to August 1992 by flagging from 8 sites in 3 regions. The frequency of B. burgdorferi infection was determined by isolation in BSK II medium. The species identity of most of the isolates was confirmed with the immunofluorescence method. 67 B. burgdorferi strains were isolated from 8 sites; the prevalence ranged from 2.8% to 7.9%. The overall isolation percentage for adult male ticks was 6.4% (7.5% for females, 5.3% for males); for nymphs, 3.8%. No statistically significant association of the prevalence was observed with either pasture or off-pasture habitats nor with specific geographic region/regions. Prevalence figures were roughly of the same magnitude in areas and parts of the country known to differ in their incidence of human borreliosis. An additional 294 ticks, mainly engorged females, were collected from places outside the main study sites. Of the 7 positive ticks 3 were engorged females, originating from a cow, a dog and a cat, respectively. The results in general demonstrate that tick populations in various parts of Finland quite commonly harbour B. burgdorferi.

R. Tanskanen, VMD, Department of Microbiology and Epizootology, College of Veterinary Medicine, Box 6, FIN-00581 Helsinki, Finland

INTRODUCTION

Ixodes ricinus-borne diseases have long been recognized in Finland. The earliest identifications of Lyme borreliosis in Finland by serology and isolation methods were made in the mid-1980s (1, 2). The annual number of serologically diagnosed/verified human cases at present is about 530 (Kosunen T., personal communication).

The Åland islands, southwest of the mainland, constitute a well known endemic area for Lyme borreliosis (3, 4). Cases (1, 5, 6) and seroprevalence data (7) however, have also been reported from various regions of the Finnish mainland. The distribution of Ixodes ricinus in Finland has been described summarily (8) and for selected places also in some detail (9); for climatological reasons, the tick occurs regularly only in the southern half of the country.

Ticks had not been studied earlier in Finland regarding frequency of B. burgdorferi infection. We carried out such a study with ticks collected in 1992 from 6 areas (8 sites) located in 3 separate regions of the country; ticks were also gathered from a few other locations.

MATERIALS AND METHODS

In Fig. 1 and Table I, the regions, areas and sites of collection of ticks are identified and characterized. The 3 main regions are Åland (area A), the coastal region near the town of Kotka (area B) and the territory close to the southeastern border (areas C and D). Both Åland and the area near Kotka are known to have a relatively high endemic occurrence of human Lyme borreliosis (4, Seppälä I., personal communication). Although cases are also encountered in eastern Finland, their incidence has been estimated to be definitely lower than that in areas A and B.

Most of the specific areas and sites of collection were selected on the grounds of knowledge of the nearby occurrence of human erythema migrans (EM) cases. In areas A and B, several cases had been recorded; in area C only 1 case, occuring 7 years previously, had been brought to our attention. For area

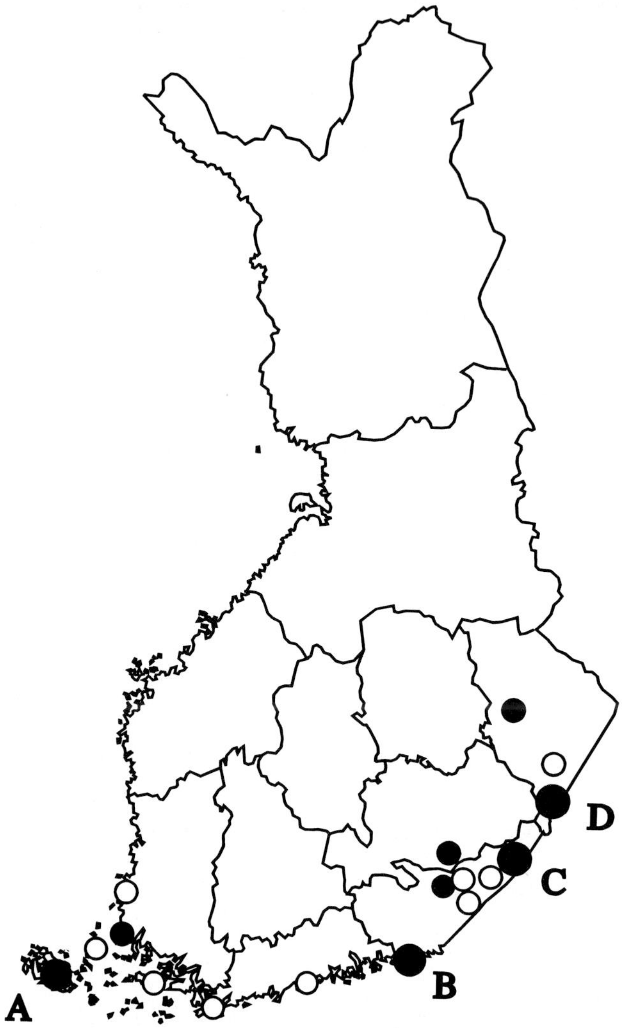

Fig 1. Regions, areas and sites of collection of Ixodes ricinus. The 8 sites of the main study are located in 3 regions; in one of them within 2 separate areas, C and D. Locations of 4 areas or close clusters of areas (A–D) of the main study are indicated with (●). The symbols for additional collection sites are: (●) B. burgdorferi infection detected, (○) not detected. Some of the additional collection sites (see also Table III) are close to the main sites, and thus cannot be indicated by separate symbols.

and site C the criterion of selection was 2 clinically suspected cases of bovine neuroborreliosis on a farm in 1990. In addition, odd ticks were collected from several locations (see Fig. 1).

Collection in June to August 1992 was performed mainly by flagging. The collection periods by area were as follows: A, late June and late August; B, early and late August; C and D, late July and mid-August. A smaller number of engorged females, picked up from domestic animals, were also included in the material. The latter originated mainly from places other than the main sites of collection. The ticks were placed in small glass or plastic tubes with a blade of grass. They were stored at 4°C until dissected.

The detection of Borrelia burgdorferi in ticks was attempted by the culture method, using the Barbour-Stoenner-Kelly medium (BSK II) (10). Rifampin and phosphomycin were added to final concentrations of 50 and 100 μg/ml, respectively (11). Six ml of the medium was aseptically dispensed into sterile 7 ml polystyrene tubes (Falcon 2027, Becton Dickinson, Rutherford, N.Y.). The tubes were stored at 4°C until used, not exceeding 4 weeks. Each lot of medium was tested for freedom from contaminants and ability to support the growth of B. burgdorferi type strain B31 (ATCC 52210).

The period of preparation of the ticks for the isolation trials and the starting of the trials extended from July to November 1992. Female ticks were dissected as described by Anderson et al. (12). After washing the tick in series in isopropyl alcohol, H_2O_2 and PBS, 30 s in each, the dorsum was removed

Table I. *Characterization of main sites for collection of ticks by flagging, in the summer of 1992*

Region	Area (community)	Site of collection: Code	Area (ha)	Characteristics of the site
Island of Åland	Ytternäs[a]	A1a	2.0	Horse farm; pasture; grass-fields with hazel bush and deciduous trees.
	Ytternäs	A1b	2.0	Horse farm; off-pasture; deciduous woodland with hazel bushes.
	Ringsböle[b]	A2a	5.5	Beef cattle farm; pasture; mainly grass-field, with less bush and trees than in A1a.
	Ringsböle	A2b	1.5	Beef cattle farm; off-pasture; woodland with mixed trees and bushes.
Vicinity of Kotka town	Mussalo	B1	2.5	Seaside resort, surrounded with pine wood; especially a nearby damp grove.
	Hevossaari	B2	17.0	Inhabited island; woodland with mixed trees, bilberry undergrowth.
Territory close to the southeastern border of Finland	Ulponniemi[c]	C	6.5	Lakeshore and nearby mixed trees woods with alder bushes.
	Kesälahti	D	4.0	Old pasture in pinewood with alder bushes, including nearby lakeshore

[a] Ca. 5 km from Mariehamn.
[b] Ca. 20 km from Mariehamn.
[c] In Parikkala.

and the midgut portion extracted and transferred to the culture tube. In the case of engorged females, the whole gut package with its contents was transferred.

Using the technique of Johnson et al. (13), males and nymphs were placed, after washing, in a sterile mortar containing 0.5 ml of BSK II medium and ground with a pestle. An additional 0.5 ml of medium was added. The suspension was transferred to the culture tube.

The cultures were incubated at 33°C. The first examination with a dark-field microscope, ×400 or ×1,000, was made after 2 to 4 weeks. When borrelia was detected, subcultures were made and part of the primary culture was frozen at −72°C, with 10% glycerol. Negative cultures were re-examined after an additional 4 weeks or were transferred at that time to 4°C for later examination. The latest re-examinations took place after 5 to 6 months' storage at 4°C. A total of 100 microscopic fields were searched before accepting a negative result.

In the early stage of the studies, all isolates growing adequately (as the great majority did) in pure or contaminated cultures were examined with the immunofluorescence method, direct or indirect (14). In the direct test the conjugate used was a FITC-labelled goat anti-borrelia sp. immunoglobulin (Kirkegaard & Perry); in the indirect method a self-prepared bovine anti-B31 hyperimmune serum and a FITC-labelled rabbit anti-cow immunoglobulin (Dakopatts) were the reagents. Quite frequently the monoclonals H5332 and H9728 (courtesy of Dr. A. G. Barbour) with the appropriate conjugate were also applied. Statistical calculations were performed with the chi-squared method.

RESULTS

1,504 Ixodes ricinus ticks (1,091 adults and 413 nymphs) were examined; 1,210 of them originated from the main sites of the study. Table II shows the results for these sites. B. burgdorferi was found in all of them. The observed prevalences ranged from 2.8% for site C to 7.9% for site A1b. The overall rates of infection for females, males and nymphs in the sites listed were 7.5%, 5.3% and 3.8%, respectively; the average rate 5.5%. The difference

Table II. *Isolation of 67 B. burgdorferi strains from 1210 ticks originating from 8 main sites of study*

Site of collection, by code[a]	Positive ticks/ticks examined (%) Females	Males	Nymphs	TOTAL
A1a	6/58 (10.3%)	2/53 (3.8%)	1/41 (2.4%)	9/152 (5.9%)
A1b	7/42 (16.6%)	6/63 (9.5%)	4/109 (3.7%)	17/214 (7.9%)
total (%)	(13.0%)	(6.9%)	(3.3%)	(7.1%)
A2a	0/3	0/2	8/140 (5.7%)	8/145 (5.5%)
A2b	4/49 (8.2%)	1/54 (1.9%)	2/75 (2.7%)	7/178 (3.9%)
total (%)	(7.7%)	(1.8%)	(4.7%)	(4.6%)
A, total (%)	(11.2%)	(5.2%)	(4.1%)	(6.0%)
B1	2/57 (3.5%)	3/73 (4.1%)	0/11	5/141 (3.5%)
B2	6/59 (10.2%)	2/41 (4.9%)	0/14	8/114 (7.0%)
total (%)	(6.9%)	(4.4%)		(5.1%)
C	3/64 (4.7%)	1/77 (1.3%)	0/1	4/142 (2.8%)
D	2/67 (3.0%)	7/56 (12.5%)	0/1	9/124 (7.3%)
TOTAL	**30/399 (7.5%)**	**22/419 (5.3%)**	**15/392 (3.8%)**	**67/1210 (5.5%)**

[a] Decoding, see Table I; location, see Fig. 1.

between females and males was not statistically significant whereas that between females and nymphs was ($p < 0.05$).

In Åland, the prevalence of B. burgdorferi was slightly higher for the tick population from the horse-keeping farm than from the farm with beef cattle. The difference was not statistically significant. (The prevalence figure for farm A2 may have been somewhat influenced by the death during storage, shortly preceding the preparation, of 60–80 nymphs; 2 isolations were made from them.) Within farms, the prevalence differences between pasture and off-pasture areas were likewise not significant. Females were found to be infected more frequently than males ($p \sim 0.05$) and adults more frequently than nymphs ($p < 0.05$). A new horse hand on farm A1 contracted EM during the summer.

Table III gives the isolation results for 294 ticks originating from outside the main study areas or sites. As shown in Fig. 1, 6/7 isolations were from eastern Finland, the northernmost from Polvijärvi. Three out of 144 engorged females were found to be positive; they had been picked up from a cow, a dog and a cat, respectively.

Of the 676 cultures prepared from ticks collected from the main study sites in Åland, and recorded appropriately, 208 were contaminated. The borrelia isolation rates were almost the same for the contaminated and non-contaminated cultures, 6.25% (13/208) and 6.0% (28/468), respectively.

DISCUSSION

The study was carried out with the isolation method only. The objective of securing a larger number of B. burgdorferi sensu lato strains for further characterization was decisive for the adoption of this approach. The laborious nature of this method has apparently largely precluded its more extensive use in tick infection prevalence studies, which instead have been conducted with dark-field microscopy and/or the immunofluorescence (IF) technique. Consequently, comparisons between isolation and other techniques regarding sensitivity are still largely lacking, a fact which affects the evaluation of the present results in a wider context.

Table III. *Isolation of 7 B. burgdorferi strains from 294 ticks collected from outside the main study sites*

Area of collection, community	Collection by flagging			Collection from animals		
	Females[a]	Males	Nymphs	Females	Males	Total
Puumala	0/4	1/3				1/7
Parikkala	1/2					1/2
Kustavi	0/5	0/3	1/4			1/12
Savitaipale	1/32	0/26	0/5			1/63
Other communities[b]	0/14	0/8	0/12			0/34
Parikkala				1/9[d]	0/1	1/10
Kesälahti				1/17[e]	0/6	1/23
Polvijärvi				1/13[f]	0/3	1/16
Other communities[c]				0/105	0/22	0/127
Total	**2/57**	**1/40**	**1/21**	**3/144**	**0/32**	**7/294**

[a] Positive ticks/n.
[b] Includes communities (no. of ticks): Åland (22), Saari (2), Ruokolahti (10).
[c] Includes Kitee (2), Uusikaupunki (34), Kustavi (4), Nauvo (13), Hanko (1), Taipalsaari (12), Lappeenranta (2), Ruokolahti (57), Helsinki (2).
[d] From a cat.
[e] From a dog.
[f] From a cow.

The comparability of these techniques is an issue in our ongoing prevalence studies with ticks collected during the summer of 1993. The preliminary results concerning unfed adults and nymphs indicate on average an approximately 1/3 lower relative sensitivity for the isolation method, as used by us, in comparison with dark-field microscopy (unpublished data). In 1992, contamination of the culture did not appear to reduce the isolation rate.

The techniques of preparation differed between females on the one hand and males and nymphs on the other. The comparable prevalence figures for both females and males do not suggest any significant sensitivity differences between the 2 methods.

The prevalence figures for the Finnish study sites, including those for the Åland islands, are in general somewhat lower than the proportions of infected ticks in populations studied in neighbouring Sweden, in Estonia or the St. Petersburg region in Russia (15), as reviewed by Gern et al. (16). The same conclusion applies to comparisons with results from Central Europe (16). It is currently uncertain to what extent the result may be attributable to a lower sensitivity of the isolation method used.

The validity of prevalence comparisons between the main sites of the present study is obviously unaffected by the methodology. The major finding, that no conspicuous differences in prevalence were detected both between regions and between sites studied, was unexpected. The hypothesis had been that the eastern areas, with a low incidence of reported human cases, would correspondingly reveal relatively low frequencies of borrelia infection in their tick populations. The results seem to contradict the hypothesis. Wherever they are examined, tick populations appear to harbour B. burgdorferi. The tick-related factors associated with the incidence of human borreliosis will more probably be found in such measures as the absolute frequency of infected ticks or the occurrence in an area of some particular genospecies or serotypes. Åland is known for its high incidence of primary Lyme disease, and also for frequent tick bites among the population (4). Our immunological characterization of the strains isolated suggests the existence of region-specific serotype differences (to be published). An association between certain serotypes and human pathogenicity has been indicated (17).

One of the issues which the present study has tried to settle was whether the prevalence of B. burgdorferi in the tick population is affected by the presence of large domestic animals in the area. Three of the collection sites (A1a, A2a and D) were pastures; the rest – some of them the adjacent off-pasture areas – were areas and sites not frequented by large domestic animals. The assumption had been that if, as has been demonstrated (18), a significant proportion of Ixodes ricinus larvae and nymphs can feed on large animals which appear not to function as sources of infection for ticks (own unpublished data from studies with experimental cattle), the prevalence of B. burgdorferi among the ticks of the pasture ecosystem would decline. No statistically significant suggestion of such an effect could be revealed in these limited studies. As regards incompetence as a reservoir host for B. burgdorferi, a comparable negative role among large wild animals has been indicated in the case of certain species of deer (19–21). Another aspect of the matter is that the presence of large animals increases the density of tick populations of pasture areas, which in turn tends to increase the absolute number of infected ticks on them, and consequently also the risk of infection.

Three of the isolations were made from engorged females, detached from a cow, a dog and a cat respectively. The result is noted because only very few such isolations have, to our knowledge, been reported earlier (22, 23); we have previously experienced difficulties in attempts to isolate B. burgdorferi from engorged females (unpublished data).

The present results give the first indication, and demonstration, that Ixodes ricinus populations in Finland are quite commonly infected with B. burgdorferi. The geographical distribution of borrelia in ticks appears largely to resemble that of bovine babesiosis and tick-borne fever (24) and to be quite different, i.e. wider, from that for the arbovirus causing human meningoencephalitis (25). The distribution difference between borrelia and arbovirus may reflect the different density demands of small mammal maintenance populations. The question of the possible contribution to the occurrence of B. burgdorferi, as competent reservoir hosts, of animals other than species of mice and voles, such as the Norway rat on Monhegan Island (26), is a further distribution-related question which still remains unanswered.

ACKNOWLEDGEMENTS

We thank Prof. Peter Wahlberg MD, former Head of the Åland Central Hospital for the selection of collection sites in the Åland islands and for other invaluable support. The technical assistance of Ms Tiina Palomäki and Mr Petri Muranen is gratefully acknowledged.

REFERENCES

1. Kovanen J, Schauman K, Valpas J. Bannwarth's syndrome and Lyme disease in Finland. Scand J Infect Dis 18: 421–424, 1986.
2. Marttila R, Panelius M. Bannwarth's syndrome – a spirochetal meningoradiculitis [in Finnish, with English summary]. Duodecim 101: 1191–1197, 1985.
3. Wahlberg P. Incidence of tick-bite in man in Åland Islands: reference to the spread of Lyme borreliosis. Scand J Infect Dis 22: 59–62, 1990.
4. Wahlberg P, Granlund H, Nyman D, Panelius J, Seppälä I. Late Lyme borreliosis: epidemiology, diagnosis and clinical features. Ann Med 25: 349–352, 1993.
5. Sonck CE. Erythema chronicum migrans with multiple lesions. Acta Derm Venereol (Stockh) 45: 34–36, 1965.
6. Schauman K, Kovanen J, Seppälä I. Lyme borreliosis in Finland 1986–1988. Biomed Pharmacother 43: 427–430, 1989.

7. Seppälä IJT, Kroneld R, Schauman K, Forsen K-O, Lassenius R. Diagnosis of Lyme borreliosis: Nonspecific serological reactions with Borrelia burgdorferi sonicate antigen caused by IgG2 antibodies. J Med Microbiol 40, 1994.
8. Öhman C. The geographical and topographical distribution of Ixodes ricinus in Finland. Acta Soc Fauna Flora Fenn 76: 1–26, 1961.
9. Brummer-Korvenkontio M. The ecology and virus isolations from ticks in Finland. Proc 1st Int Congr Parasitol, Roma 2: 1044–1045, 1966.
10. Barbour AG. Isolation and cultivation of Lyme disease spirochetes. Yale J Biol Med 57: 521–525, 1984.
11. Barbour AG. Laboratory aspects of Lyme borreliosis. Clin Microbiol Rev 1: 399–414, 1988.
12. Anderson JF, Magnarelli LA, Burgdorfer W, Barbour AG. Spirochetes in Ixodes dammini and mammals from Connecticut. Am J Trop Med Hyg 32: 818–824, 1983.
13. Johnson S, Klein G, Schmid G, Bowen G, Feeley J, Schulze T. Lyme disease: a selective medium for isolation of the suspected etiological agent, a spirochete. J Clin Microbiol 19: 81–82, 1984.
14. Burgdorfer W, Lane RS, Barbour AG, Gresbrink RA, Anderson JR. The western black-legged tick, Ixodes pacificus: a vector of Borrelia burgdorferi. Am J Trop Med Hyg 34: 925–930, 1985.
15. Korenberg E, Kovalevski Y, Kuznetsova R. Evidence of Lyme disease in the north-western USSR and the first results of this study. Med Parazitol (Mosk) 1: 45–48, 1988.
16. Gern L, Burgdorfer W, Aeschlimann A, Krampitz HE. The ecology of Lyme borreliosis in Europe. In: Weber K, Burgdorfer W, eds. Aspects of Lyme borreliosis. Berlin, Heidelberg: Springer-Verlag, 59–69, 1993.
17. Wilske B, Preac-Mursic V, Göbel UB, Graf B, Jauris S, Soutschek E, Schwab E, Zumstein G. An OspA serotyping system for Borrelia burdorferi based on reactivity with monoclonal antibodies and OspA sequence analysis. J Clin Microbiol 31: 340–350, 1993.
18. Arthur DR. Ticks and disease. Oxford: Pergamon Press, 236–269, 1962.
19. Telford SR, Mather TN, Moore SI, Wilson ML, Spielman A. Incompetence of deer as reservoir of the Lyme disease spirochete. Am J Trop Med Hyg 39: 105–109, 1988.
20. Jaenson TGT, Tålleklint L. Incompetence of roe deer as reservoirs of the Lyme borreliosis spirochete. J Med Entomol 29: 813–817, 1992.
21. Lacombe E, Rand PW, Smith RP. Disparity of Borrelia burgdorferi infection rates of adult Ixodes dammini on deer and vegetation. J Infect Dis 167: 1236–1238, 1993.
22. Anderson JF, Magnarelli LA. Spirochetes in Ixodes dammini and Babesia microti on Prudence Island, Rhode Island. J Infect Dis 148: 1124, 1983.
23. Anderson JF, Magnarelli LA. Ixodes dammini and Borrelia burgdorferi in northern New England and upstate New York. J Parasitol 73: 419–421, 1987.
24. Tuomi J. Studies in epidemiology of bovine tick-borne fever in Finland and a clinical description of field-cases. Ann Med Exp Fenn 44: 1–62, 1966.
25. Tuomi J, Brummer-Korvenkontio M. Antibodies against viruses of the tick-borne encephalitis group in cattle sera in Finland. Ann Med Exp Fenn 43: 149–154, 1965.
26. Smith RP, Rand PW, Lacombe EH, Telford SR, Rich SM, Piesman J, Spielman A. Norway rats as reservoir hosts for Lyme disease spirochetes on Monhegan Island, Maine. J Infect Dis 168: 687–691, 1993.

Submitted December 10, 1993; accepted January 31, 1994

sillit och pneumoni — AZITROMAX®
(azithromycin)

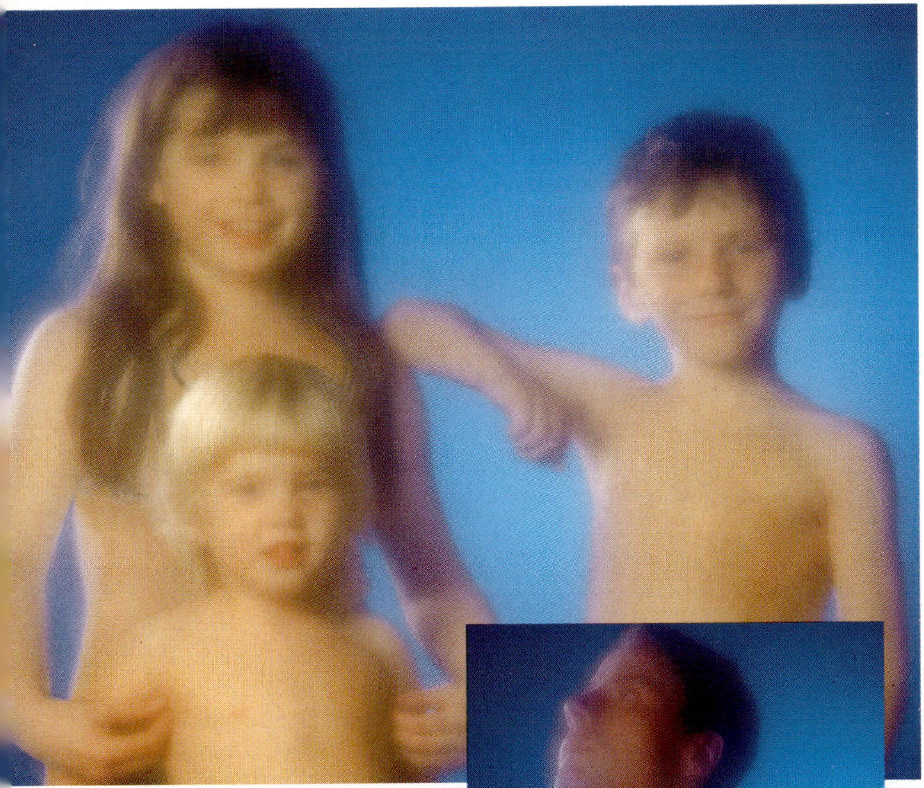

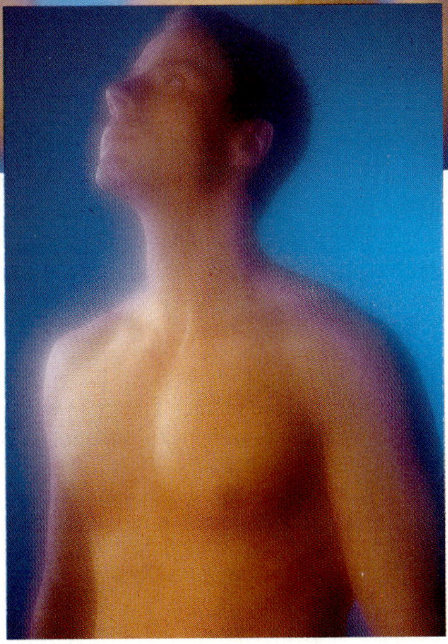

T M. Am J Med 1991; 91 (Suppl 3A): 23S-26S.
. et al. JAC 1993; 31 (Suppl E): 89-94.
Am J Med 1991; 91 (Suppl 3A): 31S-355.
R. J Int Med Res 1991; 19: 373-383.
P et al. Eur J Clin Microbiol Inf Dis 1991; 10 (5): 437-439.
vitz G and Wood R G.
in Microbiol Inf Dis 1991; 10 (10): 872-877.
ald S et al. J A C 1990; 25 (Suppl A): 123-126.
s S Am J Med 1991; 91 (Suppl 3A): 40S-45S.

Pfizer

Pfizer AB, Box 501, 183 25 Täby, Tel. 08-473 63 00

S-93 AZI-21 CEDERBLOM

Scand J Infect Dis 26: 358–360, 1994

SHORT COMMUNICATION

Mycoplasma pneumoniae Lacks Immunologically-Active Eukaryotic Actin-Like Antigens

NEVIO CIMOLAI

From the Division of Medical Microbiology, Department of Pathology, University of British Columbia, Vancouver, British Columbia, Canada

Mycoplasma pneumoniae was tested for immunologically active eukaryotic actin-like antigens with the use of both polyclonal and monoclonal anti-actin antibodies. No reactivity was demonstrable. Monoclonal antibody OC2F5, which reacts with a M. pneumoniae antigen that co-migrates with actin in one-dimensional sodium dodecyl sulphate polyacrylamide electrophoresis, did not recognize actin. Organism-specific actin antigens are not likely to be responsible for the development of smooth muscle antibodies during acute M. pneumoniae infection.

N. Cimolai, MD, Rm. 2G6, Department of Pathology, B.C.'s Children's Hospital, 4480 Oak Street, Vancouver, British Columbia, Canada V6H 3V4

INTRODUCTION

Mycoplasma pneumoniae is a common cause of community-acquired respiratory infection but has also been associated with a spectrum of extra-respiratory manifestations involving rheumatological, neurological, and dermatological systems, among others (1). Whereas direct infection by viable bacterium and the associated immune response are believed to be responsible for the respiratory disease, it is unclear which mechanisms of pathogenesis are most important in the development of non-respiratory illnesses. Nevertheless, auto-antibody formation has been suggested to account for the latter.

The findings of smooth muscle antibodies in patients with acute M. pneumoniae infection (2), and the recognition of structures resembling actin in M. pneumoniae (3–5) have led some to hypothesize that bacterial actin-like antigens could trigger an immune response to human tissue. Whereas Rodwell et al. (6) published evidence which would detract from this hypothesis, Gobel and colleagues (7) have recently restimulated interest by their finding of actin-related DNA sequences and proteins from another mycoplasma, M. genitalium, which at this time is recognized as the mycoplasma species most closely related to M. pneumoniae.

Given the availability of anti-actin immunological probes, it was determined whether immunologically active actin-like antigens were present in M. pneumoniae.

MATERIALS, METHODS AND RESULTS

Lysates of M. pneumoniae whole cells were resolved by sodium dodecyl sulphate polyacrylamide gel electrophoresis (SDS-PAGE) as detailed elsewhere (8). In addition, control bovine muscle actin (Sigma, MO, USA) and sterile mycoplasma growth media (Hayflick's) were resolved by the same methods. After SDS-PAGE, transfer to nitrocellulose was performed to provide a solid substrate for immunoblotting. The nitrocellulose was blocked with 1% skim milk/PBS (pH 7.4) overnight at 4°C. On the following day, portions of nitrocellulose containing actin, M. pneumoniae lysate, and sterile mycoplasma growth media were probed with 3 antibodies: (*a*) a muscle actin-specific monoclonal antibody HHF35 that recognizes alpha- and gamma-actin variants which are present in skeletal, cardiac, and smooth muscle (9); (*b*) rabbit polyclonal anti-actin (chicken backmuscle; Miles Scientific, IL, USA); and (*c*) monoclonal antibody OC2F5 which recognizes an antigen of M. pneumoniae which co-migrates with actin in one-dimensional SDS-PAGE (8). The anti-actin monoclonal antibody was utilized in a 1 : 1000 dilution

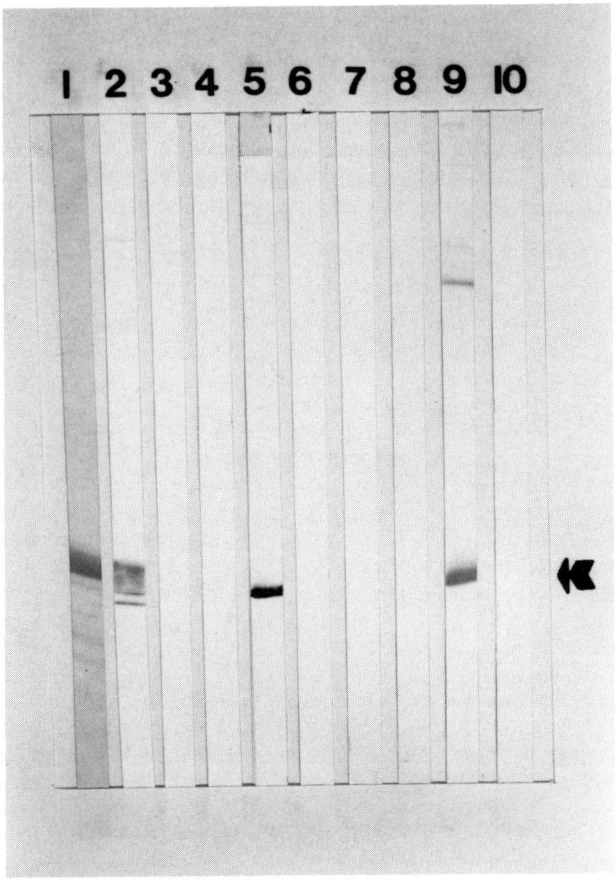

Fig. 1. Antibody reactivity with actin, M. pneumoniae, and mycoplasma growth medium. *Lane 1:* actin stained with Amido Black. *Lanes 2, 3, 4:* monoclonal antibody HHF35 was used to probe actin, M. pneumoniae, and growth media respectively. *Lanes 5, 6, 7:* polyclonal anti-actin antibody was used to probe actin, M. pneumoniae, and growth medium respectively. *Lanes 8, 9, 10:* monoclonal antibody OC2F5 was used to probe actin, M. pneumoniae, and growth medium respectively. *Arrow:* the migration level of actin and the sites with immunological reactivity.

in PBS. A biotin-labelled anti-mouse antibody and an avidin-peroxidase antibody were then employed for detection. The polyclonal anti-actin antibody was used in a 1 : 1000 dilution and then detected with a goat anti-rabbit peroxidase-labelled antibody. Monoclonal antibody OC2F5 was used as previously described.

Fig. 1 illustrates the reaction pattern of the various antibodies. Both the polyclonal and the monoclonal antibodies recognized actin only. Monoclonal antibody OC2F5 identified only the 42 kD band within the M. pneumoniae profile. Growth media were not recognized by any of the antibodies.

DISCUSSION

These findings refute the hypothesis that eukaryotic actin-like antigens are present in M. pneumoniae and that they are available to stimulate anti-mammalian actin antibodies. They do not exclude, however, that such autoantibodies might develop on the basis of polyclonal B cell stimulation or by some other unknown mechanism which may or may not be related to specific bacterial antigens.

Gobel et al. (7) have found an immunologically active actin-like antigen in M. genitalium by means of monoclonal anti-chicken muscle actin. Given the high sequence homology among actin isotypes and the fact that we used a polyclonal anti-chicken muscle actin as a probe, it is unlikely that our findings represent an artifact due to a narrow spectrum of reactivity of our immunological probes.

Biberfeld and Sterner (2) previously demonstrated that low titres ($\leq 1/80$) of anti-smooth muscle antibodies of both IgG and IgM developed in patients with M. pneumoniae infection. Their absorption experiments revealed that these antibodies had the same specificity as anti-smooth muscle antibodies from patients with active chronic hepatitis, the latter of which were believed to be anti-actin. Their finding, that M. pneumoniae does not absorb out anti-smooth muscle antibodies, is also consistent with our results.

The possibility should be considered that smooth muscle antibodies may arise whereby the specificity may be another non-actin antigen. For example, Bretherton et al. found evidence of IgM autoantibody to intermediate filaments (10). Future studies should confirm the association of M. pneumoniae infections and smooth muscle antibodies, and furthermore, should delineate the antigens which are recognized by these antibodies.

ACKNOWLEDGEMENT

I thank Richard Mah for helpful discussions.

REFERENCES

1. Fernald GW. Immunologic mechanisms suggested in the association of M. pneumoniae infection and extrapulmonary disease: a review. Yale J Biol Med 56: 475–479, 1983.
2. Biberfeld G, Sterner G. Smooth muscle antibodies in Mycoplasma pneumoniae infection. Clin Exp Immunol 24: 287–291, 1976.
3. Neimark HC. Extraction of an actin-like protein from the prokaryote Mycoplasma pneumoniae. Proc Natl Acad Sci USA 74: 4041–4045, 1977.
4. Meng KE, Pfister RM. Intracellular structures of Mycoplasma pneumoniae revealed after membrane removal. J Bacteriol 144: 390–399, 1980.
5. Gobel U, Speth V, Bredt W. Filamentous structures in adherent Mycoplasma pneumoniae cells treated with nonionic detergents. J Cell Biol 91: 537–543, 1981.
6. Rodwell AW, Rodwell ES, Archer DB. Mycoplasmas lack a protein which closely resembles alpha-actin. FEMS Microbiol Lett 5: 235–238, 1979.
7. Gobel UB, Muller MM, Maas R. Actin-related DNA sequences and proteins from motile mycoplasmas: a molecular puzzle. Bakteriol Microbiol Hyg [A] Suppl 20: 337–344, 1990.
8. Cimolai N, Bryan LE, To M, Woods DE. Immunological cross-reactivity of a Mycoplasma pneumoniae membrane-associated protein antigen with Mycoplasma genitalium and Acholeplasma laidlawii. J. Clin Microbiol 25: 2136–2139, 1987.
9. Tsukada T, Tippens D, Gordon D, Ross R, Gown AM. HHF35, a muscle actin-specific monoclonal antibody. I. Immunocytochemical and biochemical characterization. Am J Pathol 126: 51–60, 1987.
10. Bretherton L, Toh BH, Jack I. IgM autoantibody to intermediate filaments in Mycoplasma pneumoniae infections. Clin Immunol Immunopathol 18: 425–430, 1981.

Submitted August 31, 1993; accepted January 21, 1994

Scand J Infect Dis 26: 361–367, 1994

REVIEW ARTICLE

Proteus mirabilis Bacteremia: A Review of 176 Cases During 1980–1992

CHATRCHAI WATANAKUNAKORN[1,2] and SRIRAM C. PERNI[2]

From the [1]Department of Internal Medicine, Infection Disease Section, St. Elizabeth Hospital Medical Center, Youngstown, Ohio, and [2]The Northeastern Ohio Universities College of Medicine, Rootstown, Ohio, USA

Patients with Proteus mirabilis bacteremia at a large community teaching hospital during a 13-year period (1980–1992) were retrospectively reviewed. There were 176 patients whereof 44 (25%) had polymicrobial bacteremia. The median age of patients was 75 years and 64.2% were 70 years or older. Of the patients 56.8% came from a nursing home, 64.2% had an indwelling Foley catheter, and 20.5% nosocomial bacteremia. The most common source of bacteremia was the urinary tract (52.8%) whereas the lower respiratory tract was an uncommon source. Hypotension was present in 30.1% of patients. The overall mortality rate was 29.0% with an attributable mortality rate of 25.6%. The mortality rate of polymicrobial bacteremia (38.6%) was higher than that of monomicrobial bacteremia (25.8%). For patients with monomicrobial bacteremia, significant increase in mortality was found in patients who had nosocomial infection ($p < 0.02$), whose source of bacteremia was other than the urinary tract ($p < 0.01$), who had ultimately fatal underlying conditions ($p < 0.01$), who had hypotension ($p < 0.001$), who had increase in serum creatinine ($p < 0.05$), or who had increase in serum bilirubin ($p < 0.05$).

C. Watanakunakorn, MD, St. Elizabeth Hospital Medical Center, 1044 Belmont Avenue, Youngstown, Ohio 44501-1790, USA

INTRODUCTION

Among different Proteus species, Proteus mirabilis causes bacteremia in a significant number of patients (1–10). However, bacteremia due to P. mirabilis has not been a subject for detailed analysis in recent literature (11–14). For the past several years, we have studied bacteremia due to specific bacterial pathogens in our hospital (15–25). In the present study, we reviewed the clinical and laboratory data on all patients with bacteremia due to P. mirabilis in our hospital during 1980–92. The epidemiology, demography, important clinical and laboratory features, treatment and outcome were analyzed.

MATERIALS AND METHODS

St. Elizabeth Hospital Medical Center is a large community hospital, one of several major teaching hospitals of the Northeastern Ohio Universities College of Medicine. Inpatients from whose blood cultures grew P. mirabilis between January 1, 1980 and December 31, 1992 were identified from blood culture log-books. Medical records of these patients were reviewed and pertinent data recorded. Statistics on the number of patients admitted during the study period were obtained from the hospital administration.

Blood cultures were done by using the radiometric blood culture analyzer (BACTEC, Johnson Laboratories, Cockeysville, MD, USA). P. mirabilis was identified and speciated according to standard methods. Antimicrobial susceptibility tests were done according to the standard disc diffusion method (26) and/or the automatic methods: MS-2 (Abbott Laboratories, Dallas, TX, USA) (27), or the Auto-Microbic System (AMS; Vitek, Inc., Hazelwood, MO, USA) (28).

A patient was considered to have **P. mirabilis bacteremia** when a) P. mirabilis was grown from 2 or more blood cultures; b) P. mirabilis was grown from 1 blood culture and from another clinical source; or c) P. mirabilis was grown from 1 blood culture in a clinically septic patient with no other infection.

 ISSN 0036-5548

Bacteremia was considered **nosocomial** if the positive blood culture was obtained after 48 h of hospital admission, and there was no evidence of P. mirabilis infection at the time of admission from the community or from a nursing home.

A body site was considered the source of bacteremia if P. mirabilis was isolated from a culture of that site obtained within 48 h of the blood culture that grew P. mirabilis.

Bacteremia was considered **polymicrobial** when one or more bacterial species in addition to P. mirabilis was grown in blood cultures taken during the 48 h period (29).

Underlying conditions of patients were classified according to the criteria of McCabe and Jackson (30). A **rapidly fatal** underlying condition was defined as one in which death was likely within 6 months. An **ultimately fatal** underlying condition was defined as one in which death was likely within 5 years. A **non-fatal** underlying condition was defined as one in which death was unlikely within 5 years. A patient with more than one underlying condition was classified according to the most serious underlying condition.

Sepsis was defined according to the criteria of the American College of Chest Physicians/Society of Critical Care Medicine Consensus Conference Committee Report as follows: the presence of 2 or more of the following conditions as a result of infection: a) temperature $>38°C$ or $<36°C$; b) heat rate >90 beats per min; c) respiratory rate >20 beats per min; and d) white blood cell count $>12{,}000$/cu mm or $<4{,}000$/cu mm, or $>10\%$ immature (band) forms (31). Hypotension was defined as a decrease in blood pressure to $<90/60$ mm Hg (32).

Antimicrobial therapy was evaluated on day 1 and day 3 of the first positive blood culture. A patient was considered to have received appropriate antimicrobial therapy when the P. mirabilis was proved subsequently to be susceptible in vitro to the antimicrobial agent the patient received.

Statistical analysis was done by the chi-square test with Yates' correction.

RESULTS

During the 13-year study period, 176 patients had P. mirabilis bacteremia that fulfilled the study criteria. No patient had nore than 1 episode of bacteremia due to P. mirabilis. The prevalence of P. mirabilis bacteremia was 0.54 per 1,000 admissions (average 0.44 and 0.69 per 1,000 admissions for the first 7 years and last 6 years respectively).

There were 87 male and 89 female patients. The ages of patients ranged from 19 to 89 years with a median of 75 years; 113 patients (64.2%) were 70 years or older. 100 patients (56.8%) came from a nursing home. There were 36 cases (20.5%) of nosocomial bacteremia. Table I lists the duration of hospitalization before onset of nosocomial bacteremia which occurred as early as during the first week and as late as after the 4th week.

There were 44 cases (25%) of polymicrobial bacteremia. In 33 patients, there was 1 additional bacterium. Two additional bacteria were found in 9 patients and 5 additional bacteria were found in 2 other patients. Table II lists bacteria isolated from blood cultures of patients with polymicrobial bacteremia. The most common isolates were Escherichia coli, Klebsiella pneumoniae, coagulase-negative staphylococci and enterococci.

Table I. *Duration of hospitalization before onset of nosocomial bacteremia due to Proteus mirabilis*

Days from admission to bacteremia[a]	No. of patients	Cumulative percent of patients
3–7	13	36.1
8–14	5	50.0
15–21	2	55.6
22–28	6	72.2
≥29	10	100.0

[a] Range 3–203 days, median 14 days.

Table II. *Other bacteria isolated from blood cultures of patients with bacteremia due to Proteus mirabilis and polymicrobial bacteremia*

Bacteria	No. of isolates
Escherichia coli	10
Klebsiella pneumoniae	8
Coagulase-negative staphylococci	8
Enterococci	7
Providentia stuartii	6
Staphylococcus aureus	4
Pseudomonas aeruginosa	3
Morganella morganii	2
Alpha-hemolytic streptococci	3
Group B streptococcus	2
Other species	8

No patients had rapidly fatal underlying conditions. Ultimately fatal underlying conditions were found in 24 patients; 152 patients had either non-fatal or no underlying conditions. 113 patients (64.2%) had an indwelling Foley catheter and 13 patients had stones in the urinary tract. The sources of P. mirabilis bacteremia are listed in Table III. There were no cases of infective endocarditis. The urinary tract accounted for 52.8% of the cases. Sepsis was found in 142 patients (80.7%) and hypotension in 53 patients (30.1%).

Table IV lists the antimicrobial susceptibility of P. mirabilis strains that were tested. P. mirabilis strains were susceptible to a variety of antimicrobial agents with the exception of tetracycline. Considering only patients with monomicrobial bacteremia (132 patients), the majority of patients (98, 74.2%) received appropriate antimicrobial therapy on the day the positive blood culture was obtained and before the blood culture result was known. By day 3 of the first positive blood culture, 93.2% (123 patients) had received appropriate antimicrobial therapy.

The overall mortality rate was 29.0% (51 of 176 patients) with an attributable mortality rate of 25.6% (45 patients). The mortality rate of polymicrobial bacteremia (38.6%) was higher than that of monomicrobial bacteramia (25.8%). Factors which could possibly influence mortality of monomicrobial bacteremia are listed in Table V. Significant increase in mortality was found in patients who had nosocomial infection, whose source of bacteremia was other than the urinary tract, who had ultimately fatal underlying conditions or who had hypotension, increases in serum creatinine or serum bilirubin.

Table III. *Sources of bacteremia due to Proteus mirabilis*

Source	Monomicrobial ($n = 132$)	Polymicrobial ($n = 44$)	Total ($n = 176$)
Urinary tract	72 (54.5%)	21 (47.7%)	93 (52.8%)
Decubitus and wounds	11 (8.3%)	4 (9.1%)	15 (8.6%)
Lower respiratory tract	6 (4.5%)	2 (4.5%)	8 (4.5%)
Urine and decubitus[a]	5 (3.8%)	2 (4.5%)	7 (4.0%)
Other sources	13 (9.8%)	4 (9.1%)	17 (9.7%)
Unknown	25 (18.9%)	11 (25.0%)	36 (20.5%)

[a] Cultures of both urine and decubitus grew identical P. mirabilis.

Table IV. *Antimicrobial susceptibility of Proteus mirabilis*

Antimicrobial agents	No. susceptible/No. tested	% susceptible[a]
Ceftizoxime	85/85	(100)
Amikacin	65/65	(100)
Kanamycin	36/36	(100)
Ceftazidime	14/14	(100)
Gentamicin	174/175	(99.4)
Tobramycin	70/71	(98.6)
Ciprofloxacin	67/69	(97.1)
Trimethoprim-sulfamethoxazole	160/166	(96.4)
Chloramphenicol	55/58	(94.8)
Cefoxitin	53/56	(94.6)
Cefuroxime	34/36	(94.4)
Cefazolin	106/113	(93.8)
Carbenicillin	88/96	(91.7)
Cephalothin	51/57	(89.5)
Mezlocillin	103/116	(88.8)
Aztreonam	44/50	(88.0)
Ticarcillin	22/25	(88.0)
Imipenem	55/63	(87.3)
Ampicillin	139/167	(83.2)
Piperacillin	38/50	(76.0)
Tetracycline	1/31	(3.2)

[a] Fully susceptible according to break points of methods used.

DISCUSSION

Bacteremia caused by P. mirabilis is fairly common in a community hospital. Its prevalence of 0.54 per 1,000 admissions in our hospital is higher than that of bacteremia caused by group A streptococci (0.18 per 1,000 admissions) (22), serratia (0.18 per 1,000 admissions) (19), enterobacter (0.30 per 1,000 admissions) (18), and group B streptococci (0.37 per 1,000 admissions) (15), but lower than that of bacteremia caused by alpha-hemolytic streptococci (0.66 per 1,000 admissions) (25), klebsiella (0.76 per 1,000 admissions) (21), Streptococcus pneumoniae (0.97 per 1,000 admissions) (23), enterococcus (1.20 per 1,000 admissions) (24), pseudomonas (1.41 per 1,000 admissions) (20), and Staphylococcus aureus (1.72 per 1,000 admissions) (17).

The median age of our patients was 75 years. The majority of patients with proteus bacteremia in the late 1960s at the Boston City Hospital also were 70 years or older (13). The 20.5% of our cases that had nosocomial bacteremia was much lower than the 52.1% in the study from Boston City Hospital (13). This is perhaps because of improvement in hospital infection control practices. However median days to the occurrence of nosocomial P. mirabilis bacteremia remain the same, namely 14 days (13). The 20.5% cases of polymicrobial bacteremia in our study was similar to the 19.4% in a study from Israel (14). For comparison, in our hospital, polymicrobial bacteremia was 20%, 21%, 28% and 34% in bacteremia caused by serratia, pseudomonas, klebsiella and enterobacter respectively (18–21). The most common co-isolate was E. coli, similar to finding in the study from Israel (14).

The urinary tract was the most common source of bacteremia caused by P. mirabilis, unchanged from findings in the 1960s at Johns Hopkins Hospital and Boston City Hospital (12, 13). Indwelling Foley catheter had been recognized as an important predisposing factor (13). Stones in the urinary tract have been known to be a predisposing factor in urinary tract

Table V. *Risk factors versus mortality in monomicrobial Proteus mirabilis bacteremia (132 patients)*

Factor	Mortality no./total no. (%)
Sex	
Male	19/68 (27.9)
Female	15/64 (23.4)
Age	
<70 years	14/46 (26.1)
≥70 years	22/86 (25.6)
Acquisition of bacteremia	
Community or Nursing home	22/103 (21.4)[a]
Nosocomial	12/29 (41.4)[a]
Source of bacteremia	
Urinary tract	12/74 (16.2)[b]
Others	22/58 (37.9)[b]
Underlying condition	
Ultimately fatal	10/19 (52.6)[b]
Non-fatal or none	24/113 (21.2)[b]
Sepsis	
Present	29/105 (27.6)
Absent	5/27 (18.5)
Hypotension	
Present	20/38 (52.6)[c]
Absent	14/94 (14.9)[c]
Serum creatinine	
<176.8 μmol/L	13/71 (18.3)[d]
≥176.8 μmol/L	19/55 (34.5)[d]
Total serum bilirubin	
<34.2 μmol/L	25/110 (22.7)[d]
≥34.2 μmol/L	5/11 (45.5)[d]
Platelets	
$<150{,}000 \times 10^9$/L	7/24 (29.2)
$\geq 150{,}000 \times 10^9$/L	18/82 (22.0)
Antimicrobial therapy	
Day 1: appropriate	23/98 (23.4)
inappropriate	11/34 (32.4)
Day 3: appropriate	30/123 (24.4)
inappropriate	4/9 (44.4)

[a] $p < 0.02$.
[b] $p < 0.01$.
[c] $p < 0.001$.
[d] $p < 0.05$.

infection caused by proteus organisms. Therefore it is not surprising to find 13 patients with urinary tract stones in our study. The lower respiratory tract was not a common source of bacteramia due to P. mirabilis (12, 13). Although pneumonia due to proteus organisms has been described, it is uncommon (33). For comparison, in our hospital, the lower respiratory tract was the most common source of bacteremia caused by enterobacter, serratia and pseudomonas and almost as common as the urinary tract as the source for bacteremia caused by klebsiella (18–21).

The finding that P. mirabilis strains were susceptible to almost all antimicrobial agents tested except tetracycline was as expected. P. mirabilis is known to be intrinsically resistant to tetracycline (10). In a study on antimicrobial resistance, among members of Enterobacteriaceae, P. mirabilis strains were the most susceptible to different antimicrobial agents (35). Resistance to ampicillin and piperacillin was more common than other antimicrobial agents as in our study (35). In contrast, a report from Israel shows that most P. mirabilis strains isolated from blood cultures in a hospital in Tel Aviv were resistant to many antimicrobial agents including aminoglycosides, broad-spectrum penicillins and older cephalosporins (14).

The overall mortality of 29.0% for bacteremia caused by P. mirabilis was much lower than that in the 1960s (12, 13). In our hospital, mortality of bacteremia caused by P. mirabilis was lower than that caused by klebsiella (37%), serratia (52%), pseudomonas (61%) and enterobacter (69%) (18–21). Even though most patients received appropriate antimicrobial therapy on the day the first positive blood culture was done, the mortality rate was still significant. The risk factors that adversely affected the outcome namely, nonsocomial infection ultimately fatal underlying conditions, hypotension, elevated serum creatinine and bilirubin have been previously reported (17–21).

In summary, the majority of patients with P. mirabilis bacteremia in this study were elderly, came from a nursing home, did not have fatal underlying conditions, had an indwelling Foley catheter with urinary tract infection as the source of bacteremia, had the clinical picture of sepsis, received prompt antimicrobial therapy and survived. About one-quarter of the patients however, did die of infection.

REFERENCES

1. Maiztegui JI, Biegeleisen JZ Jr, Cherry WB, Kass EH. Bacteremia due to gram-negative rods. A clinical, bacteriologic, serologic and immunofluorescent study. N Engl J Med 272: 222–229, 1965.
2. Freid MA, Vosti KL. The importance of underlying disease in patients with gram-negative bacteremia. Arch Intern Med 121: 418–423, 1968.
3. DuPont HL, Spink WW. Infections due to gram-negative organisms: an analysis of 860 patients with bacteremia at the University of Minnesota Medical Center, 1958–1966. Medicine 48: 307–322, 1969.
4. Myerowitz RL, Medeiros AA, O'Brien TF. Recent experience with bacillemia due to gram-negative organisms. J Infect Dis 124: 239–245, 1971.
5. Bryant RE, Hood AF, Hood CE, Koenig MG. Factors affecting mortality of gram-negative rod bacteremia. Arch Intern Med 127: 120–128, 1971.
6. Kreger BE, Craven DE, Carling PC, McCabe WR. Gram-negative bacteremia. III. Reassessment of etiology, epidemiology and ecology in 612 patients. Am J Med 68: 332–343, 1980.
7. Lynch JM, Hodges GR, Clark GM, Dworzack DL. Gram-negative bacteremias. Analysis of factors for clinical assessment of gentamicin resistance. Arch Intern Med 141: 582–586, 1981.
8. Bryan CS, Reynolds KL, Brenner ER. Analysis of 1,186 episodes of gram-negative bacteremia in non-university hospitals: the effects of antimicrobial therapy. Rev Infect Dis 5: 629–638, 1983.
9. McCue JD. Improved mortality in gram-negative bacillary bacteremia. Arch Intern Med 145: 1212–1216, 1985.
10. Uzum O, Akalin HE, Hayran M, Unal S. Factors influencing prognosis in bacteremia due to gram-negative organisms: evaluation of 448 episodes in a Turkish University Hospital. Clin Infect Dis 15: 866–873, 1992.
11. Spittel JA, Martin WJ, Geraci JE, Nichols DR. Bacteremia owing to proteus organisms. A method of treatment. Mayo Clin Proc 29: 225–228, 1954.
12. Lewis J, Fekety FR. Proteus bacteremia. Johns Hopkins Med J 124: 151–156, 1969.
13. Adler JL, Burke JP, Martin DF, Finland M. Proteus infections in a general hospital. II. Some clinical and epidemiological characteristics. With analysis of 71 cases of proteus bacteremia. Ann Intern Med 75: 531–536, 1971.
14. Berger SA. Proteus bacteremia in a general hospital 1972–1982. J Hosp Infect 6: 293–298, 1985.
15. Gallagher PG, Watanakunakorn C. Group B streptococcal bacteremia in a community-teaching hospital. Am J Med 78: 795–800, 1985.
16. Malone DA, Wagner RA, Myers JP, Watanakunakorn C. Enterococcal bacteremia in two large community-teaching hospitals. Am J Med 81: 601–606, 1986.

17. Watanakunakorn C, Chan SJ, DeMarco DG, Palmer JA. Staphylococcus aureus bacteremia: significance of hyperbilirubinemia. Scand J Infect Dis 19: 195–203, 1987.
18. Watanakunakorn C, Weber J. Enterobacter bacteremia: a review of 58 episodes. Scand J Infect Dis 21: 1–8, 1989.
19. Watanakunakorn C. Serratia bacteremia: a review of 44 episodes. Scand J Infect Dis 21: 477–483, 1989.
20. Gallagher PG, Watanakunakorn C. Pseudomonas bacteremia in a community teaching hospital. Rev Infect Dis 11: 846–852, 1989.
21. Watanakunakorn C, Jura J. Klebsiella bacteremia: a review of 196 episodes during a decade (1980–1989). Scand J Infect Dis 23: 399–405, 1991.
22. Burkert T, Watanakunakorn C. Group A streptococcal bacteremia in a community teaching hospital – 1980–1989. Clin Infect Dis 14: 29–37, 1992.
23. Watanakunakorn C, Greifenstein A, Stroh K, Jarjoura DG, Blend D, Cugino A, Ognibene AJ. Pneumococcal bacteremia in three community teaching hospitals from 1980 to 1989. Chest 103: 1152–1156, 1993.
24. Watanakunakorn C, Patel R. Comparison of patients with enterococcal bacteremia due to strains with and without high-level resistance to gentamicin. Clin Infect Dis 17: 74–78, 1993.
25. Watanakunakorn C, Pantelakis J. Alpha-hemolytic streptococcal bacteremia: a review of 203 episodes during 1980–1991. Scand J Infect Dis 25: 403–408, 1993.
26. Barry AL, Thornsberry C. Susceptibility tests: diffusion tests procedures, Chapter 111. In: Balows A, Hausler WJ Jr, Herrmann KL, Isenberg HD, Shadomy HL, eds. Manual of Clinical Microbiology. 5th ed. Washington DC: Am Soc Microbiol, 1117–1125, 1991.
27. Thornsberry C, Anhalt JP, Washington JA II, McCarthy LR, Schoenknecht FD, Sherris JC, Spencer HJ. Clinical laboratory evaluation of the Abbott MS-2 automatic antimicrobial susceptibility testing system: report of a collaborative study. J Clin Microbiol 12: 375–390, 1980.
28. Backes BA, Cavalier SJ, Rudrik JT, Britt EM. Rapid antimicrobial susceptibility testing of gram-negative clinical isolates with the Auto Microbic System. J Clin Microbiol 19: 744–747, 1984.
29. Roselle GA, Watanakunakorn C. Polymicrobial bacteremia. JAMA 242: 2411–2413, 1979.
30. McCabe WR, Jackson GG. Gram-negative bacteremia. I. Etiology and ecology. Arch Intern Med 110: 847–855, 1962.
31. The ACCP/SCCM Consensus Conference Committee. Definitions for sepsis and organ failure and guidelines for the use of innovative therapies in sepsis. Chest 101: 1644–1655, 1992.
32. Kreger BE, Craven DE, McCabe WR. Gram-negative bacteremia. IV. Re-evaluation of clinical features and treatment in 612 patients. Am J Med 68: 344–355, 1980.
33. Tillotson JR, Lerner AM. Characteristics of pneumonias caused by Bacillus proteus. Ann Intern Med 68: 287–294, 1968.
34. Farmer JJ III, Kelly MT. Enterobacteriaceae, Chapter 36. In: Balows A, Hausler WJ Jr, Herrmann KL, Isenberg HD, Shadomy HL, eds. Manual of Clinical Microbiology. 5th ed. Washington DC: Am Soc Microbiol, 360–683, 1991.
35. Ellner PD, Fink DJ, Neu HC, Parry MF. Epidemiologic factors affecting antimicrobial resistance of common bacterial isolates. Antimicrob Agents Chemother 25: 1668–1674, 1987.

Submitted January 17, 1994; accepted March 19, 1994

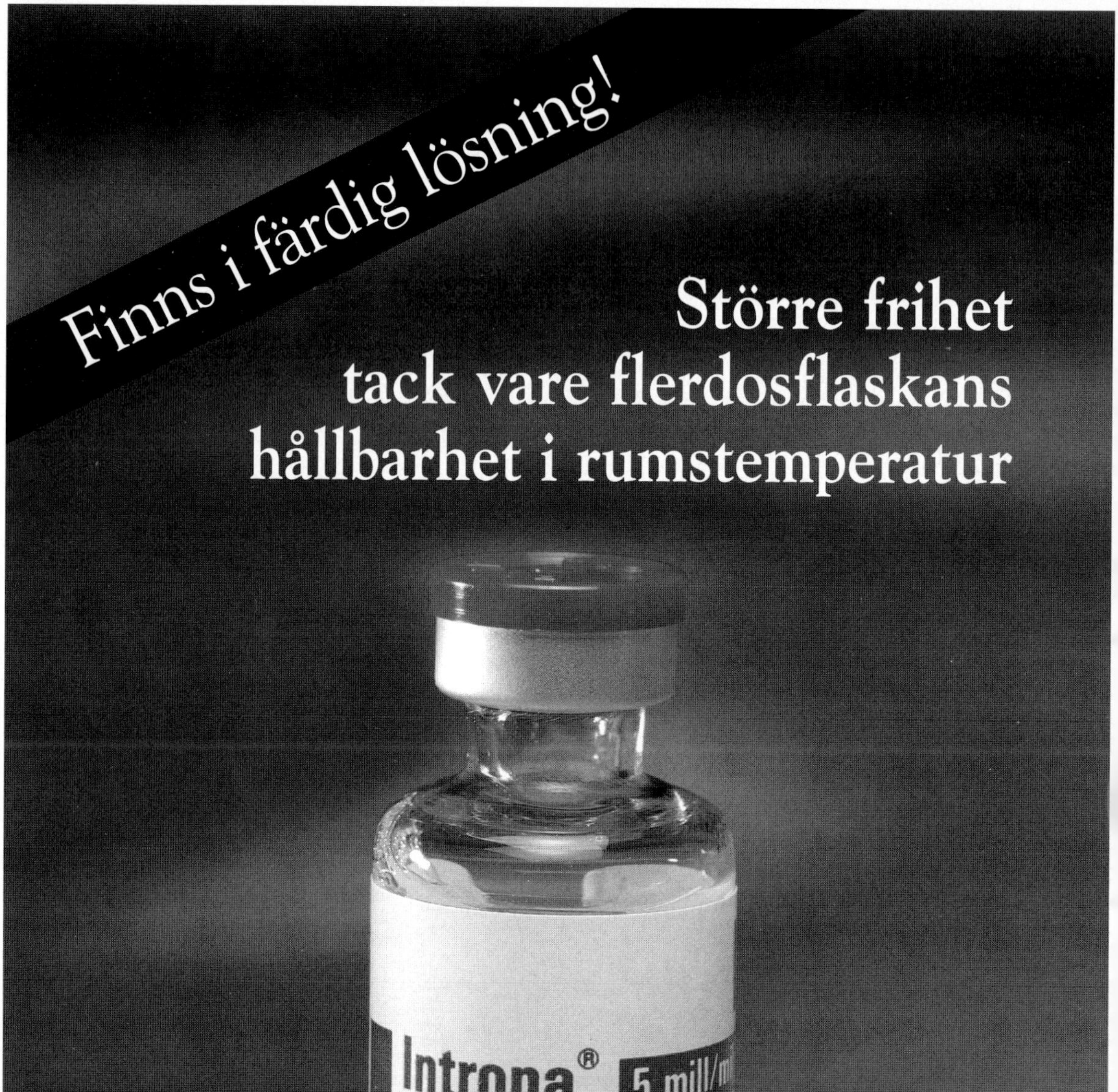
Finns i färdig lösning!
Större frihet
tack vare flerdosflaskans
hållbarhet i rumstemperatur
Introna®
5 mill/m
Schering-Plough
Introna är ett alfa
2b interferon,
se vidare Fass.
Schering-Plough
Tel. nr.: 08-670 89 00

Scand J Infect Dis 26: 369–373, 1994

Cytomegalovirus Disease of Late Onset Following Renal Transplantation: A Potentially Fatal Entity

ANNETTE BOEHLER, ANDREAS SCHAFFNER, FRANCO SALOMON and GERALD KEUSCH

From the Department of Internal Medicine, University Hospital, Zürich, Switzerland

CMV disease (CMVD) is a recognized problem of the early post-transplant period (PTP) in renal transplant recipients. Information on CMVD in the late (≥ 2 years) PTP is scarce. We have observed 5 cases of CMVD during late (3–8 years) PTP during the last 15 years. Three of these patients died from CMVD. One of the patients with late-onset CMVD recovered spontaneously from mild pneumonitis, 1 patient with severe CMVD after therapy with ganciclovir/anti-CMV-IgG. CMVD was ascribed to primary infection in 4/5 patients, and transmission was attributed to blood products in 2 cases. At the time of CMVD, 4/5 patients were on stable immunosuppression with azathioprine/prednisone; 1 patient who died had received prednisone pulses 1 month prior to CMVD. Late onset CMVD is an underreported disease in renal transplant recipients, which warrants preventive measures and consideration of antiviral therapy.

A. Böhler, MD, Department of Medicine, University Hospital, CH-8091 Zürich, Switzerland

INTRODUCTION

CMVD is a major problem in patients with organ transplants, occurring usually within the first 6 months after transplantation. This is due to transmission of CMV by transplanted organs and/or by blood products at a time when immunosuppressive therapy is most intensive. In contrast to CMVD, which occurs during the first months after transplantation, and which has been well characterized (1–4), the significance and course of CMVD occurring late in the post-transplant period has received little attention. In our review of the literature we encountered only 4 case reports of such 'late-onset' CMVD occurring ≥ 2 years after kidney transplantation (5, 6). We describe here 5 cases of CMVD occurring ≥ 2 years after renal transplantation, seen between 1974 and 1991 at a single transplant centre among 1,168 kidney recipients. Our observations indicate that 'late-onset' CMVD – even if occurring during minimal chronic immunosuppression – is a potentially fatal condition justifying anti-CMV therapy as well as preventive measures.

MATERIALS AND METHODS

Patients

At the university hospital, Zürich, 1,168 kidney transplantations have been performed between 1974 and 1991. After their hospital stay for transplantation, all patients were followed up as outpatients. Based on the charts and histopathological slides, bone marrow aspirates and autopsy records all patients who developed CMVD ≥ 2 years after transplantation were analysed.

Immunosuppression

Between 1974 and 1983, immunosuppression consisted of azathioprine and prednisone. After 1983 a triple therapy with cyclosporine A, azathioprine and prednisone was used.

Definitions

The diagnosis of CMVD was based on a clinical setting compatible with CMVD and one or more of the following criteria: seroconversion and/or positive CMV-culture in previously seronegative individuals, and/or histopathological findings of CMVD.

Diagnostic procedures

A complement fixation assay (Virion, Rüschlikon, Switzerland) was used to detect anti-CMV-IgG and anti-CMV-IgM antibodies until 1985. Subsequently an ELISA method was used to detect anti-CMV-IgG antibodies. Anti-CMV-IgM antibodies were determined with microcapture ELISA assay (Medac, Hamburg, Germany). After 1984, organ donors and recipients were routinely screened for anti-CMV-antibodies, using an agglutination test for total anti-CMV-IgG antibodies (CMV-Scan, Becton Dickinson). CMV was isolated from blood, urine, or pharyngeal specimens by short-term culture of human fibroblasts, followed by detection of early antigen by immunofluorescence. Before 1985, isolation of CMV was based on standard culture.

CASE REPORTS

All cases are summarized in Table I. As an example of a fatal outcome (case 3) and of restitution (case 5), 2 cases are described in greater detail.

Table I. *Five cases of 'late-onset' CMV disease after kidney transplantation*

	Case number (age; sex)				
	1 (55 yrs; m)	2 (45 yrs; m)	3 (46 yrs; m)	4 (30 yrs; f)	5 (58 yrs; f)
Years after transplantation	4	3	6	6	8
CMV-diagnosis	IgG and IgM antibodies	Positive virus culture in CSF in seronegative individual	Seroconversion	Seroconversion, CMV early antigen in urine	Seroconversion, CMV early antigen in urine and pharyngeal secretion
Autopsy	Pneumonitis, inclusion bodies in lung	Pneumonitis, encephalitis inclusion bodies in lung	Pneumonitis, encephalitis inclusion bodies in lung, bowel and liver		
Type of infection	Reactivation or primary inf.	Primary infection	Primary infection	Primary infection	Primary infection
Presumed mode of acquisition	Unknown	Blood transfusions	Blood transfusions	Unknown	Unknown
Immunosuppression	Azathioprine + prednisone	Azathioprine + prednisone	Azathioprine + prednisone, 3 methylpred-nisolone pulses	Azathioprine + prednisone	Azathioprine + prednisone
Laboratory findings					
lowest blood count					
Hb (g/l)	57	66	58	66	66
Lc ($\times 10^9$/l)	3.4	1.9	3.0	1.5	0.77
Trc ($\times 10^9$/l)	72	40	38	84	23
DIC	No	No	Yes	No	Yes
Liver function tests	Normal	Elevated	Elevated	Normal	Elevated
Hematophagic histiocytosis	–	+	+	–	+
Organs involved	Lung	Lung, brain, liver	Lung, liver, bowel, brain	Lung	Lung, liver
Concomitant infections	Bacterial pneumonia	Urinary tract infection, hepatitis B	–	Urinary tract infection	Hepatitis B
Anti-CMV-treatment	None	None	None	None	Ganciclovir anti-CMV-IgG
Clinical outcome	Dead	Dead	Dead	Alive	Alive

Case 3

A 39-year-old man had received a cadaveric renal transplant for terminal renal failure after glomerulonephritis. Five months after transplantation, CMV-serology was negative. Six years after transplantation the patient developed tertiary hyperparathyroidism and a parathyroidectomy was performed. Because of postoperative bleeding he received 5 units of red cells and 2 units of fresh frozen plasma. 14 days later an increased serum creatinine was noted. A transplant biopsy revealed vascular rejection, which was treated with methylprednisolone pulses. CMV-antibody titres were again negative. One month after surgery the patient was admitted to hospital because of fever, anorexia, cough, dyspnea and diarrhea. On physical examination he appeared severely ill with fever up to 39.1°C and hepatosplenomegaly. A chest X-ray demonstrated bilateral pleural effusions and echocardiography showed pericardial effusion. Broad-spectrum antibiotics were given initially, though all cultures of blood, urine, sputum, and stool obtained prior to therapy were negative for pathogenic bacteria and fungi. The patient developed progressive anemia, leukopenia, thrombocytopenia and DIC and developed signs of meningeal irritation and became obtunded. CSF examination shows pleocytosis (380/3 cells) but no bacteria or virus. A bone marrow smear and biopsy revealed marked hypocellularity. Among hemopoietic cells, only the megakaryocyte count appeared normal. The number of macrophages was markedly increased, however, and most of them had ingested red cells, neutrophils, and platelets. CMV-seroconversion with positive anti-CMV-IgM and -IgG titres were documented. The patient deteriorated rapidly, with fever, unconsciousness, respiratory failure, myotonic contractions, gastrointestinal bleeding, and renal failure. He died on the 12th hospital day with multiorgan failure.

At autopsy the cerebral findings included perivascular lymphocytic infiltrates in the brain stem, basal ganglia, cerebellum and a number of small nodes consisting of neuroglia. Widespread pneumonitis and numerous large cells with haloed intranuclear inclusions were found in the lungs, liver and bowel.

This patient illustrates the development of a generalized lethal CMVD 6 years after transplantation acquired through blood products. Leukopenia, anemia, thrombocytopenia together with the findings of hematophagic histiocytosis in the bone marrow were attributed to a CMV-triggered reactive hemophagocytic syndrome.

Case 5

A 50-year-old woman had received a cadaveric renal transplant for terminal renal failure due to chronic glomerulonephritis. The CMV serology of the donor had been positive, the serology of the recipient negative. Within the first month after transplantation there was an acute rejection crisis that was successfully treated with steroid pulses. The CMV serology remained negative. Eight years after transplantation the patient was admitted to the hospital with a 10-day history of fever up to 40°C, headache, fatigue, myalgias, nonproductive cough, and a rise in serum creatinine. On admission, hepatosplenomegaly, labial herpes, mild scleral icterus, and rales were found over both lung bases. A chest X-ray showed a right-sided subpulmonal pleural effusion. The patient was treated empirically with broad-spectrum antibiotics and low-dose heparin because of laboratory findings for DIC. The clinical course deteriorated. The leukocyte and thrombocyte counts decreased alarmingly. Bone marrow aspirate and biopsy were hypocellular and showed the typical signs of hematophagic histiocytosis. The serum levels of ferritin and transcobalamin II were clearly elevated as consequence of an increased activity of the mononuclear phagocyte system as is typical of hemophagocytic syndrome (7, 8). Bacterial and fungal cultures of blood, urine and sputum remained sterile. CMV was cultured from the throat lavage fluid and urine. Antibacterial therapy was discontinued and intravenous therapy with ganciclovir and a commercial anti-CMV-hyperimmunoglobulin (Cytotect, Biotest, Germany) was administered. The clinical and hematological abnormalities resolved and the serum creatinine level returned to normal. The previously negative CMV serology became positive: the sample obtained at hospitalization was for a first time positive for anti-CMV-IgM. A second sample collected at discharge showed in addition conversion for anti-CMV-IgG. The patient was discharged on the 31st hospital day.

This patient contracted CMV 8 years after renal transplantation. As a consequence of the CMVD, the patient also developed a hemophagocytic syndrome, which resolved promptly and completely after the start of antiviral therapy.

RESULTS

Among the 1,168 kidney transplant recipients, a diagnosis of CMVD of late onset (≥ 2 years after transplantation) was made in 5 patients, all occurring between 3 and 8 years after kidney transplantation and presenting a clinical setting compatible with CMVD. The diagnosis was confirmed in 3 cases by seroconversion (primary infection) in addition to the isolation of CMV in urine specimens from 2 patients and in pharyngeal secretion in 1. In 1 patient with presumed primary infection, CMV was isolated from the cerebrospinal fluid (Case 2, Table I). In 1 case the diagnosis rested on persistently elevated anti-CMV-IgG and anti-CMV-IgM antibody titres in addition to findings of CMVD with severe pneumonitis and inclusion bodies at autopsy (Case 1, Table I). Three of the 5 patients died. Two patients were discharged, 1 after anti-CMV therapy and 1 after spontaneous recovery.

Late-onset CMVD contributed notably to lethal CMVD in the 1,168 patients. A total of 30 patients died of CMVD, 27 patients within 6 months after transplantation with early onset CMVD, 3 patients died 3 or more years after transplantation, with late-onset CMVD.

DISCUSSION

Our observations in 5 patients with severe CMVD occurring ≥2 years after renal transplantation indicate that CMVD is a serious threat to kidney transplant recipients, not only in the early post-transplant period but also during chronic stable immunosuppression. In the past the problem of CMVD occurring late after kidney transplantation has only been rarely encountered. Linnemann et al. (5) reported 2 cases of lethal CMVD with fever, pneumonitis and hepatitis occurring more than 1 year after kidney transplantation. One of these 2 patients had a primary infection, and in 1 patient it was not clear whether the disease was the consequence of a reactivation, or a reinfection. None of the patients had received blood transfusion and the route of transmission remained unknown. Two other cases of late onset CMVD were described by Rubin and Tolkoff-Rubin (6). In both patients the virus was thought to have been transmitted sexually. To our knowledge, no other cases of CMVD occurring more than 2 years after solid organ transplantation have been reported in detail in the literature.

For the physicians caring for patients with solid organ transplants it is important to appreciate the potential threat arising from CMVD in the late PTP. From the few reports available and from our own observations it is apparent that primary CMV infection in the late PTP can cause CMVD of a severity comparable to that acquired in the early PTP. Three of our patients, and 2 reported previously, died of organ complications to CMVD. Usually CMV infections occur within the first 6 months after transplantation (1–4) and the morbidity and mortality of CMVD is increased after the use of immunosuppressive therapy with methylprednisolone pulses, and antilymphocyte globulins for rejection crisis (4). It is therefore not self-evident that 2 of the 5 patients observed here and 2 patients reported in the literature died during a phase of late stable immunosuppression. The third patient who died had received rejection therapy with methylprednisolone pulses in the preceding month. At the time of the onset of CMVD all 5 patients received immunosuppression with azathioprine and prednisone. Four of the 5 patients were transplanted when cyclosporine A did not belong to the routine immunosuppressive regimen and afterwards under stable clinical conditions the treatment of these patients was not extended to a triple therapy. One patient (case 4) received triple therapy which was discontinued because of biopsy-proven cyclosporine-induced nephrotoxicity. It is not known if the incidence of late onset CMVD is influenced by an additional immunosuppression with cyclosporine and statistical analysis was not helpful in settling this question in the present study. It is worth noting that while all our patients with late onset CMVD received double immunosuppression, the dosage of prednisone and azathioprine was the same as those used in triple therapy.

Primary infections with CMV in transplant recipients take a more severe course than does a reactivated infection (9) or infection with a new CMV strain in a patient with an established immune response due to previous infection (10). Accordingly it is not surprising that 4/5 patients (our 3 patients and 2 described in the literature) with lethal CMVD of late onset had primary infection. In the other patient, the retrospectively available data did not allow us to determine whether he had suffered from primary infection or reactivation.

In contrast to the patients described here primary infection in the normal adult host is usually asymptomatic or associated with a mononucleosis-like disease. Organ dysfunction as a consequence of pneumonia, myocarditis or encephalitis is a rarity (11). We can nevertheless not exclude that more benign forms of primary CMV infection did occur in our population of transplant recipients in the late PTP, that escaped our attention.

Because immunosuppression is most intensive in the early PTP and the degree of immunosuppression is thought to be responsible for the severe course of CMVD at that time, one could be tempted to expect that CMVD of late onset, occurring during minimal chronic immunosuppression, would take a less severe course. The observed series and previous reports indicate that attention must be paid to the fact that CMVD even years after solid organ transplantation can take a serious or even fatal course, presenting with organ dysfunction such as pneumonitis, or hepatitis, or encephalitis, or the hematophagic histiocytosis syndrome, in consequence of CMV infection in transplant patients (12, 13).

In conclusion, our experience with CMVD occurring ≥ 2 years after renal transplantation indicates that CMVD is not only a problem of the early PTP. Physicians caring for CMV-negative solid organ transplant recipients as well as these patients themselves should be aware of this problem in order 1) to take measures to avoid CMV infections through blood products from CMV-antibody-positive donors, and sexual contacts, and 2) to consider, diagnose and specifically treat CMVD of late onset in transplant patients with unexplained fever, particularly if accompanied by pancytopenia, activated coagulation, and organ dysfunction.

REFERENCES

1. Ho M. Cytomegalovirus. In: Mandell GL, Douglas RG, Bennett JE, eds. Principles and practice of infectious diseases, 3rd ed. New York: Churchill Livingstone, 1159–1171, 1990.
2. Rubin RH, Wolfson JS, Cosimi AB, Tolkoff-Rubin NE. Infection in the renal transplant recipient. Am J Med 70: 405–411, 1981.
3. Rubin RH. Infection in the renal and liver transplant patient. In: Rubin RH, Young LS, eds. Clinical approach to infection in the compromised host, 2nd ed. New York and London: Plenum Medical Book Company, 557–622, 1988.
4. Ho M. Cytomegalovirus infection and indirect sequelae in the immunocompromised transplant patient. Transplant Proc 23 (Suppl 1): 2–7, 1991.
5. Linnemann CC, Dunn CR, First MR, Alvira M, Schiff GM. Late onset of fatal cytomegalovirus infection after renal transplantation. Arch Intern Med 138: 1247–1250, 1978.
6. Rubin RH, Tolkoff-Rubin NE. The problem of cytomegalovirus infection in transplantation. In: Morris PJ, Tilney NL, eds. Progress in transplantation. Edinburgh: Churchill Livingstone, vol 1, 89–114, 1984.
7. Esumi N, Ikushima S, Todo S, Imashuku S. Hyperferritinemia in malignant histiocytosis and virus-associated hemophagocytic syndrome. N Engl J Med 316: 346–347, 1987.
8. Fehr J, De Vecchi P. Transcobalamin II: A marker for macrophage/histiocyte proliferation. Am J Clin Pathol 84: 291–296, 1985.
9. Rubin RH. Impact of cytomegalovirus infection on organ transplant recipients. Rev Infect Dis 12 (Suppl 7): S754–766, 1990.
10. Grundy JE, Super M, Sweny P, Moorhead J, Lui SF, Berry NJ, Fernando ON, Griffiths PD. Symptomatic cytomegalovirus infection in seropositive kidney recipients: Reinfection with donor virus rather than reactivation of recipient virus. Lancet 2: 132–135, 1988.
11. Cohen JL, Corey GR. Cytomegalovirus infection in the normal host. Medicine 64: 100–114, 1985.
12. Risdall RJ, McKenna RW, Nesbit ME, Krivit W, Balfour HH Jr, Simmons RL, Brunning RD. Virus-associated hemophagocytic syndrome. A benign histiocytic proliferation distinct from malignant histiocytosis. Cancer 44: 993–1002, 1979.
13. Reiner AP, Spivac JL. Hematophagic histiocytosis. A report of 23 new patients and review of the literature. Medicine 76: 369–388, 1988.

Submitted December 28, 1993; accepted March 12, 1994

Scand J Infect Dis 26: 375–378, 1994

Screening for Congenital Cytomegalovirus Infection among Preterm Infants Born before the 34th Gestational Week in Finland

SANGITA PANHANI and KIRSTI M. HEINONEN

From the Department of Neonatology, Children's Hospital, Kuopio University Hospital, Kuopio, Finland

83 infants born before 34 weeks of gestation between 1989 and 1990 and cared for at a neonatal intensive care unit in Kuopio, Finland, were screened for congenital cytomegalovirus (CMV) infection, defined as a positive culture from the sample of urine taken on the first day after birth. Four infants were infected and excreted CMV in the urine. The overall incidence of CMV excretors was 4.8%. The incidence was 1/13 infants born before 28 weeks' gestation and 3/70 infants born between 28 and 34 weeks of gestation. The 4 CMV excretors were followed up for 12–25 months. Two children had normal psychomotor and mental development but exhibited decreasing head growth during follow-up. The other 2 developed severe psychomotor retardation, retinopathy of prematurity, chorioretinitis, and microcephaly. The long-term morbidity was associated not only with congenital CMV infection but to prematurity as well. The incidence of congenital CMV excretors in this preterm population seemed to be higher than reported previously among unselected live-born infants. Early diagnosis of congenital CMV infection would seem to be important in view of forthcoming new therapeutic regimes in the near future.

K. M. Heinonen, MD, Children's Hospital, Kuopio University Hospital, P.O. Box. 1777, FIN-70211 Kuopio, Finland

INTRODUCTION

Cytomegalovirus (CMV) is the most frequent cause of congenital infection in humans. The majority of infected infants lack clinical signs at birth and are identified through screening programs (1). Excretion of CMV in first-day urine is a marker for congenital CMV infection. The incidence of congenital CMV infection ranges between 0.5% and 1.3% in all live births in populations studied (2, 3). Congenital CMV infections are estimated to occur in 1% of all births in developed countries (4), and are associated with a clinical spectrum ranging from inapparent symptoms to severe neurological problems, sensorineural deafness and microcephaly, as documented elsewhere (5–7). The incidence of congenital CMV infection in selected high-risk populations – especially in pre-term infants – is not very well known.

In the present report we describe the results of a 1-year screening of preterm infants born before 34 weeks of gestation, by showing excretion of CMV in urine on the first day of life, and comment on the follow-up of CMV excretors.

MATERIAL AND METHOD

Between 1989 and 1990, a 12-month period, a urine sample for CMV detection was taken during the first day of life from all infants born preterm before the 34th gestational week and admitted to the Neonatal Intensive Care Unit, Children's Hospital, University Hospital, Kuopio, Finland. The value of early CMV excretion in urine as an indicator of perinatal infection has been described previously (8, 9). CMV was detected in MRC-5 cells inoculated with urine specimens by using low-speed centrifugation and a monoclonal anti-CMV antibody (provided by DuPont®, USA) to an early antigen and incubated for 72 h (9).

In all, 83 preterm infants were examined.

RESULTS

Four cases excreting CMV in urine soon after birth were detected during this screening. Their clinical characteristics are reported in Table I. The overall incidence of CMV excretors in this group of preterm infants was 4.8%. The incidence of CMV excretors was 1/13 infants born before 28 weeks, and 3/70 between 28 and 34 weeks of gestation.

The clinical characteristics of the preterm CMV excretors were similar to those of prematurity-associated morbidity in general. Three out of 4 preterm CMV excretors had moderate to severe respiratory distress syndrome (RDS) and consequently, bronchopulmonary dysplasia (BPD). There was no perinatal/neonatal mortality. Long-term follow-up showed post-neonatal death, at 16 months of age in case no. 1 who was premature with a very low birth weight. Case no. 1 developed convulsions, severe mental and motor handicap, retinopathy of prematurity, severe myopia and necrotizing enterocolitis for which she was operated on several times. Cases 2 and 4 were alive and had no mental or motor retardation and no visual complications. Case no. 3 developed spastic diplegia and chorioretinitis but had normal mental development and was alive at 25 months of age (last examination). Congenital rubella virus and Toxoplasma gondii infections were ruled out.

None of the infants had classical signs of congenital CMV infection at birth (jaundice, hepatosplenomegaly, petechiae, microcephaly). Cases 1 and 3 had repeated hearing examinations performed with screening audiometry (40 dB), during the first year of life, case no. 2 had a hearing examination with pure-tone free-field audiometry (range 30–50 dB) at the age of 1 and 2 years, and case no. 4 underwent pure-tone free-field audiometry (range 30–50 dB) at 1 year, all with normal results. In all cases, antenatal head growth was appropriate, as standardized head circumferences at birth were close to the mean (Table I). During follow-up, however, all infants had decreasing head growth, as indicated by reduction of standardized head circumference values by 1 to 3 standard deviations below the mean (Table II). Cases 1, 2 and 3 were thus definitely microcephalic.

Table I. *Neonatal characteristics in 4 preterm CMV excretors*

	Case 1	Case 2	Case 3	Case 4
Gestational age	23 weeks	29 weeks	32 weeks	33 weeks
Delivery	Vaginal	Cesarean	Cesarean	Cesarean
Sex	Female	Female	Female	Female
Birth weight	610 g	1,390 g	1,895 g	1,780 g
Head circumference at birth, SD units	0.1	−0.3	0.4	−0.25
Apgar	2/3	5/7	7/8	5/6
CMV-uria	1st day	1st day	1st day	1st day
RDS[a]	yes	yes	no	yes
Surfactant	given	no	no	no
Respirator therapy	50 days	9 days	1 day	12 days
O_2 therapy	4 months	2 months	3 days	1 month
BPD[b]	yes	yes	no	yes
Brain ultrasound	Haemorrhage in thalamus	normal	normal	normal
Convulsions	present	no	no	no

[a] Respiratory distress syndrome.
[b] Bronchopulmonary dysplasia.

Table II. *Data on long-term follow-up in 4 CMV excretors*

	Case 1	Case 2	Case 3	Case 4
Age at last examination	16 months	24 months	25 months	12 months
Mental handicap	Severe	No	No	No
Motor retardation	Spastic tetraplegia	No	Spastic diplegia	No
Visual examination	ROP[a]	No	Chorioretinitis	No
Hearing examination	Normal[c]	Normal[c]	Normal[c]	Normal[c]
Head circumference, SD units	−3.0	−2.9	−2.1	−1.2
Gastrointestinal complication	NEC[b] Ilestomy	No	No	No
Outcome	Died at 16 months	Alive	Alive	Alive

[a] Retinopathy of prematurity.
[b] Necrotizing enterocolitis.
[c] Cases 1 and 3 on repeated testing with screening audiometry, (40 dB) during the first year. Case 2 with pure-tone free-field audiometry, (range 30–50 dB) at 1 and 2 years. Case 4 with pure-tone free-field audiometry, (range 30–50 dB) at 1 year.

DISCUSSION

The number of congenital CMV excretors in this preterm population seemed to be greater than reported previously among unselected live born infants (2, 3). The perinatal course and clinical examination of preterm CMV excretors was undistinguishable from that of non-excreting prematures, and thus does not allow early identification of these cases. The early morbidity of CMV excretors was similar to that associated with prematurity. It is possible, however, that CMV infection may have contributed markedly to the severity of morbidity. Although head size was normal at birth, all CMV excretors exhibited decreasing head growth from birth, and 3/4 cases developed microcephaly during follow-up.

We suggest that the presence of congenital CMV infection as documented at birth in preterm infants is associated with abnormal brain growth in infancy. Screening of preterms for cytomegaloviruria soon after birth (and follow-up of excretors) may thus be worthwile. If not diagnosed at birth by screening (which is preferable), congenital CMV infection should be investigated in any preterm infant with decreasing growth of head circumference. Early identification of CMV-infected infants will be even more important in the near future thanks to new therapeutic agents (e.g, ganciclovir) are currently being evaluated.

REFERENCES

1. Starr JJ, Bart RD, Gold E. Inapparent congenital cytomegalovirus infection. N Engl J Med 282: 1075–1078, 1970.
2. Harris S, Ahlfors K, Ivarsson S, Lernmark B, Svanberg L. Congenital cytomegalovirus infection and sensorineural loss. Ear-Hear 5: 352–355, 1984.
3. Hicks T, Fowler K, Richardson M, Dahle A, Adams L, Pass R. Congenital cytomegalovirus infection and neonatal auditory screening. J Pediatr 123: 779–782, 1993.
4. Alford CA, Stagno S, Pass RF, Britt WJ. Congenital and perinatal cytomegalovirus infections. Rev Infect Dis 12 (Suppl 7): S745–753, 1990.
5. Ramsey ME, Miller E, Pecham CS. Outcome of confirmed symptomatic congenital cytomegalovirus infection. Arch Dis Child 66: 1068–1069, 1991.
6. Williamson WD, Percy AK, Yow MD, Gerson P, Catlin FI, Koppelman ML, Thurber S. Asymptomatic congenital cytomegalovirus infection. Audiologic, neuroradiological and neurodevelopmental abnormalities during first year. Am J Dis Child 144: 1365–1368, 1990.

7. Ahlfors K, Ivarsson SA, Bjerre I. Microcephaly and congenital cytomegalovirus infection: a combined prospective and retrospective study of a Swedish infant population. Pediatrics 78: 1058–1063, 1986.
8. Balcarek KB, Warren W, Smith RJ, Lyon MD, Pass RF. Neonatal screening for congenital cytomegalovirus infection by detection of virus in saliva. J Infect Dis 167: 1433–1436, 1993.
9. Curt AG, Thomas FS, Elizabeth AS, Gary RP. Rapid detection of cytomegalovirus in MRC-5 cells inoculated with urine specimens by using low speed centrifugation and monoclonal antibody to an early antigen. J Clin Microbiol 19: 917–919, 1984.

Submitted December 29, 1993; accepted April 17, 1994

Scand J Infect Dis 26: 379–382, 1994

Hemolysis and Autoantibodies to Triosephosphate Isomerase in a Patient with Acute Hepatitis A Virus Infection

KLAUS RITTER, ANGELA UY, SUSANNE RITTER and REINER THOMSSEN

From the Department of Medical Microbiology, Georg-August-University of Göttingen, Göttingen, Germany

Having returned from a holiday in Southeast Europe, a 30-year-old German woman developed acute hepatitis. Hepatitis A virus (HAV) infection was diagnosed serologically. During the course of the infection, hemolysis was found. IgM antibodies against triosephosphate isomerase (IgM anti-TPI) were detected in the patient's serum from the acute phase of the HAV infection. Affinity purified IgM anti-TPI from the serum reduced the enzyme activity in vitro and caused an increased ^{51}Cr release from erythrocytes. IgM anti-TPI is assumed to be one of the causative agents of hemolysis in HAV infection.

K. Ritter, MD, PhD, Medizinische Mikrobiologie der Universität, Kreuzbergring 57, D-37075 Göttingen, Germany

INTRODUCTION

Cases of severe hemolytic anemia in serologically confirmed acute hepatitis A virus (HAV) infection have only occasionally been published (1–3). The mechanisms leading to hemolysis are hitherto unknown. Since HAV infections are frequently accompanied by a significant increase in IgM in the serum (4), with the IgM consisting partly of autoantibodies (5), the underlying mechanisms of the hemolytic disorder are likely to be found here.

We present here a patient who developed hemolysis during the course of an HAV infection. In serum from this patient, autoantibodies to triosephosphate isomerase (TPI) were detected. These autoantibodies have recently been found by us in patients with infectious mononucleosis accompanied by hemolytic anemia (6, 7).

CASE REPORT

Five days after a 4-week stay in Southeast Europe, a 30-year-old woman presented with clinical symptoms and signs of acute hepatitis. Acute HAV infection was confirmed by a positive IgM anti-HAV test. The hepatic enzymes showed derangement of the liver function: ASAT, 18.3 µkat/l; ALAT, 32.2 µkat/l; γGT, 0.78 µkat/l. The hemoglobin was 131 g/l, the WBC 7.4×10^9/l, the thrombocyte count 286×10^9/l, and the reticulocyte count 0.1%.

Within a period of 16 days the patient developed anemia, in the course of which the hemoglobin level dropped from 131 to 96 g/l. Prominent signs of hemolysis were found: LDH, 14.8 µkat/l; haptoglobin, 0; reticulocyte count, 4.2%. Haptoglobin values remained very low for 3 weeks. No drugs known to cause hemolysis had been given. Intermittent fever up to 39°C lasted 2 weeks.

The direct Coombs test was negative. Without treatment, the hemoglobin concentration rose to 105 g/l a month after the appearance of symptoms. Body temperature dropped to 36.8°C. Six months later, there was no evidence of residual hepatic abnormality. Hemoglobin value, reticulocyte count, LDH, and haptoglobin had all returned to normal.

MATERIAL AND METHODS

Serological investigations

Sera for follow-up serological investigations were stored at −25°C. IgM and IgG antibodies against HAV were determined according to standard protocols. Performance of the Coombs test, purification of TPI, isolation and determination of the autoantibodies against TPI, and the ^{51}Cr release assay for detection of the hemolytic effect of anti-TPI antibodies on erythrocytes have been described recently (7).

 ISSN 0036-5548

Inhibition of TPI

The inhibitory activity of anti-TPI antibodies on TPI was determined by applying the method Yoshida and Miwa had used for phosphoglycerate kinase (8). Briefly, the autoantibodies were adjusted to 1μg/ml in 0.15 M NaCl. 20 μl TPI (0.17 μkat/l) was added to increasing volumes (10, 20, 30, 40, 50 μl) of the antibody solution. Triethanolamine buffer was added to each test well to obtain a final volume of 200 μl. After incubation for 18 h at 4°C, the TPI activity was measured using the optic assay described by Michal (9). The activity of TPI in relation to antibody volumes was recorded in a diagram.

RESULTS

The patient presented developed acute HAV infection complicated by hemolytic anemia. In the patient's serum, autoantibodies to TPI were detected. The autoantibodies belonged to the IgM class, which is known to be increased in acute HAV infections. Fig. 1 presents the development of autoantibodies to TPI, the total IgM, hemoglobin, and ALAT levels.

At the onset of the HAV infection, the anti-TPI titre was 1,200, and the LDH level had increased to 6.3 μkat/l. The elevated LDH levels were due to hemolysis, since they rose concomitant to the fall in hemoglobin, whereas the ALAT levels fell during the further course of the disease.

Autoantibodies to TPI reached their maximum titre 1,600 a few days after the onset of symptoms, declining to 1:800 on the 16th day. During this period the hemoglobin value dropped to 96 g/l and the reticulocyte count gradually rose to 2.4%. Haptoglobin was not detectable at that time.

Fig. 1 presents the autoantibody levels over a period of 6 months, showing that the fall in anti-TPI autoantibodies parallels a rise in the hemoglobin value. At a control 6 months later, neither signs of hemolysis, nor autoantibodies to TPI were detectable.

The effect of anti-TPI antibodies was measured on erythrocytes as well as on TPI. TPI was purified chromatographically and after SDS polyacrylamide gel electrophoresis showed no

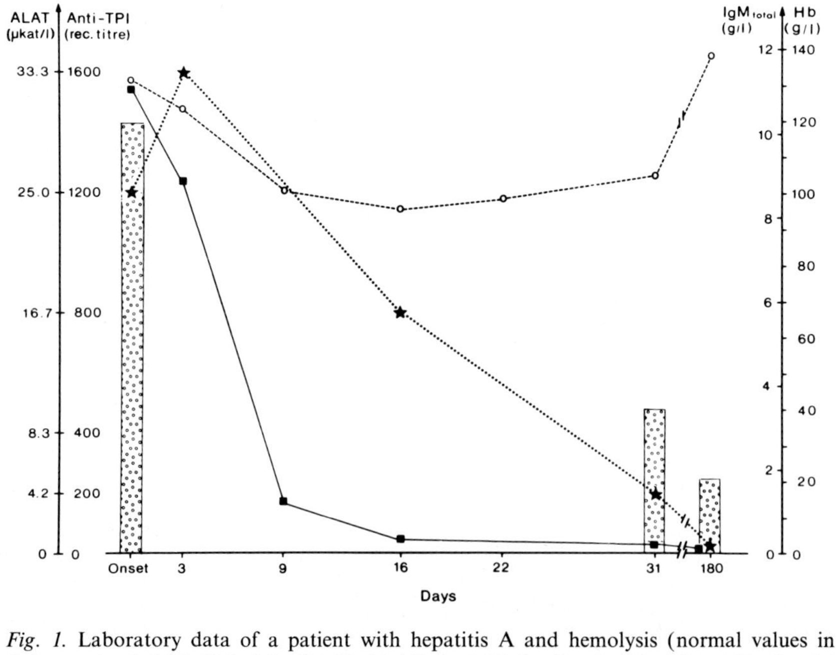

Fig. 1. Laboratory data of a patient with hepatitis A and hemolysis (normal values in parentheses). Column: total IgM (0.6–2.8 g/l); ■ ALAT (≤0.37 μkat/l); ○ Hb (120–160 g/l); ★ IgM anti-TPI (1: <50).

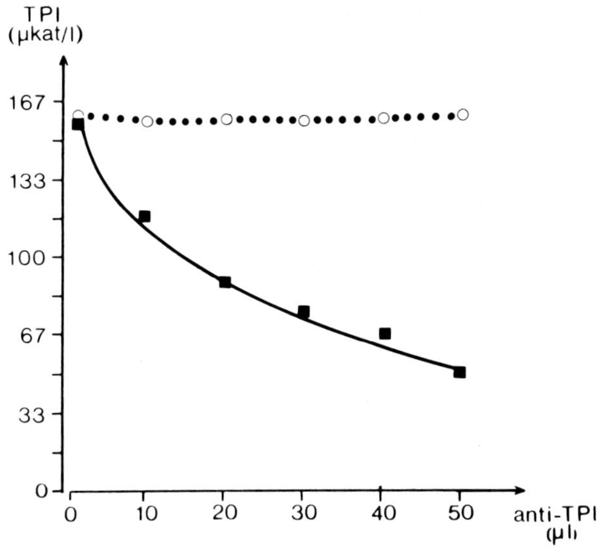

Fig. 2. Inhibition of TPI by increasing amounts of anti-TPI. *Ordinate*: activity of TPI; *abscissa*: amount of anti-TPI. ■ anti-TPI from the patient's serum taken on day 3 of the clinical disease; ○ patient's serum taken 6 months later.

contamination with erythrocyte proteins in Coomassie blue staining. In vitro, the affinity-purified antibodies from the patient's serum induced a specific ^{51}Cr release of 24% from her own erythrocytes. However, the hemoglobin release observed was very weak.

Fig. 2, presenting the enzyme activity of anti-TPI antibodies as a function of the amount of antibody added, shows that anti-TPI antibodies were able to inhibit the activity of TPI. At first the highly avid antibodies react by inducing a quick reduction of the enzyme activity presented by the rapidly declining part of the curve, whereas antibodies of a lower avidity only possessing a low inhibitory effect on TPI are responsible for the flattening of the curve. The patient's serum taken 6 months after the acute illness did not show any inhibitory activity on TPI.

DISCUSSION

Reports on hemolysis during acute HAV infection have been published repeatedly, yet its mechanisms have hitherto not been elucidated. In this context the detection of antibodies to TPI, an enzyme acting in the Embden-Meyerhoff pathway, in a patient with acute HAV infection is remarkable.

Our patient gradually developed hemolytic anemia with the hemoglobin value decreasing to 96 g/l within 3 weeks. Antibodies to TPI isolated from the patient's serum in vitro became bound to marked erythrocytes and induced a ^{51}Cr release, while complement was activated. TPI is indeed a cytoplasmatic enzyme, but it may come into contact with the cell membrane via the cytoskeleton (10). Initial binding to its antigen on the membrane may lead to a disturbance of membrane function, allowing the penetration of the autoantibody into the cell. The intracellular antibody may bind to TPI and injure the enzyme function. Damage of the enzyme function may in turn reduce the osmotic resistance of the erythrocytes. Furthermore, in hereditary lack of TPI, a reduced osmotic resistance and a shortened erythrocyte survival time have been found (11). We assume that the gradual fall in hemoglobin and the development of hemolysis is caused by an inhibition of TPI by the antibody. The incompleteness of the inhibition as evidenced by the flat part of the titration curve, may be due to the low affinity portion of the autoantibody. The antibodies to TPI belong to the IgM class. A switch to IgG was not observed at any time during or after the acute HAV infection. Since IgM anti-TPI was detectable for a short period only, it first seemed likely that the increased release of TPI from the injured liver cells had led to the activation of self B cell clones. Anti-TPI antibodies, however, have not been detected in other cases of liver damage due to infectious agents, drugs, or alcohol abuse.

It has earlier been suggested that the Kupffer cells of the liver play an important role as a barrier against the entry of bacterial products such as LPS into the bloodstream via the portal vein (12). The disturbance in this filter effect of the reticuloendothelial system in the liver during the course of acute HAV infection allows the penetration of bacterial LPS, leading to an unspecific B cell stimulation. This is considered to be the cause of the marked increase in IgM in acute HAV infection (13). The production of IgM anti-TPI may also be explained by the T-cell independent activation of self B cell clones by lipopolysaccharides.

ACKNOWLEDGEMENT

This work was supported by the Deutsche Forschungsgemeinschaft (Ri 677/1-1).

REFERENCES

1. Hara K, Tagawa K, Unuma T. Acute hemolysis associated with hepatitis A. Gastroenterol Jpn 20: 611–615, 1985.
2. Gundersen SG, Bjoerneklett A, Bruun JN. Severe erythroblastopenia and hemolytic anemia during a hepatitis A infection. Scand J Infect Dis 21: 255–228, 1989.
3. Lyons DJ, Gilvarry JM, Fielding JF. Severe haemolysis associated with hepatitis A and normal glucose-6-phosphate dehydrogenase status. Gut 31: 838–839, 1990.
4. Dietz WH, Porcell O, Moon TE, Peters CJ, Purcell RH. IgM levels and IgM-mediated immune responses in patients with acute hepatitis A, acute hepatitis B and chronic HB antigenaemia. Clin Exp Immunol 23: 69–72, 1976.
5. Horejsi J, Jezkova Z, Pencev J. Incidence and significance of autoantibodies in subjects recovering from the infectious hepatitis. Tidsskrift voor Gastro-Enterologie 13: 26–33, 1970.
6. Ritter K, Brestrich H, Nellen B, Kratzin H, Eiffert H, Thomssen R. Autoantibodies against triosephosphate isomerase. A possible clue to pathogenesis of hemolytic anemia in infectious mononucleosis. J Exp Med 171: 565–570, 1990.
7. Geurs F, Ritter K, Mast A, Van Maele V. Successful plasmapheresis in corticosteroid-resistant hemolysis in infectious mononucleosis: Role of autoantibodies against triosephosphate isomerase. Acta Haematol 88: 142–146, 1992.
8. Yoshida A, Miwa S. Characterization of a phosphoglycerate kinase variant associated with hemolytic anemia. J Hum Genet 26: 378–384, 1974.
9. Michal G. D-fructose 1,6 bisphosphate, dihydroxyacetone phosphate and D-glyceraldehyde 3-phosphate. In: Bergmeyer HU, Bergmeyer I, Grassl M, eds. Methods of enzymatic analysis, vol IV. Weinheim: Verlag Chemie, 1984, 342–350.
10. Tillmann W, Cordua A, Schröter W. Organization of enzymes of glycolysis and of glutathione metabolism in human red cell membranes. Biochim Biophys Acta 382: 157–171, 1975.
11. Eber SW, Dünnwald M, Belohradsky BH, Bidlingsmaier F, Schievelbein H, Weinmann HM, Krietsch WKG. Hereditary deficiency of triosephosphate isomerase in four unrelated families. Eur J Clin Invest 9: 195–202, 1979.
12. Knook DL, Barkway C, Sleyster EC. Lysosomal enzyme content of Kupffer and endothelial liver cells isolated from germ free and clean conventional rats. Infect Immun 33: 620–622, 1981.
13. Miller HFA, Legler, K Thomssen R. Increase in immunoglobulin M antibodies against gut bacteria during acute hepatitis A. Infect Immun 40: 542–547, 1983.

Submitted October 19, 1993; accepted March 6, 1994

Scand J Infect Dis 26: 383–389, 1994

Long-term Histological Outcome in Patients with Chronic Hepatitis C Treated Repeatedly with Interferon alpha-2b without Sustained Response

OLLE REICHARD,[1] HAND GLAUMANN[2,3] and OLA WEILAND[2]

From the Departments of Infectious Diseases, [1]Danderyd Hospital, and [2]Huddinge Hospital, and the [3]Department of Pathology, Huddinge Hospital, Karolinska Institute, Stockholm, Sweden

Nine patients with chronic hepatitis C who responded with normal or near-normal serum alanine aminotransferase (s-ALT) levels during an initial interferon alpha-2b treatment course, but who had subsequent relapses with elevated s-ALT levels after treatment cessation, were retreated once (3 patients) or twice (6 patients). The liver histological findings before the first and after the last treatment course were compared. The mean follow-up time between the initial and the follow-up assessment was 44 months (range 34–53). The histological findings were classified as chronic persistent hepatitis (CPH), chronic active hepatitis (CAH) or cirrhosis (Ci) by using a numerical scoring system assessing each portal zone separately. In the initial biopsy, 2 patients were classified as having CPH and 7 as having CAH, 2 of whom with signs of cirrhosis. According to the conventional classification, 4/9 (44%) patients improved after treatment, 3/9 (33%) remained unchanged, and 2/9 (22%) deteriorated. The mean histological scores for the necro-inflammatory parameters: portal inflammation, piecemeal necrosis, spotty necrosis and fibrosis improved, but the changes did not reach statistical significance. We conclude that repeated interferon alpha-2b treatment courses are probably beneficial in patients with chronic hepatitis C who show a non-sustained response to interferon, since studies on the natural course of chronic hepatitis C have indicated a progressive deterioration of the histological picture in many untreated patients, most marked among those with CAH.

O. Reichard, MD, Department of Infectious Diseases, Karolinska Institute, Danderyd Hospital, S-182 88 Danderyd, Sweden

INTRODUCTION

During the natural course of a chronic hepatitis C virus (HCV) infection, liver histology deteriorates over time in many patients (1–3). Patients with chronic active hepatitis (CAH) in particular seem to run an increased risk of developing liver cirrhosis and in the long-term perspective probably also hepatocellular carcinoma (2–5).

About half of the patients with chronic HCV infection treated with interferon will achieve normal serum alanine aminotransferase (s-ALT) levels during treatment (6–8), and most of these will have a simultaneous loss of HCV RNA from serum with a concomitant improvement of the liver histology (9–11). About half of the responders will relapse, however, with elevated s-ALT levels and reappearance of HCV RNA in serum, once the treatment is withdrawn (10, 12).

Whether or not further treatment courses in these non-sustained responders are beneficial on a long-term basis has not yet been elucidated. When retreated with interferon, non-sustained responders usually respond again, but with a subsequent relapse once more when treatment is discontinued (13). The long-term clinical and histological outcome after repeated interferon treatment courses is not known. In this study we evaluated the liver histological findings in a group of patients with non-sustained response after repeated interferon alpha-2b treatment courses by comparing the microscopic findings before the initial treatment with those after the last treatment.

 ISSN 0036-5548

PATIENTS AND METHODS

Patient characteristics

Patients with chronic HCV who had participated in a controlled interferon trial in 1988–89 (8) with a complete or partial s-ALT response but with relapse after treatment cessation, and who had the same outcome during 1 or 2 additional treatment courses with interferon alpha-2b, were included in the study. All patients had a complete response with a normal s-ALT level on treatment cessation after at least 1 of the courses. The patient material consisted of 8 men and 1 woman with a mean age of 59 years (range 38–75) at start of the first treatment. Blood transfusions were the mode of transmission in all patients and the mean disease duration prior to the first treatment was 54 months (range 26–180). All patients were found anti-HCV positive by a second generation ELISA (Abbott Laboratories, North Chicago, USA) confirmed by a second generation RIBA (Chiron Corp., Emeryville, USA), and all were found HCV RNA positive, when analysed by the polymerase chain reaction (PCR) method, as described earlier (13, 14). All patients gave verbal informed consent to participate, and the studies were approved by the Medical Ethics Committee at the Karolinska Institute.

Treatment regimens

Interferon alpha-2b (Introna®, Schering-Plough), 3 MU 3 times weekly, was given subcutaneously for 36 weeks (first treatment, 1988), 12 weeks (second treatment, 1989) (15) and 24 weeks (third treatment, 1991) (13).

Treatment response

Complete response was defined as a normalization of the s-ALT level (≤ 0.70 µkat/l) on treatment cessation and partial response as a $>50\%$ decrease in the s-ALT value compared with the mean pre-study value or a decrease in the s-ALT level to <1.05 µkat/l on treatment cessation. A non-sustained response was considered if the s-ALT level relapsed to pre-treatment values after treatment cessation.

Histological evaluation

A liver biopsy was performed in all patients according to a slightly modified Menghini technique within 12 months prior to the first treatment course and 6 months after cessation of the third. The biopsies were not read in pairs, and without knowledge of the patient's identity. The histological changes were assessed both in a conventional manner as chronic persistent hepatitis (CPH), chronic active hepatitis (CAH), CAH with signs of cirrhosis (CAH/Ci) or inactive cirrhosis (Ci), as recommended by an International group (16), and by using a numerical scoring system with respect to portal inflammation, piecemeal necrosis, spotty necrosis, and fibrosis (11, 17, 18). Briefly, the numerical scores for portal inflammation, piecemeal necrosis and fibrosis, respectively, were defined as follows: 0 = no portal inflammation, piecemeal necrosis or fibrosis; 1 = mild portal inflammation, piecemeal necrosis engaging isolated small positions of hepatocytes at the portal tract/parenchymal border, and fibrous portal expansion; 2 = moderate portal inflammation, piecemeal necrosis engaging 10–25% of the hepatocytes at the portal tract/parenchymal border, and fibrosis with incomplete septa; 3 = marked portal inflammation, piecemeal necrosis engaging 25–50% of the hepatocytes at the portal tract/parenchymal border, and fibrosis with complete septa; 4 = occurrence of lymphoid follicles, piecemeal necrosis engaging 50–100% of the hepatocytes at the portal tract/parenchymal border, and fibrosis with at least 2 nodule formations. The spotty necrosis score was defined as the number of areas of necrotized hepatocytes in the liver parenchyma in each field of vision (magnification $\times 100$). The mean value for each of these 4 categories from all portal zones and fields of vision in each patient constituted the score. Each portal zone was thus scored separately, a procedure that allows more subtle changes to be detected. It was possible to examine 10 or more portal areas in nearly all liver specimens.

Statistical methods

Statistical analyses were made with Wilcoxon's signed rank test.

RESULTS

The liver histological findings prior to the first treatment course and at follow-up 24 weeks after the third course, the s-ALT levels prior to and after the first, second and third treatment period, and the HCV RNA in serum prior to and after the third treatment course for each patient are presented in Table I.

Table I. *Liver histological findings, s-ALT levels and serum HCV-RNA in 9 patients with chronic hepatitis C, all of whom had a complete or partial biochemical response during repeated interferon alfa-2b treatment courses*

CPH = chronic persistent hepatitis, CAH = chronic active hepatitis, Ci = cirrhosis.

Patient no.	Liver histology prior to first treatment	S-ALT levels[a]							Serum HCV-RNA, third treatment			Liver histology at follow-up after third treatment
		First treatment		Second treatment		Third treatment						
		Start	Stop	Start	Stop	Start	Stop	Follow-up	Start	Stop	Follow-up	
1	CAH/ci	1.68	0.85	4.08	0.17	1.36	1.92	4.47	Pos	Pos	Pos	CAH/ci
2	CPH	1.84	0.93	Not done		0.61[b]	0.29	2.39	Pos	Neg	Pos	CAH
3	CAH	1.52	0.31	1.49	0.40	1.17	0.56	1.90	Pos	Neg	Pos	CPH
4	CAH	1.75	0.42	1.40	0.25	1.67	0.61	1.56	Pos	Pos	Pos	CPH
5	CAH	3.96	0.44	1.38	0.59	2.98	0.39	2.75	Pos	Neg	Pos	CPH
6	CAH	3.20	1.19	1.48	0.43	2.63	1.58	1.87	Pos	Pos	Pos	CAH
7	CPH	1.13	0.93	Not done		1.54	0.55	0.88	Pos	Pos	Pos	CAH
8	CAH	1.29	0.66	Not done		3.70	1.59	4.33	Pos	Neg	Pos	CAH
9	CAH/ci	1.89	0.63	4.14	0.48	1.37	0.24	1.29	Pos	Neg	Pos	CPH/ci
Mean		**2.03**	**0.71**	**2.33**	**0.39**	**1.89**	**0.86**	**2.38**				

[a] Normal level ≤0.7 μkat/l.

[b] Patient no. 2 had fluctuating ALT levels, at treatment within the normal range but raised levels between 1.39–1.24 μkat/l the months preceding treatment initiation.

During the first treatment course, 5 patients had a complete s-ALT response, whereas 4 responded partially. Four of the complete responders had a complete response also during the second and third treatment courses, whereas 1 had a partial response. Of the 4 partial responders during the first treatment course, 2 had a complete response during the second but a non-response during the third, and 2 a complete response during the third. Thus, 4 patients had a complete response during all three treatment courses, whereas 3 patients had a complete response during 1/2 and 2 patients during 1/3 treatment courses (Table I).

Serum HCV RNA was analysed at treatment start, on cessation, and 12 weeks after treatment during the third treatment course. All patients were HCV RNA positive at treatment start and follow-up, whereas 5/9 were negative on treatment cessation, 4 of whom had a complete s-ALT response and 1 who had a partial s-ALT response. Two patients were HCV RNA positive on treatment cessation despite a complete s-ALT response (Table I).

The mean follow-up time between the initial and follow-up biopsies was 44 months (range 34–53 months). The initial biopsy showed CPH in 2 patients, CAH in 5 and CAH/Ci in 2. By using the conventional classification 4/9 (44%) patients showed improved category, in 3/9 (33%) there was no change and 2/9 (22%) deteriorated when the histological findings before the first treatment course were compared with those 24 weeks after the third (Table I).

The individual scores for the necro-inflammatory parameters: portal inflammation, piecemeal necrosis, spotty necrosis, and fibrosis, before the first treatment and at follow-up after the last treatment, are presented separately, together with the mean values, in Fig. 1a–d. The mean histological score decreased for all parameters when the liver biopsies were compared. However, the changes did not reach statistical significance. The histological scores showed evidence of improvement of the lesions in most patients. Thus, 7/9 (78%), 5/9 (56%), 6/9 (67%) and 6/9 (67%) had improved portal inflammation, piecemeal necrosis, spotty necrosis, and fibrosis scores, respectively.

DISCUSSION

Nearly half of patients with chronic HCV infection who initially respond to interferon treatment will have a non-sustained response after treatment cessation. Why this is so, is not known at present. Recent studies suggest that prolonged interferon treatment periods might reduce the relapse rate (9, 19). Repeated treatment courses or continuous interferon treatment have both been suggested as ways of treating patients with non-sustained response. The long-term histological outcome after repeated interferon treatment courses in such patients has not been evaluated before.

All patients in our study had a complete s-ALT response, at least during 1 treatment course, but all relapsed also after being retreated. Most of the responding patients became HCV RNA negative in serum, at least during the third treatment course, in accordance with the findings in responding patients in earlier studies (9, 10). Two patients were HCV RNA positive in serum on completion of the third treatment, although their s-ALT levels were normal. As described earlier (13), HCV RNA replication was suppressed during treatment also in these 2 patients, although not totally eradicated. However, none of our patients had eradicated completely HCV RNA as they all had a relapse with elevated ALT levels and reappearance of HCV RNA in serum after cessation of the last treatment. Moreover, HCV RNA (detected by PCR) in serum has also been found, for instance in hepatocytes and mononuclear peripheral blood leukocytes (20, 21), cells in which HCV can reside during interferon treatment and later cause relapses after treatment withdrawal. Furthermore, Balart et al. (22) have shown that although HCV RNA becomes undetectable in both serum and liver during interferon treatment, relapses can still occur, with reappearance of HCV RNA, once treatment is discontinued.

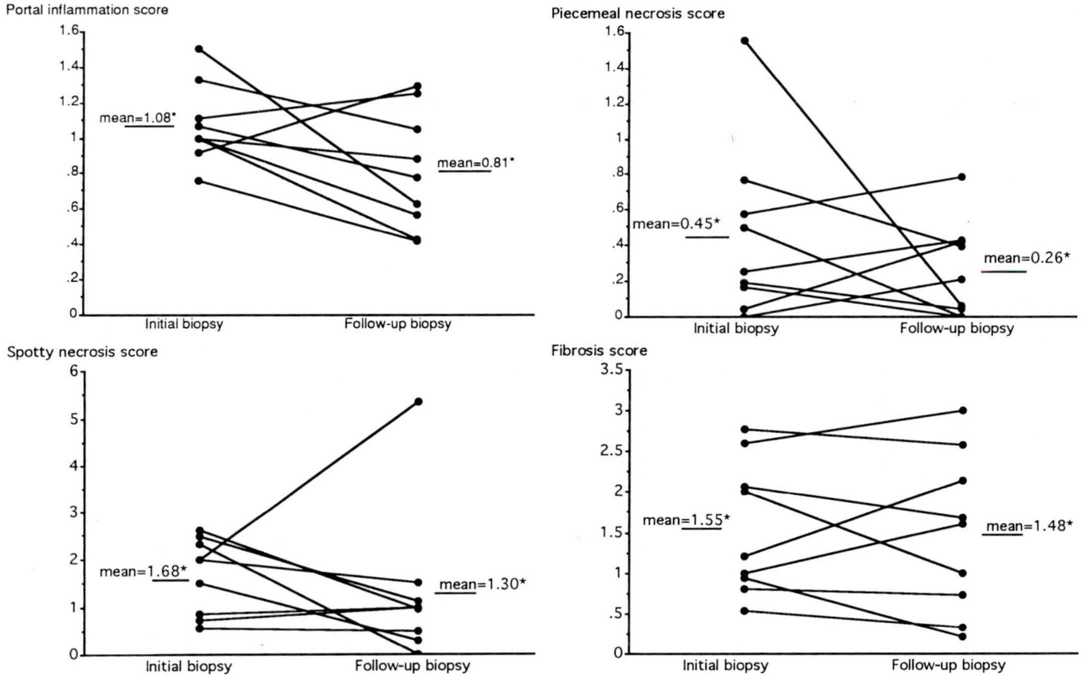

Fig. 1. Liver histology scores (for explanation, see Patients and Methods section), individuals and mean, before first and after last treatment period in 9 patients who responded in a non-sustained fashion to repeated interferon alpha-2b treatment courses. * — * = not significant.

Prospective studies have indicated that histological changes in the liver of many chronic HCV patients who do not receive interferon treatment worsen over time. Thus, Tremolada et al. (3) found that 21/65 (32%) patients with chronic hepatitis C studied for a mean of 90 months after the acute infection had developed liver cirrhosis. Di Bisceglie et al. (1) observed 39 patients for a mean of 116 months. During this time 8 (20%) developed cirrhosis, and 2 of them died of liver failure. Mattsson et al. (2) studied 19 patients with chronic post-transfusion non-A, non-B hepatitis histologically during a mean follow-up of 37 months by using almost the same numerical scoring system for their evaluation as we have used in the present study. During this period, a significant deterioration in the fibrosis score was found, while no significant change was noted in the portal inflammation, spotty necrosis or piecemeal necrosis scores. The progression of the fibrosis score was most marked in patients with CAH in the initial biopsy.

The mean interval between the time of infection and the initial liver biopsy was 52 months in our study. During this time, 7/9 (78%) patients had developed CAH, 2 of whom also had signs of cirrhosis. In contrast to results obtained in previous studies, the histological pictures in most patients improved or remained unchanged during the 44-month follow-up period, during which time the patients received repeated interferon treatment courses, as judged by both the conventional histological classification and by the numerical scoring system. The mean score for all 4 necro-inflammatory parameters thus decreased, though not significantly.

This study was open, small, non-randomized and uncontrolled. Consequently, no definite conclusion on the final outcome as compared with the natural course in untreated patients can be drawn. However, in view of the problems involved in performing controlled studies, it is unlikely that such studies with sufficient numbers of patients needing repeated interferon courses due to non-sustained response will be available in the near future. Until proven otherwise, it appears from the results presented that repeated courses of interferon alfa in non-sustained responders will certainly retard further histological deterioration, at least in a 5-year perspective.

REFERENCES

1. Di Bisceglie A, Goodman Z, Ishak K, Hoofnagle, J, Melpolder J, Alter H. Long-term clinical and histopathological follow-up of chronic post transfusion hepatitis. Hepatology 14: 969–974, 1991.
2. Mattsson L, Weiland O, Glaumann H. Long-term follow-up of chronic post-transfusion non-A, non-B hepatitis: clinical and histological outcome. Liver 8: 184–188, 1988.
3. Tremolada F, Casarin C, Alberti A, Drago C, Tagger A, Ribero ML, Realdi G. Long-term follow-up of non-A, non-B (type C) post-transfusion hepatitis. J Hepatol 16: 273–281, 1992.
4. Wejstål R, Widell A, Norkrans G. Hepatitis C virus infection with progression to hepatocellular carcinoma: A report of five prospectively followed patients in Sweden. Scand J Infect Dis 25: 417–420, 1993.
5. Tsukuma H, Hiyama T, Tanaka S, Nakao M, Yabuuchi T, Kitamura T, Nakanishi K, Fujimoto I, Inoue A, Yamazaki H, Kawashima T. Risk factors for hepatocellular carcinoma among patients with chronic liver disease. N Engl J Med 328: 1797–1801, 1993.
6. Di Bisceglie A, Martin P, Kassianides C, Lisker-Melman M, Murray LWJ, Goodman Z, Banks S, Hoofnagle J. Recombinant interferon alfa therapy for chronic hepatitis C. A randomized, double-blind, placebo-controlled trial. N Engl J Med 321: 1506–1510, 1989.
7. Davis G, Balart L, Schiff E, Lindsay K, Bodenheimer H, Perillo R, Carey W, Jacobson I, Payne J, Dienstag J, VanThiel D, Tamburro C, Lefkowitch J, Albrecht J, Meschievitz C, Ortego T, Gibas A, and the hepatitis interventional therapy group. Treatment of chronic hepatitis C with recombinant interferon alfa. A multicenter randomized, controlled trial. N Engl J Med 321: 1501–1506, 1989.
8. Schvarcz R, Weiland O, Wejstål R, Nokrans G, Fryden A, Foberg U. A randomized controlled open study of interferon alpha-2b treatment of chronic non-A, non-B posttransfusion hepatitis: no correlation of outcome to presence of hepatitis C virus antibodies. Scand J Infect Dis 21: 617–625, 1989.
9. Reichard O, Foberg U, Frydén A, Mattsson L, Norkrans G, Sönnerborg A, Wejstål R, Yun ZB, Weiland O. High sustained response rate and clearance of viremia in chronic hepatitis C following treatment with interferon alpha-2b for 60 weeks. Hepatology 19: 280–285, 1994.
10. Shindo M, Di Bisceglie A, Cheung L, Wai-Kuo Shih J, Cristiano K, Feinstone S, Hoofnagle J. Decrease in serum hepatitis C viral RNA during alpha-interferon therapy for chronic hepatitis C. Ann Intern Med 115: 700–704, 1991.
11. Schvarcz R, Glaumann H, Weiland O, Norkrans G, Wejstål R, Frydén A. Histological outcome in interferon alpha-2b treated patients with chronic posttransfusion non-A, non-B hepatitis. Liver 11: 30–38, 1991.
12. Tine F, Magrin S, Craxi A, Pagliaro L. Interferon for non-A, non-B chronic hepatitis. A meta-analysis of randomised clinical trials. J Hepatol 13: 192–199, 1991.
13. Weiland O, Zhang Y, Widell A. Serum HCA RNA levels in patients with chronic hepatitis C given a second course of interferon alpha-2b treatment after relapse following initial treatment. Scand J Infect Dis 25: 25–30, 1993.
14. Yun ZB, Lindh G, Weiland O, Johansson B, Sönnerborg A. Detection of hepatitis C virus (HCV) RNA by PCR related to HCV antibodies in serum and liver histology in Swedish blood donors. J Med Virol 39: 57–61, 1993.
15. Weiland O, Schvarcz R, Wejstål R, Norkrans G, Frydén A. Therapy of chronic posttransfusion non-A, non-B hepatitis with interferon alpha-2b: Swedish experience. J Hepatol 11: 57–62, 1990.
16. International group. Acute and chronic hepatitis revisited. Lancet 2: 914–919, 1977.
17. Knodell RG, Ishak KG, Black WC, Chen TS, Craig R, Kaplowitz N, Kiernan TW, Wollman J. Formulation and application of a numerical scoring system for assessing histological activity in asymptomatic chronic active hepatitis. Hepatology 1: 431–435, 1981.
18. Mattsson L, Weiland O, Glaumann H. Application of a histological scoring system for assessment of histological outcome in patients with chronic posttransfusion non-A, non-B hepatitis with or without antibodies to hepatitis C. Liver 10: 257–263, 1990.

19. Hoofnagle JH, Di Bisceglie AM, Shindo M. Antiviral therapy of hepatitis C – present and future. J Hepatol 17: 130–136, 1993.
20. Bartolomé J, Castillo I, Quiroga JA, Navas S, Carreno V. Detection of hepatitis C RNA in serum and peripheral blood mononuclear cells. J Hepatol 17: 90–93, 1993.
21. Takehara T, Hayashi N, Mita E, Hagiwara H, Ueda K, Katayama K, Kasahara A, Fusamoto H, Kamada T. Detection of the minus strand of hepatitis C virus RNA by reverse transcription and polymerase chain reaction: Implications for hepatitis C virus replication in infected tissue. Hepatology 15: 387–390, 1992.
22. Balart LA, Perrillo R, Roddenberry J, Regenstein F, Shim KS, Shieh C, Taylor B, Dash S, Gerber MA. Hepatitis C RNA in liver of chronic hepatitis C patients before and after interferon alfa treatment. Gastroenterology 104: 1472–1477, 1993.

Submitted December 10, 1993; accepted March 7, 1994

Scand J Infect Dis 26: 393–397, 1994

Age Specific Prevalence of Antibodies against Chlamydia pneumoniae in Iceland

SIGURDUR EINARSSON[1], HELGI K. SIGURDSSON[1], SOLVEIG D. MAGNUSDOTTIR[1], HELGA ERLENDSDOTTIR[2], HARALDUR BRIEM[2,3] and SIGURDUR GUDMUNDSSON[1,2,3]

From the [1]University of Iceland Medical School, [2]Clinical Microbiology Laboratory and [3]Department of Medicine, Borgarspitalinn, Reykjavik, Iceland

Chlamydia pneumoniae is a newly recognized common cause of respiratory tract infections. The aim of this study was to examine its prevalence in Iceland. The study was based on 1020 serum samples from individuals 0–99 years old. The samples were divided into 10-year age groups. IgG and IgM antibodies were determined with microimmunofluorescence assay. An IgG titer ≥ 32 and IgM titer ≥ 16 were considered positive.

The prevalence of positive IgG titer in the study population was $53 \pm 16\%$ (mean ± SD, age group range 14–66%). Neither seasonal nor gender-based difference in IgG antibody prevalence was demonstrated. It was lowest in the youngest group, 0–9 years old ($p < 0.001$), but rose linearly to age 70 ($p < 0.005$). 34 samples were IgM positive on initial testing; most from the older age groups. 12 were rheumatoid factor positive as well. After treatment with caprine antihuman IgG antibodies all became negative.

The prevalence of C. pneumoniae infections is high in Iceland according to these results and similar to that in neighbouring countries. The presence of IgM rheumatoid factor may cause false positive tests for pathogen-specific IgM by immune complex binding with pathogen-specific IgG, thereby requiring its removal before testing.

S. Gudmundsson, MD, PhD, Department of Medicine, University of Iceland Medical School, Landspitalinn, 101 Reykjavik, Iceland

INTRODUCTION

Chlamydia pneumoniae is a newly discovered pathogen which is a common cause of upper and lower respiratory tract infections and capable of causing severe pneumonia (1). However, most infections are probably asymptomatic (2–4). The organism was first isolated from the conjunctiva of a child in Taiwan in 1965, but indicated as a respiratory pathogen initially in 1980 (5) and first isolated from acute respiratory tract disease in 1983 (1, 5). Recent studies indicate that C. pneumoniae is a common cause of community acquired and nosocomial pneumonia (6, 7). In studies from Scandinavia and Seattle, Washington antibodies against C. pneumoniae were demonstrated in 50–60% of individuals older than 10 years (4, 8) but rarely in children younger than 5 years (1, 9, 10).

Herein we present the results of a prevalence study of IgG and IgM antibodies in a cohort of 1020 Icelandic subjects, ranging in age from 0 to 99 years.

MATERIALS AND METHODS

Serum samples

A collection of serum samples from approximately 5000 individuals had been accumulated at the Clinical Chemistry and Haematology Laboratories at Borgarspitalinn during the period of March 1989 to May 1990. The serum samples were from surplus blood drawn at the departments for any reason during this period. The sera were initially collected for a study of the prevalence of HIV infection in the Icelandic population. Personal identification had been removed from the specimens and the information available on each specimen was date of collection, age and gender. The samples were stored at −70°C. They were initially separated into 4 groups according to season of collection. A total of 889 samples from this collection were selected at random so that the samples were relatively evenly divided between 10-year age cohorts and season of collection. The 889 samples were transferred and stored at −30°C until analysis. In the original 5000 sample collection there were relatively few specimens from the age groups 0–9 and 90–99. In order to achieve our goal of approximately 100 subjects in each age group, a further 47 serum samples were obtained from residents aged 90–99 at a nursing facility in Reykjavik (Hrafnista Nursing Home) and 84 surplus depersonalized serum samples from children aged 0–9 attending the in- and outpatient services at the Pediatric Department at Landspitalinn, Reykjavik. These samples were stored at −30°C until analysed. The samples from the nursing facility were collected during 2 weeks in April 1992 and the samples from the children from December 1991 to May 1992. The final cohort thus consisted of 1020 subjects and was divided according to age of the individuals into ten 10-year age groups.

Microimmunofluorescence assay

Antibodies against C. pneumoniae were detected by microimmunofluorescence (11, 12). The procedure is based on binding of antibodies in the test serum samples to C. pneumoniae elementary bodies commercially prepared by the Washington Research Foundation, Seattle, USA, by infecting HeLa-229 cell clone with C. pneumoniae strain TW 183. The antigen is provided on glass-slides. Serial 2-fold dilutions of the serum samples in question were applied to the slides. Initial screening was done with separate 1/16 dilution for IgM and 1/32 for IgG. Fluorescein conjugates of anti-human specific immunoglobulins (IgM or IgG) were then applied to the slides and Evans blue used as a counter stain. Finally the samples were examined in a fluorescence microscope (Leitz Laborlux D, type 020-435-037, Ernst Leitz Wetzlaar GMBH, Germany). Antibody response was considered positive for IgM if it was detected in ≥1/16 dilution and positive for IgG if detected in ≥1/32 dilution (13).

Rheumatoid factor

The presence of IgM rheumatoid factor (RF) can cause false positive determination of IgM antibodies (14, 15). All IgM positive samples (34) were analyzed for IgM RF by ELISA method (15). Positive IgM samples were also further diluted up to 1/512 and reanalysed after treatment with caprine anti-human IgG antibodies (GullSORB^{TN}, Gull Laboratories, Salt Lake City, Utah, USA).

Statistical methods

Statistical evaluation was done by chi square test and test for trend in proportions (16). Confidence intervals were calculated by binomial distribution (17).

RESULTS

The 1020 samples were divided into 10 age groups each containing from 84 to 107 samples (mean ± SD: 102 ± 7). Male/female ratio of the whole study group was 498/522 (1.0/1.05), and was equal in all age groups except the first, 0–9 year olds (male/female: 47/37 = 1.0/0.8) and the last, 90–99 year olds (male/female: 35/70 = 1.0/2.0).

The prevalence of IgG antibodies in the 10 age groups is shown in Fig. 1. The mean prevalence (±SD) of IgG was 53 ± 16% (range 14–66%). Neither was any overall gender difference evident, with 54% of males and 52% of females being IgG positive, nor any gender difference between individual age groups, with male/female ratios of the percentage of IgG positive individuals in each age group ranging from 0.97 to 1.09 (p = N.S.). IgG antibody was least prevalent, 14%, in the youngest age group (0–9 year olds) but the prevalence rose significantly up to age 70, and was 66% in the 60–69 year age group ($p < 0.001$; Fig. 1). The mean (±SD) prevalence of IgG antibodies in the older age groups, 70–99 year olds, was 60 ± 6%, with a significantly lowest prevalence (55%) among the 80–89 year group ($p < 0.05$). The prevalence of IgG antibodies was 67% (38/57) in the samples from the 90–99 year old individuals recruited from the Hrafnista nursing home and 65% (31/48) in the serum bank samples (p = N.S.).

34 samples were IgM positive whereof 12 were RF positive as well. After treatment of the 34 sera with caprine anti-human IgG, IgM was detected in low titer (1/16, below cutoff limits) in 2 sera only. Both were IgM RF positive.

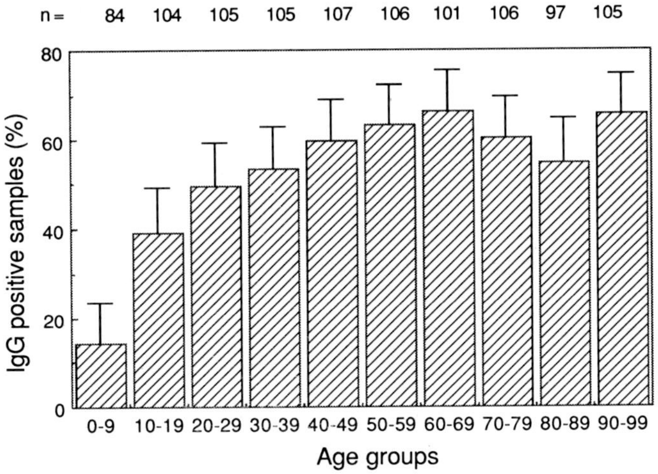

Fig. 1. Percentage of subjects in each age group with circulating IgG antibody. n = number of subjects tested in each age group; bars denote 95% confidence intervals.

DISCUSSION

A high mean prevalence of IgG antibodies against C. pneumoniae, 53%, was demonstrated in this study. In a recent Dutch study a prevalence of 80% was reported (10), but prevalence similar to the one reported herein has been observed in Seattle, Washington, and Denmark (1, 6). The mean prevalence of IgG antibodies among subjects aged >70 years was 60%, with a lowest prevalence in the 80–89 year age group, the significance of which is probably doubtful. No difference was observed between the 65 original serum samples in the oldest age group (65% prevalence) and the serum samples obtained from the 47 nursing home residents (67% prevalence).

Similar to observations by others (1, 9, 10) the prevalence in children less than 10 years of age in this study was low (14%). In fact, antibody was detected in only one individual less than 5 years of age, a 3 month old child who probably had maternally acquired antibodies.

The most prominent increase in IgG prevalence was between the first 3 age groups (0–9, 10–19 and 20–29 years; Fig. 1). Thus, it is likely that most individuals acquire their C. pneumoniae infection during the second and third decades of life. However, the alleged high incidence of new infection in these age groups was not represented by the presence of IgM antibodies in the study. The reason for this is not entirely clear, but is probably related to the method of collecting the samples, which were from serial surplus blood drawn for any reason, without any relation to respiratory or other symptoms of infection. This study was a prevalence study and was not designed to provide information on incidence of C. pneumoniae infection.

No gender related difference was observed in the prevalence of antibody against C. pneumoniae in this study, neither for the whole group of samples nor for individual age groups. Similarly, in a recent study from Japan, Kobayashi et al. (18) reported a similar prevalence of C. pneumoniae antibodies in females (26.7%) and males (26.1%). In contrast, antibodies has been found to be 10–25% more prevalent in males than females in several other recent studies (1, 4, 5).

When both pathogen-specific IgG and RF are present in an IgM negative serum sample, they may interfere with the detection of IgM and cause a false positive result (14, 15). RF is usually an IgM class, anti-IgG antibody that can bind with the pathogen-specific IgG in the sample to form an immune complex. The complex becomes a reactive site for the μ-chain specific conjugate producing a false positive result for IgM (19). Treatment of the sample with anti-human antibodies (e.g. caprine antibodies as done in this study) eliminates this interference by an immunoprecipitation reaction with the pathogen-specific IgG in the serum sample.

The prevalence of IgM RF increases with advancing age (20, 21). Of those 34 that were initially IgM positive in our study 32 were older than fifty and 18 were older than eighty. Most probably those were false positive because of rheumatoid factor. In a recent study from the Netherlands it was similarly demonstrated that IgM RF can interfere with C. pneumoniae microimmunofluorescence determination (14).

In conclusion, C. pneumoniae is a common illness in Iceland as in other neighbouring countries, with more than 50% of the population exhibiting serological evidence for the disease. Most primary infections are probably acquired between 10 and 30 years of age, but high prevalence of IgG antibodies in advancing age groups may be maintained by reinfections. Since the presence of rheumatoid factor may cause false-positive determinations of IgM, removal of interfering pathogen-specific IgG is essential prior to IgM testing, at least in age groups where the presence of RF is common.

ACKNOWLEDGEMENTS

We thank Dr. Þ. Jónsson and Professor H. Valdimarsson determination of rheumatoid factors and excellent discussions.

REFERENCES

1. Grayston JT. Infections caused by Chlamydia pneumoniae strain TWAR. Clin Infect Dis 15: 757–763, 1992.
2. Kleemola M, Saikku P, Visakorpi R, Wang SP, Grayston JT. Epidemics of pneumonia caused by TWAR, a new Chlamydia organism, in military trainees in Finland. J Infect Dis 157: 230 236, 1988.
3. Saikku P, Ruutu P, Leinonen M, Panelius J, Tupasi TE, Grayston JT. Acute lower respiratory tract infection in Filipino children associated with Chlamydia TWAR antibody. J Infect Dis 158: 1095–1097, 1988.
4. Grayston JT, Campbell LA, Kuo CC, Mordhorst CH, Saikku P, Thom DH, Wang SP. A new respiratory tract pathogen; Chlamydia pneumoniae, strain TWAR. J Infect Dis 161: 618–625, 1990.
5. Saikku P, Wang SP, Kleemola M, Brander E, Rusanen E, Grayston JT. An epidemic of mild pneumoniae due to an unusual strain of Chlamydia psittaci. J Infect Dis 151: 832–839, 1985.
6. Grayston JT, Diwan VK, Cooney M, Wang SP. Community and hospital acquired pneumonia associated with Chlamydia TWAR infection demonstrated serologically. Arch Intern Med 149: 169–173, 1989.
7. Sundelöf B, Gnarpe J, Gnarpe H, Grillner L, Darougar S. Chlamydia pneumoniae in Swedish patients. Scand J Infect Dis 25: 429–433, 1993.
8. Grayston JT, Mordhorst CH, Bruu AL, Vene S, Wang SP. Countrywide epidemics of Chlamydia pneumoniae strain TWAR in Scandinavia, 1981–1983. J Infect Dis 159: 1111–1114, 1989.
9. Puolakkainen M, Ukkonen P, Saikku P. The seroepidemiology of Chlamydiae in Finland over the period 1971 to 1987. Epidemiol Infect 1102: 287–295, 1989.
10. Stolk-Engelaar MVM, Peeters MF. Heeft Clamydia TWAR betekenis in Nederland? Ned Tijdschr Geneeskd 134: 1094–1097, 1990.
11. Wang SP, Kou CC, Grayston JT. Formalinized C. trachomatis organisms as antigen in the microimmunofluorescence test. J Clin Microbiol 10: 259–261, 1979.
12. Wang SP, Grayston JT. Micro-immunofluorescence serology of Chlamydia trachomatis. In: de la Maza LM, Peterson EM, eds. Medical virology III. Amsterdam: Elsevier Science Publishing, 87–118, 1984.
13. Saikku P, Mattila K, Nieminen MS, Huttunen JK, Leinonen M, Ekman MR, Makelä PH, Valtonen V. Serological evidence of an association of a novel Chlamydia, TWAR, with chronic coronary heart disease and acute myocardial infarction. Lancet 2: 983–986, 1988.

14. Verkooyen RP, Hazenberg MA, Van Haaren GH, van den Bosch JM, Snijder RJ, van Helden HP, Verbrugh HA. Age related interference with Clamydia pneumoniae microimmunofluorescence serology due to circulating rheumatoid factor. J Clin Microbiol 30: 1287–1290, 1992.
15. Jónsson Þ, Árnason JA, Valdimarsson H. Enzyme-linked immunosorbent assay (ELISA) screening test for detection of rheumatoid factor. Rheumatology 6: 199–204, 1986.
16. Byron WB, Hollander M, Statistics; A Biomedical Introduction. New York: John Wiley & Sons, 211–215, 1977.
17. Snedecor GW, Cochran WG. Statistical Methods. Ames, Iowa: The Iowa State University Press, 107–135, 1980.
18. Kobayashi S, Morishita T, Miyake T, Fukushi H, Hirai K, Ishihara Y, Isomura S. Prevalence of Chlamydia pneumoniae in Japan. J Infect Dis 163: 417–418, 1991.
19. Shirodaria PV, Fraser KB, Stanford F. Secondary fluorescent staining of virus antigen by rheumatoid factor and fluorescein-conjugated anti-IgM. Ann Rheum Dis 32: 53–57, 1973.
20. Allander E, Björnsson OJ, Kolbeinsson A, Ólafsson Ó, Sigfússon N, Þorsteinsson J. Rheumatoid factor in Iceland: A population study. Int J Epidemiol 1: 211–223, 1972.
21. Dequeker J, van Noyen R, Vandepitte J. Age-related rheumatoid factors – incidence and characteristics. Ann Rheum Dis 28: 431–435, 1969.

Submitted October 13, 1993; accepted March 14, 1994

Scand J Infect Dis 26: 399–402, 1994

Moraxella catarrhalis – An Uncommon Cause of Community-acquired Pneumonia in Swedish Children

BO A. CLAESSON[1] and MAIJA LEINONEN[2]

From the [1]Department of Infectious Diseases, University of Göteborg, Göteborg, Sweden, and the [2]National Public Health Institute, Helsinki, Finland

In 284 Swedish children with community-acquired, roentgenologically verified pneumonia, antibodies to Moraxella (Branhamella) catarrhalis were determined in paired serum samples with an enzyme immunoassay using a whole-cell antigen preparation from 10 strains of M. catarrhalis. Only 9 children (3%) had significant increases in antibodies to M. catarrhalis. Among these 9 children, 11–39 months of age, 6 had serologic evidence of concurrent infection with other respiratory pathogens such as S. pneumoniae, non-capsulated H. influenzae, RS virus and adenovirus. In 6 (67%) of the 9 children with antibody response and in 74 (27%) of the 275 children without antibody response to M. catarrhalis, nasopharyngeal cultures yielded growth of this bacterium. M. catarrhalis seems to be a common commensal in the upper respiratory tract, but a rare cause of pneumonia in children.

B. A. Claesson, MD, University of Göteborg, Department of Infectious Diseases, Östra Sjukhuset, S-416 85 Göteborg, Sweden

INTRODUCTION

Several bacterial species are capable of colonizing the nasopharynx, particularly in children. It is therefore difficult to assess their importance as etiological agents of lower respiratory tract infections. Moraxella (Branhamella) catarrhalis has often been regarded as a harmless commensal in the upper respiratory tract but it is nowadays generally accepted that it can cause otitis media and sinusitis and also be involved in pneumonia and bronchitis (1–6). Only rarely has M. catarrhalis been isolated from blood or other normally sterile body fluids and then mainly in patients with predisposing conditions (2).

In 17–36% of healthy Swedish preschool children, M. catarrhalis can be recovered from nasopharyngeal specimens (7, 8). In children with pneumonia, it is for practical reasons seldom possible to obtain sputum samples for cultures to establish the etiological agent. Bacterial findings in the upper respiratory tract do not necessarily correlate with findings in the lower respiratory tract, which limits the value of nasopharyngeal cultures (9). Serologic diagnosis of M. catarrhalis infections has not been used routinely because of the difficulty of identifying a common antigen of the immunologically heterogeneous strains. However, serum antibodies to the antigen prepared from different M. catarrhalis strains have been measured in a few studies to evaluate the role of the organism as an etiological agent of lower respiratory tract infections in children (4, 5). To elucidate the pathogenic role of M. catarrhalis in community-acquired childhood pneumonia, we determined serum antibodies against the bacterium in paired serum samples from 284 Swedish children with community-acquired pneumonia.

PATIENTS AND METHODS

To determine the etiology of community-acquired pneumonia in children, 336 Swedish children with roentgenologically verified pneumonia were enrolled in a prospective study. From all patients, of whom 167 were hospitalized and 169 were treated as outpatients, paired serum samples were obtained. Nasopharyngeal cultures were taken from 326 children and blood cultures from 127 children. The children had no severe underlying conditions and were between 1 month and 15 years old (median, 3 years). The first serum sample was obtained within 14 days (median, 4 days) after onset of symptoms and the second 2–7 weeks later. Antibodies were determined against 3 pneumococcal antigens, Haemophilus influenzae type b, Legionella pneumophila, Mycoplasma pneumoniae, Chlamydia species and 6 viruses. These results have been published previously (10). In 38 patients with growth of non-capsulated Haemophilus influenzae in the nasopharynx, serum antibodies against the homologous strain were analysed and the results have been reported earlier (11).

In this study, paired serum samples were available from 284 of the 336 children. Antibody concentrations against M. catarrhalis in acute and convalescent serum samples were analysed with an enzyme immunoassay, using a whole-cell preparation of 10 different strains of M. catarrhalis as antigen in the assay (1). A 3-fold increase in antibodies was defined as significant. Cultures were performed from nasopharyngeal specimens and M. catarrhalis was identified by the typical oxidase-positive colonies on blood agar plates (7).

RESULTS

Only 9 (3%) of the 284 children with pneumonia had a serum antibody response to M. catarrhalis. Table I shows the characteristics of these patients. Their ages ranged between 11 and 39 months. Mean value of C-reactive protein (CRP) was 59 mg/l (range, 0–200) and 5 children had CRP values >30 mg/l. None of them had otitis media. Six of these 9 children had serologic evidence of co-infection with other respiratory pathogens: S. pneumoniae, non-capsulated H. influenzae, respiratory syncytial (RS) virus and adenovirus, and 2 children also had concurrent culture-verified pertussis. Table II shows the numbers of children with significant antibody increases (positive serology) and children in whom M. catarrhalis was isolated from the nasopharynx (positive culture). In 6 (67%) of the 9 children with serologic evidence of M. catarrhalis infection, the organism was isolated from nasopharyngeal specimens. Among all 284 children, nasopharyngeal cultures yielded growth of M. catarrhalis in 80 (28%) of the cases and 74 (93%) of these were serology-negative.

Table I. *Characteristics of the 9 patients with significant antibody increases against M. catarrhalis*

Patient no.	Age (months)	Culture (nasopharynx)	Concurrent infection (serology)	CRP (mg/l)
1	11	M. catarrhalis S. pneumoniae H. influenzae	No	8
2	14	M. catarrhalis S. pneumoniae B. pertussis	Adenovirus	Neg.
3	18	H. influenzae	H. influenzae S. pneumoniae	75
4	20	M. catarrhalis S. pneumoniae B. pertussis	RS virus	35
5	20	S. pneumoniae	No	Neg.
6	21	M. catarrhalis S. pneumoniae	RS virus	35
7	24	S. pneumoniae	RS virus	185
8	25	M. catarrhalis S. pneumoniae	S. pneumoniae	200
9	39	M. catarrhalis	No	15

Table II. *Comparison between serology and nasopharyngeal cultures for M. catarrhalis in 284 children with pneumonia*

Serology	Number of children	Number of children with culture results: Positive	Number of children with culture results: Negative
Positive	9	6	3
Negative	275	74	201
Total	284	80	204

DISCUSSION

In this study, serum antibody increases against M. catarrhalis could be demonstrated in only 9 (3%) out of 284 children with pneumonia, suggesting the infection to be caused by M. catarrhalis. These findings are similar to those obtained in studies of Finnish children with lower respiratory tract infections (4, 5).

Antibodies to M. catarrhalis of maternal origin can be detected in sera from newborns, the concentrations decreasing during the first months of life, but with age there is a gradual increase in serum antibodies (12). Serum antibody concentrations seem to be inversely correlated with nasopharyngeal carriage of the bacterium (12). The development of serum antibodies may reflect antigenic stimulation by carriage of the bacterium in oropharynx or by respiratory infections (1). It has previously been reported that serum antibody responses to M. catarrhalis occur in children with otitis media caused by M. catarrhalis but not in children with otitis media caused by other bacteria (1). The significant rises in serum antibodies in 9 of the children with pneumonia studied here suggest the probable pathogenic role of M. catarrhalis in the pulmonary infections. Moreover, none of these 9 children had otitis media.

Six of the 9 children with infection caused by M. catarrhalis also had serologic evidence of concurrent infections with other bacteria and viruses. Mixed etiology of lower respiratory tract infections in children has been reported in several studies (4, 5, 10, 11). However, it is not concurrently possible to determine the importance of the different organisms in mixed infections in the development of the clinical symptoms.

In as many as 28% of the children with pneumonia, M. catarrhalis was isolated from the nasopharynx, but only 3% of the children had serologic evidence of M. catarrhalis infection. Thus, the rate of nasopharyngeal carriage did not correlate with the serologic responses to the bacterium, also suggesting that carriage itself does not elicit serum antibody responses. Furthermore, it has previously been shown that isolation of another potential respiratory pathogen, S. pneumoniae, in upper airways of children does not indicate pneumococcal infection in the lower airways (9). These findings invalidate the use of nasopharyngeal cultures in the etiological diagnosis of pneumonia in children.

In conclusion, M. catarrhalis is apparently a common commensal of the upper respiratory tract in children but seems to be only rarely the etiological agent of community-acquired pneumonia in otherwise healthy children.

REFERENCES

1. Leinonen M, Luotonen J, Herva E, Valkonen K, Mäkelä PH. Preliminary serologic evidence for a pathogenic role of Branhamella catarrhalis. J Infect Dis 144: 570–574, 1981.

2. Catlin BW. Branhamella catarrhalis: an organism gaining respect as a pathogen. Clin Microbiol Rev 3: 293–320, 1990.
3. Hager H, Verghese A, Alvarez S, Berk SL. Branhamella catarrhalis respiratory infections. Rev Infect Dis 9: 1140–1149, 1987.
4. Nohynek H, Eskola J, Laine E, Halonen P, Ruutu P, Saikku P, Kleemola M, Leinonen M. The causes of hospital-treated acute lower respiratory tract infection in children. Am J Dis Child 145: 618–622, 1991.
5. Korppi M, Heiskanen-Kosma T, Jalonen E, Saikku P, Leinonen M, Halonen P, Mäkelä PH. Aetiology of community-acquired pneumonia in children treated in hospital. Eur J Pediatr 152: 24–30, 1993.
6. Darelid J, Löfgren S, Malmvall B-E. Erythromycin treatment is beneficial for longstanding Moraxella catarrhalis associated cough in children. Scand J Infect Dis 25: 323–329, 1993.
7. Brorson J-E, Malmvall B-E. Branhamella catarrhalis and other bacteria in the nasopharynx of children with longstanding cough. Scand J Infect Dis 13: 111–113, 1981.
8. Söderström M, Hovelius B, Schalén C. Decreased absence due to infectious diseases in children at two day care centres over an eight-year interval. Acta Pædiatr Scand 79: 454–460, 1990.
9. Korppi M, Katila M-L, Kalliokoski R, Leinonen M. Pneumococcal finding in a sample from upper airways does not indicate pneumococcal infection of lower airways. Scand J Infect Dis 24: 445–451, 1992.
10. Claesson BA, Trollfors B, Brolin I, Granström M, Henrichsen J, Jodal U, Juto P, Kallings I, Kanclerski K, Lagergård T, Steinwall L, Strannegård Ö. Etiology of community-acquired pneumonia in children based on antibody responses to bacterial and viral antigens. Pediatr Infect Dis J 8: 856–862, 1989.
11. Claesson BA, Lagergård T, Trollfors B. Antibody response to outer membrane of noncapsulated Haemophilus influenzae isolated from nasopharynx of children with pneumonia. Pediatr Infect Dis J 10: 104–107, 1991.
12. Ejlertsen T, Thisted E, Østergaard PA, Renneberg J. Antibodies to Branhamella catarrhalis in children determined by ELISA. [Abstract 962]. Program and abstracts of the 6th European Congress of Clinical Microbiology and Infectious Diseases. Seville, Spain, March 28–31, 1993.

Submitted October 27, 1993; accepted March 21, 1994

Scand J Infect Dis 26: 403–405, 1994

Non-typhoid Salmonella Meningitis

JOHN KAVALIOTIS[1], ASIMINA TSIAOUSI[1], DEMETRIS PAPAVASILIOU[1] and ATHINA KANSOUZIDOU[2]

From the [1]Department of Paediatrics and the [2]Laboratory of Bacteriology, Infectious Diseases Hospital, Thessaloniki, Greece

The epidemiological, clinical and laboratory findings in 8 cases of meningitis due to non-typhoid salmonella were analyzed. Seven out of 8 patients were infants < 12 months old, 2 of whom died, 2 presented with recurrent meningitis. Three infants had reversible neurological sequelae on discharge, not found during follow-up in any. Conversely, one 2-month-old patient who was considered normal on discharge developed severe growth and mental retardation during follow-up.

J. Kavaliotis, MD, Department of Paediatrics, Infectious Diseases Hospital, 13 Gr Lambraki St, 546 38 Thessaloniki, Greece

INTRODUCTION

Non-typhoid salmonella meningitis is a rare clinical entity (1, 2) which occurs mainly during early infancy (6). Although during the last few years a remarkable increase in salmonellosis has been observed worldwide (4, 5), the number of salmonella meningitis cases has not shown a parallel increase. Nevertheless, all paediatricians should be aware of this complication of salmonellosis, in view of the potentially serious problems which can ensue.

This study presents our experience of meningitis caused by non-typhoid salmonella.

MATERIALS AND METHODS

Charts of patients with salmonella meningitis during the last 25 years (1968–92) were reviewed. The diagnosis of salmonella meningitis was based on characteristic findings in the cerebrospinal fluid (CSF) compatible with bacterial meningitis and also the isolation of Salmonella spp. from CSF. All patients with meningitis at our Department have a regular long-term follow-up. During the last 14 years this has been done by one of us (J.K.). The follow-up period for our 8 patients was 4–7 years. The sensitivity testing of Salmonella spp. to antibiotics was based on the Bauer-Kirby method (6).

Treatment

Therapy included 2 of the following antibiotics: ampicillin, chloramphenicol, gentamicin, cefotaxime and cotrimoxazole. In all cases the duration of treatment was 4 weeks.

RESULTS

During the study period, 2,015 patients with bacteriologically proven bacterial meningitis were hospitalized at our Department. Eight cases of non-typhoid salmonella meningitis (0.4%), (5 males and 3 females) were seen. Of the 2,015 cases, 46 were caused by bacteria other than the classical pathogens of meningitis (viz. N. meningitidis, H. influenzae, S. pneumoniae). In this group, non-typhoid Salmonella spp. were the main causative agents (8/46, 17.3%).

Seven patients were below 7 months of age (one only 18 days old) and 1 was 10 years old.

Clinical findings

The clinical findings of the patients were: fever (7/8), diarrhea (6/8), seizures (5/8), vomiting (3/8), respiratory distress (2/8), peripheral nerve palsy (2/8).

In 6 patients the meningitis was preceded by an acute gastroenteritis. Two patients had acute otitis media concomitant with the meningitis. None of the patients had any serious predisposing factor (i.e. prematurity, cerebral disease, etc).

Table I. *Clinical data of 8 cases of non-typhoid salmonella meningitis*

N: normal, AB: abnormal, CSF: cerebrospinal fluid, CT: computerized tomography, AMP: ampicillin, CEFOT: cefotaxime, CHLOR: chloramphenicol, COTRIM: cotrimoxazole, GENT: gentamycin.

Case no.	Salmonella species	CT	Treatment	Outcome	Neurolgic sequelae	Number of recurrences	Outcome during follow-up
1	Salmonella spp.	No	AMP + CHLOR	Cure	Hydrocephalus	+ 2	–
2	Salmonella typhimurium	No	AMP + GENT	Death	Hydrocephalus	+ 2	–
3	Salmonella spp.	No	AMP +	Death	–	–	–
4	Salmonella enteritidis	AB	CEFOT + COTRIM	Cure	Subdural effusion	–	Normal
5	Salmonella infantis	N	AMP + COTRIM	Cure	–	–	Normal
6	Salmonella westerstede	AB	AMP + COTRIM	Cure	Subarachnoid effusion	–	Normal
7	Salmonella infantis	N	AMP + COTRIM	Cure	–	–	Normal
8	Salmonella spp.	AB	AMP + COTRIM	Cure	–	–	Growth + mental retardation

Table I shows the strains of salmonella isolated, the antibiotic treatment, the results of computerized tomography (CT), the therapeutic outcome, and the findings at follow-up.

All salmonella strains were sensitive to the antibiotics used. The strain in the last was moderately sensitive to ampicillin. Resistant non-typhoid Salmonella spp. to ampicillin have presented a remarkable increase during recent years (1989 onwards), reaching 30% in 1993.

Computerized tomography (CT) was performed on 5 patients. In 3 of them the CT revealed: subdural effusion and ventricular dilatation (patient no. 4), subarachnoidal purulent effusion (patient no. 6), subarachnoidal and ventricular dilatation (patient no. 8). The conditions had resolved completely during follow-up in all 3.

Two patients each suffered 2 recurrences of meningitis, of whom 1 died during the second relapse. There was one further death (altogether 2 (25%)).

Three (37.5%) patients had neurological sequelae on discharge, which resolved in all 3 during follow-up. On the other hand a 2-month-old patient who was assumed to be clinically well on discharge, was diagnosed as having motor and mental retardation at follow-up.

Table II shows certain blood and CSF findings in our patients.

Table II. *Laboratory findings in non-typhoid salmonella meningitis*

	Range	Mean
White blood cells ($\times 10^9$/l)	3–15	9.51
Hemoglobin (mmol/l)	1.27–1.78	1.48
Cerebrospinal fluid		
cells ($\times 10^6$/l)	1500–6500	3300
protein (g/l)	1.36–7.5	2.95
glucose (mmol/l)	0.28–3.16	1.3

DISCUSSION

Although CNS involvement is not a common complication of non-typhoid salmonella infections (7), salmonella meningitis may be a serious problem under certain circumstances, especially during the neonatal period and in early infancy, when an increased incidence of bacteremia is observed (8, 9).

An increase in salmonella infections has been observed during recent years in Greece. Whether or not this increase will result in an increased rate of meningitis as well, is unknown. In our material, 3 cases occurred during a single year (1988), whereafter no new case has occurred, even though the number of salmonella cases is still increasing.

The frequency of the disease in Northern Greece (0.4%) is lower than that reported from other countries (0.8–6%) (8, 10, 11). The mortality rate was low (25%) as well (1, 8, 12, 13).

The 2 patients who died were treated with ampicillin and an aminoglycoside. It is not known to what extent this therapeutic regimen accounted for the high mortality rate. Nevertheless, the use of newer cephalosporins (1, 7, 14) and cotrimoxazole (15) has evidently reduced the mortality rate. Today, both cefotaxime and ceftriaxone are optimal drugs for salmonella meningitis, by virtue of their excellent CSF penetration. Cotrimoxazole is very useful especially in cases of specific drug allergy or resistance to chloramphenicol. The recommended duration of treatment should be 4 weeks (16).

REFERENCES

1. Bryan JP, Rocha H, Scheld WM. Problems in salmonellosis: rationale for clinical trials with newer β-lactam agents and quinolones. Rev Infect Dis 8: 189–207, 1986.
2. Cherubin CE, Corrado ML, Nair SR, Gombert ME, Landesman S, Humbert G. Treatment of Gram-negative bacillary meningitis: role of the new cephalosporin antibiotics. Rev Infect Dis 4(Suppl): 453–464, 1982.
3. CDC. Reported isolates of salmonella from cerebrospinal fluid in the United States, 1968–1979. J Infect Dis 143: 504–506, 1981.
4. Sharp JCM. Salmonellosis and eggs. BMJ 297: 1557–1558, 1988.
5. Telzak EE, Budnick LD, Greenberg MS, Blum S, Shayegani M, Benson CE, Schultz S. A nosocomial outbreak of Salmonella enteritidis infection due to the consumption of raw eggs. N Engl J Med 323: 394–397, 1990.
6. Bauer AW, Kirby WMM, Sherrif KC, Turck M. Antibiotic susceptibility testing by standarized simple disk method. Am J Clin Pathol 45: 493–496, 1966.
7. Kinsella TR, Yogev R, Shulman ST, Gilmore R, Chadwick EG. Treatment of Salmonella meningitis and brain abscess with the new cephalosporins: two case reports and a review of the literature. Pediatr Infect Dis J 6: 476–480, 1987.
8. Davis RC. Salmonella sepsis in infancy. Am J Dis Child 135: 1096–1099, 1981.
9. Bassa A, Parras F, Reina J, Villar E, Gil J, Alomar P. Non-typhi salmonella bacteremia. Infection 17: 290–293, 1989.
10. Appelbaum PC, Scragg J. Salmonella meningitis in infants. Lancet 1: 1052–1053, 1977.
11. Geisler PJ, Nelson KE, Levin S, Reddi KT, Moses VK. Community-acquired purulent meningitis: a review of 1,316 cases during the antibiotic era, 1954–1976. Rev Infect Dis 2: 725–745, 1980.
12. Denis F, Badiane S, Chiron JP, Sow A, Diop Mar I. Salmonella meningitis in infants. Lancet 1: 910, 1977.
13. West SE, Goodkin R, Kaplan A. Neonatal Salmonella meningitis complicated by cerebral abscesses. West J Med 127: 142–145, 1977.
14. Soe GB, Overturf GD. Treatment of typhoid fever and other systemic salmonelloses with cefotaxime, ceftriaxone, cefoperazone, and other newer cephalosporins. Rev Infect Dis 9: 719–736, 1987.
15. Murphy TF, Fernald GW. Trimethoprim-sulfamethoxazole therapy for relapses of Salmonella meningitis. Pediatr Infect Dis J 2: 465–468, 1983.
16. Hayani KC, Pickering LA. Salmonella infections. In: Feigin RD, Cherry JD, eds. Textbook of pediatric infectious diseases, 3rd ed. Philadelphia: WB Saunders Co., 620–636, 1992.

Submitted February 24, 1994; accepted April 17, 1994

Scand J Infect Dis 26: 406–410, 1994

Cluster of Multiresistant Escherichia coli O78:H10 in Greater Copenhagen

BENTE OLESEN[1,2], HANS JØRN KOLMOS[2], FRITS ØRSKOV[1] and IDA ØRSKOV[1]

[1]From the International Escherichia and Klebsiella Centre (WHO), Statens Seruminstitut, and the [2]Department of Clinical Microbiology, Hvidovre Hospital, University of Copenhagen, Copenhagen, Denmark

A multiresistant, lactose-negative Escherichia coli O78:H10 was isolated from 19 patients in Greater Copenhagen over a period of 8 months. At least 14 cases were community-acquired. 18 isolates originated from urine cultures and 1 from a faecal sample. 13 patients were predisposed to urinary tract infection (UTI) and 11 patients showed clinical signs of UTI. This is the first report of E. coli O78:H10 causing human disease. The cluster was probably food-borne, but the source was not identified. This cluster of identical disease associated E. coli was only uncovered because of its multiresistance and lactose-negative phenotype.

B. Olesen, MD, The International Escherichia and Klebsiella Centre (WHO), Statens Seruminstitut, Artillerivej 5, DK-2300 Copenhagen S, Denmark

INTRODUCTION

In 1988 a year-long community-acquired outbreak of diseases caused by a multiresistant Escherichia coli, O15:K52:H1, was reported from South-East London (1). Most of the patients had urinary tract infections (UTI), but several had severe complications.

In 1991 a somewhat similar cluster due to a multiresistant E. coli serotype O78:H10 was recorded in Greater Copenhagen. The cluster included 18 patients with UTI and 1 patient with diarrhea. Food-borne disease outbreaks of diarrhea caused by verotoxigenic strains of E. coli have been reported regularly (2), however community-acquired outbreaks of E. coli causing extra-intestinal diseases are rare. Consequently, and due to the fact that serotype O78:H10 has not previously been associated with human disease, we considered it of interest to describe this cluster in greater detail. In the present paper we present clinical and epidemiologic data of the cluster, together with a bacteriological characterization of the E. coli strains isolated.

MATERIALS AND METHODS

Clinical and epidemiological investigations

On April 19th 1991, 3 strains of E. coli, all lactose negative and with a similar unusual sensitivity pattern, were isolated in urine specimens sent to the Clinical Microbiological Department at Hvidovre Hospital from general practitioners in the Municipality of Copenhagen. All strains were resistant to ampicillin, chloramphenicol, streptomycin, sulphonamides, tetracyclines and trimethoprim, but were sensitive to cefuroxime, gentamicin, netilmicin and ciprofloxacin. Serotyping of the 3 strains showed that all were O78:H10, an uncommon serotype.

An epidemic connection between the strains was suspected, and the other 4 Clinical Microbiological Departments in Greater Copenhagen (Rigshospitalet, Herlev, Frederiksberg and Bispebjerg hospitals) were asked to refer clinical isolates of multiresistant lactose-negative E. coli to Statens Seruminstitut for serotyping. In addition 500 stool samples taken from patients in the Municipality of Copenhagen and sent to the Clinical Microbiological Department at Hvidovre Hospital for detection of parasites, were screened for the presence of the epidemic strain. A total of 72 strains of lactose-negative multiresistant E. coli were received for further investigation over the next 20 months.

As it seemed probable that the outbreak could be food-borne and as it is known from the literature that strains of serogroup O78 can cause septicaemia in calves (10), 10 strains of E. coli serotype O78 isolated from calf spleens at Statens Veterinære Serumlaboratorium were included in the investigation.

 ISSN 0036-5548

Clinical data of patients were obtained from general practitioners and case records. Since the first isolated strains were cultured from outpatients living in the same area of Copenhagen, epidemiological data concerning foodstuffs, shops and eating habits were obtained from the 3 patients themselves. However, as it became obvious that the outbreak was not limited to a small geographical area and no link was found concerning shops and foodstuffs, no further interviews were carried out. A strain was defined as community-acquired if it originated from an out-patient who had not recently been admitted to hospital, or from a hospitalized patient who had been admitted for less than 48 h.

Bacteriological investigations

Antibiotic susceptibility was determined by the agar diffusion technique using blood agar from Statens Seruminstitut Copenhagen and Neo-sensitabs® from Rosco Diagnostica, Tåstrup, Denmark (3). Faecal samples were screened for the presence of multiresistant lactose-negative E. coli, using bromthymol blue lactose agar and Rosco Neosensitabs containing chloramphenicol and tetracycline. The analysis of O, K and H antigens was carried out as previously described (4). Biotyping including 14 carbohydrates was carried out according to Kauffmann (5). The strains were tested for haemagglutination of human, bovine, sheep and guinea-pig red blood cells with and without 2% mannose on ice. Examination for P fimbriation was carried out with the PF test, Orion Diagnostica, Espoo, Finland. Fimbrial extracts were examined by rocket immunoelectrophoresis with fimbria antisera F7-F16 (6). Production of haemolysin was detected on 5% washed sheep blood-agar plates after 24 h incubation. The isolates were investigated for the presence of plasmids by the method of Kado and Liu (7). Detection of heat-labile enterotoxin (LT) was performed according to Sack and Sack (8). Heat-stable enterotoxin (ST) was assayed in microtitre wells in the form of a competitive EIA technique using the Oxoid VET-RPLA Kit. Verotoxin (VT) was tested according to Konowalchuk et al. (9).

RESULTS

19 out of 72 (26%) E. coli strains investigated had the serotype O78:H10. No K antigen was present. All 19 strains had the same antibiotic susceptibility pattern and were isolated from 19 patients over a period of 8 months (Fig. 1). 18 strains originated from urinary cultures and one from faeces. The distribution of strains according to local microbiological laboratories was: Herlev 8, Hvidovre 7, Rigshospitalet 3, Frederiksberg 1 and Bispebjerg 0. None of the 10 veterinary strains resembled the human isolates, since they were all non-motile and differed regarding both sensitivity and biotype.

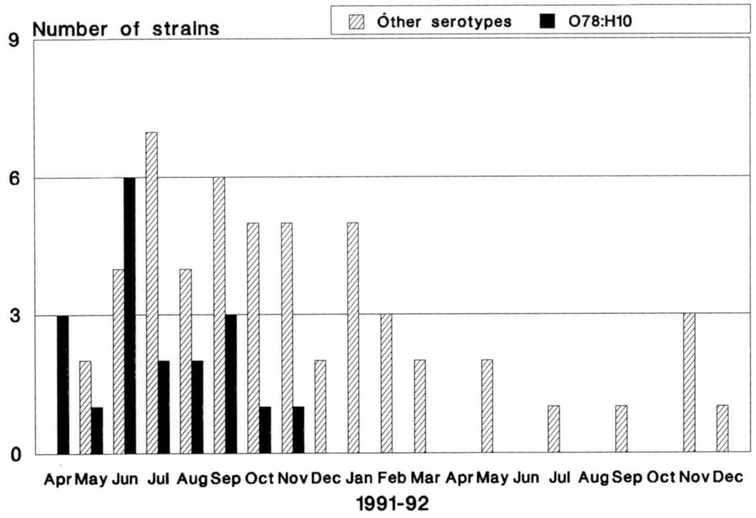

Fig. 1. E. coli strains of serotype O78:H10 isolated during 1991–92 in Greater Copenhagen.

Patients

In 15 females and 3 males (median age 59 years, range 4 months–87 years) E. coli O78:H10 was cultured from the urine (Table 1). The concentration of bacteriae was in all cases $\geq 10^5$ bacteria/ml urine. 11 patients showed obvious clinical signs of UTI; 7 patients were cultured for other reasons. 13 patients were predisposed to UTI (Table 1). Two patients were receiving antimicrobial prophylaxis bacause of recurrent UTI, 7 had received antibiotic treatment for UTI and 1 for pneumonia within the past 3 months. The single faecal strain

Table I. *Clinical data of patients with urinary tract infection caused by E. coli serotype O78:H10 in Greater Copenhagen, Denmark in 1991. The patients are listed in chronological order*

Case no.	Sex/age (years)	Reason for culture	Predisposition to UTI
1	F/76	Fatigue, dizziness	None
2	F/16	Control	Malformation of the urinary tract, recurrent UTI, trimethoprim prophylaxis
3	F/21	Neurological disease	Residual urine
4	F/27	Control	Recent UTI treated with pivampicillin
5	F/79	Symptoms of UTI	Diabetes and uraemia
6	F/1	Stomach ache and growth problems	None
7	F/60	Symptoms of UTI	Breast cancer treated with prednisolone
8	F/28	Symptoms of UTI	None
9	F/58	Symptoms of UTI	Recurrent and recent UTI treated with sulfonamides
10	F/84	Symptoms of UTI	Residual urine, urethral catheter, recent treatment with penicillin
11	F/65	Symptoms of UTI	Residual urine, recent UTI treated with nitrofurantoin
12	F/70	Symptoms of UTI	Residual urine, intermittent urethral catheter, recurrent UTI, trimethoprim prophylaxis
13	F/87	Symptoms of UTI	Treatment with prednisolone, recent UTI treated with sulfonamides and nitrofurantoin
14	M/4 mths	Control	Recurrent UTI, recent UTI treated with trimethoprim, amoxicillin and mecillinam
15	F/74	Control	Recent UTI treated with sulfonamides
16	M/4 mths	Symptoms of UTI	Malformation of the urinary tract, recurrent and recent UTI treated with sulfonamides, ampicillin, and trimethoprim-sulfa-methoxazole
17	M/30	Symptoms of UTI	None
18	F/69	Symptoms of UTI	None

originated from an AIDS patient with chronic diarrhea who had been treated with trimethoprim-sulfamethoxazole after a Pneumocystis carinii pneumonia in 1989. Faeces had numerous times been examined for bacteria and parasites causing enteritis, but all tests had proved negative. Two patients with UTI also had diarrhea (patients 8 and 12). 13 patients received antibiotics for their actual UTI. None of the patients developed bacteraemia.

At least 14 cases were community-acquired, whereas 5 strains were possibly of nosocomial origin. Three of the latter 5 were cultured from patients admitted to different units of the same hospital. The 2 remaining strains were cultured from patients at 2 different hospitals. The 14 community-acquired cases occurred in patients living in different parts of Greater Copenhagen, except for 1 patient living in the southern part of Sealand.

E. coli strains

All 19 strains had the same unusual biotype, being rhamnose- and lactose-negative. All isolates showed mannose-sensitive haemagglutination with guinea-pig red cells, suggesting the presence of type-1 pili. 11 strains, of which 5 were obtained from the patients with no predisposition to UTI, showed mannose-resistant haemagglutination (MRHA) of human, sheep and bovine erythrocytes. The results of the P fimbria specific agglutination (PF) test with these 11 strains could not be interpreted, as agglutination occurred in both the PF reagent and the control reagent. The remaining 8 strains showed a negative result in haemagglutination and PF test. Examination of fimbrial extracts with antisera to P fimbriae, F antigen number 7-16, showed a negative reaction. The positive MRHA test indicated the presence of fimbriae which were probably not P fimbriae. None of the strains produced VT, ST or LT enterotoxin. All isolates possessed a plasmid of approximately 32 megadaltons. None of the strains produced haemolysin.

DISCUSSION

From 1956 to 1990, only 30 strains of O78:H10 were found among the thousands received at the WHO Escherichia Centre at Statens Seruminstitut from all over the world. These strains could be divided into 7 biotypes and none were multiresistant. The 19 strains isolated during 8 months within a limited geographical area is thus an obvious cluster of an uncommon strain. The serogroups O78:H11 and O78:H12 (11) have frequently been isolated from cases of human enterotoxigenic diarrhea, but O78:H10 has not been reported earlier in association with human or animal disease.

We were unable to find any epidemiological connection between the patients infected by E. coli O78:H10, but it very likely existed. Probably the strains of this type were widely distributed in the community during the period investigated. This is supported by the fact that UTI-predisposed patients were infected with the strain without having any obvious epidemiological connection. A large number of patients without predisposing factors may have been colonized in the intestine without developing signs of infection. Probably the cluster was food-borne.

It is interesting that 13 out of 18 patients were predisposed to UTI, and that 11 out of 19 patients had received antibiotics within 3 months before E. coli O78:H10 was isolated. Since all O78:H10 strains were multiresistant, it is likely that they were selected from the faecal flora because of treatment with antibiotics. Since none of the strains had P-fimbriae, which is a common virulence factor in E. coli causing UTI, it seems natural that they were able to cause UTI mainly in predisposed patients. Two patients with UTI and 1 AIDS patient had diarrhea. However, as none of the strains produced ST, LT or VT, it is doubtful whether E. coli O78:H10 was the cause of the diarrhea.

This minor cluster of E. coli O78:H10 was only noticed because of the characteristic resistance pattern and the fact that the strains did not ferment lactose. Even a major cluster of a sensitive lactose-fermenting E. coli belonging to an epidemic clone could be overlooked in the routine laboratory. The present data, together with the O15:K52:H1 data from London, point to the possibility that similar clusters of extra-intestinal E. coli infections may be more common than expected. Since E. coli strains in Denmark have few acquired resistance characters, the antibiogram is of little use for epidemiological purposes. As general detailed typing of all E. coli is not feasible, one suggestion could be to use a more discriminating biotyping system in routine laboratories to indicate relationships among sequential isolates of cultures from individual patients. To confirm a suspected cluster of epidemiologically related E. coli, the strains could be examined for O, H and K antigens at a reference laboratory.

ACKNOWLEDGEMENTS

We thank the departments of clinical microbiology at Rigshospitalet and Herlev, Frederiksberg and Bispebjerg Hospitals for providing strains and data from patients and Statens Veterinære Serumlaboratorium for providing strains from calves.

REFERENCES

1. Phillips I, Eykyn S, King A, Gransden WR, Rowe B, Frost JF, Gross RJ. Epidemic multiresistant Escherichia coli infection in West Lambeth Health District. Lancet I: 1038–1041, 1988.
2. Karmali MA. Infection by verocytotoxin-producing Escherichia coli. Clin Microbiol Rev 2: 15–38, 1989.
3. Casals JB, Pringler N. Antibacterial, -fungal sensitivity testing using neosensitabs. 9th ed. Taastrup: Rosco Diagnostica, 1991.
4. Ørskov F, Ørskov I. Serotyping of Escherichia coli. In: Bergan T, ed. Methods in microbiology. Vol. 14. London: Academic Press, 43–112, 1984.
5. Kauffmann F. Enterobacteriaceae. Copenhagen: Munksgaard, 1954.
6. Ørskov I, Ørskov F. Serologic Classification of Fimbriae. In: Jann K, Jann B, eds. Bacterial Adhesins. Berlin Heidelberg: Springer-Verlag, 71–90, 1990.
7. Kado CI, Liu ST. Rapid procedure for detection and isolation of large and small plasmids. J Bacteriol 145: 1365–1373, 1981.
8. Sack DA, Sack RB. Test for enterotoxigenic Escherichia coli using Y1 adrenal cells in miniculture. Infect Immun 11: 334–336, 1975.
9. Konowalchuck J, Speirs JI, Stavric S. Vero response to a cytotoxin of Escherichia coli. Infect Immun 18: 775–779, 1977.
10. Ørskov I, Ørskov F, Jann B, Jann K. Serology, chemistry and genetics of O and K antigens of Escherichia coli. Bacteriol Rev 41: 667–710, 1977.
11. Ørskov F, Ørskov I. Special Escherichia coli serotypes among enterotoxigenic strains from diarrhea in adults and children. Med Microbiol Immunol 162: 73–80, 1976.

Submitted November 3, 1993; accepted April 10, 1994

Scand J Infect Dis 26: 411–416, 1994

Polymicrobial and Recurrent Bacteremia with Shigella in a Patient with AIDS

MÁR KRISTJÁNSSON[1,3]*, BRANT VINER[2,3] and JOEL N. MASLOW[1,3]

From the Infectious Diseases Section and the Medical Service, [1]VA Medical Center, [2]Boston City Hospital and [3]the Department of Medicine, Boston University School of Medicine, Boston, MA, USA

Shigella gastroenteritis is uncommon among HIV seropositive patients and may be complicated in some patients by bacteremia; S. flexneri being the most frequently detected serogroup. While recurrent Salmonella bacteremia is common among HIV-seropositive patients, recurrent Shigella bacteremia is not. We report here an HIV-seropositive patient with Shigella gastroenteritis, polymicrobial bacteremia due to S. flexneri and S. boydii, and recurrent gastroenteritis and bacteremia with S. boydii. Relapsing infection with the same strain of S. boydii was determined using pulsed field gel electrophoresis. Thus, HIV-seropositive patients who develop Shigella infections may require prolonged treatment and/or suppressive therapy, similar to those infected with Salmonella. Patients who develop recurrent disease should be suspected as having polymicrobial bacteremia since the incidence of this may be underestimated among patients with AIDS, particularly those with concurrent gastroenteritis.

J. Maslow, MD, PhD, Research Service (151), VA Medical Center, 150 South Huntington Avenue., Boston, MA 02130, USA

INTRODUCTION

Gastroenteritis is a common complication of HIV-seropositive patients with bacterial pathogens documented in only a minority of cases, and Shigella species being a particularly uncommon cause of diarrheal illness (1). Bacteremia, an uncommon complication of Shigella gastroenteritis in immunocompetent patients (2–4), may be more prevalent among HIV-seropositive patients (5). Whereas recurrence of bacteremia with Salmonella is common among HIV-seropositive patients (6), recurrence of bloodstream infection secondary to Shigella species has been reported for only 1 patient to date (5). We report an HIV-seropositive patient with Shigella gastroenteritis, polymicrobial bacteremia due to S. flexneri and S. boydii, and recurrent gastroenteritis and bacteremia with the same strain of S. boydii.

CASE REPORT

A 36-year-old Haitian male was admitted to another hospital because of non-bloody, watery diarrhea of 6 months duration. At the time of admission, the patient reported a 20 kg weight loss and voluminous diarrhea (2–4 litres per 24 h). There was no history of injecting drug use, blood transfusions, homosexual contact, contact with prostitutes, or male prostitution. The patient's wife and 2 children were healthy, with no history of recent diarrheal illness. The patient had recently emigrated to Boston from Haiti, with no other known travel history. The patient was febrile with a rectal temperature of 38.1°C. Microscopic examination of the stool for ova and parasites revealed Cryptosporidia; examination for occult blood was negative. Blood and stool cultures obtained on the first hospital day yielded S. flexneri. A serologic test for HIV-1 was positive. A repeat blood culture obtained on the second hospital day yielded S. flexneri; while another specimen of blood obtained an hour later yielded S. boydii. All of the isolates were susceptible to all antibiotics tested. The patient was treated with ceftriaxone for 10 days with resolution of fever, although his diarrhea persisted. Stool cultures obtained

* Present author address: Már Kristjánsson, MD, Department of Medicine, Borgarspítali, 108 Reykjavík, Iceland.

 ISSN 0036-5548

on the 9th and 12th days of hospitalization yielded no growth. On the 15th day of hospitalization the patient was transferred to Boston City Hospital (BCH).

On admission to BCH, the patient appeared cachectic and was afebrile. Occult blood was detected in a sample of the patient's stool and cryptosporidia were detected on microscopic examination. Culture of the stool yielded S. boydii with identical antibiotic susceptibilities to the prior isolate except for resistance to ampicillin. The CD4+ lymphocyte count was 10×10^6/L. Sigmoidoscopy revealed mild inflammation on direct examination with chronic inflammation detected histologically. The following day the patient became febrile. Bilateral interstitial infiltrates were evident on a radiogram of the chest, and a gallium scan revealed diffuse pulmonary uptake consistent with a diagnosis of Pneumocystis carinii pneumonia. Treatment with parenteral trimethoprim-sulfamethoxazole and oral zidovudine was initiated with clinical improvement and resolution of fever; no treatment specific for cryptosporidia was prescribed. The patient's diarrhea persisted. A specimen of stool obtained on the 25th day after his initial hospitalization (the 10th day at BCH) yielded no growth. On the 26th hospital day the patient was noted to be lethargic, tachypneic, tachycardic, hypotensive, and febrile; blood and stool cultures yielded no growth. Repeat blood cultures on the 29th hospital day yielded S. boydii resistant to ampicillin, cephalothin, piperacillin, trimethoprim-sulfamethoxazole, and chloramphenicol. Treatment with ceftriaxone resulted in resolution of fever. Specimens of blood obtained in the 35th and 39th hospital days yielded no growth. The patient and his family decided against further therapeutic interventions, and he expired on the 44th hospital day.

MATERIAL AND METHODS

At both hospitals specimens of blood were directly inoculated into bottles with nutrient broth (Septi-Check, Roche Laboratories, Nutley, NJ). At the first hospital, samples of stool were inoculated onto numerous media including Eosin Methylene Blue (EMB) agar, trypticase-soy agar with 5% sheep's blood, Hektoen Enteric agar, and Mackonkey-sorbital agar (all purchased from Adam's Scientific, West Warwick, RI); at BCH stool samples were inoculated onto EMB agar, xylose-lysine-desoxychocolate agar, and Salmonella-Shigella agar (all purchased from Becton Dickinson, Cockeysville, MD).

The case isolates included one isolate of S. flexneri and 3 isolates of S. boydii (Table I). Serotyping of the case isolates was performed at the Massachusetts State Laboratory (MSL), Enteric Division. Antisera was purchased from commercial suppliers (Centers for Disease Control, Atlanta, GA; Difco, Detroit, MI; and Roche Laboratories). Only a single colony from each available specimen was isolated for species determination, antibiotic susceptibility, and serotype analysis by each clinical microbiology laboratory. Control isolates included 4 isolates of S. flexneri and 6 isolates of S. boydii (Table I).

Whole cellular DNA was isolated as previously described (7) and subjected to restriction digestion with either *Xba*I or *Sfi*I (New England Biolabs, Beverly, MA). The resultant restriction fragments were resolved in 1% agarose gels (SeaKem GTG, FMC Bioproducts, Rockland, ME) by pulsed field gel electrophoresis (PFGE) in 0.5X TBE buffer in a CHEF DRII apparatus (BioRad, Richmond, CA) at 200 V, 15°C, and switch times of 1–40 s ramped linearly (7). The gels were stained with ethidium bromide (0.5 μg/ml) and photographed over UV light.

RESULTS

The Shigella isolates from 4/6 of the case patient's positive cultures were available for analysis and included the initial bloodstream isolates of S. flexneri (serotype 6) and S. boydii, the stool isolate of S. boydii obtained upon admission to BCH, and the bloodstream isolate of S. boydii (all S. boydii were serotype 4) obtained on the 29th day of hospitalization (isolates 1–4, respectively). Both stool samples yielding S. flexneri and S. boydii, respectively, were discarded at the time of analysis.

Analysis by PFGE (Fig. 1) showed that the 3 isolates of S. boydii from the case patient (isolates 2–4) were indistinguishable except the bloodstream isolate from the culture on hospital day 29 (isolate 4) yielded 2 additional fragments detected at 10 and 50 kb. The latter isolate was resistant to trimethoprim-sulfamethoxazole, chloramphenicol, and piperacillin. *Sfi*I digests of these isolates revealed an additional fragment at ~70 kb for this last isolate (data not shown). The PFGE pattern of the S. flexneri from the case patient (isolate 1) was markedly different from that of the S. boydii isolates.

Table I. *Isolates included in the present study*

Isolate[a]	Species	Serotype	Source[b]
1	S. flexneri	6	Case patient, bloodstream isolate, day 1[c], MSL
2	S. boydii	4	Case patient, bloodstream isolate, day 2, MSL
3	S. boydii	4	Case patient, fecal isolate, day 15, BCH
4	S. boydii	4	Case patient, bloodstream isolate, day 29, BCH
5	S. boydii	4	Clinical fecal isolate, MSL
6	S. boydii	2	Clinical fecal isolate, MSL
7	S. flexneri	1	Clinical fecal isolate, MSL
8	S. flexneri	2	Clinical fecal isolate, MSL
9	S. boydii	2	Clinical fecal isolate, BCH
10	S. boydii	2	Clinical fecal isolate, BCH
11	S. flexneri	6	Serotype reference strain, CSL
12	S. boydii	4	Serotype reference strain, CSL
13	S. flexneri	6	Type strain (No. 10125) S. flexneri serotype 6, ATCC
14	S. boydii	4	Type strain (No. 9210) S. boydii serotype 6, ATCC

[a] The isolate numbers correspond to those in Fig. 1.
[b] The laboratories providing isolates for analysis are: Boston City Hospital (BCH), Massachusetts State Laboratory (MSL), Connecticut State Laboratory (CSL), and American Type Culture Collection (ATCC).
[c] The days of hospitalization for the index patient are counted from the initial day of admission; the patient was transferred to BCH on hospital day 15.

Comparison of the index and control isolates by PFGE showed that except for 1 isolate of serotype 4 S. boydii and 2 isolates of serotype 2 S. boydii, the control isolates differed from each other and from the index isolates (Fig. 1). A control isolate of serotype 4 S. boydii (isolate 5), indistinguishable from the first 2 index isolates of S. boydii, was cultured from the stool of a child 3 months prior to the index patient's admission. Two isolates of S. boydii serotype 2 (isolates 8 and 9), indistinguishable by PFGE, were cultured from 2 patients treated concurrently on the same ward at BCH.

DISCUSSION

Shigella species are an uncommon cause of gastroenteritis and acute diarrheal syndrome in the United States, and have only rarely been reported to affect HIV-seropositive individuals. In immunocompetent patients, diarrheal disease with Shigella is usually self-limited, with ~4% of episodes complicated by bacteremia (2, 4). Prior to 1963, a total of 101 cases of Shigella bacteremia were recorded (8). Since 1963, approximately 200 additional cases have been reported (3, 4, 9). The single most important factor predisposing to the development of bacteremia is the age of the patient with an ~6 : 1 ratio in the number of pediatric to adult cases (4). Other conditions predisposing to Shigella bacteremia are those associated with impaired immune function such as malnutrition (4, 9) and severe liver or renal disease (9). Bacteremia as a complication of Shigella gastroenteritis in HIV-seropositive individuals has been reported for 14 patients (10, 11) and may be more prevalent among patients with AIDS since in one series, 3 of 8 patients developed bacteremia as a complication of dysentery (5).

This case represents the first report of S. boydii bacteremia in a patient with AIDS. In both HIV-seropositive and -seronegative individuals, S. flexneri and S. dysenteriae are the most prevalent serogroups isolated from blood cultures (40–55% and 25–44% of cases, respec-

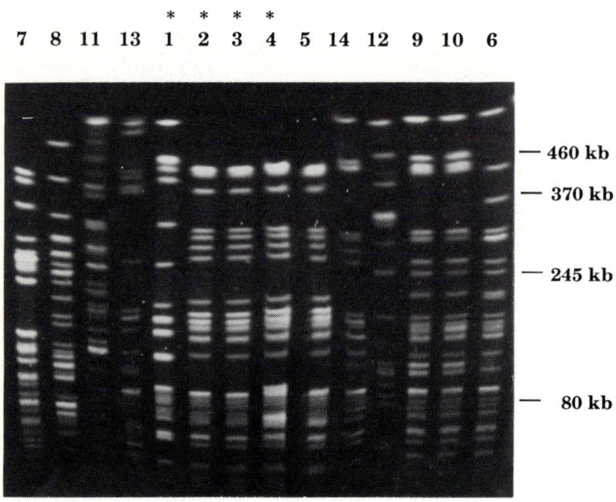

Fig. 1. Pulsed field gel electrophoresis to resolve *Xba*I restriction fragments of 14 strains of Shigella. Isolates 1–4, cultured from the case patient (indicated by the * above the isolates), represent serotype 6 S. flexneri (isolate 1) and serotype 4 S. boydii (isolates 2–4). The control isolates of S. flexneri and S. boydii are as listed in Table I. Isolate 5, cultured from the stool of a child was indistinguishable from the index isolates 2 and 3. Although there was no known epidemiological relationship between these individuals, the case patient had recently emigrated from Haiti and the family of the child (who lived 20 miles south of Boston and had no known travel outside of the Boston metropolitan area) was from the Dominican Republic, both countries on the island of Hispanõla. The 2 isolates of serotype 2 S. boydii that were indistinguishable (isolates 9 and 10) were cultured within a 2 day period from 2 inpatients at Boston City Hospital, suggesting possible nosocomial transmission.

tively) with only rare cases of S. boydii bacteremia (2–4% of cases) (3, 4, 9). Overall, the prevalence of bloodstream isolates parallels the prevalence of gastrointestinal isolates (4).

The patient reported here experienced simultaneous bloodstream infection with S. flexneri and S. boydii. Since only a single colony from each primary culture was submitted for species identification and both stool samples had been discarded at the time of analysis, we were unable to document the presence of multiple species in any of the samples. Further, the use of broth culture techniques for specimens of blood would favour the selection of a single strain. Polymicrobial bacteremia with Shigella has been reported in association with Pseudomonas aeruginosa (4), Salmonella typhimurium (10), and 2 cases involved 2 species of Shigella: S. flexneri and S. sonnei (2). The finding of polymicrobial bacteremia is not surprising since patients with diarrheal disease not infrequently have multiple stool pathogens. For example, of 20 patients with AIDS and diarrheal disease, 3 had 2 or more bacterial faecal pathogens, including 1 patient with S. flexneri and S. typhimurium (1). Also, for 3 of 82 immunocompetent patients with Shigella sepsis, culture of a stool sample yielded Shigella expressing a different serotype from the bloodstream isolate (4). Also, among patients with AIDS, polyclonal bacteremia with Mycobacterium avium complex has been described for ~20% of patients (12). Thus, the prevalence of polymicrobial or polyclonal bacteremia, particularly among HIV-seropositive patients, are likely to be underestimated.

To confirm that our patient had relapsing bloodstream infection with S. boydii, we analyzed the isolates using PFGE. The index isolates were indistinguishable from each other except that 1 isolate differed by 2 additional bands which may reflect the acquisition of 1 or 2 plasmids, consistent with the finding of additional antibiotic resistances in this isolate.

Although recurrence of bacteremia with Salmonella species among HIV-seropositive patients is not uncommon (6), recurrent bacteremia with Shigella has been previously reported for only 1 patient (5), while recurrent gastroenteritis has been reported for 4 patients (5, 13–15).

The optimal treatment regimen for Shigella bacteremia in patients with AIDS is difficult to determine from the case report literature. Our patient was initially treated for 10 days with ceftriaxone. Other agents that have been used include ampicillin, cefoxitin, trimethoprim-sulfamethoxazole, chloramphenicol, and ciprofloxacin (11). Relapsing disease (either bacteremia or gastroenteritis) has been documented for all therapies except chloramphenicol. Since 2 of the 14 cases of Shigella bacteremia were associated with relapsing infection, it may be prudent to treat immunosuppressed patients with prolonged antibacterial regimens similar to cases of Salmonella bacteremia.

In summary, this report documents an HIV-seropositive patient with polymicrobial bacteremia due to S. flexneri and S. boydii and recurrent bacteremia with the same strain of S. boydii. Patients who are HIV-seropositive and develop Shigella infections may require prolonged treatment and/or suppressive therapy, similar to those patients infected with Salmonella. Patients with AIDS who develop bloodstream infections, particularly those secondary to gastroenteritis, may be infected with multiple pathogens. In cases where patients do not respond to standard therapy or those with apparent reinfection with a different stool pathogen, the possibility of polymicrobial disease should be considered.

ACKNOWLEDGMENTS

The authors would like to thank the clinical microbiology laboratories at Boston City Hospital and Goddard Memorial Hospital, the Massachusetts State Laboratory, Enteric Division, and Donald Low of the Connecticut State Laboratory for providing bacterial isolates; Diane Levine for technical assistance; and Maura Fagan, MD, Anita Barry, MD, and Robert D. Arbeit, MD, for helpful discussions.

Financial support: MK is a Fogarty Fellow of the National Institutes of Health; JNM is supported in part by the Medical Research Program, Department of Veterans Affairs, Washington, D.C.

REFERENCES

1. Smith PD, Lane HC, Gill VJ, Manischewitz JF, Quinnan GV, Fauci AS, Masur H. Intestinal infections in patients with the acquired immunodeficiency syndrome (AIDS): etiology and response to therapy. Ann Intern Med 108: 328–333, 1988.
2. Barrett-Connor E, Connor JD. Extraintestinal manifestations of shigellosis. Am J Gastroenterol 53: 234–245, 1970.
3. Martin T, Habbick BF, Nyssen J. Shigellosis with bacteremia: a report of two cases and a review of the literature. Pediatr Infect Dis 2: 21–26, 1983.
4. Struelens MJ, Patte D, Kabir I, Salam A, Nath SK, Butler T. Shigella septicemia: prevalance, presentation, risk factors, and outcome. J Infect Dis 152. 784–790, 1985.
5. Nelson MR, Shanson DC, Hawkins D, Gazzard BG. Shigella in HIV infection. AIDS 5: 1031–1032, 1991.
6. Jacobs JL, Gold JWM, Murray HW, Roberts RB, Armstrong D. Salmonella infections in patients with the acquired immunodeficiency syndrome. Ann Intern Med 102: 186–192, 1985.
7. Maslow JN, Slutsky AM, Arbeit RD. The application of pulsed field gel electrophoresis to molecular epidemiology. In: Persing DH, Smith TF, Tenover FC and White TJ, eds. Diagnostic molecular microbiology: principles and applications. Washington DC: American Society of Microbiology 563–572, 1993.
8. Faucon R, Ducloux M. Septicemies A Shigella. Med Trop 24: 537–545, 1964.
9. Morduchowicz G, Huminer D, Siegman-Igra Y, Drucker M, Block CS, Pitlik SD. Shigella bacteremia in adults: a report of five cases and review of the literature. Arch Intern Med 147: 2034–2037, 1987.

10. Alonso C, Sanchez F, Mirelis B, Josep C. Simultaneous Shigella and Salmonella septicemia in an AIDS patient. Clinical Microbiology Newsletter 14: 134–135, 1992.
11. Hüebner M, Czerwenka W, Gruner E, von Graevenitz A. Shigellemia in AIDS patients: case report and review of the literature. Infection 21: 52–54, 1993.
12. Arbeit RD, Slutsky A, Barber TW, Maslow JN, Niemczyk S, Falkinham JO III, O'Conner GT, von Reyn CF. Genetic diversity among strains of Mycobacterium avium causing monoclonal and polyclonal bacteremia in patients with AIDS. J Infect Dis 167: 1384–1390, 1993.
13. Blaser MJ, Hale TL, Formal SB. Recurrent shigellosis complicating human immunodeficiency virus infection: failure of pre-existing antibodies to confer protection. Am J Med 86: 105–107, 1989.
14. Simor AE, Poon R, Borczyk A. Chronic Shigella flexneri infection preceding development of acquired immunodeficiency syndrome. J Clin Microbiol 27: 353–355, 1989.
15. Bell ET, Rotterdam HZ, Tapper ML. Simultaneous shigellosis and cytomegalovirus colitis in patients with acquired immunodeficiency syndrome. In: International Conference on the Acquired Immunodeficiency Syndrome. Atlanta, 1985.

Submitted February 17, 1994; accepted April 17, 1994

Scand J Infect Dis 26: 417–425, 1994

An outbreak of Legionnaires' Disease in a Swedish Hospital

JOHAN DARELID[1], LARS BENGTSSON[3], BENGT GÄSTRIN[4], HANS HALLANDER[4], STURE LÖFGREN[2], BO-ERIC MALMVALL[1], ANN-MARGRETH OLINDER-NIELSEN[1] and ANN-CHRISTIN THELIN[3]

From the Departments of [1]Infectious Diseases and [2]Clinical Bacteriology, Ryhov Hospital, Jönköping, [3]Värnamo Hospital, and the [4]National Bacteriological Laboratory, Stockholm, Sweden

We report a nosocomial outbreak of Legionella pneumophila serogroup (sg) 1 infection at the general hospital, Värnamo, Sweden. From December 1990 to February 1991, 28 patients and 3 staff fell ill with pneumonia and 3 died. L. pneumophila sg 1 together with several other Legionellae were isolated from the hot water supply to 17 of 20 hospital wards, probably being spread by aerosolization via shower nozzles. Raising the hospital's hot water temperature from 45°C to 65°C, together with heat disinfection of the shower equipment, arrested the outbreak within a week. Keeping the hot water temperature ≥ 60°C without chlorination eliminated L. pneumophila from > 75% of the wards. During a period of 2 years after the outbreak we have diagnosed only 1 case of nosocomial legionellosis at the hospital despite an active surveillance program.

J. Darelid, MD, Department of Infectious Diseases, Länssjukhuset Ryhov, 551 85 Jönköping, Sweden

INTRODUCTION

Nosocomial spread of Legionella pneumophila resulting in Legionnaires' Disease (LD) is reported worldwide (1). Nosocomial LD can appear as sporadic cases (2, 3) or as outbreaks (4, 5). Hospital water systems or air-conditioning equipment invariably seem to be involved in the spread of the L. pneumophila bacteria. Transmission of L. pneumophila to patients is believed to involve inhalation of organisms from contaminated water (1, 6, 7).

Nosocomial LD has not attracted much attention in the Scandinavian countries (8). The only reported outbreak took place at Huddinge Hospital in Stockholm, with a cluster of 5 cases of LD in renal transplant patients (9). The present paper describes a nosocomial outbreak of LD at Värnamo General District Hospital which was opened in 1974 and has 450 beds on 20 wards encompassing surgery, internal medicine, geriatrics and psychiatry, housed in 3 different but interconnected buildings. An association with the hospital hot water system was investigated. As several pneumonic cases of other origin were admitted to the hospital during the same period, diagnostic laboratory criteria were studied in greater detail.

MATERIAL AND METHODS

I. The outbreak

On January 10, 1991, a 54-year-old man with severe pneumonia was referred from Värnamo Hospital to the Department of Infectious Diseases at the County Central Hospital in Jönköping for further treatment. On clinical grounds, LD was suspected. The same day it was reported that a patient with severe pneumonia from Värnamo had died at another hospital.

On January 12, a 67-year old woman from an orthopedic ward, with a pneumonia not responding to cephalosporin treatment and 5 days later a patient with betalactam-resistant pneumonia, treated on a ward for internal medicine at Värnamo Hospital were both referred to the Infectious Diseases Department at Jönköping.

On January 18, the Värnamo District Infections Control Committee was informed. So far, 4 cases of pneumonia were reported from Värnamo town, 2 of which appeared to be nosocomially acquired. All clinicians in the district were alerted and asked to send sputum, urine and blood samples for legionella diagnosis in all cases of pneumonia.

Between January 24 and 28 another 3 patients, all linked with Värnamo Hospital, were suspected of suffering from LD. An epidemiological survey was performed and the hospital's water system was investigated.

On January 30, the first microbiologically verified legionella infection was documented. Two days later the survey showed that all suspected cases of LD during the previous month had been treated at the hospital (either ambulatory or as in-patients).

On February 4, it seemed probable that patients treated in all hospital buildings were at risk. The Hospital Board, all staff and the public were informed and water cultures were immediately obtained, before raising the hospital hot water temperature from 45 to 65°C.

Altogether 31 persons with LD were nosocomially infected at Värnamo Hospital during the period December 1990 to February 1991, of whom 3 were staff. LD cases seemed to appear anywhere in the hospital: 8 were found on surgical wards, 16 on wards for internal medicine or geriatrics, 3 on psychiatric wards, 3 at the physiotherapy unit and 1 case in the maintenance department. The longitudinal time sequence of the epidemic is presented in Fig. 1. During an 8-week period there were about 4 new cases every week. In 20 patients LD was suspected during the stay in hospital but in 11 patients LD was not detected until a retrospective investigation of all cases of hospital-acquired pneumonia could be made.

The number of patients with a diagnosis of pneumonia treated at Värnamo Hospital, month-by-month during the 2 years prior to and the half year following the outbreak, is illustrated in Fig. 2. There is a conspicuous peak in January 1991.

II. Case definition

Case definition for nosocomial pneumonia was fever >38.0°C and pulmonary infiltrates visualized by chest X-ray. In the absence of roentgenography, pneumonia was diagnosed when body temperature

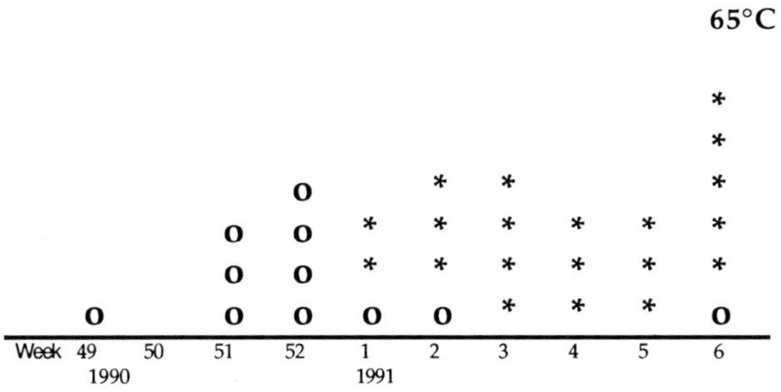

Fig. 1. Week of onset for 31 cases of Legionnaires' Disease in 1990–91 at Värnamo Hospital. *, Case diagnosed during hospital stay. ○, Case detected by the retrospective investigation. 65°C, Hospital hot water temperature raised to 65°C.

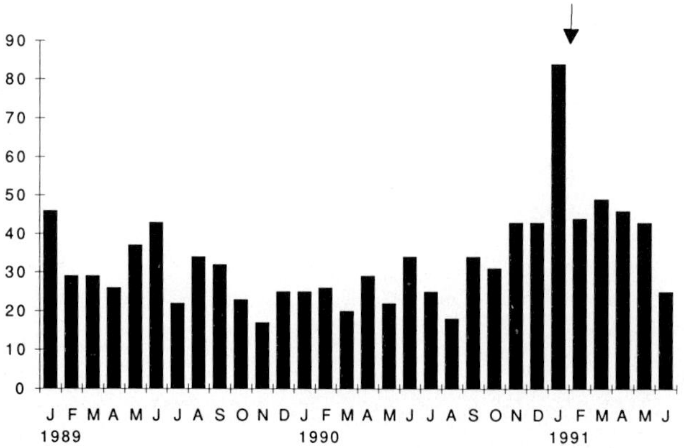

Fig. 2. Number of patients with a diagnosis of pneumonia at Värnamo Hospital, 1989–91. Arrow indicates when the hospital hot water temperature was raised to 65°C.

exceeded 38.5°C, together with cough and signs on auscultation of an inflammatory or consolidatory process in the lung. The pneumonia was considered nosocomial if it developed >2 days after admission to hospital, or within 14 days of discharge.

Case definition for legionella pneumonia was a positive culture, or a positive urinary antigen test, or positive serology (4-fold titre change or single titre ≥ 64 to L. pneumophila sg 1). A single titre of ≥ 64 was accepted as a diagnostic marker, as only 1/96 sera from patients seeking acute medical care at Värnamo Hospital for reasons other than pulmonary disease had a titre of ≥ 64. Among sera from staff at Värnamo Hospital, 5/258 (2%) showed the same level (unpublished data).

III. Bacteriological methods

Water was sampled randomly from tap sites in the shower rooms on the wards. Specimens were concentrated on 0.45 μm black filters (047 ANC Sartorius) and acid treated before culture at the Microbiological Laboratory in Jönköping on buffered charcoal yeast extract agar (BCYEα, Oxoid Ltd, England) (10), and incubated (35°C, 5% CO_2) for 48 h.

Sputum was acid treated and cultured at the NBL on $BCYE_{\alpha}$ (Difco, Detroit, MI, USA) with and without polymyxin B (Pfizer) 80,000 IU/l and cefamandole (Lilly) 4 mg/l. All plates were incubated in a plastic bag at 37°C for 7 days. Isolated strains were typed by agglutination with specific polyclonal rabbit antisera produced at the National Bacteriological Laboratory (NBL), Stockholm, Sweden. Epidemiological typing was performed at the central Public Health Laboratory, London, UK, using an International Monoclonal Antibody Subgrouping Panel as well as Restriction Fragment Length Polymorphism (RFLP).

Biopsies were examined at the NBL by indirect immunofluorescence (Genetic Systems Inc, Seattle, WA, USA) to detect L. pneumophila antigen in tissues.

Antigen of L. pneumophila sg 1 in urine was detected by a radio-immunoassay (Equate, Binax Inc, Portland, ME, USA).

Antibody titres were determined at the NBL using indirect immunofluorescence with heat-killed legionella bacteria in normal chicken yolk sac as antigen. For screening, the antigens were distributed in three groups: A) L. pneumophila sg 1, B) L. pneumophila sg 2–8, and C) L. micdadei, L. bozemanii and L. longbeachae, and tested with sera in the dilutions 1/32–1/128. In most cases, > 2 sera were available as evidence of seroconversion. In the absence of a 4-fold titre change, the second serum was chosen to represent the antibody level.

IV. The patients

All the patients had been exposed to the hospital's hot water between 2 and 11 days prior to the onset of the disease. Seven persons had undergone a surgical procedure just before contracting their nosocomial infection. The age of the afflicted individuals ranged between 32 and 87 years (mean age 66); 61% were males

The underlying diseases are shown in Table I. The 3 staff members and 5 of the patients, 2 of whom had visited the hospital for a minor diagnostic procedure, had been healthy previously. One of these 5, a 50-year-old woman, died. The 3 afflicted subjects among the staff had all been using the hospital

Table I. *Major underlying conditions in 31 patients from a nosocomial outbreak of Legionnaires' Disease*

Condition	Patients *n*
Previous healthy	8
Cardiovascular disease	8
Alcoholic abuse	3
Diabetes mellitus	3
Paraparesis	1
Chronic pulmonary disease	2
Steroid therapy	4
Renal insufficiency	2
Total	31

showers within 10 days of onset of their pneumonia. The proportion of smokers was 7/24 where this was reported (29%). 11 persons (35%) lived inside the municipal water supply area of Värnamo town.

The pneumonia was diagnosed by X-ray in 30 patients and was bilateral in 7. Severe hypoxia requiring respiratory aid developed in 4 patients. Pneumonia without respiratory symptoms was diagnosed in 1 patient. Central nervous system manifestations were seen in 11 patients (35%). Hallucination and disorientation in space and time were common symptoms. Vomiting, diarrhea or abdominal pains occurred in 5 (14%), and moderate muscular symptoms in 4 (11%) patients.

Microbiological findings

The distribution of the different positive findings among the 31 individuals comprising the outbreak is described in detail in Table II.

Sputa were cultured from 10 patients and L. pneumophila sg 1 was recovered in 1 case. The subgroup of the strain was characterized as 'benidorm like' with RFLP pattern 84. Bacterial antigen was detected in lung tissue from 1 of the patients who died.

The urinary antigen test showed a positive result in 11/18 tested patients.

By serological testing we found 16 with a significant titre increase, 4 significant titre reductions and 9 single positive titres ≥ 64.

One patient had a concomitant 4-fold titre increase against group B (L. pneumophila sg 2–8). No significant titre changes against group C antigens were detected.

Serum samples from 26 patients were analysed for antibodies to Mycoplasma pneumoniae, Chlamydia psittaci, C. pneumoniae and Influenza A & B, using routine tests (NBL), but without any significant findings.

Treatment

23 patients were treated with erythromycin orally or intravenously for >7 days and in the 5 most severely ill, rifampicin was added. Two patients received doxycycline.

Three patients died from their nosocomial LD; 2 of them were given erythromycin in an inadequate dose or very late in the disease, and 1 patient who was not diagnosed until after death had received betalactam antibiotics only.

L. pneumophila was suspected as the causative agent by the treating physician in 16/31 (52%) patients.

V. Efforts to stop the outbreak

Before the first case was microbiologically verified, all hospital physicians were informed and instructed to obtain blood, urine and sputum samples from all patients with pneumonia treated in the Värnamo district. All cases of pneumonia were also reported to the hospital infection control nurse.

When the epidemiological data indicated that LD cases were involved in a nosocomial outbreak, efforts were made to trace the source of infection. As there were no cooling towers or air humidifiers functioning at the hospital area during the time of the outbreak and as cases were diagnosed on different

Table II. *Diagnostic findings in 31 patients from an outbreak of nosocomial pneumonia due to L. pneumophila serogroup 1*

L. pneumophila serogroup 1 diagnosis	Patients *n*
Growth in sputum + Antigen/urine + 4-fold titre change	1
Antigen/lung tissue[a] + Antigen/urine	1
Antigen/lung + 4-fold titre change	7
Antigen/urine + Single titre 256	1
Antigen/urine	1
4-fold titre change	12
Single titre 256	2
Single titre 128	4
Single titre 64	2
Total	31

[a] Lung tissue from postmortem examination.

wards throughout the entire hospital, the hot water system was suspected. The Hospital Board, hospital staff and the public were informed. Water was then sampled from the various wards and the hospital's hot water temperature was increased from 45° to 65°C (113° to 149°F) to achieve a tap temperature > 60°C. All shower hoses were heat-disinfected and taps and showers in the hospital were flushed with hot water for 5 min. Within 3 months all the shower hoses and shower nozzles were replaced. The flushing was repeated weekly until November 1992.

VI. Hospital water supply

Fig. 3 gives a schematic overview of the hospital's hot water system. Municipal water from deep drilled wells is sand-filtered (but not chlorinated) before delivery to the hospital. From a main tap, water passes through a deionizing filter and is thereafter heated in a heat exchanger to 90–110°C by the municipal heating system. Heated water is stored in a 15,000 litre horizontally placed cyclindrical accumulator at temperatures ranging from 72° to 82°C. On delivery to the hospital buildings, stored water was mixed with municipal cold water via a valve to reach 45 ± 3°C. Thus the water temperature in the hotwater pipes and taps on the wards was measured at 43°C when the outbreak occurred. No blind loops have been found in the hospital's water system.

During September and October 1990 a leak was noted in the heat exchanger, allowing water from the municipal hot water system to pass to the hospital hot water system. A new heat exchanger was installed at the end of November 1990.

VII. Legionella in water

Cultures sampled before the hot water temperature had been increased grew L. pneumophila sg 1 from 13/20 wards in the hospital. The number varied between 1 and 1500 colony forming units (cfu)/100 ml water (mean value 565 cfu).

Repeated cultures from the hot water system have continued to be positive for L. pneumophila but the amount of bacteria and the number of wards with growth of L. pneumophila sg 1 have gradually decreased (Table III). Five representative strains of L. pneumophila sg 1 were subtyped and found indistinguishable from the patient isolate.

VIII. Monitoring of nosocomial pneumonia after the outbreak

After the index cases had been identified in January 1991, all cases of pneumonia treated at the hospital from February to April 1991 were analysed in the search for evidence of LD. During the rest of 1991, only cases of pneumonia where legionella was suspected were analysed. In January 1992 a prospective continuing serological survey was initiated to assess the occurrence of nosocomial LD.

The last cases of LD linked to Värnamo Hospital fell ill within 1 week of increasing the water temperature.

After the outbreak, physicians in Värnamo have become very aware of the possibility of new cases of nosocomial LD. In 1991, serum samples were analysed for legionella antibodies in more than 500 cases as were sputum and urine samples from 120 patients.

As a result of the survey initiated in January 1992, we have so far (Jan. 1993) identified 54 nosocomial cases of pneumonias at the hospital. All have been clinically and serologically evaluated for LD and 1 patient, with mild pneumonia on a surgical ward in Oct. 1992, showed a fourfold rise in titre to L. pneumophila sg 1 (unpublished data).

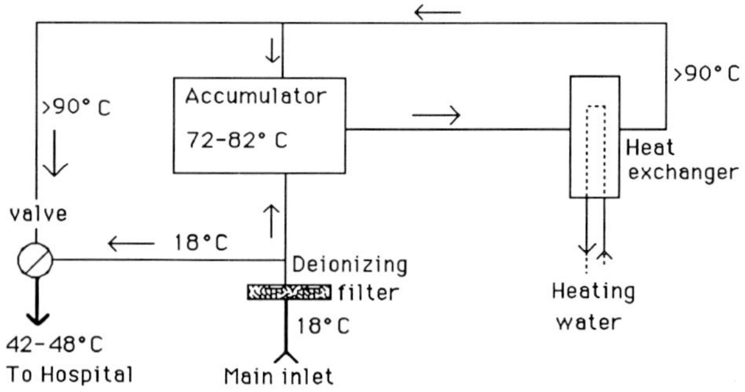

Fig. 3. Diagram of the water heating system at Värnamo Hospital during the outbreak of Legionnaires' Disease in 1990–91.

Table III. *Growth of legionellae in water samples from 20 wards at Värnamo Hospital, 1991–93*

	1991 Feb 4	1991 Feb 27	1991 Aug 28	1992 Apr 7	1993 May 3
Hospital hot water temperature	45°C	65°C	65°C	65°C	65°C
No. of wards with growth of any Legionella species[a]	13	15	16	10	12
Cfu[b]/100 ml					
Range	5–1,500	4–2,000	2–115	1–250	3–140
Mean	565	256	28	46	76
No. of wards with growth of L. pneumophila sg 1	13	15	2	1	3

[a] L. pneumophila sg 1–8, L. micdadei, bozemanii and L. longbeachae.
[b] Colony forming units, cfu.

DISCUSSION

The hospital water system

The incidence of nosocomial LD varies geographically (1, 7). This can give a false impression of security as absence of reports may only reflect a lack of diagnostic efforts. This unusually large outbreak in a small hospital in a Nordic country indicates that nosocomial LD is a worldwide threat.

The hospital's hot water system is the usual source of infection in nosocomial outbreaks (11). We found that several serogroups of L. pneumophila grew in large numbers in all water samples from the showernozzles. However, L pneumophila sg 1 was the only one verified as the agent in the aetiology of the pneumonia. Heavily contaminated water, to which all patients and staff were exposed, seems to be the probable vehicle, as cases were detected all over the hospital and among many previously healthy individuals. Therefore we believe that transmission was due to aerosols from the showers containing legionella.

Contamination of hospital water distribution systems ($>30\%$ of samples colonized), has been correlated to low water temperature, old water heaters and large-volume hot water tanks (12). Temperature is probably the most critical parameter (11), although occurrence of protozoa also seems crucial for legionella multiplication (11, 13). Värnamo Hospital has a non-chlorinated water system and the hot water tank is comparatively large (15,000 l). During the outbreak the temperature of the water used on the hospital wards was ≤ 43°C, which is a very suitable environment for multiplication of legionella bacteria. Slime in abundance was found in the shower equipment, which was partly of plastic material. It is therefore not surprising that legionellae could be cultured from water specimens on the majority of the wards.

Patient characteristics

In this nosocomial outbreak of LD the lack of severe underlying diseases in most of the patients is striking and the number of cigarette smokers and patients with a chronic lung disease was small, compared with other outbreaks (4, 14). Conceivably, conditions for legionella growth in this water system may have created a high bacterial virulence or the possibility of a large infecting dose from the contaminated aerosol.

LD was suspected before initiating therapy in 52% of the patients, demonstrating the difficulty of distinguishing LD from other pneumonias on clinical grounds (14, 15). In the Värnamo outbreak the crucial role of adequate antibiotic treatment is also evident. All 25 patients who had been treated with erythromycin or doxycyline for >7 days survived, compared with 3 deaths among the 6 inadequately treated patients.

Microbiological findings

The recovery of legionella from sputum in this outbreak was poor (one positive sample of 10 cultured), even though recommended methods were used.

In the majority of cases the bacteriological diagnosis was based on positive serology. A reproducible fourfold increase or decrease in titre between acute and convalescent sera was found in 20 cases. Urinary antigen was positive in 8 of these, indicating a much higher sensitivity than culture. The reactivity pattern of the monoclonal antibody subgrouping panel most closely resembled that for isolates of the 'benidorm' subgroup although it did not exactly match this pattern. Similarly the RFLP profile was new.

Preventive measures

Hospital outbreaks of LD emanating from the hot water supply can be controlled by thermal eradication, chlorination and by good plumbing practices, eliminating dead spaces in the system (7, 11). Control measures such as ultraviolet light, ozonization, metal ionization and water filtration require more intricate technical equipment (16) and are preferably chosen when complete eradication over a considerable period of time is desired. These systems are often included in preventive strategies confined to a section of a hospital where high-risk patients are treated (9, 16).

Continuous long-term hyperchlorination can control epidemic disease, but may exacerbate corrosion in the system (16, 17). High chlorine-residue levels are needed (18) and yet intracellular legionellae can survive in such an environment (19). Environmental hazards from the carcinogenic by-products of chlorination are another drawback of this method (17). Supplemental chlorination confined to the hot water system and the use of silicates in the plumbing system are reported to reduce these risks (20). However, a protective efficacy of 88% for nosocomial LD has been attained without chlorination (21).

We were facing a situation where the low water temperature seemed an obvious risk factor in a large-water distribution system. Keeping the hot water temperature at 45°C was in accordance with the recommendations of the housing authorities in Sweden. Our main goal was to arrest the outbreak, not necessarily to eradicate all bacteria. Raising the hot water temperature to 65°C therefore seemed to be the safest and least complicated method to start with (22). When, as a result of this, an immediate decline in the number of nosocomial pneumonias could be seen, we chose to emphasize surveillance rather than additional eradication. The preliminary results of the ongoing survey indicate that chlorination may not be necessary when trying to avoid new clusters of nosocomial LD in this type of hospital without specialised wards for nephrology, oncology, bone marrow and organ transplantation.

Regular flushing of showers has proved effective in reducing legionellae below detectable levels in shower nozzles (23). Our suspicion was early focused on contaminated aerosols which motivated the flushing of all showers at the hospital and the replacement of the shower equipment. We have thus far no reported mishaps of scalding among patients or staff despite a hot water temperature of 60–62°C measured at the most distal sites from the hospital plumbing system.

Why did the outbreak start?

The incidence of pneumonias treated at the hospital during 1988–91 (Fig. 3) contradicts any major outbreak (though a system for clinical and serological surveillance was lacking). The conditions favouring legionella colonization of the hospital's water system have been similar for several years and sporadic cases of nosocomial LD have probably been overlooked.

The leakage of hot water from the municipal heating system through the heat exchanger is an interesting observation. This could have favoured a growth of virulent strains of L. pneumophila by adding nutritional factors to the hot water system (24). Immediate raising of the hot water temperature seemed to arrest the epidemic, or at least promote its decline. Furthermore, after 6 months the occurrence of L. pneumophila sg 1, the strain causing the documented infections in this outbreak, had demonstrably diminished (Table III). This suggests that the temperature level rather than the lack of chlorination was the major risk factor in this hospital water system.

CONCLUSIONS

To reduce the risk of nosocomial LD in this type of hospital, the hot water temperature should be kept at $\geq 65°C$.

Legionella should be included in the initial diagnostic and therapeutic approach to all cases of hospital-acquired pneumonia.

A geographic selection of the reference population may increase the sensitivity of the serological diagnosis of L. pneumophila sg 1 infections.

If nosocomial legionellosis is discovered, preventive measures against bacterial spread from the hospital water system should be considered and all individuals at risk should be identified.

When a major outbreak is suspected, immediate information of the hospital administration, the staff and the public is vital as is an epidemiological mapping of all suspected cases. In this situation, the treatment of all nosocomial pneumonias should include an antibiotic effective against L. pneumophila, as nosocomial LD is a potential threat not only to patients suffering from immunosuppression.

ACKNOWLEDGEMENTS

We are most grateful to Professor Richard Birtles at Central Public Health Laboratory, London, England, who kindly performed the epidemiological typing of the legionella strains.

REFERENCES

1. Edelstein PH. Nosocomial Legionnaires' disease: a global perspective. J Hosp Infect (Suppl A) 11: 182–188, 1988.
2. Marrie TJ, MacDonald S, Clarke K, Haldane D. Nosocomial legionnaires' disease: Lessons from a four-year prospective study. Am J Infect Control 19: 79–85, 1991.
3. Meenhorst PL, Reingold AL, Groothuis DG, Gorman GW, Wilkinson HW, McKinney RM, Feeley JC, Brenner DJ, van Furth R. Water-related nosocomial pneumonia caused by Legionella pneumophila serogroups 1 and 10. J Infect Dis 152: 356–364, 1985.
4. O'Mahony MC, Stanwell-Smith RE, Tillett HE, Harper D, Hutchison JGP, Farrell ID, Hutchinson DN, Lee JV, Dennis PJ, Duggal HV, Scully JA, Denne C. The Stafford outbreak of Legionnaires' disease. Epidemiol Infect 104: 361–380, 1990.
5. Kirby BD, Snyder KM, Meyer RD, Finegold SM. Legionnaires' disease: Report of sixty-five nosocomially acquired cases and review of the literature. Medicine 59: 188–205, 1980.
6. Muder RR, Yu VL, Woo AH. Mode of transmission of Legionella pneumophila. Arch Intern Med 146: 1607–1612, 1986.
7. Hart CA, Makin T. Legionella in hospitals: a review. J Hosp Infect (Supply A) 18: 481–489, 1991.
8. Bernander S, Kallings I, Nordström K. Legionellainfektioner diagnostiserade i sluten vård i Västmanland. Läkartidningen 87: 4429–4431, 1990 [In Swedish].
9. Wilczek H, Kallings I, Nyström B, Hoffner S. Nosocomial Legionnaires' disease following renal transplantation. Transplantation 43: 847–851, 1987.
10. Edelstein PH. Comparative study of selective media for isolation of Legionella pneumophila from potable water. J Clin Microbiol 16: 697–699, 1982.

11. Epidemiology, prevention and control of legionellosis: Memorandum from a WHO meeting. Bull W H Organ 68: 155–164, 1990.
12. Alary M, Joly JR. Factors contributing to the contamination of hospital water distribution systems by Legionella. J Infect Dis 165: 565–569, 1992.
13. Fields BS, Sander GN, Barbaree JM, Morrill WE, Wadowsky RM, White EH, Feeley JC. Intracellular multiplication of Legionellae pneumophila from amoebae isolated from hospital hot water tanks. Current Microbiol 18: 131–137, 1989.
14. Roig J, Aguilar X, Ruiz J, Domingo C, Mesalles E, Manterola J, Morera J. Comparative study of Legionnella pneumophila and other nosocomial-acquired pneumonias. Chest 99: 344–350, 1991.
15. Yu VL, Kroboth FJ, Shonnard J, Brown A, McDearman S, Magnussen M. Legionnaires' disease: New clinical perspective from a prospective pneumonia study. Am J Med 73: 357–361, 1982.
16. Muraca PW, Yu VL, Goetz A. Disinfection of water distribution systems for Legionella: A review of application procedures and methodologies. Infect Control Hosp Epidemiol 11: 79–88, 1990.
17. Helms CM, Massanari RM, Wenzel RP, Pfaller MA, Moyer NP, Hall N. Legionnaires' disease associated with a hospital water system. JAMA 259: 2423–2427, 1988.
18. Pankhurst CL, Philpott-Howard JN, Hewitt JH, Casewell MW. The efficacy of chlorination and filtration in the control and eradication of Legionella from dental chair water systems. J Hosp Infect 16: 9–18, 1990.
19. Kilvington S, Price J. Survival of Legionella pneumophila within cysts of Acanthamoeba polyphaga following chlorine exposure. J Appl Bacteriol 68: 519–525, 1990.
20. Snyder MB, Siwicki M, Wireman J, Pohlod D, Grimes M, Bowman-Riney S, Saravolatz LD. Reduction in Legionella pneumophila through heat flushing followed by continuous supplemental chlorination of hospital hot water. J Infect Dis 162: 127–132, 1990.
21. Struelens MJ, Maes N, Rost F, Deplano A, Jacobs F, Liesnard C, Bornstein N, Grimont F, Lauwers S, McIntyre MP, Serruys E. Genotypic and phenotypic methods for the investigation of nosocomial Legionella pneumophila outbreak and efficacy of control measures. J Infect Dis 66: 22–30, 1992.
22. Schulze-Röbbecke R, Jung KD, Pullman H, Hundgeburth J. Sanierung eines mit Legionella pneumophila kontaminierten Krankenhaus-Warm-wassersystems. Zbl Hyg 190: 84–100, 1990.
23. Makin T, Hart CA. The efficacy of control measures for eradicating legionella in showers. J Hosp Infect 16: 1–7, 1990.
24. Spriggs DR. Legionella, Microbial ecology, and inconspicuous consumption. J Infect Dis 155: 1086–1087, 1987.

Submitted October 13, 1993; accepted April 12, 1994

Vilken antibiotikabehandling väljer Du vid bukinfektioner?

Kombinationsbehandling

Monoterapi

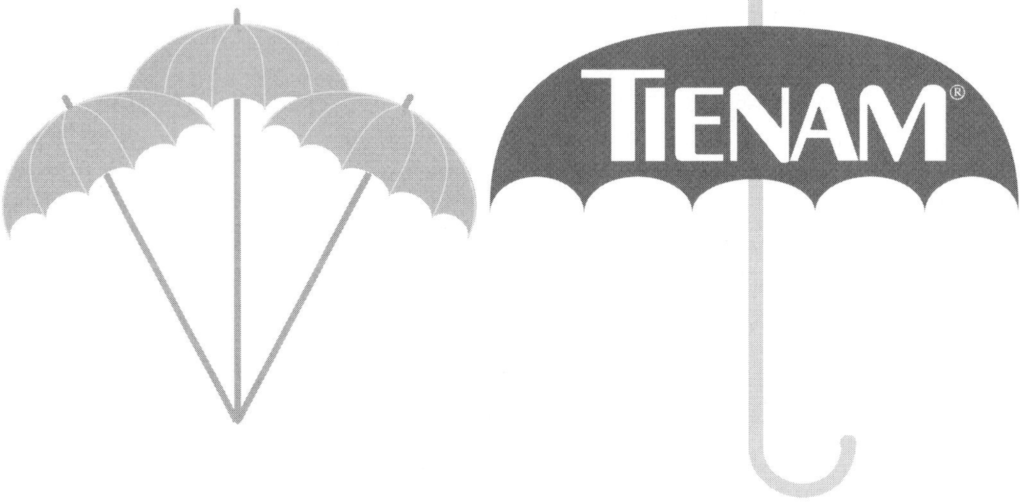

- TIENAM®* –initialterapi vid bukinfektioner
- TIENAM®* kan förkorta vårdtiden jämfört med kombinationsbehandling [1,2,3].

Ref

1 Guerra J G et al. Imipenem/cilastatin VS, gentamicin/clindamycin for the treatment of moderate to severe infections in hospitalized patients. Rev Infect Dis 1985; 7:463–470

2 Heseltine PNR et al. Imipenem therapy for perforated gangrenous appendicitis. Surg Gynecol Obstet 1986; 162: 43–48

3 Gonzenbach H R, Simmen HP, Amgwerd R. Imipenem (N–F–Thienamycin) versus netilmicin plus clindamycin:A controlled and randomized comparison in intra abdominal infections. Ann Surg 1987; 205(3): 271–275

Scand J Infect Dis 26: 427–434, 1994

Seroconversion for Lyme borreliosis Among Dutch Military

KOEN VOS[1,2], ALJE P. VAN DAM[1], HERMAN KUIPER[1], HANS BRUINS[2], LODEWIJK SPANJAARD[1] and JACOB DANKERT[1]

From the Departments of [1]Medical Microbiology, University of Amsterdam, Amsterdam and [2]Military Health Service, Utrecht, The Netherlands

Few prospective studies for Lyme borreliosis (LB) have been conducted among subjects at risk to acquire this disease during their work when wearing well-defined protective clothing against tick-bites. We prospectively compared the rate of seroconversion and the occurrence of clinical manifestations of LB among 2 groups of Dutch military. The at risk-group worked predominantly outdoors, and the control-group conducted predominantly indoor activities. During outdoor work, the at risk-group wore long sleeves, long trousers, closed around the ankles and high boots. Initial serum samples from 2158 military were collected immediately after entering the service. From 932 military (at risk-group: 469, control-group: 463) a second sample was drawn 9 to 12 months later. Sera were tested for IgG and IgM antibodies by ELISA. Four persons (0.9%) in the at risk-group and 10 persons (2.2%) in the control-group seroconverted for IgG and/or IgM antibodies against B. burgdorferi. This difference was not statistically significant. Only 1 person who had seroconverted had noticed an erythema migrans. In conclusion, military performing outdoor activities have a low risk for infection with B. burgdorferi, most likely because they wear protective clothing. Among seroconverted persons clinical manifestations of Lyme borreliosis occurred rarely.

A. P. van Dam, MD, Department of Medical Microbiology, University of Amsterdam, Meibergdreef 15, 1105 AZ Amsterdam, The Netherlands

INTRODUCTION

Lyme borreliosis is a tick-borne infection caused by the spirochete Borrelia burgdorferi. In Europe the disease is transmitted through the tick Ixodes ricinus. In the Netherlands the percentage of I. ricinus infested with B. burgdorferi varies from 1 to 20% (1). In human populations living in areas endemic for Lyme borreliosis and among persons involved in outdoor-work, the prevalence of clinical Lyme borreliosis, as well as the prevalence of antibodies to B. burgdorferi is higher compared to control groups (2–5). Prospective studies among Swiss orienteers and among Dutch forestry workers showed an increased incidence of positive Lyme serology (6, 7).

Protective clothing is an effective preventive measure against tick bites (8, 9). For military personnel, clothing instructions are usually strict and include the use of long sleeves, long pants and high boots. This uniform contrasts to the clothes worn by most people involved in leisure activities. Bowen et al. (10) showed that also among persons who worked at a military facility, outdoor work was associated with an increased risk for clinical Lyme borreliosis. However, in this retrospective study no details were given on clothing instructions for persons working outdoors in this military facility.

To evaluate whether military personnel is at risk for acquiring Lyme borreliosis despite their protective clothing, we prospectively assessed the incidence of seroconversion and clinical Lyme borreliosis among a cohort of recruits entering the military service in the Netherlands. A group of persons who had mainly outdoor activities and who wore protective clothes during this work was compared with a group with mainly indoor tasks.

MATERIALS AND METHODS

Study groups

In the Netherlands every 2 months about 6,500 young men join the military for about 14 months (situation in 1991). All 1,639 persons who started their military service in January and March 1991 and who would train extensively outdoors during their service as infanterists or commandos were asked to participate voluntarily in the seroepidemiological study. Of this group, 905 persons (55%) were willing to participate in the study (at risk-group). As a control-group 2,349 persons who started their military service at the same moment and who would be mainly functioning indoors were asked to join the study. This group consisted of office-workers, technicians and cooks. Of this group, 1,253 persons (53%) were willing to participate voluntarily in the study.

In both groups the age ranged from 18 to 28 years (median age: 20.6). All persons were male. Persons of both groups were stationed all over the country. Following informed consent all the participants received information about Lyme borreliosis and a blood sample was drawn.

In November or December 1991, which was 9 to 12 months after the first blood had been drawn and after the end of the tick bite season, participants were asked by their superiors to give a second blood sample. At that time 260 subjects already had left the service. Of the remaining 1,898 military, 932 permitted us to collect a second blood sample. Of them, 469 persons belonged to the at risk-group and 463 to the control-group. Blood samples were centrifuged and serum samples were stored at −20°C prior to the assay for antibodies.

At the time the second blood sample was drawn the participants were asked to complete a questionnaire. The questions were whether participants had been bitten by ticks in 1991, and if so, at which geographical location; whether during this year they had noticed a red circular rash which had slowly increased in diameter and which had possibly disappeared afterwards (suggesting erythema migrans); whether they had had joint swellings, and whether they had been treated for Lyme disease during 1991.

The military who showed seroconversion for Lyme borreliosis were interviewed 2 to 3 months after the second blood sample was collected. These persons were also asked to undergo physical examination.

In addition all military doctors were requested to report all cases of Lyme borreliosis to the Military Health Service.

Serology

The sera were tested for IgG and IgM antibodies against B. burgdorferi with an enzyme linked immunosorbent assay (ELISA) as previously described (11). Shortly, antigen was purified from B. burgdorferi strain PKo, a German skin isolate (provided by courtesy of V. Preac-Mursic, Max von Pettenkofer-institut, Munich), as described by Hansen et al. (12) with some modifications as reported previously (11). The resulting protein preparation consisted of flagellin and the 23kD OspC. Sera were tested at a 1/1,000 dilution in duplicate. A titration curve of 5 dilutions of a positive serum, originating from a patient with acrodermatitis chronica atrophicans, 2 sera reacting borderline positive, originating from asymptomatic forestry workers, a negative control serum and a buffer control were included on every plate. For every ELISA plate a standard curve was constructed correlating the measured ODs of these 9 samples with average ODs for these samples over all plates by linear regression analysis. Corrected ODs for tested serum samples were obtained using this standard curve. Extinctions exceeding the average OD plus 3 standard deviations (SD) of all 2,158 initially drawn serum samples were defined as positive. Extinctions between 2 and 3 SDs above the average extinction were considered borderline, whereas extinctions below the average OD plus 2 SDs were regarded negative. If the second serum sample reacted borderline or positive, paired sera were retested on the same plate. Seroconversion was defined as a shift from both negative IgG- and IgM-ELISA in the first serum sample to a positive IgG- or IgM-ELISA in the serum sample collected 9–12 months later.

To determine the sensitivity of the ELISA in early Lyme borreliosis we tested serum samples from 48 patients with erythema migrans. 28 persons of this group (58%) reacted positively for IgG and/or IgM antibodies against B. burgdorferi (11), yielding a sensitivity of 58%. This sensitivity is similar to the result published by Hansen et al. (13).

To obtain additional evidence for the specificity of seroconversion shown by ELISA, paired sera of seroconverters were tested by Western blotting. Blotting was performed as described earlier (7). As conjugates we used anti-human IgG alkaline phosphatase (Promega, Madison, WI, USA, 1:7,500 in phosphate-buffered saline containing 0.1% Tween-20 (PBST)) or anti-human IgM, conjugated to peroxidase (Tago, Burlingame, CA, USA, 1:500 in PBST). Developing was performed with 66 µl nitro blue tetrazolium solution and 33 μl 5-bromo-4-chloro-3-indolyl phosphate solution (Promega) in 10 ml 100 mM Tris/HCl (pH 9.5), 100 mM NaCl, 5 mM $MgCl_2$ if alkaline phosphatase was used as a conjugate. For HRP-conjugated anti-IgM, 100 μg/ml 4-chloro-1-naphtol (Sigma) in PBS containing 0.003% H_2O_2 was used.

The subjects who had seroconverted were tested with the VDRL and TPHA assays.

Skin biopsy and culturing of B. burgdorferi

From one person who had seroconverted and who recalled an erythema, a 4 mm skin punch biopsy was taken at the site where this person had noticed the erythema. Culture of B. burgdorferi from this specimen and further characterization of this strain by reactivity with monoclonal antibodies and rRNA gene restriction analysis was performed as described elsewhere (14).

Statistical analysis

For dichotomous variables, two-by-two tables were constructed and the 95% confidence intervals (CIs) to odds ratios (ORs) were calculated. When the upper and lower limits of the 95% CI enclose 1, no statistically significant difference is present.

RESULTS

Initial seroprevalence of antibodies against B. burgdorferi

Among 2,158 subjects entering the military service 66 subjects (3.1%) had antibodies against B. burgdorferi. The initial seroprevalence of the at risk-group as well as of the control-group was 3.1%. In total 35 (1.6%) had IgG antibodies and 32 (1.4%) had IgM antibodies. One person had both IgM and IgG antibodies.

Rate of seroconversion

Among 932 persons from whom paired serum samples were available 14 (1.5%) subjects had seroconverted for IgM and/or IgG antibodies against B. burgdorferi within one year. Four of these 14 persons belonged to the at risk-group; they all developed only IgM antibodies (Fig. 1, sector A). 10 persons who seroconverted belonged to the control-group: 4 seroconverted for IgM and 6 for IgG antibodies (Figs. 1 and 2, sector A). None of the 14 persons converted for IgM as well as for IgG antibodies. The results from four subjects shifting from a borderline to a positive ELISA, thus not fulfilling the criteria for seroconversion, are shown in sector B of Figs. 1 and 2.

Two of the 932 persons showed IgM antibodies and 15 persons showed IgG antibodies for B. burgdorferi in both serum samples (Figs. 1 and 2, sector C). One person had both IgM and IgG antibodies in both serum samples. Seven persons had IgM antibodies against B. burgdorferi in the first but not in the second serum sample; none of them had developed IgG antibodies. Three persons had IgG antibodies in the first serum sample only (sector D in Figs. 1 and 2).

By means of the Western Blot technique, further evidence for seroconversion was found in 9 of the 14 seroconverted subjects. In 5 of the 6 persons who seroconverted for IgG antibodies measured by the ELISA, specific antibodies against B. burgdorferi could be detected in the second serum sample by appearance of new reactive bands (Fig. 3, lanes 1–5). In 1 of the 8 persons who seroconverted for IgM antibodies measured in the ELISA, new reactive bands in the second serum sample could be detected in the Western blot (Fig. 3, lane 8), whereas the second serum samples from 3 persons showed a considerable increased reactivity with the 41 kD band (lanes 7, 9 and 10).

None of the sera of the seroconverted subjects were positive in the VDRL or TPHA assays.

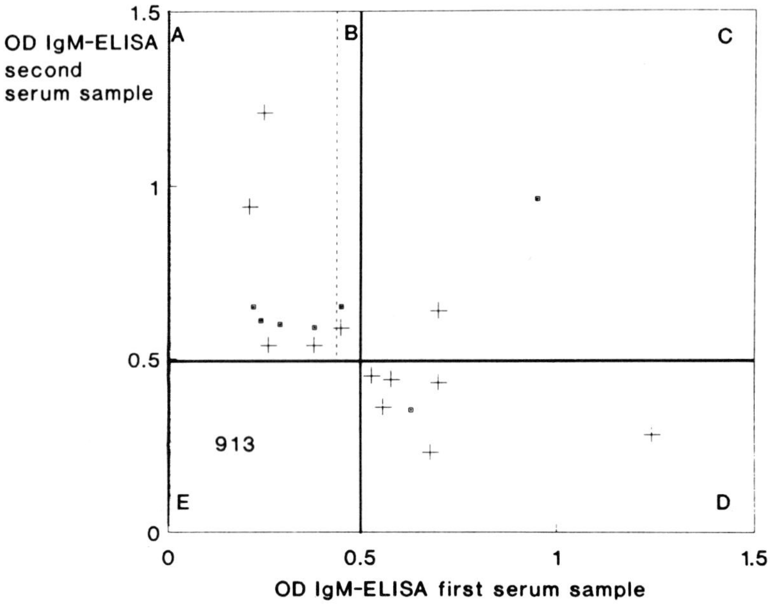

Fig. 1. IgM antibodies in paired serum samples from 932 military. The persons who seroconverted for antibodies against B. burgdorferi are indicated in sector A. Sector B depicts persons whose initial serum sample was borderline and therefore did not fulfil the criterium for seroconversion. Sector C includes persons who persistently had a positive serology. In sector D the persons who had antibodies in the first, but not in the second serum sample are depicted. The military who had no B. burgdorferi antibodies in both serum samples are shown in sector E. A + indicates a person of the at risk-group; a ● indicates a person of the control-group.

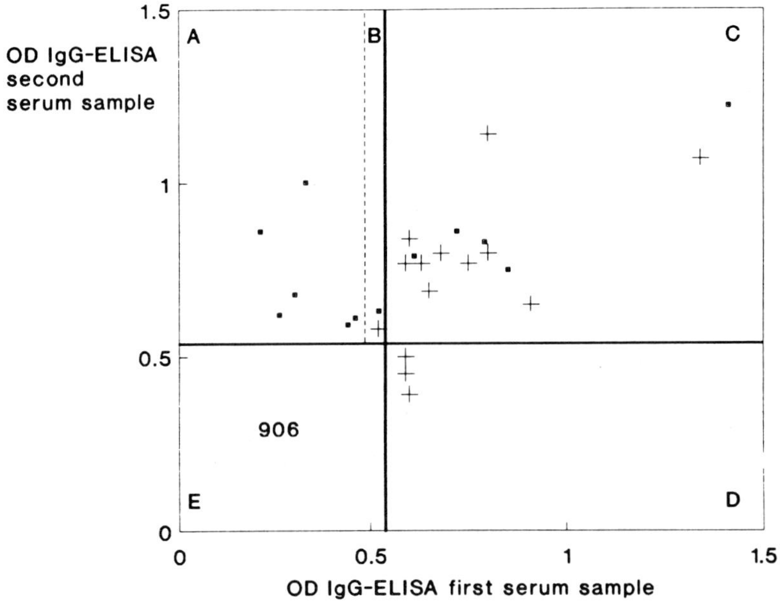

Fig. 2. IgG antibodies in paired serum samples from 932 military. A–E: see Fig. 1. A + indicates a person of the at risk-group; a ● indicates a person of the control-group.

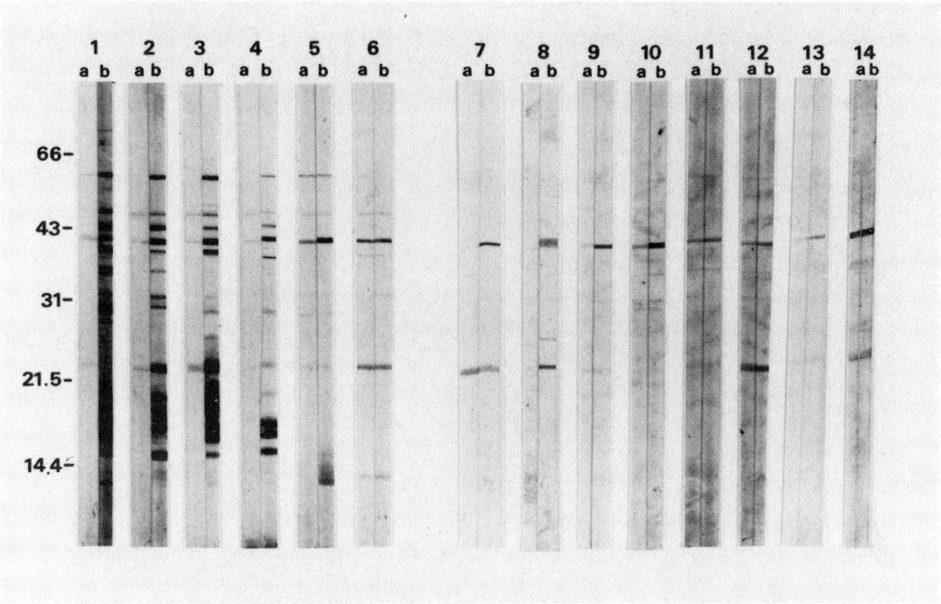

Fig. 3. Western blot results using paired sera of the 14 military who seroconverted for IgG (persons 1–6) or IgM (persons 7–14) antibodies against B. burgdorferi by ELISA. a: first serum sample, b: second serum sample. The position of molecular weight markers (kDa) which were run in parallel is shown at the left.

Results of questionnaire

Questionnaires were completed by 453 persons (97%) of the persons of the at risk-group and 442 persons (95%) of the control-group. 29 tick bites were reported in the at risk-group whereas 12 tick bites were reported in the control-group (OR: 2.45 CI 1.11–5.16 $p = 0.008$).

Six persons of the at risk-group and 13 persons of the control-group had noticed an erythema (difference not significant). None of these skin-rashes had been diagnosed by a physician and none of these persons had been treated for Lyme disease. Only 1 person with an erythema, belonging to the control-group, seroconverted for antibodies (IgG) against B. burgdorferi.

Clinical manifestations among seroconverted military

Two to 3 months after taking the second serum sample 9 of the 14 persons who seroconverted for Lyme borreliosis were interviewed and physically examined; the other 5 persons were interviewed by telephone.

Only 1 of the 14 subjects who had seroconverted had noticed an erythema, which he also had reported in the questionnaire. At the time of the physical examination, the erythema had disappeared and no other symptoms of LB were present, although no antibiotic treatment had been given. For this person a skin biopsy was taken 6 months after disappearance of the erythema migrans at the site of the former lesion and B. burgdorferi was cultured from this skin biopsy. This strain, designated A84S, was characterized as belonging to group VS461 by rRNA gene restriction analysis and reactivity with monoclonal antibodies as reported in detail elsewhere (14). The soldier was treated with 100 mg doxycycline twice daily for 14 days. A control biopsy, taken 1 month later, yielded no spirochetes.

The other persons who had seroconverted reported no clinical manifestations suggesting that Lyme borreliosis had occurred. In addition, the physical examinations revealed no abnormalities possibly related to Lyme borreliosis.

During the whole study period, no cases of Lyme borreliosis were reported by the physicians who cared after the study population.

DISCUSSION

In this study we assessed the rate of seroconversion for Lyme borreliosis among Dutch military in an at risk-group conducting field training and in a control-group performing predominantly in-door jobs. The at risk-group consisting of commandos and infantry performed their training in forests in areas endemic for ticks. The results show no significant difference in clinical and asymptomatic Lyme borreliosis between the 2 groups. The most likely explanation for this lack of difference between both groups is the fact that military always wear their training-uniform during field training: long sleeves, long pants and high boots. The frequency of seroconversion in the entire study group (1.5%) was lower than reported for Swiss orienteers (8%) (6) and Dutch forestry workers (5%) (7), persons which are probably less well protected by their clothing.

Additional evidence that seroconversion demonstrated by ELISA indeed represented an increase in antibodies against B. burgdorferi was obtained by Western blotting in 5 out of 6 persons who developed IgG antibodies, but only in 4 out of 8 persons who developed IgM antibodies. Therefore, the number of persons who seroconverted may have been overestimated in this study. The IgM ELISA seems to be less specific in comparison to the IgG assay. This can also be drawn from the fact that none of 7 persons who initially had IgM antibodies, developed IgG antibodies during the study. However, we did not obtain clinical data on these persons and therefore we do not know whether they had been treated with antibiotics before they entered the army. Early treatment of persons with Lyme borreliosis can interfere with the development of IgG antibodies against B. burgdorferi (15).

Only 29 (6.5%) of 447 persons of the at risk-group reported tick bites. This is a very low number in comparison to Swiss orienteers and Dutch forestry workers, of whom 78% (6) and 55% (5) recalled tick bites. Nonetheless, the number of tick bites was significantly higher in the at risk-group than in the control-group. Despite this finding the prevalence of Lyme borreliosis in both groups was similar. In previous investigations a poor correlation between tick bites and prevalence of antibodies against B. burgdorferi was demonstrated (6, 16). Various reasons may be related to this finding, such as the variation of the percentage of ticks infested with B. burgdorferi (1), the duration of the tick-attachment, on which transmission of B. burgdorferi to man is dependent (17), and finally the fact that a tick bite is often not noticed. Of the 14 persons in this study who seroconverted for Lyme borreliosis only 2 recalled a tickbite.

In the control-group the number of cases with erythema ($n = 13$) was higher than in the at risk-group ($n = 6$) but the difference was not statistically significant. Since only 1 out of these 19 persons seroconverted, whereas none of them had been treated for Lyme disease, most probably the majority of the skin lesions were not an erythema migrans.

Our study strengthens the view that in Europe infection with B. burgdorferi is predominantly asymptomatic. In this study, only 1 (7%) of the 14 persons with a seroconversion showed clinical manifestations of early Lyme borreliosis, in the form of an erythema migrans. In the U.S.A. a higher frequency of clinical Lyme borreliosis in persons having antibodies against B. burgdorferi has been reported. Retrospectively, Smith et al. (2) found that 14 (52%) out of 27 seropositive persons recalled past symptoms of Lyme borreliosis; 7

of them reported a rash, suggestive for erythema migrans. Steere et al. (18) estimated that 50% of infected persons on Great Island, Massachusetts were symptomatic; 70% of the symptomatic persons reported erythema migrans. Hanrahan et al. (19) found 8 symptomatic persons, all with erythema migrans, among 21 persons who were seropositive or who had seroconverted. These studies indicate that about 25–35% of seropositive persons living in endemic areas for Lyme borreliosis in the United States have had symptoms of early Lyme borreliosis. In contrast, European studies report much lower rates of symptomatic infection among seropositive persons. In a recent Swedish study, only 6 (7%) of 90 persons with antibodies against B. burgdorferi reported clinical manifestations of Lyme borreliosis; only 2 of them had had erythema migrans (16). Gustafsson et al. found also frequently asymptomatic seropositive persons among Swedish persons living in or visiting endemic areas for Lyme borreliosis (20) or practising orienteering (21). Fahrer et al. (6) showed that only 1 (1.6%) of 63 Swiss orienteers who had a significant increase in IgG antibodies developed signs of Lyme borreliosis; this person recalled an erythema migrans. Clement et al. (22) reported that 18 of 488 U.S. military, conducting frequent outdoor activities in Southern Germany, seroconverted for Lyme borreliosis in 1 year. None of them had shown clinical symptoms of Lyme borreliosis during the follow-up period of 6 to 9 months. The frequency of clinical Lyme borreliosis among seropositive Dutch forestry workers was 7/43 (16%) (7). Five of these 7 persons reported a history of erythema migrans. In addition, seroconversion was observed in 5 initially seronegative forestry-workers. Two of these 5 persons had clinical manifestations during the 1 year follow-up period but none of them met case definition criteria for Lyme borreliosis. The difference between the frequency of clinical manifestations among subjects in the North American continent and Europe may be due to differences in pathogenicity among the various B. burgdorferi genospecies (14, 23, 24). It is possible that asymptomatic infections are more often caused by genospecies only occurring in Europe.

In conclusion, Dutch military personnel training in areas where Borrelia-infested ticks occur, can not be regarded as a high-risk group to acquire Lyme borreliosis. Most likely, their clothing gives sufficient protection.

REFERENCES

1. Nohlmans MKE, De Boer R, Van Den Bogaard AEJM, Blaauw AAM, Van Boven CPA. Voorkomen van Borrelia burgdorferi in Ixodes ricinus in Nederland. Ned Tijdschr Geneeskd 134: 1300–1303, 1990.
2. Smith PF, Benach JL, White DJ, Stroup DF, Morse DL. Occupational risk of Lyme disease in endemic areas of New York State. Ann NY Acad Sci 539: 289–301, 1988.
3. Neubert U, Münchhoff P, Völker B, Reimers CD, Pflüger KH. Borrelia burgdorferi infections in Bavarian forest workers. Ann NY Acad Sci 539: 476–479, 1988.
4. Nadal D, Wunderli W, Briner H, Hansen K. Prevalence of antibodies to Borrelia burgdorferi in forestry workers and blood donors from the same region in Switzerland. Eur J Clin Microbiol Infect Dis 8: 992–995, 1989.
5. Kuiper H, De Jongh BM, Nauta AP, Houweling H, Wiessing LG, Moll van Charante AW, Spanjaard L. Lyme borreliosis in Dutch forestry workers. J Infect 23: 279–286, 1991.
6. Fahrer H, Van der Linden SM, Sauvain M-J, Gern L, Zhioua E, Aeschlimann A. The prevalence and incidence of clinical and asymptomatic Lyme borreliosis in a population at risk. J Infect Dis 163: 305–310, 1991.
7. Kuiper H, Van Dam AP, Moll van Charante AW, Nauta AP, Dankert J. One year follow-up study to assess the prevalence and incidence of Lyme borreliosis among Dutch forestry workers. Eur J Clin Microbiol Infect Dis 12: 413–418, 1993.
8. Schwartz BS, Goldstein MD. Lyme disease in outdoor workers: risk factors, preventive measures and tick removal methods. Am J Epidemiol 131: 877–885, 1990.
9. Lane RS, Manweiler SA, Stubbs HA, Lennette ET, Madigan JE, Lavoie PE. Risk factors for Lyme disease in a small rural community in northern California. Am J Epidemiol 136: 1358–1368, 1992.

10. Bowen SG, Schulze TL, Hayne C, Parkin WE. A focus of Lyme disease in Monmouth County, New Jersey. Am J Epidemiol 120: 387–394, 1984.
11. Kuiper H, Devriese PP, De Jongh BM, Vos K, Dankert J. Absence of Lyme borreliosis among patients with presumed Bell's palsy. Arch Neurol 49: 940–943, 1992.
12. Hansen K, Hindersson P, Strandberg Pedersen N. Measurement of antibodies to the Borrelia burgdorferi flagellum improves serodiagnosis in Lyme disease. J Clin Microbiol 26: 338–346, 1988.
13. Hansen K, Åsbrink E. Serodiagnosis of erythema migrans and acrodermatitis chronica atrophicans by the Borrelia burgdorferi flagellum enzyme-linked immunosorbent assay. J Clin Microbiol 27: 545–551, 1989.
14. Van Dam AP, Kuiper H, Vos K, Widjojokusumo A, Spanjaard L, De Jongh BM, Ramselaar ACP, Kramer MD, Dankert J. Different genospecies of Borrelia burgdorferi are associated with distinct clinical manifestations in Lyme borreliosis. Clin Infect Dis 17: 708–717, 1993.
15. Craft J, Fischer DK, Shimamoto GT, Steere AC. Antigens of Borrelia burgdorferi recognized during Lyme disease. Appearance of a new immunoglobulin M response and expansion of the immunoglobulin G response late in the illness. J Clin Invest 78: 934–939, 1986.
16. Berglund J, Eitrem R. Tick-borne borreliosis in the archipelage of southern Sweden. Scand J Infect Dis 25: 67–72, 1993.
17. Piesman J, Mather TN, Sinsky RJ, Spielman A. Duration of tick attachment and Borrelia burgdorferi transmission. J Clin Microbiol 25: 557–558, 1987.
18. Steere AC, Taylor E, Wilson ML, Levine JF, Spielman A. Longitudinal assessment of the clinical and epidemiological features of Lyme disease in a defined population. J Infect Dis 154: 295–300, 1986.
19. Hanrahan JP, Benach JL, Coleman JL, Bosler EM, Morse DL, Cameron DJ, Edelman R, Kaslow RA. Incidence and cumulative frequency of endemic Lyme disease in a community. J Infect Dis 150: 489–496, 1984.
20. Gustafson R, Svenungsson B, Gardulf A, Stiernstedt G, Forsgren M. Prevalence of tick-borne encephalitis and Lyme borreliosis in a defined Swedish population. Scand J Infect Dis 22: 297–306, 1990.
21. Gustafson R, Forsgren M, Gardulf A, Granström M, Svenungsson B. Antibody prevalence and clinical manifestations of Lyme borreliosis and tick-borne encephalitis in Swedish orienteers. Scand J Infect Dis 25: 605–611, 1993.
22. Clement J, Leirs H, Armour V, Ward D, Groen J, Osterhaus A, Kunz C. Exposure to Borrelia burgdorferi and tick-borne encephalitis (TBE) virus of US troops in South-Germany. Vth International conference on Lyme borreliosis 335: A57, 1992. (abstract)
23. Wilske B, Preac-Mursic V, Göbel UB, Graf B, Jauris S, Soutschek E, Schwab E, Zumstein G. An OspA serotyping system for Borrelia burgdorferi based on reactivity with monoclonal antibodies OspA sequence analysis. J Clin Microbiol 31: 340–350, 1993.
24. Assous MV, Postic D, Paul G, Névot P, Baranton G. Western blot analysis of sera from Lyme borreliosis patients according to the genomic species of the Borrelia strains used as antigens. Eur J Clin Microbiol Infect Dis 12: 261–268, 1993.

Submitted December 3, 1993; accepted March 23, 1994

Scand J Infect Dis 26: 435–445, 1994

Serum IgG Antibody Responses to Shigella Invasion Plasmid-coded Antigens Detected by Immunoblot

AN LI[1], CHUN R. ZHAO[1], ERIK EKWALL[2] and ALF A. LINDBERG[1]

From the Departments of [1]Clinical Bacteriology, and [2]Infectious Diseases, Karolinska Institute, Huddinge Hospital, Huddinge, Sweden

Serum IgG antibody responses to Shigella invasion plasmid-coded antigens (Ipa) from 58 Shigella flexneri, S. sonnei, and S. dysenteriae infected Swedish patients were investigated by immunoblot technique. Intense responses to most components of Ipa (Ipas A, B, C, D, and VirG – virulence determinant on *SalI* fragment G of the plasmid) were evident in sera from S. flexneri infected patients. The strongest response was to Ipa B and the weakest, to Ipa D. In contrast, there were weaker responses to Ipas A, B, C, and VirG but none at all to Ipa D in sera from S. sonnei infected patients. After absorption of the Ipa-positive sera by Ipa expressing strains of S. flexneri and S. sonnei, most IgG antibodies to components of Ipa were removed in sera absorbed by S. flexneri, but IgG antibodies to Ipas – especially to Ipa D – were only slightly reduced in sera absorbed by S. sonnei, suggesting that Ipa D in S. sonnei may not be exposed on the S. sonnei cell surface.

A. A. Lindberg, MD, Karolinska Institute, Department of Clinical Bacteriology F82, Huddinge Sjukhus, S-141 86 Huddinge, Sweden

INTRODUCTION

Since the discovery that invasion of epithelial cells by shigellae depends on the presence of a 120–140 MDa plasmid (1, 2) the pathogenesis of shigellosis has become better understood. Invasion is closely related to expression of antigens coded on a large invasion plasmid which appears to be conserved in different species of virulent Shigella and enteroinvasive Escherichia coli (3–5). The invasion plasmid-coded antigens (Ipas) B, C and D have been found to be related with the invasive phenotype (6, 7), whereas another plasmid-coded antigen VirG (Ics A, virulence determinant on *SalI* fragment G of the plasmid) is responsible for the intra- and inter-cellular spread of the bacteria (8). The function of Ipa A is not yet understood. Recently, an additional gene, *ipa*H, was reported to be present in multiple copies in both the plasmid and chromosome (9). The 60 kDa Ipa H protein is suggested to act through its leucine-rich motif to inhibit thrombin-induced platelet aggregation, thereby muting the platelet-mediated inflammatory response and facilitating dissemination of Shigella in host tissues (10). A number of chromosome and plasmid genes modulating the surface expression of the Ipas have also been reported (11–14).

However, only limited information is available regarding the immunogenicity of Ipa in humans (15–17). In our previous study on serum antibody responses to shigella lipopolysaccharides and to Ipa in shigella-infected patients by enzyme immunoassay (EIA) (18), we observed that IgG antibody responses to Ipa in sera from S. flexneri infected patients appeared to be more pronounced than responses in sera from S. sonnei infected patients. However, since we used an aqueous extract with Ipa we could not define which component(s) of the Ipa the antibodies were elicited against. In this communication we qualitatively characterized the serum IgG antibody responses to the Ipas by sodium dodecylsulfate polyacrylamide gel electrophoresis (SDS-PAGE) and Western blot.

MATERIALS AND METHODS

Serum collection

The patient sera were from the collection of Shigella-infected Swedish patients used in our previous serum EIA study (18). Serum was separated immediately after the collection of blood and stored in aliquots at −70°C until used. A single one serum sample was collected between 3 weeks and 3 months after the onset of dysentery in each patient. Altogether there were 24, 32 and 2 samples from Shigella flexneri-, S. sonnei-, and S. dysenteriae-infected patients, respectively. Sera from 38 healthy Swedish blood donors served as controls.

Bacterial strains and their cultivation

Cell lysates of S. flexneri serotype 5 strains M90T and M90T55 (19) were used as Ipa antigens for detecting serum IgG antibody responses. Strain M90T harbours the 140 MDa invasion plasmid and expresses Ipas. Strain M90T55 has lost the invasion plasmid and therefore lacks Ipas. Cell lysates of M90T and M90T55 were run simultaneously in all SDS-PAGE and Western blot experiments throughout the study.

The expression of Ipa antigens from 22 S. flexneri, 26 S. sonnei and 2 S. dysenteriae isolates from the Shigella-infected patients was examined. Two additional S. flexneri and 6 additional S. sonnei strains from the patients were rough. Two smooth S. boydii strains from the Department's strain collection were also tested. Each isolate was first cultured on Congo-red plates. Congo-red-positive colonies, indicative of cell invasiveness and Ipa-expression (20), were inoculated and cultivated to exponential phase in Penassay broth (OD 0.8 at 600 nm). For S. flexneri, S. dysenteriae and S. boydii, 10 ml of the broth from each strain was centrifuged and the pellet washed once with phosphate-buffered saline (PBS) and suspended in 0.5 ml sampling buffer. For S. sonnei, in order to reduce the number of plasmid-negative rough segregants, the broth was kept at 4°C overnight, then 10 ml of unsedimented bacterial suspension was centrifuged, washed and finally suspended in sampling buffer. The number of Congo-red-positive colonies ranged from 95% to 100% (mean 98%) for S. flexneri, S. dysenteriae and S. boydii. For S. sonnei the corresponding figures were 80–99% (mean 93%).

Supernatants of each culture broth of 2 S. flexneri and 2 S. sonnei strains from the patients were examined to ascertain whether the Ipas secreted by the bacteria were consistent with the immune responses elicited them and water extracts of Ipas from E. coli Sp10, an E. coli K12 strain with the invasion plasmid (2), and from E. coli J53 (lacking the invasion plasmid) (2) were also investigated for their Ipa contents.

Sodium dodecylsulfate polyacrylamide gel electrophoresis (SDS-PAGE) and Western blot

SDS-PAGE with 14% acrylamide was used *ad modum* Oaks et al. (15) and Pál et al. (19). Ipa polypeptides separated on the gel were blotted on nitrocellulose sheets, cut to strips and incubated with human serum overnight at 20°C. We used sera diluted 1:50 after titration experiments had shown that at this dilution both strong and weak IgG responses could be detected (unpublished data). The strips were finally incubated for 1 h with alkaline-phosphatase labelled protein A (Sigma, St. Louis, Mo., USA) followed by development in 50 mM Tris-HCl substrate solution.

Evaluation of Western blots

Antibody responses to plasmid coded antigens of M90T were seen in the form of bands with reported molecular weights: VirG, 120 kDa; Ipa A, 78 kDa; Ipa B, 62 kDa; Ipa C, 43 kDa; Ipa D, 38 kDa; and Ipa H, 60 kDa, and by their absence from the strips containing antigens of M90T55 (lacking the plasmid). A serum sample from a S. flexneri 2a infected patient who had IgG antibodies to all the Ipa components was used as a positive control. Results of serum responses were scored visually on the basis of the presence and intensity of stained bands at the positions corresponding to the positive control on strips where Ipas from cell lysate of M90T had been applied and the absence of staining at the same position on strips where proteins from cell lysate of M90T55 had been applied. The intensity of staining was defined as: 1) negative, score 0; 2) weak positive staining, score 1; 3) moderate positive staining, score 2; 4) strong positive staining, score 3. The blots were read blind by 2 independent investigators. Some minor inconsistent results were jointly re-examined.

Serum antibody absorption

Congo-red-positive colonies of S. flexneri 2a and S. sonnei were each grown on 3 Congo-red agar plates at 37°C for 30 h, harvested, and suspended in PBS. The suspension was adjusted to OD 0.8 at 600 nm and a 150 ml suspension of each strain was centrifuged at 800 × *g* at 4°C for 30 min. The pellet was suspended in an aliquot of 3 ml serum (1:50 dilution with 0.1% NaN_3). The mixture was incubated on a roller mixer at 20°C for 2 h. Following centrifugation, the absorbed serum was incubated with a nitrocellulose strip onto which SDS-PAGE separated Ipa antigens from S. flexneri strain M90T (plasmid positive) had been blotted. After incubation the strip was stained with the protein A conjugate and developed as described above. Ten aliquots of each of the 10 sera from S. flexneri infected patients, with strong staining to major Ipa components (VirG, Ipas A, B, C, and D) and 10 aliquots of each of the 5 sera from S. sonnei infected patients with relatively strong staining to Ipas were absorbed with each of 5 Congo-red-positive strains of S. flexneri 2a and 5 Congo-red-positive S. sonnei – all collected from these patients. Aliquots of each of the 15 unabsorbed sera were used to stain the nitrocellulose strip for comparison of the staining pattern with the counterparts absorbed. Positive and negative controls were included in each assay.

Statistical method

The intensity of staining of Ipa bands by sera from S. flexneri and S. sonnei infected patients was compared, using the Mann-Whitney U-test.

RESULTS

Serum IgG antibody responses to Ipa

In sera from S. flexneri infected patients 10/24 had detectable antibodies against all 5 components of Ipa (VirG, Ipas A, B, C, and D). Another 7 had antibodies against all components but Ipa D (Table I). The staining to Ipa B was the strongest, as judged by the intensity (mean score ± SD 2.0 ± 1.3), followed by Ipa A, Ipa C (mean scores 1.6 ± 1.1 and 1.5 ± 1.1, respectively), and VirG and Ipa D the weakest (mean scores 1.0 ± 0.8 and 1.0 ± 1.2, respectively) (Fig. 1). The mean number of positive bands to the 5 components was 3.25 (calculated from all S. flexneri infected patients).

In sera from 32 S. sonnei infected patients, no patient had antibodies to all 5 components. 13/32 sera had antibodies to 2 or 3 of the five components. 18 had responses to Ipa B, 8 to Ipa A, 6 to Ipa C and 5 to VirG, respectively. No staining reaction to Ipa D was seen. Ipa B showed the strongest staining (mean score 1.3 ± 1.3), followed by Ipas A, C, and VirG (mean scores 0.3 ± 0.4, 0.2 ± 0.5, and 0.2 ± 0.4, respectively). Thus the staining was much weaker than seen in sera from S. flexneri infected patients (Table I, Fig. 1). The mean number of bands to the 5 components of Ipa was only 1.16 ($p < 0.01$ compared with the mean number of bands in sera from S. flexneri infected patients).

Sera from the 2 S. dysenteriae infected patients showed strong staining to all 5 components of Ipa (Table I).

Table I. *Serum IgG antibody responses to invasion plasmid-coded antigens (Ipa) in Shigella flexneri, Shigella sonnei and Shigella dysenteriae infected Swedish patients detected by immunoblot*

Patients infected with	No. of persons	VirG (+)[a]	VirG Score[b]	Ipa A (+)	Ipa A Score	Ipa B (+)	Ipa B Score	Ipa C (+)	Ipa C Score	Ipa D (+)	Ipa D Score	Total (+)[c]	Total Score
S. flexneri	24	17	1.0 ± 0.8	17	1.6 ± 1.1	17	2.0 ± 1.3	17	1.5 ± 1.1	10	1.0 ± 1.2	17	1.4 ± 0.4
S. sonnei	32	5	0.2 ± 0.4	8	0.3 ± 0.4	18	1.3 ± 1.3	6	0.2 ± 0.5	0	0	18	0.4 ± 0.5
S. dysenteriae	2	2	3.0	2	3.0	2	3.0	2	3.0	2	2.5	2	2.9 ± 0.2
Blood donors	38	0	0	1	0.03	2	0.1	3	0.1 ± 0.4	1	0.05	5	0.1 ± 0.1
Significance (p)[d]		<0.01/<0.05		<0.01/<0.01		<0.05/<0.01		<0.01/>0.05		<0.01/>0.05		<0.01/<0.01	

(Column group heading: Serum IgG antibody responses to)

[a] Represents the number of samples positive to the defined antigen.

[b] Represents the mean score ± 1SD from all of the patients or blood donors. Scores are defined as: 0 = negative; 1 = weakly positive; 2 = moderately positive; 3 = strongly positive.

[c] Samples with a positive staining to at least one component of the Ipa are defined as positive.

[d] Significance was calculated by comparing the intensity of staining to each Ipa component between sera from S. flexneri- and sera from S. sonnei-infected patients/between sera from S. sonnei-infected patients and sera from blood donors.

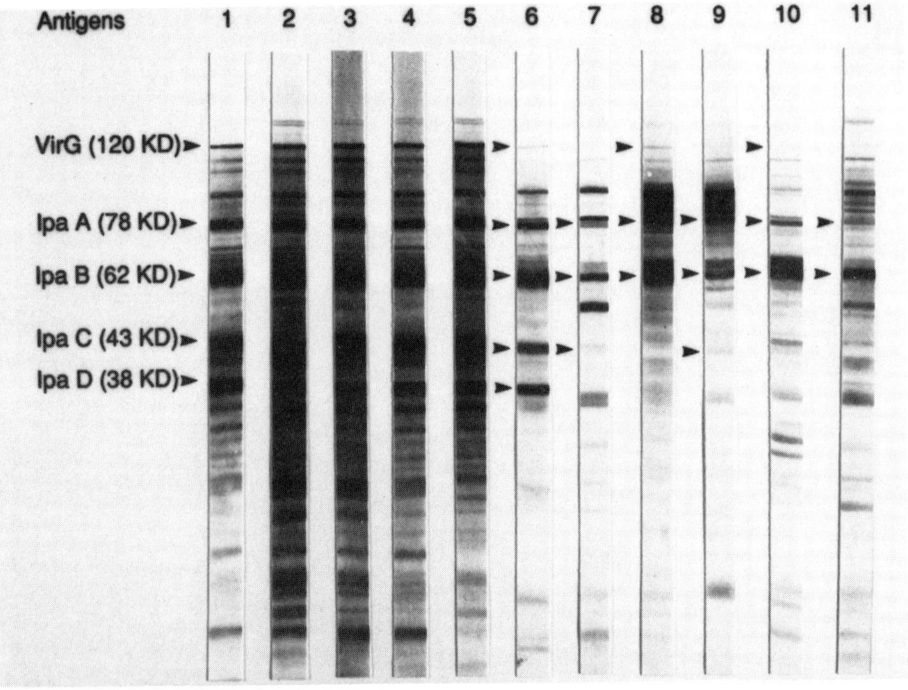

Fig. 1. Serum IgG antibody responses to Shigella invasion plasmid-coded antigens (Ipa) in S. flexneri and S. sonnei infected Swedish patients. Ipa from cell lysate of S. flexneri 5 invasion plasmid-positive strain M90T was used as antigen. Lane 1: positive control serum; lanes 2–6: sera from S. flexneri infected patients which were positive to all 5 components of Ipa; lanes 7–11: sera from S. sonnei infected patients. Arrowheads indicate positive staining to components of Ipa.

All serum samples which in our previous study were shown to have positive IgG titres to Ipa in EIA (18) also showed positive staining in the immunoblots. The immunoblots also detected 8 weak anti-Ipa responses (one for S. flexneri and 7 for S. sonnei) not seen in EIA for serum IgG (Table II).

Staining of Ipa bands was found in 5/38 serum samples (13.2%) from healthy blood donors which served as controls (Table I, Fig. 2). The mean number of bands to the 5 components was 0.18 ($p < 0.01$ compared with that in sera from either S. flexneri- or S. sonnei-infected patients). Three blood donors had antibodies to one of the 5 components but the other 2 had antibodies to Ipas B and C. These 2 sera were shown to have positive IgG titres against Ipa when tested with EIA (EIA data not shown).

Staining of Ipa after absorption of sera by live S. flexneri and S. sonnei

After absorption of 10 aliquots of 10 sera positive in immunoblot and EIA from S. flexneri infected patients by either of 5 S. flexneri and 5 S. sonnei isolates, staining to Ipa B was completely removed. The number of positive sera and the intensity of staining to Ipa C were greatly reduced (the mean intensity of staining dropped from 2.5 ± 0.7 to 0.2 ± 0.4 and 0.3 ± 0.4 in sera absorbed by S. flexneri and S. sonnei, respectively). Staining to Ipa A was also reduced in sera absorbed by both species (mean intensity of staining dropping from 2.5 ± 0.5 to 1.1 ± 0.7 and 1.2 ± 0.5 in sera absorbed by S. flexneri and S. sonnei, respectively). In aliquots absorbed by S. flexneri the staining to VirG and Ipa D was abolished in 18 of the 50 aliquots and in the rest the intensity of staining was greatly reduced (mean

Table II. *Responders in serum IgG to Ipa in S. flexneri and S. sonnei infected patients detected by EIA and immunoblot*

	S. flexneri infected patients			S. sonnei infected patients		
		Immunoblot			Immunoblot	
Relative EIA titre	Number of responders	Mean no. of bands	Mean score of staining	Number of responders	Mean no. of bands	Mean score of staining
<250	3/4[a]	4.3 ± 0.4	1.4 ± 0.2[b]	6/13	2.0 ± 0.7	0.6 ± 0.2
250–500	6/6	4.5 ± 0.5	1.8 ± 0.2	5/5	2.0 ± 0.9	0.8 ± 0.2
>500	7/7	4.9 ± 0.4	2.5 ± 0.4	0	0	0

[a] Number of responders detected by EIA/number of responders detected by immunoblot whose EIA titres were within the defined category. All responders in EIA were positive in immunoblot.
[b] Mean score ± 1SD is presented. The definition of scores is as in Table I. Serum IgG antibody responses to VirG, Ipas A, B, C, and D were counted.

$$\text{Mean score of staining} = \frac{\sum (\text{individual total score} \div 5)}{\text{number of responders}}$$

staining intensity dropped from 1.8 ± 0.6 to 0.7 ± 0.6 for VirG and from 2.4 ± 0.7 to 1.0 ± 0.9 for Ipa D, respectively). In aliquots absorbed by S. sonnei the staining to VirG and Ipa D was only slightly weakened (mean staining intensity dropped from 1.8 ± 0.6 to 1.1 ± 0.6 for VirG and from 2.4 ± 0.7 to 2.0 ± 0.8 for Ipa D, respectively) and the bands disappeared in only a few cases (Table III, Fig. 3).

In the 5 sera from S. sonnei infected patients there was no VirG or Ipa D staining before absorption. Mean intensity of staining to Ipas A, B and C before absorption was 0.6 ± 0.5, 2.4 ± 0.4 and 0.6 ± 0.8, respectively). After absorption by both species, staining to Ipas B and

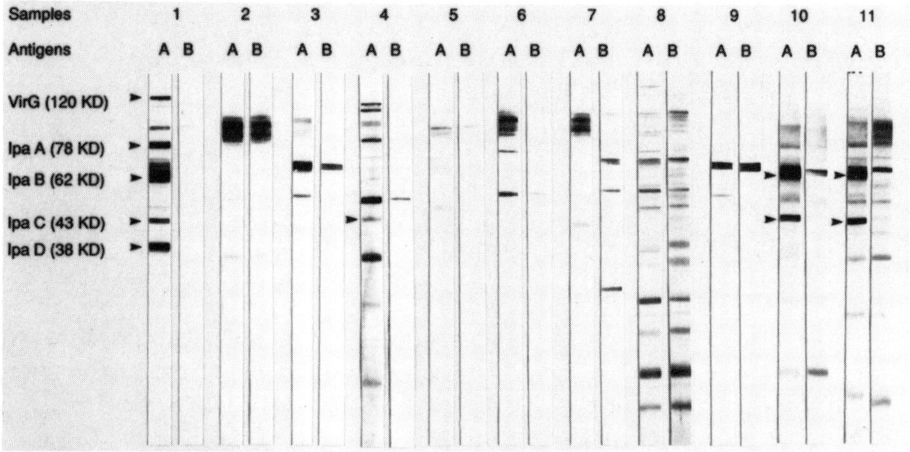

Fig. 2. Serum IgG antibody responses to Ipas in healthy Swedish blood donors. Lane 1: positive control serum; lanes 2–11: sera from blood donors. (A) IgG antibodies to Ipas from lysate of virulent S. flexneri 5 strain M90T (invasion plasmid positive). (B) IgG antibodies to proteins from lysate of avirulent S. flexneri strain M90T55 (invasion plasmid negative). Positive staining to Ipas in blood donors is indicated with an arrowhead.

Table III. *Comparison of antibody responses to Ipa after absorption by each 5 strains of Congo red positive, live S. flexneri and S. sonnei with aliquots of 10 sera from S. flexneri infected patients who had IgG antibodies to most of the Ipa antigens*[a]

	Before absorption		After absorption with S. flexneri		After absorption with S. sonnei		Significance[d]
Antigen	No. of (+) bands	Intensity of staining	No. of (+) bands[b]	Intensity of staining[c]	No. of (+) bands	Intensity of staining	(p-value)
Vir G	50	1.8 ± 0.6	32/50	0.7 ± 0.6	42/50	1.1 ± 0.6	<0.05
Ipa A	50	2.5 ± 0.5	42/50	1.1 ± 0.7	46/50	1.2 ± 0.5	>0.05
Ipa B	50	2.8 ± 0.4	0	0	0	0	>0.05
Ipa C	50	2.5 ± 0.7	9/50	0.2 ± 0.4	14/50	0.3 ± 0.4	>0.05
Ipa D	50	2.4 ± 0.7	32/50	1.0 ± 0.9	45/50	2.0 ± 0.8	<0.01
Ipa H[e]	DD[f]	DD	20/50	1.1 ± 1.4	20/50	1.1 ± 1.4	>0.05

[a] 10 aliquots of each of the 10 sera were absorbed by 10 live strains of 5 S. flexneri and 5 S. sonnei.
[b] Mean number of positive bands after absorption with S. flexneri or S. sonnei

$$= \frac{\sum (\text{individual total bands in 5 aliquots} \div 5)}{10}$$

[c] Mean intensity of staining $\pm$ 1SD is presented

$$\text{Mean intensity of staining after absorption} = \frac{\sum (\text{individual total scores in the 5 aliquots} \div 5)}{10}$$

[d] The intensity of staining after absorption by S. flexneri was compared with that after absorption by S. sonnei.
[e] Serum aliquots from 4 samples were positive after absorption by S. flexneri and S. sonnei.
[f] DD: difficult to determine.

C was not detectable. Staining to Ipa A was weakened (mean intensity of staining dropped to 0.4 ± 0.5 in sera absorbed by either species).

We noted that before absorption the staining to Ipa B was seen as a broad band in positive sera and it was impossible to distinguish Ipa B (62 kDa) from Ipa H (60 kDa). The absorption by live S. flexneri and S. sonnei abolished staining to Ipa B and rendered Ipa H staining identifiable (Fig. 3). All sera positive to Ipa B were therefore subjected to absorption with a Congo-red-positive S. flexneri 2a strain to identify Ipa H. Six, two and one sera from S. flexneri, S. sonnei, and S. dysenteriae infected patients, respectively, had positive staining to Ipa H. All these sera showed intense staining to the major components of Ipa. The intensity of Ipa H staining was slightly weaker than the mixed bands of Ipa B and H before absorption (Table III, Fig. 3).

Detection of Ipas in patient isolates of S. flexneri, S. sonnei and S. dysenteriae

In immunoblot, all the 50 Congo-red-positive patient isolates of S. flexneri, S. sonnei, and S. dysenteriae and 2 strains of S. boydii expressed the 5 components of Ipa (VirG, Ipas A, B, C, and D) (Fig. 4). There were no visible differences in intensity of staining when using the positive control serum. In lysates from 2 rough S. flexneri and 3 rough S. sonnei strains, expression of Ipa was, as expected, only seen in the single S. flexneri Congo-red-positive strain (Fig. 4).

Staining of separated and blotted water extracts of Ipa from E. coli Sp10 and J53 with the positive control serum showed that the extract from Sp10 (invasion plasmid positive)

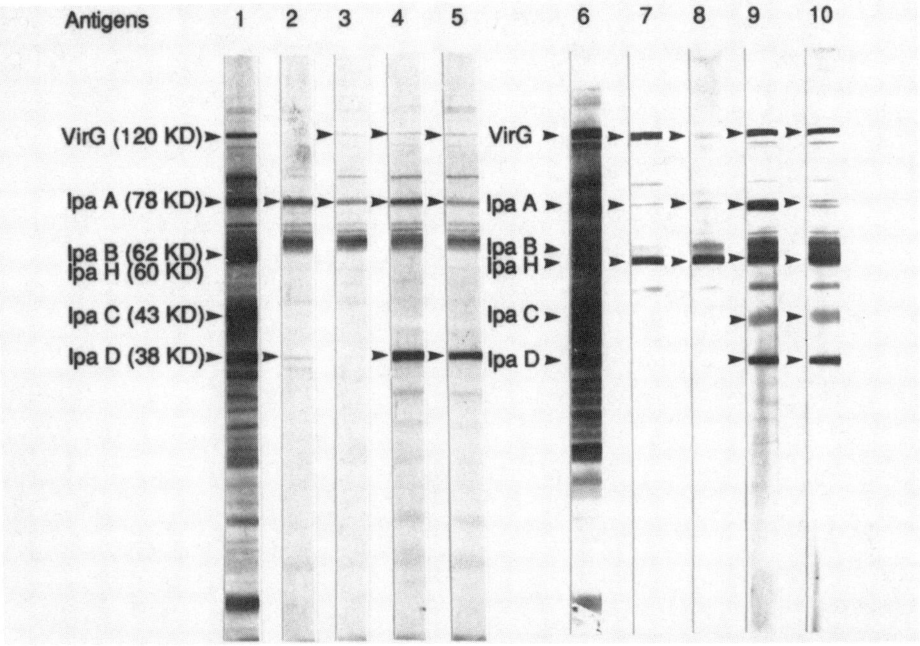

Fig. 3. Serum IgG antibody responses to Ipa after absorption of positive sera from S. flexneri infected patients by Congo-red-positive, live S. flexneri 2a and S. sonnei. Ten aliquots of each of the 10 sera from S. flexneri infected patients wee absorbed with Congo-red-positive bacteria of S. flexneri 2a (5 strains) and S. sonnei (5 strains). Lane 1: staining of the unabsorbed Ipa-positive serum (anti-Ipa H antibody negative); lanes 2, 3: staining of the positive serum after absorption by Congo-red-positive strains of S. flexneri 2a; lanes 4, 5: staining of the positive serum after absorption by Congo-red-positive strains of S. sonnei; lane 6: staining of another unabsorbed Ipa-positive serum (anti-Ipa H antibody positive); lanes 7, 8: staining of the positive serum after absorption by Congo-red-positive strains of S. flexneri 2a; lanes 9, 10: staining of the positive serum after absorption by Congo-red-positive strains of S. sonnei. Arrowheads indicate positive staining.

contained Ipas B, C, D and Ipa H and less Ipa A. Ipa C appeared to be the most abundant. No VirG was found. The water extract of J53 (invasion plasmid negative) did not contain any Ipa.

Staining of supernatants of S. flexneri broth showed Ipa A, B, C and D bands. Staining of supernatants of S. sonnei broth showed Ipa B, C and weak D bands, the richest component being Ipa C. None of the strains secreted detectable VirG (Fig. 5).

DISCUSSION

In a previous study we analysed the antibody responses to Ipa by EIA and found that the serum IgG antibody responses in S. flexneri infected patients were significantly greater than in S. sonnei infected patients (18). This raised the question whether there were any differences in the expression of Ipa between the 2 species. Analysis of cell lysates of S. flexneri and S. sonnei by immunoblot using Ipa-positive serum showed that the Ipas A, B, C, D and VirG could be clearly distinguished and that qualitatively there appeared to be no difference in Ipa content between the patient isolates of S. flexneri and S. sonnei (Fig. 4). However, analysis of the Ipa-positive sera subsequent to absorption with whole, live S. flexneri and S. sonnei showed that Ipa B appeared to be the most abundant cell surface antigen, as judged by the total disappearance of stained Ipa B bands after absorption with either S. flexneri or S.

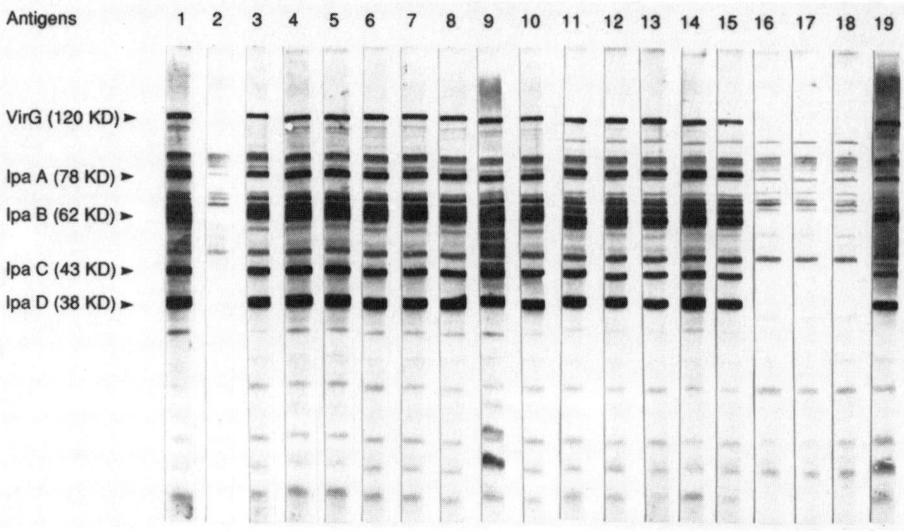

Fig. 4. Detection of Ipas from strains of S. flexneri, S. sonnei, S. dysenteriae and S. boydii. An anti-Ipa-positive serum was used to detect Ipas. All strains (unless specified) were Congo-red-positive. Lane 1: lysate from S. flexneri type 5 invasion plasmid-positive strain M90T; lane 2: lysate from S. flexneri type 5 invasion plasmid-negative strain M90T55; lane 3: S. boydii; lanes 4 and 5: S. dysenteriae type 1 and type 3; lanes 6–10: strains of S. flexneri; lanes 11–15: strains of S. sonnei; lanes 16, 17: strains of rough and Congo-red-negative S. sonnei; lane 18: rough and Congo-red-negative S. flexneri; lane 19: rough but Congo-red-positive S. flexneri. Note: one of the rough mutants (no. 19) is still Ipa-positive.

sonnei (Fig. 3). Ipa C seems to be another major Ipa expressed on cell surface in both species, as evidenced by the significantly reduced intensity of staining to Ipa C after absorption. However, absorption only partly reduced the intensity of staining of Ipa A, which we interpret to mean that it is not readily accessible on the cell envelope (Table III). Antibodies to VirG and especially to Ipa D, in contrast, were much better absorbed by S. flexneri but much less absorbed by S. sonnei.

The immunoblot also demonstrated that the serum IgG responses to all the Ipas elicited by S. flexneri were stronger than those elicited by S. sonnei (Fig. 1). The most striking differences were that staining of VirG was only seen in 5/32 sera from S. sonnei infected patients vis-à-vis 17/24 sera from S. flexneri infected patients ($p < 0.01$ when the numbers of positive stains were compared) and staining of Ipa D was only seen in sera from S. flexneri infected patients. This agrees with the results of the absorption using whole, live bacterial cells, which indicates that S. flexneri may have more VirG and Ipa D accessible than S. sonnei. The intensity of staining indicated that Ipa B induced the strongest IgG responses and those to Ipa D and Ipa H the weakest.

Our observations suggest that some components of Ipa in S. sonnei, Ipa D in particular, may be less exposed on the cell surface than in S. flexneri. Either less Ipa D is synthesized or it may be partly masked by other surface component(s) such as LPS. At present we have no quantitative data to favour either hypothesis, but the observation of similar intensities of staining of Ipa D in broth-grown S. flexneri and S. sonnei suggests that the difference may be in accessibility rather than in quantities of Ipa D synthesized. Another hypothesis is that S. sonnei is less able to multiply intracellularly than S. flexneri, and hence quantitatively less antigen is presented to the immune system in S. sonnei infected patients.

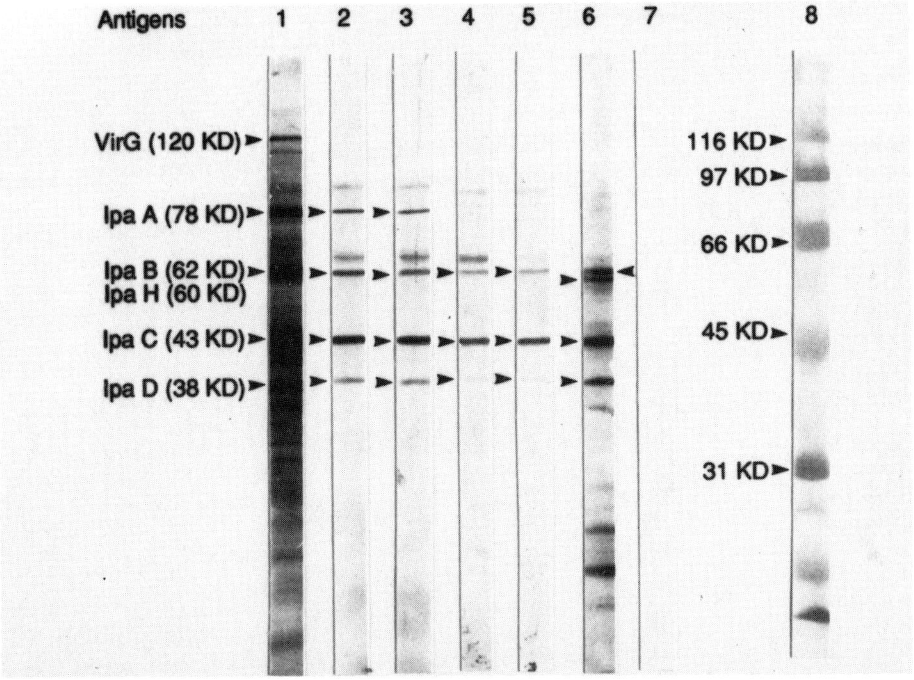

Fig. 5. Detection of Ipas in supernatants of bacterial culture and in water extracts of Sp10 and J53. An anti-Ipa-positive serum was used to detect Ipas. Lane 1: lysate from S. flexneri 5 invasion plasmid-positive strain M90T; lanes 2, 3: Ipas in supernatants of 2 strains of Congo-red-positive S. flexneri bacterial culture; lanes 4, 5: Ipas in supernatants of 2 strains of Congo-red-positive S. sonnei bacterial culture; lane 6: water extract of E. coli K12 strain Sp10 (invasion plasmid positive); lane 7: water extract of E. coli K12 strain J53 (invasion plasmid negative); lane 8: standard molecular markers. Positive staining is marked by an arrowhead. Lane 6: water extract of E. coli K12 strain Sp10 contained Ipa H as well as Ipas B, C, and D.

The essential roles of various Ipas in the pathogenesis of shigellosis have been studied: Ipas B, C, and D are responsible for epithelial cell invasion and the subsequent escape from the phagosome (6, 7, 21–23) and VirG for intra- and inter-cellular spread (8). S. flexneri may be able to invade and multiply more easily than S. sonnei, which subsequently results in more severe damage to the colonic tissue. The hypothesis has some credence in the observations that S. flexneri infections are often more severe than S. sonnei infections (24–28). However, Ipas are not the only virulence factors in shigellae; factors such as lipopolysaccharide and Shiga or Shiga-like toxin are of importance for the pathogenesis.

By studying the Ipa contents in water extracts and in bacterial culture supernatants we demonstrated that Ipas B, C, D and H are associated with the cell membrane and can easily be extracted by water. Ipa C appears to be the main component of Ipas, being loosely associated and/or secreted by the bacteria (Fig. 5). VirG, on the other hand, may be more firmly associated with the cell envelope, or less prone to dissolve in water. Our observation on Ipa contents in shigella culture supernatants is consistent with the finding of Ipa secretion in supernatants of S. flexneri Ipa mutants (22).

The observation in the immunoblots that the serum antibody responses to Ipas were mainly against Ipa B is consistent with the study performed on the sera from Chilean and North American populations (17).

We also found that by immunoblot more positive cases could be detected than by EIA (35 by immunoblot versus 27 by EIA). However, all that were detected only by immunoblot were weak responders (mean intensity of staining 0.8 ± 0.3) (Table II). A similar observation was made by Oberhelman et al. (16). In a comparison of the two assays, EIA is easy to perform, results can be obtained within 24 h and it is convenient for mass samples. EIA is therefore the first choice for clinical use. Immunoblotting can be seen as a supplementary means, allowing more detailed study of responses to individual Ipa components.

ACKNOWLEDGEMENTS

This study was supported by the Swedish Medical Research Council (grant no. 16x-656) and the Swedish Agency for Research Cooperation with Developing Countries (SAREC).

REFERENCES

1. Sansonetti PJ, Kopecko DJ, Formal SB. Shigella sonnei plasmids: evidence that a large plasmid is necessary for virulence. Infect Immun 34: 75–83, 1981.
2. Sansonetti PJ, Kopecko DJ, Formal SB. Involvement of a plasmid in the invasive ability of Shigella flexneri. Infect Immun 35: 852–860, 1982.
3. Hale TL, Sansonetti PJ, Schad PA, Austin S, Formal SB. Characterization of virulence plasmids and plasmid-associated outer membrane proteins in Shigella flexneri, Shigella sonnei, and Escherichia coli. Infect Immun 40: 340–350, 1983.
4. Sansonetti PJ, d'Hauteville H, Ecobichon C, Pourcel C. Molecular comparison of virulence plasmids in Shigella and enteroinvasive Escherichia coli. Ann Microbiol (Paris) 134A: 295–318, 1983.
5. Sansonetti PJ, Hale TL, Oaks V. Genetics of virulence in enteroinvasive Escherichia coli. In: Schlessinger D, ed. Microbiology-1985. Washington, DC: Amer Soc Microbiol, 74–77, 1985.
6. Maurelli AT, Baudry B, d'Hauteville H, Hale TL, Sansonetti PJ. Cloning of plasmid DNA sequences involved in invasion of Hela cells by Shigella flexneri. Infect Immun 49: 164–171, 1985.
7. Baudry B, Maurelli AT, Clerc P, Sadoff JG, Sansonetti PJ. Localization of plasmid loci necessary for the entry of Shigella flexneri into Hela cells, and characterization of one locus encoding four immunogenic polypeptides. J Gen Microbiol 133: 3403–3413, 1987.
8. Bernardini ML, Mounier J, d'Hauteville H, Coquis-Rondon M, Sansonetti PJ. Identification of *ics*A, a plasmid locus of Shigella flexneri that governs bacterial intra- and intercellular spread through interaction with F-actin. Proc Natl Acad Sci USA 86: 3867–3871, 1989.
9. Venkatesan MM, Buysse JM, Kopecko DJ. Use of Shigella flexneri *ipa* C and *ipa* H gene sequences for the general identification of Shigella spp. and enteroinvasive Escherichia coli. J Clin Bacteriol 27: 2687–2691, 1989.
10. Ventatesen MM, Buysse JM, Hartman AB. Sequence variation in two Ipa H genes of Shigella flexneri 5 and homology to LTG-like family of proteins. Mol Microbiol 5: 2435–2445, 1991.
11. Sakai T, Sasakawa C, Yoshikawa M. Expression of four virulence antigens of Shigella flexneri is positively regulated at the transcriptional level by the 30 kilodalton virF protein. Mol Microbiol 2: 589–597, 1988.
12. Yamada M, Sasakawa C, Okada N, Makino S-I, Yoshikawa M. Molecular cloning and characterization of chromosomal virulence region *kcp*A of Shigella flexneri. Mol Microbiol 3: 207–213, 1989.
13. Maurelli AT, Sansonetti PJ. Identification of a chromosomal gene controlling temperature-regulated expression of Shigella virulence. Proc Natl Acad Sci USA 85: 2820–2824, 1988.
14. Allaoui A, Sansonetti PJ, Parsot C. MxiD, an outer membrane protein necessary for the secretion of the Shigella flexneri Ipa invasins. Mol Microbiol 7: 59–68, 1993.
15. Oaks EV, Hale TL, Formal SB. Serum immune response to Shigella protein antigens in Rhesus monkeys and humans infected with Shigella spp. Infect Immun 53: 57–63, 1986.
16. Oberhelman RA, Kopecko DJ, Salazar-Lindo E, Gotuzzo E, Buysse JM, Venkatesan MM, Yi A, Fernandez-Prada C, Guzman M, León-Barúa R, Sack RB. Prospective study of systemic and mucosal immune responses in dysenteric patients to specific Shigella invasion plasmid antigens and lipopolysaccharides. Infect Immun 59: 2341–2350, 1991.
17. Van De Verg LL, Herrington DA, Boslego J, Lindberg AA, Levine M. Age-specific prevalence of serum antibodies to the invasion plasmid and lipopolysaccharide antigens of Shigella species in Chilean and North American populations. J Infect Dis 166: 158–161, 1992.

18. Li A, Rong ZC, Ekwall E, Forsum U, Lindberg AA. Serum antibody responses to Shigella lipopolysaccharides and invasion plasmid coded antigens in Shigella infected Swedish patients. Scand J Infect Dis 25: 569–577, 1993.
19. Pál T, Newland JW, Tall BD, Formal SB, Hale TL. Intracellular spread of Shigella flexneri associated with the KcpA locus and a 140-kilodalton protein. Infect Immun 57: 477–486, 1989.
20. Maurelli AT, Blackmon B, Curtiss R III. Loss of pigmentation in Shigella flexneri 2a is correlated with loss of virulence and virulence-associated plasmid. Infect Immun 43: 397–401, 1984.
21. Sasakawa C, Kamata K, Sakai T, Makino S, Yamada M, Okada N, Yoshikawa M. Virulence-associated genetic regions comprising 31 kilobases of the 230-kilobase plasmid in Shigella flexneri 2a. J Bacteriol 170: 2480–2484, 1988.
22. Ménard R, Sansonetti PJ, Parsot C. Nonpolar mutagenesis of the *ipa* genes defines IpaB, IpaC, and IpaD as effectors of Shigella flexneri entry into epithelial cells. J Bacteriol 175: 5899–5906, 1993.
23. High N, Mounier J, Prevost MC, Sansonetti PJ. IpaB of Shigella flexneri causes entry into epithelial cells and escape from the phagocytic vacuole. EMBO J 11: 1991–1999, 1992.
24. Keusch GT. Shigellosis. In: Evans AS, Feldman HA, eds. Bacterial Infections of Humans. New York: Plenum Press, 487–509, 1982.
25. Stoll BJ, Glass RI, Huq MI, Khan MU, Banu H, Holt J. Epidemiological and clinical features of patients infected with Shigella who attended a diarrheal disease hospital in Bangladesh. J Infect Dis 146: 177–183, 1982.
26. Halpern Z, Dan M, Giladi M, Schwartz I, Sela O, Levo Y. Shigellosis in adults: epidemiological, clinical, and laboratory features. Medicine 68: 210–217, 1989.
27. Bennish ML, Harris JR, Wojtyniak BJ, Struelens M. Death in shigellosis: incidence and risk factors in hospitalized patients. J Infect Dis 161: 500–506, 1990.
28. Hossaim MA, Albert MJ. Effect of duration of diarrhoea and predictive values of stool leukocytes and red blood cells in the isolation of different serogroups or serotypes of Shigella. Trans Roy Soc Trop Med Hyg 85: 664–666, 1991.

Submitted January 12, 1994; accepted March 7, 1994

Scand J Infect Dis 26: 446–452, 1994

Clinical Outcome of Acute Otitis Media Caused by Pneumococci with Decreased Susceptibility to Penicillin

BEATRIX BARRY[1], PIERRE GEHANNO[1], MARC BLUMEN[1] and ISABELLE BOUCOT[2]

From the [1]Hôpital Bichat-Claude-Bernard, and [2]Hôpital Necker, Paris, France

Raw data from 4 clinical studies involving pre-inclusion paracentesis were pooled to assess demographic characteristics and clinical outcome of acute otitis media (AOM) due to S. pneumoniae with decreased susceptibility to penicillin (SpRP). Children in the age range 3 months to 10 years were treated with β-lactam antibiotics for 10 days. 54 children with SpRP AOM were compared with 182 children with penicillin-susceptible pneumococcal (SpSP) (AOM). The groups were found comparable with regard to sex, age at first AOM, and frequency of earlier bouts of AOM. SpRP AOM was significantly more frequent before age 18 months (40/54 versus 85/166 in the SpSP group; $p = 0.003$) and associated with more clinical failure on days 4–10 (10/54 versus 14/166; $p = 0.03$). These results suggest that the antibiotic treatment used to treat AOM in children under 18 months should be reconsidered in areas with a high incidence of SpRP.

B. Barry, MD, Service d'Oto-Rhino-Laryngologie, Hôpital Bichat-Claude Bernard, 46 rue Henri Huchard, F-75877 Paris cedex 18, France

INTRODUCTION

The emergence of pneumococci with decreased susceptibility to penicillin (SpRP) differs from one country to another, but it is on the increase in many parts of the world. It is associated with pharyngeal carriage serotypes and is a particularly frequent cause of upper respiratory tract infections in children. In Hungary, such strains accounted for 70% of all S. pneumoniae isolated from ear, nose, throat, and sinus swabs in 1988–89 (1). Similarly, they accounted for 33% of S. pneumoniae middle ear (ME) isolates in a children's hospital in the USA in 1989 (2) and for 22% of S. pneumoniae ME isolates in France in 1990 (3). Empirical treatment of acute otitis media (AOM) should take these strains into account, but multiresistance frequently limits the number of alternative oral antibiotics.

The clinical impact of S. pneumoniae with decreased susceptibility to penicillin in AOM is unknown. We therefore compared the demographic characteristics and clinical outcome in children with AOM due to SpRP with that in children with AOM caused by penicillin susceptible pneumococci.

PATIENTS AND METHODS

Enrolment and assignment

This study was based on raw data from 4 comparative phase III trials of β-lactams in pediatric AOM. The studies were randomized and compared an oral cephalosporin (cefprozil, cefposoxime-proxetil, ceftibuten, cefuroxime-axetil) with a reference drug (co-amoxiclav, cefaclor, and cefixime) in children over 3 months. In 2 studies the children were aged from 3 months to 10 years, whereas in the more recent studies only children from 6 months to 3 years were enrolled (Table I).

These consecutive studies were performed by the same investigators in Paris and its suburbs. The environmental conditions and sample collection, transport and culture were the same.

Ambulatory children with perulent AOM were included with their guardians' informed consent. AOM was diagnosed on the basis of otalgia, irritability and/or fever associated with a bulging tympanic membrane on otoscopic examination or, in the first 2 studies, with rupture of the tympanic membrane <24 h previously. Children who had received antibiotics in the month prior to enrolment, and those who had chronic otitis media with effusion or a history of hypersensitivity to β-lactams were excluded.

Table I. *Characteristics of the 4 clinical studies*

Study no.	Antibiotic evaluated	Comparative drug	No. of investigators	Total no. pats	Age range
1	Cefprozil	Co amoxi-clav	35	361	6 months–10 years
2	Cefpodoxime -proxetil	Co amoxi-clav	35	229	3 months–10 years
3	Ceftibuten	Cefaclor	28	287	6 months–3 years
4	Cefuroxime-axetil	Cefixime	30	215	6 months–3 years

Middle-ear sample collection

At enrolment, purulent middle-ear (ME) effusion was collected by paracentesis into a Teflon catheter after disinfection of the external auditory tract. In the first 2 studies, children with spontaneous otorrhea starting <24 h previously were included and accounted for 25% of samples. The catheter containing the ME aspirate was immediately transferred in transport medium (TGV Biomerieux) to the microbiology laboratory for culture. Bacterial isolates were identified by standard methods. Pneumococci were screened for penicillin susceptibility by the oxacillin disk diffusion method. A repeat sample was obtained if initial treatment failed.

Antibiotic susceptibility testing

The 54 SpRP and SpSP strains were selected on the basis of oxacillin resistance detected by using an oxacillin disk (5 μg). In the first study, penicillin resistance was screened for retrospectively and MICs to β-lactams and penicillin are not available. In the other studies MICs of benzyl penicillin and β-lactam agents for the corresponding strains were determined by an agar dilution method, using Mueller-Hinton agar supplemented with 5% horse blood. For MIC testing, suspensions with a turbidity equivalent to an 0.5 McFarland standard were prepared by suspending growth from blood agar plates in 5 ml brain–heart infusion broth. A final inoculum of 10^4–10^5 CFU/spot was applied to a blood–agar plate, using a Steers replicator and incubated overnight at 37°C in an atmosphere with 10% CO_2. Ten penicillin-susceptible strains as well as S. aureus ATCC 25923 and E. coli ATCC 25922 were included as quality control strains (4). The CMI was defined as the lowest antibiotic concentration which completely inhibited bacterial growth. Erythromycin susceptibility of the strains was not determined in study 2. The SpRP strains were serotyped by latex agglutination (Statens Serum Institute, Copenhagen, Denmark) in studies 3 and 4.

Treatment and follow-up

Antibiotics were randomly assigned and administered for 8–10 days. A phone contact was established on day 3–4 to evaluate the clinical outcome and to decide whether an intermediate visit was necessary; if so, a second ME sample was obtained and the antibiotic regimen was modified if clinical failure was apparent. All the children were evaluated clinically and otoscopically on day 10 after starting therapy. A clinical evaluation and a tympanometry were carried out on day 30. The results were categorized as follows:

On day 10:

–Clinical cure was defined as the disappearance of clinical symptoms and recovery of a normal otoscopic tympanic appearance.

–Improvement was defined by disappearance of clinical symptoms, but persistence of tympanic inflammation.

–Failure was defined by persistence of symptoms and a bulging tympanic membrane or otorrhea.

On day 30:

–Clinically satisfactory response: as defined on day 10.

–Early recurrence: clinical evidence of AOM with fever and pain and a bulging tympanic membrane, or

–disappearance of acute symptoms, but persistent ME effusion with a flat tympanometric curve.

Data analysis

We selected children with pneumococcal otitis media from the 4 studies. The children with otitis media due to SpRP were compared with the children with penicillin-susceptible (MIC < 0.1 μg/ml) pneumococcal otitis media. Demographic data were collected from case report forms and from questionnaires sent to parents. Treatment efficacy was based on clinical outcome on day 10 and on the persistence of ME effusion on day 30. One child in the SpRP group did not complete the treatment course because of adverse events and was not evaluable for clinical response. As the number of children in each treatment arm in the SpRP group was small, clinical outcome was evaluated for all the treatments as a whole. Clinical outcome was also stratified according to age. Isolation of >1 pathogen, the patients' history of otitis and day-care attendance were analysed on the basis of available data.

Results are expressed as means ± SD and the 95% confidence interval for n patients. Category data were analysed with the χ^2-test. Continuous data were analysed by comparison of the means. P-values ≤ 0.05 were considered significant.

RESULTS

Prevalence of SpRP AOM

The proportion of SpRP isolates in ME aspirates gradually increased from one study to the next (Table II) to 37% in the last study, performed in 1991–92.

During the course of the 4 studies, 236 children had a pneumococcal AOM. 182 isolates were penicillin-susceptible and 54 had decreased susceptibility to penicillin.

Demographic characteristics (Table III)

The mean age in the SpRP group was 19 ± 16 months (CI 95%: 13.2–22.4). Children in this group were significantly younger than those in the SpSP group. 74% were <18 months old, compared with only 51% in the SpSP group ($p = 0.003$) (Table IV). Day-care attendance was not significantly more frequent in the SpRP group ($p = 0.06$). There was no difference between the 2 groups in terms of the sex ratio, age at first AOM, or the number of episodes of AOM in the previous 12 months. 12/30 children (40%) in the SpRP group and 29/68 (30%) in the SpSP group had their first episode of AOM during the study ($p = 0.81$).

Circumstances of Sp isolation

SpSP were isolated from ME effusion before initiation of therapy. Only 1 child had an early recurrence, during which an SpSP was isolated. SpRP were isolated from ME effusion before initiation of therapy in 54 children. During the 4 studies, 4 SpRP were isolated after the

Table II. *Incidence and age of children with pneumococcal acute otitis media in the studies*

Period	Cases of pneumococcal AOM[b]	Cases of SpRP[a] n	(%)	Mean age ±SD (months) [CI 95%]
Nov 89–May 90	50	7	(14)	28 ± 21 [21.2–34.0]
June 90–Oct 90	40	7	(18)	40 ± 26 [31.6–48.2]
Nov 90–Oct 91	75	15	(20)	17 ± 9 [15.1–19.5]
Nov 91–May 92	67	25	(37)	15 ± 8 [13.3–7.1]

[a] Pneumococci with decreased penicillin susceptibility.
[b] Acute otitis media.

Table III. *Demographic data according to penicillin susceptibility*

	SpRP	SpSP	p
Age < 18 months	74% (n = 54)	51% (n = 166)	0.003
Sex ratio (M/F)	1 (n = 54)	1.16 (n = 166)	0.63
Age at first AOM (months)	8.9 ± 3.6 (n = 31)	9.8 ± 4.6 (n = 67)	1
Day-care attendance	72% (n = 42)	56% (n = 108)	0.06
No. of AOM in previous 12 months	1.6 ± 1.6 (n = 42)	1.4 ± 1.5 (n = 108)	0.37

Table IV. *Age distribution of penicillin-resistant (SpRP) and susceptible (SpSP) strains*

Age (months)	SpRP n (%)	SpSP n (%)
6–12	28 (52)	55 (33)
12–18	12 (22)	30 (18)
18–24	5 (9)	13 (8)
24–36	5 (9)	35 (21)
36–60	2 (4)	13 (8)
60–124	2 (4)	20 (12)
Total	54 (100)	166 (100)

initiation of therapy, 2 on the seventh day of therapy with cephalosporins, one 7 days after the end of treatment with a cephalosporin, and one 9 days after the end of treatment with co-amoxiclav.

SpRP was the only pathogen isolated in ME effusion from 30 children (56%). Other pathogens were associated in 24 cases (44%), of which Haemophilus influenzae was the most common (16/21: 76%, 38% of which were β-lactamase producers). Only 1 associated pathogen, a Pseudomonas aeruginosa, was resistant to the allocated regimen. SpSP strains were associated with other pathogens in 74 of the 166 samples (45%). The proportions of infections with more than 1 agent were thus comparable in the 2 groups ($p = 0.98$). Haemophilus influenzae was also the pathogen most frequently associated (48/72) with SpSP otitis, and only 25% of strains were β-lactamase producers.

Microbiological data

Among SpRP strains, 31/47 (66%) were erythromycin resistant, whereas only 46/133 (35%) of SpSP strains were erythromycin resistant ($p = 0.0002$). Available data on MICs of SpRP strains to penicillin and to the cephalosporins studied are detailed in Table V. Five serotypes were recovered among 40 SpRP strains tested. The predominant serotypes were 23 (60%), 9 (15%) 19 (13%), 14 (8%), and 6(5%).

Clinical outcome

The 2 children from whom SpRP was isolated during treatment were cured after a change in antibiotic regimen on day 7. The 2 children with early recurrence of SpRP were cured

Table V. *MICs (μg/ml) of SpRP strains to penicillin and β-lactams studied*

No. of strains with MIC

Study		0.06	0.125	0.25	0.5	1	2	4	8	16	32	64
	Penicillin	–	1	3	1	1	1	–	–	–	–	–
2	Amoxicillin	–	3	2	–	1	1	–	–	–	–	–
	Cefpodoxime--proxetil	–	2	–	4	–	–	1	–	–	–	–
	Penicillin	–	4	2	5	3	1	–	–	–	–	–
3	Cefaclor	–	–	–	–	3	1	3	1	2	5	–
	Ceftibuten	–	–	–	–	–	–	–	–	2	3	10
	Penicillin	–	4	3	1	5	11	1	–	–	–	–
4	Cefuroxime--axetil	1	1	3	2	5	2	10	1	–	–	–
	Cefixime	–	–	2	–	2	1	3	4	13	–	–

Table VI. *Efficacy of β-lactams in the treatment of AOM caused by pneumococci with decreased susceptibility to penicillin and susceptible pneumococci*

	SpRP AOM	SpSP AOM	*p*
Failures	10/53 (19%)	14/166 (8%)	0.03
Otitis media with effusion on day 30	13/43 (30%)	32/152 (21%)	0.21

without changing the treatment. Among 53 clinically evaluable children from whom SpRP were isolated before starting treatment, 43 were cured or improved by day 10. Clinical failure occurred in 10 cases (19%), between day 4 and day 10. A repeat aspiration was performed in only 3 cases, yielding SpRP in 2 cases and Pseudomonas aeruginosa in 1 (previously associated with SpRP). A clinical cure was obtained after a change in treatment in 6 cases and with no change in 3. One of these patients was lost to follow-up. Most (9/10) clinical failures occurred in children <18 months of age and the mean age of the children in whom treatment failed was 13 ± 8 months.

The clinical response was significantly better in the SpSP group in which treatment only failed in 8% of cases (14/166) (Table VI). The mean age of the children in whom treatment failed was 11 ± 6 months in this group. Among the children aged ≤ 18 months, the rate of clinical failure was 23% in the SpRP group and 15% in the SpSP group ($p = 0.29$).

Persistent ME effusion on day 30, despite clinical improvement on day 10, was observed in 13/43 cases (30%; mean age: 22 ± 26 months) in the SpRP group, and 32/152 (21%; mean age: 20 ± 12) in the SpSP group.

DISCUSSION

The increasing prevalence of penicillin-resistant S. pneumoniae in AOM in the 4 successive studies is in keeping with the results of epidemiological studies published by the French Centre National de Reference du Pneumocoque (5). However, our results reflect the epidemiology in Paris and its suburbs, and probably over-estimate the incidence of SpRP in France as a whole.

The analysis of demographic data suggests that SpRP are preferentially isolated from children <18 months. Day-care attendance is a well-known risk factor for AOM and seems to be involved in infection by penicillin-resistant strains, whereas a past history of otitis does not. SpRP are strongly associated with carriage serotypes and their pathogenicity could be discussed. The results of this study support a causal role of these strains in AOM, as the frequency of multiple pathogens in ME effusion was similar in the 2 groups. Moreover, clinical failure occurred even when SpRP was the only organism isolated. In only 1 case was the failure related to an associated pathogen, a Pseudomonas aeruginosa resistant to the allocated treatment.

The rate of failure of β-lactam therapy was significantly greater when a penicillin-resistant strain was involved. These results suggest that β-lactam antibiotics are not suitable for the treatment of penicillin-resistant pneumococcal AOM. However they consider β-lactams as a whole and do not take into account the differences between compounds with regard to penicillin-resistance suggested by microbiological data (6). The dosages of antibiotics administered in these studies are those recommended by French regulatory authorities under standard conditions. Data from animal studies suggest that moderately increased dosages, especially of amoxicillin, could be sufficient to treat penicillin-resistant AOM (7), but clinical confirmation is necessary.

The poor efficacy of treatment in the SpRP group could also be related to the lower age of the children in the SpRP group, as young age is a risk factor for failure (8). However, when only children <18 months were considered, the rate of clinical failure tended to be higher in the SpRP group (23% vs. 15%); although this difference was not statistically significant ($p = 0.19$) it is of value in the context of AOM, where self-limited infection can be a limiting factor when studying treatment efficacy (9).

Persistent ME effusion did not appear to be age-related. It seemed more common in the SpRP group, but no statistical difference could be found.

CONCLUSION

Penicillin-resistant pneumococcal AOM is associated with a higher risk of clinical failure after β-lactam treatment than is SpSP AOM. These strains are more frequently encountered in children <18 months of age and are associated with more clinical failures at this age. It is therefore probably necessary to adapt empirical treatment of AOM in children <18 months in areas where the prevalence of SpRP is high. Clinical and experimental studies of higher dosages of β-lactams and other families of antibiotics are required in this context.

REFERENCES

1. Marton A, Gulyas M, Munoz R, Tomasz A. Extremely high incidence of antibiotic resistance in clinical isolates of Streptococcus pneumoniae in Hungary. J Infect Dis 163: 542–548, 1991.
2. Ford LK, Mason EO, Kaplan SL, Lamberth LB, Tillmanand J. Factors associated with middle ear isolates of Streptococcus pneumoniae resistant to penicillin in a children's hospital. J Pediatr 119: 941–944, 1991.
3. Geslin P, Fremaux A, Sissia G. Evolution de la résistance des pneumocoques responsables des infections des voies respiratoires en France. Med Mal Infect 22 spécial: 74–86, 1992.
4. Boucot I., Poyart-Salmeron C., Bingen E., Lambert-Zechowsky N., Berche P., Veron M. In vitro activity of 9 oral and parenteral B-lactam agents against penicillin resistant pneumococci isolated from community-acquired acute otitis media. 32nd Interscience Conference of Antimicrobial and Chemotherapy, Poster no. 1026, Anaheim, 1992.

5. Société de Pathologie Infectieuse de Langue Française (SPILF). Fourth Consensus Conference on Antimicrobial Therapy: respiratory tract infections. Med Mal Inf 22: 47–50, 1992.
6. Michel J, Dickman D, Greenberg Z, Bergner-Rabinowitz S. Serotype distribution of penicillin-resistant pneumococci and their susceptibilities to seven antimicrobial agents. Antimicrob Agents Chemother 23: 397–401, 1983.
7. Barry B, Muffat-Joly M, Gehanno P, Pocidalo JJ. Increased dosage of amoxicillin in the treatment of experimental middle ear otitis due to penicillin-resistant streptococcus pneumoniae. Antimicrob Agents Chemother 37: 1599–1603, 1993.
8. Harsten G, Prellner K, Heldrup J. Treatment failure in acute otitis media. A clinical study of children during their first three years of life. Acta Otolaryngol (Stockh) 108: 253–258, 1989.
9. Marchant CD, Carlin SA, Johnson CE, Shurin PA. Measuring the comparative efficacy of antibacterial agents for acute otitis media: "the Pollyanna phenomenon". J Pediatr 120: 72–77, 1992.

Submitted January 10, 1994; accepted March 27, 1994

Scand J Infect Dis 26: 453–457, 1994

Effect of Erythromycin Treatment on Antibody Responses in Pertussis

GUNNAR GRANSTRÖM[1] and MARTA GRANSTRÖM[2]

From the Departments of [1]Infectious Diseases, Danderyd Hospital, Danderyd, and [2]Clinical Microbiology, Karolinska Hospital, Stockholm, Sweden

The effect of erythromycin treatment on antibody responses to Bordetella pertussis filamentous haemagglutinin (FHA) and pertussis toxin (PT) was investigated in convalescent blood samples from 105 children with pertussis. Erythromycin had been given to 59 children, median age 3.2 years (range 0.3–9.9) on median day 7 (range 11–14) after onset of disease while the remaining 46 children, age 3.45 (0.6–8.1) were untreated. No significant differences in IgG antibody concentration were noted to FHA by ELISA and to PT, neither by NT nor by ELISA, but a tendency towards lower median titers was seen to both antigens and by both type of assays in the erythromycin-treated group. Similarly, early erythromycin treatment i.e. within 7 days of onset of symptoms, did not influence significantly of the development of the antibody responses but tended to lead to lower titer levels. A significant response to PT and FHA was found in about 90% of blood samples, irrespective of treatment. All 56 children with culture-confirmed B. pertussis infection had a significant response to PT. The study has thus shown a slight but not significant effect of erythromycin treatment on antibody responses in pertussis.

G. Granström, MD, PhD, Department of Infectious Diseases, Danderyd Hospital, S-182 88 Danderyd, Sweden

INTRODUCTION

Erythromycin is the most commonly used antibiotic therapy against Bordetella pertussis. The drug is generally considered to be efficient in clearing the bacterium from the nasopharynx (1–3). When given to full blown clinical cases, erythromycin has been found inefficient to change the clinical course in all but one study (1, 2, 4–6). The effect of erythromycin given in early stages of the disease or as prophylaxis might be more benefical but the effect is questioned, due to conflicting outcome in clinical studies (4, 7, 8).

Eradication of the B. pertussis from the nasopharynx represents a mean of reducing transmission of the disease on an individual basis. Antibiotic treatment and prophylaxis of contacts to proven or suspected cases of perussis has been recommended (9, 10). In Sweden with no general immunisation against pertussis since 1979, erythromycin therapy represents an important part of the strategy to minimise B. pertussis exposure of infants, the group with the highest rate of severe disease (10). Erythromycin to infants below 6 months of age is recommended as prophylaxis upon suspicion of exposure and as treatment for clinical disease recognised as pertussis. Treatment of infants 6–12 months of age is recommended for clinical disease alone while above 12 months of age, treatment is recommended only if the child could be a source of infection for an infant.

The concern that erythromycin treatment, especially when given early, will inhibit or decrease antibody responses to B. pertussis antigens is common. The aim of the present study was, therefore, to investigate the antibody responses to 2 major antigens of B. pertussis, pertussis toxin and filamentous haemagglutinin, in children with pertussis in relation to erythromycin treatment.

MATERIALS AND METHODS

Patients

The patients were identified in an earlier study to have pertussis by positive culture and/or serology (11, 12). In that study, 300 patients presenting with cough and with clinical or epidemiological indications of pertussis were included and 163 patients were diagnosed to have pertussis by nasopharyngeal culture and/or serology in paired blood samples. The serological diagnosis was based on significant titer rises to B. pertussis FHA, PT and lipopolysaccharide (LPS). The study population in the present investigation was restricted to children and to those with a disease duration of ≤ 14 days at the first visit and, for the erythromycin-treated group, to treatment given within ≤ 14 days after onset of symptoms (including 2 cases treated prior to symptoms). The median (range) age of these 105 children was 3.3 years (0.3–9.9) and the first visit with blood sampling was made on median day 7 (range 1–14, mean ± SD 7.3 ± 3.5) after onset of symptoms, as stated by the parents. The second, convalescent blood sample was drawn on median day 47 (range 34–138, mean ± SD 51.6 ± 16.6) after onset of disease.

Erythromycin treatment

Erythromycin aethyl succinate was given in a dose of 40 mg/ kg of body weight/day for 10 days.

Antibody assays

Enzyme-linked immunosorbent assay (ELISA). Purified pertussis toxin (1 μg/ ml) and FHA (2 μg/ ml) were used as antigens and serum samples were screened at a 1 : 500 dilution (11). Further dilutions were made by 2-fold dilution steps when necessary. ELISA IgG titers were expressed as the mean A 405 value of triplicate determinations multiplied by the serum dilution factor. A significant titer rise was defined as at lease a 2-fold change in titers between the 2 samples.

Neutralisation test (NT)

Two-fold patient serum dilutions from an initial 1 : 2 dilution and 4 cytopathogenic units of PT were used (11). After a 3-hour incubation of the mixture, Chinese hamster ovary (CHO) cells were added and the plates incubated for 48 h. The neutralising effect of antibodies on the clustering induced by PT was read in an inverted microscope. The neutralisation titers were expressed as the reciprocal of the highest serum dilution giving a 100% neutralisation of the clustering. A significant titer rise was defined as at least a 4-fold increase between samples.

Statistical analysis

Comparisons were made by Mann-Whitney's rank-sum test.

RESULTS

Erythromycin treatment had been given to 59 children on median day 7 (range day 11–14) of illness while the 46 remaining children were untreated. The age of the treated children was 3.2 (0.3–9.9) years and of the untreated was 3.45 (0.6–8.1) ($p = 0.2345$). The diagnosis was confirmed by culture in 40 patients in the erythromycin group and in 18 patients in the untreated group (including 1 case of B. parapertussis in each group), respectively ($p = 0.005$). The convalescent blood samples were drawn on median day 46 (range 35–121) and 50.5 (34–138) after onset of disease for the treated and untreated groups, respectively ($p = 0.1776$).

The response to pertussis toxin measured by NT and ELISA and to filamentous haemagglutinin by ELISA are shown in Table I. A comparison between titer levels showed no significant effect of erythromycin on the antibody concentrations in the convalescent samples. 12 (11.4%) of the 105 children (including the 2 cases of B. parpertussis infection) had no significant response to PT by neither NT nor ELISA, 5/59 in the treated group and 7/46 in the untreated group (data not shown). 11 (10.4%) children showed no significant response to FHA, 6/59 in the treated group and 5/46 in the untreated group.

Confining the analysis to only children with culture-confirmed B. pertussis infection, the 39 treated children had a median age of 3.7 years and the 17 untreated children of 3.8 years and the convalescent samples were drawn on median day 42 in both groups. The median anti-PT response by NT was 8 (range <2–512) in the treated group while untreated children had a median of 32 (range <2–256) ($p = 0.4634$). The corresponding data for anti-PT by ELISA was 2,240 (125–32,640) and 4,560 (300–27,840) ($p = 0.2256$) and for anti-FHA 125 (25–

Table I. *Effect of erythromycin treatment on antibody responses to B. pertussis antigens in children with ≤ 14 days of disease at the first visit*

Erythromycin treatment	No.	IgG antibody titers in convalescent blood samples: Pertussis toxin (PT) Neutralisation test (NT) Median (range)	Pertussis toxin (PT) ELISA Median (range)	Filamentous haemagglutinin (FHA) ELISA Median (range)
Yes[a]	59	8 (<2–512)	1000 (20–32,640)	130 (20–5,600)
No	46	16 (<2–1,024)	1000 (40–27,840)	187.5 (20–2,160)
p value		0.0675	0.8156	0.2221

[a] Treatment given ≤ 14 days after onset of symptoms.

5,600) and 210 (45–1420), respectively ($p = 0.1783$). All children in both groups had a significant antibody response to PT by NT and/or ELISA while 5 children (4 in the treatment group) had no significant anti-FHA response.

In order to further investigate the possible negative effects of erythromycin treatment on antibody responses, analysis was restricted to children treated within ≤ 7 days after onset of disease in the erythromycin group. The 37 treated children had median antibody concentrations to PT by NT of 8 (<2–512) ($p = 0.2314$), by ELISA of 1000 (40–16160) ($p = 0.8036$) and to FHA by 150 (25–5,600) ($p = 0.4524$) in their convalescent sample as compared to the untreated group (Table I).

The subgroup with a disease duration of ≤ 7 days and treated within ≤ 7 days of illness, is shown in Table II. No significant differences were found. Finally, an analysis within the group of treated children, comparing those ($n = 37$) who had received erythromycin ≤ 7 days after onset of disease to those ($n = 22$) who had received treatment > 7 days after onset showed no significant differences in antibody levels in the convalescent samples, with p values ranging from 0.3084 (for NT to PT) and 0.9375 (for ELISA to PT).

Table II. *Effect of erythromycin treatment on antibody responses to B. pertussis antigens in children with ≤ 7 days of disease at the first visit*

Erythromycin treatment	No.	IgG antibody titers in convalescent blood samples: Pertussis toxin (PT) Neutralisation test (NT) Median (range)	Pertussis toxin (PT) ELISA Median (range)	Filamentous haemagglutinin (FHA) ELISA Median (range)
Yes[a]	36	8 (<2–512)	1000 (40–16,160)	145 (25–5,600)
No	26	8 (<2–1,024)	990 (40–10,080)	207.5 (20–2,160)
p value		0.8109	0.3599	0.1304

[a] Treatment given ≤ 7 days after onset of symptoms.

DISCUSSION

The present study has compared the antibody responses to 2 major antigens of B. pertussis in convalescent sera from 105 children with pertussis where 1 group of 59 children was treated with erythromycin and the other group of 46 children was untreated. No significant differences in response rates or titer levels were found.

The present study can be criticized for being open and non-randomised but the ideal placebo-controlled, double blind design is excluded for ethical reasons. We have, however, tried to avoid introducing a bias by including only children and only with the same and short disease duration prior to medical contact. A comparison was also made in the smaller, culture-confirmed group of children with B. pertussis infection and showed the same results as in the main study group. With these precautions, the risks for a bias in the study should at least be minimised.

Our finding of an anti-PT response in about 90% of patients, irrespective of treatment, indicates that this response is not inhibited by erythromycin but that such a response is not invariably present in all cases of pertussis. The question whether erythromycin treatment, especially when given early, will inhibit antibody responses to B. pertussis antigens has been addressed in a few earlier studies. We have reported a case of reinfection in an erythromycin-treated patient with no anti-PT response (13). Others have also described cases, both treated and untreated, with no response to PT (14, 15). Zackrisson et al. found an anti-PT response in 90% and 84% of treated and untreated pertussis patients of all age groups, respectively (16).

The height of antibody responses to PT and FHA in relation to antibiotic treatment has, to our knowledge, not been investigated earlier. We found no definite effect of erythromycin treatment on titer levels but did note a trend towards lower titers. If high antibody concentrations will result in a longer protection, then the finding may have some clinical relevance but even in such a case, a lack of significant differences indicate that the effect might be small.

The issue of antibodies and protective antibody concentrations against B. pertussis is still somewhat unclear but most studies support the view that the 2 antibody responses investigated in the present study are the most important in pertussis. With regard to the relative importance of the 2 antibody responses, a comparison of antibodies in predisease samples from adults with pertussis to age-matched controls showed that antibodies to both PT and FHA were significantly lower in the predisease samples of the patients (17). Titer distribution, however, was significantly lower only to PT, indicating a major role for this antibody in protection. Other studies, comparing reports of clinical pertussis to antibody concentrations, also indicate that antibodies to PT are better correlated to clinical disease and, presumably, to protection than antibodies to FHA, which could also reflect infection with B. parapertussis (18, 19).

In conclusion, we have found no signs of inhibited antibody responses to pertussis toxin (PT) and filamentous haemagglutinin (FHA) by erythromycin treatment in children with pertussis and no significant differences in antibody concentrations in the convalescent samples. On the other hand, there was a trend towards lower antibody levels in the treatment group and the need for treatment has to be weighted also against further negative effects of erythromycin i.e. the problem of resistance in other respiratory pathogens.

REFERENCES

1. Bass JW, Klenk EL, Kotheimer JB, Linnemann CC, Smith MHD. Antimicrobial treatment of pertussis. J Pediatr 75: 768–781, 1969.
2. Baraff LJ, Wilkins J, Wehrle PF. The role of antibiotics, immunizations and adenoviruses in pertussis. Pediatrics 61: 224–230, 1978.

3. Trollfors B. Effect of erythromycin and amoxycillin on Bordetella pertussis in the nasopharynx. Infection 6: 228–230, 1978.
4. Halsey N, Welling MA, Lehman RM. Nosocomial pertussis: A failure of erythromycin treatment and prophylaxis. Am J Dis Child 134: 521–522, 1980.
5. Henry RL, Dorman DC, Skinner JA, Mellis CM. Antimicrobial therapy in whooping cough. Med J Aust 2: 27–28, 1981.
6. Bergquist S-O, Bernander S, Dahnsjö H, Sundelöf B. Erythromycin in the treatment of pertussis: a study of bacteriologic and clinical effects. Ped Infect Dis J 6: 458–461, 1987.
7. Altemeier WA, Ayoub EM. Erythromycin prophylaxis for pertussis. Pediatrics 59: 623–625, 1977.
8. Granström G, Sterner G, Nord C-E, Granström M. Use of erythromycin to prevent pertussis in newborns of mothers with pertussis. J Infect Dis 155: 1210–1214, 1987.
9. Linnemann CC, Nasenbeny J. Pertussis in the adult. Ann Rev Med 28: 179–185, 1977.
10. Trollfors B. Whooping cough-aspects of pathogenesis and treatment. Acta Otolaryngol 407: 33–39, 1984.
11. Granström G, Wretlind B, Salenstedt CR, Granström M. Evaluation of serologic assays for diagnosis of whooping cough. J Clin Microbiol 26: 1818–1823, 1988.
12. Granström G, Wretlind B, Granström M. Diagnostic value of clinical and bacteriological findings in pertussis. J Infection 22: 17–26, 1991.
13. Granström M, Granström G, Gillenius P, Askelöf P. Neutralizing antibodies to pertussis toxin in whooping cough. J Infect Dis 151: 646–649, 1985.
14. Burstyn DG, Baraff LJ, Peppler MS, Leake RD, St. Geme Jr., J, Manclark CR. Serological response to filamentous hemagglutinin and lymphocytosis-promoting toxin of Bordetella pertussis. Infect Immun 41: 1150–1156, 1983.
15. Trollfors B, Krantz I, Sigurs N, Taranger J, Zackrisson G, Roberson R. Toxin-neutralizing antibodies in patients with pertussis, as determined by an assay using Chinese hamster ovary cells. J Infect Dis 158: 991–998, 1988.
16. Zackrisson G, Krantz I, Lagergård T, Larsson P, Sekura R, Sigurs N, Taranger J, Trollfors B. Antibody response to pertussis toxin in patients with clinical pertussis measured by enzyme-linked immunosorbent assay. Eur J Clin Microbiol Infect Dis 7: 149–154, 1988.
17. Granström M, Granström G. Serological correlates in whooping cough. Vaccine 11: 445–448, 1993.
18. Zackrisson G, Krantz I, Lagergård T, Larsson P, Sekura R, Taranger J and Trollfors B. Antibody response to pertussis toxin in patients with clinical pertussis measured by enzyme-linked immunosorbent assay. Eur J Clin Microbiol Infect Dis 7: 149–154, 1988.
19. Mark A, Granström M. Cumulative incidence of pertussis in an unvaccinated preschool cohort based on notifications, interview and serology. Eur J Epidemiol 7: 121–126, 1991.

Submitted February 22, 1994; accepted April *25, 1994*

Scand J Infect Dis 26: 459–467, 1994

Immunity from Diphtheria, Tetanus, Poliomyelitis, Measles, Mumps and Rubella among Adults in Lithuania

BO ANDREASSEN RIX[1], ALFONSAS ZHOBAKAS[3], CARSTEN HENRIK WACHMANN[2], VYTAUTAS BAKASENAS[4] and TOVE RØNNE[1]

From the Departments of [1]Epidemiology and [2]Biostatistics, Statens Seruminstitut, Copenhagen, Denmark, the [3]Center of Hygiene, Panevezyr and the [4]Republican Immunization Centre, Vilnius, Lithuania

Health authorities have estimated a low immunity level against diphtheria, tetanus, poliomyelitis, measles, mumps and rubella among adults in Lithuania due to less than optimal vaccine quality. The aim of this study was to evaluate the level of immunity by blood sampling 100 young women, 50 young men and 50 middle-aged men and from the immunization history by questionnaire. Lack of protection against diphtheria was found in 0%, 2% and 46% of the young women, young men and middle-aged men respectively. The corresponding data for tetanus were 0%, 0% and 10%. It was found that 85% of the women had antibodies to all 3 types of polioviruses vs. 80% of the young men and 56% of the middle-aged men. A sub-protective antibody level against measles was found in 12% of the women, 22% of the young men, but in none of the middle-aged men. A protective titre of rubella antibodies was found among 94% of the young, pregnant women. It can be concluded that the level of immunity in Lithuania is comparable to that in Western Europe for the same age groups and that the launching of adult vaccination programs in Eastern Europe should be preceded by sero-epidemiological studies.

B. Andreassen Rix, MD, Department of Epidemiology, Statens Seruminstitut, Artillerivej 5, DK-2300 Copenhagen S, Denmark

INTRODUCTION

In Lithuania, diphtheria-pertussis-tetanus vaccine was introduced in 1956, oral polio vaccine (OPV) in 1957, measles vaccine in 1964 and mumps vaccine in 1985. Vaccination against rubella has not been a part of the routine program and implementation of a vaccination program against rubella is considered very urgent by the health authorities. All vaccines used in the immunization program in Lithuania have until recently (1991) been purchased in the former USSR. As the potency of these vaccines was considered to be low, the vaccination program until 1991 consisted of 22 vaccinations at 18 different ages.

The incidences of the diseases vaccinated against were only: 6 cases of diphtheria, 13 of tetanus and 2,279 of measles in the 5-year period 1987–91 and no cases of poliomyelitis since 1972, in a population of approx. 4 million. However, vaccination coverage among children in Lithuania has declined during recent years. Vaccination coverage against measles has declined among children aged 1 year from 94% in 1988 to 86% in 1991, against diphtheria and tetanus (3 doses) from 86% to 75% and against polio (3 doses) from 84% to 80% (1, 2). It has been estimated that in 1992 only 73–78% of children were immunized against these diseases before the age of 1 (2).

Against this background and a higher prevalence of some of these diseases in neighbouring countries, the health authorities in Lithuania have now adopted a national immunoprophylaxis program in accordance with the recommendations of the World Health Organization (3). According to this program, a first 2-year-period will be used to summarize the results of immunoprophylactic efforts, to decide on a monitoring system for immunization and to organize a cold chain vaccine supply. Revaccination against tetanus at 26, 36, 46 and 56 years of age, against diphtheria in areas where the disease is reported among adults and vaccination of girls against rubella at 16–17 years of age are being considered.

The aim of the present study was to assess immunity from and immunization levels against diphtheria, tetanus, poliomyelitis, measles, mumps and rubella among adults as a background to recommendations for vaccination programs.

MATERIALS AND METHODS

Serum samples from 100 young, pregnant women and 50 middle-aged men (policemen) at local health centres in Vilnius and from 50 young men at a military camp 100 km outside Vilnius, Lithuania were sent to Statens Seruminstitut in Copenhagen, Denmark, for analysis. The sera were tested for antibodies to measles, mumps and rubella by in-house ELISA tests developed at Statens Seruminstitut. Samples were considered positive for rubella IgG antibodies if they had ≥ 15 IU/ml. The serum concentration of diphtheria antitoxin was determined by an in vitro neutralization assay, while the serum concentration of tetanus antitoxin was determined by a modified ELISA (4). A serum antitoxin concentration of 0.01 IU/ml was considered protective. Sera were tested for neutralizing antibodies to polio virus types 1, 2 and 3, and a titre of 1 : 4 was considered protective. At the time of blood sampling, a questionnaire was completed concerning sex, age and previous vaccination against measles, diphtheria, tetanus and poliomyelitis as reported by the test person or documented in vaccination records. A history of measles, mumps, rubella, diphtheria, tetanus and poliomyelitis as well as age at vaccination or disease were also recorded.

STATISTICAL ANALYSIS

The χ^2-test and Fisher's test were used to evaluate differences in immunity in different test groups and regression analysis was used to evaluate immunity as a function of time since the previous vaccination. The significance level chosen was 5%.

RESULTS

The median age in the study groups was 22.4 years (range: 20–27 years) for the young women, 19.5 years (range: 19–22) for the young men and 44.9 years (range: 39–54) for the middle-aged men.

Vaccination against and immunity to diphtheria and tetanus

97% of young women and 92% of young men reported or had documented records of having been vaccinated 4 times or more against both diseases. 2% of women reported 1–3 vaccinations, while 1% of women and 8% of young men reported no vaccination at all, $p =$ n.s. Middle-aged men reported significantly fewer vaccinations: 0–2 against diphtheria and 0–3 against tetanus, $p < 0.00001$. Young women had vaccination records for ≥ 1 vaccination in 20% of cases, versus 10% among young men and 0% among middle-aged men ($p < 0.05$ *versus* women).

Titres of serum antitoxin against diphtheria and tetanus are presented in Figs. 1 and 2. No young women and 2% of the young men had a serum diphtheria antitoxin concentration below protective level (0.01 IU/ml). Middle-aged men had significantly lower protection, as 46% had a diphtheria antitoxin concentration below protective level, $p < 0.00001$. Also significantly more middle-aged men (32%) had serum diphtheria antitoxin concentrations between 0.01 and 0.1 IU/ml, compared with young women (24%) and young men (6%), $p < 0.005$. Comparing young women and young men, significantly more women had titres below 0.1 IU/ml, $p < 0.05$.

None of the young age groups had an antibody titre against tetanus below the protective level (0.01 IU/ml), while significantly more middle-aged men (10%) had titres below this level, $p = 0.002$. Also significantly more middle-aged men (46%) had titres between 0.01 and 0.1 IU/ml compared with young women (9%) and young men (4%), $p < 0.00001$.

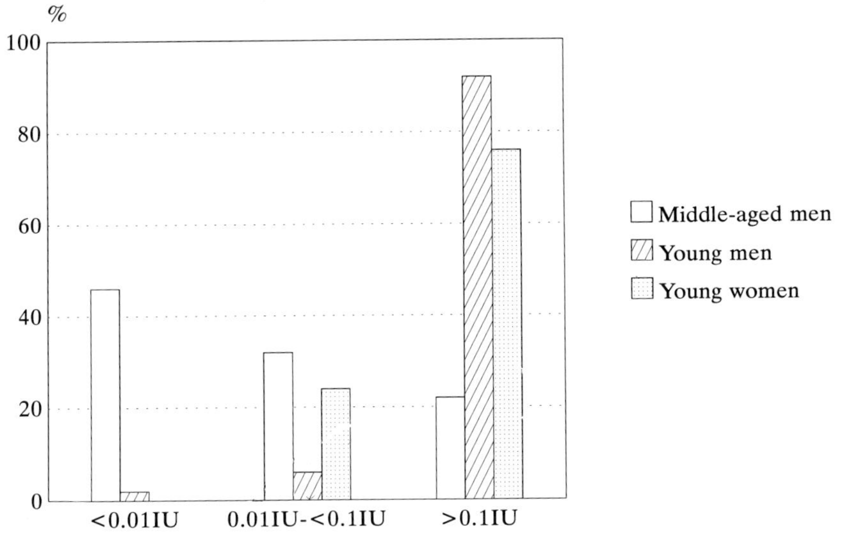

Fig. 1. Distribution of diphtheria antitoxin titres by age and sex. A titre <0.01 IU/ml is considered unprotective.

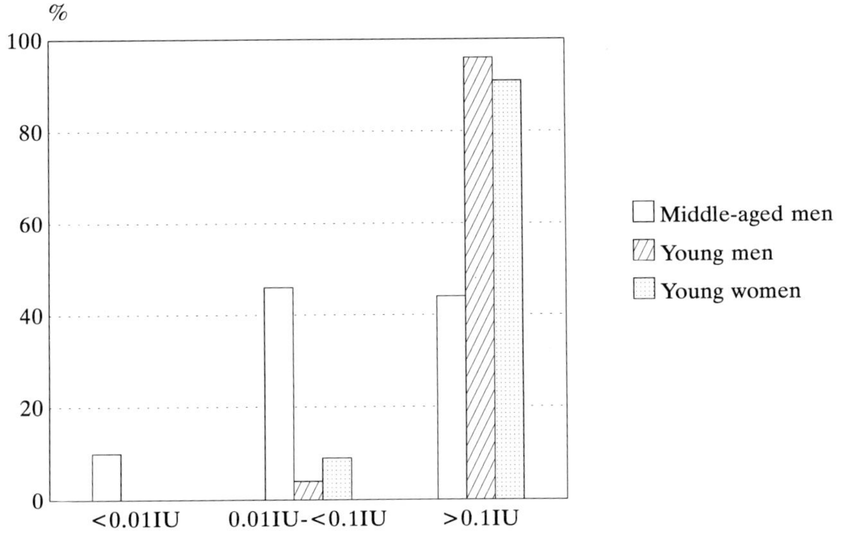

Fig. 2. Distribution of tetanus antitoxin titres by age and sex. A titre <0.01 IU/ml is considered unprotective.

Figs. 3 and 4 show titres of antibodies in relation to time since previous diphtheria and tetanus vaccinations. The median interval for both was 7.9 years in young women (range: 5–20 years) and 4.4 years in young men (range: 2–8), $p = 0.0001$. Among middle-aged men, the median interval since last vaccination was 29.1 years (range: 24–35) against diphtheria and 26.7 years (range 21–34) against tetanus. Within each group the antibody titres against

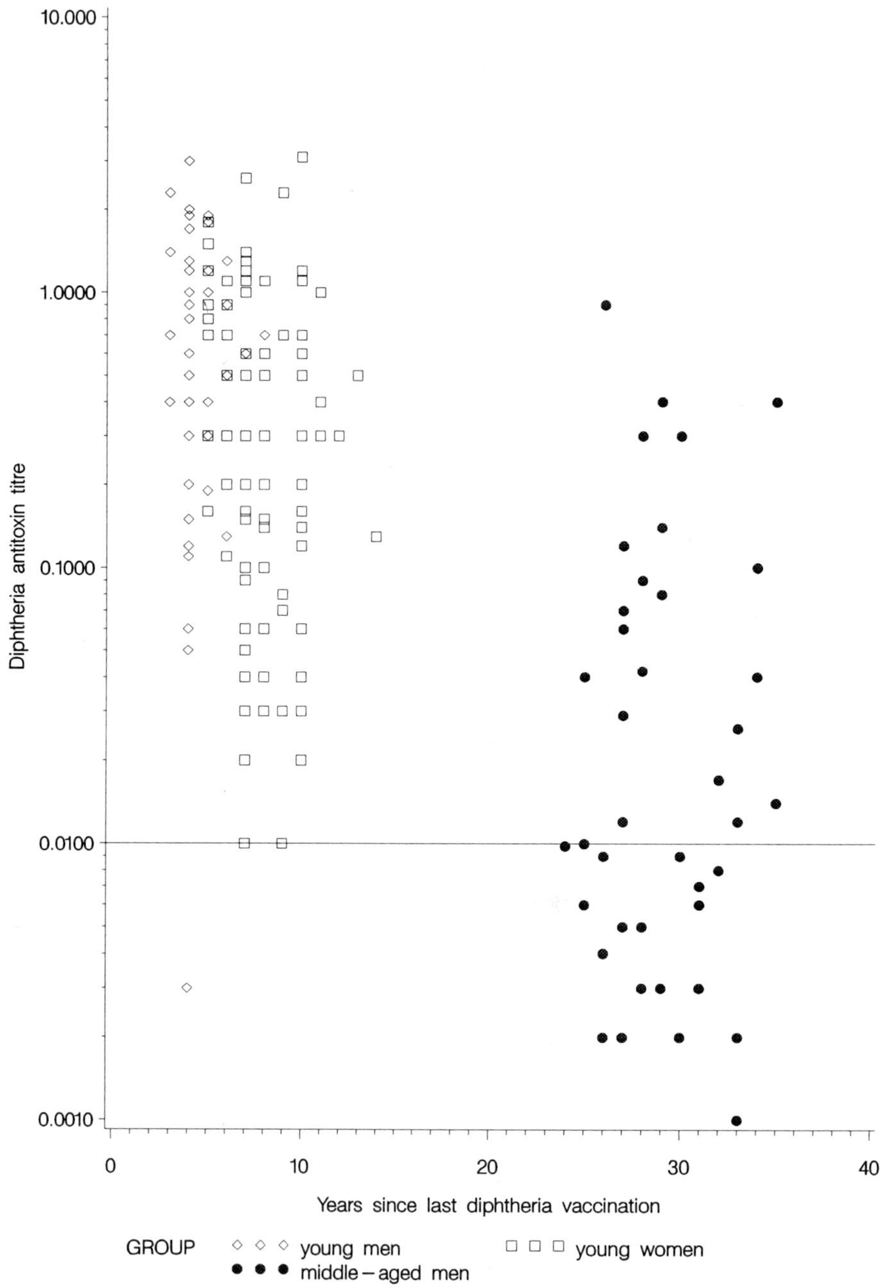

Fig. 3. Diphtheria antitoxin titre in relation to interval since latest diphtheria vaccination. A titre <0.01 IU/ml is considered unprotective.

diphtheria and tetanus did not vary significantly over time since last vaccination, but vis-à-vis pregnant young women and young men with the same number of vaccinations together, the titre of antibodies to diphtheria did fall significantly over time, $p < 0.05$. This was not the case when comparing the titre of antibodies to tetanus.

Regression analysis comparing all groups together showed a significant decline in antibody titre against diphtheria and tetanus in relation to time since last vaccination, $p = 0.0001$.

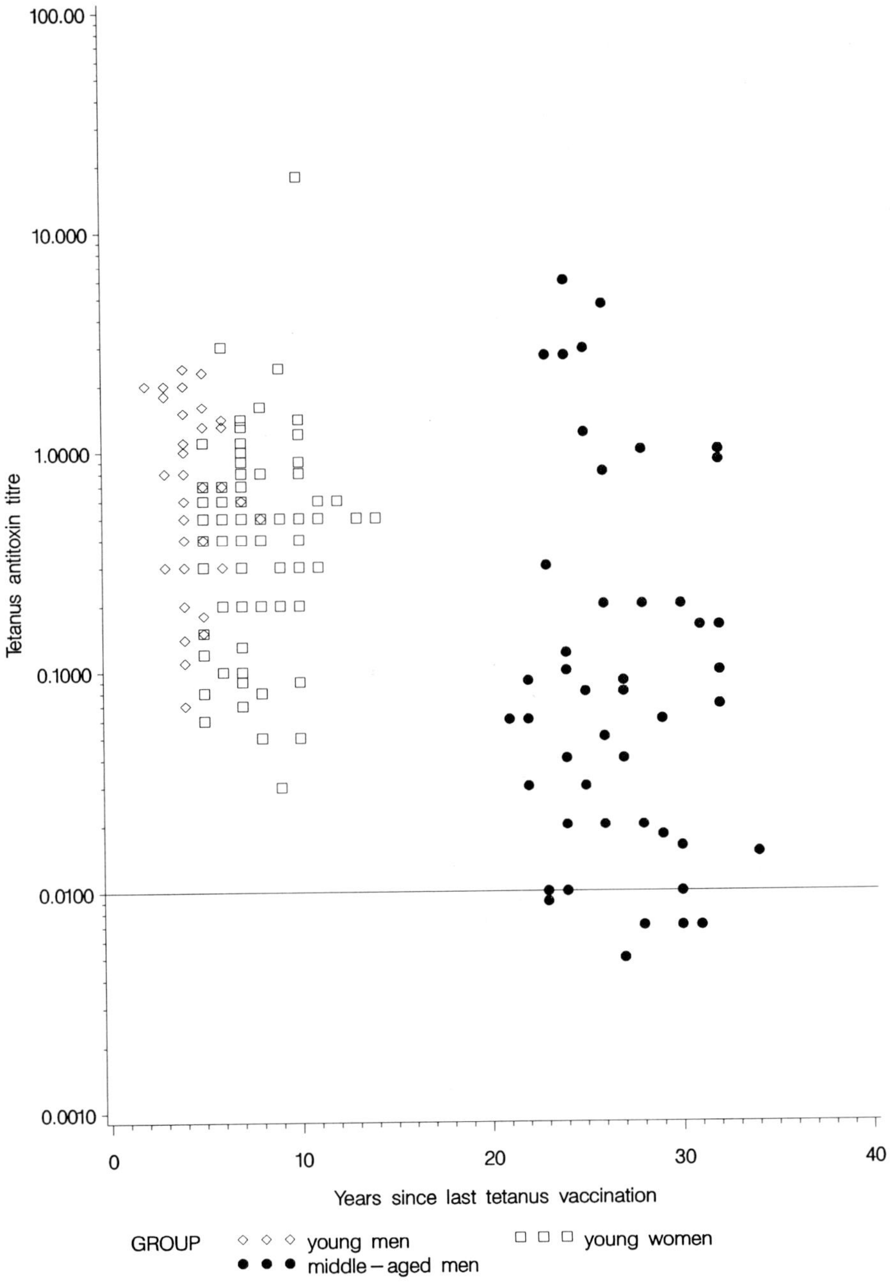

Fig. 4. Tetanus antitoxin titre in relation to interval since latest tetanus vaccination. A titre <0.01 IU/ml is considered unprotective.

Middle-aged men had significantly lower titres of antibodies to the 2 diseases, a significantly longer interval since last vaccination and reported fewer vaccinations.

The titres of antibodies to diphtheria and tetanus did not differ from the documented or self-reported vaccination record. Among young women and young men, only 6 persons reported <4 vaccinations against diphtheria and tetanus, but all these persons had protective levels of antibodies.

Vaccination and immunity from polio

Four or more polio vaccinations were reported by 99% of young women, 92% of young men, but by none of the middle-aged men, $p < 0.00001$. Among middle-aged men, 66% reported 1–2 vaccinations and 34% no vaccinations.

Fig. 5 shows the proportions of young women, young men and middle-aged men lacking a protective antibody concentrations against polio types 1, 2 and 3 (titre <1:4). More middle-aged men than young men or women had titres to polio type 1 below the protective level ($p = 0.018$). The protective level against polio type 2 among young women was significantly better than among young and middle-aged men, $p = 0.008$. As for polio type 3, middle-aged men tended to be less well protected than younger age groups (p = n.s.). 85% of young women had antibodies to all 3 types of poliovirus vs. 80% of young men and 56% of middle-aged men, $p < 0.0005$. No young woman was totally unprotected, while 8% young men and 4% middle-aged men were unprotected, p = n.s.

The median time since last vaccination against polio was 8.6 years (range: 5–19) for young women, 5.5 years (range: 5–8) for young men and 28.5 years (range: 16–34) for middle-aged men, $p = 0.0001$. There was no significant correlation between titre of antibodies against polio <1:4 and time since last polio vaccination in any test group. Regression analysis showed no association between time since last vaccination and antibody titre in young women and young men considered together. Regression analysis of titre and time since last vaccination among all showed a significant decline over time in titre of antibodies against polio types 1 and 2, but not 3, $p < 0.05$.

Persons with a documented record of vaccination did not have a better immunity than persons with a self-reported vaccination record. Among young women and young men only 5 persons did not report vaccination against polio and only 2 persons reported <5 vaccinations. All these persons had antibodies at a protective level. Among middle-aged men, the level of protection did not vary according to number of vaccinations reported.

Vaccination and immunity against measles

It was found that 96% of young women, 92% of young men, but no middle-aged men reported vaccination against measles, $p < 0.00001$. A level of antibodies against measles

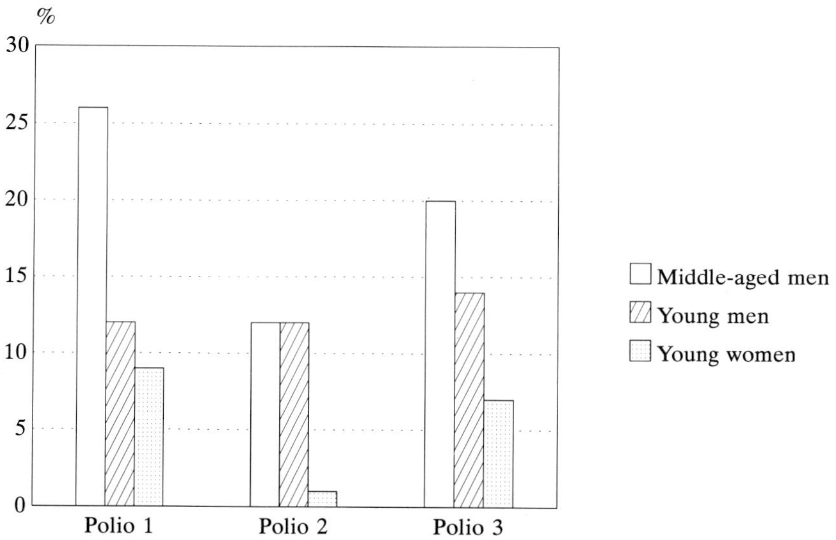

Fig. 5. Proportions of subjects with antibody titres below 1:4 against polio types 1, 2 and 3.

below protective level was found in 12% of young women, 22% of young men and none of middle-aged men, $p < 0.005$.

The median time since vaccination against measles was 20.6 years (range: 7–26) among young women and 18.5 years (range: 15–21) among young men, $p = 0.0022$. The level of protection did not vary significantly with time since vaccination. Of young women and men reporting having had a vaccination at the age of 1 year, 22% of young women and 0% of young men reported having caught measles later in life. No correlation between level of protection and documented record of vaccination was found for the young age groups. The 20 women reporting measles had had the disease 1 to 11 years after vaccination.

Immunity against mumps

Vaccination against mumps was not reported or documented. In this study 14% of pregnant women, 14% of soldiers and 4% of policemen had a titre of antibodies below the protective level, p = n.s. Clinical mumps was reported by 43% of young women, 30% of young men and 28% of middle-aged men. The protective level of antibodies against mumps did not correlate significantly to a history of disease.

Immunity against rubella in young women and young men

Information about vaccination against rubella was not reported or documented. Of young, pregnant women, 94% and of young men 90% had a protective level of antibodies to rubella, p = n.s. Of 6 young women negative for rubella IgG antibodies, 5 did not report rubella in the past. 28% of the young women but none of the young men reported a history of rubella.

DISCUSSION

The Lithuanians examined in this study lived in or near the capital and therefore the results reflect primarily immunity in the urban population. However, Lithuania has a national immunization program and the vaccination coverages in non-urban areas might not differ much from urban areas. In this study, the reported coverage of vaccination among young men and women was high, more than 90% reporting >3 vaccinations against diphtheria, tetanus and polio, a rate similar to or higher than reported from Denmark (5). Middle-aged men reported fewer or no vaccinations at all and this could be explained by the fact that all these men were born at least 3 years before the introduction of the vaccination program. Also, recall bias could play a role. If our results represent the situation in general among Lithuanians, the immunization program in Lithuania before 1991 was well established, especially in the younger age groups.

Young women and young men in this study were well protected against diphtheria and tetanus, with antitoxin concentrations higher than reported from Denmark and Sweden but similar to levels reported from Israel (5–9). The Soviet vaccine against diphtheria and tetanus has a lower potency than vaccines used in Western Europe. Thus the diphtheria vaccine holds 10–20 Lf of toxoid per ml compared with 50 Lf in the Danish vaccine for children, while the amount of tetanus toxoid is 5–10 IE compared with 40 IE in the Danish vaccine. The fact that younger adult groups in Lithuania seem better protected against diphtheria and tetanus than similar groups in Denmark can be due to the number of vaccinations and the rather short interval since last vaccination in this study.

In the middle-aged men, represented by policemen in this study, nearly half had a diphtheria antitoxin concentration below the protective level and 10% were not protected against tetanus. Concerning diphtheria, these rates are similar to or higher than those reported from Denmark (10, 11) and concerning tetanus similar to or lower than those reported from Denmark, Sweden and Israel (10, 12, 13). Thus men in the age group around

45 years in Lithuania seemed to be well protected against tetanus in this study, while the proportion of Lithuanian men in this age group susceptible to diphtheria was rather high. Susceptibility to diphtheria should be evaluated in relation to risk of exposure. During 1987–91, 1 case of diphtheria on average was reported per year. In 1992, WHO reported 9 cases of diphtheria in Lithuania (14).

Comparing subjects with the same number of vaccinations among young men and women, a significant fall-off in serum antitoxin concentration was only found concerning diphtheria antitoxin. This could either be a result of a fall-off effect since last vaccination, or be due to the fact that the female gender as such might be a factor of significant importance regarding antitoxic immunity against diphtheria (11). No women older than 27 years were tested for antibodies in this study, but one could have expected that the proportion of susceptible women around 45 years of age would be higher than among men of the same age group.

In the younger age groups of some 20 years of age, about 90% had a protective level of antibodies to each of polio types 1, 2 and 3. The proportion of middle-aged men protected against polio types 1 and 3 was smaller (74% vs. 80%), but they also reported fewer vaccinations. The relatively high level of protection in the older age group, even among the reportedly unvaccinated, might be explained by immunization from wild strains of poliovirus in the prevaccination era, or circulation of polio vaccine virus, or by recall bias. These rates of protection are, however, similar to rates reported from Denmark, Germany and Italy (15–17).

The coverage of vaccination against measles in Lithuania in individuals born after measles vaccine was included in the program exceeded 90% in this study, i.e. comparable to the coverage among children in Denmark. Immunity to measles was found in about 90% of young women, 80% of young men and all the middle-aged men. These rates are similar to or slightly lower than reported from the USA, Denmark and Sweden (18–21). One-fourth of young women in the present study had had measles after vaccination, but the distribution of intervals between vaccination and measles does not allow of conclusions as to whether the failure was of primary or secondary nature. It is noteworthy that all cases appeared within an 11-year period after vaccination, indicating primary failure, or at least that the period of protection was relatively short.

Our study showed that about 85% of the younger adults and about 95% of the older men had protective antibodies to mumps without vaccination. These rates are equal to or higher than those reported from the USA, Denmark and Sweden (19–21). Children in Lithuania have been immunized against mumps since 1985. The vaccine efficacy is unknown, but the disease has been rare in recent years. The level of protection in adults in Lithuania does not indicate any need for an adult vaccination program, but it is crucial that the vaccination program for children is effective.

A large proportion of the young, pregnant women (94%) had a protective level of rubella IgG antibodies. This rate is higher than reported from the USA (19), but similar to those reported from Great Britain (22) and Australia (23).

From our study it can be concluded that immunity from diphtheria, tetanus, poliomyelitis, measles, mumps and rubella among adults in Lithuania is to some extent comparable to immunity in some countries in Western Europe. A low immunity level due to the low quality of previously used vaccines should not *a priori* be taken for granted, as demonstrated by the immunity from diphtheria and tetanus in young adults. It is therefore important to evaluate immunity in serological studies before planning new vaccination program including adult age groups.

ACKNOWLEDGEMENTS

Many thanks to B. Böttiger, C. H. Mordhorst, Department of Virology, K. Bro-Jørgensen, Department of Virus vaccine and I. Heron, Department of Bacteria vaccine, all at Statens Seruminstitut, for undertaking the analyses and for assistance in connection with evaluating the results.

REFERENCES

1. Republican Immunization Center. Immunization against six target diseases in Lithuania. Vilnius, 1991.
2. National programme on immunization in the Republic of Lithuania, 1992–1996. Vilnius, 1992.
3. National immunoprophylaxis programme of the Republic of Lithuania, 1991.
4. Simonsen O, Schou C, Heron I. Modifications of the ELISA for the estimation of tetanus antitoxin in human sera. J Biol Stand 15: 143–157, 1987.
5. Simonsen O, Kjeldsen K, Heron I. Immunity against tetanus and effect of revaccination 25–30 years after primary vaccination. Lancet 2: 1240–1242, 1984.
6. Simonsen O, Klærke M, Klærke A, Bloch AV, Hansen RB, Hald N, Hau C, Heron I. Revaccination of adults against diphtheria. II: combined diphtheria and tetanus revaccination with different doses of diphtheria toxoid 20 years after primary vaccination. APMIS, Sect C 94: 219–225, 1986.
7. Kjeldsen K, Simonsen O, Heron I. Immunity against diphtheria 25–30 years after primary vaccination in childhood. Lancet 1: 900–902, 1985.
8. Christenson B, Böttiger M. Serological immunity to diphtheria in Sweden in 1978 and 1984. Scand J Infect Dis 18: 227–233, 1986.
9. Cohen D, Katzenelson E, Green M, Slepon R, Bercovier H, Danon Y. Prevalence and correlates of diphtheria toxin antibodies among young adults in Israel. J Infect 23: 117–121, 1991.
10. Simonsen O. Vaccination against tetanus and diphtheria. Evaluations of immunity in the Danish population, guidelines for revaccination, and methods for control of vaccination programmes. Dan Med Bull 36: 24–47, 1989.
11. Simonsen O, Kjeldsen K, Bentzon MW, Heron I. Susceptability to diphtheria in populations vaccinated before and after elimination of indigenous diphtheria in Denmark – a comparative study of antitoxic immunity. APMIS, Sect C 95: 225–231, 1987.
12. Christenson B, Böttiger M. Epidemiology and immunity to tetanus in Sweden. Scand J Infect Dis 19: 429–435, 1987.
13. Matzkin H, Regev S, Kedem R, Nili E. A study of factors influenzing tetanus immunity in Israeli male adults. J Infect 11: 71–78, 1985.
14. Diphtheria in Europe in 1992. WHO Europe, 25.3 1993.
15. Petersen I. Vaccination against polio in Denmark. Ugeskr Læger 147: 265–268, 1985 [In Danish].
16. Maass G, Doerr HW. Study on immunity against poliomyelitis in Germany. Dtsch Med Wochenschr 111: 1670–1676.
17. Santoro R, Lombardi F, Novello F, Amato C, Ruggeri FM, Grandolfo ME, Annesi I, Cortellessa CM, Timperi F, Inglese R. Serum antibodies to poliomyelitis in Italy. Bull WHO 62: 591–595, 1984.
18. Wallace MR, Hooper G. Immunity to measles during pregnancy. Clin Infect Dis 14: 1262–1263, 1992.
19. Kelley PW, Petrucelli BP, Stehr-Green P, Erickson RL, Mason CJ. The susceptibility of young adult Americans to vaccine-preventable infections. A national serosurvey of US recruits. JAMA 266: 2724–2729, 1991.
20. Glikmann G, Petersen I, Mordhorst C-H. Prevalence of IgG-antibodies to mumps and measles in non-vaccinated children. Dan Med Bull 35: 185–187, 1988.
21. Christenson B, Böttiger M. Changes of the immunological patterns against measles, mumps and rubella. A vaccination programme studied 3 to 7 years after the introduction of a two-dose schedule. Vaccine 9: 326–329, 1991.
22. Noah ND, Fowle SE. Immunity to rubella in women of childbearing age in the United Kingdom. BMJ 297: 1301–1304, 1988.
23. Menser MA, Hudson JR, Murphy AM, Upfold LJ. Epidemiology of congenital rubella and results of rubella vaccination in Australia. Rev Infect Dis 7 (Suppl 1): 37–41, 1985.

Submitted November 9, 1993; accepted March 3, 1994

Scand J Infect Dis 26: 468–470, 1994

Seroconversion after Additional Vaccine Doses to Non-responders to Three Doses of Intradermally or Intramuscularly Administered Recombinant Hepatitis B Vaccine

JOHAN STRUVE[1], BO ARONSSON[2], BERTIL FRENNING[3], MARIANNE FORSGREN[4] and OLA WEILAND[1]

From the [1]Departments of Infectious Diseases and [4]Clinical Virology, Karolinska Institute, Huddinge Hospital, Huddinge, the [2]Department of Bacteriology, Stockholm County Council Central Microbiological Laboratory, Stockholm, and the [3]Department of Occupational Health Services, Western District, Sabbatsbergs Hospital, Stockholm, Sweden

Hospital staff members who failed to respond (anti-HBs < 10 IU/l) after 3 doses of a recombinant hepatitis B (HBV) vaccine (given either as 20 μg intramuscularly ($n = 8$) or 2 μg intradermally ($n = 15$)) received 1 or 2 additional doses by the same route as the initial vaccination. After the first additional dose, 12/23 responded with anti-HBs levels ≥ 10 IU/l and after the second, another 2/5 responded, corresponding to a total response rate of 61%. No significant difference was seen in the response rate according to vaccination route, gender, age, or whether the vaccinee was a smoker or not. In this limited study some 50% of non-responders to 3 intradermal or intramuscular doses of recombinant HBV vaccine seroconverted after an additional 1–2 doses given by the same route as the initial vaccination, suggesting that additional doses can be administered by the same route as the initial one.

J. Struve, MD, Department of Infectious Diseases I 73, Huddinge Hospital, S-141 86 Huddinge, Sweden

INTRODUCTION

In clinical practice with heterogeneous groups of vaccinees, such as hospital staff, a variable proportion will not respond to a standard regimen of 3 doses of recombinant HBV vaccine. The proportions of non-responders (anti-HBs level < 10 IU/l) have varied between 0 and 14% after intramuscular (i.m.) (1–4) and 3–45% after intradermal (i.d.) vaccination (4–9). Non-responding vaccinees constitute a practical problem with regard to subsequent management and counselling, especially where risks for exposure to HBV are frequent. Additional vaccine doses have been recommended in order to achieve seroconversion to protective anti-HBs levels, but this is sparsely documented with recombinant HBV vaccines. In small series, response rates have ranged between 59 and 88% following a standard i.m. and 0–28% after an i.d. vaccination scheme, respectively (3, 5, 10, 11).

In the present study we report on our experience of additional doses given to hospital staff who failed to respond to 3 doses of i.d. or i.m. administered recombinant HBV vaccine.

MATERIALS AND METHODS

In a previous investigation we compared the anti-HBs response after 3 doses of recombinant HBV vaccine (Engerix B®, SmithKline Beecham) given either as 2 μg i.d. or 20 μg i.m. at 0, 1 and 6 months. In that trial 52/595 (8.7%) failed to respond (anti-HBs < 10 IU/l) (4). Additional vaccine doses and serologic follow-up were accepted by 23 of these non-responders, 15 i.d. and 8 i.m. vaccinees. Their median age was 41 years (range 22–66 years), 14/23 (61%) were women and 15/23 (65%) were smokers.

A fourth vaccine dose given by the same route as the first 3 doses was offered within a year after the 3rd dose and a fifth to those still not responding to the fourth. Serum was drawn 1 month after each dose and analysed for anti-HBs (AUSAB IMX, Abbot) together with samples from 1 month after the third dose.

The study was approved by the Ethics Committee at the Karolinska Institute.

 ISSN 0036-5548

Table I. *The anti-HBs response after a fourth hepatitis B vaccine dose given to hospital personnel who failed to reach an anti-HBs level ≥ 10 IU/l after 3 doses of a recombinant hepatitis B vaccine given either as 2 μg intradermally (i.d.) or 20 μg intramuscularly (i.m.)*

Anti-HBs level after 3 doses	No. of subjects	Anti-HBs (IU/l) level after a fourth HBV vaccine dose							
		0		1–9		10–99		100–999	
		i.d.	i.m.	i.d.	i.m.	i.d.	i.m.	i.d.	i.m.
0	20	6	2	1	1	7	2	0	1
1–9	3	1	0	0	0	0	2	0	0

RESULTS

The anti-HBs levels achieved after the 4th vaccine dose are reported according to vaccination route and level after the 3rd dose in Table I. The response rate (anti-HBs level ≥ 10 IU/l) was 12/23 (52%) after the 4th dose. Another 2/5 responded to a 5th dose, giving a total response rate of 14/23 (61%). No significant difference was noted in response rates after the 4th dose between i.d. and i.m. vaccination (7/15 vs 5/8 responders), between men and women (3/9 vs 9/14), or between smokers and non-smokers (7/15 vs 5/8) by univariate analysis (χ^2 with Yates' correction or Fisher's exact test when appropriate). The median age was 43 years (range 29–66 years) among responders and 41 (range 22–64 years) among non-responders. The geometric mean anti-HBs level among seroconverters (GMT) became slightly higher after i.m. than i.d. (29 vs 19 IU/l) vaccination, among non-smokers than smokers (47 vs 15 IU/l), but was the same for women and men (23 vs 22 IU/l). As shown in Table I, 10/20 (50%) anti-HBs negative and 2/3 with a level 1–9 IU/l after the first 3 doses responded to the fourth dose.

DISCUSSION

This study although limited in size, is to our knowledge the first where the response to additional doses given to non-responders after i.d. and i.m. vaccination with recombinant HBV vaccine are compared. We found that 47% of i.d. and 62% of i.m. vaccines not responding to 3 doses of recombinant HBV vaccine achieved a protective anti-HBs level when a 4th vaccine dose was given by the same route. These figures are consistent with previous uncontrolled studies with recombinant vaccines (3, 5), but better than the 15–25% response rate reported after additional vaccination of i.m. vaccinees with plasma-derived vaccines (12). In one study of low responders to recombinant i.d. vaccination, no effect on the GMT was seen after an additional i.d. dose (11). We found a trend toward a better response among non-smokers and i.m. vaccinees than among smokers and i.d. vaccinees, as previously reported during primary vaccination (4, 13). Our findings must be interpreted cautiously however, due to the limited size of this study, and need to be confirmed in a larger study.

Our data suggested that the likelihood of a non-responder to the initial 3-dose scheme to seroconvert after 1 or 2 additional doses is in the same order of magnitude after vaccination by the i.d. and i.m. routes. This important information needs to be confirmed in a larger series because it will have a major impact on any cost-effectiveness analysis of i.d. HBV vaccination. If additional i.d. vaccine doses can be used in non-responders to i.d. vaccination, we (in agreement with others, (7) but as opposed to others (11)) still believe that i.d. vaccination can be used as a cost reducing strategy for certain groups of vaccinees (young, women, non-smokers) even if a greater proportion of i.d. than i.m. vaccinees will require additional doses and post-vaccination testing.

We conclude that approximately half of non-responders to a 3-dose scheme of an i.m. or i.d. administered recombinant HBV vaccine achieved protective anti-HBs levels after an additional 1–2 doses and suggest that additional vaccination can be carried out by the same route as the initial vaccination, even if low-dose i.d. vaccination has been used.

REFERENCES

1. Halliday ML, Rankin JG, Bristow NJ, Coates RA, Corey PNJ, Strickler AC. A randomized double-blind clinical trial of a mammalian cell-derived recombinant DNA hepatitis B vaccine compared with a plasma derived vaccine. Arch Intern Med 150: 1195–1200, 1990.
2. Hoffman F, Berthold H. Zur Hepatitis-B-Gefährrtung des Krankenhauspersonals. Med Welt 40: 1294–1301, 1989.
3. Rogan PD, Duguid KM. Immunisation of staff of a regional blood transfusion centre with a recombinant hepatitis B vaccine. J Infect 22: 5–9, 1991.
4. Struve J, Aronsson B, Frenning B, Granath F, von Sydow M, Weiland O. Intramuscular versus intradermal administration of a recombinant hepatitis B vaccine: A comparison of response rates and an analysis of factors influencing the antibody response. Scand J Infect Dis 24: 423–429, 1992.
5. Morris CA, Oliver PR, Reynolds F, Selkon JB. Intradermal hepatitis B immunization with a yeast-derived vaccine: serological response by sex and age. Epidemiol Infect 103: 387–394, 1989.
6. Wiström J, Settergren B, Gustafsson Å, Juto P, Norrby RS. Intradermal vs intramuscular hepatitis B vaccinations. JAMA 264: 181–182, 1990.
7. Parish D, Muecke H, Joiner T, Pope W, Hadler S. Immunogenicity of low-dose intradermal recombinant hepatitis B vaccine. South Med J 84: 387–394, 1991.
8. Anonymous. Inadequate immune response among public safety workers receiving intradermal vaccination against hepatitis B-United States, 1990–1991. MMWR 40: 569–572, 1991.
9. Bryan J, Sjogren M, Perine P, Legters L. Low-dose intradermal and intramuscular vaccination against hepatitis B. Clin Infect Dis 14: 697–707, 1992.
10. Jilg W, Schmidt M, Deinhardt F. Four-year experience with a recombinant hepatitis B vaccine. Infection 17: 70–76, 1989.
11. Gonzales ML, Usandizaga M, Alomar P, Salva F, Martin F, Erroz M, Lardinois R. Intradermal and intramuscular route for vaccination against hepatitis B. Vaccine 8: 402–405, 1990.
12. Recommendations of the Immunization Practices Advisory Committee (ACIP). Hepatitis B virus: a comprehensive strategy for eliminating transmission in the United States through universal child-hood vaccination. MMWR 40: 1–25, 1991.
13. Coleman P, Shaw F, Hadler S, Margolis H, Serovich J. Intradermal hepatitis B vaccination in a large hospital employee population. Vaccine 9: 723–727, 1991.

Submitted November 3, 1993; accepted March 3, 1994

Scand J Infect Dis 26: 471–475, 1994

Immune Status and Booster Effects of Low Doses of Tetanus Toxoid in Swedish Medical Personnel

BENGT BJÖRKHOLM[1], MARTIN WAHL[1], MARTA GRANSTRÖM[2] and LARS HAGBERG[1]

From the [1]Department of Infectious Diseases, Göteborg University, Östra Hospital, Göteborg and the [2]Department of Clinical Microbiology, Karolinska Hospital, Stockholm, Sweden

Of 102 medical staff at a Swedish hospital, 81% had tetanus antitoxin titres ≥0.01 IU/ml in 1984–85. The unprotected individuals (antitoxin titre <0.01 IU/ml) were all >30 years of age. Of this group, one-third lacked a protective antibody level against tetanus toxin. Low booster doses of tetanus toxoid (0.75 or 1.9 Lf) were given to 66 vaccinees with a history of previous basic vaccination and no history of booster vaccination within the previous 5 years. The median titre increased from 0.26 IU/ml before to 3.3 IU/ml after vaccination. Low doses of tetanus toxoid may thus still provide an adequate immune response when given as a booster vaccination to individuals with a reliable history of basic immunization.

B. Björkholm, MD, Göteborg University, Department of Infectious Diseases, Östra Sjukhuset, S-416 85 Göteborg, Sweden

INTRODUCTION

Tetanus is a very rare disease in most industralized countries thanks to extensive vaccination programmes. Tetanus toxoid vaccine is often combined with other vaccines, such as vaccines against diphtheria and pertussis. A booster dose of tetanus and diphtheria toxoid to adults and older children in Sweden was earlier given with 0.5 ml of a combined vaccine containing 7.5 Lf tetanus toxoid/ml and a very small diphtheria toxoid component (1 Lf/ml). After an outbreak of diphtheria in 1984–85 in Sweden, studies on diphtheria immunity and vaccination were conducted, resulting in changes in the recommended doses of diphtheria toxoid (1–3). Currently in Sweden, 0.25 ml of a vaccine with 7.5 Lf tetanus and 30 Lf diphtheria toxoid/ml is recommended as booster dose. Amended recommendations resulted in an increased dosage of diphtheria toxoid, but a lowering of the previously recommended booster dose of tetanus toxoid from 3.75 Lf to 1.9 Lf. The present study was initiated to analyse the effects of low tetanus toxoid doses on the serological response and on the adverse reactions in persons with a history of previous basic immunization.

MATERIAL AND METHODS

102 individuals, aged 19–65 years (13 males and 89 females) on the medical staff at Östra Hospital, Göteborg, participated in the study. Three different aspects of tetanus immunity and effects of tetanus vaccination were studied among the vaccinees.

(1) Immunity among medical staff. Serum specimens were collected in 1984–85 from 102 participants and antitoxin levels against tetanus toxin were examined.

(2) Serological response to low booster doses of tetanus toxoid. 69 of the participants who reported a history of >2 previous tetanus immunizations and no booster vaccination within the last 5 years, were boostered with combined vaccines containing diphtheria and low doses of tetanus toxoid (0.75 or 1.9 Lf); 43 (mean age 32 years, range 19–57) received 0.75 Lf tetanus and 2.5 Lf diphtheria toxoid (0.1 ml DT) and 26 (mean age 44 years, range 27–66) received 1.9 Lf tetanus and 6.25 Lf diphtheria toxoid (0.25 ml DT). Serum samples for antitoxin determination were taken before and 1 month after vaccination.

(3) Adverse reactions to the diphtheria-tetanus toxoid booster doses. Adverse reactions were registered by the vaccinees on a record form during the week after immunization. Systemic reactions were assessed by registration of body temperature and signs of malaise such as general discomfort, headache and inability to work. Local reactions were measured by questions on occurrence of tenderness, redness or swelling and by the extent of these reactions. Local reactions of clinical significance were defined as redness or swelling >5 cm.

Vaccine

Regular DT vaccine from the National Bacteriological Laboratory (NBL) in Stockholm (lots 68, 69, 70, 71, 72 and 73) was used. It contained 25 Lf diphtheria toxoid and 7.5 Lf tetanus toxoid/ml. The toxoid components had a purity for tetanus of 1500–2100 Lf/mg Protein-N and of 1800–2100 Lf/mg protein-N for diphtheria toxoid.

Antibodies to tetanus toxin

Antibodies to tetanus toxin were measured by enzyme-linked immunosorbent assay (ELISA). Tetanus toxoid (NBL, Stockholm) was diluted in 0.05 M glycine-HCl buffer (pH 3) to a concentration of 2 Lf/ml and 100 μl/well were used for coating of 96-well microplates overnight at room temperature (22°C). Serum samples were tested in 10-fold dilutions between 10^{-1} and 10^{-4} and the dilution(s) giving OD (optical density) values between 0.2 and 0.9 were used to determine the antibody concentration against the standard. The standard, a human immunoglobulin against tetanus (250 IU/ml, NBL) calibrated against the WHO standard by the mouse assay, was titrated in 9 2-fold dilution steps from 0.1 IU/ml.

Statistics

For statistical analyses the Mann-Whitney test was used to evaluate the serological results. Comparison between groups with regard to adverse reactions was made with χ^2-test with Yates' correction.

RESULTS

Of the 102 medical personnel, 19 (19%) had tetanus antitoxin titres below the level considered to give protection (0.01 IU/ml). The pool of non-protected persons was found in the age groups 31–49 (31%) and 50–65 (33%), while none of 42 vaccinees ≤30 years of age had a titre <0.01 IU/ml (Table I). All non-protected persons were females.

Pre- and postvaccination tetanus antitoxin levels in 69 vaccinees given a low booster dose of tetanus toxoid (0.75 or 1.9 Lf) in combination with diphtheria toxoid are shown in Table II. Prior to booster vaccination, 53 (77%) of the vaccinees had a protective antibody level (≥0.01 IU/ml). Of the 16 (23%) vaccinees with prevaccination titres below <0.01 IU/ml, all but 3 (1 in the 0.75 Lf group and 2 in the 1.9 Lf group) developed a protective antibody level 1 month after vaccination. These 3 non-responders, all women, were 34, 56 and 57 years old and had pre- and postvaccination titres ≤0.003 IU/ml. They were regarded as previously not having received basic immunization when their vaccination histories were re-examined and were thus excluded from further evaluation.

Table I. *Tetanus antitoxin titres in 102 sera from medical staff*

		No. (%) with antitoxin titre		
Age (yrs)	No.	<0.01 (IU/ml)	0.01–0.09 (IU/ml)	≥0.1 (IU/ml)
18–30	42	0 (0)	2 (5)	40 (95)
31–49	39	12 (31)	8 (20)	19 (49)
50–65	21	7 (33)	5 (24)	9 (43)
	102	19 (19)	15 (15)	68 (66)

Table II. *Distribution of pre- and postvaccination tetanus antitoxin titres in individuals vaccinated with 0.75 or 1.9 Lf of tetanus toxoid*

Antitoxin titre (IU/ml)	No. of persons: Before vaccination	No. of persons: After vaccination
<0.01	16	3
0.01–0.09	11	4
0.1–0.9	15	11
1.0–4.9	23	30
≥5.0	4	21
	69	69

The median titre for the 66 vaccinees regarded as responders increased from 0.26 IU/ml (range 0.002–17) to 3.3 IU/ml (range 0.042–45) ($p < 0.001$). The prevaccination titres were slightly higher in the 0.75 Lf tetanus toxoid group than in the 1.9 Lf tetanus toxoid group, median titre 1.2 IU/ml (range 0.002–5.6) and 0.094 IU/ml (range 0.002–17) ($p < 0.05$), respectively. There was no significant difference in postvaccination titres between the 0.75 Lf and 1.9 Lf groups, with median titres 2.9 IU/ml (range 0.042–34) and 2.25 IU/ml (range 0.042–33), respectively.

55 of 66 vaccinees (83%) answered the questionnaire on adverse reactions, 36 in the 0.75 Lf group and 19 in the 1.9 Lf group. A total of 15 (27%) reported clinically significant adverse reactions, i.e. systemic reaction and or local reaction (redness or swelling) >5 cm. Seven of 36 (19%) in the 0.75 Lf group reported clinically significant adverse reactions. Eight of 19 (42%) vaccinated with 1.9 Lf tetanus toxoid reported clinically significant adverse reactions. Although twice as many reported significant reactions to the 1.9 Lf dose, the groups were small and the difference was not statistically significant.

No relation between adverse reactions and prevaccination or postvaccination titres was found. For vaccinees without adverse reactions, the prevaccination median titre was 0.24 IU/ml (range 0.002–5.6) and for vaccinees with clinically significant adverse reactions the prevaccination median titre was 0.20 IU/ml (range 0.002–5.2) (ns). The post-vaccination median titre was 3.3 IU/ml (range 0.072–25) for vaccinees without adverse reactions. For those with clinically significant adverse reactions the post-vaccination median titre was twice as high, 6.9 IU/ml (range 0.42–45), but the difference was not statistically different due to the small size of the groups.

DISCUSSION

Medical staff, of whom 87% were women, were found to be well protected against tetanus when 30 years old or younger. On the other hand, one-third of staff older than 30 years lacked antitoxin titres regarded as protective (≥0.01 IU/ml). Since the 1950s, all infants in Sweden are offered vaccination with tetanus toxoid. The vaccination programme has a high coverage rate which has been confirmed by serological findings previously (4). In older age groups, especially among women, absence of measurable protective antibodies against tetanus toxin has been found to be common in the Swedish population (4). The present study has thus shown that these findings are equally relevant for medical staff, a somewhat unexpected observation since medical staff are generally considered to be better monitored and more aware of immunizations, than the general population.

An antitoxin level of 0.01 IU/ml has been suggested to be protective against tetanus, based on both experimental and human studies (5–10). Some studies have, however, indicated that tetanus can occur in the presence of higher antitoxin levels (11, 12). On the other hand previously immunized individuals with antitoxin titres below the 0.01 IU/ml level may have an immunologic memory. In these cases, a rechallenge with a sufficient amount of antigen, natural or by vaccination, will result in a rapid increase in antitoxin levels (8, 13).

Doses of ≥5 Lf tetanus toxoid have often been recommended as booster vaccination (10). Few studies analysing the serologic response of lower doses of booster to adults have been performed. In a study from the early 1960s, Volk et al. showed a good serologic response to 2 Lf tetanus toxoid as booster to teenagers, 7 and 13 years after primary vaccination (14). In another study from the same period, 12 of 20 previously well immunized vaccines reacted with a serologic response to a dose as low as 0.2 Lf toxoid (15). These individuals had previously received basic immunization and at least 1 booster injection. Recently, a Swedish tetanus booster study in children has shown good serologic results with 0.75 and 1.9 Lf tetanus toxoid combined with diphtheria toxoid (16).

Low tetanus toxoid booster doses of 0.75 and 1.9 Lf resulted in high antitoxin levels in the adults in our study. These levels can be expected to give reliable protection for a long time. The 3 individuals who did not reach protective antibody levels had probably no previous basic immunization and were mistakenly included in the booster study. All had prevaccination antitoxin titres below detection level, and the titres remained unchanged after booster vaccination. When we re-examined their vaccination histories, these individuals were found to be uncertain about their previous basic tetanus vaccination.

We have earlier shown that adverse reactions to combined diphtheria and tetanus vaccines in Sweden were frequent and correlated mostly to the tetanus toxoid component (1). One possible reason for the high rate of adverse reactions to tetanus toxoid is the vaccine production method. In contrast to diphtheria vaccine, the tetanus toxoid is purified after formaldehyde treatment. Inactivation of crude or half-purified preparations of tetanus toxin by formalin prior to purification leads to the incorporation of foreign compounds into the toxoid, which may be responsible for adverse reactions (10, 17).

In a previous study we found that a dose of 0.75 Lf tetanus toxoid gave a lower rate of adverse reactions than a dose of 3.75 Lf, 20% and 34% respectively (1). Adverse reactions at a rate of 26% in the present study are in agreement with these data. Reducing the dose of tetanus toxoid as booster dose for adults from 3.75 Lf to 0.75–1.9 Lf decreased the rate of adverse reactions and still resulted in an adequate immune response. The current Swedish recommendation of 1.9 Lf tetanus toxoid for booster vaccination seems thus to concur with these two major objectives of immunization policy.

REFERENCES

1. Björkholm B, Wahl M, Granström M, Hagberg L. Immune status and booster effects of low doses of diphtheria toxoid in Swedish medical personnel. Scand J Infect Dis 21: 429–434, 1989.
2. Björkholm B, Granström M, Wahl M, Hedström C-E, Hagberg L. Adverse reactions and immunogenicity in adults to regular and increased dosage of diphtheria vaccine. Eur J Clin Microbiol 6: 637–640, 1987.
3. Björkholm B, Granström M, Wahl M, Hedström C-E, Hagberg L. Increased dosage of diphtheria toxoid for basic immunization of adults. Eur J Clin Microbiol 8: 701–705, 1989.
4. Christenson B, Böttiger M. Epidemiology and immunity to tetanus in Sweden. Scand J Infect Dis 19: 429–435, 1987.
5. McComb J, Dwyer R. Passive-active immunization with tetanus immunoglobulin (human). N Engl J Med 268: 857–862, 1963.

6. Edsall G. Specific prophylaxis of tetanus. JAMA 171: 417–427, 1959.
7. Tasman A, Huygen FJA. Immunization against tetanus of patients given injections of antitetanus serum. Bull WHO 26: 397–407, 1962.
8. Scheibel I. The uses and results of active tetanus immunization. Bull WHO 13: 381–394, 1955.
9. Sneath PAT, Kerslake EG, Scruby F. Tetanus immunity: the resistance of guinea pigs to lethal spore doses induced by active and passive immunization. Am J Hyg 25: 464–476, 1937.
10. Bizzini B: Tetanus. In: Germanier R, ed. Bacterial vaccines. Orlando: Academic Press, 37–68, 1984.
11. Goulon M, Girard O, Grosbuis, S, Desormeau JP, Capponi MF. Les anticorps antitetaniques. Nouv Presse Medicale 1: 3049–3050, 1972.
12. Passen EL, Andersen BR. Clinical tetanus despite a protective level of toxin-neutralizing antibody. JAMA 255: 1171, 1986.
13. Ullberg-Olsson K, Eriksson E. Active immunization against tetanus in man. Eur Surg Res 7: 249–258, 1975.
14. Volk VK, Gottshall RY, Andersson HD, Top FH, Bunney WE, Serfling RE. Antigenic response to booster dose of diphtheria and tetanus toxoids: seven to thirteen years after primary inoculation of noninstitutionalized children. Public Health Rep 77: 185–194, 1962.
15. McComb JA, Levine L. Adult immunization II. Dosage reduction as a solution to increasing reactions to tetanus toxoid. New Engl J Med 265: 1152–1153, 1969.
16. Christenson B, Böttiger M. Immunity and immunization of children against tetanus in Sweden. Scand J Infect Dis 23: 643–647, 1991.
17. Relyveld EH, Henocq E, Bizzini B. Studies on untoward reactions to diphtheria and tetanus toxoids. Dev Biol Stand 43: 33–37, 1979.

Submitted January 19, 1994; accepted March 21, 1994

Scand J Infect Dis 26: 479–485, 1994

Detection of Candida albicans DNA in Serum by Polymerase Chain Reaction

ERJA CHRYSSANTHOU[1], BIRGER ANDERSSON[2], BJÖRN PETRINI[1], SVEN LÖFDAHL[3] and JAN TOLLEMAR[4]

From the [1]Department of Clinical Microbiology, Karolinska Hospital, [2]Calab Medical Laboratories, the [3]Department of Bacteriology, Swedish Institute for Infectious Disease Control, and the [4]Department of Transplantation, Huddinge Hospital, Karolinska Institute, Stockholm, Sweden

Polymerase chain reaction (PCR) was applied in order to improve the diagnosis of disseminated candidosis. A nested PCR technique with 2 primer pairs was used to increase the sensitivity. We were able to detect Candida DNA in serum and tissue samples from experimentally infected mice as well as in serum samples from candidemia patients and patients with deep-seated Candida infection. Our PCR could detect as little as 1 pg Candida albicans DNA. The PCR method was more sensitive than culture in both the mouse experiments and the patients with deep candidosis (5/7 were PCR positive and 0/7 blood culture positive), and of similar sensitivity in candidemia patients (11/17 were PCR positive and 15/17 blood culture positive). The relatively short processing time of PCR, when compared with culturing, its sensitivity, as well as the possibility of using serum samples for analysis, all helped improve the diagnostics in deep-seated candidosis and candidemia.

E. Chryssanthou, BS, Department of Clinical Microbiology, Karolinska Hospital, Box 70470, S-10726 Stockholm, Sweden

INTRODUCTION

Candida albicans is the most common cause of fungal infection encountered in the immunocompromised patient (1). Candida species are also sometimes involved in hospital-acquired infections (2). Diagnosis of disseminated candidosis is often difficult to establish, as the only sign of infection may be prolonged fever refractory to broad-spectrum antibacterial treatment (1). Routine blood cultures are insensitive to fungal detection, but the development of special fungal blood culture systems has improved the detection of candidemia (3, 4). Among patients with autopsy verified disseminated candidosis, 73% had blood cultures positive with the Isolator system (5). However, blood cultures are slow to turn positive: mean interval to recovery of yeasts was 3.4–5.0 days, depending on method (4, 5). Moreover, fungal blood cultures can remain negative despite widespread dissemination of Candida in internal organs, and during antifungal therapy.

Polymerase chain reaction (PCR) has been applied to detect Candida DNA in various clinical specimens (6–8). Buchman et al. (9) developed a PCR method to detect Candida DNA isolated from whole blood. His PCR primers were selected from a single-copy gene sequence encoding cytochrome P-450 L1 A1 and the detection level of the PCR was 12 Candida cells. The advantages of PCR are the relatively short processing time as well as its high sensitivity and specificity. We have developed a nested PCR technique which detects naked Candida DNA in serum, thereby reducing cumbersome sample preparation from whole blood.

MATERIALS AND METHODS

Serum samples

Mouse sera were obtained from experimental groups as described below. Serum samples were obtained from patients at Swedish hospitals and PCR analysis for Candida DNA was performed retrospectively. 17 sera were obtained from patients with candidemia, 7 from transplant patients and 6 control sera from transplant patients who died of causes other than Candida infection (for details, see Tables III and IV).

Strains

For the specificity study, control DNA preparations were made from C. albicans ATCC 26790, C. albicans ATCC 56881, C. tropicalis ATCC 750, C. parapsilosis ATCC 7330, C. glabrata ATCC 15126, C. kefyr ATCC 28838, C. lusitaniae ATCC 427020, C. guilliermondii ATCC 6260 and C. krusei ATCC 6258.

PCR primers

DNA oligonucleotide primers were selected from the sequenced Candida gene encoding the cytochrome P450 L1 A1 (lanosterol 14 α-demethylase) (10). The outer pair was 5′-CATAACTCAATATGGCTATT-3′ and 5′-CTTTTGACGACATGATTCGA-3′ which correspond to bases 137 to 156 and the complement of bases 361 to 381 (9). The primers were expected to amplify a fragment of 244 bp. The inner pair consisted of 5′-TTGTTGAAACTGTCATTGATG-3′ and 5′-TCCAATAAAACACTAATGGAGC-3′ which correspond to bases 155 to 175 and the complement of bases 289–310 and the expected amplicon was of 155 bp. The primers were synthesized by Scandinavian Gene Synthesis AB (Köping, Sweden).

Amplification

The first PCR was carried out in a total volume of 50 μl containing 10 mM Tris-Cl [pH 8.3], 50 mM KCl, 2 mM $MgCl_2$, 0.4 mM of each nucleotide, 1.25 U of Amplitaq (all reagents were supplied by Perkin-Elmer Cetus, Norwalk, CT), 1 μM of each primer (outer primer pair) and 23 μl of sample DNA. The DNA amplification was initiated with a 5 min denaturation step at 94°C followed by 35 cycles at 94°C for 60 s, 55°C for 60 s, 72° for 2 min and a final 10 min extension step at 72°C. The second (nested) PCR was carried out in a total volume of 50 μl containing 10 mM Tris-HCl [pH 8.3], 50 mM KCl, 1.5 mM $MgCl_2$, 0.04 mM of each nucleotide, 1.25 U of Amplitaq and 0.5 μM of each primer (inner primer pair). One μl from the first PCR reaction was added as template. After 5 min of denaturation, 35 cycles at 94°C for 30 s, 45°C for 30 s, 72°C for 30 s followed by a final 10 min extension step at 72°C were performed. Negative (water) and positive (1 pg of C. albicans DNA) controls were included with each PCR run.

The amplified DNA (10 μl) was analysed by electrophoresis in 4% agarose (Nu Sieve 3:1; FMC Bioproducts, Rockland, ME) in 1 × TBE buffer, run at 120 V for 30 min. Gels were stained with ethidium bromide (1 mg L^{-1}). Samples giving a fragment of 155 bp were regarded as positive.

Yeast DNA preparation

Candida strains were grown overnight in 8 ml yeast-peptone-dextrose broth at 37°C on a rotatory shaker (100 rev. min^{-1}). Of each cell suspension, 1.5 ml was pelleted, washed twice in PBS and resuspended in 500 μl lysis buffer (50 mM Tris-HCl [pH 7.5], 10 mM EDTA, 0.5% β-mercaptoethanol and zymolyase (ICN Biomedicals, Lisle) 0.3 mg/ml) and incubated at 37°C for 60 min on a shaker. Sodium dodecyl sulphate and proteinase K (Boehringer Mannheim, Germany) were added to a final concentration at 1% and 50 μg/ml respectively and the mixture was incubated at 56°C for 60 min. The mixtures were boiled for 5 min and DNA was extracted with an equal volume of phenol-chloroform-isoamyl alcohol; 25:24:1 (Sigma) and finally extracted with chloroform-isoamyl alcohol; 24:1. The DNA was harvested by ethanol precipitation and dissolved in deionised autoclaved water. 0.5 μg of template DNA was used in PCR.

Yeast DNA extraction from serum

DNA was extracted from 500 μl of serum. Proteinase K and SDS were added to a final concentration at 15 μg/ml and 1% respectively and the mixture was incubated at 37°C for 60 min on a shaker. The samples were then boiled for 5 min, chilled to 4°C and phenol-chloroform-isoamyl alcohol extracted and ethanol precipitated as described above.

Sensitivity studies

To determine the level of sensitivity of this PCR assay, C. albicans ATCC 26790 DNA was diluted in water and PCRs were performed with 1 ng, 0.1 ng, 10 pg, 1 pg and 0.1 pg of genomic DNA.

Mouse model of systemic candidosis

In the first experiment, 12 male albino BALB/c mice were immunosuppressed with a non-lethal, single dose of 4.0 Gy of X-irradiation on day −3. On day 0, 10 mice were injected via the lateral tail vein with various inocula (from 10^3 to 10^7) of C. albicans ATCC 26790 yeast cells in 200 μl of buffered saline. Two control mice were injected with 200 μl of buffered saline only. Blood samples for culture and PCR were drawn after 15 min and 1 to 7 days post-inoculation. Sera for PCR were processed as described above.

In the second experiment, 7 male BALB/c mice were immunosuppressed as above. On day 0, 6 mice were injected with 10^5 of C. albicans yeast cells. A control mouse was injected with saline as above. Blood for culture was drawn from mouse no. 1 after 30 min. The animal was then sacrificed and kidneys, spleen and liver were removed. One-half of the organs was weighed and homogenized in 500 μl of buffered saline and 300 μl of the homogenate was cultured on Sabouraud dextrose agar plates and incubated overnight at 37°C. The other half of the organs was quick-frozen at −70°C for histology and PCR analysis. For histological examination, tissue sections were cut and stained with Periodic Acid Schiff (PAS) for detection of fungal elements. For PCR analysis, sections of tissue were suspended in 1 ml of digestion buffer (100 mM NaCl, 10 mM Tris-HCl [pH 8.0], 25 mM EDTA, 0.5% SDS and 0.1 mg ml^{-1} proteinase K) and incubated overnight at 37°C on a rotatory shaker (40 rev. min^{-1}) and then extracted with phenol-chloroform-isoamyl alcohol. Finally, DNA was collected by ethanol precipitation and dissolved in deionised water. The remaining 5 infected mice and the control mouse were sampled and processed as above on days 1 to 7 post-inoculation.

RESULTS

Sensitivity and specificity of the system

The sensitivity of PCR when using the outer primer pair was 10 pg of C. albicans DNA. The nested PCR detected 1 pg of C. albicans DNA. The specificity of the test was examined using DNAs from other clinically relevant Candida species as templates. The 155 bp fragment was only amplified from C. albicans strains and not from other Candida species.

Mouse model of systemic candidosis

Systemic candidosis was induced in immunosuppressed mice in order to find out if PCR could be applied to detect Candida DNA in serum and tissues. A summary of PCR, blood and tissue cultures and histology results is given in Tables I and II. Our results from the first experiment showed that Candida DNA was detected by PCR in assayed sera with increasing doses of injected Candida cells (Table I). With lower doses of Candida (group 10^3 and 10^4) blood cultures and PCR were negative throughout the experiment.

In groups 10^5, 10^6 and 10^7, only the first blood cultures, drawn 15 min post-inoculation, were positive and turned negative during the following days. The PCR was more sensitive than blood culture and was positive days 2 to 4 in group 10^5, days 0 and 1 in group 10^6 (mice died day 2) and day 0 in group 10^7 (mice died day 1), (Fig. 1). The sera from control mice

Table I. *Analysis of blood samples from mice inoculated i.v. with Candida albicans*

+ = positive, − = negative, * = cfu/ml, † = dead.

	Number of Candida cells per mouse											
	10^3		10^4		10^5		10^6		10^7		Controls	
Day	Culture	PCR	Culture	PCR	Culture	PCR	Culture	PCR	Culture	PCR	Culture	PCR
0	−	−	−	−	4 × 10^2*	−	2.5 × 10^3	+	2.8 × 10^4	+	−	−
1	−	−	−	−	−	−	−	+	†		−	−
2	−	−	−	−	−	+	†				−	−
3	−	−	−	−	−	+					−	−
4	−	−	−	−	−	+					−	−
7	−	−	−	−	−	−					−	−

Table II. *Mouse model of systemic candidosis: analysis of organs following an i.v. dose of* 10^5 *Candida yeast cells*

+ = positive, − = negative, nd = not done.

		Culture				PCR			Histology
Mouse no.	Day	Blood cfu/ml	Kidney	Spleen	Liver	Kidney	Spleen	Liver	in kidney tissue
1	0	52	+	+	+	+	−	+	+
2	1	−	+	+	+	+	+	+	+
3	2	−	+	+	+	+	nd	nd	+
4	3	−	+	+	+	+	nd	nd	+
5	4	−	+	+	+	+	nd	nd	−
6	7	−	+	+	+	+	nd	nd	+
Control	7	−	−	−	−	−	nd	nd	−

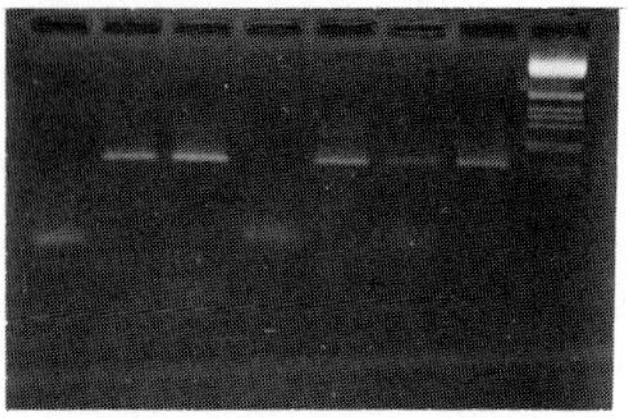

Fig. 1. PCR of sera from mice experimentally infected with different doses of Candida albicans: Lane 1: 10^5 Candida cells, day 0; Lane 2: 10^6 Candida cells, day 0; Lane 3: 10^7 Candida cells, day 0; Lane 4: 10^5 Candida cells, day 1; Lane 5: 10^6 Candida cells, day 1; Lane 6: 10^5 Candida cells, day 2; Lane 7: 10^5 Candida cells, day 3; Lane 8: 1-Kb DNA size standard.

were negative for both Candida DNA and blood cultures. The controls in which C. albicans DNA was added or omitted proved positive and negative, respectively.

In the second set of experiments we studied whether our PCR method could be used to detect Candida DNA extracted from mouse organs (Table II). Cultures from kidneys, spleen and liver were positive for Candida in all 6 infected mice. Kidney sections from each mouse were assayed and yielded the expected PCR product in all specimens. Two liver and 1 spleen specimen were also PCR positive. The control mouse was culture-, histology- and PCR-negative.

Clinical samples

Clinical data and results of blood culture and PCR in patients of the human candidemia group are summarized in Table III. Nine of the 11 PCR-positive patients had positive blood culture for Candida around the time of PCR sampling. Two patients with detectable Candida DNA had negative blood cultures but deep Candida infection and clinically suspected candidemia, respectively.

Six blood culture-positive sera failed to give positive results on PCR. These negative results may have been due to technical difficulties in sample preparation. The fact that blood samples for culture and PCR analysis were not taken the same day complicates the evaluation of these results.

In the human transplantation group, all 7 patients had autopsy-verified deep Candida infections, despite negative blood cultures. Five of the 7 samples were PCR-positive and 2 gave negative PCR results (Table IV). Serum for PCR analysis was taken 1–7 days before

Table III. *Candida PCR in candidemia patients*

+ = positive, − = negative.

Patient (sex)	Age (years)	Clinical background	Candida blood culture	PCR in serum
1(M)	50	Perforated ulcus ventriculi	+	+
2(M)	70	Cholecystectomia	+	+
3(F)	46	Candidemia	+	+
4(M)	46	Diabetes	+	+
5(M)	78	Urinary tract infection	+	+
6(M)	74	Deep Candida infection	−	+
7(F)	71	Lymphoma, suspected candidemia	−	+
8(M)	83	Candidemia	+	+
9(M)	67	Diabetes	+	+
10(F)	23	Neurosurgery	+	+
11(F)	30	Central venous catheter	+	+

Table IV. *Candida PCR in transplant patients*

+ = positive, − = negative, BMTX = bone marrow transplantation, LTX = liver transplantation, CML = chronic myeloic leukemia, AML = acute myeloic leukemia.

			Candida culture		
Patient (sex)	Age (years)	Clinical background	Autopsy material	Blood before death	PCR in serum before death
1(F)	49	Myeloma, BMTX	+	−	+
2(F)	62	LTX	+	−	+
3(F)	39	CML, BMTX	+	−	+
4(M)	49	CML, BMTX	+	−	−
5(F)	11	Fanconi anemia BMTX	+	−	+
6(M)	39	Lymphoma	+	−	−
7(M)	36	AML, BMTX	+	−	+

death in 6 cases and 84 days before in 1 case. The sera from the control group gave negative PCR results (Fig. 2).

DISCUSSION

The diagnosis of deep or disseminated Candida infection is difficult clinically and at the laboratory. The clinical diagnosis is often circumstantial and a result of exclusion of other causes of fever or absence of effect of antibacterial treatment (11). Interpretation of serological tests is complicated by the presence of background antibody levels against Candida antigens and the differentiation between invasive and superficial Candida infection

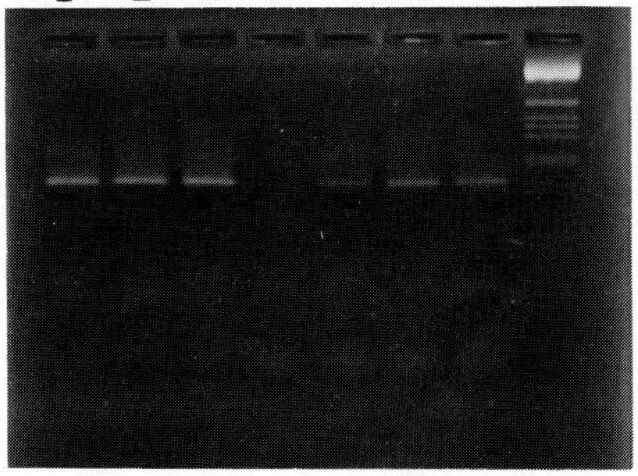

Fig. 2. PCR of clinical serum samples: Lanes 1, 2, 3: samples from patients with positive Candida blood culture; Lane 4: negative control sample from patient with autopsy verified Aspergillus infection; Lanes 5, 6, 7: samples from patients with autopsy verified deep Candida infection; Lane 8: 1-Kb DNA size standard.

is difficult (12). Blood cultures are not very sensitive to disseminated candidosis. Even in autopsy-verified candidosis, negative outcome of blood cultures is reportedly as high as 56% (13). Since the mortality rate in disseminated candidosis can be reduced with early antifungal therapy (14), it is essential to introduce new and faster diagnostic tools for deep Candida infection. PCR has improved the diagnostic sensitivity in a variety of infections (15–17). We therefore developed a Candida-specific nested PCR system with outer primers as described by Buchman (9) and inner primers designed by using the search algorithm of Primer Detective (18). Our nested PCR was specific for C. albicans and the 155 bp fragment was not detected from any other analysed Candida species. DNA fragments other than the 155 bp segment were amplified from C. tropicalis and C. lusitaniae and showed faint bands on UV visualization. The sensitivity of the nested PCR was 1 pg of genomic DNA.

We ascertained in a mouse model the usefulness of our PCR system and found that it had better sensitivity than blood cultures. As an improvement of the diagnostic procedure we showed that Candida DNA could be detected in serum from infected mice, thus eliminating the need for tedious DNA isolation from whole blood. Moreover, our PCR was shown to be useful to detect Candida DNA in mouse tissue sections.

In a group of patients with candidemia, PCR was of similar sensitivity as blood cultures. In another group of transplant patients with negative fungal blood cultures but autopsy-proven candidosis, PCR in serum taken before death was positive in 5/7 cases. Thus PCR in serum proved to be a sensitive tool to detect deep and disseminated candidosis. Considering that PCR can be performed within 2 days, we conclude that it can be a useful diagnostic procedure for deep/disseminated Candida infections.

REFERENCES

1. Dupont B. Clinical manifestations and management of candidosis in the compromised patient. In: Warnock DW, Richardson MD, eds. Fungal infection in the compromised patient. Chichester: John Wiley & Sons, 56–83, 1991.
2. Weber DJ, Rutala WA. Epidemiology of hospital-acquired fungal infections. In: Holmberg K, Meyer R, eds. Diagnosis and therapy of systemic fungal infections. New York: Raven Press, 1–24, 1989.
3. Murray PR, Spizzo AW, Niles AC. Clinical comparison of the recoveries of bloodstream pathogens in septi-chek brain heart infusion broth with saponin, septi-chek tryptic soy broth, and the isolator lysis-centrifugation system. J Clin Microbiol 5: 901–905, 1991.
4. Wilson ML, Davis TE, Mirrett S, Reynolds J, Fuller D, Allen SD, Flint KK, Koontz F, Barth Reller L. Controlled comparison of the BACTEC high-blood-volume fungal medium, BACTEC plus 26 aerobic blood culture bottle, and 10 milliliter Isolator blood culture system for detection of fungemia and bacteremia. J Clin Microbiol 4: 865–871, 1993.
5. Telenti A, Roberts GD. Fungal blood cultures. Eur J Clin Microbiol Infect Dis 9: 825–831, 1989.

6. Hopfer RL, Walden P, Setterquist S, Highsmith WE. Detection and differentiation of fungi in clinical specimens using polymerase chain reaction (PCR) amplification and restriction enzyme analysis. J Med Vet Mycol 31: 65–75, 1993.
7. Crampin AC, Matthews RC. Application of the polymerase chain reaction to the diagnosis of candidosis by amplification of an HSP 90 gene fragment. J Med Microbiol 3: 233–238, 1993.
8. Sugita Y, Kanaizuka I, Nakajima H, Ibe M, Yokota S, Matsuyama S. Detection of Candida albicans DNA in cerebrospinal fluid. J Med Vet Mycol 31: 343–358, 1993.
9. Buchman TG, Rossier M, Merz W, Charache P. Detection of surgical pathogens by in vitro DNA amplification. Part I. Rapid identification of Candida albicans by in vitro amplifica- of a fungus-specific gene. Surgery 108: 338–347, 1990.
10. Lai MH, Kirsch DR. Nucleotide sequence of cytochrome P450 L1A1 (lanosterol 14 α-demethylase) from Candida albicans. Nucleic Acids Res 17: 804, 1989.
11. Jones J. Laboratory diagnosis of invasive candidiasis. Clin Microbiol Rev 1: 32–45, 1990.
12. de Repentigny L. Serodiagnosis of candidiasis, aspergillosis, and cryptococcosis. Clin Infect Dis 14 (Suppl 1): 11–12, 1992.
13. de Repentigny L, Reiss E. Current trends in immunodiagnosis of candidiasis and aspergillosis. Rev Infect Dis 6: 301–312, 1984.
14. Rantala A, Niinikoski J, Lehtonen OP. Yeasts in blood cultures: impact of early therapy. Scand J Infect Dis 21: 557–561, 1989.
15. Spreadbury C, Holden D, Aufauvre-Brown A, Bainbridge B, Cohen J. Detection of Aspergillus fumigatus by polymerase chain reaction. J Clin Microbiol 3: 615–621, 1993.
16. Wakefield AE, Pixley FJ, Banerji S, Sinclair K, Miller RF, Moxon ER, Hopkin JM. Detection of Pneumocystis carinii with DNA amplification. Lancet 336: 451–453, 1990.
17. Forbes BA, Hicks KES. Direct detection of Mycobacterium tuberculosis in respiratory specimens in a clinical laboratory by polymerase chain reaction. J Clin Microbiol 7: 1688–1694, 1993.
18. Lowe T, Sharefkin J, Yang SQ, Dieffenbach CW. A computer program for selection of oligonucleotide primers for polymerase chain reaction. Nucleic Acids Res 18: 1757–1761, 1990.

Submitted February 14, 1994; accepted March 24, 1994

Scand J Infect Dis 26: 486–488, 1994

CASE REPORT

Encephalopathy Associated with Salmonella enteritidis Infection

KATHERINE MARTIN, MICHAEL SHARLAND and EDWARD GRAHAM DAVIES

From the Department of Child Health, St. George's Hospital Medical School, Cranmer Terrace, London, England

A 15-year-old boy who presented with a short history of a diarrhoeal illness associated with encephalopathic features is described. Salmonella enteritidis phage type 4 was cultured from his stool. Although encephalopathy in the absence of CNS infection or electrolyte disturbance is well described in enteric fever, it is very rare in infections with non-typhoidal Salmonella serotypes and has not previously been described in association with S. enteritidis infection.

K. Martin, Department of Child Health, St. George's Hospital Medical School, Blackshaw Road, London SW17 0RE, England

INTRODUCTION

Encephalopathy complicating salmonella infections has been described almost exclusively in association with typhoidal disease (1, 2). We would like to report the association of an acute encephalopathy with non invasive salmonella infection due to Salmonella enteritidis phage type 4. This particular organism is the commonest reported Salmonella spp isolated in human disease in England and Wales and the number of isolates has risen sharply from 2,979 in 1986 (17.5% of all Salmonella isolates) to 16,981 in 1992 (over 50% of isolates) (3).

CASE REPORT

A previously healthy 15-year-old boy of Asian origin presented with an 18 h history of fever, diarrhoea and vomiting, and a 12 h history of confusion. His parents observed that he had not been talking, did not seem able to recognise them and had been incontinent of faeces in his bed. There was no history of convulsions, trauma or substance abuse and no previous history of confusional states. There had been no recent travel outside the United Kingdom and no family members had suffered any similar illness.

On examination he was confused and uncooperative. He had a swinging pyrexia with a temperature of up to 40°C. Heart rate was 120/min, respiratory rate 25/min and blood pressure was 130/80 mmHg. His mucous membranes were dry and there was loss of skin turgor, but capillary return was normal. His eyes were open spontaneously. He was not oriented in time, place or person and he was uttering incomprehensible sounds but no recognisable words. He was responding to commands inconsistently. He was therefore assessed to have a Glasgow coma scale (4) score of 11 out of 15 (eye opening 4 out of 4, best verbal response 2 out of 5, best motor response 5 out of 6). This confusional state was present even when he became afebrile. Fundi were normal and there was no meningism. Examination of the cranial nerves revealed no deficit. Muscle power and tone were normal. Tendon reflexes were not elicited. Both plantar responses were flexor. General examination was otherwise unremarkable.

Full blood count revealed a haemoglobin of 154 g/l, white cell count of 14.8×10^9/l with 82% polymorphonuclear leucocytes. Platelet count was 224×10^9/l. Coagulation screen was normal. Arterial pH was 7.37 with a base deficit of 3.9 mmol/l. PaO_2 was 13.6 kPa in air and $PaCO_2$ was 4.4 kPa. Plasma sodium was 138 mmol/l, potassium 4.0 mmol/l, urea 7.4 mmol/l and creatinine 128 μmol/l. Plasma glucose was 6.3 mmol/l. Plasma alanine transaminase was 0.42 μkat/l (reference range 0–0.75 μkat/l), gamma-glutamyl transferase 0.25 μkat/l (reference range 0–1.0 μkat/l), bilirubin 39 μmol/l and albumin 41 g/l. Plasma lactate was 3.8 mmol/l (reference range: 0.6–2.4 mmol/l) and ammonia <10 μmol/l (reference range <50 μmol/l).

A provisional diagnosis of meningo-encephalitis was made. Intravenous cefotaxime and acyclovir were commenced. Cranial computerised axial tomography without contrast showed no focal lesion. Lumbar puncture produced clear, colourless CSF with a pressure of 25 cm of water. CSF microscopy revealed less than 3×10^6 WBC/l and 9×10^6 RBC/l. CSF glucose was 5.6 mmol/l (concurrent plasma glucose was 6.9 mmol/l) and protein 0.17 g/l. Gram stain of the CSF was normal and culture was sterile. Stool cultures grew S. enteritidis phage type 4. Blood cultures taken before commencement of antibiotics were sterile. No virus was detected from tissue culture of CSF, stool, throat swab. Enteroviral IgM and mycoplasma IgM were negative. Serum complement fixation tests demonstrated titres of less than 64 for adenovirus, mumps soluble antigen, measles, herpes simplex and varicella zoster virus.

Intravenous ciprofloxacin was commenced on the second day of admission after isolation of Salmonella from the stools. Two days after admission the patient was alert and oriented in time, place and person, with a Glasgow coma scale score of 15 out of 15. He continued to have profuse diarrhoea with a maximum stool volume of more than 3 litres per day for a total of 8 days. Arterial blood pressure, peripheral perfusion and serum electrolytes remained normal with intravenous fluid replacement. 11 days after admission the patient was completely well. His diarrhoea had resolved and stool cultures were sterile. He has subsequently remained well.

DISCUSSION

Neuro-psychiatric manifestations are well recognised in enteric fever. Studies in Africa and India show that confusional states or delirium are relatively common (23 to 57%) with semi-coma or coma less common (3.6 to 7.7%) (1, 2). However these features appear to be less common in other countries. Hoffman (5) found neuro-psychiatric complications in only 5% of 105 patients with typhoid fever during the Florida outbreak in 1973. In some cases encephalopathy may be caused by meningo-encephalitis or electrolyte derangement, but in others encephalopathic features occur in their absence.

The role of endotoxaemia in the pathogenesis of the symptoms of enteric fever is uncertain. Nag et al. (6) detected endotoxin by the chick embryo assay method in 6 out of 6 patients with typhoid encephalopathy but in none of 5 controls with uncomplicated typhoid fever. Studies using the limulus amoebocyte gelation test to detect endotoxin have produced conflicting results. Magliulo (7) reported a positive limulus test in 9/14 patients with typhoid fever and 13/25 patients with other salmonelloses. The test was negative in all patients 1 week later when afebrile and recovering from the disease. Butler (8) failed to detect endotoxin using this method in 21 patients with typhoid fever, 6 of whom had associated delirium.

Encephalopathy is very rare in infections with non typhoidal Salmonella serotypes. Meningo-encephalitis due to S. enteritidis is rare and occurs almost exclusively in infants (9). Encephalopathy manifested by a depressed level of consciousness and delirium in the presumed absence of CNS infection has been reported in association with Salmonella choleraesuis infection (10), but the CSF findings were compatible with a partially treated meningitis. There was no evidence of direct CNS infection in the patient presented here. As the encephalopathic features in this child remained when he became afebrile, it is possible that his toxic confusional state could have been due to S. enteritidis endotoxaemia. Apart from this one case there are no previous reports in the literature of encephalopathy associated with non typhoidal salmonella infection.

The severity of the encephalopathy in the case described is cause for concern in the light of the increasing incidence of infection with S. enteritidis phage type 4.

REFERENCES

1. Osuntokun BO, Bademosi O, Ogunremi K, Wright SG. Neuropsychatric manifestations of typhoid fever in 959 patients. Arch Neurol 27: 7–13, 1972.

2. Khosla SN, Srivastava SC, Gupta S. Neuro-psychiatric manifestations of typhoid. J Trop Med Hyg 80: 95–98, 1977.
3. PHLS-SVS Update on Salmonella infection 14, 1993.
4. Teasdale G, Jennett B. Assessment of comma and impaired consciousness: a practical scale. Lancet 2: 81–84, 1974.
5. Hoffman TA, Ruiz CJ, Counts GW, Sachs JM, Nitzkin JL. Waterborne typhoid fever in Dade County, Florida. Am J Med 59: 481–487, 1975.
6. Nag AK, Saha K, Mehrotra AN, Ray D. Endotoxemia in Typhoid Encephalopathy. Indian J Med Res 63: 1273–1279, 1975.
7. Magliulo E, Scevola D, Fumarola D, Vaccaro R, Bertotto A, Burberi S. Clinical Experience in Detecting Endotoxaemia with the Limulus Test in Typhoid Fever and other Salmonella Infections. Infection 4: 21–24, 1976.
8. Butler T, Bell WR, Levin J, Linh NN, Arnold K. Typhoid fever: Studies of Blood Coagulation, Bacteraemia and Endotoxaemia. Arch Intern Med 138: 407–410, 1975.
9. Saphra I, Winter JW. Clinical manifestations of salmonellosis in man. An evaluation of 7779 human infections identified at the New York Salmonella Center. N Engl J Med 256: 1128–1134, 1957.
10. Daras M, Blankfein R, Singh BM. Salmonella choleraesuis encephalopathy. NY State J Med 80: 1606–1607, 1980.

Submitted January 13, 1994; accepted March 20, 1994

Scand J Infect Dis 26: 489–490, 1994

CASE REPORT

Salmonella paratyphi – an Unusual Cause of Primary Septic Arthritis of the Hip

GEOFFREY J. STRANKS and MAGNUS I. McLAREN

From the Department of Orthopaedics, Queen Alexandra Hospital, Cosham, Portsmouth, Hampshire, England

Salmonella paratyphi is an extremely rare cause of primary septic arthritis of the hip, especially in the U.K. The presentation is no different from other causative organisms. A case is described illustrating that uncommon organisms can cause septic arthritis and that for successful treatment correct organism identification is paramount.

G. J. Stranks, FRCS (Ed), "Rivendell", Chase Grove, Waltham Chase, Hampshire, SO32 2LF, England

INTRODUCTION

Septic Arthritis occurs very rarely after infection with salmonella, even in endemic areas. It then most often occurs in patients with osteomyelitis who are immunocompromised to some degree due to malignancy, diabetes, rheumatoid diseases or who have sickle cell disease. We report here a case of salmonella primary septic arthritis of the hip.

CASE REPORT

A 66-year-old Caucasian woman presented with a 2 month history of right sided groin and buttock pain following a perforated duodenal ulcer. She was diabetic controlled on oral medication. On admission she had severe pain on any right hip movement. X-ray of the right hip showed marked destruction of the femoral head which had not been present on a previous X-ray taken 6 weeks before (Fig. 1). Her Erythrocyte Sedimentation Rate was 70. A needle aspiration and washout of the right hip was performed. Salmonella parathyphi B was isolated and grown from all specimens obtained from the hip. All blood, urine and stool cultures were negative. There was no history of fever or gastrointestinal disturbance apart from the perforated duodenal ulcer so no clear source for the infection could be established. She was treated with 6 week course of Ciprofloxacin (intravenously for 5 days 200 mg b.d. then orally 500 mg b.d.) prior to a further aspiration and washout of the right hip. No organisms were grown. The Erythrocyte Sedimentation Rate returned to normal. The destruction to the hip was so severe that a right sided cemented total hip replacement was performed. A further 6 week course of prophylactic antibiotics was given.

After 2 years she is fully mobile, pain free and there is no radiological evidence of hip loosening.

DISCUSSION

Salmonella causing osteomyelitis and more particularly a destructive arthropathy is rare and not widely reported in the literature (1). It is especially uncommon in the United Kingdom. A bacteraemia with or without any gastrointestinal disturbance is known to occur with salmonella infections and, in association with the diabetes, is the most likely mechanism by which the infection occurred in this case. The bacteraemia may have occurred at the time of the perforated duodenal ulcer as there was no history of fever or enteric symptoms.

The clinical and radiological presentations of salmonella osteomyelitis or septic arthritis are no different from other infective causes. Relapse of infection and development of chronic sepsis has been reported to be a problem with salmonella infections after initial treatment (2).

 ISSN 0036-5548

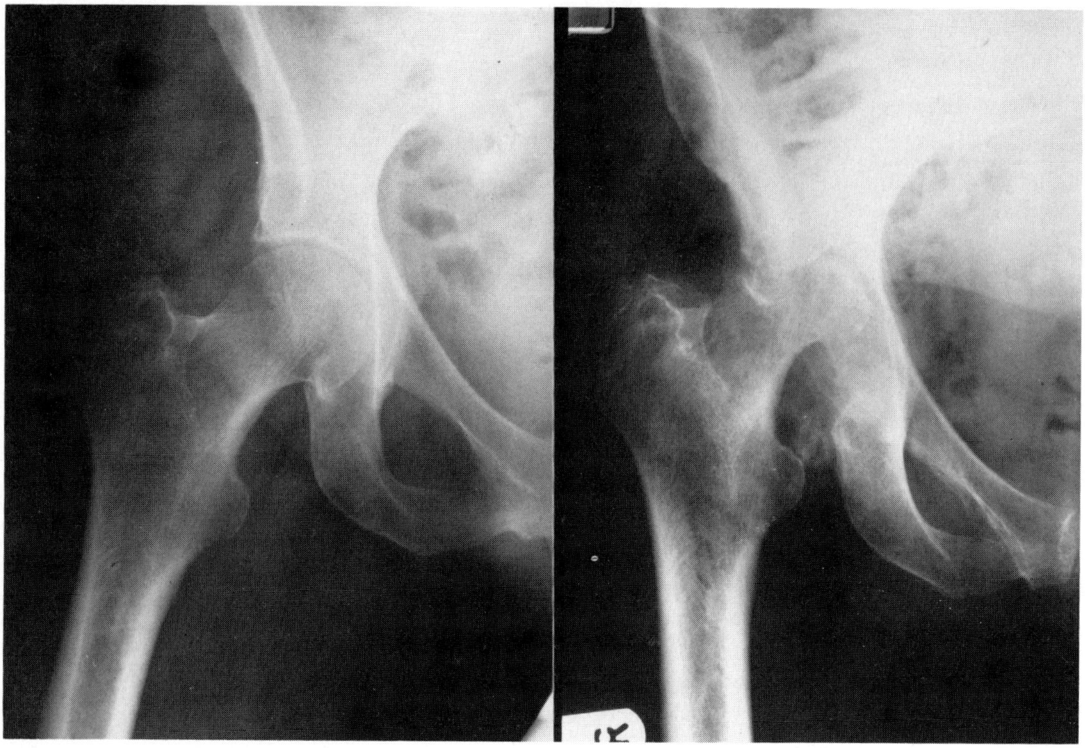

Fig. 1. Right hip 6 weeks before and on admission.

It has also been reported as causing infection post total hip replacement especially where a patient is a possible carrier (3). Correct organism identification and treatment with appropriate antibiotics until the Erythrocyte Sedimentation Rate is normal is therefore extremely important especially if joint replacement is contemplated. Prophylactic antibiotics at the time of surgery must also reflect the antibiotic sensitivity of the salmonella and if there are any signs of early loosening of the prosthesis, reactivation of the salmonella infection must be excluded.

REFERENCES

1. Morgan MG, Forbes KJ, Gillespie SG. Salmonella septic arthritis: a case report and review. J Infect 21: 195–203, 1990.
2. Govender S, Chotai PR. Salmonella Osteitis and Septic Arthritis. J Bone Joint Surg [Br] 72-B: 504–506, 1990.
3. Samra Y, Shakred Y, Maier MK. Nontyphoid Salmonellosis in Patients with Total Hip Replacement. Rev Infect Dis 8: 978–983, 1986.

Submitted February 21, 1994; accepted March 28, 1994

Scand J Infect Dis 26: 491–492, 1994

CASE REPORT

A Case of Haemorrhagic Fever with Renal Syndrome Complicated by Spleen Haemorrhage

OLEG A. ALEXEYEV[1], VJACHESLAV G. MOROZOV[1], ANDREI G. EFREMOV[2] and BO SETTERGREN[3]

From the [1]Department of Infectious Diseases, Samara's Medical University, the [2]Division of Computer Tomography, Diagnostic Center, Samara, Russia, and the [3]Department of Infectious Diseases, Umeå University Hospital, Umeå, Sweden

A case of haemorrhagic fever with renal syndrome (HFRS) complicated by spleen haemorrhage is described. The patient developed progressive anaemia, hypotension and signs of preshock. Computerized tomography demonstrated extensive haematoma in the spleen and splenectomy was performed. This case confirms previous reports that HFRS caused by Puumala virus may be associated with severe haemorrhagic manifestations.

B. Settergren, MD, PhD, Department of Infectious Diseases, Umeå University Hospital, S-90185 Umeå, Sweden

INTRODUCTION

Haemorrhagic fever with renal syndrome (HFRS) is an acute viral zoonosis with worldwide distribution (1). The hallmark of this disease is the triad of fever, acute renal failure and various haemorrhagic signs. Puumala virus associated HFRS occurs chiefly in Europe and is generally characterized by mild haemorrhagic manifestations (2, 3). However, several reports have shown that the disease may be associated with severe haemorrhage (3–5). We report a case of HFRS complicated by a spleen hematoma.

CASE REPORT

A 45-year-old male was admitted to the Department of Infectious Diseases, Clinics of the Medical Institute, Samara, Russia on the 4th day after onset of the disease. On admittance he complained of fever (38.4°C), headache, abdominal and flank pain, oliguria (150 ml/24 h) and thirst.

His blood pressure was 100/80 mmHg and pulse rate 80/min. Laboratory findings were: massive proteinuria (16.5 g/l), haematuria, and increased concentration of blood urea nitrogen, 20.9 mmol/l (normal value <8.5). During the following days he became afebrile and diuresis was restored. On the 8th day of disease, left flank and chest pain occurred and the patient became hypotonic (blood pressure 80/60 mmHg). Laboratory analysis revealed progressive anaemia (Hb 110/g/l and 84 g/l on days 4 and 10 after onset of disease, respectively). The thrombocyte count was slightly decreased ($90{,}000 \times 10^9$/l). Intra-abdominal bleeding was suspected. Computerized tomography (CT) revealed extensive subcapsular bleeding (8×22 cm) in the spleen (Fig. 1). Splenectomy was performed. Histological investigation revealed a parenchymal haematoma.

The patient was discharged 6 weeks after hospitalization, in good clinical condition. Since the patient came from a highly endemic area, HFRS was suspected and sera were tested for specific IgG antibodies by an indirect immunofluorescence assay using Puumala virus grown in Vero E6 cells as antigen (6). Analysis of acute and convalescence phase sera revealed a 4-fold increase in IgG antibody titre to Puumala virus strain CG-1820; titres were 1/40 and 1/512, respectively. In addition, Puumala virus specific IgM was demonstrated in the acute-phase sample by use of a μ-capture ELISA.

DISCUSSION

To the best of our knowledge this is the first case of HFRS caused by Puumala virus complicated by a spleen haemorrhage. The patient had suffered severe renal failure and developed progressive anaemia and hypotension accompanied by pain in the left flank and

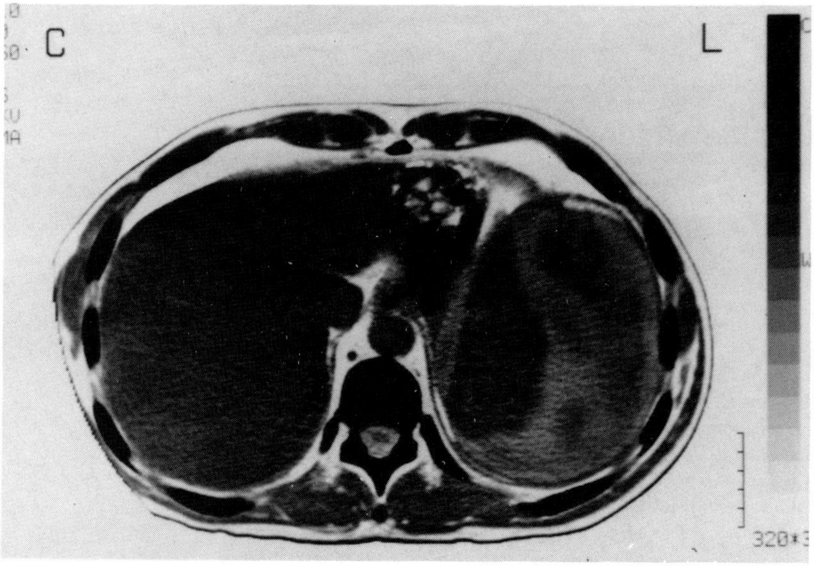

Fig. 1. CT scan showing an excessive haematoma in the spleen.

chest. Clinically the patient was in preshock. A spleen haematoma was verified by computerized tomography, and a splenectomy was performed.

In Europe, most cases of HFRS are caused by Puumala virus and the disease is generally associated with a benign course. However, severe clinical manifestations such as renal haematoma (3), disseminated intravascular coagulation (4) and cerebral haemorrhage (7) have been reported. The mechanisms leading to haemorrhage during HFRS are not fully understood, but thrombocytopenia, platelet dysfunction, changed coagulation factors, and increased capillary fragility may all contribute (8). In conclusion, this case confirms that HFRS caused by Puumala virus may be associated with severe haemorrhagic manifestations, as previously reported for HFRS caused by other hantaviruses.

REFERENCES

1. Lee HW, Lee PW, Baek LJ, Chu YK. Geographical distribution of hemorrhagic fever with renal syndrome and hantaviruses. Arch Virol (Suppl 1): 5–18, 1990.
2. Settergren B. Nephropathia epidemica (hemorrhagic fever with renal syndrome) in Scandinavia. Rev Infect Dis 13: 736–744, 1991.
3. Roshchupkin VI, Suzdaltsev AA. Hemorrhagic fever with renal syndrome. Kuibyshev: Saratov University, 1–104, 1990 [in Russian].
4. Settergren B, Norrby R, Näslund U, Wadell G. Case of epidemic nephropathy associated with disseminated intravascular coagulation. Lancet 2: 1419, 1983.
5. Zeier M, Zöller L, Weinreich T, Padeberg-Wolf E, Andrassy K, Ritz E. Severe hemorrhagic complications from infection with nephropathia epidemica strain of hantavirus. Clin Nephrol 38: 190–192, 1992.
6. Lee HW, Lee PW, Johnson KM. Isolation of the etiologic agent of Korean hemorrhagic fever. J Infect Dis 137: 298–308, 1978.
7. Settergren B, Leschinskaya E, Zagidullin I, Faslyeva R, Khunafina D, Niklasson B. Hemorrhagic fever with renal syndrome: comparison of clinical course in Sweden and the Western Soviet Union. Scand J Infect Dis 23: 549–552, 1991.
8. Cosgriff TM. Mechanisms of disease in hantavirus infection: pathophysiology of hemorrhagic fever with renal syndrome. Rev Infect Dis 13: 97–107, 1991.

Submitted January 12, 1994; accepted March 20, 1994

Scand J Infect Dis 26: 493–494, 1994

CASE REPORT

Mixed Bacteremia with Vibrio metschnikovii in an 83-year-old Female Patient

HJØRDIS HARDARDOTTIR,[1] KJELL VIKENES,[2] ASBJØRN DIGRANES,[1] JØRGEN LASSEN[3] and ALFRED HALSTENSEN[2]

From the Departments of [1]Microbiology and Immunology, the Gade Institute, [2]Medicine, Haukeland Hospital, Bergen, and of [3]Bacteriology, National Institute of Public Health, Oslo, Norway

An 83-year-old woman suddenly fell ill and was admitted to the hospital on suspicion of a heart attack. After admission she developed high fever, chills and malaise. Vibrio metschnikovii and Staphylococcus hominis were isolated from 2 separately obtained blood cultures. One of the cultures also yielded Escherichia coli. The patient's condition improved rapidly after treatment with ampicillin intravenously. To our knowledge, this is the fourth reported case of V. metschnikovii bacteremia in humans.

K. Vikenes, MD, Department of Heart Disease, Haukeland Hospital, N-5021 Bergen, Norway

INTRODUCTION

Like other species of the genus Vibrio, Vibrio metschnikovii is widely distributed in the aquatic environment and has been frequently recovered from rivers, estuaries and sewage (1). The organism has also been isolated from blood, urine, feces and other clinical specimens, but only 3 cases of well-documented human infections have been reported. The present report describes a bacteremic case in an elderly female patient.

CASE REPORT

On March 25, 1992, an 83-year-old woman fell abruptly ill; on her way to the shop she fainted and remained unconscious for about 1–2 min. She complained of chest pain and was admitted to the hospital on suspicion of a heart attack. On admission, her blood pressure was 155/75 mmHg, pulse rate 70/min and body temperature 37°C. No cyanosis, edema or jaundice was observed.

Physical examination revealed a systolic murmur at the base of the heart, compatible with an aortic stenosis. The electrocardiogram showed no signs of myocardial infarction.

Cardiac enzyme values in serum were evaluated, but the pattern was not typical of myocardial infarction. The peripheral blood leukocyte count was 14×10^9/l, the erythrocyte sedimentation rate 17 mm and the serum C-reactive protein 6 mg/l.

Shortly after admission, the patient developed high fever, chills and malaise. Two blood cultures were drawn 1.5 h apart and a urine specimen was collected. Treatment with ampicillin intravenously was initiated, whereupon the patient's condition rapidly improved.

METHODS

The Bactec NR 660 system (Becton Dickinson, MD, USA) was used for blood cultures; Bactec Plus 26 medium for aerobic culture and Bactec Plus 27 medium for anaerobic culture. The blood volume in each bottle was 8–10 ml. Both blood cultures (4 bottles) yielded Staphylococcus hominis and a pleomorphic Gram-negative rod which could not be identified by conventional methods. One of the blood cultures (2 bottles) also grew Escherichia coli. The unidentified Gram-negative rod was submitted to the National Institute of Public Health, Oslo, where it was identified as a V. metschnikovii. The diagnosis was later confirmed at the Department of Clinical Bacteriology, Culture Collection, University of Göteborg, Göteborg, Sweden.

 ISSN 0036-5548

The V. metschnikovii and E. coli isolates were both fully susceptible to ampicillin, cephalosporins, fluoroquinolones and netilmicin. The Staphylococcus hominis isolate did not produce beta-lactamase and was susceptible to cephalosporins, clindamycin, vancomycin and netilmicin.

DISCUSSION

Although V. metschnikovii has been recovered from clinical specimens, human infection caused by this organism is a rarity (2, 3). V. metschnikovii requires only a small amount of sodium for growth. It grows well on non-selective media such as blood agar and should not be easily overlooked in bacteriological laboratories. Like most of the Vibrio species, V. metschnikovii is halophilic, but it is differentiated from other Vibrio species of clinical importance by its negative oxidase and nitrate reductase reactions.

In our patient, V. metschnikovii was isolated together with S. hominis in both blood cultures and also with E. coli in one of the cultures. The potential role of the different isolates is questionable, and the clinical significance of V. metschnikovii is difficult to assess. However, the patient had a clinical picture of a serious systemic infection, V. metschnikovii was isolated from 2 separately obtained blood cultures, and it is not likely that the cultures could have been contaminated with a marine vibrio from the skin of the patient or from the hospital environment.

Most infections caused by marine vibrios are associated with exposure to seawater or seafood. The original source in our case is not known; the patient had not been abroad recently and had not consumed uncooked seafood. An association between V. metschnikovii and gallbladder disease has been reported (2). In our patient, the gallbladder had been removed several years previously, and blood cultures drawn at that time proved negative.

The patient had no predisposing diseases such as malignancy, diabetes or immunoglobulin deficiency syndrome. She was readmitted several months later for other reasons; blood cultures drawn on that occasion did not show any growth.

To our knowledge, only 3 cases of V. metschnikovii bacteremia have previously been described. Our report provides further evidence that this organism can cause serious infections in humans.

REFERENCES

1. Lee JV, Donovan TJ, Furniss AL. Characterization, taxonomy, and emended description of Vibrio metschnikovii. Int J Syst Bacteriol 28: 99–111, 1978.
2. Jean-Jacques W, Rajashekaraiah KR, Farmer III JJ, Hickman FW, Morris JG, Kallick CA. Vibrio metschnikovii bacteremia in a patient with cholecystitis. J Clin Microbiol 14: 711–712, 1981.
3. Hansen W, Freney J, Benyagoub H, Letouzey M-N, Gigi J, Wauters G. Severe human infections caused by Vibrio metschnikovii. J Clin Microbiol 31: 2529–2530, 1993.

Submitted November 2, 1993; accepted March 24, 1994

Scand J Infect Dis 26: 495–497, 1994

CASE REPORT

Bacteroides fragilis Arthritis in a Sickle Cell-Thalassaemia Patient

KOSTAS KONSTANTOPOULOS, ATHINA AVLAMI, KYRIAKI DEMARONGONA, GIANNIS SIDERIS, LITSA REKOUMI, JOANNA STEFANOU, ERSI VOSKARIDOU and DIMITRIS LOUKOPOULOS

From the First University Department of Medicine and the Department of Microbiology, Laikon Hospital, Athens, Greece

Anaerobic arthritis due to Bacteroides fragilis was diagnosed in a 33-year-old patient with prolonged fever suffering from sickle cell/thalassaemia. The causative agent was isolated from blood and purulent synovial fluid from both knee joints. A combination of chloramphenicol plus metronidazole treatment proved effective. Anaerobic arthritis has not previously been described in patients with sickle cell disease, and may reflect the well-known susceptibility of these patients to pathogens.

K. Konstantopoulos, MD, First University Department of Medicine, Laikon Hospital, 11527 Athens, Greece

INTRODUCTION

Anaerobic septic arthritis represents a rather uncommon event in clinical practice. Although underestimation of undiagnosed cases cannot be excluded, the proportion of arthritides due to anaerobic bacteria seems to be less than 1% in large series. In the reported cases, the commonest causative factors documented were anaerobic cocci and clostridium species (1). We report a case of anaerobic arthritis in a Greek patient suffering from sickle-cell/thalassaemia, a condition of well-known susceptibility to certain infections. To the best of our knowledge this seems to be the first case of anaerobic arthritis reported in the literature on sickle cell disease.

CASE REPORT

A 33-year-old Greek male was admitted to our hospital with a febrile and painful crisis of sickle cell/thalassaemia. The crisis started 3 days before his admission; he complained of pain in the legs, especially his knees and ankles, and also of headache and rigour. His body temperature ranged between 38.5° and 40°C during the day.

The sickle cell/thalassaemia had been diagnosed when he was 4 years old. The course of his disease was mild. There was a history of pulmonary tuberculosis which had been diagnosed 2 years before and successfully treated with a standard anti-TBC regimen; there was also a history of ulcerative colitis confirmed by colonoscopy and biopsy some 12 months before his present admission. The latter disease seemed to be in remission for the last few months; however, the patient was taking sulfasalazine perorally and a steroid retention enema was applied on a daily basis.

On clinical examination he looked pale and slightly jaundiced. No signs of mental confusion, meningitis or neurological pathology were evident. The spleen was palpable 12 cm below the left costal margin; no lymph nodes were palpable. The physical examination was otherwise normal. The laboratory values on admission were: haematocrit, 26%; haemoglobin, 81.5 g/l; ESR, 110 mm/1 h; WBC, 18.3×10^9/l (differential count: neutrophils 78%, lymphocytes 12%, monocytes 8%, eosonophils 1%, basophils 1%); platelets, 220×10^9/l.

The patient was treated with ampicillin (4 g/d) plus amikacin (1 g/d). Blood cultures were taken prior to instituting antibiotics. Two days later, his left knee joint became tender, swollen and erythematous

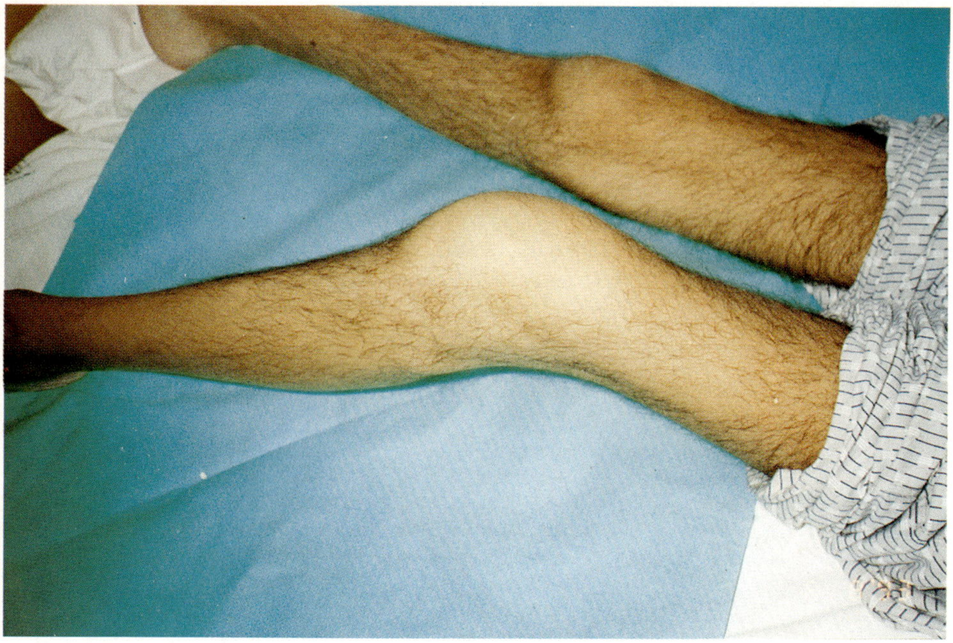

Fig. 1. Local signs of left knee arthritis.

(Fig. 1). Following a 2-day observation and as the knee became worse, some 80 ml of viscous and yellowish purulent fluid was aspirated from the joint. There were 80,000 WBCs/mm^3, 95% of which were segmented neutrophils; a Gram strain revealed occasional negative bacilli.

The patient's medication was changed to chloramphenicol 3 g, co-trimoxazole 320/1600 mg and ciprofloxacin 1 g/day. Following isolation of the pathogen, Bacteroides fragilis, from both the blood culture and the synovial fluid culture, he was treated with metronidazole 3 g/d and chloramphenicol 3 g/d for 28 days.

One day later, during the above antibiotic treatment, the right knee joint developed similar local symptoms and findings. Aspiration yielded purulent fluid; following appropriate culture, a B. fragilis strain was also isolated. During the following days, there was some evidence of inflammatory involvement in several other joints; however, the local signs were less severe and a gradual remission was noted. The knee x-ray was normal throughout the illness. Five weeks after admission, the patient was discharged from the hospital in fairly good condition.

Bacteriology

The Bacteroides fragilis strain was isolated from blood and synovial fluid by Bactec NR-730 (Becton-Dickinson Diagnostics, MD, USA) in the anaerobic bottle. Isolation and identification was conducted according to the Wadworth Anaerobic Bacteriology Manual (2). Bacterial growth was recorded by the third day of incubation for the synovial fluid culture and by the fifth day of incubation for the blood cultures.

Susceptibility testing was conducted in the laboratory by microbroth dilution (Sensititre anaerobic plate) to the following antimicrobials (MIC, Minimal Inhibitory Concentration, mg/l): Benzyl penicillin, 8; timentin, 95/4; augmentin, 8/4; piperacillin, 4; cefoxitin, 64; cefoperazone, 64; moxalactam, 0.25; imipenem, <0.5; clindamycin, 0.25; doxycycline, 4; metronidazole, 32.

The confirmation of susceptibility results by a reference laboratory (Huddinge Hospital, Stockholm) revealed the following MIC values: Benzyl penicillin, 8; OSV ampicillin 4, cefoxitin 32, imipenem 0.15, clindamycin 0.25, chloramphenicol 4, metronidazole 1, erythromycin 2. This discrepancy as far as MIC for metronidazole is concerned, may have been due to the method applied at our laboratory (microbroth dilution).

DISCUSSION

There is accumulating evidence of a greater incidence of certain infections in patients with sickle cell disease. Salmonella, Streptococcus pneumoniae and Haemophilus influenzae are the commonest pathogens reported (3), whereas other pathogens are relatively more common in this disease than in the general population, viz. E. coli and probably malaria (3, 4). Agents such as mycoplasma and several viruses, apart from their higher incidence among sickle cell patients, are also assumed to have unusual clinical features in this group (3, 5). Osteomyelitis in sickle cell anaemia is a common complication (6); and septic arthritis is also increasingly recognized (7).

The precise mechanism of the susceptibility of sickle cell patients to infection is still unclear; probably, it has to do with defective splenic function which commences early in life. On the other hand, abnormalities in complement, immunoglobulins and leukocytes are also reported. Vaso-occlusion resulting in the formation of necrotic tissue which harbours certain pathogens is a further contibuting factor. It should be emphasized that the double heterozygotes sickle cell anaemia/thalassaemia patients are as prone to infection as are homozygous sickle cell anaemia subjects (3, 5); However, it seems necessary to learn much more about the mechanisms underlying the susceptibility of this group to infections.

In general, the involvement of anaerobes as infectious agents in sickle cell patients is rather uncertain. The cases reported are few and the relevant literature is limited. In particular, we are unaware of any data on cases of anaerobic arthritis in sickle cell anaemia patients. However, the demanding conditions for isolation of anaerobes may have produced false-negative results and underestimation of the true incidence of anaerobes as a cause of septic arthritis (8). Furthermore, it is evident that more clinical and epidemiological data are necessary before one can connect sickle cell anemia with B. fragilis. It is also fairly obvious that facilities for isolation and identification of anaerobes must be available in centres dealing with patients of this group.

ACKNOWLEDGEMENT

The authors wish to thank Professor Carl Erik Nord for his kind help.

REFERENCES

1. Fitzgerald RH, Rosenblatt JE, Tenney JH. Anaerobic septic arthritis. Clin Orthop 164: 141–148, 1982.
2. Sutter VL, Citron DM, Edelstein MAC, Finegold SM. Wadsworth Anaerobic: Bacteriology Manual. 4th ed. Star Publishing Co 1985, Belmont CA.
3. Serjeant GR. Sickle cell disease. Oxford: Oxford University Press, 1985.
4. Robinson MG, Halpern C. Infections, Escherichia coli and sickle cell anemia. JAMA 230: 1145–1148, 1974.
5. Weatherall DJ, Clegg JB. The Thalassaemia Syndromes. 3rd ed. Oxford: Blackwell, 1981.
6. Bennet OM, Namnyak SS. Bone and joint manifestations in sickle cell anaemia. J Bone Joint Surg [Br] 72: 494–499, 1990.
7. Sankaran-Kutty M, Sadat-Ali M, Kutty MK. Septic arthritis in sickle cell disease. Int Orthop 12: 255–257, 1988.
8. Rosenkranz P, Lederman MM, Gopalakrishna KV, Ellner JJ. Septic arthritis caused by Bacteroides fragilis. Rev Infect Dis 12: 20–30, 1990.

Submitted December 10, 1993; accepted March 30, 1994

Scand J Infect Dis 26: 498–501, 1994

CASE REPORT

Air Crescent sign and Fatal Haemoptysis in Pulmonary Mucormycosis

ROELF S. DYKHUIZEN[1], KEITH N. KERR[2] and RICHARD L. SOUTAR[3]

From the Department of [1]Infectious Diseases, City Hospital, and the Departments of [2]Pathology and [3]Haematology, Aberdeen Royal Infirmary, Aberdeen, Scotland

A case of invasive pulmonary mucormycosis complicated by fatal, massive haemoptysis in a patient with acute myeloid leukaemia is reported. This patient represents the twelfth reported case of fatal haemoptysis due to mucormycosis. The other 11 cases are reviewed and the aetiology of cavity formation and massive haemoptysis is discussed. The development of the air crescent sign on chest radiograph is an important clinical indicator of potentially fatal haemoptysis and should lead to appropriate antifungal and surgical therapy.

R. S. Dykhuizen, MD, The Infection Unit, City Hospital Urquhart Road, Aberdeen AB9 8AU, Scotland

INTRODUCTION

The term "mucormycosis" encompasses a group of infections caused by fungi belonging to classes within the order Mucorales, namely Rhizopus, Absidia, and Mucor. These fungi are ubiquitous but rarely cause disease in the normal host. Infection arises where normal immune defences are ineffective as occurs in diabetes mellitus, chemotherapy induced neutropenia and in chronic renal failure.

We report a patient who developed a pulmonary infiltrate during chemotherapy for acute myeloid leukaemia (AML). Despite clinical improvement with antimicrobial therapy, which included antifungal therapy, the patient died suddenly from fatal, massive haemoptysis. Post-mortem examination revealed a large cavity filled with necrotic sequestrum of lung parenchyma which was infiltrated by Mucorales. The aetiology and bronchial pathology of published reports on similar cases is reviewed.

CASE REPORT

A 51 year old man became pyrexial on day 1 after induction chemotherapy for acute myeloid leukaemia (AML, FAB Type M 5a).

Chest radiograph and microbiological investigations were not contributory and the patient was treated empirically with broad spectrum antibacterial agents. High dose fluconazole was added on day 7 because of persistence of the pyrexia. On day 11 crepitations were noted over the right upper lobe, without radiographic abnormality. The patient developed pleuritic chest pain and a cough with streaky haemoptysis. Fluconazole was replaced by amphotericin B and high dose co-trimoxazole was added. From day 20 onwards the patient's bone marrow regenerated from chemotherapy. Chest radiograph now showed consolidation of the right upper zone. Bronchoscopy on day 29 showed oedematous mucosa of the right upper lobe bronchus, but no other abnormality. Histopathological examination of biopsy, brushings and washings revealed features of pneumonitis only. Staining for fungi, Pneumocystis carinii and acid fast bacilli was negative.

The pyrexia settled on day 31 and bone marrow biopsy on day 32 proved the AML to be in remission. Chest radiographed showed an air crescent in the consolidation of the right upper zone (see Fig. 1). Two consecutive sputum samples on day 34 and 35 were positive on immunofluorescence for P. carinii. Antimicrobial therapy was stopped apart from co-trimoxazole which was continued orally. The patient was allowed home on day 37 and was readmitted 6 days later for consolidation chemotherapy. He appeared well clinically and was apyrexial. Eight hours after readmission he suddenly collapsed with exsanguinating haemoptysis and died despite attempts at resuscitation.

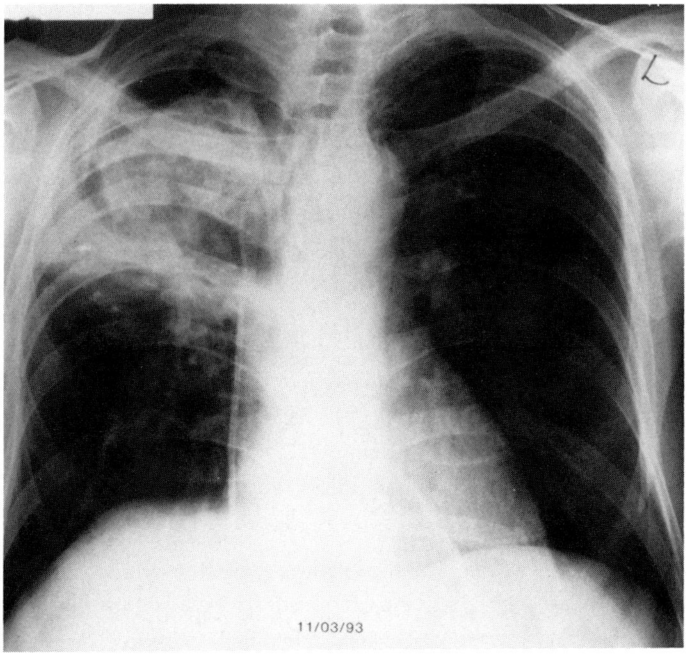

Fig. 1. The air crescent sign which appeared on chest radiograph 13 days after regeneration of bone marrow from chemotherapy and 10 days before fatal haemoptysis.

At autopsy there was fresh blood in the larynx, trachea and widespread aspiration of blood in both lungs. The apical segment of the right upper lobe was the site of an 8 × 6 × 5 cm cavity which was filled with a haemorrhagic sequestrum of lung parenchyma and blood clot. The cavity was surrounded by fibrosis and organising pneumonic consolidation. Histological examination of the sequestrum showed widespread vascular infiltration by broad, non septate fungal hyphae with right angled branches, characteristic of the Mucorales. The cavity wall showed intensive infiltration of neutrophil polymorphs, focal necrosis and haemorrhage. Despite widespread tissue sampling there was no evidence of fungus in the lungs outside the cavity.

DISCUSSION

Clinical manifestation of invasive mucormycosis is categorised as rhinocerebral, pulmonary, widely disseminated, gastrointestinal, cutaneous and miscellaneous. The predilection for one of these types of presentations differs for each of the predisposing conditions. Patients with diabetes mellitus most often develop rhinocerebral mucormycosis and neutropenic leukaemic patients typically present with pulmonary or disseminated manifestations of the disease. Invasive mucormycosis is usually fatal without specific therapy. The hallmarks of successful treatment are early diagnosis, systemic antifungal therapy, aggressive surgical debridement, and control of the underlying disease (1).

Cavity formation with development of the air crescent sign on the chest radiograph (2–4) and fatal massive haemoptysis (2–10) are recognized, but rare, complications of invasive pulmonary mucormycosis. This patient represents the twelfth reported case of fatal massive haemoptysis due to mucormycosis. In 8 of the other 11 cases the arterial-bronchial communication also involved the right bronchial tree, with a predominance of upper lobe involvement. No explanation for this preponderance is apparent and it may be no more than a chance occurrence (see Table I).

Table I. *Fatal haemoptysis due to mucormycosis: predisposing conditions and site of bleeding*

Case	Underlying disease	Steroids	Chemo-therapy	Renal-failure	Clinical condition prior to fatal haemorrhage	Site of mucorales
Winston (5), 1965	diabetes	no	no	no	improved	R-middle lobe
Reich (2), 1970	diabetes	no	no	chronic	deteriorated	R-upper lobe[a]
Bragg et al. (4), 1973	diabetes	no	no	no	unknown	R-upper lobe[a]
Murray (6), 1975	diabetes	no	no	acute	improved	R-upper lobe
Murray (6), 1975	leukaemia	no	yes	no	improved	R-upper lobe
Donohue et al. (7), 1980	diabetes	no	no	chronic	improved	R-middle lobe
Donohue et al. (7), 1980	diabetes	no	no	no	well, stable	L-hilum
Watts (8), 1983	leukaemia	no	yes	no	improved	L-upper lobe
Passamonte et al. (9), 1985	none	yes	no	acute	improved	R-upper lobe
Yagihashi et al. (10), 1991	glom. nephr	no	no	dialysis	well, stable	R-lower lobe
Harada et al. (3), 1992	leukaemia	no	yes	chronic	improved	L-upper lobe[a]
present report	leukaemia	no	yes	no	improved	R-upper lobe[a]

[a] Air crescent sign.

Death was sudden and unexpected in 10/12 patients. One patient's clinical condition was not reported and another had been deteriorating prior to the fatal haemoptysis. In 8 patients host defences had returned after an episode of severe illness and/or leucopenia. Reporting on pulmonary cavitation and massive haemoptysis in invasive pulmonary aspergillosis, Albeda et al. (11) concluded that recovery from granulocytopenia was associated with pulmonary cavitation and massive haemoptysis. An acute inflammatory reaction to necrotic lung parenchyma invaded by fungus develops, causing separation of dead from viable lung and creating a cavity with a necrotic "lung ball': the air crescent on chest radiograph. The tissue-destructive power of the neutrophils shows little intrinsic ability to differentiate between foreign and host antigens (12), which may lead to destruction of bloodvessels, explaining the association of massive haemoptysis with return of host defence mechanisms. In our case haemoptysis took place 23 days after recovery of the bone marrow from chemotherapy.

Six of the 12 reported patients had diabetes mellitus, 4 had leukaemia, 1 was on renal replacement therapy for chronic renal failure and 1 patient's host defence mechanisms were impaired by hyperglycaemia, acute renal failure and corticosteroid administration. The high prevalence of diabetes as the underlying disease in patients with pulmonary mucormycosis who suffered fatal haemoptysis contrasts with those without fatal haemoptysis, where leukaemia is the predominant predisposing condition (1). This shift may be due to differences in availability of neutrophils to cause tissue destruction. In 4 cases the air crescent sign appeared on chest radiograph prior to the fatal haemorrhage. The appearance of this sign is a clinical index for initiating surgical therapy because of the attendant risk of catastrophic haemoptysis even after appropriate medical antifungal therapy has been administered.

REFERENCES

1. Lehrer RI, Howard DH, Sypherd PS, Edwards JE, Segal GP, Winston DJ. Mucormycosis. Ann Intern Med 93: 93–108, 1980.
2. Reich J, Renzetti AD. Pulmonary phycomycosis. Am Rev Resp Dis 102: 959–964, 1970.
3. Harada M, Manabe T, Yamashita K, Okamoto N. Pulmonary mucormycosis with fatal massive haemoptysis. Acta Pathol Jpn 42: 49–55, 1992.
4. Bragg DG, Janis B. The roentgenographic manifestations of pulmonary opportunistic infections. AJR Am J Roentgenol 11: 798–809, 1973.

5. Winston RM. Phycomycosis of the bronchus. J Clin Pathol 18: 729–731, 1965.
6. Murray WM. Pulmonary mucormycosis with massive fatal haemoptysis. Chest 68: 65–68, 1975.
7. Donohue JF, Scott RJ, Walker DH, Bromberg PA. Phycomycosis: A cause of bronchial obstruction. South Med J 73: 734–736, 1980.
8. Watts WJ. Bronchopleural fistula followed by massive fatal haemoptysis in a patient with pulmonary mucormycosis. Arch Intern Med 143: 1029-1030, 1983.
9. Passamonte PM, Dix JD. Nosocomial pulmonary mucormycosis with fatal massive haemoptysis. Am J Med Sci 289: 65–67, 1985.
10. Yagihashi S, Watanabe K, Nagia K, Okudiara M. Pulmonary mucormycosis presenting as massive fatal haemoptysis in a haemodialytic patient with chronic renal failure. Klin Wochenschr 69: 224–227, 1991.
11. Albeda SM, Talbot GH, Gerson SL, Miller GT, Cassileth PA. Pulmonary cavitation and massive haemoptysis in invasive pulmonary aspergillosis. Am Rev Respir Dis 31: 115–120, 1985.
12. Weiss SJ. Tissue destruction by neutrophils. N Engl J Med 320: 365–376, 1989.
13. De Souza R, MacKinnon S, Spagnola SV, Fossieck BE Jr. Treatment of localised pulmonary phycomycosis. South Med J 72: 609–612, 1979.
14. Zagoria RJ, Choplin RH, Karstaedt N. Pulmonary gangrene as a complication of mucormycosis. AJR Am J Roentgenol 144: 1195–1196, 1985.
15. Silver SF, Grymaloski MR, Bosken CH, Paré PD, Müller ML. Pulmonary consolidation with an air crescent sign in an immunocompromised woman. J Can Assoc Radiol 40: 167–169, 1989.

Submitted February 4, 1994; accepted March 10, 1994

Scand J Infect Dis 26: 503–510, 1994

REVIEW ARTICLE

Peptostreptococcal Infection in Children

ITZHAK BROOK

From the Department of Pediatrics, Georgetown University School of Medicine, Washington, D.C., USA

680 Peptostreptococcus sp. (Ps) were recovered from 598 (34%) of 1,750 specimens obtained from 554 patients. They included 103 Ps asaccharolyticus, 74 Ps magnus, 56 Ps prevotii, 51 Ps micros, 46 Ps anaerobius, 11 Ps morbilorium, and 10 Ps saccharolyticus. Most infections were polymicrobial (in 553 instances or 92%) but in 45 (8%), Ps were recovered in pure culture. Most Ps were isolated from abscesses (237), ears (104), peritoneal fluid (95), lung infections (66), bone (30) and sinuses (24). Predisposing conditions were present in 224 (40%) children. These were previous surgery (54), immunodeficiency (43), malignancy (35), trauma (34), diabetes (23), prematurity (22), steroid therapy (19), foreign body (10) and sickle-cell anemia (7). The organisms most commonly isolated with Ps were Bacteroides sp. (276, including 190 B. fragilis group), Prevotella sp. (159), Fusobacterium sp. (122), Escherichia coli (114), and Staphylococcus aureus (97). Antimicrobial therapy was administered to all but 14 patients. Surgical drainage or correction of pathology was performed in 307 (56%) patients. 10 patients (2%) died of their infection. These data illustrate the importance of Ps and suggests their enhancing potentials in infection in children

I. Brook, MD, P.O. Box 70412, Chevy Chase, MD 20813-0412, USA

INTRODUCTION

Interest in the role of anaerobic bacteria in pediatric infections has increased in recent years. Most of the attention has been directed at the role of Bacteroides sp., while other groups of bacteria such as Peptostreptococcus sp. (Ps) were not studied as intensely. Ps are the second most common anaerobic bacteria isolated from clinical specimen (1). Although these organisms infrequently cause infections by themselves, they were found to enhance the virulence of other aerobic and anaerobic bacteria in mixed infections (2).

This paper summarizes the author's experience over a period of 15 years in the recovery of Ps from infections in children. Some of the data was published earlier in separate articles describing the role of anaerobic bacteria in pediatric infections (3). However, the role of Ps was not highlighted in any of these studies, as they were considered to be easily treated with penicillins. Furthermore, this overview includes cases not previously presented that were seen after these studies were completed.

PATIENTS AND METHODS

The children included in the study were studied by the author between June 1973 and June 1988. They were seen in the following hospitals: University of California Medical Center, Los Angeles County Medical Center, and Serra Memorial Hospital in Los Angeles, and Fairview State Hospital, Costa Mesa, California; Children's Hospital National Medical Center and South-East Community Medical Center in Washington, D.C.; and the Naval Medical Center in Bethesda, Maryland.

The clinical microbiology laboratory records were reviewed to identify patients infected with Ps. The available case histories of all patients from whom Ps had been isolated were reviewed to ascertain the

---

The opinions and assertions contained herein are those of the writer alone and are not to be construed as official or reflecting the views of the Navy Department or the naval services at large.

 ISSN 0036-5548

presence and site of infection, associated microorganisms, disease process, and possible predisposing and associated conditions.

The microbiology laboratories accepted only specimens that were properly collected and submitted in a transport medium appropriate for anaerobic bacteria. Specimens accepted for processing were those collected in a fashion that avoided contamination by the normal skin or mucus surface flora (4). These were specimens obtained during surgery, aseptic aspiration of body fluids, or needle or biopsy aspiration of abscesses or body cavities. Aspirates of lungs were obtained by transtracheal aspiration or biopsy, and urine was collected by suprapubic aspiration. When possible, pus and fluids were collected and transported in syringes. Tissues were transported in oxygen-free gassed-out tubes or in small volumes of thioglycolate broth. When possible, specimens were hand delivered. Most specimens, except blood, were submitted in Port-a-Cul transport swab or liquid systems (BBL, Cockeysville, MD). However, no exact record of the transport media used is available. Blood was collected aseptically from patients suspected of having bacteremia and was inoculated (10%, vol/vol) into 1 bottle each of 2 commercially obtained broth media, 1 under vacuum and 1 with CO_2.

The specimen material was inoculated onto pre-reduced vitamin K_1-enriched Brucella blood agar, an anaerobic blood agar plate containing kanamycin and vancomycin, an anaerobic blood plate containing colistin sulfate and naladixic acid, and an enriched thioglycolate broth (containing hemin, sodium carbonate, and vitamin K_1) (4–6). It was then incubated in GasPak jars (BBL) and examined at 48 and 96 h.

Plates that showed growth were held until the organisms were processed and identified. All cultures that showed no growth were held for at least 5 days. Organisms were identified by the API anaerobic system (Analytab Products, Plainview, NY) or by the Minitek system (BBL). In addition to these tests, when complete identification was not possible by the above methods, other carbohydrate tests (Scott Laboratories, Fiskeville, RI) and gas-liquid chromatography (4) were performed as needed, to identify the organisms. The criteria for identification were according to previously published guidelines (4, 6).

RESULTS

Of the 1,750 specimens studied for anaerobic bacteria, 680 Ps were recovered from 598 (34%) specimens obtained from 554 patients. Patients' ages ranged from 1 day to 18 years (mean 8 years, 2 months), and 302 (55%) were males. Clinical records were not available from 16 additional cases. These were not included in the final analysis. The 680 Ps included 103 Ps asaccharolyticus, 74 Ps magnus, 56 Ps prevotii, 51 Ps micros, 46 Ps anaerobius, 11 Ps morbilorum, and 10 of Ps saccharolyticus (Tables I and II). The ratio of recovery of all Ps sp. was similar among all infection sites.

Most infections were polymicrobial (in 553 instances), but in 45 (8%), Ps were recovered in pure culture. Most Ps isolated were recovered from abscesses (237 of 680 isolates, or 35%), ears (104, or 17%), peritoneal fluid (95, or 14%), and lung (66, 10%).

Predisposing or underlying conditions were present in 224 (40%) patients. A single condition was noted in 203 instances, 2 conditions were observed in 19, and three in 2 patients. The predisposing conditions were previous surgery (in 54 cases), immunodeficiency (43), malignancy (35), trauma (34), diabetes (23), prematurity (22), steroid therapy (19), foreign body (10) and sickle cell anemia (7).

There were 1,342 other bacterial isolates recovered, mixed with Ps in the 553 specimens with polymicrobial flora, 574 anaerobes and 768 facultative anaerobes or aerobes. The number of other isolates in these infections varied between 1 to 6 (average 2.4 isolates/per specimen, 1.0 anaerobe and 1.4 facultative or aerobes). The organisms most commonly isolated with Ps were Bacteroides sp (276 isolates, including 190 B. fragilis group), Prevotella sp. (159), (including 40 P. melaninogenica, 20 P. intermedia, and 12 P. oralis, Fusobacterium sp. (122), Escherichia coli (114), Staphylococcus aureus (97) and alpha hemolytic streptococci (78).

Most S. aureus isolates were isolated from abscesses, and E. coli from intra-abdominal infection, and skin and soft tissue infection proximal to the rectal area.

Table I. *Incidence of* Peptostreptococcus *sp. in 598 specimens obtained from children*

	Number of Specimens					Number of isolates						
	total	with Ps	with Ps alone	total Ps	Ps sp.	Ps asacch.	Ps morbil.	Ps prevotii	Ps sacch.	Ps anaerobius	Ps micros	Ps magnus
Abscesses	538	205	6	237	95	57	3	22	4	19	15	22
Bites	39	25		27	18	4						5
Blood	34	6	5	6	2	1	1			1		1
Burn	180	22	1	27	10	6	2	3				6
Conjunctivitis	148	24	7	29	27			1		1		
Decubitus ulcers	59	19		22	10		1	2		4	3	2
Empyema	72	8	2	8	4					1	1	2
Omphalitis	25	4		4	2			1		1		
Otitis (acute)	218	26	15	28	19	1		2		1	2	3
Otitis (chronic)	94	36	4	38	21	4		3		3	2	5
cholesteatoma	24	10		13	6	1		2	1	2	1	
mastoiditis	24	18		20	10	2		2	1		2	3
Otitis (serous)	23	4	1	5		3		1			1	
Peritonitis	115	82		95	51	8	3	2	1	3	15	12
Pneumonia	80	60	1	66	40	5		7	2	6	4	2
Osteomyelitis	27	26	1	30	10	5		5		3		7
Sinusitis	45	22	2	24	4	5	1	3	1	1	5	4
Urinary tract	5	1		1		1						
Total	1750	598	45	680	329	103	11	56	10	46	51	74

Table II. *Incidence of* Peptostreptococcus *sp. (Ps) in 205 abscesses from children*

Abscesses	No. of specimens	No. of abscesses with Ps	No. of abscesses with Ps alone	Total Ps	Number of isolates: Ps sp.	Ps asacch.	Ps morbil.	Ps prevotii	Ps sacch.	Ps anaerobius	Ps micros	Ps magnus
Abdomen	40	21		23	5	7	1	3		2	3	2
Breast	14	2		2		1						1
Buttocks	15	11		12	4	3		3		2		
Cervical	53	8	1	9	4	3					1	1
Dental	15	7		8	3			1			4	
Hand	25	3		3	2	1						
Fingers	20	6		7	4	2					1	
Head	31	9	1	10	2	5		1			1	1
Intracranial	39	16	1	18	8	3		2		1	1	3
Liver	8	2		2						1		1
Leg	28	5		5	3	1				1		
Lung	10	8		13	5	2		2	1	2	1	
Neck	36	5	1	7	2	1		3		1		
Paronychia	33	20		23	12	6						5
Parotid	5	2	1	2	1							1
Perirectal	28	13		15	6	4	1	2				2
Peritonsillar	18	14		16	8	2		1	1	2		2
Placental	25	14		14	4	7		3				
Renal	10	2		2		1					1	
Retropharyngeal	14	13		18	7	3		1	2	3	1	1
Scalp	23	5		6	3	2						1
Spleen	11	2	1	2						1		1
Subphrenic	14	10		12	8	3	1					
Trunk	17	2		2	1					1		
Vulvovaginal	6	5		6	3					2	1	
Total	538	205	6	237	95	57	3	22	4	19	15	22

Of the 598 specimens, 205 (34%) were from abscesses (Table I). The most common abscesses harboring Ps were oropharyngeal (34), extremities and fingers (34), rectal area (24), abdominal (21), intracranial (16), and cervical head and neck (13). The most common other organisms that were also recovered in abscesses mixed with Ps were Fusobacterium sp. (55), B. fragilis group (54), S. aureus and E. coli (42 each).

Of the 27 Ps isolated from bites, 18 were recovered from human origin and 9 from animal bites. They were isolated from bites of all body parts and were mostly mixed with S. aureus and Fusobacterium sp.

Of the 6 Ps recovered from blood, 5 were isolated in pure culture, and 1 was recovered with B. fragilis in a child with intra-abdominal abscess. The 5 single isolates were found in 4 patients with head and neck infections (2 sinusitis and one peritonsillar abscess and one subdural empyema) and 1 patient with a burn of the head.

Of the 27 burns, all except 1 were recovered with other organisms. Nine isolates were recovered from the upper extremities isolates, 6 from the oral area, 9 from the lower extremities and 3 from the anal area. The most common other organism mixed with Ps were Staphylococcus sp.

Of the 29 conjunctival isolates, 7 were recovered in pure culture, and the others were mixed with Staphylococcus sp., Propionibacterium acnes, and Streptococcus pneumoniae.

Of the 22 isolates from decubitus ulcers, 8 were recovered from scalp, 7 from the hand, 5 from the buttocks, and 22 from the leg ulcers. The most common other isolates were Bacteroides sp. and Enterobacteriaceae.

Of the 8 empyema isolates, 2 were recovered in pure culture, 4 were found mixed with S. aureus and 2 with Fusobacterium sp.

The 4 omphalitis isolates were all recovered mixed with other flora.

Of the 28 isolates of acute otitis media and 5 with serous otitis, 16 were recovered in pure culture, and the others were mixed with S. aureus, Haemophilus influenzae and S. pneumoniae.

Of the 71 isolates found in chronic otitis media and its complications (including mastoiditis and cholesteatoma), 4 were recovered in pure culture, and the others were mixed with other bacteria, mostly H. influenzae, S. aureus, and Prevotella sp.

The 95 peritoneal isolates were recovered from 82 children, all mixed with other bacteria, mostly B. fragilis group, E. coli and Enterococcus sp. 66 patients presented with peritonitis after ruptured appendix, 7 after trauma, 6 after rupture of viscus, and 3 had spontaneous peritonitis.

Of the 66 isolates from aspiration pneumonia, 65 were mixed with other organisms, mostly of oral flora origin (viz., Fusobacterium sp., Prevotella spp.).

Of the 30 osteomyelitis isolates, 29 were mixed with other flora. The single isolate was recovered from the temporal bone and the blood from a patient with chronic mastoiditis. 13 of the isolates were recovered from osteomyelitis of the orofacial bones associated with mastoiditis, 3 from maxillary and mandibular bones associated with periodontal abscess, 5 from the coccyx or occipital areas associated with decubitus ulcer, 7 from fingers (originating from bites), and 1 from the tibia following trauma.

Of the 24 chronically infected sinus isolates, 2 were found in pure culture in chronic maxillary sinusitis, and the others were mixed with other organisms, mostly Fusobacterium sp. and Prevotella sp.

The single urinary isolate was mixed with Eubacterium adolescentis from a 7-year-old girl with lower urinary tract infection.

Systemic antimicrobial therapy was given to all patients, except 8 with burns and 6 with conjunctivitis. Surgical drainage or correction of pathology was performed in 307 (56%) of the patients. The antimicrobials administered were clindamycin (in 131 instances), amoxicillin or ampicillin (92), penicillin (86), cefazolin (52), cefoxitin (49), chloramphenicol (46), ureidopenicillin (44), beta-lactam resistant penicillin (26), erythromycin (25), metronidazole (18), trimethropim-sulfa (16) and aminoglycosides (188). 10 patients (2%) died of their infection, 4 with pneumonia, 3 with peritonitis and 1 each with burn, bacteremia, and intracranial abscess.

DISCUSSION

This retrospective study demonstrated the importance of Ps in a variety of infections in children. The 680 isolates of Ps were recovered from 598 (34%) of 1,750 specimens submitted for culture for anaerobic bacteria. This review of clinical specimens confirms the importance of Ps as a common organism generally isolated mixed with other bacteria, especially in abscesses (mostly abdominal, intracranial, oropharyngeal and of the fingers), pneumonia, otolaryngological infections, bites, burns and osteomyelitis.

Anaerobic cocci have been most often reported in older studies either as 'anaerobic streptococci' or 'anaerobic Gram-positive cocci'. These organisms were previously divided into Peptococcus sp. and Peptostreptococcus sp. However, they are currently all named Peptostreptococcus sp. and further divided according to species primarily on the basis of their metabolic products. The species most commonly isolated in adults as well as in children are magnus, asaccharolyticus, anaerobius, prevotii, and micros (1, 3, 7).

Anaerobic cocci are part of the normal flora of the mouth, upper respiratory tract, intestinal tract, vagina and skin. Their presence has been documented in adults in a variety of syndromes including endocarditis, brain abscesses, puerperal sepsis, traumatic wounds, and postoperative necrotizing fasciitis (7). They have been recovered in pediatric infections in subcutaneous abscesses, decubitus ulcers and burns around the oral and anal area, brain abscesses, intra-abdominal infections, and bacteremia (3). These organisms are predominant isolates also in all types of respiratory infections, including chronic sinusitis, mastoiditis, acute and chronic otitis media, aspiration pneumonia, and lung abscess (3). Generally they are recovered mixed with other aerobic or anaerobic organisms, but in many cases they are the sole pathogen recovered. This may be of particular significance in cases of bacteremia (3, 7).

The organisms recovered in polymicrobial infections that include Ps vary and depend on the location and the circumstances leading to the infection. Most polymicrobial infections originate from the mucus flora adjacent to the infected site. B. fragilis group and Enterobacteriaceae predominate in abdominal and rectal infections, while pigmented Prevotella and Porphyromonas and Fusobacterium sp. predominate in infection in and around the oropharynx.

Ps mixed with other bacteria are frequently recovered from infections at different sites in the body (3, 7). Many of these infections are synergistic (8, 9), and the role of Ps in these infections and their effect on their aerobic or anaerobic counterparts was studied in animal models (2, 8–15). The criteria for establishing in vivo synergy between Ps and other organisms were judged by induction of sepsis (8, 9, 11, 12), mortality (13), and abscesses (10, 14, 15).

The mutual enhancement of growth of each bacterial component in mixed infections in subcutaneous (s.c.) abscesses (2) was also evaluated (2). The bacterial growth of the strict anaerobic and facultative or aerobic bacteria-inducing abscesses was enhanced much more than the growth of Ps. Although Ps strains reached the same number in mixed infections as they did in single infections, the other bacteria grew at a faster rate in mixed infection with

Ps than when injected alone (2). The promotion of growth of the flora associated with Ps therefore supports the pathogenic role of Ps in mixed infections.

We have evaluated the relative importance of 20 strains of Ps to anaerobic, aerobic, and facultative organisms, using a s.c. abscess model in mice (15). The relationship between the Ps and the other bacteria was determined by observing the effect of antimicrobial therapy directed against one or both organisms present in the abscess. Of the 70 different combinations, Ps were relatively more important than the other species in 6 combinations, equally important in 35, and less important in 29. The Ps most often found to be equal to or more important than the other bacteria were P. magnus and P. anaerobius. Proteus mirabilis, E. coli, and S. aureus were frequently found to be of greater importance than Ps.

The mutual enhancing potential of Ps and other bacteria that are commonly recovered mixed with them in clinical infection demonstrates the pathogenic potential of these organisms. The enhancing effect noted between these different bacterial strains may be due to protection from phagocytosis and intracellular killing (16), production of essential growth factors (17), and lowering of oxidation/reduction potentials in host tissues (18).

The virulence of Ps as determined by the ability to induce s.c. abscess was correlated to the presence of a capsule (14). Of 22 Ps studied, only the 11 heavily encapsulated isolates (>50% of the cells, were encapsulated) induced abscesses. However, when the other 11 isolates were injected with Bacteroides sp. or facultative and aerobic bacteria, abscesses formed in 8 of the 11 combinations. Over 50% of the Ps cells recovered from the mixed infections were encapsulated. Encapsulation also occurred in Ps injected with capsular material or with formalin-killed cells of K. pneumoniae or capsule-positive Bacteroides sp. After acquisition of capsules, these Ps strains induced abscesses by themselves on reinoculation in mice. The implication of capsular polysaccharide as a factor associated with virulence is not unique to Ps. This phenomenon has also been described in aerobic streptococci, B. fragilis (19), and Prevotella melaninogenica (20), where the capsular material was shown to inhibit phagocytosis (21). Although the presence of capsular material may be one of the important virulence mechanisms of Ps, other yet undetermined factors may influence their synergistic role in mixed infection.

Management of polymicrobial infections caused by aerobic and anaerobic bacteria including Ps requires, in addition to surgical correction and drainage of pus, the administration of antimicrobials. These agents should be effective against both aerobic and anaerobic bacterial components of the infection (22), including Ps, and other more resistant anaerobic bacteria. When such therapy is not given, the infection may persist and complications may occur (23). Ps are almost uniformly susceptible to penicillins. However, Ps are generally resistant to imidazoles (24) (metronidazole, tinidazole, and ornidazole). Antimicrobial therapies that provide coverage for infections that include Ps as well as penicillin-resistant anaerobes (i.e., B. fragilis group) are clindamycin, imipenem, the combination of a penicillin and a beta-lactamase inhibitor or cefoxitin. Therapy against resistant aerobic or facultative bacteria such as Enterobacteriaceae or S. aureus may also be needed when these organisms are present.

ACKNOWLEDGEMENTS

The author acknowledges the laboratory assistance of the staff of the Microbiology Laboratories at the University of California Medical Center, Los Angeles County Medical Center, and Serra Memorial Hospital in Los Angeles, California; Children's Hospital National Medical Center and South-East Medical Center in Washington, D.C., the Navy Hospital in Bethesda, Maryland; and the editorial assistance of Ms. J. Pietrafitta.

REFERENCES

1. Brook I. Recovery of anaerobic bacteria from clinical specimens in 12 years at two military hospitals. J Clin Microbiol 26: 1181–1188, 1988.
2. Brook I. Enhancement of growth of aerobic, anaerobic, and facultative bacteria in mixed infections with anaerobic and facultative gram-positive cocci. J Surg Res 45: 222–227, 1988.
3. Brook I. Pediatric Anaerobic Infection: Diagnosis and Management, 2nd ed. St. Louis: Mosby Co., 1989.
4. Sutter VL, Citron DM, Edelstein MAC, Finegold SM. Wadsworth Anaerobic Bacteriology Manual, 4th ed. Belmont, Ca: Star Publishing, 1985.
5. Lennette EH, Balows A, Hausler WJ Jr, Shadomy HG, eds. Manual of Clinical Microbiology, 4th edn. Washington DC: American Society for Microbiology, 1985.
6. Holdeman LV, Cates EP, Moore WEC, ed. Anaerobe Laboratory Manual, 4th ed. Blacksburg: Virginia Polytechnic Institute and State University, 1977.
7. Finegold SM. Anaerobic Bacteria in Human Disease. New York: Academic Press Inc., 1977.
8. Hite KE, Locke M, Hesseline HC. Synergism in experimental infections with nonsporulating anaerobic bacteria. J Infect Dis 84: 19, 1949.
9. Meleney F, Olpp S, Harvey HD, Jern H. Peritonitis. II. Synergism of bacteria commonly found in peritoneal exudates. Arch Surg 25: 709–721, 1932.
10. Brook I, Walker RI. Infectivity of organisms recovered from polymicrobial abscesses. Infect Immun 42: 986–989, 1983.
11. Kelly MJ. Mixtures of aerobic and anaerobic human pathogens: A rapid 4-plate counting technique. Br J Exp Pathol 58: 4478–4483, 1977.
12. Altemeier WA. The pathogenicity of the bacteria of appendicitis peritonitis. Surgery 11: 374–378, 1942.
13. Brook I, Hunter V, Walker RI. Synergistic effect of Bacteroides, Clostridium, Fusobacterium, anaerobic cocci, and aerobic bacteria on mortality and induction of subcutaneous abscesses in mice. J Infect Dis 149: 924–928, 1984.
14. Brook I, Walker RI. The role of encapsulation in the pathogenesis of anaerobic gram-positive cocci. Can J Microbiol 31: 176–180, 1985.
15. Brook I, Walker RI. Pathogenicity of anaerobic gram-positive cocci. Infect Immun 48: 320–324, 1984.
16. Ingham HR, Tharagonnet D, Sisson PR, Selkon JB, Codd AA. Inhibition of phagocytosis in vitro by obligate anaerobes. Lancet 2: 1252–1254, 1977.
17. Lev M, Keudell KC, Milford AF. Succinate as a growth factor for Bacteroides melaninogenicus. J Bacteriol 1098: 175–178, 1971.
18. Mergenhagen SE, Thomard JC, Scherp HW. Studies on synergistic infections. I. Experimental infections with anaerobic streptococci. J Infect Dis 103: 33–44, 1957.
19. Onderdonk AB, Kasper DL, Cisneros DL, Bartlett JG. The capsular polysaccharide of Bacteroides fragilis as a virulence factor: Comparison of the pathogenic potential of encapsulated strains. J Infect Dis 136: 82–89, 1977.
20. Brook I, Gillmore JD, Collbaugh JC, Walker RI. Pathogenicity of encapsulated Bacteroides melaninogenicus group, Bacteroides oralis and Bacteroides ruminicola in abscesses in mice. J Infect Dis 7: 281–286, 1983.
21. Okuda K, Takazoe I. Antiphagocytic effects of the capsular structure of a pathogenic strain of Bacteroides melaninogenicus. Bull Tokyo Dent Coll 16: 99–104, 1973.
22. Weinstein WM, Onderdonk AB, Bartlett JG, Gorbrach SL. Antimicrobial therapy of experimental intraabdominal sepsis. J Infect Dis 132: 282–286, 1975.
23. Solomkin JS, Meakins JL, Allo MD, Dellinger EP, Simmons RL. Antibiotics trials in intraabdominal infection: an initial evaluation of study design and outcome reporting. Ann Surg 200: 29–39, 1984.
24. Sutter VL, Finegold SM. Susceptibility of anaerobic bacteria to 23 antimicrobial agents. Antimicrob Agents Chemother 10: 736–752, 1976.

Submitted January 3, 1994; accepted March 7, 1994

Scand J Infect Dis 26: 511–516, 1994

HIV-Seropositive Rate and HIV Test Activity Among STD Clinic Attendees In Bergen, Norway

KÅRE-STEINAR TVEIT, ALAN NYFORS and ARVID NILSEN

From the Section of Venereology, Department of Dermatology, Haukeland University Hospital, Bergen, Norway

We wanted to determine the HIV seropositive rate and to study the connection between previous HIV testing, acceptance of HIV testing and sexual behaviour among STD clinic patients in Bergen, Norway. Patients attending the STD clinic in 1986–93 requesting HIV testing were registered, and all patients visiting the clinic in April–June 1989 received a questionnaire and were asked if they wanted to be HIV tested. The overall HIV seropositive rate was 0.4% (14/3805); in homo-/bisexual men: 2.9% (8/278); IVDUs: 0.4% (1/236) and in heterosexual non-IVDUs: 0.2% (5/3291). Among the 599 individuals offered anonymous HIV testing, 42.2% were HIV tested and 69.2% did not object to HIV-testing. IVDUs/prostitutes ($p < 0.001$), customers of prostitutes ($p < 0.001$), homo-/bisexuals ($p < 0.01$), and patients receiving blood transfusion ($p < 0.05$) had all been HIV tested more frequently than 'other heterosexuals'. Respondents reporting casual sex, casual sex abroad, infection with STDs, and a greater number of partners were more frequently HIV tested and also accepted HIV testing more frequently than respondents without such behaviour, indicating that there is some rationale behind the decision to be tested.

K.-S. Tveit, MD, Department of Dermatology, Haukeland University Hospital, N-5021 Bergen, Norway

INTRODUCTION

In Norway on 31st December 1993, a total of 1,337 persons (seropositive rate 31.3/100,000) were tested HIV positive according to test (1). The total number of HIV-infected persons has been estimated at 1,500–2,000, including those already identified (2). Since August 1983, the Norwegian health authorities have noted sociodemographic variables and collected information regarding sexual behaviour in all AIDS cases (3), and from 1986 such information has been collected for HIV-infected persons as well (4).

By the end of December 1992, 833,041 clinical HIV-tests had been carried out in a population of 4.2 million (2). In addition, 175,000 blood donors, 126,940 soldiers and 437,124 pregnant women had been HIV-tested (2). Together, in these 3 groups, after more than 2 million HIV tests, 27 HIV-infected individuals who were unaware of their HIV-positive status have been identified (blood donors: 6; pregnant: 18; military personnel: 3) (2) indicating that Norway is still a low prevalence area for HIV. In 1985, 28.9 HIV-positive samples were identified per 1,000 tests performed (5), and this ratio fell to 0.9 per 1,000 in 1990 (5).

Because of the high prevalence of high risk behaviour of STD clinic attendees, these clinics have been suggested as appropriate for HIV surveillance and for monitoring the possible spread of HIV infection among heterosexuals (6). We therefore undertook a study to determine the seropositive rate of HIV-infected persons, to study the connection between previous HIV testing, HIV testing at their present attendance and sexual behaviour among STD clinic patients.

PATIENTS AND METHODS

All patients attending the STD clinic voluntarily and requesting HIV testing in the period 1986–93, were recorded. We registered whether the patients were homosexuals, intravenous drug users (IVDUs) or heterosexual non-IVDUs. Information about the patients was coded before the blood samples were sent to the laboratory.

 ISSN 0036-5548

In another study, we approached all new patients (606) visiting the STD Clinic at the University Hospital in Bergen, Norway, in April–June 1989, and 599 (98.8%) agreed to participate. The study was voluntary and anonymous. The inclusion criteria were that the patient wanted to be examined for any STD, and that it was the first attendance for that particular reason. A questionnaire, printed in Norwegian, was given to the patient after the preliminary medical anamnesis and clinical examination had been completed.

Respondents themselves reported whether they were homosexual or bisexual, had any experience with intravenous drugs/ever received money for sex, paid for sex between 1985 and 1989, and whether they had received a blood transfusion. Patients with no such history were classified as 'other heterosexuals'.

The respondents reported sexual behaviour (previous/present casual sexual contacts, casual sex abroad between 1985 and 1989, number of sexual partners the last year, previous years and if they used a condom when having casual sex). Casual sexual partner was defined as any other sexual partner other than their married sexual partner, cohabiting sexual partner or boy-/girlfriend. The distinction between previous and present casual sexual practice was set to 1 month preceding their attendance at the STD clinic now. The respondents were to report all STDs that had been diagnosed up to the present attendance. Candida albicans was not included. Self-reported perceived high-risk behaviour is a subjective definition of their perceived risk of becoming HIV-infected (perception of susceptibility) and was given 2 alternatives ('yes', have had high risk sexual activity, and 'do not know', if high risk/'no' high-risk sexual activity).

The respondents reported if they had ever been HIV-tested or would agree to being HIV-tested at the present visit. Previous HIV testing and their acceptance of testing at the present visit were tested for correlation to their sexual behaviour.

For statistical analyses, the χ^2-method was used (7); a p-value of <0.05 was significant. Statistical analyses were performed using Statview package designed for Macintosh (8).

RESULTS

At the STD Clinic, from 1986 to 1993, we registered 35 HIV-infected subjects, of whom 21 (homosexuals: 6; IVDUs: 8; heterosexual non-IVDUs: 7) were known to be HIV-positive before attending the Clinic. Among these, 13 (61.9%) had been found to be HIV-positive before 1987, while those identified at the Clinic were tested HIV-positive from 1988 and onwards. Altogether we have performed 3,805 tests (men: 2,737; women: 1,068) from 1986 – as of 1st January 1994. The retest activity has been 18.5%; 707/3,805 (homosexuals: 49.3%; IVDUs: 40.7%, and heterosexual non-IVDUs: 14.3%). The overall HIV-seropositive rate has been 0.4% (14/3,805), the majority being homo-/bisexual men (2.9%, 8/278), while few IVDUs (0.4%; 1/236) and heterosexual non-IVDUs (0.2%, 5/3,291; men: 0.2%, 4/2,273; women: 0.1%, 1/1,018) have been identified. There has been no annual increase in HIV-positive persons from 1988 to 1994.

Sexual behaviour and previous HIV testing (all respondents: 599)

Altogether 42.2% (253/599) of the respondents (men: 42.3%; women: 42.0%) were previously HIV tested. Compared with 'other heterosexuals' (176/480; 36.7%), IVDUs/prostitutes (17/21, 81%, $p < 0.001$), customers of prostitutes (37/62, 59.7%, $p < 0.001$), homo-bisexuals (15/22, 68.2%, $p < 0.01$), and transfused patients (14/23, 60.9%, $p < 0.05$) had all undertaken the HIV test more frequently.

Individual reporting previous casual sexual practice, casual sex abroad, STD infection, more sexual partners previous years and perceived high-risk sexual behaviour had more frequently been HIV tested than those without such behaviour (Table I). To correct for the bias caused by 'traditionally high risk groups' in behaviour at risk for HIV infection, the HIV test activity 'other heterosexuals' was correlated to their sexual behaviour. Respondents reporting other sexual behaviour variables (Table I) and perceived high-risk sexual behaviour had more frequently been HIV tested than those without such behaviour. There was no connection between using a condom with a casual sexual partner and earlier HIV test activity.

Table I. *Sexual behaviour and previous HIV testing*

A) All respondents: Sexual Behaviour	HIV tested	Not HIV tested	*P*-value
Previous casual sexual practice[a]	185/198 (93.4%)	243/283 (85.9%)	$p < 0.01$
Casual sex abroad, 1985–1989	131/253 (51.8%)	114/346 (33.0%)	$p < 0.001$
More sexual partners previous years[a]	169/250 (67.6%)	189/335 (56.4%)	$p < 0.01$
Ever infected with STD	154/253 (60.9%)	164/346 (47.4%)	$p < 0.01$
Self-reported high risk sexual behaviour	81/252 (32.1%)	65/345 (18.8%)	$p < 0.001$
B) 'Other Heterosexuals'			
Previous casual sexual practice[a]	119/131 (90.8%)	213/251 (84.9%)	NS[b]
Casual sex abroad, 1985–1989	70/176 (39.8%)	86/304 (28.3%)	$p < 0.01$
More sexual partners previous years[a]	106/175 (60.6%)	159/295 (53.9%)	NS[b]
Ever infected with STD	100/176 (56.8%)	141/304 (46.4%)	$p < 0.05$
Self-reported high-risk sexual behaviour	44/174 (25.1%)	50/303 (16.5%)	$p < 0.05$

[a] Respondents reporting 'do not know' have been excluded.
[b] NS: Not statistically significant.

Accepting HIV testing now (all respondents)

Altogether 413/597 (69.2%) of the respondents did not object to HIV-testing at their present visit (homo-/bisexuals: 86.4%; customers of prostitutes: 79%; transfused patients: 73.9%; 'other heterosexuals': 67%, and IVDUs/prostitutes: 66.7%). We did not identify any new HIV-positive individuals. There was little difference in acceptance among respondents who were tested before (183/252; 72.6%) and respondents never previously tested (230/345; 66.7%). Among those accepting HIV testing, 183/413 (44.3%) had been tested before, compared with 69/184 (37.5%) of the respondents who did not agree to be tested. Altogether, 482/597 (80.7%) of the patients had been tested previously or accepted testing now. In Table II we see that few homo-/bisexuals, men with paid sexual partner and IVDUs had never been tested, either previously or now. All blood transfusion patients had been tested either previously or now.

Respondents reporting present casual sexual practice, casual sex abroad, 2 or more sexual partners last year, and perceived high-risk sexual behaviour, agreed to being HIV tested at the present visit more frequently than did respondents without such behaviour (Table III). Also among the 'other heterosexuals', we saw an increased acceptance of HIV testing today among the respondents reporting these sexual behaviour variables or perceived high-risk sexual behaviour (Table III).

Table II. *Risk groups for HIV infection and previous/present acceptance of HIV testing*

		Yes/Yes	No/Yes	Yes/No	No/No
'Other heterosexuals'	$n = 478$	26.6%	40.4%	10.0%	23.0%
Homo-/bisexuals	$n = 22$	59.1%	27.3%	9.1%	4.5%
IVDUs/Prostitutes	$n = 21$	57.1%	9.5%	23.8%	9.5%
Paid sexual partner	$n = 62$	43.5%	35.5%	16.1%	4.8%
Received blood transfusion	$n = 23$	34.8%	39.1%	26.1%	0

Table III. *Agreeing to HIV testing in the present study*

A) All respondents: Sexual Behaviour	HIV tested	Not HIV tested	*P*-value
Casual sex abroad, 1985–1989	186/413 (45.0%)	59/184 (32.1%)	$p < 0.01$
≥2 sexual partners last year	257/413 (62.2%)	81/182 (44.5%)	$p < 0.001$
Present casual sex practice (yes/no)	242/413 (58.6%)	79/184 (42.9%)	$p < 0.001$
Self-reported high risk sexual behaviour	116/412 (28.2%)	30/183 (16.4%)	$p < 0.01$
B) 'Other Heterosexuals'			
Casual sex abroad, 1985–1989	115/320 (35.9%)	41/158 (26%)	$p < 0.05$
≥2 sexual partners last year	189/320 (59.1%)	67/158 (42.4%)	$p < 0.001$
Present casual sexual practice (yes/no)	178/320 (55.6%)	61/158 (38.6%)	$p < 0.001$
Self-reported high-risk sexual behaviour	73/319 (22.9%)	21/157 (13.4%)	$p < 0.05$

DISCUSSION

At our STD Clinic, few individuals were found to be HIV-positive during an 8-year period of voluntary HIV testing. Most HIV-positive individuals (8 persons) were homosexuals, in accordance with other studies (6, 9–11). Among the patients offered HIV testing, the traditionally high-risk groups had been HIV tested far more frequently than 'other heterosexuals'. We also found a clear correlation between different sexual behaviour variables including self-reported perceived high-risk behaviour and the respondents' past and present acceptance of HIV testing, indicating that there must be some rationale behind the decision to be tested.

In USA there has been a 20-fold increase in HIV prevalence among STD clinic attendees from 1979 to 1989 with recent increases most marked among women, teenagers and blacks (12). Another American study from 1988 to 1989, showed an HIV prevalence among STD clinic attendees ranging between 0 and 38.5% (9). Studies from STD clinics all over Europe show a great variation in HIV-seropositive rates (excluding known seropositives) between homo-/bisexuals (0% in Finland and Sweden, 10.2% in Britain, 21.8% in Germany and 54.1% in Portugal), IVDUs (0% in Finland, and Sweden, 31.6% in Italy and 45.4% in Spain) and heterosexual non-IVDUs (0.1% in Denmark and Greece, 0.2% in Britain, 0.5% in The Netherlands, 1.1% in Italy and 3.3% in Spain) (11).

In an English study of female STD clinic attendees, only 25% had previously been HIV tested, of whom 2.7% were positive, indicating that people with a high risk of acquiring HIV infection have been tested more often than others (13). The tested women also reported a higher frequency of vaginal intercourse (13). Among pregnant women in France there was a significantly higher risk perception among women who had already been HIV tested than in those who had not been tested (14).

HIV testing can only become an important sero-epidemiological tool if the acceptance of testing is high in the group being tested. One obstacle to getting valid data is that if people being HIV tested are linked to their test results, many will not participate and may have different seroprevalence rates from participants (15). At the STD clinics the acceptance has been found to vary from 9% to 90.5% (10, 15, 16); in this study, 69% agreed to being HIV tested. Thus, when high-risk behaviour studies that link testing results to participants are carried out, unlinked testing of non-participants (control groups) should also be conducted to determine the true overall seroprevalence rates (15, 16). This was not done in the present study.

While the debate over the merits of mandatory testing versus voluntary testing may never be resolved, some experts in the fields of medicine, public health, and law favour voluntary and confidential testing as the most appropriate vehicle to encourage the reduction of behaviour that results in the transmission of HIV (15, 17).

It has been demonstrated that when HIV antibody testing protocols were changed by offering anonymous rather than confidential (names recorded) testing, the demand for testing increased by 125% in the 'gay' male community and by 50% overall (18).

Moreover, poorly designed screening policies may create irrational fears in the general public and promote unnecessary and unethical coercive attitudes toward people with HIV (19). We believe therefore that STD clinics are important surveillance centres for HIV seroprevalence and incidence because STD clinics serve persons whose behaviour places them at risk for acquiring HIV infection. In the future, one should have in mind why a person wants to undertake an HIV test because, as we have seen in this study, there was a clear correlation between different sexual behaviour variables and acceptance of HIV testing. One should also strongly encourage return for post-test counselling, even if the test result is negative, and finally the testing procedure should be voluntary and anonymous.

ACKNOWLEDGEMENT

This study received financial support from the University of Bergen, Norway.

REFERENCES

1. Hasseltvedt V, Nilsen Ø, Lystad A. HIV-situasjonen i Norge pr. 31. desember 1993. MSIS-rapport. Meldesystem for Infeksjons-sykdommer. Statens Institutt for Folkehelse, Norge 21: 3, 1993 [in Norwegian].
2. Nilsen Ø, Lystad A, Hasseltvedt V. HIV-infeksjon – en vurdering av den epidemiologiske situasjonen i Norge. MSIS-rapport. Meldesystem for Infeksjons-sykdommer. Statens Institutt for Folkenhelse, Norge 21: 9, 1993 [in Norwegian].
3. Lystad A. AIDS – Overvåking og kontroll. MSIS. Meldesystem for Infeksjons-sykdommer. Statens Institutt for Folkenhelse, Norge 24: 1985 [in Norwegian].
4. Lystad A, AFIM. Kartlegging av HIV-infeksjon ved hjelp av melding om påvist HIV-antistoff. MSIS. Meldesystem for Infeksjons-sykdommer. Statens Institutt for Folkenhelse, Norge 38: 1986 [in Norwegian].
5. Nilsen Ø, Lystad A, Hasseltvedt V. HIV/AIDS – en vurdering av den epidemiologiske situasjonen. MSIS-rapport. Meldesystem for Infeksjons-sykdommer. Statens Institutt for Folkehelse, Norge 19: 12, 1991 [in Norwegian].
6. Cannon RO, Schmid GP, Moore PS, Pappaioanou M. Human immunodeficiency virus (HIV) seroprevalence in persons attending STD clinics in the United States, 1985–1987. Sex Transm Dis 16: 184–189, 1989.
7. Siegel S. Non parametric Statistics for the Behavioral Sciences. Tokyo: McGraw-Hill, 1959.
8. StatView™. The graphic statistics utility for the Macintosh™. Calabasas, CA: Brainpower, 1985.
9. McCray E, Onorato IM. The Field Services Branch. Sentinel surveillance of human immunodeficiency virus infection in sexually transmitted disease clinics in the United States. Sex Transm Dis 19: 235–241, 1992.
10. Fennema JS, van Ameijden EJ, Coutinho RA, van Doornum GJ, Henquet CJ, van den Hoek JA. HIV prevalence among clients attending a sexually transmitted disease clinic in Amsterdam: the potential risk for heterosexual transmission. Genitourin Med 69: 23–28, 1993.
11. The European Study Group. European Community Concerted Action on HIV seroprevalence among sexually transmitted disease patients in 18 European sentinel networks. AIDS 7: 393–400, 1993.
12. Quinn TC, Groseclose SL, Spence M, Provost V, Hook EW 3d. Evolution of the human immunodeficiency virus epidemic among patients attending sexually transmitted disease clinics: a decade of experience. J Infect Dis 165: 541–544, 1992.
13. Sherr L, Strong C. Safe sex and women. Genitourin Med 68: 32–35, 1992.

14. Moatti J-P, Le Gales C, Seror V, Papiernik E, Henrion R. Social acceptability of HIV screening among pregnant women. AIDS Care 2: 213–222, 1990.
15. Hull HF, Bettinger CJ, Gallaher MM, Keller NM, Wilson J, Mertz GJ. Comparison of HIV-antibody prevalence in patients consenting to and declining HIV-antibody testing in an STD clinic. JAMA 260: 935–938, 1988.
16. Chiasson MA, Stoneburner RL, Lifson AR, Hildebrandt DS, Ewing WE, Schultz S, Jaffe HW. Risk factors for Human Immunodeficiency Virus type 1 (HIV-1) infection in patients at a sexually transmitted disease clinic in New York City. Am J Epidemiol 131: 208–220, 1990.
17. Osborn JE. Sounding board – AIDS: politics and science. N Engl J Med 318: 444–447, 1988.
18. Fehrs LJ, Foster LR, Fox V. Trial of anonymous versus confidential human immunodeficiency virus testing. Lancet 2: 379–381, 1988.
19. Dab W, Moatti J-P, Bastide S, Abenhaim L, Brunet J-B. Misconceptions about transmission of AIDS and attitudes toward prevention in the French general public. AIDS 3: 433–437, 1989.

Submitted March 7, 1994; accepted June 6, 1994

Scand J Infect Dis 26: 517–522, 1994

Danish AIDS Patients 1988–1993: A Recent Decline in Pneumocystis carinii Pneumonia as AIDS-defining Disease Related to the Period of Known HIV Positivity

ELSE SMITH[1] and MARIANNE K. ORHOLM[2]

From the [1]Department of Epidemiology, Statens Seruminstitut, Copenhagen, and the [2]Department of Infectious Diseases, Rigshospitalet, University of Copenhagen, Denmark

The frequency of PCP among adult Danish AIDS patients notified in 1988–93 was higher among patients tested HIV-positive less than 4 months prior to AIDS than among those known to be positive for >1 year. Among the latter, the proportion with PCP decreased significantly over the period, from 45.3% in 1988 to 22.0% in 1993, while no such trend was found among patients tested positive for HIV less than 4 months before AIDS was diagnosed. The incidence of PCP as an AIDS-defining disease has decreased, most likely due to the use of PCP prophylaxis.

E. Smith, MD, Department of Epidemiology, Statens Seruminstitut, Artillerivej 5, DK-2300 Copenhagen, Denmark

INTRODUCTION

In most developed countries the major AIDS-defining disease has been Pneumocystis carinii pneumonia (PCP), being diagnosed in about 50% of such patients (1–3). In Denmark, notification of AIDS cases to the Health Authorities has been mandatory since 1983. The first Danish AIDS patient was diagnosed in 1981 and the country now has the sixth highest cumulated incidence rate for AIDS in Europe: 260.8 per million inhabitants at the end of December 1993 (4).

In Denmark, secondary PCP prophylaxis has been in use since the very beginning of the AIDS epidemic. Since 1991, primary PCP prophylactic treatment has been given to HIV-infected persons with a low CD4-cell count.

The objective of this study was to evaluate the relation between the period of known HIV positivity before AIDS and the incidence of PCP as an AIDS-defining disease among Danish AIDS patients.

MATERIAL AND METHODS

All notified adult AIDS cases in Denmark diagnosed in 1988–93 and reported by March 31st, 1994 were included. In Denmark, an AIDS notification is followed by a standard questionnaire including among other items, data on risk behaviour, date of first HIV-positive test and date of AIDS diagnosis. Data on AIDS-defining disease(s) are collected through a standardized list. More than one disease can be reported per patient. All data are computerized. No data on treatment are available.

We looked for changes in the prevalence of PCP as an AIDS-defining disease in the period 1988–93, since the case definition used for the Danish national surveillance of AIDS has followed that defined by the Center for Disease Control (CDC), including the 1987 revision (5) which was introduced on January 1st 1988 (6), and since the use of zidovudine has been recommended for all HIV-infected persons with compromised immunology, since 1987. We also compared the incidence of PCP among persons diagnosed as HIV-antibody-positive less than 4 months before they were diagnosed with AIDS, versus persons known to be HIV-positive >1 year before the AIDS diagnosis.

Since January 1st, 1988 diagnosis of PCP has been verified according to the CDC classification criteria microbiological (silver or Giemsa staining and/or immunofluorescence) or by clinical signs and symptoms.

Statistical methods

Frequencies were compared by Fisher's exact test and trends were analysed using the χ^2-test. P-values below 0.05 were considered significant.

RESULTS

By December 31st, 1993, a total of 1,109 adult patients had been diagnosed with AIDS in the 6-year period 1988–93 and notified to the Danish Health Authorities: 1,022 men (92.2%) and 87 women (7.8%). The men were older than the women, the median age being 39 years (range: 20–76 years) among men and 34 years (range: 21–77 years) among women ($p < 0.05$).

Overall, 799 (72.0%) of the patients were homo/bisexual men, 155 (14.0%) were heterosexuals without i.v. drug use and 79 (7.1%) were i.v. drug users (IVDUs). Over the study period the number of annually diagnosed AIDS patients has increased from 125 in 1988 to 218 in 1993. Homo/bisexual men have represented a decreasing proportion of the AIDS patients: from 80.8% diagnosed in 1988 to 74.0% in 1991 and 67.9% in 1993 ($p < 0.005$ for trend). In the same period the proportion classified as heterosexuals has increased from 8.8% in 1988, to 14.2% in 1991 and to 17.0% in 1993 ($p < 0.05$ for trend).

The reporting delay, i.e. the interval between the date of AIDS diagnosis and the date of received notification at the surveillance unit, was significantly constant over the study period. This lag was a median 24 days (range: 1–1,118 days). However, the delay was consistently shorter for cases with PCP as AIDS-defining disease than for cases without PCP. Overall, the median delay was 20 days (range: 1–928 days) for cases with PCP compared with 28 days (range: 1–1,118 days) for cases without PCP ($p < 0.0001$).

A total of 456 patients (41.1%) had PCP as AIDS-defining disease. The frequency of PCP was 41.5% among male AIDS patients and 36.8% among female patients (not significant). PCP was the major AIDS-defining disease within each transmission group except among IVDUs, among whom esophageal candidiasis was the most frequent disease (45.6%), PCP being ranked second (20.3%). The diagnosis of PCP was verified microbiologically in 91% of the reported cases and by clinical signs and symptoms in 9%.

For 992 out of the 1,022 men (97.1%) and for all 87 women, the date of first HIV-positive test was known. The median interval between first positive HIV test and diagnosis of AIDS was 1,004 days (range: 0–4,599 days) among men and 641 days (range: 0–3,445 days) among women. Overall, 323 persons (29.1%) had a positive HIV-antibody test <4 months before being diagnosed as having AIDS. We found no significant trend over time in this proportion. However, among patients notified in 1993 the proportion tested <4 months before AIDS diagnosis dropped to 22%, chiefly among male cases, being as low as 19% among homo/bisexual men.

The proportion of those tested HIV-antibody-positive <4 months before being diagnosed as having AIDS varied, however, with the mode of transmission (Table I). Among homo/bisexual men, 26.7% were tested within 4 months of being diagnosed with AIDS, a proportion higher among heterosexually infected cases (48.7%) ($p < 0.00001$) and lower among IVDUs (14.5%) ($p < 0.05$). The same tendency was found within each calendar year.

In the study period 1988–93 the proportion of patients with PCP as AIDS-defining disease decreased from 46.4% among patients diagnosed in 1988 to 47.5% in 1991 and to 30.3% in 1993 ($p < 0.0001$ for trend) (Table I). A similar trend was found among both homo/bisexual men ($p < 0.01$ for trend) and heterosexuals without i.v. drug use ($p < 0.05$ for trend). However, the proportion of patients with PCP was higher among those tested <4 months prior to the AIDS diagnosis than among those known to have been positive for >1 year (54.8% versus 35.4%, $p < 0.00001$); a difference that was found in each calendar year, although the significance of the difference varied over the period. The same tendency was found among homo/bisexual men, among whom PCP was diagnosed in 57.2% of those tested within 4 months of being diagnosed as having AIDS compared to 36.0% among those known to be positive for >1 year ($p < 0.0001$).

Table I. *Number of patients with PCP as AIDS-defining disease among notified adult Danish AIDS patients, distributed by duration of period of known HIV-positivity before AIDS, mode of transmission and year of AIDS diagnosis, 1988–1993*

Interval between 1st positive HIV test and AIDS, and mode of transmission	Year of AIDS diagnosis 1988 No. PCP/Total	1989 No. PCP/Total	1990 No. PCP/Total	1991 No. PCP/Total	1992 No. PCP/Total	1993 No. PCP/Total	1988–1993 No. PCP/Total	(%)
All patients	58/125	74/171	97/194	97/204	64/197	66/218	456/1109	(41.1)
<4 months, $n = 323$	20/40	29/49	35/60	40/68	29/59	23/47	177/323	(54.8)
>1 year, $n = 704$	34/75	40/107	60/129	50/120	32/123	33/250	249/704	(35.4)
Homo/bisexual men, $n = 799$	53/101	60/129	71/140	68/151	36/120	44/148	332/799	(41.6)
<4 months, $n = 208$	19/32	23/30	24/42	24/46	15/30	13/28	119/208	(57.2)
>1 year, $n = 533$	31/63	33/88	46/94	37/91	20/92	25/105	192/533	(36.0)
Heterosexuals, $n = 155$	3/11	7/21	17/24	19/29	16/33	14/37	76/155	(49.0)
<4 months, $n = 74$	1/5	3/11	7/9	11/16	9/18	7/15	38/74	(51.4)
>1 year, $n = 69$	1/3	4/9	9/14	8/12	5/12	5/19	32/69	(46.4)
I.v. drug user, $n = 79$	1/6	2/8	3/16	4/15	4/15	2/19	16/79	(20.3)
Other, $n = 76$	1/7	5/13	6/14	6/9	8/19	6/14	32/76	(42.1)

Among patients known to be HIV-positive >1 year before being diagnosed as having AIDS, the proportion of patients with PCP as AIDS-defining disease decreased over the period, from 45.3% in 1988 to 22.0% in 1993 ($p < 0.0001$ for trend). This decrease was due mainly to a decline in the incidence among homo/bisexual men, among whom the decline was from 49.2% in 1988 to 23.8% in 1993 ($p < 0.001$).

Among patients tested as HIV-positive <4 months before the AIDS diagnosis, we found no statistically significant trend in the frequency of patients with PCP as AIDS-defining disease from 1988 to 1993, either in the whole group or within the different transmission categories.

DISCUSSION

We have studied the incidence of PCP as AIDS-defining disease among Danish AIDS patients in the 6-year period 1988–93. PCP was the single most frequent AIDS-defining disease throughout the period. However, the incidence has declined significantly over the years, being the AIDS-defining disease in only one-third of all notified AIDS patients in 1993. Since the number of new AIDS patients has been almost stable during the last 4 years, we also found a decrease in the absolute number of PCPs, from 97 cases in 1990 and 1991, to 66 in 1993.

Furthermore, we found that this decrease in occurrence was almost entirely due to a decrease among patients known to be HIV-positive >1 year. The incidence of PCP among persons tested positive less than 4 months prior to the AIDS diagnosis was statistically unchanged.

These observations indicate an effect of prophylactic treatment and an unchanged epidemiology of P. carinii. With respect to PCP it seems to be 'an advantage' to have been known to be HIV-positive for a longer period of time before the diagnosis of AIDS is set.

The reporting delay did not change over the study period but was shorter among cases with PCP, compared with cases without PCP. Therefore, the presented frequencies of PCP among cases diagnosed in later years are most likely overestimated, if anything.

The overall reporting of AIDS cases in Denmark is estimated to be close to 100% (3). The vast majority of patients are followed in out-patient clinics at Departments of Infectious Diseases from the day they are tested HIV-antibody positive. As long as they present no medical problems they are seen for clinical examination and blood-analyses including a CD4 cell count every half year. If the patients present symptoms and/or signs of the HIV infection they are seen more often. Since the very beginning of the AIDS epidemic, patients who had survived an attack of PCP were given secondary prophylactic treatment due to the high incidence of relapses (7–11). In the late 1980s it was found in cohort studies that patients with a CD4 cell count $<200 \times 10^6$/l ran a high risk of contracting PCP (12, 13); hence primary prophylaxis was recommended for this group of patients (14). Several studies have since shown a significant prophylactic effect of both aerosol pentamidine and trimethoprim-sulfamethoxazole (TMP-SMX) (15–17). In Denmark, treatment has been TMP-SMX (80 mg/400 mg twice daily) or aerosol pentamidine given 60–150 mg biweekly. The results of this study clearly demonstrate the impact of this prophylactic strategy.

The patients are furthermore offered zidovudine when the immune system becomes depressed. Although this drug may delay the development of opportunistic infections for months, it cannot prevent the infections (18, 19). Hence, treatment with zidovudine, which was introduced in the mid-1980s, seems to be without significance for the recent decrease in PCP incidence observed in this study. Graham et al. (20) followed a cohort of 2,145 HIV-1 seropositive men and 371 who seroconverted during a study period 1986–90. They examined the effect of zidovudine and PCP prophylaxis on the probability of progression to AIDS and found a significant reduction in rates of progression for participants starting with $< 350 \times 10^6$/l CD4 lymphocytes. In multivariate log-linear models, virtually all the treatment effect was attributed to zidovudine. However, when they restricted the analysis of the independent effect of PCP prophylaxis on progression rates to PCP to transitions in zidovudine users only, PCP prophylaxis was found to be significantly protective.

Other studies have reported a decline in the overall PCP incidence. Peters et al. (21) observed a drop in the proportion of patients who developed PCP, from 56% in 1984 to 24% in 1989, whereas the frequency of PCP as index diagnosis remained stable during the period. This result may reflect the effect of secondary PCP prophylaxis, and that primary prophylaxis was not yet a routine treatment.

Chien et al. (22) found a significant reduction in the total number of PCP hospital admissions when comparing two 1-year periods before and after the start of the Toronto aerosol pentamidine program.

Wall and co-workers (23) also found a decline in the incidence of PCP as initial AIDS-defining disease from 1989 to 1992, and – exactly as in the present study – the decline was observed entirely among patients aware of their seropositivity, which means that they were more likely to have received PCP prophylaxis.

In conclusion, the incidence of PCP as AIDS-defining disease has decreased, most likely due to primary PCP prophylaxis. Since we observed no decrease among patients unaware of their HIV-infection, we have no reason to believe in any change in P. carinii epidemiology or virulence. In the future we may concentrate on the use and development of prophylaxis against other opportunistic infections.

REFERENCES

1. Selik RM, Starcher ET, Curran JW. Opportunistic diseases reported in AIDS patients: Frequencies, associations and trends. AIDS 1: 175–182, 1987.
2. Klatt EC. Diagnostic findings in patients with acquired immune deficiency syndrome AIDS. J Acquir Immune Defic Syndr 1: 459–465, 1988.
3. Smith E, Orholm M. Trends and patterns of opportunistic diseases in Danish AIDS patients 1980–1990. Scand J Infect Dis 22: 665–672, 1990.
4. European Center for the Epidemiological Monitoring of AIDS. AIDS surveillance in Europe. Quarterly Report no. 40. Paris, March 1994.
5. Center for Disease Control. Revision of the CDC surveillance case definition of the acquired immunodeficiency syndrome. MMWR Morb Mortal Wkly Rep 36: Suppl. S-15, 1987.
6. Smith E, Mathiesen L, Skinhøj P, Seefeldt T, Isager H. Impact of the 1987 AIDS case definition in Denmark: a follow-up study 2 years after its adoption. Scand J Infect Dis 24: 293–299, 1992.
7. Glatt AE, Chirgwin K, Landesman SH. Treatment of infections associated with human immunodeficiency virus. N Engl J Med 318: 1439–1448, 1988.
8. Rankin JA, Collman R, Daniele RP. Acquired immunodeficiency syndrome and the lung. Chest 94: 155–164, 1988.
9. Masur H, Lane C, Kovacs JA, Allegra CJ, Edman JC. Pneumocystis carinii pneumonia: from bench to clinic. Ann Intern Med 111: 813–826, 1989.
10. Montaner JSG, Lawson LA, Gervais A, Hyland RH, Chan CK, Falutz JM, Renzi PM, MacFadden D, Rachlis AR, Fong IW. Aerosol pentamidine for secondary prophylaxis of AIDS-related Pneumocystis carinii pneumonia. Ann Intern Med 114: 948–953, 1991.
11. Jensen BN, Nielsen TL, Lerche B, Jensen TH, Backer V, Mathiesen L, Nielsen JO, Skinhøj P. Prevention of Pneumocystis carinii pneumonia relapse by aerosolised pentamidine, 60 mg biweekly, using an acorn system 22 nebuliser. Scand J Infect Dis 22: 533–536, 1990.
12. Masur H, Ognibene FP, Yarchoan R, Shelhamer JH, Baird BF, Travis W, Suffredini AF, Deyton L, Kovacs JA, Falloon J. CD4 counts as predictors of opportunistic pneumonias in human immunodeficiency virus (HIV) infection. Ann Intern Med 111: 223–231, 1989.
13. Phair J, Muñoz A, Detels R, Kaslow R, Rinaldo C, Saah A, and the Multicenter AIDS Cohort Study Group. The risk of Pneumocystis carinii pneumonia among men infected with human immunodeficiency virus type 1. N Engl J Med 322: 161–165, 1990.

14. Center for Disease Control. Guidelines for prophylaxis against Pneumocystis carinii pneumonia for persons infected with human immunodeficiency virus. MMWR Morb Mortal Wkly Rep 38: Suppl. S-5, 1989.
15. Jensen BN, Nielsen TL, Backer V, Nelsing S, Simonsen L, Flaschs H, Gaub J, Højlyng N, Nielsen JO, Mathiesen L, Skinhøj P. Low dose aerosol pentamidine for primary prophylaxis of Pneumocystis carinii pneumonia: A controlled, randomized trial. J Acquir Immune Defic Syndr 6: 472–477, 1993.
16. Hirschel B, Lazzaran A, Chopard P, Opravil M, Furrer H-J, Rüthmann S, Vernazza P, Chave J-P, Ancarani F, Gabriel V, Heald A, King R, Malinverni R, Marten J-L, Mermillod B, Nicod L, Simoni L, Vivirito MC, Zerboni R and the Swiss Group for Clinical Studies on AIDS. A controlled study of inhaled pentamidine for primary prevention of Pneumocystis carinii pneumonia. N Engl J Med 324: 1079–1083, 1991.
17. Fischl MA, Dickinson GM, La Voie L. Safety and efficacy of sulfamethoxazole and trimethoprim chemoprophylaxis for Pneumocystis carinii pneumonia in AIDS. JAMA 259: 1185–1189, 1988.
18. Fischl MA, Richman DD, Grieco MH, Gottlieb MS, Volberding PA, Laskin OL, Leedom JM, Groopman JE, Mildvan D, Schooley RT, Jackson GG, Durack DT, King D, and the AZT Collaborative Working Group. The efficacy of azidothymidine (AZT) in the treatment of patients with AIDS and AIDS-related complex. A double-blind, placebo-controlled trial. N Engl J Med 317: 185–191, 1987.
19. Concorde: MRC/ANRS randomised double-blind controlled trial of immediate and deferred zidovudine in symptom-free HIV infection. Lancet 343: 871–881, 1994.
20. Graham NM, Zeger SL, Park LP, Phair JP, Detels R, Vermund SH, Ho M, Saah AJ and the Multicenter AIDS Cohort Study. Effect of zidovudine and Pneumocystis carinii prophylaxis on progression of HIV-1 infection to AIDS. Lancet 338: 265–269, 1991.
21. Peters BS, Beck EJ, Coleman DG, Wadsworth MJH, McGuinness O, Harris JRW, Pinching AJ. Changing disease patterns in patients with AIDS in a referral centre in the United Kingdom: the changing face of AIDS. BMJ 302: 203–207, 1991.
22. Chien S-M, Rawji M, Mintz S, Rachlis A, Chan CK. Changes in hospital admissions pattern in patients with human immunodeficiency virus infection in the era of Pneumocystis carinii prophylaxis. Chest 102: 1035–1039, 1992.
23. Wall PG, Porter K, Noone A, Goldberg DJ. Changing incidence of Pneumocystis carinii pneumonia as initial AIDS defining disease in the United Kingdom. AIDS 7: 1523–1525, 1993.

Submitted February 17, 1994; accepted June 6, 1994

Scand J Infect Dis 26: 523–533, 1994

Markers of Immune Stimulation in the Cerebrospinal Fluid During HIV Infection: A longitudinal study

MAGNUS GISSLÉN[1], FRANCESCA CHIODI[3], DIETMAR FUCHS[4], GUNNAR NORKRANS[1], BO SVENNERHOLM[2], HELMUT WACHTER[4] and LARS HAGBERG[1]

From the Departments of [1]Infectious Diseases and [2]Virology, University of Göteborg, and [3]Virology, Karolinska Institute, University of Stockholm, Sweden, and the [4]Institute of Medical Chemistry and Biochemistry and Ludwig-Boltzman-Institute for AIDS Research, University of Innsbruck, Austria

Markers of immune stimulation were studied in 76 sequential cerebrospinal fluid (CSF) samples from 19 patients infected with HIV-1 without antiretroviral treatment during observation periods ranging from 22 months to 6 years. Eight of these patients were further followed with 14 CSF samples for 3–24 months of zidovudine treatment. During the course of HIV-1 infection, the mean CSF neopterin and β_2-microglobulin (β2M) concentrations increased from 12.7 to 20.4 nmol/l ($p < 0.01$) and from 1.93 to 2.17 mg/l ($p < 0.05$), respectively, while the mean peripheral CD4 + T cell count decreased from 624 to 320 cells × 10^6/l ($p < 0.001$). The IgG index, reflecting intrathecal immunoglobulin production, increased from 0.72 to 0.92 ($p = 0.08$). The number of patients with CSF pleocytosis did not change significantly during follow-up (8/19 at baseline, 7/19 at endpoint). In the 8 patients followed up during antiretroviral treatment, a significant reduction in mean CSF levels of neopterin and β2M (−48% and −32%, respectively, $p < 0.01$) was seen after 3–12 months on zidovudine. We suggest that a gradual increase in immune stimulation reflected by the rising CSF concentrations of neopterin and β2M indicates that HIV-1 infection in the central nervous system is progressive even in neurologically asymptomatic stages.

L. Hagberg, MD, PhD, Department of Infectious Diseases, University of Göteborg, S-416 85 Göteborg, Sweden

INTRODUCTION

In the long-term perspective, HIV-1 infection is devastating for the immune system and for the central nervous system (CNS). The immune system mounts protection against HIV in the peripheral blood during the early phases of infection but cannot eliminate the invader, which is actively replicating in lymphoid tissues (1). In the cerebrospinal fluid (CSF), positive HIV isolations or positive HIV polymerase chain reaction tests (2, 3) indicate spread of the virus to CNS in the majority of HIV-infected patients. Activated CSF monocytes, increased intrathecal immunoglobulin production, and increased CSF concentrations of general markers of immune stimulation, such as neopterin and β-2 microglobulin (β2M), have been reported in all stages of HIV infection (4–6). In peripheral blood, the CD4+ cell count has been the marker most often used to determine the progress of infection, although both neopterin and β2M each had nearly as much statistical power to predict the probability of developing AIDS (7). It is far more difficult to follow a HIV-1 infection in CNS than in peripheral blood, since CSF, the fluid closest to the CNS, is obtained by lumbar puncture. Since, in addition, CSF cells are sparse and fragile, characterization of CSF T-cells is difficult and has not been properly evaluated. To explore the potential value of other markers of immune stimulation and infectious activity, we have followed neopterin and β2M concentrations, monocytic cell counts, IgG index, p24 antigen, and HIV isolations for 2–6 years in annually collected CSF samples from 19 HIV-seropositive patients who had no HIV-associated symptoms at the study start.

MATERIALS AND METHODS

Patients

19 HIV-seropositive patients, aged 21–65 years (mean age 38.6), at CDC stage II or III (8) and not undergoing antiretroviral treatment entered the study during 1985–89 for planned participation until June 1993 (Table I). The study group included 13 homosexual or bisexual males, 3 heterosexual males, 2 men infected in connection with drug abuse, and 1 woman infected by blood transfusion. Clinical neurological examination by a specialist in neurology showed that all but 1 of the patients were neurologically asymptomatic at inclusion. The exception was a patient with previous drug abuse in whom signs of peripheral polyneuropathy were regarded as not HIV-related.

As long as the patients did not receive antiretroviral treatment, i.e. during periods of 22 months to 6 years (mean 42.8 months), CSF samples were collected at about 1 year intervals (mean number of lumbar punctures 4.1, range 3–7). After initiation of zidovudine treatment, further CSF samples were obtained from some participants. A first post-treatment sample was collected after 3–12 months (mean 6.1) of zidovudine treatment in 8 patients, and 6 patients agreed to a second sample after 1–2 years of treatment. The daily dose of zidovudine varied between 400 and 1200 mg (mean 740 mg). Seven of the patients also participated in a study of CSF indolamine and catecholamine concentrations before and after zidovudine treatment (unpublished data).

CSF samples from 14 patients with AIDS (9 with pneumocystis carinii pneumonia (PCP), 1 with Kaposi's sarcoma, 1 with both PCP and Kaposi's sarcoma, 2 with wasting syndrome, and 1 with extrapulmonary tuberculosis) but not undergoing antiviral treatment were collected during the same period as the study group. The CSF analyses were performed after completed acute treatment of the opportunistic infection.

CSF samples

Approximately 20–25 ml of CSF was collected from each patient. After cell counting, a portion of the first 12 ml was centrifugated, and proteins were assayed by isoelectric focusing in polyacrylamide gel with silver staining (9). Neopterin was measured by a commercially available radio-immunoassay (neopterin, IMMU test, Henning-Berlin, Germany) (10) and β2M by an enzyme-linked immunosorbent

Table I. *Clinical data in 19 HIV-seropositive patients*

Patient	Sex	Age (years)	CDC stage: first control	CDC stage: last control	Follow-up time (months)	No. of lumbar punctures	Reason for leaving the study
1	M	65	II	II	50	5	Zidovudine treatment
2	M	61	II	II	26	3	Zidovudine treatment
3	M	57	II	III	55	5	Zidovudine treatment
4	M	53	II	II	33	3	Remained until endpoint
5	M	50	III	IV C1	26	4	Zidovudine treatment
6	M	47	III	III	38	4	Cerebral infarction
7	M	47	II	IV C2	22	3	Zidovudine treatment
8	M	46	II	II	33	3	Death, ruptured spleen
9	M	40	III	IV E	27	3	Zidovudine treatment
10	F	37	II	II	65	6	Zidovudine treatment
11	M	31	II	II	77	7	Remained until endpoint
12	M	28	II	II	37	4	Refused further participation
13	M	28	II	II	25	3	ddI treatment
14	M	27	II	III	42	3	Refused further participation
15	M	25	II	III	63	4	Remained until endpoint
16	M	25	II	IV A	48	3	Zidovudine treatment
17	M	25	II	II	74	4	Zidovudine treatment
18	M	24	II	II	42	4	Zidovudine treatment
19	M	21	II	IV C2	31	5	Zidovudine treatment

assay (11). Normal reference values at the laboratory were <8.8 nmol/l in serum, and <4.2 nmol/l in CSF for neopterin and <2.4 mg/l in serum and 2.2 mg/l in CSF for β2M. The p24 HIV antigen was analysed with an enzyme-linked immunosorbent assay (Abbot Laboratories). IgG index was calculated as (IgG-CSF/IgG-serum)/(albumin-CSF/albumin-serum). Nested polymerase chain reaction (PCR) for detection of CMV was done in CSF from the final samples collected from the follow-up patients and has been described elsewhere (12). Both primers were from the fourth exon of the CMV IEA 1 gene located in the ECO RI J fragment of the strain CMV AD169 (13). The sensitivity of the PCR analysis was 5 fg of CMV DNA, corresponding to 20 genomes. The peripheral CD4+ cell count was measured by direct immunofluorescence on a flow cytometer. The Wasserman reaction and veneral disease research laboratory test (VDRL) were performed on sera.

The CSF samples for HIV isolations were analysed in Stockholm (Department of Virology, Karolinska Institute) during 1985 to August 1989 and in Göteborg during September 1989–93 (Department of Virology, University of Göteborg). Having the analyses made locally shortened the transportation time from 7–9 h to less than 2 h.

From 5 to 8 ml of CSF was used for virus isolations. The cells of the CSF were collected by low-speed centrifugation (1200 × *g*, 10 min). The cell-free CSF was then centrifugated at 100,000 *g* for 30 min to pellet any free virus particles. The cells and pelleted material were inoculated together onto $5–20 \times 10^6$ healthy donor peripheral blood mononuclear cells (PBMC), which had been pretreated for 3 days with phytohemagglutinin (PHA; Difco, 2.5 μg/ml). The cultures were grown in the RPMI medium supplemented with 10% fetal calf serum, 10% T cell growth factor between 1985 and Aug 1989 (Cellular products, Buffalo, NY, USA), or 100 units of interleukin-2 between Sept 1989 and 1993 (Proleukin, EuroCetus, Amsterdam, Netherlands), 2 μg/ml polybrene, and antibiotics. Five μg/ml hydrocortisone acetate was added to the cultures between Sept 1989 and 1993. The cultures were monitored twice a week to determine reverse transcriptase activity and cytopathic changes, between 1985 and Aug. 1989. Positive cultures were confirmed by indirect immunofluorescence using monoclonal antibodies to the HIV core proteins p24 (2). The cultures supernatants were assayed twice a week for HIV antigen with the p24 antigen capture ELISA (Abbot) between Sept. 1989 and 1993.

The study was approved by the Research Ethics Commitée at the University of Göteborg, Sweden.

Statistics

Paired samples were analysed by means of the Wilcoxon sign rank test; independent samples by means of Mann-Whitney U-test. Fisher's exact test was used for the comparison of unpaired proportions.

RESULTS

Clinical follow-up

Clinical data are reported in Table I. One patient was unwilling to remain in the study after 37 months, and another dropped out after 42 months. One patient died of a ruptured spleen after suffering from spleen enlargement of unknown origin for 4 months. One patient with diabetes mellitus and hypertension had an acute cerebral infarction and was withdrawn from further study. 12 patients receiving antiretroviral therapy were withdrawn from the basic follow-up study as soon as the treatment was started. Three patients not undergoing antiretroviral treatment remained in the study until June 1993.

Five patients progressed from CDC stage II or III to CDC stage IV during the study. The HIV-related complications responsible for this change in CDC classification were PCP (case 5), hairy cell leukoplakia (cases 7 and 19), weight loss (case 16), and uveitis (case 9). These 5 patients were treated with zidovudine. In 7 further patients, antiretroviral therapy with zidovudine or didanosine was started because of decreased number of peripheral CD4+ cells.

Laboratory follow-up

Laboratory values are given in Table II. During the study period without antiretroviral treatment, the peripheral CD4+ cells decreased ($p < 0.001$), while the concentrations of

Table II. *Laboratory data at the first control and after 22–77 months in 19 HIV-seropositive patients and 14 patients with AIDS*

n.s. = not significant.

	Follow-up patients ($n = 19$)					AIDS-patients ($n = 14$)		
	First control		Last control					
	Mean	Range	Mean	Range	Significant change	Mean	Range	Significant difference[a]
CD4+ peripheral cells ($\times 10^6$/l)	624	320–2130	320	39–1450	$p < 0.001$	59	10–340	$p < 0.001$
S-β_2 microglobulin (mg/l)	2.76	1.5–4.1	3.76	1.5–5.1	$p < 0.01$	4.70	3.0–10.9	n.s.
CSF-β_2 microglobulin (mg/l)	1.93	1.0–3.6	2.17	1.1–3.8	$p < 0.05$	3.73	2.1–7.5	$p < 0.01$
S-neopterin (nmol/l)	15.1	3.4–28.0	22.7	7.8–55.9	$p < 0.01$	41.4	18.1–85.3	$p < 0.01$
CSF-neopterin (nmol/l)	12.7	1.3–29.2	20.4	6.7–47.7	$p < 0.01$	28.0	8.8–57.0	$p < 0.05$
CSF-IgG index	0.72	0.45–1.72	0.92	0.41–2.43	n.s.	0.64	0.40–1.00	n.s.
Albumine quotient	6.44	2.9–13.6	6.28	3.5–10.1	n.s.	7.04	3.2–19.9	n.s.
No. of patients with CSF pleocytosis ($> 5 \times 10^6$/l)	8/19		7/19		n.s.	0/14		$p < 0.05$

[a] Significant difference compared with follow-up patients (last control).

neopterin increased in CSF ($p < 0.01$) as well as in serum ($p < 0.01$). The CSF and serum concentrations of β2M increased ($p < 0.05$ each). An elevated IgG index (>0.70) was found in 5 patients at the start, as compared with 10 patients at the end of the study. The mean IgG index increased from 0.72 to 0.92 ($p = 0.08$, not significant). The albumin quotient, indicating blood-brain barrier disturbances, did not change significantly and was elevated (>6.0–8.0, age dependent) in the same 5 patients at the start as at the end of the study. Eight patients had CSF pleocytosis ($>5 \times 10^6$/l) at the start compared with 7 at the end of the study. None of the patients in the follow-up study had a CSF-positive HIV-1 p24 antigen test, and none had a positive PCR-CMV test in CSF at the final check-up.

The AIDS patients had significantly lower CD4+ cell counts ($p < 0.001$) and significantly higher CSF neopterin and β2M concentrations than the study group had at any time during the study period ($p < 0.05$). None of the AIDS patients had CSF pleocytosis. No positive p24 HIV antigen test was found in CSF.

HIV isolations

The results of the CSF HIV isolations are given in Table III. Positive HIV isolates in CSF were registered in 8/17 patients with non contaminated CSF cultures at study start and in 13/19 at the final examination. 16/19 follow-up patients (84%) had at least 1 positive HIV isolation in CSF. The 3 patients without positive CSF-isolation tests (cases 4, 11, and 12) were tested 3, 7 and 3 times respectively, giving negative cultures; one CSF sample could not be determined because of contamination. Patient no. 11, with 7 negative CSF isolation tests, had a peripheral CD4+ count of $1,000 \times 10^6$/l after more than 6 years of follow-up, while patients 4 and 12 had CD4+ counts of 500 and 480×10^6/l, respectively, at the end of the

Table III. *CSF-HIV isolations in 76 sequential samples from 19 patients*

	Yearly lumbar puncture no.						
Patient no.	1	2	3	4	5	6	7
1	+	–	–	+[a]	+[a]		
2	–	+[a]	–[a]				
3	–	+	–	+[a]	+[a]		
4	–	–[a]	–[a]				
5	+	–	+	–			
6	–	+	+	+			
7	+	+	+				
8	+	–	+				
9	+	–	+				
10	–	+	–	+	–[a]	–[a]	
11	–	–	–	–	–[a]	–[a]	–[a]
12	C[b]	–	–	–			
13	+[a]	+[a]	+[a]				
14	+	+	+[a]				
15	–	–	–	+[a]			
16	C	–	+[a]				
17	+	+	+[a]	+[a]			
18	–	–	+[a]	+[a]			
19	–	–	+	+	+		

[a] Virus isolation performed at Department of Virology, University of Göteborg, while the other CSF samples were isolated at the Department of Virology, Karolinska Institute, University of Stockholm.
[b] C = Contaminated sample.

study. HIV isolations in blood sampled on the same dates as the CSF isolations were positive in 1 of 3 tests, 2 of 7 tests, and 2 of 4 tests in patients 4, 11, and 12, respectively. In the zidovudine-treated group, HIV was isolated in 7 of 13 available CSF samples.

The differing patterns of immune stimulation seen during this longitudinal study are demonstrated by the specific cases described below and in Table IV.

Patient no. 10 – few laboratory signs of CSF immune stimulation

A 37-year-old female who was infected by blood products in April 1985. The first CSF sample was obtained 16 months later. Her CSF concentrations of β2M, CSF cells, and IgG index remained normal throughout the study. There was a slow increase in CSF neopterin concentrations (from 3.8 to 9.5 nmol/l, regression line $y = 9.07 \times -2.11$, $r^2 = 0.81$, $p < 0.05$). After zidovudine treatment CSF neopterin concentration decreased to 5.4 nmol/l. HIV isolation from CSF was positive in 2 of 6 samples.

Patient no. 15 – laboratory signs of biphasic CSF immune stimulation

A 25-year-old homosexual male who in 1986 had an acute aseptic meningitis 3 weeks after a period of fever and enlarged lymph glands. This was later found to be a serologically verified, primary HIV-1 infection. The first CSF study sample was obtained 4 months after the acute infection. The CSF neopterin and β2M concentrations and the CSF cell counts

Table IV. *CD_4 peripheral cells, CSF concentrations of β_2-microglobulin (β2M) and neopterin, and IgG-index during follow-up in 3 HIV-seropositive patients*

Time after primary infection (months)	CD4+ ($\times 10^6$/l)	CSF-β2M (mg/l)	CSF-neopterin (nmol/l)	IgG index	CSF-HIV isolation
Patient no. 10					
16	325	1.2	3.8	0.56	–
30	400	1.1	4.1	0.57	+
42	372	1.8	3.7	0.50	–
56	271	1.4	5.0	0.50	+
69	290	1.8	7.7	0.53	–[a]
81	242	1.8	9.5	0.52	–[a]
Zidovudine treatment					
95	180	1.4	5.4	0.56	–[a]
Patient no. 15					
4	750	2.1	17.7	0.5	–
16	623	1.3	8.3	0.48	–
30	612	1.8	12.0	0.63	–
67	370	2.5	23.4	1.2	+[a]
Patient no. 18					
19	700	1.6	10.9	0.76	–
34	530	1.8	17.1	1.26	–
51	350	2.2	17.3	2.36	+[a]
62	182	1.8	18.3	2.43	+[a]
Zidovudine treatment					
74	290	1.2	11.5	1.89	–[a]
Reference value	>340	<2.2	<4.2	<0.7	–

[a] Virus isolation performed at the Department of Virology, University of Göteborg, while the other CSF samples were isolated at the Department of Virology, Karolinska Institute, University of Stockholm.

Table V. *Percentage change from mean pretreatment baseline values to post-zidovudine (ZDV) treatment values*

	3–12 months post ZDV ($n = 8$)		1–2 years post ZDV ($n = 6$)	
CD_4 peripheral cells ($\times 10^6$/l)	+7.6%	n.s.	−21%[a]	n.s.
S-β_2-microglobulin (mg/l)	−18%	n.s.	−23%[a]	n.s.
CSF β_2-microglobulin (mg/l)	−32%	$p < 0.01$	−40%[a]	n.s.
S-neopterin (nmol/l)	−7.6%	n.s.	−14%	n.s.
CSF-neopterin (nmol/l)	−48%	$p < 0.01$	−51%	n.s.
CSF-IgG index	−17%	n.s.	−4.9%	n.s.
Albumin quotient	+13%	n.s.	−11%	n.s.

[a] One sample missing.

were initially elevated but decreased after 1 to 2 years. Thereafter, the CSF neopterin concentration increased again. The IgG index kept increasing throughout the observation period. HIV isolation was positive in 1 of 4 CSF samples.

Patient no. 18 – steady increase in CSF immune stimulation

A 24-year-old homosexual male with a serologically verified, primary infection in 1986. The first CSF sample was obtained 19 months later. During the next 3 years, the patient was healthy, but showed a relatively rapid decrease in peripheral CD4+ cells, increasing concentrations of CSF neopterin, and gradually increasing IgG index as signs of immunostimulation in the CSF. The CSF β2M concentrations did not increase above the reference value at the laboratory. After 12 months of zidovudine treatment, CSF neopterin concentrations decreased to the same level as that seen on admission to the study. HIV isolation was positive in 2 of 4 CSF samples.

Effect of zidovudine treatment

The effect of zidovudine treatment was analysed in 8 patients. The CSF neopterin and β2M concentrations decreased with 48% and 32% respectively ($p < 0.01$) during the first year of zidovudine treatment and remained at the lower level during the second year of treatment as well (Table V). During the same period, the peripheral CD4+ cell counts were continuously decreasing (−21%). The number of patients with CSF pleocytosis in this group decreased from 6 to 8 during the last 6–12 months before treatment to 3 of 8 at start of treatment, to 1 of 8 after 1 year of treatment, and to 0 of 6 after 2 years of zidovudine treatment.

DISCUSSION

The gradual increase in neopterin and β2M concentrations seen in CSF over time in HIV infection suggests a progressive, active infection in the CNS, even in patients without overt neurological or psychiatric symptoms. Opportunistic infections concomitant with HIV infection may complicate the interpretation of CSF patterns in later stages of disease. Most patients in the follow-up study were not, however, in an advanced stage of disease, and there were no signs of cytomegalovirus infection, (the opportunistic infection that has attracted most attention as a cause of dementia) in the CNS, as determined by negative PCR tests at the final check-ups. The increased immune stimulation in CSF was therefore ascribed to the HIV infection.

The interval between HIV transmission and development of AIDS often exceeds 10 years (14, 15). Thus a follow-up time of 2–6 years, as in this study, gives insufficient information about the natural course of immune activity in the CSF throughout the course of HIV infection. Furthermore, most patients were excluded before they had reached the AIDS stage because of interference by antiretroviral treatment. Today it is almost impossible to conduct longitudinal studies without interference by antiviral drugs for longer than in the present study, as treatment traditions have changed towards earlier antiviral regimens. Our longitudinal study group was therefore compared with a group of AIDS patients not given antiviral treatment, who had attended the Department of Infectious Diseases in Göteborg, during the same period of time.

Neopterin is a product derived largely from macrophages stimulated by interferon-gamma (16), and β2M is a low-molecular-weight protein that forms the light chain of class I major histocompatibility complex antigen. Both substances are unspecific biochemical indicators of immune stimulation and have been shown to be surrogate markers for progression of the HIV-1 infection (7). Several reports have been published, showing increased CSF neopterin and β2M levels in HIV infection in early and more advanced stages of the disease (5, 6, 17, 18), in HIV encephalitis (19), and in opportunistic CNS infections (18, 20), but few longitudinal studies have been performed. Elovaara et al. have, however, shown gradually increasing CSF concentrations of β2M in neurologically healthy HIV-1-infected individuals (21). The present study confirms this finding and shows that CSF neopterin also follows the course of HIV infection.

Although β2M and neopterin concentrations often correlate, they do not measure exactly the same activation mechanisms of the immune system. Whether neopterin or β2M is the more sensitive general immune activity marker in CSF could not be determined from this study because of the small number of subjects, but changes in the neopterin concentrations (vis-à-vis the β2M) seemed to develop earlier during the course of infection. When measuring CSF concentrations of different biochemical products, the risk of diffusion or transport over the blood-brain barrier must be considered. It is unlikely, however, that the increased CSF neopterin and β2M concentrations merely reflect the serum concentrations. Intrathecal origin of neopterin and β2M was suggested by the fact that the CSF concentrations were higher than the serum concentrations in 3 of 19 cases for β2M and in 9 of 19 for neopterin, on admission. At the last check-up, none of the patients had a higher β2M concentration in CSF than in serum, while 8 patients still had a higher neopterin concentration in CSF than in serum. Passive diffusion is more likely for proteins such as β2M, than for a small and polar molecule such as neopterin. However, no correlation between CSF and serum β2M concentrations was found in patients with HIV dementia (19). It has been estimated that only 2.5% of the CSF neopterin concentration originates from serum (18), which speaks for neopterin as a marker of immune stimulation in CSF.

HIV isolations in CSF proved positive at least once in over 80% when the patients were followed longitudinally, a finding previously seen in a smaller number of patients (2). The finding of 3 patients with repeatedly negative CSF isolations suggests that there may be HIV-positive individuals without HIV infection in the CNS, or that the negative cultures may be due to the difficulty of isolating small amounts of virus in the laboratory. The latter suggestion was found to be most probable, as all the repeatedly CSF culture-negative patients showed at least one sign of immune stimulation in CSF, such as increased neopterin, CSF pleocytosis, or intrathecal immunoglobulin production. The rate of virus replication has been associated with neopterin concentration and with the severity of HIV infection (22). Although there was a tendency towards more positive isolations in the last samples than at the beginning of the follow-up study, the results were inconsistent, and the change in transportation during the study most certainly affected the results. Furthermore, there were minor changes in cultivation technique and a change in screening procedure during the study. Following zidovudine treatment, 7 of 13 CSF samples were still isolation positive. HIV virus isolation, without determining replicative capacity, was found not to be a useful method for monitoring the infectious course. Also p24 antigen was a poor marker of viral burden in CSF, since all follow-up patients and all AIDS patients were CSF p24 antigen-negative. To monitor the viral load in CSF, development of reliable quantitative assays, such as a quantitative polymerase chain reaction test, would be preferable.

The pattern of CSF immunostimulation over time differed between individuals. Some had very few signs of immunostimulation in spite of positive HIV isolations. When followed over a couple of years, however, CSF neopterin concentrations were seen to increase slowly, as shown in patient no. 10. Other patients had a biphasic pattern of immunostimulation, as illustrated by patient no. 15 who had an aseptic meningitis with CSF pleocytosis, and increased CSF neopterin and β2M levels in association with a primary HIV infection. After that, normalization of CSF neopterin and β2M occurred over 1–2 years, but a new increase followed thereafter. The IgG index in this patient increased steadily. A third pattern was an increased CSF neopterin concentration shortly after a primary HIV infection, with further increases over the following years, and was correlated to a relatively rapid reduction of peripheral CD4+ cells, as illustrated by patient no. 18. Since in most cases it was difficult to obtain a CSF sample close to the primary infection, a biphasic pattern might have been present even in these cases.

The results of the CSF analysis in the AIDS patients with markedly elevated neopterin and β2M concentrations, but without pleocytosis and few signs of intrathecal immunoglobulin production, indicate cytokine production, but an inability to mount a cellular response. In previous cross-sectional studies, CSF pleocytosis and intrathecal IgG production have been seen to increase in the early to middle stages of the disease and then return to normal values (17, 23). In the present longitudinal study, we also found a tendency (not significant) toward an increase in IgG index over time in the follow-up group, where the majority had not reached the AIDS stage.

Immune stimulation has been suggested as one of several important factors in the pathogenesis of the AIDS dementia complex. An elevated neopterin concentration indicates interferon gamma stimulation (16). Interferon gamma induces degradation of tryptophan and increased concentrations of degradation products such as the potentially neurotoxic N-formyl-kynurenin and quinolinic acid (24). In fact, the concentration of quinolonic acid has been correlated to degree of AIDS dementia (25). Neopterin as a surrogate marker for this whole process might thus reflect an important pathogenic mechanism.

Zidovudine has been shown to be clinically effective on HIV-related neurological symptoms (26), and the distribution through the blood-brain barrier has proved to be fairly good (27). In two studies, zidovudine treatment significantly decreased CSF neopterin and β2M concentrations after 2 months (18, 19) and 4–8 months (28), but it is at present not known for how long this effect will last. In serum, the effect of zidovudine was more persistent on neopterin than on β2M concentrations (29). Whether this is true also in CSF could not be determined in our small number of subjects. The zidovudine effect on the CSF parameters studied could either be a specific antiretroviral response in the CNS, or the result of an unspecific anti-inflammatory activity of the drug. Regardless of the mechanism involved, the reduced immune activity following zidovudine treatment must be interpreted as beneficial for the patient. Effective anti-retroviral therapy should inhibit HIV stimulation and, in consequence, reduce the immunostimulation associated with it. Analyses of surrogate markers in CSF, such as neopterin and β2M, indicate that the HIV-CNS infections (which most HIV-1 infected patients suffer from) are not latent infections, but active, progressive processes. These results may have important implications when deciding on antiretroviral treatment.

REFERENCES

1. Pantaleo G, Graziosi C, Demarest JF, Butini L, Montroni M, Fox CH, Orenstein JM, Kotler DP, Fauci A. HIV infection is active and progressive in lymphoid tissue during the clinically latent stage of disease. Nature 362: 355–358, 1993.
2. Chiodi F, Keys B, Albert J, Hagberg L, Lundeberg J, Uhlén M, Fenyö E-M, Norkrans G. HIV-1 is present in the cerebrospinal fluid of the majority of infected individuals. J Clin Microbiol 30: 1768–1771, 1992.
3. Sönnerborg A, Johansson B, Strannegård Ö. Detection of HIV-1 DNA and infectious virus in cerebrospinal fluid. AIDS Res Hum Retroviruses 7: 369–373, 1991.
4. Hagberg L, Norkrans G, Larsson M, Forsman A, Svennerholm L. Cytological and immunoglobulin findings in cerebrospinal fluid of symptomatic and asymptomatic human immunodeficiency virus seropositive patients. Infection 16: 13–18, 1988.
5. Fuchs D, Chiodi F, Albert J, Åsjö B, Hagberg L, Hausen A, Norkrans G, Reibnegger G, Werner ER, Wachter H. Neopterin concentrations in cerebrospinal fluid and serum of individuals infected with HIV-1. AIDS 3: 285–288, 1989.
6. Sönnerborg A, von Stedingk L-V, Hansson L-O, Strannegård Ö. Elevated neopterin and β2-microglobulin levels in blood and cerebrospinal fluid occur early in HIV-1 infection. AIDS 3: 277–283, 1989.
7. Fahey JL, Taylor JMG, Detels R, Hofmann B, Melmed R, Nishanian P, Giorgi JV. The prognostic value of cellular and serological markers in infection with HIV. N Engl J Med 322: 166–172, 1990.
8. Centers for Disease Control: Classification system for human T-lymphotropic virus type III/lymphadenopathy-associated virus infection. MMWR Morb Mortal Wkly Rep 35: 334–339, 1986.
9. Wikkelso C, Andersson M, Andersson R, Blomstrand C. Isoelectric focusing followed by silver staining. A suitable method for investigation of cerebrospinal fluid protein. Eur Neurol 23: 306–312, 1984.
10. Werner ER, Bichler A, Daxenbichler G, Fuchs D, Fuith LC, Hausen A, Hetzel H, Reibnegger G, Wachter H. Determination of neopterin in serum and urine. Clin Chem 33: 62–66, 1987.
11. Bjerrum OW, Birgens HS. Measurement of β2-microglobulin in serum and plasma by an enzyme-linked immunosorbent assay (ELISA). Clin Chim Acta 155: 69–76, 1986.
12. Studahl M, Ricksten A, Sandberg T, Elowson S, Säll C, Herner S, Bergström T. Cytomegalovirus infection of the central nervous system in non-compromised patients. Acta Neurol Scand (in press).
13. Akrigg A, Wilkinson GWG, Oram JD. The structure of the major immediate early gene of human cytomegalovirus strain AD169. Virus Res 2: 107–121, 1985.
14. Rutherford GW, Lifson AR, Hessol NA, Darrow WW, O'Malley PM, Buchbinder P, Barnhart JL, Bodecker TW, Cannon L, Doll LS, Holmberg SD, Harrison JS, Rogers MF, Werdeger D, Jaffe HW. Course of HIV-1 infection in a cohort of homosexual and bisexual men: an 11 year follow up study. BMJ 301: 1183–1188, 1990.
15. Ward JW, Bush TJ, Perkins HA, Lieb LL, Allen JR, Goldfinger D, Samson SM, Pepkowitz SH, Fernando LP, Holland PV, Kleinman SH, Grindon AJ, Garner PA, Rutherford GW, Holmberg SD. The natural history of transfusion-associated HIV infection: factors influencing progression to disease. N Engl J Med 321: 947–952, 1989.
16. Huber C, Batchelor JR, Fuchs D, Hausen A, Lang A, Niederwieser D, Reibnegger G, Swetley P, Troppmair J, Wachter H. Immune response-associated production of neopterin release from macrophages primarily under control of interferon-gamma. J Exp Med 160: 310–316, 1984.
17. Lucey DR, McGuire SA, Clerici M, Hall K, Benton J, Butzin CA, Ward WW, Shearer G, Boswell N, Hendrix CW. Comparison of spinal fluid β2-microglobulin levels with CD4+ T cell count, in vitro T helper cell function, and spinal fluid IgG parameters in human immunodeficiency virus type 1. J Infect Dis 163: 971–975, 1991.
18. Bogner JR, Junge-Hülsing B, Kronawitter U, Sadri I, Matuschke A, Goebel F-D. Expansion of neopterin and $beta_2$-microglobulin in cerebrospinal fluid reaches maximum levels early and late in the course of human immunodeficiency virus infection. Clin Investig 70: 665–669, 1992.
19. Brew BJ, Bhalla RB, Morris P, Sidtis JJ, Keilp JJ, Sadler AE, Gallardo H, McArthur JC, Schwartz MK, Price RW. Cerebrospinal fluid β2-microglobulin in patients with AIDS dementia complex: an expanded series including responses to zidovudine treatment. AIDS 6: 461–465, 1992.

20. Brew BJ, Bhalla RB, Morris P, Gallardo MS, McArthur JC, Schwartz MK, Price RW. Cerebrospinal fluid neopterin in human immunodeficiency virus type 1 infection. Ann Neurol 28: 556–560, 1990.
21. Elovaara I, Nykyri E, Poutiainen E, Hokkanen L, Raininko R, Suni J. CSF follow-up in HIV-1 infection: Intrathecal production of HIV-specific and unspecific IgG, and beta-2-microglobulin increase with duration of HIV-1 infection. Acta Neurol Scand 87: 388–396, 1993.
22. Fuchs D, Albert J, Åsjö B, Fenyö EM, Reibnegger G, Wachter H. Association between serum neopterin concentrations and in vitro replicative capacity of HIV-1 isolates. J Infect Dis 160: 724–725, 1989.
23. Marshall DW, Brey RL, Cahill WT, Houk RW, Zajac RA, Boswell RN. Spectrum of cerebrospinal fluid findings in various stages of human immunodeficiency virus infection. Arch Neurol 45: 954–958, 1988.
24. Heyes MP, Rubinow D, Lane C, Markey SP. Cerebrospinal fluid quinolinic acid concentrations are increased in acquired immunodeficiency syndrome. Ann Neurol 26: 275–277, 1989.
25. Heyes MP, Brew BJ, Martin A, Price RW, Salazar AM, Sidtis JJ, Yergey JA, Mouradian MM, Sadler AE, Keilp J, Rubinow D, Markey SP. Quinolinic acid in cerebrospinal fluid and serum in HIV-1 infection: Relationship to clinical and neurological status. Ann Neurol 29: 202–209, 1991.
26. Yarchoan R, Brouwers P, Spitzer AR, Grafman J, Safai B, Perno CF, Larson SM, Berg G, Fishl M, Wichman A, Thomas RV, Brunetti A, Schmidt PJ, Myers CE, Broder S. Response of human immunodeficiency virus-associated neurological disease to 3′-azido-3′-deoxythymidine. Lancet 1: 132–135, 1987.
27. Yarchoan R, Klecker RW, Weinhold KJ, Markham PD, Lyerly HK, Durack DT, Gelmann E, Nusinoff Lehrman S, Blum RM, Barry DW, Shearer GM, Fishl MA, Mitsuya H, Gallo RC, Collins JM, Bolognesi DP, Myers CE, Broder S. Administration of 3′-azido-3′-deoxythmidine, an inhibitor of HTLV-III/LAV replication, to patients with AIDS or AIDS related complex. Lancet 1: 575–580, 1986.
28. Hagberg L, Norkrans G, Andersson M, Wachter H, Fuchs D. Cerebrospinal fluid neopterin and β-2 microglobulin levels in neurologically asymptomatic HIV-infected patients before and after initiation of zidovudine treatment. Infection 20: 313–315, 1992.
29. Bass HZ, Hardy D, Mitsuyasu RT, Taylor JMG, Wang X, Fishl MA, Spector SA, Richman DD, Fahey JL. The effect of zidovudine treatment on serum neopterin and β2-microglobulin levels in mildly symptomatic, HIV-type 1 seropositive individuals. J Acquir Immune Defic Syndr 5: 215–221, 1992.

Submitted February 16, 1994; accepted April 20, 1994

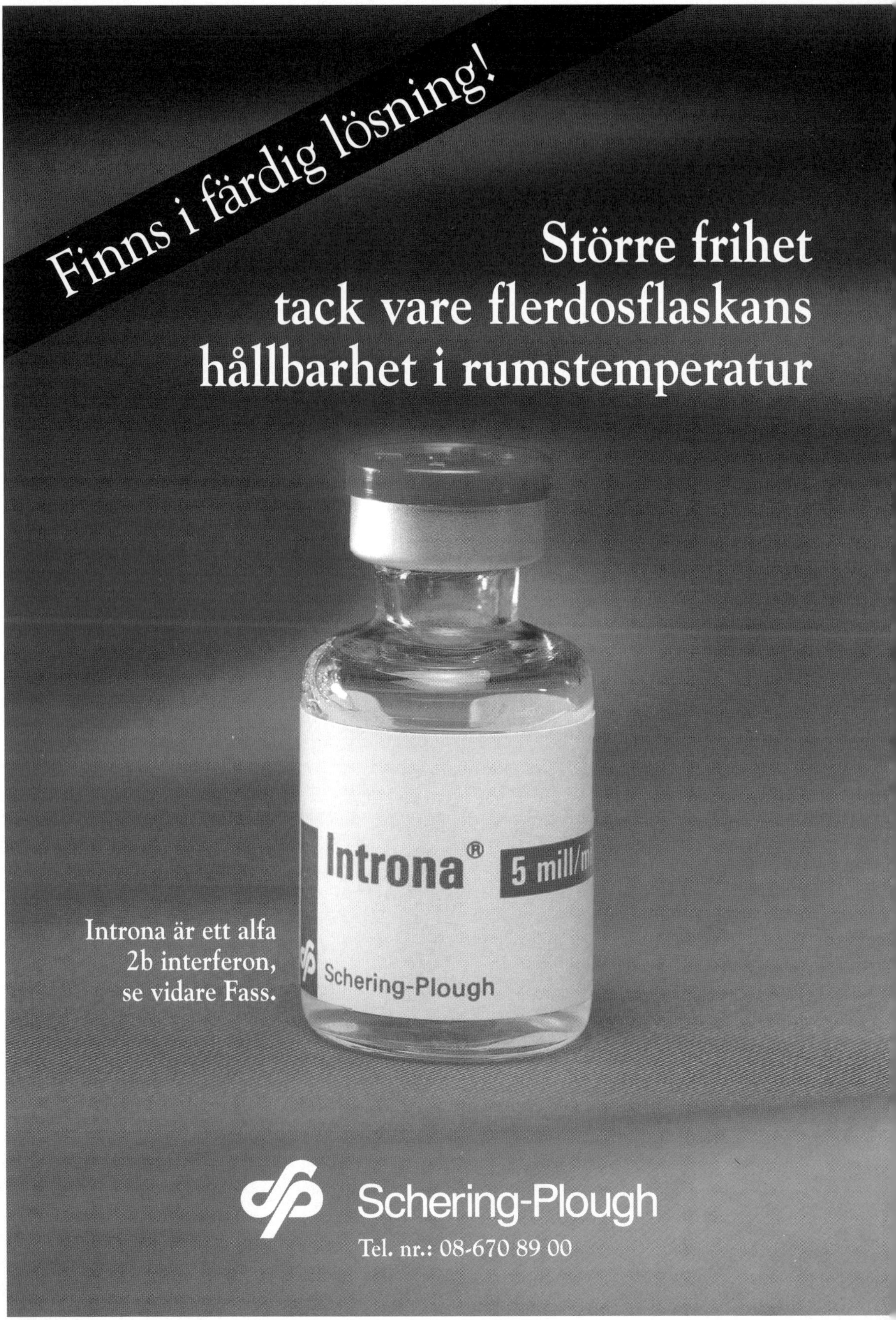
Finns i färdig lösning!
Större frihet
tack vare flerdosflaskans
hållbarhet i rumstemperatur
Introna®
Schering-Plough
Introna är ett alfa
2b interferon,
se vidare Fass.
Schering-Plough
Tel. nr.: 08-670 89 00

Scand J Infect Dis 26: 535–541, 1994

Clindamycin in Persisting Streptococcal Pharyngotonsillitis after Penicillin Treatment

ARNE ORRLING[1], ANNA STJERNQUIST-DESATNIK[1], CLAES SCHALÉN[2] and CARL KAMME[2]

From the Departments of [1]Oto-Rhino-Laryngology and [2]Medical Microbiology, University Hospital, Lund, Sweden

239 patients with streptococcal pharyngotonsillitis completed treatment with phenoxymethyl penicillin 12.5 mg per kg body weight b.i.d. for 10 days. At examination after completing therapy, throat specimens from 53 patients (22%) yielded growth of group A streptococci of the same T-type as the initial culture (bacterial treatment failure). 20 of these 53 (38%) had symptoms and signs of tonsillitis (clinical and bacterial treatment failure). 48 of the patients with bacterial failure were randomly allocated to phenoxymethyl penicillin or clindamycin in an open design; 22 of them received a second course of phenoxymethyl penicillin for 10 days and 26 were given clindamycin, 6.5 mg per kg body weight b.i.d. (children) or 300 mg t.i.d. (adults) for 10 days. After completing their treatment, 14 of 22 patients (64%) given phenoxymethyl penicillin harboured the same T-type as in the previous two cultures, while group A streptococci were not recovered from any of the 26 patients receiving clindamycin. In patients with clinical failure after phenoxymethyl penicillin treatment, a new course with this drug is not motivated. In that situation clindamycin seems to be an efficient choice.

A. Stjernquist-Desatnik, MD, PhD, Department of Oto-Rhino-Laryngology, University Hospital, S-221 85 Lund, Sweden

INTRODUCTION

Group A streptococci (GAS) constitute a major cause of acute pharyngotonsillitis, accounting for 30–50% of all cases (1, 2). Since, in untreated patients, the acute episode may develop into non-suppurative complications, e.g. rheumatic fever or acute glomerulonephritis, antibiotic treatment of streptococcal tonsillitis is indicated. Also, the severity and duration of the acute episode will be ameliorated by antibiotics such as phenoxymethylpenicillin, the preferred treatment in Sweden (3). Although strains resistant to phenoxymethyl penicillin have not so far been encountered in clinical specimens, high rates of clinical and/or bacterial failure (5–25%) following 10-day phenoxymethyl penicillin treatment have been reported (4, 5). Furthermore, a second course of phenoxymethyl penicillin is known to result in treatment failure even more often, in some cases necessitating tonsillectomy (6).

Several factors possibly contributing to the treatment failure have been suggested: poor patient compliance or reinfection from the environment might account for some cases. Penicillin tolerance or delayed killing of streptococci has been suggested by some investigators, but they were unable to confirm this in a later study (7, 8). Eradication of the normal throat flora, in particular alpha-streptococci with inhibitory activity against group A streptococci, by phenoxymethyl penicillin might increase the likelihood of treatment failure (9). In a recent study, administration of alpha-streptococci into the throat following penicillin treatment thus seemed to reduce the number of unhealed cases (10). Finally, selection of betalactamase-producing bacterial species in the throat by penicillin may lead to treatment failure due to inactivation of the drug (11, 12, 13); favourable results of treatment of streptococcal pharyngotonsillitis with betalactamase-stable cephalosporins, may support this view (14).

In previous reports, treatment of recurrent streptococcal pharyngotonsillitis with clindamycin versus to phenoxymethyl penicillin appeared significantly more favourable (15, 16).

In the present investigation, clindamycin was compared with phenoxymethyl penicillin in patients with clinical and/or bacterial failure of GAS pharyngotonsillitis following phenoxymethyl penicillin treatment.

MATERIAL AND METHODS

Patients

Patient or parental consent to therapy was obtained for the participants. The study was approved by the Medical Ethics Committee of the University of Lund. Consecutive patients with acute tonsillitis and a positive throat culture for GAS, examined by the same physician (A.O.), were enrolled. Their age range was 2–62 years (median 9, mean 15.2, SD 13.3 years). Patients hypersensitive to clindamycin or phenoxymethyl penicillin, with gastrointestinal or renal disease, pregnant or nursing, were not included in the investigation.

Bacterial treatment failure was defined as presence of GAS of the same T-type as the original isolate within 2 weeks of completing antibiotic treatment. **Clinical and bacterial treatment failure** was defined as above, combined with clinical symptoms and signs of pharyngotonsillitis. **Reinfection** was defined as occurrence of a new T-type within 2 weeks of completing of treatment.

Treatment regimen

From June 1990 to June 1992, 278 patients with acute streptococcal pharyngotonsillitis were treated with oral phenoxymethyl penicillin, 12.5 mg/kg bodyweight b.i.d. for 10 days. Of these, 239 subjects fulfilled the inclusion criteria by taking the drug as prescribed. At 4–6 days after completing their therapy, and later if symptoms recurred, the patients were re-examined and another specimen for culture was obtained. Patients with bacterial treatment failure, regardless of symptoms, were randomized to either phenoxymethyl penicillin (Calciopen^{R}) 12.5 mg/kg body weight b.i.d. or clindamycin (Dalacin^{R}) 6.5 mg/kg bodyweight t.i.d. (children) or 300 mg t.i.d. (adults) for 10 days. The randomization was performed by the patient by blindly drawing a number indicating one of the drugs. The result of the randomization was known to one of us (A.O). At 4–6 days after cessation of treatment, patients were again examined and a throat specimen collected. The patients were informed to return in case of recurrence of symptoms; in those cases, a new examination, including throat culture, was performed. Patient compliance was checked by thorough interview by the physician. In addition, patients were carefully informed about the importance of taking the drug for no less than 10 days and told that the prospects of failure would otherwise increase. It was emphasized that bacterial failure alone was the reason for further treatment.

Bacteriological investigation

Culture specimens were obtained from the throat by rotating a sterile cotton swab along both tonsils. The specimens were transported in a modified Stuart agar medium, inoculated onto horse-sheep blood agar and incubated anaerobically for 18–20 h. Beta-haemolytic streptococci were diagnosed by bacitracin susceptibility and enhanced haemolysis on horse blood agar by sodium nucleate, or serologically grouped. Strains were T-typed by slide agglutination (Chemapol, Prague). Laboratory staff were not informed about the treatment regimen of individual patients.

According to the number of colonies, growth of GAS was classified as sparse (0–10 CFU), moderate (10–100 CFU) or abundant (>100 CFU).

Statistical method

The χ^2-test with Yates' correction was used. *P*-values below 0.05 were considered significant.

RESULTS

Outcome of initial treatment

At examination within 2 weeks following the initial treatment with phenoxymethyl penicillin, specimens from 53 out of 239 patients (22%) yielded GAS of the same T-type as the initial culture (bacterial treatment failure), whereas in 3 cases another T-type was recovered (reinfection). Most of the isolates from patients with bacterial treatment failure belonged to T-types 28, 4, 12 or 1. These four T-types were also predominant among the 239 primary isolates (Table I).

Table I. *T-types of group A streptococci before treatment and after the first and second failure after phenoxymethyl penicillin*

		T-type							
Culture	No.	1	2	4	12	21	25	28R	NT
First	180	10	3	48	25	1	13	50	30
Second	53	7		12	11		1	14	8
Third	14			2	3			4	5

Of the 53 patients with bacterial treatment failure, 20 (38%) had symptoms and signs of pharyngotonsillitis. In 43 of the patients, abundant growth of GAS was found, whereas growth was recorded as moderate or sparse in 8 and 2 cases, respectively.

Outcome of retreatment

Of the 53 patients with bacterial treatment failure, 25 were randomized to phenoxymethyl penicillin and 28 to clindamycin. Five of the patients were excluded, 3 from the penicillin group and 2 from the clindamycin group, due to failure to return for check-up within the stipulated time. Thus, 48 patients (median 6.0, mean 9.5, SD 10.0 years) were evaluated, of whom 22 received phenoxymethyl penicillin and 26 clindamycin. There was no difference in age or sex between the groups. A somewhat larger proportion, 12 of 22 of the patients allocated to penicillin, had clinical symptoms and signs of pharyngotonsillitis, as compared with 8 of 26 allocated to clindamycin ($p > 0.05$).

After the second treatment, 14/22 patients (64%) receiving phenoxymethyl penicillin harboured the same T-type as in the previous two throat cultures, while GAS were not recovered from any of 26 patients receiving clindamycin ($p < 0.001$). Of the 14 patients with bacterial treatment failure, 4 had clinical symptoms and signs of pharyngotonsillitis (Table II). Most of the positive specimens yielded abundant or moderate growth of GAS, 8 and 5, respectively, whereas sparse growth occurred in one case. Side effects included a slight gastro-intestinal disturbance occurring in some cases, but showing no difference between the penicillin and clindamycin groups, and in no case was treatment discontinued.

Table II. *Eradication of group A streptococci from the throat by clindamycin or phenoxymethyl penicillin following initial penicillin treatment failure*

Treatment	Antibiotic (No. treated)	Bacteriological treatment failure No (%)	Clinical + bacteriological treatment failure No (%)
Initial	Phenoxymethyl penicillin (239)	53 (22%)	20 (8%)
Retreatment	Phenoxymethyl penicillin (22)	14 (64%)[a]	4 (18%)[b]
	Clindamycin (26)	0	0

[a] $p < 0.001$ vs. clindamycin treatment.
[b] N.S. (non-significant).

DISCUSSION

The present results demonstrated clindamycin to be effective in eradicating GAS in patients with treatment failure following a 10-day course of phenoxymethyl penicillin for verified GAS pharyngotonsillitis. This outcome was in accordance with a study by Brook & Hirokawa (16) showing clindamycin to be superior in this respect to both penicillin and erythromycin. Tanz et al. (17) reported clindamycin to be superior to benzathine penicillin combined with rifampin in eradicating GAS from the throat in chronic carriers of GAS.

The bacterial treatment failure rate, 22% after the first and 64% after the second course of phenoxymethyl penicillin, was in agreement with other studies (6, 18). In only 3 out of 56 cases were we able to diagnose reinfection rather than treatment failure, by the appearance of GAS of a new T-type, following the initial treatment. Since most GAS strains in the closest family members could be identical to the type carried by the patient being studied, the distinction between treatment failure and reinfection by the same serotype is not always possible. By obtaining a follow-up throat culture as soon as 4 days after cessation of treatment, the risk of including patients with reinfection was minimized. This was supported by the fact that reinfection was not found among any of the patients receiving clindamycin.

At the second visit, 20 out of 53 patients with bacterial failure showed signs of pharyngotonsillitis. Since abundant growth of GAS was noted in most of the cases, irrespective of signs or symptoms at follow-up culture, a chronic, asymptomatic carrier state among them was less likely.

One possible explanation for the good results with clindamycin might be its high penetration into the site of infection, in comparison with penicillin V (19, 20). The concentration of the antibiotic in tonsillar surface fluid rather than intracellularly may appear crucial in this context (21, 22). Furthermore, in a mouse model of streptococcal myocarditis, Stevens at al. (23) found clindamycin to be more effective than penicillin, which was ascribed to a long post-antibiotic effect of clindamycin and its independence of inoculum size. Finally, inhibition of antiphagocytic activity of streptococci by clindamycin (24) may also contribute to its high efficacy.

Beta-lactamase stable cephalosporins, such as cefadroxyl (14, 5), loracarbef (25), cefaxetil (26), cefixime (27), and cefpodoxyme (28) are reported to be superior to phenoxymethyl penicillin for primary acute streptococcal pharyngotonsillitis, and the addition of a betalactamase inhibitor, clavulanic acid, was reported to potentiate the effect of amoxycillin on recurrent tonsillitis (6). This may indicate that betalactamase-producing bacterial species in the respiratory tract flora are of significance by inactivating the penicillin. On the other hand, in a study of acute streptococcal pharyngitis, Tanz et al. (29) did not find any difference between phenoxymethyl penicillin and amoxycillin-clavulanic acid as concerns the eradication of streptococci and were also unable to demonstrate any prognostical impact of betalactamase-producing species in the throat.

In a critical evaluation of a meta analysis suggesting that oral cephalosporins are superior to penicillin for the treatment of streptococcal pharyngotonsillitis (30), only three of 19 investigations in the meta analysis were found to fulfil the criteria for a comparative analysis (31). The difference in bacterial eradication rates for penicillin and cefadroxyl or cefaclor in those studies was only 4–6%. Theoretically, a slight influence of cephalosporins on throat-resident alpha-streptococci could account for the better eradication of GAS by cephalosporins than by penicillin (14). However, since most alpha-streptococci are evidently highly sensitive to clindamycin (MIC < 0.1 mg/l in 10 random isolates at our laboratory), this cannot explain the beneficial effect of clindamycin as compared to penicillin, reported here.

Thus, neither the lesser activity of the cephalosporins against the alpha-streptococci, postulated to inhibit GAS, nor the betalactamase-producing species in the throat, potentiated during betalactam therapy, have been convincingly shown to be of any significance for the outcome of treatment of streptococcal pharyngotonsillitis. In the present investigation, phenoxymethyl penicillin was given b.i.d. according to current practice in Sweden. A brief postantibiotic effect does not seem to explain the failure rate as this is reported to be the same in patients receiving the drug twice or four times a day (32).

Clindamycin has long been implicated in eliciting pseudo-membranous colitis (PMC) and other gastro-intestinal side effects (33). In a recent survey of PMC, however, cephalosporins and penicillins were found to be comparable to clindamycin in this respect (34). In the present study, there was no difference between patients receiving phenoxymethyl penicillin or clindamycin for 10 days as regards gastro-intestinal side effects.

The risk for the emergence of resistance against macrolides and related drugs is known from Japan (35) and from Finland (36) as well as from southern Sweden (37). Resistance to macrolides in GAS is commonly mediated by a plasmid encoding methylase production and, in constitutively resistant strains, phenotypically linked to clindamycin resistance. However, clindamycin (vis-à-vis current macrolides) seldom induces methylase production in GAS and strains with low level erythromycin resistance are usually susceptible to clindamycin (36, 38).

We conclude that phenoxymethyl penicillin, by virtue of its narrow antimicrobial spectrum, low cost and absence of penicillin resistance among GAS despite many years of use, is still the drug of choice for primary tonsillitis caused by GAS. However, in patients with clinical and bacterial failure after penicillin treatment, clindamycin appears to be an appropriate alternative. The efficacy of the cephalosporins has not been clearly documented in this respect. Moreover, for the eradication of GAS in rheumatic fever, clindamycin may be a suitable choice.

Finally, by virtue of both its greater efficacy and its lower potential for the development of resistance in GAS, clindamycin seems preferable to the macrolides in cases of GAS pharyngotonsillitis and hypersensitivity to penicillin.

ACKNOWLEDGEMENT

The investigation was supported by the Medical Faculty, University of Lund, the Royal Physiographical Society, Lund, and Upjohn AB, Sweden.

REFERENCES

1. Wannamaker LW. Perplexity and precision in the diagnosis of streptococcal pharyngitis. Am J Dis Child 124: 352–358, 1972.
2. Stjernquist-Desatnik A, Prellner K, Christensen P. Clinical and laboratory findings in patients with acute tonsillitis. Acta Otolaryngol (Stockh) 104: 351–359, 1987.
3. Krober MS, Bass JW, Michels GN. Streptococcal pharyngitis. Placebo-controlled double-blind evaluation of clinical response to penicillin therapy. JAMA 253: 1271–1274, 1985.
4. Gastanaduy AS, Kaplan EL, Huwe BB, McKay C, Wannamaker LW. Failure of penicillin to eradicate group A streptococci during an outbreak of pharyngitis. Lancet 1: 498–501, 1980.
5. Strömberg A, Schwan Å, Cars O. Five versus ten days treatment of group A streptococcal pharyngotonsillitis: a randomized controlled clinical trial with phenoxymethylpenicillin and cefadroxil. Scand J Infect Dis 20: 37–46, 1988.
6. Kaplan EL, Johnson DR. Eradication of group A streptococci from the upper respiratory tract by amoxicillin with clavulanate after oral penicillin V treatment failure. J Pediatr 113: 400–403, 1988.
7. Kim KS, Kaplan EL. Association of penicillin tolerance with failure to eradicate group A streptococci from patients with pharyngitis. J Pediatr 107: 681–684, 1985.
8. Smith TD, Huskins WC, Kim KS, Kaplan EL. Efficacy of β-lactamase-resistant penicillin and

influence of penicillin tolerance in eradicating streptococci from the pharynx after failure of penicillin therapy for group A streptococcal pharyngitis. J Pediatr 110: 777–782, 1987.

9. Sanders C, Sanders E, Harrow D. Bacterial interference: effects of oral antibiotics on the normal throat flora and its ability to interfere with group A streptococci. Infect Immun 13: 808–812, 1976.
10. Roos K, Grahn E, Holm SE, Johansson H, Lind L. Interfering alpha-streptococci as a protection against recurrent streptococcal tonsillitis in children. Int J Pediatr Otorhinolaryngol 25: 141–148, 1993.
11. Brook I. The role of β-lactamase-producing bacteria in the persistence of streptococcal tonsillar infection. Rev Infect Dis 6: 601–607, 1984a.
12. Brook I. β-lactamase-producing bacteria recovered after clinical failures with various penicillin therapy. Arch Otolaryngol 110: 228–231, 1984b.
13. Tunér K, Nord CE. Emergence of beta-lactamase producing anaerobic bacteria in the tonsils during penicillin treatment. Eur J Clin Microbiol 5: 399–404, 1986.
14. Holm SE, Roos K, Strömberg A. A randomized study of treatment of streptococcal pharyngotonsillitis with cefadroxil or phenoxymethylpenicillin (penicillin V). Pediatr Infect Dis J 10: S68-S71, 1991.
15. Jensen JH, Larsen SB. Treatment of recurrent acute tonsillitis with clindamycin. An alternative to tonsillectomy? Clin Otolaryngol 16: 498–500, 1991.
16. Brook I, Hirokawa R. Treatment of patients with a history of recurrent tonsillitis due to group A beta-hemolytic streptococci. Clinical Pediatrics 24: 331–336, 1985.
17. Tanz R, Poncher J, Corydon K, et al. Clindamycin treatment of chronic pharyngeal carriage of group A streptococci. J Pediatr 119: 123–128, 1991.
18. Schwartz R, Wientzen R, Pedreira F, et al. Penicillin V for group A streptococcal pharyngotonsillitis. JAMA 246: 1790–1795, 1981.
19. Panzer J, Brown D, Epstein W, et al. Clindamycin levels in various body tissues and fluids. J Clin Pharmacol 12: 259–262, 1972.
20. Roos K, Grahn E, Ekedahl C, Holm S. Pharmacokinetics of phenoxymethylpenicillin in tonsils. Scand J Infect Dis 18: 125–130, 1986.
21. Strömberg A, Friberg U, Cars O. Concentrations of phenoxymethylpenicillin and cefadroxil in tonsillar tissue and tonsillar surface fluid. Eur J Clin Microbiol 6: 525–529, 1987.
22. Stjernquist-Desatnik A, Samuelsson P, Walder M. Penetration of penicillin V to tonsillar surface fluid in healthy individuals and in patients with acute tonsillitis. J Laryngol Otol 107: 309–312, 1993.
23. Stevens D, Gibbons A, Bergström R, Winn V. The Eagle effect revisited: efficacy of clindamycin, erythromycin, and penicillin in the treatment of streptococcal myositis. J Infect Dis 158: 23–28, 1988.
24. Gemmell CG, Peterson PK, Schmeling D, Kim Y, Mathews J, Wannamaker L, Quie PG. Potentiation of opsonization and phagocytosis of Streptococcus pyogenes following growth in the presence of clindamycin. J Clin Invest 67: 1249–1256, 1981.
25. Disney FA, Hanfling MJ, Hausinger SA. Loracarbef (LY163892) vs. pencillin V in the treatment of streptococcal pharyngi-tis and tonsillitis. Pediatr Infect Dis J 11 S: 20–26, 1992.
26. Holm SE, Henning C, Staley H, Lomberg H. A comparison of cefuroxime axetil suspension and penicillin V syrup in the treatment of recurrent streptococcal tonsillitis in children. Abstract, 18th ICC, Stockholm, Sweden, 1993.
27. Block SL, Hedrick JA, Tyler RD. Comparative study of the effectiveness of cefixime and penicillin V for the treatment of streptococcal pharyngitis in children and adolescents. Pediatr Infect Dis J 11: 919–925, 1992.
28. Portier H, Chavanet P, Waldner-Combernoux A, et al. Five versus ten days treatment of streptococcal pharyngotonsillitis: a randomized controlled trial comparing cefpodoxime proxetil and phenoxymethyl penicillin. Scand J Infect Dis 26: 59–66, 1994.
29. Tanz RR, Shulman ST, Sroka PA, Marubio S, Brook I & Yogev R al. Lack of influence of beta-lactamase producing flora on recovery of group A streptococci after treatment of acute pharyngitis. J Pediatr 117: 859–863, 1990.
30. Pichichero ME. Cephalosporins are superior to penicillin for treatment of streptococcal tonsillopharyngitis: is the difference worth it? Pediatr Infect Dis J 12: 268–274, 1993.
31. Shulman ST, Gerber MA, Tanz RR, Markowitz M. Streptococcal pharyngitis: The case for penicillin therapy. Pediatr Infect Dis J 13: 1–7, 1994.
32. Krober MS, Weir MR, Themelis NJ, van Hamont JE. Optimal dosing interval for penicillin treatment of streptococcal pharyngitis. Clin Pediatrics 29: 646–648, 1990.

33. Tedesco FJ, Barton RW, Alpers DH. Clindamycin-associated colitis. A prospective study. Ann Intern Med 81: 429–433, 1974.
34. Bartlett J G. Antibiotic-associated diarrhea. Clin Infect Dis 15: 573–581, 1992.
35. Maruyama S, Yoshioka H, Fujita K, Takimoto M, Satake Y. Sensitivity of group A streptococci to antibiotics. Am J Dis Child 133: 1143–1145, 1979.
36. Seppälä H, Nissinen A, Järvinen H, et al. Resistance to erythromycin in group A streptococci. N Engl J Med 326: 292–297, 1992.
37. Schalén C, Stjernquist-Desatnik A, Ekedahl A, Ståhl S. Erythromycin resistance in Streptococcus pyogenes in Sweden. In: Totolinn A, ed. Pathogenic streptococcii present and future. St. Petersburg: Lancer Publication, 68–69, 1994.
38. Dixon J, Lipinski A. Resistance of group A beta-hemolytic streptococci to lincomycin and erythromycin. Antimicrob Agents Chemother 1: 333–339, 1972.

Submitted January 25, 1994; accepted May 15, 1994

Världens bredaste antibiotika-sortiment.

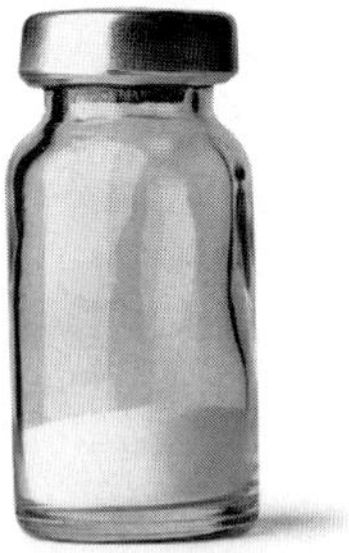

AZACTAM® (AZTREONAM)
MOT BAKTERIER.

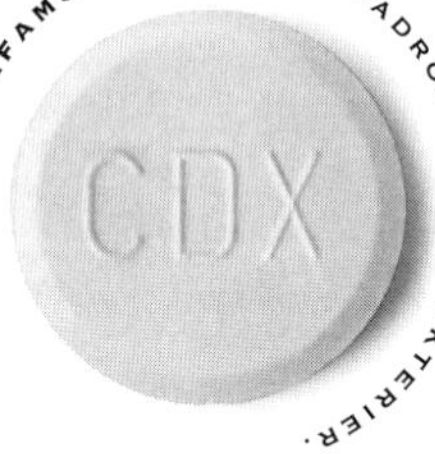

CEFAMOX® LÖSLIG (CEFADROXIL) MOT BAKTERIER.

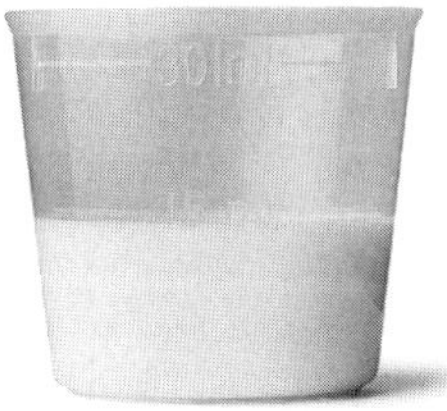

MYCOSTATIN® (NYSTATIN)
SVAMPMEDEL.

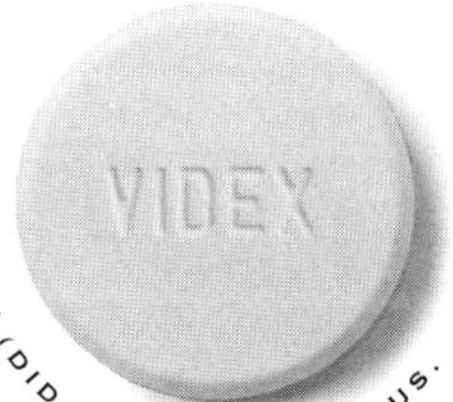

VIDEX® (DIDANOSIN) MOT VIRUS.

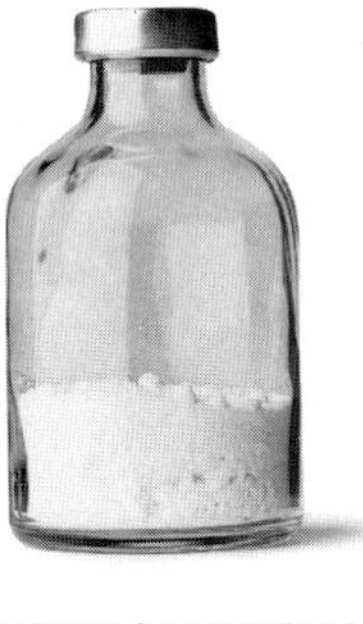

PENTREXYL® (AMPICILLIN)
MOT BAKTERIER

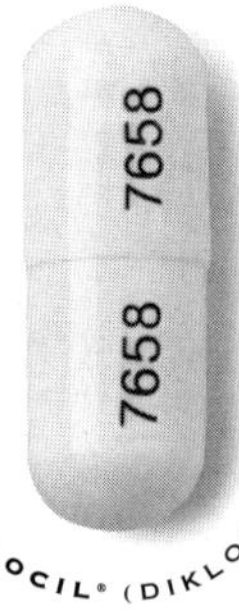

DICLOCIL® (DIKLOXACILLIN) MOT BAKTERIER.

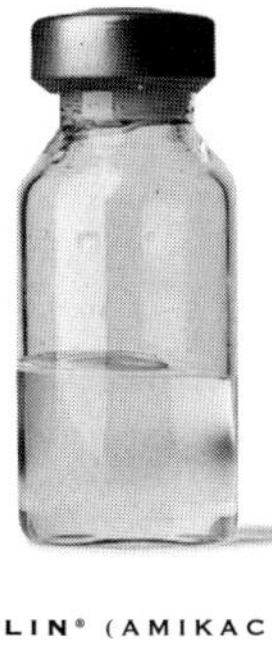

BIKLIN® (AMIKACIN)
MOT BAKTERIER.

AZACTAM (AZTREONAM). ANTIBIOTIKUM AV MONOBACTAM-TYP. INJEKTIONS- OCH INFUSIONSSUBSTANS 1G, 2 G. INDIKATIONER: INFEKTIONER ORSAKADE AV AZTREONAMKÄNSLIGA BAKTERIER, T EX SEPTIKEMI, ÖVRE URINVÄGSINFEKTIONER, KOMPLICERADE NEDRE URINVÄGSINFEKTIONER, NEDRE LUFTVÄGSINFEKTIONER ORSAKADE AV GRAMNEGATIVA BAKTERIER SAMT GONORRÉ. **BIKLIN (AMIKACIN).** BREDSPEKTRUMANTIBIOTIKUM. INJEKTIONSVÄTSKA 250 MG/ML. INDIKATIONER: INFEKTIONER AV ALLVARLIG ELLER LIVSHOTANDE KARAKTÄR SPECIELLT DÅ ETIOLOGIN ÄR OKÄND ELLER GRAMNEGATIV SEPTIKEMI BEFARAS. VID ALLVARLIGA INFEKTIONER AV OKÄND ETIOLOGI BÖR PREPARATET KOMBINERAS MED ETT BETALAKTAMANTIBIOTIKUM I AVVAKTAN PÅ ODLINGS- OCH RESISTENSBESKED. **CEFAMOX (CEFADROXIL).** ANTIBIOTIKUM AV CEFALOSPORINTYP. KAPSLAR 500 MG, TABLETTER 1G, PULVER TILL MIXTUR 100 MG/ML. INDIKATIONER: INFEKTIONER ORSAKADE AV MIKROORGANISMER KÄNSLIGA FÖR CEFADROXIL, EXEMPELVIS NEDRE OCH ÖVRE URINVÄGSINFEKTIONER, HUD- OCH MJUKDELSINFEKTIONER OCH ÄVEN ÖVRE LUFTVÄGSINFEKTIONER SÅSOM STREPTOKOCKTONSILLIT, DÄR PENICILLINBEHANDLING INTE GIVIT ÖNSKAD EFFEKT ELLER ÄR OLÄMPLIG AV ANDRA SKÄL. **DICLOCIL (DIKLOXACILLIN).** PENICILLINASSTABILT PENICILLIN. KAPSLAR 250 MG, 500 MG, PULVER TILL MIXTUR 12,5 MG/ML, INJEKTIONS- OCH INFEKTIONSSUBSTANS 0,5 G, 1 G, 2 G. INDIKATIONER: INFEKTIONER ORSAKADE AV PENICILLINASPRODUCERANDE STAFYLOKOCKER. **FUNGIZONE (AMFOTERICIN B).** ANTIBIOTIKUM MOT GENERALISERAD

Scand J Infect Dis 26: 545–551, 1994

Children with Persistent Cough – Outcome with Treatment and Role of Moraxella catarrhalis?

PETER GOTTFARB[1] and ANNELIE BRAUNER[2]

From the [1]Department of Pediatrics, Sachsska Barnsjukhuset, Dalen Clinic and the [2]Department of Bacteriology, Karolinska Hospital Stockholm, Sweden

52 children with severe cough persisting for more than 10 days were randomized to treatment with amoxycillin/clavulanic acid or placebo in a prospective double-blinded study. Clinically suspected cases of pertussis were excluded, yet 12 (23%) of the children had laboratory verified pertussis infection. The nasopharyngeal colonization showed a predominance of Moraxella catarrhalis which was isolated in 37 (71%) children. Streptococcus pneumoniae and Haemophilus influenzae were isolated in 11 (20%) and 16 (30%) children, respectively. The antibiotic-treated group had a significantly better recovery in both the pediatrician's estimation ($p = 0.02$) and the independent parental judgement ($p = 0.002$). These findings are consistent with the view that Moraxella catarrhalis could be directly involved in the pathogenesis of persistent cough in children.

P. Gottfarb, MD, Sachsska Barnsjukhuset, Dalen Clinic, S-121 87 Enskededalen, Sweden.

INTRODUCTION

The difficulty of establishing an etiological diagnosis in lower respiratory tract infection (LRI) is well known. Ethical and technical reasons limit the use of invasive techniques with which to obtain specimens from the site of infection. Nasopharyngeal samples are widely used for bacterial culture and antigen detection of respiratory viruses in the acute phase of the disease. Serology is, however, still the most useful etiological tool for diagnosing the respiratory viruses, Mycoplasma pneumoniae, Bordetella pertussis, Chlamydia species and Legionella.

To demonstrate an etiological role for common respiratory pathogens such as Streptococcus pneumonia, Haemophilus influenzae and Moraxella catarrhalis, more severe methodological difficulties are involved.

Cultures from the upper respiratory tract show a poor correlation to cultures from lung puncture in pneumonic children (1, 2). A better correlation is found when intra- or transtracheal aspiration is applied; techniques only suited for severely ill children (3, 4).

The value of blood culture is limited by low sensitivity. Methods to detect capsular bacterial antigens in serum or urine for Streptococcus pneumoniae strains and Haemophilus influenzae type b have a somewhat better, but still not defined sensitivity (1, 5).

Not surprisingly therefore, most etiological studies fail to identify the pathogen in about half of the cases (5, 6). However, by using both conventional microbiological and a variety of modern serological methods including bacterial antibody assays and detection of viral and bacterial antigens and nucleic acid, Nohynek et al. (7) were able to demonstrate an etiological agent in 70% of children with acute LRI. They concluded that bacterial infections were common (45%) in young children and previously generally underestimated.

This study dealt with a subgroup of LRI: children with persistent cough (≥ 10 days). Moraxella catarrhalis has been suggested as a possible etiological agent in these children (8, 9).

The aim of the present study was to investigate the nasopharyngeal flora in children with persistent cough and to evaluate the effects of treatment with amoxycillin/clavulanic acid.

Table I. *Points earned in the coughing score system*

No. of coughing attacks/24 h	>20	10 p
	11–20	8 p
	6–10	6 p
	1–5	4 p
	0	0 p
Coughing attacks with vomiting		2 p
Pulmonary auscultation with wheezes or rales		+ 2 p
		Total points

PATIENTS AND METHODS

Patients

Between January 1990 and April 1991, 52 children (7 months–7 years of age) were recruited by two pediatricians (P.G., E.A.) at three out-patient clinics in southern Stockholm. Inclusion criteria were a lower respiratory tract infection with cough for a minimum of 10 days. In order to exclude children with only slight or moderate symptoms, the severity of cough was evaluated according to a coughing score system and only children with 8 points or more were enrolled (Table I). Data were collected regarding allergic diseases and environmental smoking. Exclusion criteria were signs of pneumonia, or acute otitis media, or clinical suspicion of Bordetella pertussis infection.

Following oral parental consent, randomization was performed double-blinded and patients were assigned to treatment with amoxycillin/clavulanic acid (Spektramox®) 20 mg/kg/24 h or placebo for 7 days.

The parents were instructed to register the estimated number of coughing attacks every day during the following 8 days, using the same intervals of coughing attacks as shown in Table I. The parents were also asked to give a written assessment of the efficacy of treatment. The children were not given any antitussive medication.

Bacteriological methods

A nasopharyngeal sample was obtained with a cotton wire swab and transported to the laboratory in modified Stuart medium. Culture and identification of bacteria and disc diffusion testing was performed according to routine laboratory methods. Antimicrobial susceptibility testing was performed against amoxycillin 20 mg + clavulanic acid 10 mg for all Moraxella catarrhalis and Haemophilus influenzae strains. β-lactamase production was tested with nitrocefine.

Bordetella pertussis was cultured aerobically on charcoal-agar plates at 37°C. Agglutination was done with antisera from Difco Laboratories. Blood samples for serology to pertussis and mycoplasma were obtained at the first visit and 2 weeks after start of treatment. The pertussis sera were examined by ELISA and antibody response was determined against pertussis toxin (PT) IgG and IgA, filamentous hemagglutinin (FHA) IgG, IgM, IgA and lipopolysaccharide (LPS) IgG and IgM (10).

Antibodies to mycoplasma were examined on paired sera by complement fixation. A positive test was a four-fold titre increase or antibody level exceeding 40.

A second nasopharyngeal specimen was obtained at the follow-up visit from those children who were willing to cooperate. Due to the long duration of symptoms, no attempt was made at viral detection.

This study was approved by the Medical Ethics Committee at Huddinge Hospital, Stockholm.

Statistical analysis

Wilcoxon 2-sample tests were used for comparison between treatment groups, for coughing scores, clinical outcome and parents' estimation. Significance tests were performed at the 5% level and were two-sided.

RESULTS

The 52 children had a mean duration of coughing attacks of 3–4 weeks. The demographic data were similar in the two groups (Table II). Two children did not return for a follow-up visit but sent in coughing scores and parental assessment by post. One child refused

Table II. *Demographic data of 52 children (30 boys, 22 girls) with persistent cough according to treatment group*

Patients' characteristics	Amoxycillin/clavulanic acid	Placebo
Median age (years)	2.7	2.6
Community child care	70%	73%
Environmental smoking[a]	41%	46%
Heredity for atopic disease	48%	54%
History of asthma/wheezy bronch.	15%	12%
Mean duration of cough (weeks)	3–4	3–4

[a] Including home and indoor-day care.

medication. Four children (3 in the placebo group) deteriorated and received other antibiotics before follow-up had ended.

Treatment response

Treatment efficacy against cough was evaluated at a follow-up visit on days 12–14. The results are shown in Figs. 1 and 2. The pediatrician's assessment, which included an evaluation of both general and respiratory tract symptoms during the last 2 weeks and also broncho-pulmonary status, showed a significant difference between the groups, with better clinical recovery in the antibiotic group ($p = 0.02$). The parents were asked whether treatment was effective against the cough. In their opinion, children in the antibiotic group showed 71% satisfactory recovery compared with 22% in the placebo group ($p = 0.002$). A comparison between parental and doctors' estimations showed an agreement of about 85%. The pediatricians were more reluctant to deem full recovery, compared with the parents.

The improvement during treatment was first seen at the end of the treatment week with reduction of coughing attacks in the antibiotic group by days 7 and 8 compared with the placebo group (Fig. 2).

Loose stools were reported in 6 children; 3 in each treatment group. No other adverse reactions were reported.

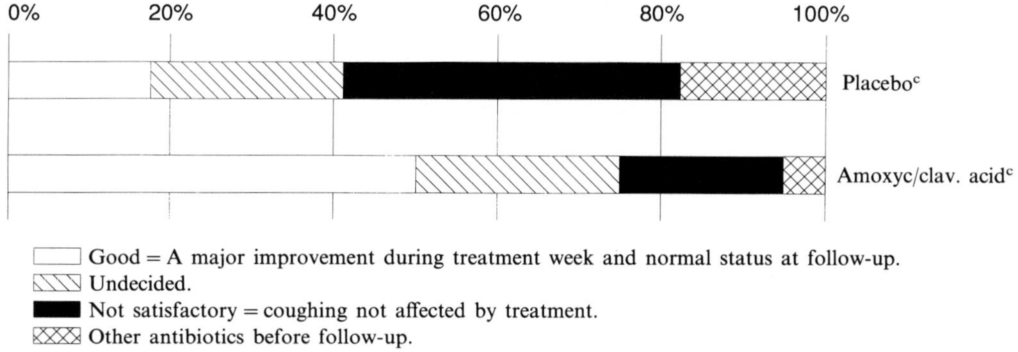

Fig. 1. Clinical outcome according to doctor's estimation[a] at follow-up Days 12–14 in 37 children[b]
[a] Clinical summary of treatment result, considering all relevant symptoms and signs.
[b] Excluded from analysis: 12 children with pertussis. Two children without follow-up visit. One child who refused medication.
[c] $p = 0.023$.

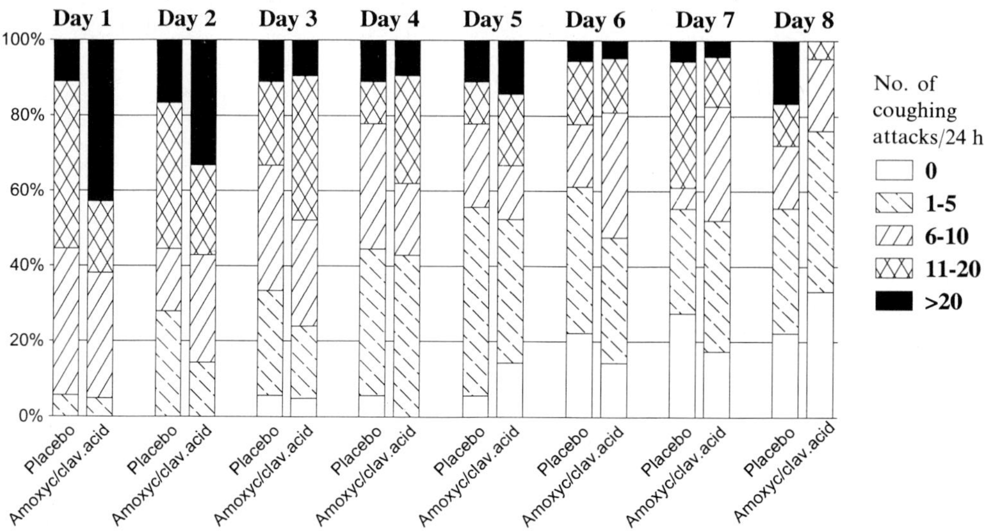

Fig. 2. No. of coughing attacks per 24 h in the amoxycillin/clav. acid and placebo groups according to home records. 39 children were analysed.

Bacteriological outcome

12 children (23%) were excluded from the efficacy analysis due to laboratory-confirmed pertussis; 4 of these children had a positive pertussis culture. One child had a positive culture of Bordetella parapertussis. 10 children had serologically verified pertussis infection. No child had laboratory-verified mycoplasma infection.

The bacterial isolates from the first nasopharyngeal specimen are shown in Table III. Pathogens were recovered from 92% of the children. Cultures revealing a single pathogen or mixed bacterial growth were found in 50% each. The predominant finding in both groups was Moraxella catarrhalis, which colonized about 70% of the children. β-lactamase producing strains constituted 54%. All isolates of Haemophilus influenzae and Moraxella catarrhalis were sensitive to amoxycillin/clavulanic acid. A comparison of treatment results

Table III. *Bacterial pathogens in the nasopharyngeal culture before treatment in 52 children according to antibiotic or placebo treatment*

Species	Amoxycillin/ clavulanic acid ($n = 26$) No. of isolates	Placebo ($n = 26$) No. of isolates	Total no. of isolates[a] (%)	No. of isolates in monoculture
Streptococcus pneumoniae	6	5	11 (21.1)	1
Haemophilus influenzae	6	10	16 (30.8)	6
β-lactamase +	3	–	3	
Moraxella catarrhalis	18	19	37 (71.2)	17
β-lactamase +	10	10	20	
Streptococcus pyogenes	–	2	2 (3.8)	2
Normal flora			2 (3.8)	
No growth			2 (3.8)	

[a] A total of 66 isolates.

between children with positive or negative Moraxella catarrhalis culture was not possible since only 8 children with follow-up data did not have a positive (single or mixed) Moraxella culture.

The nasopharyngeal specimen at the follow-up visit (day 12–14) was obtained from 28/52 children. It showed a lower average colonization in the antibiotic group compared with the placebo group. The mean number of bacterial isolates per child was 0.9 and 1.8 in each of the two groups ($p < 0.01$). Due to many refusals to the taking of a second specimen it was not possible to evaluate the elimination of specific pathogens in the nasopharynx. In the antibiotic group, 6 children had become colonized with β-lactamase-producing strains of Moraxella catarrhalis or Haemophilus influenzae, compared with one child in the placebo group.

DISCUSSION

In view of the methodological obstacles when studying etiology in respiratory infections, we chose to scrutinize the background ecology in terms of nasopharyngeal colonization. Our high colonization rate (92%) is in agreement with other studies performed on pre-school children with or without respiratory symptoms (11–13).

However, our material differs in the predominant isolation of Moraxella catarrhalis which was cultured from 70% of the children, of whom 33% had it as the sole pathogen. By comparison, most studies on pre-school children with acute otitis media or otitis media with effusion show Moraxella catarrhalis nasopharyngeal carrier rates of 30–50% (11, 12, 14). Streptococcus pneumoniae and Haemophilus influenzae have similar carrier rates. Brorson and Malmvall, who also took nasopharyngeal specimens from children with persistent cough, found a corresponding predominance of Moraxella catarrhalis, which was cultured in 66%, compared with 28% in control children without cough (8). Streptococcus pneumoniae and Haemophilus influenzae showed no difference between the groups. In a recent Swedish study with similar inclusion criteria as this study, Moraxella catarrhalis was isolated from the nasopharynx in 75% of the children. Only the elimination of this bacterium after treatment with erythromycin was correlated to clinical recovery (9).

The children in our study received amoxycillin/clavulanic acid or placebo. We found a significant clinical improvement in the antibiotic group, observed in both the parental and pediatrician's estimations. The outcome of treatment suggests that bacterial pathogens contribute to the etiology of persistent cough in children. It is well known, however, that cough is a complex symptom and that other environmental factors such as indoor-climate, smoking exposure and allergens, are of importance. 43% of the children for instance were exposed to smoke (Table II), which can be compared with a Swedish average of 30% daily smokers among middle-aged women (Institute for Tobacco Studies, 1992).

Somewhat surprisingly, we had 12 children with pertussis infection despite our efforts to exclude clinically suspected cases. This reflects the high incidence of pertussis in Sweden. Zachrisson et al. (15) have reported that 50% of non-vaccinated 4-year-old children had antibodies to Bordetella pertussis and that atypical cases were common.

The specific role of Moraxella catarrhalis remains to be defined. Previously regarded as a non-pathogen in the oro-pharyngeal flora, Moraxella catarrhalis has over the last 10–15 years emerged as a significant pathogen in broncho-pulmonary infections among adults and is considered in some areas to be the third most common cause of LRI (16, 17, 18, 4). In children the pathogenic role is most clearly documented in acute otitis media (AOM) (18, 19). Studies from the U.S.A. have reported a Moraxella catarrhalis etiology in 7–20% of AOM cases (18). In Sweden, Kamme found the corresponding figure to be 9% (20).

Leinonen et al. have demonstrated an antibody response to Moraxella catarrhalis in middle-ear and serum in children with AOM (21). Some authors have reported an etiological role in children with maxillary sinuitis (22). There are also a number of case reports on Moraxella catarrhalis pneumonia in hospital-treated children. These cases have compromising factors such as trauma requiring mechanical ventilation, prematurity, broncho-pulmonary dysplasia or neutropenia (23, 24).

Our study shows that Moraxella catarrhalis has a predominant presence in the nasopharynx among children with persistent cough and that clinical improvement results from antibiotic treatment. These circumstances lend support to the theory that Moraxella catarrhalis could be directly involved in the pathogenesis of persistent cough. In an etiological context it should be noted, however, that there was a substantial group with non-diagnosed pertussis infection in which antibiotics is less effective. Despite bacterial involvement, the majority of our children were in good general condition, which makes antibiotic treatment questionable. Nevertheless, there are children with severe cough, sleep disturbance, fretfulness and loss of appetite where treatment is worth consideration. In such cases we think it important not to disregard the pathogenic potential of Moraxella catarrhalis.

ACKNOWLEDGEMENTS

This study owes many thanks to MD Elisabeth Aldea, pediatrician, for collection of data and expert care of the children; Robbyna Svärd, clinical research scientist; Astra Läkemedel, for generous support and helpful discussions; Gunnary Englund, Astra Läkemedel, for statistical analysis; Berit Hallin for skilful preparation of the manuscript.

REFERENCES

1. Silverman M, Stratton D, Diallo A, Egler LJ. Diagnosis of acute bacterial pneumonia in Nigerian children. Arch Dis Child 52: 925–931, 1977.
2. Mimica I, Donoso E, Howard JE, Ledermann GW. Lung puncture in the etiological diagnosis of pneumonia. Am J Dis Child 122: 278–282, 1971.
3. Davidson M, Tempest B, Palmer DL. Bacteriologic diagnosis of acute pneumonia. JAMA 235: 158–163, 1976.
4. Boyle FM, Georghiou PB, Tilse MH, McCormack JG. Branhamella (Moraxella) catarrhalis: Pathogenic significance in respiratory infections. Med J Aust 154: 592–596, 1991.
5. Isaacs D. Problems in determining the etiology of community-acquired childhood pneumonia. Pediatr Infect Dis J 8: 143–148, 1989.
6. Turner RB, Lande AE, Chase P, Hilton N, Weinberg D. Pneumonia in pediatric outpatients: Cause and clinical manifestations. J Pediatr 111: 194–200, 1987.
7. Nohynek H, Eskola J, Laine E, Halonen P, Ruutu P, Saikku P, Kleemola M, Leinonen M. The causes of hospital-treated acute lower respiratory tract infection in children. AJDC 145: 618–622, 1991.
8. Brorson J-E, Malmvall B-E. Branhamella catarrhalis and other bacteria in the nasopharynx of children with longstanding cough. Scand J Infect Dis 13: 111–113, 1981.
9. Darelid J, Löfgren S, Malmvall B-E. Erythromycin treatment is beneficial for longstanding Moraxella catarrhalis associated cough in children. Scand J Infect Dis 25: 323–329, 1993.
10. Sato Y, Cowell JL, Satu H, Burstyn D, Manclark C. Separation and purification of the hemagglutinins from Bordetella pertussis. Infect Immun 41: 313–320, 1983.
11. Prellner K, Christensen P, Hovelius B, Rosén C. Nasopharyngeal carriage of bacteria in otitis-prone and non-otitis-prone children in day-care centres. Acta Otolaryngol (Stockh) 98: 343–350, 1984.
12. Hemlin C. Brauner A, Carenfelt C, Wretlind B. Nasopharyngeal flora in otitis media with effusion. Acta Otolaryngol (Stockh) 111: 556–561, 1991.
13. Vaneechoutte M, Verschraegen G, Claeys G, Weise B, Van d Abeele A. Respiratory tract carrier rates of Moraxella (Branhamella) catarrhalis in adults and children and interpretation of the isolation of M. catarrhalis from sputum. J Clin Microbiol 28: 2674–2680, 1990.

14. Kamme C, Nilsson N-I. Secretory otitis media: Microbiology of the middle ear and the nasopharynx. Scand J Infect Dis 16: 291–296, 1984.
15. Zackrisson G, Taranger J, Trollfořs B. History of whooping cough in nonvaccinated Swedish children, related to serum antibodies to pertussis toxin and filamentous hemagglutinin. J Pediatr 16: 190–4, 1990.
16. Doern GV. Branhamella catarrhalis – An emerging human pathogen. Diagn Microbiol Infect Dis 4: 191–201, 1986.
17. Feleke G, Kahn FA. Branhamella infections. Postgrad Med 85: 379–386, 1989.
18. Vergese A, Berk SL, Guest Editors. Proceedings of a Symposium; Branhamella catarrhalis – A Microbiologic an Clinical Update. Am J Med 88: 1–56, 1990.
19. Bluestone CD. Otitis media and sinusitis in children – Role of Branhamella catarrhalis. Drugs 31 (Suppl 3): 132–141, 1986.
20. Kamme C, Lundgren K. Mårdh P-A. The aetiology of acute otitis media in children. Scand J Infect Dis 3: 217–223, 1971.
21. Leinonen M, Luotonen J, Herva E, Valkonen K, Mäkelä PH. Preliminary serologic evidence for a pathogenic role of Branhamella catarrhalis. J Infect Dis 144: 570–574, 1981.
22. Wald ED, Milmore GJ, Bowen AD, Ledesma-Medina J, Salamon N, Bluestone CD. Acute maxillary sinusitis in children. N Engl J Med 304: 749–754, 1981.
23. Keren G, Bogokowsky B, Barzilay Z. Branhamella catarrhalis pneumonia in non-immunocompromised pediatric patients: Report of three cases and review of the literature. J Med 20: 65–72, 1989.
24. Berg RA, Bartley DL. Pneumonia associated with Branhamella catarrhalis in infants. Pediatr Infect Dis J 6: 569–573, 1987.

Submitted February 2, 1994; accepted June 9, 1994

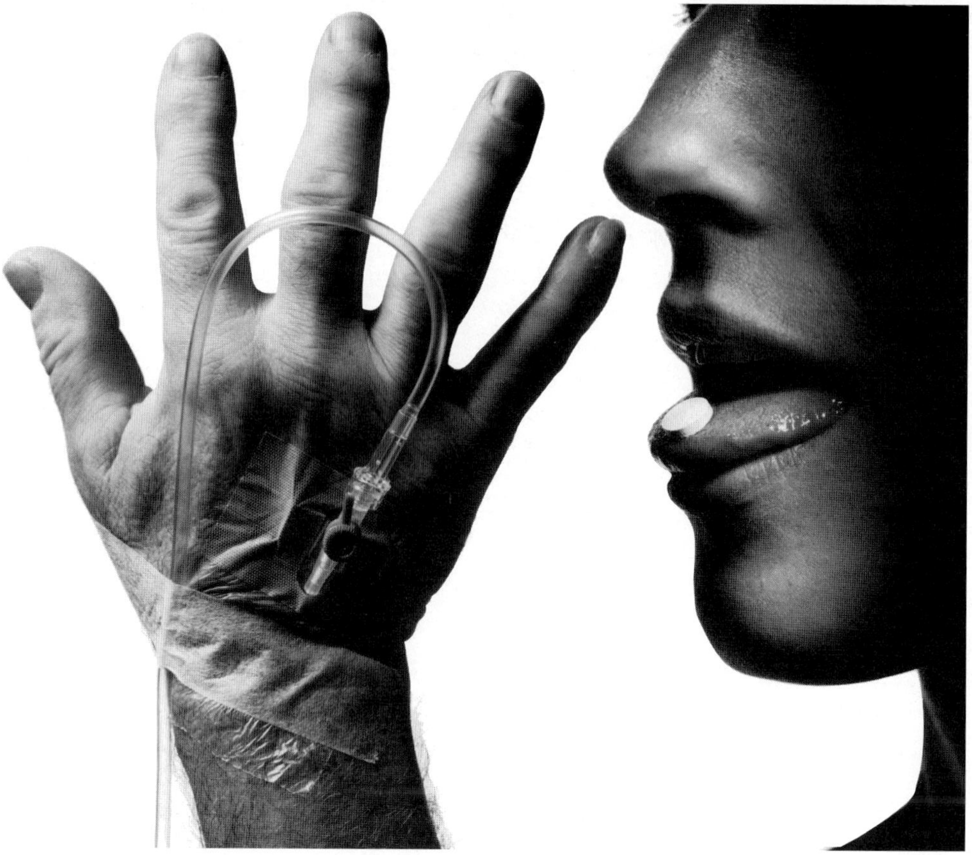
Brunkell & Strömberg

Scand J Infect Dis 26: 553–558, 1994

Significance of Isolation of Moraxella catarrhalis in Routine Cultures from the Respiratory Tract in Adults: Antibody Response Studied in a Whole Cell EIA

INGEGERD JÖNSSON[1], TORD HOLME[2] and AUD KROOK[1]

From the [1]Department of Immunology, Microbiology, Pathology and Infectious Diseases, Karolinska Institute, Huddinge Hospital, Huddinge, and the [2]Microbiology and Tumor Biology Center, Karolinska Institute, Stockholm, Sweden

The significance of the isolation of Moraxella catarrhalis from sputum or nasopharynx was studied in patients treated at an infectious disease clinic. A whole-cell enzyme immunoassay was used to detect a specific antibody response to M. catarrhalis during infection. In all, 27 patients with respiratory tract infections and 4 with other infections were studied. Titre rises were recorded in 11/23 patients with lower respiratory tract infections, whereas patients with common cold or infections elsewhere all had negative serology. In patients with acute bronchitis, 7/10 patients responded with a significant titre rise. Patients with a low titre in their acute serum sample were those who responded with a titre increase during infection. The findings indicate that isolation of M. catarrhalis from sputa and nasopharyngeal samples in adults is of value for the etiological diagnosis of acute bronchitis and other lower respiratory tract infections, and is therefore important for the choice of drug for treatment, as many isolates are resistant to β-lactam antibiotics.

I. Jönsson, MD Department of Immunology, Microbiology, Pathology and Infectious Diseases, Karolinska Institute, Huddinge Hospital I 73, S-141 86 Huddinge, Sweden

INTRODUCTION

Based on isolation of Moraxella catarrhalis from clinical specimens, this species has been increasingly recognized as a cause of bacterial lower respiratory tract infections in adult patients (1–3). However, most reported cases of pneumonia caused by M. catarrhalis are elderly patients having an underlying disease: chronic obstructive pulmonary disease, chronic bronchitis, asthma, cancer, or heart disease (1, 4). In children, most infections caused by M. catarrhalis occur in the upper respiratory tract (2). In most studies, isolation of large numbers of M. catarrhalis from the nasopharynx or sputum has been regarded as a diagnostic sign of etiology. The validity of a positive culture for the bacterium from these samples has been questioned as evidence of its etiological role in an acute infection, since it may be found with varying frequencies in healthy subjects (2, 5, 6). Serological evidence of infection is therefore of great value in frequency studies. Previous studies have indicated a very variable titre rise in paired sera during infection. Differences in the characteristics of the patient materials and in the serological methods used make it difficult to interpret and compare the results of these studies (7–10).

We have earlier studied adult patients with pneumonia and only isolated a small number of M. catarrhalis from these subjects. However, isolation of this species from respiratory tract specimens from adult patients is not uncommon. We therefore performed a prospective study over 29 months that included adult patients admitted to the Dept. of Infectious Diseases and from whom M. catarrhalis was isolated by routine procedures. Clinical findings were recorded and the serum antibody response in paired sera was analysed. The aim of the investigation was to estimate the significance of the isolation of M. catarrhalis in nasopharyngeal samples and sputa from patients with different clinical diagnoses.

MATERIALS AND METHODS

Isolation and diagnosis of bacterial strains

Sputum and nasopharyngeal samples were processed as described earlier (11). Purulent sputa were defined as those having a leukocyte to epithelial cell ratio >5. Identification of M. catarrhalis strains was done according to conventional procedures (11).

Patients and sera

In a prospective study, acute and convalescent sera were collected from patients from whom M. catarrhalis had been isolated in nasopharyngeal (nph) and/or sputum (sp) samples at Roslagstulls Hospital between February 1988 and June 1990. M. catarrhalis was found in samples from 187 patients. The clinical diagnoses were: pneumonia (30%), acute bronchitis (14%), exacerbation of chronic bronchitis (8%), upper respiratory tract infection (32%) and non-respiratory tract infection (16%). Patients from whom acute serum samples were taken within 10 days and convalescent serum samples taken ≥11 days after onset of disease were accepted for the serological study. 14 females and 17 men were included. The median age was 78 years, range 15–96 years. 12 patients had predisposing diseases: 7 had chronic pulmonary disease, 1 diabetes, 1 heart incompensation, 1 diabetes and heart incompensation, 1 malignancy and 1 alcohol abuse. Convalescent sera were collected from the 11th day up to 94 days after onset of disease (Table I).

Table I. *Culture findings and titre rises of sera taken at indicated days after onset of disease*

M.c. = M. catarrhalis, Pne = pneumococci, x = not done, neg = negative, titre rise = convalescent serum titre/acute serum titre. Patients 10, 11, 12, 13, 14, 17 and 22 had chronic pulmonary disease. Patients 1, 8, 19, 25 and 30 had other predisposing diseases.

				Days after onset of disease			
Diagnosis	No.	Nph	Sputum	Serum 1	(titre)	Serum 2	Titre rise
A. Acute bronchitis	1	M.c.	M.c.	10	(780)	94	6,3
	2	M.c.	x	4	(1540)	12	6,1
	3	M.c.	neg	9	(1480)	32	5,8
	4	M.c.	x	10	(1740)	24	3,5
	5	neg	M.c.	6	(2240)	24	1,9
	6	M.c.	x	0	(1230)	33	1,8
	7	M.c.	M.c.	3	(930)	15	1,6
	8	M.c.	x	3	(1150)	28	1,4
	9	M.c.	x	7	(7320)	74	1,1
	10	neg	Pne M.c.	8	(6310)	43	<1,0
B. Exacerbation of chronic bronchitis	11	M.c.	M.c.	6	(1630)	82	3,5
	12	x	M.c.	1	(7100)	11	1,0
	13	M.c.	neg	4	(2590)	48	<1,0
	14	M.c.	x	6	(2390)	31	<1,0
C. Pneumonia	15	M.c.	x	7	(2180)	35	2,7
	16	M.c.	M.c.	8	(750)	16	2,7
	17	Pne M.c.	Pne M.c.	5	(1080)	45	1,9
	18	neg	M.c.	7	(1380)	48	1,3
	19	M.c.	x	10	(1080)	24	1,3
	20	neg	M.c.	2	(7970)	35	1,1
	21	M.c.	x	1	(890)	30	<1,0
	22	M.c.	x	6	(4260)	28	<1,0
	23	Pne M.c.	Pne M.c.	10	(2810)	32	<1,0
D. Common cold	24	M.c.	x	7	(760)	35	1,4
	25	M.c.	x	2	(1760)	32	1,3
	26	M.c.	x	1	(8470)	18	1,1
	27	M.c.	x	7	(800)	23	<1,0
E. No respiratory infection	28	M.c.	x	7	(3420)	40	1,0
	29	M.c.	x	1	(2000)	26	< 1,0
	30	M.c.	x	5	(811)	14	<1,0
	31	M.c.	x	6	(1170)	25	<1,0

Human whole-cell enzyme immunoassay

Microtitre plates (M 129 A, Dynatech laboratories, USA) were coated with whole-cell preparations of the Moraxella catarrhalis strain RS 26 (12). Lyophilized bacteria were washed three times in phosphate-buffered saline (PBS) and suspended in 0.05 M sodium carbonate coating buffer, pH 9.6 (OD 0.01 at 600 nm). Plates were incubated at room temperature overnight, dried and kept in the dark at 4°C for ≤2 weeks before use. Before adding sera the plates were washed four times in saline containing 0.05% (v/v) Tween 20 (saline-T).

Two-fold dilutions of sera (from 1/500 to 1/16000) in PBS with 0.05% Tween 20 (v/v) were added in 100 μl amounts to each well. Plates were incubated at 37°C for 1 h and then rinsed 4 times in saline-T. Alkaline phosphatase conjugated rabbit anti-human immunoglobulin G (DAKO A/S, Copenhagen, Denmark) was used in a dilution of 1 : 750, 100 μl of which was added to each well and incubated for 90 min at 37°C. After another washing procedure, a volume of 100 μl of a 1.0 M diethanolamine substrate buffer, pH 9.8, was added to the wells, and the plates were incubated at room temperature for 40 min. The reaction was stopped by adding 50 μl of 3 M NaOH and the absorbance read at 405 nm in a Titertec Multiscan photometer (Labsystems AB, Stockholm, Sweden). Serum titres were determined at an absorbance of 0.5, where the curves had their steepest fall. In 6 sera, titres were read at 0.3 because the values were low. Acute and convalescent sera from the same patient were run in duplicate on the same microtitre plate. For each set of experiments run on the same day, at least 1 positive and 1 negative human control serum were included. An intra-assay variation <10% was accepted and thus a titre rise of ≥50% could be considered as positive. Since the interassay variation exceeded 10%, one single serum sample could not be compared with the value obtained in a test run on another day. In order to minimize this problem in comparing the levels of the acute sera of different patients, a coefficient, obtained by dividing the titre of the positive control with the median titre of all titre values (read at OD 0.5) of the positive control obtained during the study period (22 values), was used to obtain the acute serum titre recorded in Table I.

RESULTS

M. catarrhalis was isolated from 27 adult patients with symptoms of respiratory tract infections, and in 4 with other diseases (Table I); in 26 from nasopharyngeal swabs and in 11 from sputum samples, of which 8 were purulent. Seven patients had been prescribed antibiotics (5 phenoxymethyl penicillin) prior to admission. In 11/23 patients with symptoms of lower respiratory tract infection and from whom M. catarrhalis was isolated, a ≥50% titre rise was demonstrated in the enzyme immunoassay (Table I). In the patients with acute bronchitis, 7/10 patients responded, and in this group the highest titre rises were noted. The patients with common cold or infections elsewhere had no or only a slight rise in titre (Table I). In 2 patients (nos. 1 and 11) the convalescent sera were obtained after 82 and 94 days, respectively. These patients had the highest titre rises.

The titres of the acute sera are shown in Table I. There was a great variability in titres in these sera. Titres <1,500 were noted in approximately half of the sera in all groups except B (exacerbation of chronic bronchitis). Fig. 1 shows that the highest titre rises were detected among the patients with a low titre in their acute sera.

DISCUSSION

An antibody response to M. catarrhalis was seen only in patients with lower respiratory tract infection. In our study population, consisting of patients with acute bronchitis as well as patients with X-ray verified pneumonia, it was interesting to note that M. catarrhalis seemed to play a more important role in the first group. Acute bronchitis is an infection which has not been exhaustively studied from the etiological point of view, and is usually regarded as being of viral or non-infectious origin (13). Our findings can explain why some of these patients improve upon treatment with tetracycline or erythromycin.

According to other studies, M. catarrhalis is not a frequent cause of pneumonia and should not as a matter of routine be considered as a likely etiology (2, 3, 14). In this study,

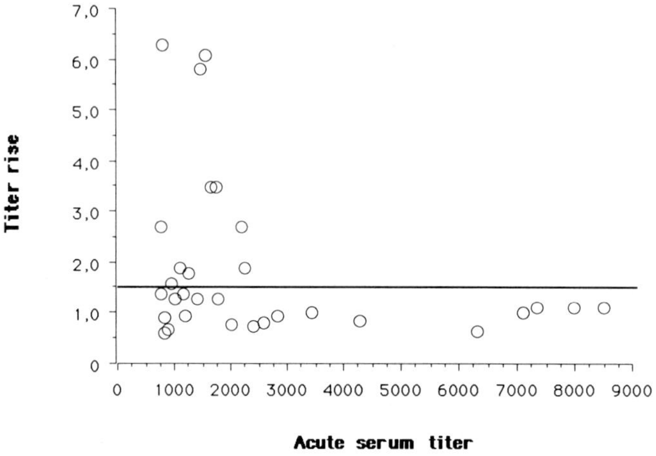

Fig. 1. Titre rise in sera from all patients from whom M. catarrhalis had been isolated, in relation to the titres in the acute sera. The titre rise is defined as the convalescent serum titre acute serum titre. The serum titre is expressed as the reciprocal value of the serum dilution.

M. catarrhalis was isolated in 40 of approximately 1,000 patients with pneumonia, treated at the clinic during the study period. Only 3/9 pneumonia patients included in the serological study had a significant titre rise against M. catarrhalis. In 3 of the remaining patients, high titres were already seen in their acute sera. Thus antibodies to M. catarrhalis do not seem to protect against a new infection. This was also suggested by Chapman et al. who found an IgG-mediated bactericidal effect against M. catarrhalis in acute sera from patients with lower respiratory tract infections (15). Three patients without significant titre rise had low titres in their acute sera. An explanation for this may be that these patients had a pneumonia of unknown etiology and were colonized by M. catarrhalis.

Previous studies of M. catarrhalis serology have been performed on sera from children, with a few exceptions (7, 16, 17). Black & Wilson (9) studied the IgG response to M. catarrhalis in adult patients with acute bronchopulmonary infections by using an immunofluorescence antibody test based on an antigen preparation of 10 different strains. They found, as in this study, higher titres in acute sera of the patients with chronic obstructive pulmonary disease (COPD), compared with patients with other diseases. They also concluded that this must not be taken as an indication that M. catarrhalis is of minor importance in patients with COPD and that in such infections other markers have to be developed to differentiate between colonization and a clinically significant isolation of M. catarrhalis. Black & Wilson also found a titre rise (2–4-fold) in 7/45 patients (25%) (9). Compared with these results, our finding of a significant titre rise in 48% was more satisfactory.

Chi et al. also investigated the antibody response during M. catarrhalis infection in 29 adult patients with different kinds of lower respiratory tract infections (10). They focused on the higher acute serum antibody rate in these patients vis-à-vis healthy controls. In only 17 patients did they have a convalescent serum and in these, 8 (47%) were positive in a M. catarrhalis EIA based on an outer membrane protein antigen.

As can be seen, there is a paucity of studies on M. catarrhalis serology in paired sera from adult patients with lower respiratory tract infection. In the few studies published, the number of patients is limited. One explanation could be the fact that M. catarrhalis is not a common isolate in patients with pneumonia. During the study period, M. catarrhalis was isolated from about 4–5% of the 400–500 patients with community acquired pneumonia treated each year, altogether 20–25 patients annually. Many of these patients were elderly and had underlying diseases. This means that it is difficult to obtain convalescent sera if they have already left the hospital. Furthermore, the problems with their underlying disease may be so severe that one forgets to collect a convalescent serum sample for a study purpose. This means that it is often difficult to obtain representative acute *and* convalescent serum samples from one and the same patient. The lack of a significant titre rise in most patients with pneumonia and exacerbations of chronic bronchitis is probably due to the high titres observed in the acute serum sample. The highest titre rise was seen in 2 patients from whom the convalescent sera were obtained approximately 3 months after the onset of the disease. This may indicate that the antibody rise comes late in some patients. However, in patient no. 2 a high titre rise was seen as early as 12 days after the onset of the disease.

Despite the fact that the number of serological studies is still limited it is now evident that M. catarrhalis is of clinical significance in lower respiratory tract infections. The findings support the view that isolation of M. catarrhalis from sputa and nasopharyngeal samples is of value for the etiological diagnosis of lower respiratory tract infections and thus is important for the choice of drug for treatment, since many isolates are resistant to β-lactam antibiotics (2, 18).

ACKNOWLEDGEMENTS

This study was supported by the Swedish Medical Research Council (Project No 8299), and grants from the Swedish Heart Lung Foundation and the Karolinska Institute.

REFERENCES

1. Slevin N, Aitken JJ, Thornley PE. Clinical and microbiological features of Branhamella catarrhalis bronchopulmonary infections. Lancet 1: 782–783, 1984.
2. Catlin BW. Branhamella catarrhalis: an organism gaining respect as a pathogen. Clin Microbiol Rev 3: 293–320, 1990.
3. Macfarlane JT, Colville A, Guion A, Macfarlane RM, Rose DH. Prospective study of aetiology and outcome of adult lower-respiratory-tract infections in the community. Lancet 341: 511–514, 1993.
4. Doern GV. Branhamella catarrhalis – an emerging human pathogen. Diagn Microbiol Infect Dis 4: 191–201, 1986.
5. Vaneechoutte M, Verschraegen G, Claeys G, Weise B, van den Abeele AM. Respiratory tract carrier rates of Moraxella (Branhamella) catarrhalis in adults and children and interpretation of the isolation of M. catarrhalis from sputum. J Clin Microbiol 28: 2674–2680, 1990.
6. Ejlertsen T. Pharyngeal carriage of Moraxella (Branhamella) catarrhalis in healthy adults. Eur J Clin Microbiol Infect Dis 10: 89, 1991.
7. Leinonen M, Luotonen J, Herva E, Valkonen K, Mäkelä PH. Preliminary serologic evidence for a pathogenic role of Branhamella catarrhalis. J Infect Dis 144: 570–574, 1981.
8. Eliasson I. Serological identification of Branhamella catarrhalis. Serological evidence for infection. Drugs 31 (Suppl 3): 7–10, 1986.
9. Black AJ, Wilson TS. Immunoglobulin G (IgG) serological response to Branhamella catarrhalis in patients with acute bronchopulmonary infections. J Clin Pathol 41: 329–333, 1988.
10. Chi DS, Verghese A, Moore C, Hamati F, Berk SL. Antibody response to P-protein in patients with Branhamella catarrhalis infections. Am J Med 88 (Suppl 5A): 25–27, 1990.
11. Jönsson I, Eriksson B, Krook A, Minimal criteria for identification of Moraxella (Branhamella) catarrhalis. APMIS 98: 954–956, 1990.
12. Jönsson I, Holme T, Krook A, Rahman M, Thorén M. Variability of surface-exposed antigens of different strains of Moraxella catarrhalis. Eur J Clin Microbiol Infect Dis 11: 29–32, 1992.
13. Gwaltney JM Jr. Acute bronchitis. In: Mandell GL, Douglas RG Jr, Bennet JE., eds. Principles and practice of infectious diseases. New York: Churchill Livingstone, 529–531, 1990.
14. Holmberg H, Krook A. Comparison of enzyme-linked immunosorbent assay with coagglutination and latex agglutination for rapid diagnosis of pneumococcal pneumonia by antigen detection in sputa. Eur J Clin Microbiol 5: 282–286, 1986.

15. Chapman AJ Jr, Musher DM, Jonsson S, Clarridge JE, Wallace RJ Jr. Development of bactericidal antibody during Branhamella catarrhalis infection. J Infect Dis 151: 878–882, 1985.
16. Faden H, Hong J, Murphy T. Immune response to outer membrane antigens of Moraxella catarrhalis in children with otitis media. Infect Immun 60: 3824–3829, 1992.
17. Brorson J-E, Axelsson A, Holm SE. Studies on Branhamella catarrhalis (Neisseria catarrhalis) with special reference to maxillary sinusitis. Scand J Infect Dis 8: 151–155, 1976.
18. Olsson-Liljequist B, Burman L, Kallings I and the Swedish Respiratory Tract Study Group. Antibiotic susceptibility of upper respiratory tract pathogens in Sweden: A seven year follow-up study including Loracarbef. Scand J Infect Dis 24: 485–493, 1992.

Submitted March 16, 1994; accepted June 6, 1994

Scand J Infect Dis 26: 559–567, 1994

Long-term Findings in Patients with Facial Palsy and Antibodies against Borrelia burgdorferi

MAGNUS ROBERG[1], PIA FORSBERG[1], ARIL FRYDÉN[1], BENGT HEDERSTEDT[3], DAG HYDÉN[2] and LARS ÖDKVIST[2]

From the Departments of [1]Infectious Diseases and [2]Oto-Rhino-Laryngology, Faculty of Health Sciences, University Hospital, Linköping, and the [3]National Bacteriological Laboratory, Stockholm, Sweden

Little is known about the long-term effects of Borrelia burgdorferi (Bb) infection in untreated patients with peripheral facial palsy. We investigated 12 patients with elevated serum Bb antibody levels, with a median follow-up time of 11 years, during which 3 of the 12 still exhibited intrathecal antibody production of antibodies against Bb flagellar antigen, and 2 of the 3 had normal serum Bb antibodies. Four of the 12 had elevated serum antibody titres at the late follow-up examination. Arthralgia, reported by 7 patients, was the single most common complaint. Four patients showed extensive oculomotor disturbances, which were not correlated to antibody titres or intrathecal antibody synthesis. In 1 of the patients with intrathecal Bb antibody production, most symptoms were eradicated by antibiotic treatment 6 years after the initial infection. We conclude that even several years after a Bb infection, intrathecal Bb antibody production can still occur in serum Bb IgG antibody negative patients with a history of facial palsy.

M. Roberg, MD, Department of Infectious Diseases, Faculty of Health Sciences, University Hospital, S-581 85 Linköping, Sweden

INTRODUCTION

Peripheral facial palsy is the single most common neurological manifestation in neuroborreliosis, occurring in some 30–60% of such patients in Europe (1, 2) and in 11% of unselected Lyme borreliosis patients in the USA (3). In Sweden, 10–20% of cases of idiopathic peripheral facial palsy are reported to be associated with Borrelia burgdorferi (Bb) infection (4–7).

Peripheral facial palsy due to Bb is probably not a homogeneous disease. Peripheral neuritis without evidence of intrathecal Bb antibody synthesis (8, 9) and the Bannwarth syndrome with evidence of intrathecal Bb antibody synthesis have been reported (2, 10, 11). Due to the lack of reliable routine methods for detecting the Bb spirochete, it has been difficult to show a definite correlation between serological findings and neurological symptoms. Cultivation of Bb is time consuming and yield is low, especially when using cerebrospinal fluid (CSF) (12). Moreover, the clinical use of the polymerase chain reaction for detection of Bb DNA in clinical samples is still unreliable (13).

In view of the shortcomings of these procedures, the most dependable method for confirming a Bb infection has thus far been to demonstrate the presence of Bb antibodies.

The Bb antibody response in serum is demonstrably very slow, and initial samples from patients with early manifestations often prove negative (2). The Bb flagellum antigen, on the other hand, provokes an early antibody response and is also more specific than the sonicate antigen (14). In most patients with neuroborreliosis, titres in CSF are usually already elevated when symptoms first appear. However, when using CSF titre values, the effects of an impaired blood-brain barrier (BBB) must be taken into account (11, 15).

In the present study, the natural clinical course was examined in untreated patients exhibiting peripheral facial palsy after initial infection diagnosed by an elevated Bb antibody titre.

MATERIALS AND METHODS

The investigation was approved by the Local Ethics Committee of the University of Linköping.

150 consecutive patients (mean age 43, range 5–89 years; 84 males) who presented with peripheral facial palsy between 1974 and 1983 were eligible. Available sera collected from 74 of these patients (mean age 43, range 5–89 years; 36 males) were analysed for antibodies against Bb.

Patients were regarded as true Bb antibody positive and included in the study if they fulfilled 1 or more of the following criteria: i) an elevated Bb flagellum ELISA titre (see below) in serum at onset; ii) an increasing Bb sonicate ELISA titre in serum (16); iii) an elevated Bb sonicate ELISA CSF titre. By using these criteria, 15 patients (20%) were found to have elevated Bb antibody levels and were offered investigation; 1 of these had died of old age, 1 could not be traced, and 1 declined the investigation. Thus, 12 antibody-positive patients (mean age at onset of disease 39 years, range 9–70 years; 3 males) agreed to a follow-up (Table I).

The remaining 59 of the original 74 'serum-available' patients (mean age 42, range 5–76 years; 32 males) were found to be antibody negative. These 59 were informed of their negative antibody results and were asked to answer a questionnaire and 31 (53%) complied with the request, while the remainder could not be traced or did not reply. The mean age and sex distribution in the seropositive group did not differ significantly from that of the seronegative group.

Initial examination

Each patient was clinically investigated within 1 week of onset of the palsy, and then regularly until the palsy had disappeared, or for a period of 1 year. Serum samples were taken at the start of the investigation and again 3–4 weeks later; all samples were stored at −20°C. A thorough ear, nose and throat (ENT) examination was performed at the same time (17).

Late follow-up examination

The 12 Bb IgG antibody positive patients who agreed to the examination were asked to describe past and present symptoms suggestive of Bb infection. Clinical examination was also carried out, as were routine blood chemistry tests (erythrocyte sedimentation rate, haemoglobin content, white blood cell and differential count, electrolytes, serum creatinine, serum electrophoresis) and electro-cardiography (ECG). Lumbar puncture was performed on all subjects except one who refused.

According to standard procedure in cases of facial palsy, neurological examination was performed, as was testing of the eighth cranial nerve. Standard audiometry and electronystagmography were also carried out.

The 31 Bb IgG antibody negative patients were asked to complete the questionnaire regarding symptoms experienced, as presented to the Bb antibody positive patients. The seronegative patients were not systematically examined or lumbar punctured.

Table I. *Data for the 12 patients positive for Borrelia burgdorferi IgG antibodies*

Patient no.	Age at onset	Duration of follow-up (years)	History of tick bite	Erythema migrans	Concomitant diseases	Oral antibiotics[a]
1	47	11	No	No		Penicillin V
2	66	14	No	No		Penicillin V
3	67	11	No	No	Confusion, diabetes	Doxycycline
4	52	11	Multiple	Yes		None
5	39	11	No	No	Diabetes	Penicillin V
6	9	11	No	No		Penicillin V
7	54	13	No	No	Back pain	None
8	21	15	No	No		Penicillin V
9	25	13	Multiple	Yes		None
10	70	13	No	No	Angina pectoris	None
11	41	6	Yes	Yes		None
12	11	8	Yes	No		Penicillin V

[a] Oral antibiotics given due to other infections during follow-up period.

Bb antibody analysis

The antibody analysis was carried out at the Swedish National Bacteriological Laboratory. Sera from the initial phase and paired serum-CSF from the late follow-up phase were analysed simultaneously for each of the patients. Initially, a Bb sonicate ELISA, described elsewhere (16), was used but when the more specific Bb flagellum ELISA (Dakopatts, Denmark) became available this was preferred. Native flagella from Bb (strain DK-1) are used in the latter technique. Titres above the cut-off (CO) were regarded antibody positive according to the manufacturer's instructions; values below CO were considered negative. The CO level for this ELISA is based on the 98 percentile for 200 blood donors. Titres are expressed as OD $\times$ dilution factor.

CSF analyses

CSF cell counting and albumin, IgG, IgA and IgM determinations were performed. Albumin, IgG and IgA were determined in unconcentrated CSF and serum by an automated immunoprecipitation technique, utilising nephelometric analysis of antigen-antibody complexes in a continuous flow system (Behring nephelometric analyser, Behringwerke, Germany). An albumin ratio reflecting BBB status was calculated as albumin ^{CSF}/albumin ^{serum}; age-dependent reference values, i.e. $<5.7 \times 10^{-3}$ (17–30 years) to $<9.0 \times 10^{-3}$ (>60 years) were used (20). IgG and IgA indices indicating intrathecal Ig production were calculated using the formula Ig ^{CSF} : Ig ^{serum}/albumin ^{CSF} : albumin ^{serum}. IgM was determined in CSF and serum by a modified ELISA (21), and the corresponding IgM index was calculated in analogy with IgG and IgA indices. In our laboratory, the upper normal value for CSF IgG index is 0.7, for IgA index 0.62, and for IgM index, 0.060.

Bb intrathecal antibody production was calculated using a similar formula, i.e. Bb IgG ^{CSF} : Bb IgG ^{serum}/albumin ^{CSF} : albumin ^{serum}. Titre index values >1.0 were considered abnormal (2, 22). Oligoclonal IgG bands obtained by electrophoresis of CSF and serum were analysed by isoelectric focusing on thin-layer polyacrylamide gel (23).

Statistical analyses

Student's 2-tailed *t*-test was used for comparing groups. Fisher's exact test was used for clinical and otoneurological data.

RESULTS

Bb antibody positive patients

The serum Bb IgG titres from initial and late follow-up phases are shown in Fig. 1 and Table II. After a median of 11 years (range 6–15 years), one-third of the initially elevated Bb titres were still positive, although significantly reduced ($P = 0.004$).

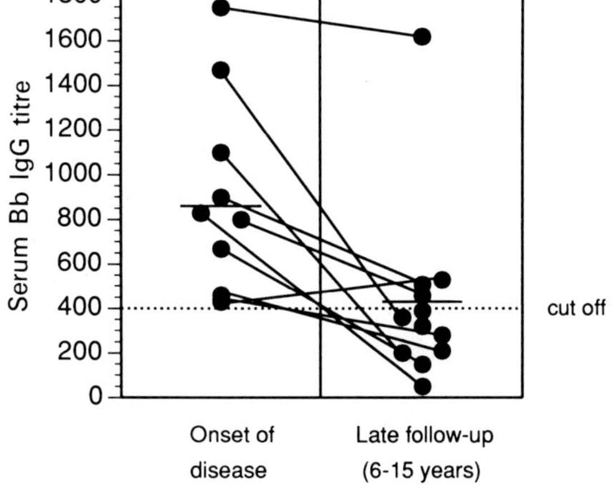

Fig. 1. Acute and late follow-up Bb flagellum IgG titres in serum. Two patients were not analysed with the flagellum ELISA in the acute phase.

Table II. *Acute and late follow-up serum Borrelia burgdorferi antibody titres and CSF antibody index values*

(Normal values are within parentheses).

	Initial Bb antibodies				Late follow-up antibodies	
	Sonicate			Flagellum	Flagellum	
Patient	IgM[a] (<800)	IgG[a] (<500)	IgG[b] (<500)	IgG[a] (<400)	IgG (<400)	CSF Bb index[c] (<1.0)
1	>2000	1210	2200	830	50	0.88
2	–	1250	–	800	460	0.12
3	880	750	1220	900	530	–
4	–	4600	3800	1470	360	1.86
5	–	4000	2800	670	150	0.85
6	–	230	1690	–	320	0.28
7	860	2000	5090	1750	1620	2.74
8	–	1090	–	430	510	0.28
9	–	890	–	460	210	0.23
10	–	550	–	440	280	0.18
11	–[d]	–[d]	–	–	390	3.96
12	–	840	6200	1100	200	0.29

[a] Acute sample.
[b] Early convalescent sample (3–4 weeks after onset).
[c] For explanation, see Methods.
[d] CSF titre: IgM 46, IgG 970.

CSF analyses

There were few pathological CSF findings in the serum-positive patients at the late follow-up. None of the patients displayed CSF pleocytosis. Only 1 patient showed evidence of a disturbed BBB, as indicated by an elevated albumin ratio; for 2 patients, oligoclonal IgG bands were found in CSF (for 1/2 also in serum); and 2 patients had elevated IgM index values.

CSF specific antibodies

Three of the 12 patients (25%) showed evidence of intrathecal Bb IgG antibody production, as indicated by an increased CSF Bb index value (Table II).

Otoneurology and neurophysiology

i) Initial examination. In 11 patients the palsy was unilateral, and in 1 bilateral. At the onset of symptoms, 5/12 patients exhibited total palsy, 5 severe palsy, 1 moderate and 1 slight palsy. All 7 patients with slight to severe palsies recovered completely, i.e. lacked sequelae, within 10 days to 10 months (mean 4.7 months). In 3/5 patients exhibiting total palsies on the initial examination, recovery was incomplete, with slight impairment of muscle activity and sequelae in terms of contractures and synkinesias.

ii) Late follow-up. The examination 6–15 years (median 11 years) after the onset of symptoms confirmed incomplete recovery in the 3 patients exhibiting contractures and synkinesias. One of the patients who had completely recovered from an initial facial palsy presented with another palsy on the contralateral side 3 years later, but she again made a complete recovery.

Audiometry showed no further hearing loss compared with the initial examination except that what could be attributed to ageing (data not shown). One patient experiencing confusion did not participate in any of the tests. None of the patients was completely normal in all otoneurological tests. Compared with our normal data, more than half of the 12 patients had pathological findings in all audiometric tests, except visual suppression during rotation. Four patients had pathological findings in all tests (Table III). No statistically significant correlation was found between the initial antibody titre and pathological otoneurological tests.

Past patient history

Four of the 12 patients could recall a pre-palsy tick bite, whereof 3 could remember an erythema migrans prior to the palsy. None of the patients had received antibiotic treatment in connection with the palsy, but 7/12 individuals had later, for other reasons, received oral antibiotics; 6 had been treated with penicillin V and 1 with oral doxycycline (100 mg daily) (Table I). No patient had received intravenous antibiotics prior to the late follow-up.

Present symptoms

Symptoms reported by the patients are shown in Fig. 2. The most frequent complaint was mild arthralgia (7 cases) though without clinical findings on examination. Three patients complained of impaired memory (nos. 1, 3 and 4) and 2 of disabling vertigo (nos. 3 and 4). Patient no. 7 had pronounced pain in the lumbosacral joints. Two patients complained of cardiac problems (angina pectoris and paroxysmal tachycardia). Altogether, the 12 patients in the seropositive group complained of 34 symptoms (average 2.8 per patient).

Clinical examination

Two patients suffered from an impaired short-term memory, and in 1 of these this was combined with a state of slight confusion. No signs of arthritis or meningitis were observed. None of the subjects produced a pathological ECG despite the fact that 2 of them had a history of cardiac symptoms.

Table III. *Otoneurological findings in 12 patients positive for Borrelia burgdorferi IgG antibodies at late follow-up*

N = normal; P = pathological; n.d. = not done.

Patient no.	Electronystagmogram	Saccadic test	Eye tracking	Visual suppression	CSF Bb index[a]
1	**P**	**P**	N	N	N
2	**P**	**P**	**P**	**P**	N
3	n.d.	n.d.	n.d.	n.d.	n.d.
4	**P**	**P**	**P**	**P**	**P**
5	N	N	**P**	**P**	N
6	N	**P**	N	N	N
7	**P**	N	**P**	N	**P**
8	N	N	P	N	N
9	**P**	**P**	**P**	**P**	N
10	**P**	**P**	**P**	**P**	N
11	**P**	N	N	N	**P**
12	**P**	N	N	N	N

[a] For explanation, see Methods.

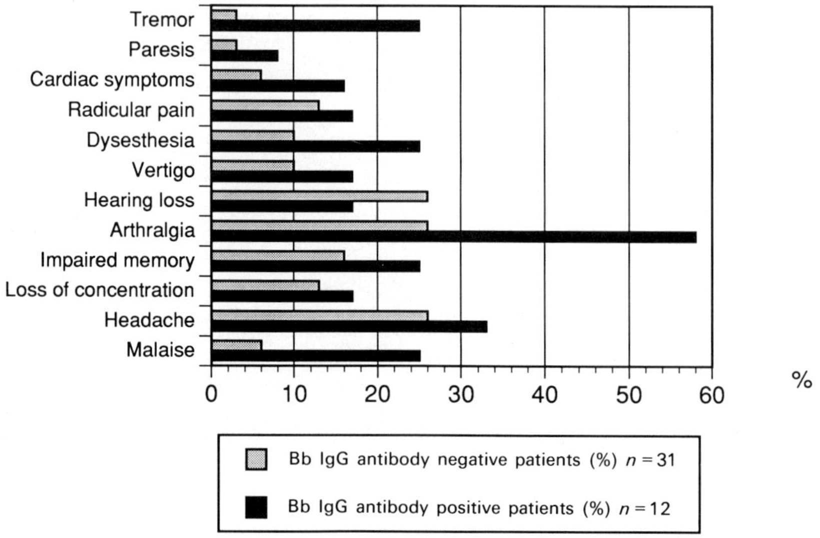

Fig. 2. Proportion of reported symptoms exhibited at late follow-up by patients positive and negative for Bb IgG antibodies.

Bb antibody negative patients

The 31 patients who returned a completed questionnaire complained of 49 symptoms (average 1.6 per patient). The most frequent complaints were moderate hearing loss, arthralgia and headache (Fig. 2).

Treatment

The 3 patients with intrathecal Bb antibody synthesis were given antibiotics, viz. benzyl penicillin 3 g t.i.d. i.v. for 10 days. Patient no. 11 subsequently improved dramatically; more precisely, malaise and symptoms of moderate arthralgia in distal finger-joints, elbows and dorsal pain and dysesthesia on the right side of the face had disappeared completely 14 days after starting treatment. Patient no. 4 had symptoms of presenile dementia and vertigo; the latter disappeared on treatment, but the dementia was essentially unaffected. Back pains felt by patient no. 7 were unaffected, whereas headache and pain on the right side of the face had abated.

DISCUSSION

The proportion of Bb serum antibody positive patients experiencing facial palsy does not seem to have changed over the last two decades, when the present result (20%) is compared with a recent prospective study (16%) (7). It is not likely that this represents a normal seroprevalence in the population in general, because seroprevalence figures of this magnitude have only been reported from high-endemic coastal areas in Sweden (24, 25). In the present patient material, a past or ongoing Bb exposure was indicated retrospectively by performing serum antibody analysis. This was done because a patient's history of tick bites and erythema migrans (EM) is an unreliable indicator of past borrelia infections and the Bb spirochete had not been described at the time of initial patient sampling. It has been reported that in chronic neuroborreliosis as few as 17% of the patients recall a preceding EM (2). A Bb sonicate ELISA was employed at the start of the investigation, but subsequently the flagellum ELISA was used as it is considered to be the most sensitive and specific IgG assay in use. The risk of crossreacting antibodies with common epitopes is also minimized with this fairly specific antigen (14). At late follow-up after a mean of 11 years, 3 of the 12 studied patients (25%) showed signs of intrathecal Bb antibody production and also clinical symptoms of chronic disease. None of these 3 had been given any antibiotics prior to the follow-up. Only 1 of the 3 was Bb antibody positive in serum. Thus, serum Bb antibody determination alone is not sufficient to diagnose an ongoing intrathecal immune response in patients with a past facial palsy. The discrepancy between the CSF Bb index and the serum antibody titre was also observed by Hammers-Berggren et al. (26). Whether or not a positive Bb antibody result represents an active disease cannot be determined on the basis of antibody synthesis alone. In the absence of reliable tests for Bb antigen, pleocytosis and clinical response to antibiotic treatment might be an indication of persistent infection.

Considering the other 9 patients positive for serum Bb antibodies, CSF findings were few and did not indicate immunological activity in the central nervous system (CNS). An explanation for this may be that the patients had recovered and the antibody production had ceased during the long follow-up period. It is also possible that a substantial proportion of the Bb-related facial palsies might have been caused by peripheral neuritis without effects in the CNS. In some cases it cannot be completely excluded that the palsies had no direct connection with the antibody findings (nos. 8–10, Table II). The proportion of subjects with intrathecal Bb synthesis varies from 3% (6) in Bell's palsy patients to 80% in patients with leuko-meningo-radiculitis (Bannwarth's syndrome) (11). This can reflect different disease manifestations but also differences in study populations. Patients investigated at ENT departments tend to exhibit less severe symptoms than those described at neurological departments; the latter cases more often involve clinical symptoms of meningitis and more extensive effects on the CNS. It is impossible to retrospectively verify the extent of the initial effects on the CNS in the present subjects, since only one of our patients underwent lumbar puncture during the acute phase. For this particular patient (no. 11), the follow-up study showed that the albumin ratio, the IgM index and the CSF Bb antibody index were still elevated. Interestingly, this patient improved most dramatically upon antibiotic treatment, indicating a persistent infection despite lack of pleocytosis.

However, in patients with neuroborreliosis Krüger et al. (27) found no or very little effect of antibiotics in 7 patients having sequelae and intrathecal Bb antibody production several years after initial infection. In a follow-up study of neuroborreliosis patients, treated with antibiotics, Hammers-Berggren (26) found that subjects with sequelae often have persistent intrathecal Bb antibody production. Although intrathecal antibody production may not be a suitable indication of active disease, determination of such production might be a useful indicator in patients with associated sequelae. This group of patients could benefit from corticosteroids, as indicated in Krüger's follow-up study (28).

Except for the dementia and confusion experienced by 2 of our subjects, the symptoms described by our patients are vague and could represent other diseases, or normal ageing. The Bb antibody-positive patients had more symptoms than the Bb antibody-negative subjects, although this difference was not statistically significant. Arthralgia was the symptom most often described in the Bb seropositive group; this ailment was less prominent in the seronegative group. Arthralgia was also reported in 2 sero-epidemiological studies conducted in Sweden (24, 25), although at a lower frequency than in our study (13–17% and 58%, respectively). The high arthralgia frequency in our seropositive group should be considered with caution due to the relatively small material.

Even though the number of apparent clinical signs in our study was limited, refined otoneurological analyses disclosed more pathological findings than could be expected from our normal material. Our finding of otoneurological disturbances agrees well with the earlier literature (29, 30). The computerized saccadic test, the tracking eye movement, and visual suppression tests are especially sensitive to disturbances in the central vestibulo-oculomotor pathways (31–33). In view of the neurotropism of the Bb spirochete, it is not surprising that many of our patients exhibited pathological neurological findings, though it cannot be excluded that some of these could have been secondary, i.e. due to other diseases.

We conclude that lumbar puncture can be a worthwhile method for demonstrating a persistent intrathecal antibody production in patients with a past peripheral facial palsy. This is true even when puncture is performed several years after the initial infection and when no serum Bb antibodies have been detected. The pathological significance of this finding calls for further evaluation.

ACKNOWLEDGEMENTS

This investigation was supported by grants from the Swedish Society of Medicine, the Swedish Multiple Sclerosis Foundation and the County Council of Östergötland.

REFERENCES

1. Ackermann R, Horstrup P, Schmidt R. Tick-borne meningopolyneuritis (Garin-Bujadoux-Bannwarth). Yale J Biol Med 57: 485–490, 1984.
2. Stiernstedt G. Tick-borne borrelia infection in Sweden. Scand J Infect Dis Suppl 45: 1–70, 1985.
3. Clark JR, Carlsson RD, Sasaki CT, Pachner AR, Steere AC. Facial palsy in Lyme disease. Laryngoscope 95: 1341–1345, 1985.
4. Olsson I, Engervall K, Åsbrink E, Carlsson-Nordlander B, Hovmark A. Tick-borne Borreliosis and facial palsy. Acta Otolaryngol (Stockh) 105: 100–107, 1988.
5. Bjerkhoel A, Carlsson M, Ohlsson J. Peripheral facial palsy caused by the borrelia spirochete. Acta Otolaryngol (Stockh) 108: 424–430, 1989.
6. Jonsson L, Stiernstedt G, Carlsson J, Strömberg A, Sjöberg O, Larsson A. Serum and cerebrospinal fluid examinations in the diagnosis of Borrelia infection in Bell's palsy. Acta Otolaryngol (Stockh) 110: 421–426, 1990.
7. Roberg M, Ernerudh J, Forsberg P, Fridell E, Frydén A, Hydén D, Linde A, Ödkvist L. Acute peripheral facial palsy: CSF findings and etiology. Acta Neurol Scand 83: 55–60, 1991.
8. Halperin JJ, Luft BJ, Volkman DJ, Dattwyler RJ. Lyme neuroborreliosis-peripheral nervous system manifestations. Brain 113: 1207–1221, 1990.
9. Halperin JJ, Golightly M. Lyme borreliosis in Bell's palsy. Neurology 42: 1268–1270, 1992.
10. Wilske B, Schierz G, Preac-Mursic V, von Busch K, Kühbeck R, Pfister HW, Einhäupl K. Intrathecal production of specific antibodies against Borrelia burgdorferi in patients with lymphocytic meningoradiculitis (Bannwarth's syndrome). J Infect Dis 153: 304–314, 1986.
11. Hofstad H, Matre R, Nyland H, Ulvestad E. Bannwarth's syndrome: serum and CSF IgG antibodies against Borrelia burgdorferi examined by ELISA. Acta Neurol Scand 75: 37–45, 1987.
12. Karlsson M, Hovind-Hougen K, Svennungsson B, Stiernstedt G. Cultivation and characterization of spirochetes from cerebrospinal fluid of patients with Lyme borreliosis. J Clin Microbiol 28: 473–479, 1990.
13. Hansen K. Laboratory diagnostic methods in Lyme borreliosis. Clin Dermatol 11: 407–414, 1993.
14. Hansen K, Hindersson P, Strandberg Pedersen N. Measurement of antibodies to the Borrelia burgdorferi flagellum improves serodiagnosis in Lyme disease. J Clin Microbiol 26: 338–346, 1988.
15. Steere AC, Berardi VP, Weeks KE, Logigan EL, Ackermann R. Evaluation of the intrathecal antibody response to Borrelia burgdorferi as a diagnostic test for Lyme borreliosis. J Infect Dis 161: 1203–1209, 1990.
16. Stiernstedt G, Granström M, Hederstedt B, Sköldenberg B. Diagnosis of spirochetal meningitis by enzyme-linked immunosorbent assay in serum and cerebrospinal fluid. J Clin Microbiol 21: 819–825, 1985.
17. Hydén D, Sandstedt P, Ödkvist LM, Prognosis in Bell's palsy based on symptoms, signs and laboratory data. Acta Otolaryngol (Stockh) 93: 407–414, 1982.
20. Tibblin G, Link H, Öhman S. Principles of albumin and IgG analysis in neurological disorders. Scand J Lab Invest 37: 385–390, 1977.

21. Forsberg P, Henriksson A, Link H, Öhman S, Reference values for CSF-IgM, CSF-IgM/S-IgM ratio and IgM index and its application to patients with multiple sclerosis and aseptic meningoencephalitis. Scand J Clin Lab Invest 44: 7–12, 1984.
22. Stiernstedt G. Svensk medicin. Svenska Läkarsällskapet. 1: 41, 1988 [in Swedish].
23. Olsson T, Kostulas V, Link H. Improved detection of oligoclonal IgG on cerebrospinal fluid by isoelectric focusing in agarose, double-antibody peroxidase labeling and avidin biotin amplification. Clin Chem 30: 1246–1249, 1984.
24. Gustavsson R, Svennungsson B, Gardulf A, Stiernstedt G, Forsgren M. Prevalence of tick-borne encephalitis and Lyme borreliosis in a defined Swedish population. Scand J Infect Dis 22: 297–306, 1990.
25. Berglund J, Eitrem R. Tick-borne borreliosis in the archipelage of southern Sweden. Scand J Infect Dis 25: 67–72, 1993.
26. Hammers-Berggren S, Hansen K, Lebech A-M, Karlsson M. Borrelia burgdorferi-specific intrathecal antibody production in neuroborreliosis. Neurology 43: 169–175, 1993.
27. Krüger H, Kohlhepp W, König S. Follow-up of antibiotically treated and untreated neuroborreliosis. Acta Neurol Scand 82: 59–67, 1990.
28. Krüger H, Reuss K, Pulz M, Rohrbach E, Pflughaupt K-W, Martin R, Mertens HG. Meningoradiculitis and encephalomyelitis due to Borrelia burgdorferi: a follow-up study of 72 patients over 27 years. J Neurol 236: 322–328, 1989.
29. Djupesland G, Degré M, Stien R, Skrede S. Acute peripheral facial palsy. Part of a cranial polyneuropathy? Arch Otolaryngol 103: 641–644, 1977.
30. Sandstedt P, Hydén D, Ödkvist LM. Bell's palsy – part of a polyneuropathy? Acta Neurol Scand 64: 66–73, 1981.
31. Baloh RW, Honrubia V, Sills A. Eye-tracking and optokinetic nystagmus. Results of quantitative testing in patients with well-defined nervous system lesions. Ann Oto Rhinol Laryngol 86: 108, 1977.
32. Hydén D, Larsby B, Ödkvist LM. Visual suppression tests in CNS diagnosis. Adv Otorhinolaryngol 30: 205–209, 1983.
33. Ödkvist LM, Jervall L, Andersson H, Larsby B, Hydén D. A computerized saccade test-clinical value. Proc NES 10: 202–208, 1983.

Submitted January 18, 1994; accepted April 20, 1994

Scand J Infect Dis 26: 569–576, 1994

The Role of Mycobacteria Other Than Tuberculosis (MOTT) in Patients with Cystic Fibrosis

KARSTEN HJELT[1], NIELS HØJLYNG[1], PETER HOWITZ[1], NIELS ILLUM[1], ERIK MUNK[1], NIELS H. VALERIUS[1], KURT FURSTED[2], KAREN N. HANSEN[1], IVAR HELTBERG[1] and CHRISTIAN KOCH[1]

From the [1]Danish Cystic Fibrosis Centre, Department of Paediatrics, Rigshospitalet, University of Copenhagen, and the [2]Department of Mycobacteria, Statens Seruminstitut, Copenhagen, Denmark

The purpose of this study was to estimate the frequency of and evaluate the clinical impact of pulmonary mycobacterial infections among cystic fibrosis (CF) patients. 185 CF patients aged 2.2–38.5 years were screened by sputum samples and by intracutaneous skin tests against tuberculin and sensitins produced from Mycobacterium chelonae subsp. abscessus, M. avium, M. intracellulare and M. scrofulaceum (the MAIS complex). The skin tests towards the sensitins in BCG-vaccinated patients ($n = 60$) were significantly influenced by the vaccination. 26 of the remaining 125 non-vaccinated patients had ≥ 1 positive skin test (95% confidence limits 15–29%). The majority reacted against the MAIS complex. However, the reactions were similar to those of healthy siblings and an age-matched control group. Moreover, the lung function, growth and HbA1c were similar among skin test positive and negative patients. Three patients had repeated positive sputum cultures, the point prevalence being 1.6% (M. intracellulare, $n = 2$ and M. chelonae subsp. abscessus, $n = 1$). During the subsequent 4 years, 4 additional patients with M. chelonae subsp. abscessus were identified. Based on clinical observations, 5 of the infected patients were considered asymptomatic, while 2 might have been symptomatic. In 1 patient, M. chelonae subsp. abscessus disappeared spontaneously. Despite intensive treatment with new antibiotics against Mycobacteria Other Than Tuberculosis (MOTT) in 4 patients, the mycobacteria were not eradicated. In conclusion, MOTT infection was rare and the clinical impact difficult to prove. Treatment should focus on clinical improvement in the individual patient suspected of suffering from significant symptomatic infection. Eradication of the bacteria should not be expected.

C. Koch, MD, Danish Cystic Fibrosis Centre, Department of Paediatrics, Rigshospitalet, DK-2100 Copenhagen, Denmark

INTRODUCTION

In the past decade an increase in the frequency of lung infections with Mycobacteria Other Than Tuberculosis (MOTT) has been observed among patients without as well as with predisposing diseases such as chronic lung disease, diabetes mellitus and treatment with steroids (1). Moreover, the clinical signs of MOTT infection may be difficult to distinguish from pulmonary infections by other microorganisms in cystic fibrosis (CF) patients (2, 3).

These observations prompted us to perform a screening study in our CF patients of the prevalence of mycobacteria in sputum and the status of skin test reactions to tuberculin and MOTT (i.e. sensitins). Moreover, sputum-positive patients were followed clinically including repeated cultures for 3–4 years, during which period our CF patients were investigated for pulmonary mycobacteria infections on the slightest clinical suspicion.

MATERIAL AND METHODS

Patients

All patients ≥ 2 years of age attending the Danish Cystic Fibrosis Centre were invited to participate in a cross-sectional screening investigation with skin test reactions and sputum analysis for mycobacteria

 ISSN 0036-5548

from 1987 to 1988. During the succeeding years the mycobacteria-positive patients were followed up and, based on clinical suspicion, other CF patients were examined for mycobacteria in sputum.

Control groups

44 healthy siblings of 38 CF patients and 100 normal, non-BCG vaccinated schoolchildren aged 7–15 years served as controls (4).

Skin tests

Intracutaneous tests (Mantoux) were carried out simultaneously with 1 unit of PPD-tuberculin (0.1 ml) and 5 units (0.1 ml) of four different sensitins produced from M. chelonae subsp. abscessus, M. avium, M. intracellulare and M. scrofulaceum (Statens Seruminstitut, Copenhagen). These four sensitins represent the most commonly isolated MOTT in Denmark (Tuberculosis Department, Statens Seruminstitut, personal communication). The skin tests were read at 72 h and expressed in mm of the largest diameter of the induration. The skin tests were performed and read by the authors.

Definitions of positive and significant skin reactions

Any induration ≥ 1 mm was considered positive. Indurations with a diameter ≥ 6 mm were defined as significant reactions (5). A primary skin reaction was defined as the largest significant skin reaction in a patient. Hence, a primary reaction could not be identified in case of equal size of ≥ 2 of the largest reactions.

Sputum analyses

Three consecutive samples of sputum were obtained on different days over a period of 3 months. Sputa were either delivered by the patients themselves or obtained by laryngeal suction as appropriate. Smears were examined after being stained with auramine-rhodamine. Sputum samples were decontaminated with a mixture of 4% oxalic acid and 5% N-acetyl-cysteine and cultured on Løwenstein-Jensen (LJ) medium. Mycobacterial isolates were identified either by a nucleic-acid hybridization kit (Gen Probe Inc, San Diego, USA) (6) or by standard biochemical tests (7). Susceptibility testing of slow-growing mycobacteria were determined on either LJ by the resistance ratio method (8) or by using the radiometric method on Bactec (9). Drug susceptibility testing of rapidly growing mycobacteria was determined using the agar disc diffusion method (10).

Lung function tests

Our patients made monthly visits to the out-patient clinic. At each visit, lung function tests were performed in patients >6 years using an electronic spirometer (Spirotron®, Dräger). Forced vital capacity (FVC) and forced expiratory volume in the first second (FEV_1) were recorded and expressed as means of the 12 values obtained during 1 year. These results were expressed as percentages of normal values for sex and height (11, 12).

Height and weight

Height and weight were transformed into percentage of the 50th percentile values for age and sex according to Danish growth charts (13).

Statistics and ethics

Non-parametric statistics were used. The statistics included median and range, Mann-Whitney test, χ^2 and Spearman's test. $p < 0.05$ (two-sided) was chosen as the level of significance. The children and their parents were provided with oral and written information, and informed consent was obtained from children >7 years of age and from all parents with children ≤ 18 years. The study was approved by the Scientific Ethical Committee of Copenhagen.

RESULTS

The screening investigation

185 (99 boys) out of 192 CF patients >2 years participated. Their ages ranged between 2.2 and 38.5 yrs (mean 15.3). None of the patients had been in contact with people with recognized tuberculosis or infection with MOTT.

Skin test reactions

The skin test results are shown in Table I. The BCG-vaccinated patients showed a significantly higher frequency of positive tests than those not vaccinated. Moreover, the profiles of the positive and significant skin tests were different in the two groups, e.g. in contrast to the BCG-vaccinated patients, the non-vaccinated group showed a higher frequency of positive reactions towards the MAIS complex than for tuberculin (positive reactions: $p < 0.003$ and significant reactions $p < 0.03$).

Skin reactions in CF patients and their healthy siblings

44 healthy siblings of 38 patients volunteered to be tested with tuberculin and the four sensitins. The frequencies of BCG vaccination were similar in the two groups and so were the frequencies of positive (36 vs. 30%) and significant skin reactions (23 vs. 30%).

Skin test reactions in CF patients and in normal children

6/56 unvaccinated patients (11%) aged 7–15 years showed ≥1 significant tests. This corresponded to the 15% positive children in the control group (4).

Relationship between pulmonary infection with P. aeruginosa and positive skin reactions

94 unvaccinated patients (75%) suffered from pulmonary infections with Pseudomonas aeruginosa. All patients but one with positive skin reactions ($n = 25$) and all patients with significant skin tests ($n = 16$) belonged to the group with P. aeruginosa infection ($p < 0.02$ and $p < 0.04$, respectively). The age of those with P. aeruginosa infection and positive skin

Table I. *Skin test reactions against tuberculin and sensitins derived from different MOTT in CF patients with and without BCG vaccination*

	(A) No BCG vaccination ($n = 125$)			(B) BCG vaccination ($n = 60$)		
	≥1 mm	≥6 mm	Primary[b] reaction	≥1 mm	≥6 mm	Primary[b] reaction
Induration[a]	n(%)[c]	n(%)[d]	n(%)	n(%)[c]	n(%)[d]	n(%)
Tuberculin	6(5)	4(3)	2(2)[e]	36(60)	29(48)	10(15)[e]
M. chelonae subsp. abscessus	6(5)	4(3)	1(1)	19(32)	14(23)	2(3)
M. scrofulaceum	20(16)	11(9)	7(6)	31(52)	24(40)	7(12)
M. intracellulare	13(10)	8(6)	2(1)	30(50)	24(40)	0(0)
M. avium	12(10)	8(6)	2(2)[f]	39(65)	32(53)	12(20)[f]
MAIS complex[g]	22(18)	14(11)	13(10)[h]	40(67)	34(57)	22(37)[h]

[a] Largest diameter of induration.
[b] The primary reaction is the largest significant skin reaction, i.e. skin induration ≥6 mm. A primary reaction could not be identified in cases where two or more of the largest reactions were of equal size.
[c, d] The frequencies of positive reactions (≥1 mm) and of significant reactions (≥6 mm) of tuberculin and the 4 sensitins were significantly lower in group A than in group B ($p < 0.0001$).
[e, f, h] The frequencies of primary reactions were significantly lower in group A than in group B (tuberculin: $p < 0.001$, M. avium and MAIS complex: $p < 0.0001$).
[g] MAIS complex: M. avium, M. intracellulare, M. scrofulaceum. The figures describe the frequencies of the different reactions towards one of more of these sensitins. A primary reaction was ascribed to the complex if one or more of these reactions were larger than those of tuberculin or M. chelonae subsp. abscessus.

Table II. *Clinical and microbiological data of patients with repeated mycobacteria positive sputum samples*

Patient	Age (yrs)	Mycobacterium spp.	Microscopy no. pos. total no.	Culture no. pos./ total no.	Follow-up (mo)	Pseudomonas[a]	Other microorg.	Chest X-ray[b]	Susceptibility[c, d] to antibiotics	Type and duration[c] of treatment	Side effects
LSP	10	M. chelonae subsp. abscessus	1/11	10/11	17	Intermittent	S. aureus	Stable. Little fibrosis			
TN[e]	29	M. intracellulare	5/11	9/11	48	Intermittent	S. aureus	Stable. Emphysema			
KS[e]	7	M. intracellulare	12/50	35/50	60	Intermittent	S. aureus	Stable. Bronchiectasia of left lower lobe.	I, E, Cl, RE synergism	0–9 mo: IEP + R or An 9–21 mo: RIEP + Cl	Adverse reaction to Ansamycin
ATJ	7	M. chelonae subsp. abscessus	6/30	29/30	36	None	S. aureus	Small infiltrations of lower lobes. Increased interstitial density. Slight fibrosis of upper lobes	period 1: A, Er period 2: A, Im, Ro	period 1: 0–5 mo: RIE, 3–5 mo: +Er period 2: 20–32 mo: RIE + Er or Ro 1 mo: i.v.A and 1 mo i.v.A + Im	None
CG	17	M. chelonae subsp. abscessus	6/19	18/19	32	Intermittent	S. aureus Aspergillus	Moderate bilateral fibrosis. Infiltrate of left upper lobe.	Period 2: resistance to A after 1 mo of treatment	period 1: 0–9 mo: RIE + 2 mo i.v.A period 2: 16–26 mo: RIE + 1 mo i.v.A +8 mo Er	None
TME	19	M. chelonae subsp. abscessus	30/55	52/55	36	Chronic	Aspergillus	Stable. Moderate bilateral fibrosis.	Before treatment: A, Ce. After: multiresistance	0–2 1/2 mo: RIE the last mo: i.v.A + Ce	None
MKA[e]	21	M. chelonae subsp. abscessus	40	13/40	36	Chronic	S. aureus	Stable. Moderate to severe fibrosis Emphysema.	Before treatment A, Ce	0–1 mo: i.v.A + Ce 1–2 mo: RIE + Cl + i.v.A. 2–3 mo: Cl	Cefoxitin caused Drug fever

[a] P. aeruginosa infection was described as chronic if the bacteria were found regularly for more than 6 months in sputum. If it was only found now and then the infection was considered intermittent.

[b] The chest X-ray description refers to the status when the mycobacteria was found. Stable chest X-ray means unchanged or only minor changes at least the previous 2 years and the follow-up period.

[c] Abbreviations: A: Amikacin, An: Ansamycin, Ce: Cefoxitin, Cl: Clofazimin, E. Ethambutol, Er: Erythromycin, Im: Imipenem, I: Isoniazid, P: Pyrazinamid, R: Rifampicin, Ro: Roxithromycin.

[d] Only the antibiotics against which sensitivity was found are listed.

[e] Patients detected by screening. The detection of the other patients was based on clinical suspicion.

tests (mean 15.6 yrs, range 6.6–29.6) was not significantly higher than the age of those with negative skin tests (mean 13.8 yrs, range 3.8–30.8).

Skin tests, lung function tests, growth and HbA1c

No differences were found between the skin test positive ($n = 26$) and the skin test negative patients ($n = 99$).

Patients with only one mycobacteria-positive sputum sample

6 patients (age 7–32 years) had mycobacteria identified only once in sputum. In the following 1–2 years, 6–20 sputum samples from these patients all proved negative. The culture results were: M. gordonae, $n = 4$ (≤ 10 CFU), M. fortuitum, $n = 1$, (< 50 CFU) and M. intracellulare, $n = 1$ (≤ 10 CFU). All samples were negative at microscopy.

Patients with repeated mycobacteria-positive sputum samples

Clinical and microbiological details are given in Table II. Three patients were diagnosed by the screening giving a point prevalence of 1.6% (95% confidence limits 0.3–5%). During the follow-up, 4 more patients were identified.

Antimycobacterial treatment. Background

Five patients were treated with antimycobacterial drugs (Table II). The basis of the treatment was the traditional antituberculosis drugs, i.e. rifampicin, isoniazide and ethambutol. These drugs were supplemented with oral erythromycin ($n = 2$) or clofazimine ($n = 2$). Four patients received an additional 1–2 months of i.v. amikacin, cefoxitin or imipenem. The treatment regime varied according to susceptibility, side effects and the patients' endurance.

Outcome. Persistence of mycobacteria

Two patients demonstrated disappearance of the mycobacteria after 9 months (MKA) and 3 years (TN), respectively. In both cases the disappearance seemed to be spontaneous. In the remaining 5 patients, mycobacteria persisted despite treatment of 4 patients.

Outcome. Clinical status

Data for FEV_1 starting 3–4 years before the diagnosis of mycobacteria and up to 5 years follow-up are shown in Fig. 1. The condition of patients KS, TME and MKA was stable and did not seem to be influenced by MOTT (Table II, Fig. 1). The antimycobacterial treatment of CG and ATJ seemed to have a positive impact on the clinical condition, with reduced sputum production and an increased sense of well-being. The X-ray improved as well. However, simultaneously the patients received treatment for infections with P. aeruginosa and pulmonary aspergillosis (CG) plus Staphylococcus aureus (CG and ATJ).

DISCUSSION

In order to evaluate the frequency and clinical impact of MOTT in CF patients, we included skin tests as a diagnostic tool. We assumed that a positive skin reaction in non-BCG vaccinated patients was due to a previous or current infection with the corresponding organism (5, 14) reflecting a specific T-cell mediated immune response (15). Previous studies have included vaccinated patients (16, 17). This seems inappropriate as we found that not only were skin reactions to tuberculin influenced by the vaccination, but so too were the reactions to the sensitins.

When the skin reactions of the non-vaccinated CF patients were compared with healthy age-matched unvaccinated children, no differences were found. Moreover, the clinical status

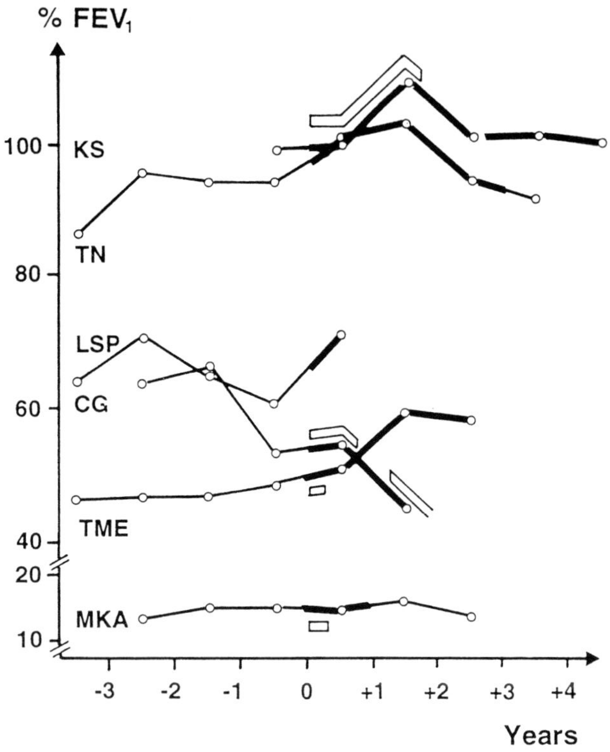

Fig. 1. The forced expiratory volume in one second as a % of standard for age and sex (%FEV_1) during 3–5 years before and after detection of MOTT in the sputum. Each circle depicts a mean value for monthly measurements obtained during one year and is placed in the middle of that year. The closed thick lines illustrate existence of MOTT in the sputum. The open bars parallel to the thick lines depict the period of antimycobacterial treatment. (One patient, aged 7 years (ATJ), was unable to perform the lung test.)

of non-vaccinated skin test positive CF patients did not differ from that of patients with negative reactions. Therefore, based on skin reactions alone, cystic fibrosis neither seemed to be a predisposing condition for infection with MOTT, nor did this infection have any clinical impact on these patients. On the other hand, we found a higher frequency of skin reactions in CF patients infected with P. aeruginosa when compared with those uninfected by this organism. P. aeruginosa is known to cause damage to lung tissue in CF patients (18) and might therefore precipitate MOTT infection.

The frequency of significant skin reactions (tuberculin and sensitins) among our vaccinated CF patients seemed to be somewhat higher than those reported by others (16, 17) but in accordance with the vaccinated control groups of these studies. Therefore, we find it unlikely that the cell-mediated immune responses towards mycobacteria in our CF patients were reduced. This is in agreement with Schiøtz (19) who found a normal immune response capacity in CF patients.

The profile of skin reactions could be influenced by the members of the patients' families (4). Therefore, the patients were compared not only with a national reference material but also with healthy siblings. No differences were found.

The prevalence of patients with persistent mycobacteria was low (1.6%). Four more patients were found during the subsequent years but the overall frequency seemed to be somewhat lower than that reported by Hjelte et al. (16). Moreover, the profile was quite different in the 2 studies, since we found M. chelonae subsp. abscessus in 5 of our patients, whereas they found none.

One patient with M. intracellulare was treated according to recent recommendations (3, 20), but the microorganism could not be eradicated. On the other hand, the patient did well despite this. Another patient demonstrated spontaneous disappearance of this bacteria.

However, M. intracellulare may lead to severe disease in CF patients as demonstrated by the case report by Kinney et al. (21). The 3 patients infected with M. avium-intracellulare in the study by Hjelte et al. (16) were reported to improve on traditional antituberculous treatment. However, neither the duration of the treatment nor the impact on the microorganism was reported.

M. chelonae subsp. abscessus disappeared spontaneously in one of our patients. However, it was not possible to eradicate the bacteria in any of the other 4 patients despite multidrug treatment, including newer antimycobacterial drugs given according to resistance pattern. Moreover, multiresistance was observed in 2 patients and development of cefoxitin and amikacin resistance was found in 1 and 2 patients, respectively. Others have also reported difficulty with eradication of M. chelonae subsp. abscessus in CF patients (22, 23) and in other patients with non-pulmonary infection (24).

The distinction between symptomatic and asymptomatic infection with MOTT (21) in CF patients with persistent positive sputum samples is difficult, as chest X-ray infiltrates may often be caused by other well-known pathogenic microorganisms in these patients. Moreover, the typical chest X-ray of pulmonary infection with M. chelonae subsp. abscessus shows a reticulonodular picture (3) which is not unusual in CF patients, especially those infected by P. aeruginosa. Wallace et al. (3) suggested that bronchial washing or even lung biopsy may be used for diagnostic purposes. However, these are invasive procedures that we find could be justified only if they lead to significant therapeutic advantages.

The significance of MOTT in CF patients has not yet been firmly established. However, in the individual patient this organism may certainly be of significance as ultimately shown by pathological studies in fatal or transplanted cases (21, 22). In order to ascertain whether an individual patient has symptomatic or asymptomatic infection, it is important to monitor closely the clinical, microbiological and radiological status prospectively. Moreover, a screening with sensitins in unvaccinated patients may be helpful later in order to demonstrate conversion in skin reactions.

Although the experience with treatment of CF patients infected with MOTT is very limited, we find it justified to treat those suspected of having significant symptoms. The aim of treatment should be clinical improvement, but eradication of the bacteria should not be expected.

ACKNOWLEDGEMENTS

This work has been supported by a grant from the National Society for Pulmonary Research. The authors thank the nurses and secretaries at the Danish Cystic Fibrosis Centre for being very helpful in the practical management of this project. Special thanks are given to the head nurse Anne Lise Hansen. Mogens Magnusson (Statens Seruminstitut) kindly provided the sensitins and has been very helpful in sharing with the authors his extensive knowledge regarding sensitins and the cutaneous reactions.

REFERENCES

1. Iseman MD. Mycobacterium avium complex and the normal host. The other side of the coin. N Engl Med J 321: 896–898, 1989.
2. Prince DS, Peterson DD, Steiner RM, Gottlieb JE, Scott R, Israel HL, Figueroa WG, Fish JE. Infection with Mycobacterium avium complex in patients without predisposing conditions. N Engl J Med 321: 863–868, 1989.
3. Wallace RJ, O'Brien R, Glassroth J, Raleigh J, Dutt A. Diagnosis and treatment of disease caused by nontuberculous mycobacteria. Am Rev Respir Dis 142: 940–953, 1990.
4. Hansen KN, Heltberg I, Hjelt K. Sensitivity to tuberculin and sensitins from atypical mycobacteria (M. chelonae subsp. abscessus, M. avium, M. intracellulare, M. scrofulaceum) in 100 Danish school children. Dan Med Bull 36: 399–401, 1989.

5. Engbæk HC, Vergman B, Bentzon MW. A prospective study of lung disease caused by Mycobacterium avium/Mycobacterium intracellulare. Eur J Respir Dis 65: 411–418, 1984.
6. Drake TA, Hindler JA, Berlin OGW, Brukner DA. Rapid identification of M. avium complex in culture using DNA probes. J Clin Microbiol 25: 1442–1445, 1987.
7. Wayne LG. The atypical mycobacteria: Recognition and disease association. Crit Rev Microbiol 12: 185–222, 1985.
8. Canetti G, Froman S, Grosset J, Hauduroy P, Langerova M, Mahler HT, Meissner G, Mitchison DA, Sula L. Mycobacteria: laboratory methods for testing drug sensitivity and resistance. Bull World Health Organ 29: 565–5678, 1963.
9. Siddiqi SH, Hawkins JE, Middlebrook G. Evaluation of a rapid radiometric method for drug susceptibility testing of Mycobacterium tuberculosis. J Clin Microbiol 13: 908–912, 1981.
10. Welch DF, Kelly MT. Antimicrobial susceptibility testing of Mycobacterium fortuitum complex. Antimicrob Agents Chemother 15: 754–757, 1979.
11. Polgar G, Promadhat V. Pulmonary function testing in children: techniques and standards. Philadelphia: Saunders, 1971.
12. Quanjer Ph H. Standardized lung function testing. Report of working party on "Standardization of lung function tests", European Community for Coal and Steel. Bull Eur Physiopathol Respir 19 (suppl 5): 1–95, 1983.
13. Andersen E, Hutchings B, Jansen J, Nyholm M. Heights and weights of Danish children. Ugeskr Læger 144: 1760–1765, 1982.
14. Del Beccaro MA, Mendelman PM, Nolan C. Diagnostic usefulness of mycobacterial skin test antigens in childhood lymphadenitis. Pediatr Infect Dis J 8: 206–210, 1989.
15. Hasløv K, Heron I. The generation of guinea pig T-cell lines reactive to antigens from Mycobacterium tuberculosis. Selected lines induce erythematous skin reactions. Scand J Immunol 29: 281–288, 1989.
16. Hjelte L, Petrini B, Källenius G, Strandvik B. Prospective study of mycobacterial infections in patients with cystic fibrosis. Thorax 45: 397–400, 1990.
17. Mulherin D, Coffey MJ, Halloran DO, Keogan MT, FitzGerald MX. Skin reactivity to atypical mycobacteria in cystic fibrosis. Respir Med 84: 273–276, 1990.
18. Høiby N, Friis B, Jensen K, Koch C, Møller NE, Støvring S, Scaff M. Antimicrobial chemotherapy in cystic fibrosis patients. Acta Pædiatr Scand Suppl 301: 75–100, 1982.
19. Schiøtz PO. Systemic and mucosal immunity and nonspecific defense mechanisms in cystic fibrosis. Acta Pædiatr Scand Suppl 301: 55–62, 1982.
20. Banks J. Treatment of pulmonary disease caused by opportunistic mycobacteria. Thorax 44: 449–454, 1989.
21. Kinney JS, Little BJ, Yolken RH, Rosenstein BJ. Mycobacterium avium complex in a patient with cystic fibrosis: disease vs. colonization. Pediatr Infect Dis J 8: 393–396, 1989.
22. Boxerbaum B. Isolation of rapidly growing mycobacteria in patients with cystic fibrosis. J Pediatr 96: 689–691, 1980.
23. Smith MJ, Efthimiou J, Hodson ME, Batten JC. Mycobacterial isolations in young adults with cystic fibrosis. Thorax 39: 369–375, 1984.
24. Wallace RJ. Swenson JM, Silcox VA, Bullen MG. Treatment of nonpulmonary infections due to Mycobacterium fortuitum and Mycobacterium chelonei on the basis of in vitro susceptibilities. J Infect Dis 152: 500–514, 1985.

Submitted February 11, 1994; accepted May 16, 1994

Scand J Infect Dis 26: 577–584, 1994

Twice Daily Cefpodoxime Proxetil Compared with Thrice Daily Amoxicillin/Clavulanic Acid for Treatment of Acute Otitis Media in Children

PIERRE GEHANNO[1], BÉATRIX BARRY[1], SERGE BOBIN[2] and CHRISTINE SAFRAN[3]

From the [1]Hôpital Bichat-Claude-Bernard, Paris, and the [2]Hôpital Kremlin Bicêtre, Le Kremlin Bicêtre, and [3]Roussel Uclaf, Romainville, France

A total of 260 children, 3 months to 11 years old (median age 24 months), with acute otitis media (AOM) received either cefpodoxime proxetil (CP) 8 mg/kg/d b.i.d. or amoxicillin/clavulanic acid (ACA) 40/10 mg/kg/d t.i.d. for 8 days. A significant difference in clinical cure rates was observed between the CP group 71/118 (60%) and the ACA group 42/105 (40%), $p = 0.003$. At the follow-up visit (20–30 days after the start of treatment), significant advantages were recorded with the CP vs. ACA therapy, in terms of satisfactory clinical response [90/111 (81%) vs 60/94 (63.8%), $p = 0.005$] residual middle ear effusion (14.4% vs 28.7%, $p = 0.01$) and normal tympanometry (78% vs 61.4%, $p = 0.017$). Compliance and adverse event frequency were the same in both treatment groups. The higher clinical cure rate and equivalent safety profile of CP indicates that it is an acceptable alternative to ACA for the treatment of AOM in children.

C. Safran, MD, Roussel Uclaf, 102 route de Noisy, F-93230 Romainville, France

INTRODUCTION

Acute otitis media (AOM) is the most common infection diagnosed by physicians who provide health care to children. Annual incidence rates ranging between 25% and 83% have been reported in preschool children in Finland and the United States (1–3).

Antimicrobial therapy for AOM is now standard practice in order to prevent suppurative complications and serous otitis, with related hearing loss and impaired speech development in infancy (1, 4, 5). Amoxicillin and, in some areas, penicillin have been regarded as first-line therapy for AOM. This situation is changing, however, due to alterations in the susceptibility patterns of the pathogens responsible for AOM.

The pathogens most commonly implicated in AOM are H. influenzae, S. pneumoniae, and M. catarrhalis. (1, 4, 6, 7). S. pneumoniae is the second most common pathogen in AOM, with an incidence of 18–36.5% (1, 8). Pneumococcus has long been considered a susceptible species but strains with reduced susceptibility to penicillin (MIC $\geq$ 0.1 mg/l) were first described in Australia and South Africa (9) and, have more recently been reported in Europe (10, 11). Pneumococci with reduced susceptibility to penicillin initially reported in Spain and Hungary were first reported in France in 1991 (12). The incidence of pneumococci with reduced susceptibility which have been isolated from acute otitis pus is currently 18–50% in France (6, 12). Strains of S. pneumoniae with reduced susceptibility to penicillin have become common within the last 15 years (4, 9–11, 13).

Recently, the proportion of β-lactamase-producing strains of H. influenzae isolated from patients with AOM has increased to 35% and the proportion in M. catarrhalis strains to 76% (6, 8, 14, 15). It is therefore desirable for the clinician treating AOM to have access to an antibiotic which is active against these three organisms which is highly resistant to hydrolysis by the β-lactamases. For treatment of AOM, a combination of a β-lactamase inhibitor and amoxicillin or a sulfonamide with a macrolide or an oral third generation cephalosporin have therefore been used.

Cefpodoxime proxetil (CP) is a new orally absorbed third generation cephalosporin. It is active against β lactamase-producing strains of H. influenzae and M. catarrhalis (16). It has an in vitro activity against penicillin susceptible S. pneumoniae similar to that of penicillin. In S. pneumoniae, strains that show intermediate susceptibility to penicillin, cefpodoxime activity is slightly weaker than that of amoxicillin (12). An oral suspension of CP for pediatric use has been found clinically efficacious in 90% of Japanese children with a AOM (17). After a single oral dose of 5 mg/kg CP suspension, the serum peak in children ranged between 1.3 and 3.4 mg/ml, with an elimination half-life of 1.4 to 2.6 h (17).

At present, the antibiotic of choice for treatment of AOM in children is amoxicillin/clavulanic acid (ACA). The extended antibacterial spectrum of cefpodoxime and its high intrinsic bactericidal activity at low concentrations suggest that it may be effective against AOM. The aim of the present study was to compare the efficacy of CP with ACA in pediatric patients with AOM.

MATERIAL AND METHODS

This trial was conducted as a multicentre, comparative, open-labeled, two-armed, parallel group study in pediatric patients with AOM. Study centres were located in France (33 centres) and Finland (2 centres). The study protocol was approved by the local Medical Ethics Committee at each investigative centre. Patients were enrolled after witnessed oral or written informed consent (according to the law in each country) obtained from the patient's parents or guardian.

Patients

Pediatric patients 3 months to 11 years of age with AOM documented by fever ($\geq 38°C$) and/or otalgia, and either abnormal otoscopic examination or presence of otorrhea due to ear drum perforation (within previous 24 h) were eligible. Both inpatients and outpatients weighing at least 7 kg and being able to undergo tympanocentesis for bacteriological culture at inclusion were enrolled.

Exclusion criteria

(*a*) Evidence of serous otitis, chronic otorrhea, cholesteatoma, or presence of tympanic tubes; (*b*) evidence of perforation of the ear drum having occurred more than 24 h prior to the start of the study; (*c*) history of allergy to β-lactams; (*d*) renal impairment, liver dysfunction, or phenylketonuria; (*e*) evidence of immunodeficiency including neutropenia (neutrophils $<1500 \times 10^9/l$) or AIDS classified as CDC score III or IV; (*f*) malabsorption syndrome, chronic vomiting, terminal neoplasia, or severe psychiatric disorder; (*g*) previous antibiotic treatment within the 48 h prior to inclusion (unless the pathogen responsible for infection was resistant in vitro to the antibiotic received); (*h*) treatment with any investigational drug within 2 weeks prior to the start of the study; (*i*) inability to fulfil the requirements of the study; and (*j*) previous participation in a clinical trial with CP.

Trial design

Patients were randomized to receive either CP or ACA for 8 days. CP was given at a dose of 8 mg/kg/day b.i.d. and ACA at a dose of 40/10 mg/kg/day t.i.d. The antibiotics were administered during or after a meal.

Prior to treatment, the complete medical and surgical history of each patient was taken by an Ear Nose and Throat (ENT) specialist. A physical examination, including the detection of signs and symptoms of AOM, was also carried out. Bacterial cultures for the identification of the pathogen(s) and in vitro susceptibility testing were obtained via a tympanocentesis or an aspirate from spontaneous otorrhea. Patients were further examined for clinical signs and symptoms of infection and for normal or abnormal tympanometry 2–3 days after the completion of therapy and at the follow-up visit one month after the end of treatment. Patients with relapse were evaluated prior to these routine examinations.

Evaluation

Patients were evaluated by a per protocol analysis and an intention-to-treat analysis. In the per protocol analysis, the response was evaluated by the investigator according to the following definitions.

Clinical response at end of treatment

Satisfactory response: disappearance of clinical signs and symptoms, plus normal tympanometry; **Unsatisfactory response**: Improvement: persistence of some clinical signs and/or tympanometric abnormalities not requiring additional antibiotic therapy; Failure: clinical signs and symptoms worsened or unchanged with requirement of additional antibiotic therapy.

Clinical response at follow-up

Satisfactory response: no new infection: i.e. the patient showed no signs or symptoms of an AOM; **Residual middle ear effusion**: otoscopic and/or tympanometric signs of serous otitis, tubal dysfunction, or persistent inflammation; **Unsatisfactory response**: signs and symptoms of a new AOM infection at the original infection site.

Bacteriological response at end of treatment

Satisfactory response: Eradication with no pathogen isolated or presumed eradication if clinical recovery; **Unsatisfactory Response**: No eradication of causative pathogen isolated from the original infection site; Partial eradication: more than one pathogen isolated in the pretreatment culture, of which at least one was eradicated and one isolated from the original site of infection at the end of treatment visit; Superinfection: one or more pathogens, different from the pathogen isolated in the pretreatment culture, were isolated, and signs and symptoms of AOM were present or reappeared. Patients who had an unsatisfactory clinical response but had no culture to document an unsatisfactory bacteriological response (i.e., no eradication, partial eradication, or superinfection) were also categorized as having an unsatisfactory response.

Bacteriological response at follow-up

Satisfactory response: no pathogen isolated or no culture obtained in the case of clinical recovery; **Unsatisfactory response**: Relapse: reappearance of the pretreatment pathogen that was eradicated at the end of treatment visit, accompanied by signs and symptoms of acute otitis media; Reinfection: the pretreatment pathogen was eradicated, but infection recurred and a pathogen other than the pretreatment pathogen was isolated. Patients who showed an unsatisfactory clinical response but had no corroborating bacterial culture were categorized as 'unsatisfactory response'.

All patients who received at least one dose of study medication and had a pre- and post-treatment evaluation were included in the intention-to-treat analysis. Only patients who were lost to follow-up after the initial visit were excluded. In the intention-to-treat analysis, all non-cured patients from the per protocol analysis, all those improved but who received any new antibiotic for a respiratory tract infection between the end of treatment and follow-up visits, all relapsers, all patients with a residual middle ear effusion at the follow-up or those who discontinued the treatment were considered failures.

Compliance

Bottles and treatment boxes of study medication were collected and the patient's follow-up card was reviewed at the end of treatment visit to assess patient compliance with the treatment regimen. Poor compliance was defined as taking less than 80% of the scheduled doses over the observed treatment period, or receiving fewer than 5 days treatment at the prescribed dose, unless the patient was considered a failure or in the presence of a resistant pathogen. In such cases, patients were excluded from the per protocol analysis as major protocol violators.

Safety

Adverse events were assessed by spontaneous reports or physical examination throughout the treatment period, at the end of treatment visit in all patients who received at least one dose of study medication. Laboratory data were examined for clinically important abnormalities based on normal ranges.

Statistics

Disposition of patients, demographic characteristics, medical history, clinical signs and concomitant diseases were compared between treatment groups for all patients. Treatment duration and evolution of clinical signs were compared between treatment groups for all patients. Bacteriological and clinical response rates were summarized by treatment group for evaluable patients and compared using the χ^2-test or Fisher's exact test. 95% confidence intervals of the difference between success rates were calculated to establish the comparability of the two treatment groups. Adverse events were summarized by treatment group and body system and compared using Fisher's exact test. Differences between treatment groups in laboratory variables, in reference to the laboratory normal ranges, were analysed using Fisher's exact test.

RESULTS

From June 1990, to April 1991, 262 patients with AOM were enrolled by 35 investigators. Of these, 260 received study medication, 131 CP and 129 ACA. Two patients in the CP group had parental consent withdrawn before receiving any drug. The mean ages of the patients treated with CP and ACA were 2.8 ± 2.3 years (range: 0.4–10.3 years) and 3.1 ± 2.7 years (range: 0.3–10.6 years) respectively. In the CP treatment group, 57.1% of the patients enrolled were males, vís-a-vís 50.4% in the ACA group. No significant differences in demographic variables were observed between the two treatment groups, and no differences with respect to distribution of clinical signs and symptoms, aggravating factors or medical history.

Pretreatment bacterial isolates

A total of 258 organisms were isolated from the pretreatment cultures (Table I). Of these, 93 were isolated from spontaneous otorrhea and 165 after tympanocentesis. No causative organism was identified in the pretreatment culture in 14% of the CP patients and 6% of the ACA patients. One CP patient had no bacteriological sample obtained at the pretreatment visit. Among all the patients, the organisms isolated at baseline were: H. influenzae (40.0% and 36.1%), S. pneumoniae (26.4% and 33.1%), S. aureus (10.4% and 8.3%), M. catarrhalis (4.0% and 7.5%), P. aeruginosa (4.8% and 6.0%), and others (14.4% and 9.0%) in the two treatment groups, respectively (Table I). Of the 98 H. influenzae isolates, 25 were β-lactamase positive.

Treatment duration

The mean duration of treatment was 8.0 ± 1.0 days in the CP treatment group, and 7.9 ± 2.2 days in the ACA treatment group.

Evaluation

Of the 262 patients enrolled in the study, 223 (118 CP and 105 ACA) were evaluable in the per protocol analysis for clinical efficacy at the end of treatment, and 205 patients (111 CP and 94 ACA) were evaluable at follow-up. The primary reason for non-evaluability across

Table I. *Pathogens isolated at baseline in patients with acute otitis media treated with cefpodoxime proxetil (n = 131) amoxicillin/clavulanic acid (n = 129)*

CP, cefpodoxime/proxetil; ACA, amoxicillin/clavulanic acid.

Pathogen	Pathogens from patients treated with CP *n*	(%)	β-lactamase positive pathogens *n*	(%)	Pathogens isolated from patients treated with ACA *n*	(%)	β-lactamase positive pathogens *n*	(%)
H. influenzae	50/125	(40.0)	11	(22)	48/133	(36.1)	14	(48)
S. pneumoniae	33/125	(26.4)			44/133	(33.1)		
S. aureus	13/125	(10.4)	10	(77)	11/133	(8.3)	8	(73)
M. catarrhalis	5/125	(4.0)	3	(60)	10/133	(7.5)	9	(90)
P. aeruginosa	6/125	(4.8)			8/133	(6.0)		
Others	18/125	(14.4)			12/133	(9.0)		

both groups was the isolation of a resistant pathogen at inclusion, accounting for 18 of the 44 (41%) reasons for non-evaluability at the end of treatment. All 14 P. aeruginosa isolates were resistant to both study drugs. In addition, 1 S. faecalis strain was resistant to CP and 3 E. cloacae strains to ACA.

For the bacteriological efficacy analysis, 195 patients (98 CP and 97 ACA) were evaluable at the end of treatment, and 143 patients (81 CP and 62 ACA) at follow-up.

Among the patients who were clinically evaluable at the end of treatment, no satistically significant differences were observed between treatment groups in terms of resolution of spontaneous otalgia, pain on pressure, fullness in the ear, purulent otorrhea, or temperature. Significantly more patients who received CP and who were evaluated for clinical efficacy had normal otoscopic examinations, as compared with those who received ACA (68.4% and 54.3%, respectively; $p = 0.031$). Similar differences were observed with respect to all of the treated patients and those who were bacteriologically evaluable: more patients who had received CP had normal otoscopic examinations at the end of treatment.

Clinical outcome

Cefpodoxime proxetil was significantly more effective in achieving clinical response than was ACA, as depicted in Table II. At the end of treatment, the cure rate among patients in the CP group (60%, 71/118) was significantly higher ($p = 0.003$) than among patients treated with ACA (40%, 42/105). In addition, significantly more CP patients than ACA patients had satisfactory clinical response rates at follow-up (81.1% vs 63.8%, respectively, $p = 0.005$) (Table II). A significantly lower rate of residual middle ear effusion was also observed in the CP than in the ACA group at follow-up (14.4% vs. 28.7%, respectively) (Table II). The CP group had normal tympanometry results significantly more often than the ACA group at the end of treatment (61.1% vs. 39.5%, $p = 0.004$) and at follow-up (78.0% vs. 61.4%, $p = 0.017$).

Bacteriological outcome

In the CP group, 100% of pathogens isolated in pretreatment cultures of evaluable patients were eradicated – or presumably eradicated – at the end of treatment visit, compared with

Table II. *Clinical response in patients with acute otitis media treated with cefpodoxime proxetil or amoxicillin/clavulanic acid*

	Cefpodoxime proxetil	Amoxicillin/clavulanic acid	p-value
Clinical Response			
End of treatment	($n = 118$)	($n = 105$)	0.003
Satisfactory	71 (60.2%)	42 (40.0%)	
Unsatisfactory	47 (39.8%)	63 (59.8%)	
– improved	41	58	
– failure	6	5	
Follow-up	($n = 111$)	($n = 94$)	0.005
Satisfactory	90 (81.1%)	60 (63.8%)	
Residual middle ear	16 (14.4%)	27 (28.7%)	
Unsatisfactory	5 (4.5%)	7 (7.4%)	
Tympanometry			
End of treatment	($n = 95$)	($n = 86$)	0.004
Normal	58 (61.1%)	34 (39.5%)	
Follow-up	($n = 91$)	($n = 83$)	0.017
Normal	71 (78.0%)	51 (61.4%)	

Table III. *Bacteriological response in patients with acute otitis media treated with cefpodoxime proxetil or amoxicillin/clavulanic acid*

Bacteriological response (per patient basis)	Cefpodoxime proxetil	Amoxicillin/ clavulanic acid
End of treatment	($n = 98$)	($n = 97$)
Satisfactory	96 (98.0%)	93 (95.9%)
Unsatisfactory	2 (2.0%)	4 (4.1%)
Clinical Failure	0	4
Superinfection	2	0
Follow-up visit	($n = 81$)	($n = 62$)
Satisfactory	78 (96.3%)	56 (90.3%)
Unsatisfactory	3 (3.7%)	6 (9.7%)
Clinical Failure	2	3
Relapse	0	1
Reinfection	1	2

96.3% in the ACA group. At the end of treatment, the bacteriological response was satisfactory in 98.0% (96/98) of patients in the CP group and 95.9% (93/97) of the ACA group (Table III). Results were similar at follow-up. Seven isolates of S. pneumoniae showed a reduced susceptibility to penicillin ($MIC > 0.12$ mg/l). One of these was resistant ($MIC = 2$) and 6 were moderately resistant ($0.12 < MIC < 2$). The in vitro activity of CP, ACA and penicillin was similar for these 7 strains, as no more than 2 dilutions of difference were observed for any of the drugs. The outcome for all 7 patients (4 in the CP group and 3 in the ACA group) was satisfactory.

Two of 262 enrolled patients were excluded from the intention-to-treat analysis as they did not receive any study medication due to parenteral refusal. Of the 260 patients included in the intention-to-treat overall efficacy analysis, satisfactory response rates were 76.3% (100/131) in the CP group and 59.7% (77/129) in the ACA group ($p = 0.004$), which confirmed the results of the per protocol analysis.

Good compliance was observed in both groups, 100% (131/131) and 97.7% (126/129) in the CP and ACA groups, respectively.

Safety

Of the 262 patients enrolled in this study, 260 received study medication and were evaluated for safety. Nine adverse events probably or possibly related to the study drugs were reported by 9 patients, 5/131 (3.8%) patients in the CP groups and 4/129 (3.1%) in the ACA group. In both treatment groups, the most common adverse events were associated with the digestive system (3 and 4 events, respectively, for CP and ACA). Except for 4 severe events reported in the ACA group, all adverse events were mild or moderate in intensity. The severe adverse events were: 2 cases of diarrhea and 1 case with increased aminotransferase levels, all considered possibly related to study drug, and 1 case of exophthalmos, considered unrelated. One CP patient and 2 ACA patients had treatment discontinued due to diarrhea, mild in the case of CP and severe in the ACA cases. No significant differences in biochemical or hematological values were seen between the treatment groups.

DISCUSSION

The results of this study indicate that CP, 8 mg/kg/day administered b.i.d., was significantly more efficacious and as safe as 40/10 mg/kg/day ACA administered t.i.d. for the treatment of AOM in children. To treat both β-lactamase-producing strains of bacteria and penicillin-resistant S. pneumoniae in AOM, ACA is usually the preferred drug among currently available antibiotics. Although treatment is generally given for 10 days (8, 18, 19), efficacy has even been shown when treatment duration has been reduced to 8 days (20, 21).

The dosage of ACA used in this study was 40/10 mg/kg/day, as recommended internationally at the time when the study was conducted. However, since then the recommended dosage for ACA has been increased in some countries (up to 80/10 mg/kg/day) for children under the age of 30 months and maintained at 40/10 mg/kg/day for children of 30 months and above. A retrospective analysis of these two age subgroups was performed, but the results showed no difference in the efficacy results in the two age groups defined by a cut-off point of 30 months. The results obtained were confirmed after adjustment for the two age groups defined.

This study demonstrated that CP, administered b.i.d. at a dose of 8 mg/kg/day for 8 days was just as or more effective than ACA administered t.i.d. at a dose of 40/10 mg/kg/day. There were no significant differences between study drugs in terms of resolution of symptoms, bacteriological response, or compliance. The results concerning clinical response, otoscopy, tympanometry, and residual middle ear effusion showed a significant advantage for CP. Thus, the proportion of patients with a complete clinical recovery was significantly larger in the CP vs ACA group at the end of treatment (60.2% vs. 40%, $p = 0.003$) and at the follow-up visit (81.1% vs. 63.8%, $p = 0.005$). These results confirm those of a study undertaken in the USA in which CP (10 mg/kg/day b.i.d.) was shown to be equally just as effective as amoxicillin/clavulanate potassium (40/10 mg/kg/day t.i.d.) for the treatment of AOM (22).

Recent data suggest that middle ear effusion may persist following AOM due to an inflammatory reaction to non-eradicated pathogens (20). Therefore, the better success rates observed with CP could be the result of a superior activity in situ, compared with ACA acid. Testing this hypothesis, however, would require invasive sampling from the middle ear of apparently healthy children which would not be ethically acceptable or compatible with the European and USA Guidelines for the clinical evaluation of anti-infective drugs (23, 24).

In agreement with the results reported in the literature, the most common pathogens in this study population were H. influenzae and S. pneumoniae, with 25% of the isolates of H. influenzae being β-lactamase positive. Thus, the results of this study should have broad applicability to AOM in children.

The intention-to-treat analysis confirmed the results of the per protocol analysis. The satisfactory response rates were significantly in favour of CP (76.3%) vís-à-vís ACA (59.7%). Thus, CP offers a significantly better overall complete clinical recovery than ACA acid, with equivalent safety in the treatment of AOM in children.

ACKNOWLEDGEMENTS

The authors acknowledge financial support and assistance in coordinating the study from Roussel Uclaf.

REFERENCES

1. Bluestone CD. Management of otitis media in infants and children: current role of old and new antimicrobial agents. Pediatr Infect Dis J 7: S129–S136, 1988.
2. Teele DW, Klein JO, Rosner B. Greater Boston otitis media study group: epidemiology of otitis media during the first seven years of life in children in Greater Boston: a prospective cohort study. J Infect Dis 160: 83–94, 1989.
3. Sipilä M, Pukander J, Karma P. Incidence of acute otitis media up to the age of 1.5 years in urban infants. Acta Otolaryngol (Stockh). 104: 138–145, 1987.

4. Karma P. Finnish approach to the treatment of acute otitis media. Report of the Finnish Consensus Conference. Ann Otol Rhinol Laryngol 96: 129: 1–29, 1987.
5. Gates GA. Otologic referral: indications and expectations. Pediatr Infect Dis J 5: 1–5, 1986.
6. Gehanno P, Boucot I, Simonet M, Bingen E, Lambert Zechovsky N, Berche P. Epidémiologie bactérienne de l'otite aiguè chez l'enfant en région parisienne de 1987 à 1991 à propos de 1232 cas. La Lettre de l'Infectiologue 6: 408–414, 1991.
7. Giebink GS. The microbiology of otitis media. Pediatr Infect Dis J 8: S18–S20, 1989.
8. Odio CM, Kusmiesz H, Shelton S, Nelson JD. Comparative treatment trial of Augmentin versus cefaclor for acute otitis media with effusion. Pediatrics 75: 819–826, 1985.
9. Jacobs MR, Koornhof HJ, Robins Browne RM, Stevenson CM, Vermaak ZA, Freiman I, Miller GB, Witcomb MA, Isaacson M, Ward JI, Austrian R. Emergence of multiply resistant pneumococci. N Engl J Med 299: 735–740, 1978.
10. Baquero F, Martinez-Beltran J, Loza E. A review of antibiotic resistance patterns of Streptococcus pneumoniae in Europe. J Antimicrob Chemother 28 (Suppl C): 31–38, 1991.
11. Klugman K. Pneumococcal resistance to antibiotics. Clin Microbiol Rev 3: 171–196, 1990.
12. Berche P., Boucot I., Duval F., Gehanno P., Lenoir G., Chiche D. Bacterial epidemiology of children with acute otitis media in France. 6th ICID, Prague. Abstract PCS 6, 1994.
13. Marlon A, Gulyas M, Munoz R, Tomasso A. Extremely high incidence of antibiotic resistance in clinical isolates of Streptococcus pneumoniae in Hungary. J Infect Dis 163: 542–556, 1991.
14. Shurin PA, Marchant CD, Kin CH. Emergence of β-lactamase producing strains of M. catarrhalis as important agents of acute otitis media. Pediatr Infect Dis J 2: 34, 1983.
15. Powel M, Koutsia-Courouzou C, Voutsinas D, Seymour A, Williams JD. Resistance of clinical isolates of H. influenzae in the United Kingdom. BMJ 295: 176, 1987.
16. Chin NX, Neu HC. In vitro activity of and oral iminomethoxy aminothiazolyl cephalosporin, R-3746. Antimicrob Agents Chemother 32: 671–677, 1988.
17. Fujii R, Meguro H, Arimasu O, Shiraishi H, Abe T, Yoshioka H, et al. Overall clinical evaluation of cefpodoxime proxetil against infections in pediatric fields. Jpn J Antibiot 42: 1439–55, 1989.
18. Gan VN, Kusmiesz H, Shelton S, Nelson JD. Comparative evaluation of Loracarbef and Amoxicillin-Clavulanate for acute otitis media. Antimicrob Agents Chemother 35:967–971, 1991.
19. Marchant CD, Shurin PA, Johnson CE, Murdell-Panek D, Feinstein JC, Fulton D, Flexon P, Carlin SA, Van-Hare GF. A randomized controlled trial of amoxicillin plus clavulanate compared with cefaclor for treatment of acute otitis media. J Pediatr 109: 891–896, 1986.
20. Gehanno P, Berche P., Boucot T. lambert-Zechovsky N., Bingen E., Gres J. J., Rollin C. Comparative efficacy and safety of cefprozil and amoxicillin/clavulanate in the treatment of acute otitis media in children. J Antimicrob Chemother 1994 (in press).
21. Cohen C, Lebeau A, Narcy P. Traitement des otities moyennes aiguès du jeune enfant par la formulation amoxicillin/acide clavulanique. Ann Pediatr 36: 49–54, 1989.
22. Mendelman PM, Dol Beccaro MA, McLinn SE and Todd WM. Cefpodoxime proxetil compared with amoxicillin-clavulanate for the treatment of otitis media. Pediatr Pharmacol Ther 121: 459–465, 1991.
23. European guidelines for the clinical evaluation of anti-infective drug products. European Society of Clinical Microbiology and Infectious Diseases. 1993.
24. USA guidelines for the evaluation of new anti-infective drugs for the treatment of respiratory tract infections. Clin Infect Dis 15, 1992.

Submitted February 8, 1994; accepted June 16, 1994

Scand J Infect Dis 26: 585–595, 1994

Comparison of Imipenem versus Cefuroxim Plus Tobramycin as Empirical Therapy for Febrile Granulocytopenic Patients and Efficacy of Vancomycin and Aztreonam in case of Failure

ZORAN ERJAVEC[1], HILLY G. DE VRIES-HOSPERS[2], HARMEN VAN KAMP[1], DICK VAN DER WAAIJ[2], MARTIN R. HALIE[1] and SIMON M. G. J. DAENEN[1]

From the Departments of [1]Haematology and [2]Medical Microbiology, University Hospital Groningen, The Netherlands

143 aplastic episodes with fever in 91 haematological patients with granulocytopenia were treated empirically in a randomized prospective study using either imipenem (Imi) or a combination of tobramycin and cefuroxim (T/C). Response after 72 h was significantly better in patients receiving Imi (44/75 vs 27/68, $p < 0.05$). This was seen especially in patients with bacteriologically proven infections where the isolated staphylococci and streptococci were more susceptible to Imi. In both groups, patients who failed to respond to the initial antibiotic therapy were given vancomycin and aztreonam (V/A). The response rate after another 72 h, measured using the same criteria as after the first 72 h, did not differ statistically between the groups. One patient in each study group died from the bacterial infection, both from Gram-positive bacteraemia. Duration of fever was significantly shorter in the Imi group (4 days vs 7 days, $p < 0.04$). Serum peak and trough concentrations of the antibiotics were comparable. Both regimens were well tolerated. Our results show that monotherapy with imipenem is superior to the combination of tobramycin and cefuroxime during the first 72 h of therapy and can be safely administered to neutropenic patients with predominantly Gram-positive infections. A combination of vancomycin and aztreonam, given when initial imipenem treatment has failed, was effective in only a few patients. Adjuvant glycopeptide therapy from the outset in the treatment of febrile granulocytopenic patients did not seem worthwhile.

Z. Erjavec, MD, Department of Haematology, University Hospital, Groningen, Oostersingel 59, 9713 EZ Groningen, The Netherlands

INTRODUCTION

Granulocytopenia from haematological disorders or their treatment is often accompanied by infections (1). Prompt empirical treatment by broad-spectrum antibiotic therapy is now standard practice (2). Combinations of an anti-pseudomonas penicillin or cephalosporin with an aminoglycoside are now the most frequently chosen treatments (3, 4). The advantages of such combinations are broad-spectrum coverage and potential synergistic interaction against most infecting organisms (5). Disadvantages include limited activity against some Gram-positive organisms and potential nephro- and ototoxicity (7). With the development of new broad-spectrum antibiotics such as ceftazidime and imipenem, monotherapy has become a feasible treatment option. So far, several studies have shown that monotherapy using either of these 2 agents seems to be as efficacious and as safe as a combination therapy (7–14).

In the past decade, Gram-positive microorganisms have become increasingly important as a cause of infections in granulocytopenic patients (15, 16). The increased use of indwelling catheters with penetration of the skin barrier, the use of oral antibiotics to selectively decontaminate the digestive tract, as well as the intensification of antileukaemic chemotherapy with cytostatics, which can cause severe mucositis, are believed to be responsible for this phenomenon. At our centre, infections by Gram-positive microorganisms are responsible for almost 75% of microbiologically documented infections. Since the introduction of selective decontamination of the digestive tract (SDD), aimed at the elimination of all aerobic Gram-negative microorganisms from the digestive tract, Pseudomonas did not seem to be a major pathogen and we used a combination of aminoglycoside and second generation cephalosporin (cefuroxime) as empirical therapy in our Department. This strategy has kept mortality from bacterial infections very low (17), yet efficacy in microbiologically documented infections, particularly of those caused by Gram-positive microorganisms, seemed to be low.

To improve the results of empirical therapy, we choose imipenem because of its broad antibacterial coverage. Reportedly (18, 19), it is also efficacious against Gram-positive isolates and gives less risk of renal side effects than other drugs. Our aim was to establish the efficacy and safety of imipenem used as monotherapy in the treatment of febrile granulocytopenic patients in which Gram-positive infections were the predominant cause of bacteriologically documented infections. In addition, we were interested in the therapeutic value of the standardized subsequent therapy with vancomycin and aztreonam given when the initial empirical treatments failed.

MATERIAL AND METHODS

The study comprised adult (>16 years) haematological patients who were suffering from granulocytopenia owing to disease or cytostatic treatment and who had fever, with or without definite signs and symptoms of an infection. Fever was defined as a single axillary reading of a temperature >38.5°C or a persistent temperature above 38°C for more than 24 h. Granulocytopenia was defined as a granulocyte count below 0.5×10^9/l, or $<1.0 \times 10^9$/l that was rapidly falling. Most of the patients (75/91) were managed in rooms with 2 or more persons without laminar air flow or high efficiency air filtration. All patients received SDD consisting of oral amphotericin-B (2 g/day) and colistin (800 mg/day), while 63 out of them also received cotrimoxazole (2,880 mg/day). Patients allergic to the latter received oral ciprofloxacin (1,000 mg/day) instead. Patients were entered only once during the same granulocytopenic episode and at least a week had to pass between the granulocytopenic episodes before a patient could be included again. Most of the patients (80/91) had a Hickman catheter. Patients were not included if they had a known allergy to one or more of the drugs in the study, severe renal failure (creatinine >450 μmol/l or clearance <10 ml/min), suspected or proven brain abscess, endocarditis or Hickman tunnel infection, or if they had received any other oral absorbable antibiotic than those used for SDD. We did not include them if they had changed SDD antibiotics within 48 h before their fever started or if any i.v. antibiotic had been given less than 7 days previously. The study was approved by the local Ethics Committee. Informed consent was obtained from every patient included.

Clinical and laboratory investigations

We examined patients daily for clinical signs of infection and obtained complete blood cell counts, serum electrolytes, kidney- and liver function tests before the start of the antibiotic therapy and daily thereafter. X-rays of the thorax and nasal sinuses were taken at the onset of the fever and afterwards as indicated by the clinical condition, i.e., persistent fever or specific complaints.

Microbiological investigations

At least 2 blood cultures were taken (one via the Hickman catheter) along with cultures from urine and possible sites of infection before the start of the antibiotic treatment. Blood cultures were further taken daily if a patient's temperature stayed above 38°C, for verification that the microbiological infection had been eradicated. Throat swabs and faeces were cultured 3 times a week for control of SDD from all patients. Invasive procedures to obtain material for microbiological investigation were performed if indicated and possible.

Culture-positive microorganisms were identified by standard laboratory techniques and their susceptibility was determined by the disc diffusion method. The susceptibility of coagulase-negative staphylococci (CNS) for cefuroxime and imipenem was related to oxacillin. Serum was collected on day 2 of treatment for peak (30 min after the end of the infusion) and trough concentrations in the serum (immediately before the next dose) for all antibiotics during the first 72 h and these were determined by HPLC.

Classification of febrile episodes

Febrile episodes were classified using the criteria of The Immunocompromised Host Society (20). **Bacteriologically documented infection** (BDI) was diagnosed when a responsible pathogen was isolated at the infection site. For coagulase negative staphylococci (CNS) at least 2 positive blood cultures were required. We judged patients to have a **clinically documented infection** (CDI) if they had fever and clinical evidence of an infection, such as cellulitis or pulmonary infiltrate(s), but when no microbiological pathogen could be isolated. We diagnosed **fever of unknown origin** (FUO) when we could not identify any clinical, radiological or bacteriological evidence of an infection and non-infectious causes had been excluded.

Treatment

Eligible patients were stratified according to whether or not they used absorbable antibiotics for SDD and randomized to receive either Imi or T/C. Imipenem was given intravenously in a dose of 12.5 mg/kg (with a maximum of 1 gram) over 60 min every 6 h. We started tobramycin treatment with a 2.5 mg/kg loading dose followed by 2 mg/kg over 30 min every 12 h and cefuroxime 15 mg/kg over 30 min every 8 h. Tobramycin dosage was adjusted according to the results of the serum assay. If the assessment was unsatisfactory, initial treatment was stopped in both study groups, and vancomycin (1 g over 60 min every 12 h) and aztreonam (2 g over 60 min every 8 h) were given. Patients who responded were treated for a minimum of 7 days, or for 5 days after resolution of fever and all signs and symptoms of infection, whichever was the longer. We gave Amphotericin-B i.v. when fungal infection was strongly suspected or proven, or when fever persisted after 6 days of antibiotic treatment.

Evaluation of responses and toxicity

The outcome of the initial antibiotic treatment was evaluated in all patients after the first 72 h (early evaluation). For patients who failed to respond after the first 72 h, the subsequent treatment was evaluated after another 72 h in the same way as after the initial course (second evaluation). Final evaluation was done when the granulocytopenia had resolved. Response was defined as disappearance of all signs, symptoms and microbiological evidence of infection as well as resolution of fever (temperature under 37.5°C measured twice within 8 h). All other patients, including the one who died from infection, were defined as failures. Patients who died of their malignant disease or as a result of another non-infectious cause were classified as having shown a good response if the original infection had resolved and no evidence of infection was present at postmortem examination. Relapse was defined as reappearance of the same infection within 7 days after discontinuation of the antibiotic treatment. Superinfection was diagnosed in patients whose infection was caused by a different organism which appeared during the treatment, or as infection at a different site if we could not isolate an organism from the original site (21). Breakthrough bacteraemia was defined as recovery of the same micro-organism from blood cultures, as found before the i.v. antibiotics were given and to which the micro-organism was susceptible in vitro.

We defined nephrotoxicity as a doubling of the initial serum creatinine concentration. Hepatic toxicity was considered proven in patients whose hepatic enzymes increased to 3 times the original value.

Statistical Methods

The χ^2-test was used to compare the categorical parameters in both study populations and Student's t-test for comparison of continuous variables. The Wilcoxon test was used for a comparison of fever days between the groups. A p-value of <0.05 was considered statistically significant.

RESULTS

Over 38 months we monitored 179 consecutive aplastic episodes in 127 patients with haematological abnormalities for inclusion in the study. 36 (20%) aplastic episodes were deemed non-evaluable, because they were retrospectively assessed as having a non-infectious cause of fever (11), protocol violations (mainly other oral antibiotics than SDD, 15), infection with Aspergillus (6), Candida (2), Mycobacterium (1), or a virus (1) from the start. After exclusion of these episodes, we were left with a total of 143 aplastic episodes with fever in 91 patients and these were assessed in the study: 115 of them were stratified in the group with absorbable SDD antibiotics and 28 in the group with only non-absorbable antibiotics. When the episodes were randomized, 75 were assigned to Imi and 68 to T/C group.

Table I gives the characteristics of the study populations. Both groups were comparable with respect to sex, haematological diagnosis, levels of neutropenia at inclusion, treatment in a laminar air flow (LAF) room (equipped with HEPA filters) and presence of an indwelling double lumen Hickman catheter. The mean age, however, was higher in the Imi group (45.1 SD $\pm$ 15.5 vs 39.2 SD $\pm$ 16.9, $p < 0.025$). More aplastic periods occurred from the treatment of acute lymphocytic leukemia (ALL) than of acute myeloid leukemia (AML) in T/C group but statistical analysis showed no difference either in the pattern or the incidence of infections between the AML and ALL groups. 75% of the patients were newly diagnosed and receiving their first course of chemotherapy. The duration of granulocytopenia and the use of the SDD antibiotics were comparable in the 2 groups, as was the distribution of BDI, CDI and FUO.

Evaluation of response

Early evaluation. We evaluated the response to the initial treatment after the first 72 h and compared the 2 groups (Table II). The Imi group responded better, measured according to the previously noted criteria (44/75 vs 27/68, $p < 0.05$). The significant difference in response was also seen in the BDI group, where only 3/21 patients responded after initial treatment with T/C (3/21 vs 14/27, $p < 0.01$). That was the case in infections caused by Streptococci as well as those caused by CNS (Table III). Gram-negative infections occurred less frequently, so that numbers were too small for any difference to emerge, but evaluation of response showed that the Imi group tended to respond better. The only breakthrough bacteraemia in

Table I. *Clinical characteristics of the patients*

Imi = Imipenem; T/C = Tobramycin/Cefuroxime; AML = acute myeloid leukaemia; ALL = acute lymphocytic leukaemia; CML = chronic myeloid leukaemia; NHL = non-Hodgkin lymphoma; AA = aplastic anaemia; others = 2 × multiple myeloma, 2 × Autologous bone marrow transplantation for NHL.

	Imi	T/C
Total no. episodes	92	87
No. of evaluable episodes	75	68
SDD absorbable and non-absorbable	61	54
only absorbable	14	14
Mean age (years, range)	45 (17–78)	39 (17–70)
Sex (M/F)	41/34	40/28
Underlying disease		
AML	48	31
ALL	12	24
CML	4	7
NHL	6	4
AA	2	1
Other	3	1
Granulocyte count at entry		
<0.5	59	52
<0.1	16	16
Duration of granulocytopenia (days < 1.0)	18	16
No. with Hickman catheter	67	60
Bacteriologically documented infection	27	21
Clinically documented infection	15	15
Fever of unknown origin	33	32

Table II. *Responses at early and second evaluation*

BDI = bacteriologically documented infection; CDI = clinically documented infection; FUO = fever of unknown origin.

	Imipenem		Tobramycin/cefuroxime	
	Early evaluation	Second evaluation	Early evaluation	Second evaluation
BDI	14/27[a] (51%)	18/27 (66%)	3/21[a] (14%)	11/21 (52%)
CDI	5/15 (33%)	7/15 (46%)	4/16 (26%)	6/15 (40%)
FUO	25/33 (75%)	28/33 (84%)	20/32 (62%)	26/32 (81%)
Total	44/75[b] (58%)	53/75 (70%)	27/68[b] (39%)	43/68 (63%)

[a] $p < 0.01$
[b] $p < 0.05$

Table III. *Responses in bacteriologically and clinically documented infections and in fever of unknown origin (FUO) at 72 h*

NB = non-bacteraemic.

	Imi	T/C
Bacteriologically documented infections		
Response 72 h (response/total)	14/27[a]	3/21[a]
Gram-pos (response/total)	10/18	2/11
Streptococcus spp.		
S. viridans	2/2	1/2
S. mitis	1/4	1/6
S. sanguis	1/1	–
CNS	6/10	0/2
Staphylococcus aureus	–	0/1
Enterococcus faecalis	0/1	–
Gram-neg (response/total)	3/4	1/5
Escherichia coli	1/2	1/1
Pseudomonas aeruginosa	1/1 (NB)	0/1
Acinetobacter	–	0/1
Enterobacter cloacae	1/1 (NB)	0/1
Gram-neg rod	–	0/1 (NB)
Polymicrobial (response/total)	1/4	0/5
Lactobacillus + Enterococcus faecalis	0/1	–
Bacteroides fragilis + CNS	–	0/2
Streptococcus viridans + CNS	0/2	0/2
Acinetobacter + Enterobacter cloacae + Enterococcus faecalis	0/1	–
Enterobacter + Pseudomonas aeruginosa (NB)	–	0/1
Clinically documented infections		
Response 72 h (response/total)	5/15	4/15
Infection site		
Lung	2/10	0/7
Sinus	2/4	3/7
Skin	1/1	–
Urogenital tract	–	1/1
Fever of unknown origin		
Response 72 h (response/total)	25/33	20/32

[a] ($p < 0.01$)

the study occurred in the T/C group – a patient who developed Pseudomonas aeruginosa sepsis. The patient survived the sepsis after we changed the initial antibiotic regimen to V/A treatment. A subgroup with polymicrobial infections showed a poor response with both initial regimens after the first 72 h of treatment. Clinically documented infections, most of them defined as pneumonia, responded poorly to both initial regimens. Evaluation of the response in patients with FUO showed comparable responses in both groups. Of 44 responders in Imi group, 2 developed fungal and 2 viral superinfection. In the T/C group, 2 fungal superinfections and 1 relapse occurred in a patient with FUO. We assessed serum peak and trough concentrations on the second day for all empirically given antibiotics in 65 episodes in both study groups. Peak serum concentrations of imipenem, cefuroxime and tobramycin were (mean values) 24.3 ± 8.3 mg/l, 35.2 ± 7.0 mg/l and 5.2 ± 3.3 mg/l, respectively. Peak concentrations of tobramycin in the T/C group were not optimal despite an initial loading dose of 2.5 mg/kg. As stated earlier, the dosage was adjusted following the assay results. Trough concentrations were 1.1 ± 1.0 mg/l for imipenem, 0.5 ± 0.3 mg/l for cefuroxime and 0.2 ± 1.3 mg/l for tobramycin. Comparison of the serum antibiotic peak concentrations between the responders and non-responders at 72 h showed no statistical difference in both groups.

Second evaluation. After the early evaluation, patients who failed to respond to the initial regimen were subsequently given V/A in both groups. The results of their response are also given in Table II. Of 31 non-responders in the Imi group, 9 responded to V/A, and in the T/C group, 16/41 non-responders responded to V/A. The significant inter-group difference in response seen following the initial treatment did not diminish after patients received the subsequent therapy (53/75 vs 43/68, $p > 0.20$). In the BDI subgroup, almost half of the failures in the T/C group responded to V/A (8/18), while one-third responded in the Imi group (4/13). Two further patients in each CDI subgroup responded to subsequent treatment, thus confirming the known poor response in this subgroup. Response in the group with FUO was the same in both groups after subsequent treatment. In each group, one patient required later treatment with an antiviral drug.

Final evaluation. Of the 91 patients we treated, 10 died from an infection, giving an infection-related mortality of 10%. Only 2 patients died from infection with a bacterial pathogen: 1 Staphylococcus aureus bacteraemia occurred in the T/C group and 1 CNS bacteraemia in the Imi group. Both pathogens were susceptible in vitro to the initial antibiotics and were subsequently treated with V/A, but both patients died 8 days after the initial antibiotic therapy was started. Remaining infection-related deaths were fungal in origin, all caused by filamentous fungi. There were 4 in each group: in the Imi group, 1 in BDI and 3 in CDI subgroup, in the T/C group 2 in CDI and 2 in the FUO subgroup. Another 5 patients died from progression of their underlying disease or fatal haemorrhage.

We gave the remaining patients who still had fever after 72 h of second treatment Amphotericin-B i.v., or earlier if fungal infection was strongly suspected or proven. Most responded shortly afterwards or simultaneously with recovery of granulocytes. Most of the superinfections that occurred in both study groups were of fungal or viral origin. CNS bacteraemia as a superinfection occurred twice in the Imi group and 4 times in the T/C group, while the only Gram-negative superinfection was bacteraemia with Xanthomonas maltophilia in the Imi group. X. maltophilia was not identified as a primary causative organism during the trial period. Because of its known resistance to Imi, as well as to cefuroxime and tobramycin, and its known ability to colonize hospitalized patients (22, 23), we evaluated the surveillance cultures during the study period. At the start, 3% of patients

Table IV. *In vitro susceptibility of isolated micro-organisms (susceptible/total number of strains)*

Cef = Cefuroxime; Tobr = Tobramycin; Imi = Imipenem; Van = Vancomycin; Aztr = Aztreonam.

	Cef	Tobr	Imi	Van	Aztr
CNS	11/16	3/16	14/16	16/16	–
Streptococci spp.	15/15	0/15	15/15	15/15	–
Enterococcus faec.	0/4	0/4	4/4	4/4	–
Pseud. aeruginosa	0/2	2/2	2/2	–	2/2
E. coli	2/2	2/2	2/2	–	2/2

had one or more positive surveillance culture showing X. maltophilia, but ultimately X. maltophilia was seen in 7% of them. We were unable to prove infection with X. maltophilia in any of these patients, so this finding reflects the increase in colonization of patients with this microorganism. The fact that we have not seen more X. maltophilia bacteriaemia cases is probably because we rigorously performed the SDD regime to eradicate of Gram-negative pathogens from the gastrointestinal tract (24). When we took all 179 monitored episodes into account and undertook an intention-to-treat analysis, patients in the Imi group again responded better than the other group (56/94 vs 36/85, $p < 0.05$, RR = 1.39, 95% CI 1.03 to 1.88). This finding was supported by the fact that duration of fever (number of fever days per patient) was also found to be significantly shorter in the Imi group (median value: 4 days (range 1–33) vs 7 days (range 1–26), $p < 0.04$).

Susceptibility of isolated micro-organisms

The susceptibility of isolated organisms to the antibiotics used is given in Table IV.

Adverse events

Generally speaking, patients tolerated the treatment well; 5 in the Imi group had nausea but none in the combination group. We did not have to stop Imi treatment in any of the patients nor did we observe any seizures (14, 25). More renal disturbances were observed in the T/C group, 4, than in the Imi group, mainly in patients who received concomitant antifungal treatment. Liver function disturbances occurred in 1 patient in the Imi and in 3 in the combination group. Two patients in the monotherapy group developed rash. Side effects did not differ significantly between the groups.

DISCUSSION

This study aimed to answer questions about the possibility of imipenem monotherapy for patients with granulocytopenia and fever during the first 72 h and about the efficacy of subsequent treatment when initial therapy failed. On the first question, overall results at the 72 h assessment showed that imipenem is more efficacious than a combination of cefuroxime and tobramycin as empirical antibiotic treatment (44/75 vs 27/68, $p < 0.05$). The difference in the response rate was most pronounced in the patients whose fever episodes were classified as having bacteriologically proven infections, mainly caused by Gram-positive bacteria (14/27 vs 3/21, $p < 0.05$).

Several explanations for the evident differences are possible: first, tobramycin peak serum concentrations were, despite the loading dose, in the low normal range. The dosage was adjusted during further treatment and we did not find any statistical difference when peak concentrations of tobramycin were compared, between the responders and non-responders in the combination group. The second, and probably most significant explanation for the observed difference is the susceptibility of isolated micro-organisms to antibiotics. Most of them were Gram-positive (70%) and therefore their susceptibility to the initial antibiotics may have influenced the outcome of the infections (Table IV). In the subgroup of BDI, 5 CNS proved to be resistant in-vitro to cefuroxime and almost all (12) to tobramycin, while only 2 were found to be resistant to imipenem.

In the case of streptococci there were no differences in in-vitro susceptibility between cefuroxime and imipenem, but all were resistant to tobramycin. These results support the finding that response rate was lower in the combination group, as is the fact that the duration of fever in each patient was longer in the T/C group. On the other hand, this did not have any influence on the infection related mortality, since none of the patients with infection caused by resistant Gram-positive bacteria died of it. The only 2 patients with bacteraemia who died, did so as a result of infection with Gram-positive strains, 1 CNS and 1 Staphylococcus aureus, both of which were susceptible in vitro to cefuroxime and imipenem. After the initial 3-day treatment, both were given vancomycin and aztreonam, without success.

The recent study by Cornelissen et al. (12) also compared imipenem with a combination of antibiotic agents consisting of a second generation cephalosporin agent and an aminoglycoside. Their results showed a higher response rate than we found in both the mono- and the combination therapy. This was perhaps due to different definitions of the response. We used strict criteria to evaluate the response. Beside clinical and microbiological eradication of the infection, the patients with fever in our study had to show a return to normal temperature. Nevertheless, as in our study, empirical imipenem treatment had a better overall efficacy. As in our study, efficacy of imipenem was better mainly because of greater susceptibility. This was especially so in the bacteriologically proven infections which were caused mostly by Gram-positive bacteria.

The overall results of the imipenem therapy itself are also comparable to those of several other studies, especially if the response at 72 h is noted (4, 8, 10, 25). This was also the case in BDI: in our study, 60% of CNS and streptococcal infections responded after 72 h of imipenem therapy. Regarding the controversy over the susceptibility of imipenem to methicillin-resistant staphylococci (18, 26), our susceptibility data showed that most of the CNS isolates were susceptible in vitro to cloxacillin, this supporting the observation that a substantial part of the CNS bacteraemias responded to empirical imipenem therapy.

Evaluation of the subsequent treatment showed no differences between the groups after a total of 6 days of antibiotic therapy (53/75 vs 43/68, $p < 0.20$). The best response to V/A was seen in the T/C group in the case of BDI, while in other subgroups additional response to V/A was slightly lower. In the Imi group, most of the BDI responded after 72 h and only 30% of the failures responded to V/A. Thus if the patients fail to respond to imipenem after an initial 72 h of treatment, the addition of or a switch to a glycopeptide-containing combination therapy is in our opinion unnecessary if clinical and microbiological circumstances have not changed. Rolston et al. (4) came to the same conclusion in their study where addition of vancomycin in failures after 48 h of initial imipenem treatment was seen as premature. Controversy still exists, however, over the exact role of glycopeptide treatment in the management of febrile patients with granulocytopenia (27). For example, in contrast to our study, some authors advocate immediate empirical glycopeptide therapy (28, 29). The potential benefit in both studies was found to be a reduced morbidity from Gram-positive infections, and even a reduced need for empirical use of toxic amphotericin-B (27). However, the largest study performed on this point (30) showed no differences between the treatment regimens (with vs without vancomycin) in the proportion of febrile patients on each trial day or in the duration of patients' fever. One drawback was vancomycin-associated toxicity which was more frequent in this group, but most importantly there was no mortality due to Gram-positive bacteraemia during the first 3 days of true empirical therapy. This finding seems to be supported by the results of our study. Most of the Gram-positive infections responded to empirical treatment with imipenem, while in the combination group, despite the resistance of most of the isolated micro-organisms to one of the given combination antibiotics, no increase in infection related mortality was seen.

Patients tolerated both antibiotic regimens well. Despite high doses of Imi, we did not observe any serious neurological disturbances or seizures (31). This was probably due to the very low incidence of renal toxicity in the Imi group and the fact that no patient had any (recorded) neurological abnormality before the Imi treatment. Superinfections, especially fungal ones, were relatively common in both groups. A possible reason for the occurrence of filamentous fungal superinfections was that most of our patients were treated in rooms not equipped with laminar air flow, while construction works were under way in the immediate surroundings of the haematology ward. This is a known risk factor in the occurrence of fungal infections (32).

In conclusion, empirical therapy with imipenem proved to be more efficacious than treatment with cefuroxime and tobramycin in patients with manifest and protracted granulocytopenia and predominantly Gram-positive infections. This finding is based mainly on the better response of patients with bacteriologically documented infections. Subsequent treatment of these patients with vancomycin and aztreonam, given when initial treatment had failed at the 72 h assessment, showed a response in a minority of these failures. We confirm the observation that there seems to be no need for immediate glycopeptide treatment in case of confirmed Gram-positive infection if the microorganisms responsible are susceptible to the given empirical therapy (30). The combination of a second generation cephalosporin and an aminoglycoside is not to be recommended as empirical therapy for granulocytopenic patients with predominantly Gram-positive infections.

ACKNOWLEDGEMENTS

The authors thank Dr E. Wattel and Dr W. J. Sluiter for their statistical assistance. This study was performed with financial support from Merck, Sharp & Dohme.

REFERENCES

1. Bodey GP, Buckley M, Sathe YS, Freireich EJ. Quantitative relationships between circulating leucocytes and infection in patients with acute leukaemia. Ann Intern Med 64: 328–340, 1966.
2. Hughes WT, Armstrong D, Bodey GP, Feld R, Mandell GL, Meyers JD, Pizzo PA, Schimpf SC, Shenep JL, Wade JC, Young LS, Yow MD. Guidelines for the use of antimicrobial agents in neutropenic patients with unexplained fever. J Infect Dis 161: 381–396, 1990.
3. Pizzo PA, Hathorn JW, Hiemenz J, Browne M, Commers J, Cotton, D. A randomized trial comparing ceftazidime alone with combination antibiotic therapy in cancer patients with fever and neutropenia. N Engl J Med 315: 552–555, 1986.
4. Rolston KV, Berkey P, Bodey GP, Anaissie EJ, Khardori NM, Joshi JH, Keating MJ, Holmes FA, Cabanillas FF, Elting L. A comparison of imipenem to ceftazidime with or without amikacin as empiric therapy in febrile neutropenic patients. Arch Intern Med 152: 283–291, 1992.
5. Klastersky J, Zinner SH. Synergistic combinations of antibiotics in Gram-negative bacillary infections. Rev Infect Dis 4: 294–301, 1982.
6. Meyer RD. Risk factors and comparisons of clinical nephrotoxicity of aminoglycosides. Am J Med 80 (Suppl 6B): 119–125, 1986.
7. Norrby SR, Vandercam B, Louie T, Runde V, Norberg B, Anniko M, Andrien F, Baudrihate M, Bow E, Burman LA, Bury J, Ezzedine H, Gigi J, Granlund M, Holm J, Lundberg S, Michaux JL,

Le Saux N, Wahlin A, Zakrisson E. Imipenem/cilastatin versus amikacin plus piperacillin the treatment of infections in neutropenic patients: a prospective, randomized multi-clinic study. Scand J Infect Dis Suppl 52: 65–78, 1987.
8. Leyland MJ, Bayston KF, Cohen J, Warren R, Newland AC, Bint AT, Cefai C, White DG, Murray SA, Barefood D, Deaney NB. A comparative study of imipenem versus piperacillin plus gentamicin in the initial management of febrile neutropenic patients with haematological malignancies. J Antimicrob Chemother 30: 843–854, 1992.
9. Liang R, Yung PY, Chau TK, Chan WK, Lam SY, So SY, Imipenem/cilastatin as initial therapy for febrile neutropenic patients. J Antimicrob Chemother 22: 765–770, 1988.
10. Liang R, Yung R, Chiu E, Chau P, Chan T, Lam W, Todd D. Ceftazidime versus Imipenem-cilastatin as initial monotherapy for febrile neutropenic patients. Antimicrob Agents Chemother 34: 1136–1134, 1990.
11. Novakova IR, Donnelly JP, de Pauw BE. Amikacin plus piperacillin versus ceftazidime as initial therapy in granulocytopenic patients with presumed bacteremia. Scand J Infect Dis 22: 705–711, 1990.
12. Cornelissen JJ, De Graeff A, Verdonck LF, Branger T, Rozenberg-Arska M, Verhoef J, Dekker AW. Imipenem versus gentamicin combined with either cefuroxime or cephalotin as initial therapy for febrile neutropenic patients. Antimicrob Agents Chemother 36: 801–807, 1992.
13. EORTC International Antimicrobial Therapy Cooperative Group. Ceftazidime combined with a short or long course of amikacin for empirical therapy of Gram-negative bacteraemia in cancer patients with granulocytopenia. N Engl J Med 317: 1692–1698, 1987.
14. Winston DJ, Ho WG, Bruckner DA, Champlin RE. Beta-lactam antibiotic therapy in febrile granulocytopenic patients. Ann Intern Med 115: 849–859, 1991.
15. Viscoli C, Van der Auwera P, Meunier F. Gram-positive infections in granulocytopenic patients: an important issue? J Antimicrob Chemother 21 (Suppl C): 149–156, 1988.
16. Johansson PJH, Sternby E, Ursing B. Septicaemia in granulocytopenic patients: a shift in bacterial etiology. Scand J Infect Dis 24: 357–360, 1992.
17. Donnelly JP, Maschmeyer E, Daenen S. Selective oral antimicrobial prophylaxis for the prevention of infection in acute leukaemia – Ciprofloxacin versus co-trimoxazole plus colistin. Eur J Cancer 28A: 873–878, 1992.
18. May G. Topics in clinical pharmacology: imipenem, a new broad spectrum antibiotic. Am J Med 296: 289–290, 1988.
19. Clissold SP, Todd PA, Campoli-Richards DM. Imipenem/Cilastatin – a review of its antibacterial activity, pharmacokinetic properties and therapeutic efficacy. Drugs 33: 183–241, 1987.
20. Immunocompromised Host Society. The design, analysis, and reporting of clinical trials on the empirical antibiotic management of the neutropenic patient. J Infect Dis 161: 397–401, 1990.
21. Klastersky J, Zinner SH, Calandra T, Gaya H, Glauser MP, Meunier F, Rossi M, Schimpf SC, Tatersall M, Viscoli C, and EORTC. Empiric antimicrobial therapy for febrile granulocytopenic cancer patients: lessons from four EORTC trials. Eur J Cancer Clin Oncol 24 (Suppl 1): S35–S45, 1988.
22. Morrison AJ, Hoffman KK, Wenzel RP. Associated mortality and clinical characteristics of nosocomial Pseudomonas maltophilia in a university hospital. J Clin Microbiol 24: 52–55, 1986.
23. Schoch PE, Cumha BA. Topics in clinical microbiology. Pseudomonas maltophilia. Infect Control 8: 169–172, 1987.
24. De Vries-Hospers HG, Sleijfer DT, Mulder NH, van der Waaij D, Nieweg HO, van Saene HK. Bacteriological aspects of selective decontamination of the digestive tract as a method of infection prevention in granulocytopenic patients. Antimicrob Agents Chemother 19: 813–820, 1981.
25. Bodey GP, Alverez ME, Jones PG, Rolston VI, Steelhamer L, Fainstein V. Imipenem-cilastatin as initial therapy for febrile cancer patients. Antimicrob Agents Chemother 30: 211–214, 1986.
26. Fan W, Del Busto R, Love M, Markowitz N, Cendrowski C, Cardenas J, Imipenem-cilastatin in the treatment of methicillin-sensitive and methicillin-resistant Staphylococcus aureus infections. Antimicrob Agents Chemother 29: 26–29, 1986.
27. Menichetti F, Del Favero A. The role of Gram-positive therapy in the neutropenic patient. J Antimicrob Chemother 27 (Suppl B): 51–60, 1991.
28. Karp JE, Dick JD, Angelopulos CP, Charache P, Green L, Burke PJ, Saral R. Empiric use of vancomycin during prolonged treatment induced granulocytopenia: randomized, double-blinded, placebo-controlled clinical trial in patients with acute leukaemia. Am J Med 81: 237–242, 1986.

29. Shenep J, Hughes W, Roberson P, Blankenship J, Baker D, Meyer W, Gigliotti F, Sixbey JW, Santana VM, Feldman S, Lott L. Vancomycin, ticarcillin and amikacin compared with ticarcillin-clavulanate and amikacin in the empirical treatment of febrile neutropenic children with cancer. N Engl J Med 319: 1053–1058, 1988.
30. EORTC and National Cancer Institute of Canada. Vancomycin added to empirical combination antibiotic therapy for fever in granulocytopenic cancer patients. J Infect Dis 163: 951–958, 1991.
31. Calandra G, Lydick E, Carrigan J, Weiss L, Guess H. Factors predisposing to seizures in seriously ill infected patients receiving antibiotics. Experience with imipenem/cilastatin. Am J Med 84: 914–918, 1988.
32. Dewhurst AG, Cooper MJ, Khan SM, Palett AP, Dathan JR. Invasive aspergillosis in immunosuppressed patients: potential hazard of hospital building work. BMJ 381: 801–804, 1990.

Submitted February 18, 1994; accepted April 20, 1994

Scand J Infect Dis 26: 599–604, 1994

Epidemiology of Toxic Shock Syndrome Toxin-1 Production in Staphylococcus aureus Strains Isolated in Denmark between 1959 and 1990

TOVE EJLERTSEN[1], ANNETTE JENSEN[1], ANNE LESTER[1] and VIBEKE THAMDRUP ROSDAHL[2]

From the [1]Department of Clinical Microbiology and [2]Division of Preventive Microbiology, Statens Seruminstitut, Copenhagen, Denmark

A total of 436 Staphylococcus aureus bacteremia strains isolated between 1959 and 1990 were tested for the production of toxic shock syndrome toxin-1 (TSST-1) by a semiquantitative reversed passive latex agglutination test. TSST-1 production was found in 147/260 (57%) of phage group I strains, excluding the "80" complex, and in 17/176 (10%) of non-group I strains. Strains of the 52, 52A, 80, 81 complex ("80" complex), constituting a subgroup of group I, did not have the same high frequency of TSST-1 production as the rest of group I strains (4% versus 57%). The "80" complex has almost disappeared in Denmark. TSST-1 production was found with the same high frequency among group I strains from the beginning (1959) and throughout the observation period. The TSST-1 production was associated with the phages 29 and/or 52, which in turn lysed 95% of group I strains. The TSST-1 production was quantitatively greater in the phage group I strains than in the non-group I strains. TSST-1 production of the bacteremia strains was not correlated to the clinical parameters: mortality, age, gender, bacterial focus, underlying diseases, or whether the infection was hospital or community acquired.

T. Ejlertsen, MD, Department of Clinical Microbiology, Aalborg Hospital, DK-9000 Aalborg, Denmark

INTRODUCTION

Toxic shock syndrome (TSS) was first described by Todd et al. in 1978 (1). In the literature they found similar sporadically reported cases in 1927, 1942, and 1960. A toxin produced by Staphylococcus aureus was suspected. In 1981, enterotoxin F (2) and pyrogenic exotoxin C (3) were described independently. The 2 exoproteins proved identical and were thereafter called Toxic Shock Syndrome Toxin 1 (TSST-1) (4, 5). TSST-1 is produced by more than 90% of S. aureus strains isolated from patients with menstruation associated TSS (2, 3, 6, 7). In S. aureus strains isolated from patients with non-menstrual TSS, the prevalence of TSST-1 production has been only 50–60% (8). TSST-1 was observed to be associated with phage group I staphylococci (1), and further investigations pointed to a close relation to S. aureus strains of phage-types 29, 52 and 29/52 (6, 9–11). Investigations concerning when and how TSST-1 production was introduced in the S. aureus population have only given rather inconclusive results due to the lack of representative S. aureus material. Altemeier et al. (12) found that strains typed with phage 29 and/or 52 occurred throughout the period 1960–80 but with an increased incidence around 1970; toxin production was, however, not detected before 1970 and they therefore concluded that acquisition of the toxic shock toxin gene took place in the early 1970s. Hayes et al. (11) tested a random sample of 281 strains from the years 1956–82 and found toxin-producing strains as early as 1957 and an increase in TSST-1 production around 1976.

In Denmark, centralized phage-typing since 1959 and the collection and storage of all blood isolates have enabled us to follow closely the changing S. aureus epidemiology, as blood isolates have been shown to represent the total S. aureus population. In the present study a representative selection of strains from the period 1959–90 have been analysed for TSST-1 production in order to establish the possible time of introduction of TSST-1 producing strains and the occurrence of these strains among isolates not directly related to TSS patients. The material has been supplemented by further strains of group I in order to analyse in greater detail the proposed correlation between 29 and 52. Correlation of TSST-1 production to a few clinical data has also been investigated.

MATERIALS AND METHODS

S. aureus isolates and epidemiological information

Since 1957 the Staphylococcus Reference Laboratory has performed centralized phage-typing for the whole of Denmark, receiving annually approximately 27,000 isolates from 18,000 patients. Since 1960 data on 1 strain per patient per year have been collected, including also phage-type pattern and site of isolation on the patient, e.g. vagina. None of the normal vaginal strains has been stored, but strains from TSS patients have been kept together with clinical information.

Since 1957 all bacteremia strains isolated from patients from the whole of Denmark have been collected and stored with clinical information (13).

None of the bacteremia strains included in this investigation were isolated from patients with recognized toxic shock syndrome. From the years 1960, 1965, 1970, 1975, 1980, 1985, and 1990, 2 × 25 bacteremia strains (25 from surviving patients and 25 from non-surviving patients) were selected, 15 representing the annual phage-type distribution and 10 additional strains from group I without the "80" complex. Each strain in the bacteremia material is given a number, and the 2 × 25 strains were picked for each year, taking the first number of the phage-type wanted; no other selection criteria except mortality were used. In 1960 and 1965 the small number of strains available allowed fewer than 2 × 10 additional group I strains to be investigated. Therefore 124 additional group I strains from the years 1959, 1961–64, and 1966–69 were investigated.

Phage-typing was performed as described previously (7). Strains of the "80" complex included strains typed with phage 80 and/or 81 and a combination of phages 52 and/or 52A with 80 and/or 81. The "80" complex is part of group I which include strains reacting with phages 29, 52, 52A, 79, and 80, alone or in combination. In the present report, S. aureus strains have been divided into strains belonging to the "80" complex and strains belonging to the rest of group I without the "80" complex.

Detection of TSST-1

The strains were tested for production of TSST-1 by means of a semiquantitative reversed passive latex agglutination kit (Oxoid^{R}) using the procedure recommended by the manufacturer. This test has been evaluated in our laboratory previously and was found to have a sensitivity of 0.94 and a specificity of 0.92 for vaginal strains isolated from patients with TSS (7). The test was performed with serial dilutions of overnight broth-culture filtrates in seven wells, from undiluted 1/1 to dilution 1/64. Reactions in the first 2 wells were regarded as positive. A positive reaction in dilution 1/8 or higher was regarded as a strong reaction indicative of a high TSST-1 production.

Statistical analysis

The χ^2-test was used to calculate significant differences between various groups.

RESULTS

Occurrence of group I strains

Fig. 1 shows the occurrence of S. aureus strains of "80" complex and rest group I in bacteremia strains and in strains isolated from all body sites. Since 1970, strains of the "80" complex have nearly disappeared, and the decline in frequency has occurred equally in the material of blood isolates and isolates from all body sites. The frequency of rest group I strains has remained fairly constant, between 12% and 18% of the total S. aureus population. The phage pattern frequencies of S. aureus strains isolated from vagina have been recorded since 1970. From 1970 to 1985 the frequency of rest group I strains was equal in the vaginal strains, the bacteremia strains, and the whole material (Fig. 1). Since 1986 the frequency of rest group I strains in vagina has fallen, but the difference is not statistically significant.

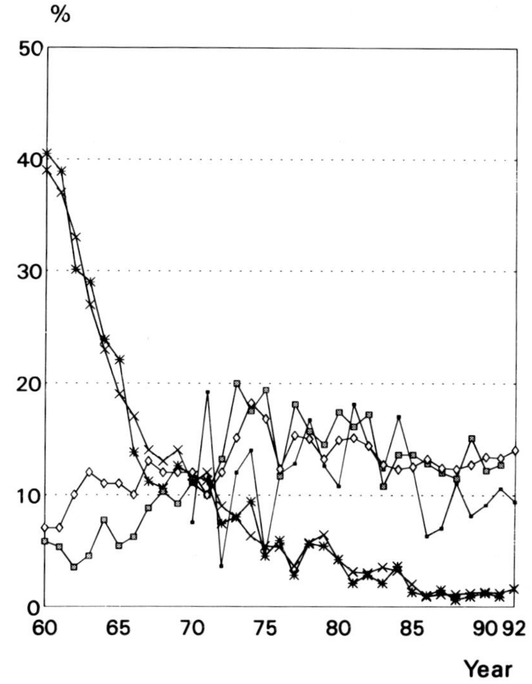

Fig. 1. Frequency of S. aureus group I strains (—◇—) and group "80" strains (—×—) in % of all S. aureus strains isolated from 1960 to 1992. Frequency of S. aureus group I strains (—■—) and group "80" strains (—*—) isolated from the blood in % of all bacteremia strains, and finally frequency of S. aureus group I strains isolated from vagina (—●—) in % of all strains isolated from the vagina.

Occurrence of TSST-1 production

436 strains were tested for TSST-1 production, 200 selected to represent the distribution of the phage-type patterns in the years investigated, supplemented with a further 236 strains of group I (Table I and Material and Methods). Altogether 164 strains were found to be producing TSST-1. The prevalence of TSST-1 production was unevenly distributed between the phage groups with the highest frequency in phage group I (56.6%), the "80" complex

Table I. *Toxic shock syndrome toxin 1 (TSST-1) production in S. aureus bacteremia strains isolated in the period 1959–69, and 1970, 1975, 1980, 1985, and 1990*

NI = Miscellaneous isolates, NT = Non-typable isolates.

Phage-type patterns of all bacteremia strains submitted in the periods investigated			S. aureus strains tested for TSST-1 production	TSST-1 positive S. aureus strains	
Phage-type pattern	No.	(%)	*n*	*n*	(%)
"80" complex	1,257	(7.0)	23	1	(4.3)
Group I	2,291	(12.9)	260[a]	147	(56.6)
Group II	2,391	(13.5)	28	2	(7.1)
Group III	3,198	(18.0)	36	3	(8.3)
83A complex	2,597	(14.6)	36	4	(11.1)
94/96 complex	2,028	(11.4)	19	2	(10.5)
Type 95	1,603	(9.0)	13	0	(0.0)
NI	1,379	(7.7)	13	3	(23.1)
NT	967	(5.4)	8	2	(25.0)
Total	17,711		436	164	

[a] See Table II.

excluded. In the "80" complex, only one strain (4.3%) produced TSST-1. The lowest frequency was found in phage-type 95 (0%). The overall frequency of TSST-1 production, excluding phage group I, was 9.7% (Table II). TSST-1 production was found from the first year tested and throughout the period. In phage group I the prevalence of TSST-1 production was evenly distributed throughout the period tested (Table II). In the other phage groups a small but significant increase in frequency of TSST-1 production was seen in the years 1970 and 1975 ($p = 0.02$).

The association between lysis by the phages 29 and 52 and TSST-1 production is shown in Table III.

The TSST-1 detection method included testing of different dilutions of the broth filtrates, allowing a semiquantitative determination of the amount of toxin produced. High titres of

Table II. *TSST-1 production in S. aureus bacteremia strains in relation to year of isolation from patients not suffering from TSS*

	Phage group I, "80" complex excluded			Other phage groups		
Isolation year	No. of strains tested	No. of strains with TSST-1	(%)	No. of strains tested	No. of strains with TSST-1	(%)
1959	11	5	(45.5)	0		–
1960–64	46	21	(45.7)	24	2	(8.3)
1965–69	83	46	(55.4)	29	1	(3.5)
1970	24	15	(62.5)	24	5	(20.8)[a]
1975	24	13	(54.2)	23	4	(17.4)[a]
1980	24	17	(70.8)	26	1	(3.9)
1985	24	13	(54.2)	24	2	(8.3)
1990	24	17	(70.8)	26	2	(7.7)
1959–90	260	147	(56.6)	176	17	(9.7)[b]

[a] $p = 0.02$. Prevalence of TSST-1 production in non-group I S. aureus strains in 1970 + 1975 compared with TSST-1 production in non-group I S. aureus strains in the rest of the period tests.
[b] $p < 0.005$. Prevalence of TSST-1 production in phage group I S. aureus strains compared with non-group I S. aureus strains in the whole period tested.

Table III. *TSST-1 production in S. aureus phage group I in relation to phage types 29, 52, and 29/52, "80" complex excluded*

Phage group I Phage type(s)	Total no. of group I strains in the years investigated (% of whole group I) N	(%)	No. of strains tested (% of group I) n	(%)	No. of strains with TSST-1 production (% of TSST-1 producing group I strains) n	(%)
29	175	(23.8)	63	(24.2)	39	(26.5)
52	139	(18.9)	51	(19.6)	24	(16.3)
29/52	141	(19.2)	68	(26.2)	47	(32.0)
29 and/or 52[a]	227	(30.8)	65	(25.0)	36	(24.5)
No 29 or 52	54	(7.3)	13	(5.0)	1	(0.7)
	736	(100)	260	(100)	147	(100)

[a] Plus other phage types in phage group L.

TSST-1 production were found in 138/147 (94%) of the TSST-1-positive phage group I strains, whereas high titres of TSST-1 production were found in only 8/17 (47%) of the TSST-1-negative non-group I strains of different phage patterns.

Occurrence of TSS

Notification of TSS has been obligatory in Denmark since 1981. 57 cases have occurred, varying between 2 and 8 cases per year in the period 1981–92. In 41 cases an S. aureus strain was isolated; 25 (61%) belonged to group I, 8 were non-typable and 8 belonged to other phage-type patterns.

Correlation between clinical data and TSST-1 production

No significant differences in frequency or quantity of TSST-1 production were found between the strains from bacteremic patients who died, compared with surviving patients. TSST-1 production was correlated neither to gender, to specific age groups, focus, nor underlying diseases. Nor was it related to whether the infection was hospital- or community-acquired.

DISCUSSION

The present study investigated production of TSST-1 among the normal S. aureus population represented by bacteremia strains as early as from 1959. Like Hayes et al. (11) we found toxin production as far back as could be tested. The investigation showed that a fairly constant frequency of TSST-1 production has occurred in Denmark through all 30 years in non-TSS related S. aureus strains.

The strong correlation of TSST-1 production to phage group I and phage-types 29, 52 and 29/52, as found by Hayes et al. (11) and Altemeier et al. (12), was confirmed in this study. In our investigation we have demonstrated that strains of phage-types 29, 52 and 29/52 were a completely predominant part of the phage group I, being present in 92.7% of all group I strains isolated from blood in the period investigated, "80" complex excluded. Only strains of the specific type 29/52 occurred with a significantly increased frequency among the TSST-1 producing strains, while among the few group I strains not typable with 29 and/or 52, only 8% produced TSST-1 toxin (1 of 13 strains).

Strains of the "80" complex were, according to our results, different from the other group I strains, as they only produced TSST-1 at a very low frequency. Furthermore, during the investigation period the "80" complex almost disappeared from Danish isolates. The present results thus suggest that these strains formed a distinct part of the group I strains. In addition to the association between phage group I and TSST-1 production, the phage group I strains showed a quantitatively greater production of TSST-1 than did the non-group I strains.

REFERENCES

1. Todd J, Fishaut M, Kapral F, Welch T. Toxic-shock syndrome associated with Phage-Group-I staphylococci. Lancet 2: 1116–1118, 1978.
2. Bergdoll MS, Crass BA, Reiser RF, Robbins BA, Davis JP. A new staphylococcal enterotoxin, enterotoxin F, associated with toxic-shock-syndrome staphylococcus aureus isolates. Lancet 2: 1017–1021, 1981.
3. Schlievert PM, Shands KN, Dan BB, Schmid GP, Nishimura RD. Identification and characterization of an exotoxin from Staphylococcus aureus associated with toxic-shock syndrome. J Infect Dis 143: 509–516, 1981.
4. Cohen ML, Graves LM, Hayes PS, Gibson RJ, Rasheed K, Feeley JC. Toxic shock syndrome: modification and comparison of methods for detecting marker proteins in Staphylococcus aureus. J Clin Microbiol 18: 372–375, 1983.

5. Staneck JL, Bonventre PF. Toxic shock syndrome: a microbiological perspective. Surv Synth Path Res 3: 38–53, 1984.
6. De Saxe MJ, Hawtin P, Wieneke AA. Toxic shock syndrome in Britain – epidemiology and microbiology. Postgrad Med J 61: 5–21, 1985.
7. Espersen F, Bæk L, Kjældgaard P, Rosdahl VT. Detection of staphylococcal toxic shock syndrome toxin 1 by a latex agglutination kit. Scand J Infect Dis 20: 449–450, 1988.
8. Garbe PL, Arko RJ, Reingold AL, Graves LM, Hayes LM, Hightower AW, Chandler FW, Broome CV. Staphylococcus aureus isolates from patients with non-menstrual toxic shock syndrome. Evidence for additional toxins. JAMA 253: 2538–2542, 1985.
9. Christensson B, Hedström S-Å. Biochemical and biological properties of Staphylococcus aureus septicemia strains in relation to clinical characteristics. Scand J Infect Dis 18: 298–303, 1986.
10. Altemeier WA, Lewis SA, Bjornson HS, Staneck JL, Schlievert PM. Staphylococcus in toxic shock syndrome and other surgical infections. Arch Surg 118: 281–284, 1983.
11. Hayes PS, Graves LM, Feeley JC, Hancock GA, Cohen ML, Reingold AL, Broome CV, Hightower AW. Production of toxic-shock-associated protein(s) in Staphylococcus aureus strains isolated from 1956 through 1982. J Clin Microbiol 20: 43–46, 1984.
12. Altemeier WA, Lewis SA, Schlievert PM, Bergdoll MS, Bjornson HS, Staneck JL, Crass BA. Staphylococcus aureus associated with toxic shock syndrome. Ann Intern Med 96: 978–982, 1982.
13. Rosendal K, Jessen O, Faber V, Bentzon MW. Frequency, phage types and antibiotic resistance of Staphylococcus aureus isolated from blood cultures in Denmark 1975–1981. Scand J Infect Dis Suppl 41: 19–26, 1983.

Submitted November 1, 1993; accepted June 6, 1994

Scand J Infect Dis 26: 605–609, 1994

Bacteremia in Patients Without Known Underlying Disorders

MIRIT AMIT[1], SILVIO D. PITLIK[2], ZMIRA SAMRA[3], HANNA KONISBERGER[2], MOSHE DRUCKER[2] and LEONARD LEIBOVICI[1]

From the [1]Department of Medicine B, the [2]Infectious Disease Unit and the [3]Microbiology Laboratory, Beilinson Medical Center and Basil & Gerald Felsenstein Medical Research Center, Petah Tiqva; and the Sackler Faculty of Medicine, University of Tel Aviv, Ramat Aviv, Israel

Of 2030 consecutive patients with bacteremia, only 102 were free from underlying disorders. 43 were males, and the median age was 66 years. The sources of infection were the urinary tract (in 48%), lower respiratory tract (13%), endocarditis (7%), biliary tract (6%) and the meninges (5%). The most common pathogens were Escherichia coli (in 45% of patients), Streptococcus pneumoniae (21%), Staphylococcus aureus (9%) and hemolytic streptococci (9%). Overall mortality rate was 13%, 4% in patients with urinary tract infection and 19% in patients with other sources. Half of the deaths occurred within 2 days of hospitalization, and 75% of them within 4 days. All patients with septic shock and all patients with meningitis died. Other factors related to mortality were residence in a nursing home, low functional capacity, advanced age, high blood urea nitrogen and creatinine and low albumin, and infections caused by Staphylococcus aureus, Neisseria meningitidis and polymicrobial infections. A protective effect of appropriate antimicrobial antibiotic therapy could not be demonstrated. In conclusion, bacteremic patients with no known underlying disorder and source of their infection other than the urinary tract should be given maximum supportive treatment and should be closely watched.

L. Leibovici, MD, Department of Medicine B, Beilinson Medical Center, 49 100 Petah Tiqva, Israel

INTRODUCTION

Most episodes of bacteremia nowadays occur in patients with underlying disorders predisposing to infection (1–3). Few patients with bacteremia have no recognizable underlying disease (3).

Mortality from bacteremia is substantial, ranging from 20% to 30% (1, 2, 4, 5). The outcome is determined by the virulence of the infecting microorganism, the integrity of the host defence mechanisms and the efficacy of the antimicrobial and supportive therapy (6–10). In the present study we prospectively surveyed all episodes of community acquired bacteremia in adults with no underlying disease, detected during 42 months at 1 hospital. The objectives of the study were to describe the clinical features, pathogens, treatment and outcome in a group of bacteremic patients without any known underlying disorder, in whom the main prognostic determinant is probably the virulence of the infecting microorganism.

PATIENTS AND METHODS

Patients

Included in the study were all adult patients, ≥18 years old, with community acquired bacteremia but without any known underlying disease, detected between March 1988 and August 1992 at The Beilinson Medical Center.

Patients were excluded from this study if they were known to be suffering from solid or hematological neoplastic diseases (solid malignancies one year or more after resection, and without evidence of recurrence were defined as 'cured'), atherosclerotic or valvular heart diseases, congestive heart failure, cerebrovascular diseases (patients ≥6 months after a cerebrovascular accident with no or minimal incapacitating residua were defined as 'cured'), hypertension, acute or chronic renal failure, diabetes mellitus, obstructive lung disease, trauma, major surgery or burns during the month before admission, liver diseases, severe dementia, bed sores, neurological disorders affecting functional state, invasive diagnostic procedures, blood or blood products transfusion, hyperalimentation or placement of a central venous line during the month before admission, urinary indwelling catheter, acute intoxication, thyroid diseases, inflammatory bowel disease, autoimmune disorders, immunodeficiency or suppression states, corticosteroid treatment for more than one day during the month before admission, drug abuse, hemoglobinopathies and skin diseases predisposing to skin infections. The episodes were detected by daily surveillance of the microbiology laboratory records. The Beilinson Medical Center is a 900-bed university hospital serving an urban population of 250,000 as a first-line facility. It is also a referral center for several hospitals in the vicinity.

Clinical and laboratory data

Data were collected from the patients' charts and the attending physicians during hospital stay and afterwards, as previously described (7, 10).

Blood cultures

A 10-ml volume of venous blood was obtained aseptically and inoculated into a two-bottle set (6B aerobic and 7D anerobic tryptic soy broth; Johnson Laboratories, Towson, MD, USA). The bottles were incubated and tested as described elsewhere (7, 10). The median number of sets obtained during one bacteremia episode was three, with a range 1–8. Microorganisms were identified by standard methods.

Organisms that are commonly recovered from the environment or the skin were judged to be contaminants unless the clinical findings, the results of cultures of material from other body sites, or the number of positive sets (≥ 2) indicated a high probability of true bloodstream infection.

Definitions

An episode was defined as **bacteremia** if positive and uncontaminated blood cultures were obtained in a case of fever >38.2°C or hypothermia <36.2°C, or septic shock (as defined below), or evidence of localized infection, or a toxic appearance.

An episode of bacteremia was defined as **community acquired** if detected within 48 h of admission to the hospital.

Empirical antimicrobial treatment was considered appropriate if the infecting microorganism was subsequently found to be susceptible in vitro to the drug administered, and if that antimicrobial drug was given intravenously during the 24 h after the first positive blood culture was taken.

Septic shock was defined as systolic blood pressure of <90 mmHg and evidence of organ hypoperfusion or disseminated intravascular coagulopathy (7). A score of 0–3 was used to define the patients **functional class**: 0, bedridden; 1, needing assistance for most daily life activities; 2, restricted activity, does not leave home; 3, full function. The **state of consciousness** was defined as: 0, deep coma; 1, coma with reaction to noxious stimuli; 2, stupor; 3, full consciousness.

Data analysis

For statistical analysis of contingency table, the X^2-test or the Fisher exact test, as indicated, was used. As most of the continuous variables were not normally distributed, their values are reported as median and range, and the statistical significance of comparisons between two classes was tested with the Wilcoxon rank-sum test. As there were few deaths, we did not perform a multivariate analysis.

RESULTS

Clinical features

Of the 2,030 adult patients with bacteremia detected between March 1988 and August 1992 at The Beilinson Medical Center, 102 (5%) had no recognizable underlying disease. Of these patients, 43 were males. The median age was 66 years (range 19–100 years). 10 patients came from nursing homes. The majority of the patients (83%) were in functional class 3. 85 were admitted to the medical departments, 14 to the surgical department, 1 to the intensive care unit and 2 to the pediatric department. 19 patients (19%) had received antimicrobial therapy before admission. Sources of infection and pathogens are detailed in Table I.

Table I. *Source of the infection in 102 patients with bacteremia and no recognizable underlying disease*

LRTI = Lower respiratory tract infection; UTI = Urinary tract infection; Biliary = Biliary system; BE = Bacterial endocarditis; Mening. = Meningitis.

	Source of infection								
Pathogen	LRTI	UTI	Biliary	BE	Mening.	Soft tissue	Other	Unknown	Mortality (%)
Staph. aureus	1	1		1	1	2	1	2	3/9 (33%)
Hemolytic strept.	2			4		3			0/9 (0%)
Strept. Gr D			1	1					0/2 (0%)
Strept. pneumoniae	8				2	1			2/11 (10%)
Meningococcus					2				2/2 (100%)
Haemophilus sp.	1						1		0/2 (0%)
E. Coli		41	3					1	3/45 (7%)
Klebsiella sp.		1	1						0/2 (0%)
Pseudomonas sp.							1		0/1 (0%)
Shigella sp.							1		0/1 (0%)
Salmonella sp.							3		0/3 (0%)
Enterobacter sp.			1	1					0/2 (0%)
Other Gram-negative		2				1	1		1/4 (25%)
Brucella sp.							2		0/2 (0%)
Anaerobes			1				1		0/2 (0%)
Polymicrobial		1	1	1		2			2/5 (40%)
Total	12	46	8	8	5	9	11	3	13/102 (13%)

Septic shock

Septic shock occurred in 9 patients, of whom all died. Mortality from septic shock accounted for 69% of all mortality cases. The causative pathogens were Staphylococcus aureus in 1 patient, Streptococcus pneumonia in 1, meningococci in 2, Escherichia coli in 2, Proteus species in 1, anaerobes in 1 and polymicrobial in 1 patient.

Sources of infection were unknown in 2 of these patients, urinary tract infection (UTI) in 2, meningitis in 3, lower respiratory tract infection in 1 and soft tissue infection in 1 patient.

Mortality

13 of the 102 patients with no known underlying disease died. Half of the deaths occurred within 2 days of admission (range 1–14 days) and 75% occurred by the fourth day.

Staphyloccus aureus was responsible for 23% (3/13) of mortality cases. Streptococcus pneumoniae, meningococci, Escherichia coli and polymicrobial infection were each responsible for 15% (2/13) of mortality cases. The 2 bacteremia cases caused by meningococci were fatal.

Sources of infection associated with high mortality rates were meningitis (38% of all mortality cases; 100% mortality in meningitis) and unknown origin (23% of all mortality cases, 60% mortality in bacteremia of unknown origin). UTI was responsible for 15% (2/13) of fatalities but only 4% (2/46) patients with UTI died.

High rates of mortality occurred in patients from nursing homes (5/10, $p = 0.001$), in patients in functional classes 0–2 (7/17, $p = 0.001$), and in patients with consciousness score 0–1 (10/12, $p = 0.001$).

Other clinical and laboratory factors associated with higher mortality rates were age (median age of patients who survived was 63 years, vs. 77 years in those who died, $p = 0.04$), blood urea nitrogen (median value of 5.4 mmol/l in survivors vs. 10 mmol/l in those who died, $p = 0.01$), albumin level (median level 36 g/l in survivors, vs. 25 g/l in those who died, $p = 0.01$) and creatinine level (median value of 92.8 μmol/l in survivors vs. 123.8 μmol/l in those who died, $p = 0.01$). There was no difference in mortality rates between patients who received appropriate empirical antimicrobial therapy (11/82 patients, 13%) and those who received inappropriate empirical therapy (2/20 patients, 10%), relative risk of 0.96, 95% confidence interval 0.81–1.13. Appropriate antimicrobial therapy was initiated after a median of 3 days (range 3–35) from the onset of the febrile disease in patients who survived, and after a median of 1 day (range 0–7) from onset of disease in patients who died of bacteremia ($p = 0.1$).

DISCUSSION

Out of 2,030 consecutive patients with bacteremia seen at our hospital, only 102 (5%) had no recognizable underlying disorder, a lower percentage than described in other studies (1–3, 8, 9). The difference can be attributed in part to the strict definition of 'no underlying disorder' used in our survey. However, over the years the proportion of bacteremic patients with no underlying disorder has changed: it is lower in later (2, 3) than in early studies (9). Geerdes et al. (3) conducted four prospective 1-year studies of bacteremia between 1979 and 1989, and showed a decrease both in total numbers and in percentage of bacteremia in patients with no underlying disease, from 73 cases (33.2% of episodes) in 1979 to 16 (5.5%) in 1989.

The definition of 'patient without known underlying disorder' is somewhat arbitrary, as not all patients underwent a uniform work-up. However, it has clinical cohesion, as this is the extent of data available to the clinician after a careful anamnesis, physical examination and appropriate investigation. It is of interest to note that the proportion of our patients without underlying disorders was similar to that reported by Geerdes et al. in 1989 (3).

The sources of infection and pathogens in our patients were similar to those in all patients with community acquired bacteremia (1, 2, 7, 8, 10). The only significant difference was a higher proportion of Escherichia coli in patients with no underlying disorder, and a lower incidence of Klebsiella bacteremia.

The most interesting findings are those related to mortality. The gross fatality rate was 13%, but in patients with a source of bacteremia other than the urinary tract it reached 19%. All bacteremic patients with septic shock or meningitis died. Half of those who died did so within 2 days, and 75% within 4 days, while the median interval to death in our bacteremic patients with underlying disease was 8 days (7, 10). We could not demonstrate any difference in mortality between patients given appropriate vs. inappropriate empiric antibiotic treatment. Though the fatality rate was low, even at the upper limit of the 95% confidence interval, the relative risk for mortality in patients given inappropriate treatment was 1.13. The difference was highly significant in patients with underlying disorders (7, 9). Moreover, antibiotic treatment had been started earlier in the patients who died.

It is probable that some of our patients had an unrecognized underlying disorder: e.g. deficiency of complement components, gammaglobulins (total or sub-fractions), or functional asplenia.

In conclusion, the proportion of bacteremic patients with no known underlying disorder nowadays is small. However, those with a source of infection other than the urinary tract have a high mortality rate, and die early in the course of their disease. Patients with septic shock or meningitis are at extreme risk to die. A significant protective effect of appropriate empiric antibiotic treatment could not be shown. In such patients we should concentrate on optimal supportive treatment during the first days of disease, preferably in an intensive care unit, especially in the groups at high risk for a fatal outcome. Further study should address the question of unrecognized underlying disorders in these patients.

REFERENCES

1. Ispahani P, Pearson NJ, Greenwood D, An analysis of community and hospital-acquired bacteremia in a large teaching hospital in the United Kindgom. Q J Med 63: 427–440, 1987.
2. Rayner BL, Willcox PA. Community-acquired bacteremia: a prospective survey of 239 cases. Q J Med 69: 907–919, 1988.
3. Geerdes HF, Ziegler D, Lode H, Hund M, Loehr A, Fangmann W, Wagner J. Septicemia in 980 patients at a university hospital in Berlin: Prospective studies during 4 selected years between 1979 and 1989. Clin Infect Dis 15: 991–1002, 1992.
4. Kreger BE, Craven DE, McCabe WR. Gram-negative bacteremia. IV. Re-evaluation of clinical features and treatment in 612 patients. Am J Med 68: 344–356, 1980.
5. Gatell JM, Trilla A, Latorre X, Almela M, Mensa J, Moreno A, Miro JM, Martinez JA, Jimenez de Anta MT, Soriano E, Garcia San Miguel J. Nosocomial bacteremia in a large Spanish teaching hospital: analysis of factors influencing prognosis. Rev Infect Dis 10: 203–210, 1988.
6. McCabe WR, Jackson GG. Gram-negative bacteremia. I. Etiology and ecology. Arch Intern Med 110: 847–855, 1962.
7. Leibovici L, Konisberger H, Pitlik SD, Samra Z, Drucker M. Bacteremia and fungemia of unknown origin in adults. Clin Infect Dis 14: 436–443, 1992.
8. Eykyn SJ, Gransden WR, Phillips I. The causative organisms of septicemia and their epidemiology. J Antimicrob Chemother 25 (Suppl C): 41–48, 1990.
9. Weinstein MP, Murphy JR, Reller LB, Lichtenstein KA. The clinical significance of positive blood cultures: a comprehensive analysis of 500 episodes of bacteremia and fungemia in adults. II. Clinical observations, with special reference to factors influencing prognosis. Rev Infect Dis 5: 54–70, 1975.
10. Leibovici L, Samra Z, Konisberger H, Kalter-Leibovici O, Pitlik SD, Drucker M. Bacteremia in adult diabetic patients. Diabetes Care 14: 89–94, 1991.

Submitted March 7, 1994; accepted May 28, 1994

Scand J Infect Dis 26: 611–614, 1994

Cost-benefit Analysis of General Vaccination against Haemophilus influenzae type b in Sweden

BIRGER TROLLFORS

From the Department of Paediatrics, University of Göteborg, Göteborg, Sweden

A cost-benefit analysis of general vaccination of infants with a conjugated Haemophilus influenzae type b (HIB) vaccine was performed. Information on incidence and prognosis of HIB meningitis and acute epiglottitis in children was obtained from nation-wide retrospective studies covering the years 1981–83, when the birth rate was approximately 93,000 per year. The annual cost for hospitalization, neurologic and auditory sequelae and parents' absence from work amounted to 54 million Swedish crowns (SEK). A mean of 6 children died every year. Inclusion of value of lives lost added SEK 72 million to the cost of disease. With vaccine prices (≈SEK 125/dose) and birth rate (≈120,000 per year) prevailing in 1993, vaccine costs would be SEK 45 million, provided that 3 doses are sufficient to offer protection close to 100%. Other costs for vaccination, e.g. physicians' and nurses' time, needles and syringes, are negligible, since the vaccine can be given at the same time as other infant vaccinations at already existing Child Health Centres. In conclusion, general vaccination of infants against HIB is cost-effective, saves lives and reduces human suffering.

B. Trollfors, MD, PhD, Department of Paediatrics, Östra hospital, S-416 85 Göteborg, Sweden

INTRODUCTION

In Sweden, all children are offered vaccination against diphtheria, tetanus and polio at 3, 5 and 12 months of age and against measles, mumps and rubella at 18 months. The vaccines are given free of charge at Child Health Centres financed by the 25 county councils. Recommendations for vaccines to be offered free of charge and vaccination schedules are issued for the whole country by the National Board for Health and Welfare but the final decisions concerning the vaccination program and its financing are taken separately by the county councils.

In 1991 and 1992, 2 vaccines against Haemophilus influenzae type b (HIB) were licensed by the Medical Products Agency. In 1992 the National Board of Health and Welfare recommended that a HIB vaccine should be offered free of charge to all infants. However, several county councils were hesitant to allocate resources for a HIB vaccine, since they are considerably more expensive than the other vaccines used for infant vaccination. Therefore the following estimates of the cost to society of invasive HIB disease was performed.

MATERIAL AND METHODS

Information on incidence, case-fatality rate, days of hospitalization and severe neurologic sequelae were obtained from 2 nation-wide studies of HIB meningitis and acute epiglottitis covering the years 1981–83 (1, 2). There was an annual mean number of 157 cases of Haemophilus influenzae (HI) meningitis and 162 cases of acute epiglottitis in 0–14-year-old children. It was assumed in this study that all cases of HI meningitis and acute epiglottitis in children were caused by HIB, even though it is known that, rarely, other serotypes of HI can cause meningitis and other organisms that HIB can cause acute epiglottitis.

Data on frequency of auditory impairment (13%) and less severe neurologic sequelae (13%) after HIB meningitis were extrapolated from a study in the Göteborg region (Greater Gothenburg) (3).

All costs are calculated in Swedish crowns (SEK). Currently there are 8 crowns to $1 US and 12 crowns to £1 Sterling.

RESULTS AND DISCUSSION

Estimated costs attributable to HIB meningitis and acute epiglottitis in children are summarised in Table I.

The background to the estimates is as follows.

1. Mortality. Six children die of HIB disease every year. It is difficult to assign a certain sum of money to the value of a life lost. In 1 cost-benefit analysis of HIB vaccination, death was not included among costs (4), whereas one American study (5, 6) applied the sum of 1.875 million $US for the death of a child (1987). The Swedish Road Administration used a similar sum, SEK 12 million (1993), for the value of a life lost, regardless of age, when making analyses for investments to reduce road traffic accidents. However, in strict financial terms, the loss to society must be greater if a young healthy adult dies, when investment in education has been completed, than in the case of a small child who has not yet 'cost' much in investments, or an elderly person who has retired from work. The sum of SEK 12 million is used in this analysis, but costs for death are reported separate from other costs.

2. Hospitalization during acute disease. The cost for one day of hospitalization is estimated to SEK 4,000 per day, based on information from 10 departments of paediatrics and otorhinolaryngology. Costs for hospitalization of children with meningitis and acute epiglottitis are probably higher than the average cost of hospitalization of a child, but this has not been considered in this analysis.

3. Neurologic sequelae. The cost for care of a child with severe neurologic sequelae (combinations of severe mental retardation, para- or tetraplegia, blindness, convulsive disorders) at an institution is estimated to SEK 0.9 million per year (personal communication, Ass. Prof. Mårten Kyllerman, Annedalskliniken, Department of Paediatrics, Göteborg). The countrywide study (1) showed that about 2 children per year develop neurologic sequelae of such severity that chronic care at an institution or equivalent care in the home is necessary. It is not known for how long children with such severe neurologic damage survive. In this analysis, costs for 10 years per child have been included.

Furthermore, the study from Göteborg (3) shows that about 13% of children with HIB meningitis develop less severe neurologic sequelae (e.g. hydrocephalus, monoplegia, mental retardation, psychiatric disturbances). This would mean about 20 cases for the whole

Table I. *Estimated annual costs for children 0–14 years with HIB meningitis and acute epiglottitis*

1. Deaths: 6 children × SEK 12 million = SEK 72 million
2. Hospitalization during acute disease:
   2,500 days × SEK 4,000 = SEK 10 million
3. Neurologic sequelae:
   Long-term care at institution:
   2 children × 10 years × SEK 900,000 = SEK 18 million.
   Less severe sequelae:
   20 children × SEK 400,000 = SEK 8 million
4. Auditory impairment:
   20 children × SEK 750,000 = SEK 15 million
5. Parents' absense from work due to care of child with:
   Meningitis: 3,300 days × SEK 600 = SEK 2 million
   Epiglottitis: 1,100 days × SEK 600 = SEK 0.7 million
   Death or severe brain damage:
   1,400 days × SEK 600 = SEK 0.8 million

country. A study from the USA estimated a cost of $50,000 per child (1985) for this type of neurologic sequela (6). In the absence of Swedish estimates, this figure has been used arbitrarily for the present calculation.

4. *Auditory impairment.* Auditory impairment following HIB meningitis can vary from slight unilateral to profound bilateral (3). Total costs for education of a deaf child are estimated to SEK 2.25 million during childhood and adolescence (personal communication, Prof. Ulf Rosenhall, Department of Audiology, Karolinska Hospital, Stockholm). An average cost of SEK 0.75 million per child with auditory impairment, irrespective of degree, has been used in the analysis in order to avoid overestimation of disease-induced costs.

5. *Absence from work* costs SEK 600 per day estimated from a mean monthly income of SEK 13,000 plus 40% employers' taxes (7). It has not been studied for how long parents of children with HIB infections are absent from work. Based on personal experience the following conservative estimate was made. Children with HIB meningitis: 3 weeks; with acute epiglottitis: 1 week; who die or develop serious neurologic sequelae: 6 months.

In summary, total costs of invasive HIB disease in children (excluding deaths) exceed SEK 54 million per year. To this should be added the costs of deaths, which can amount to SEK 72 million, if the sum of SEK 12 million is appropriate. Furthermore, the following HIB induced costs should be considered.

Other HIB induced costs

1. *Other manifestations of invasive HIB disease in children.* HIB can cause septicaemia, pneumonia, cellulitis, arthritis and osteomyelitis. Extrapolating data from a study in Göteborg (3), there should be at least 35 cases of such HIB infections in the whole country, but the true number is probably higher, since cultures from the blood are often not obtained from these children.

2. *HIB disease in adults.* There are about 120 cases of acute epiglottitis in adults each year in Sweden and at least 50% of them are caused by HIB (2). HIB causes meningitis in about 5 adults every year (1) and can also cause other disease manifestations. Since it will probably not be known for several decades whether general vaccination of infants against HIB will reduce HIB infections in adults, these figures should currently not be included in a cost-benefit analysis. It is possible, however, that vaccination of infants will reduce HIB disease in adults, as vaccination reduces the carriage of HIB in the respiratory tract (8), which should in turn limit the spread of the organism.

Vaccine efficacy

Data from two controlled prospective studies show that HIB conjugate vaccines are considerably more than 90% effective (9, 10). However, some cases will occur even after general vaccination, e.g. in infants who have not yet been vaccinated or who have received only one dose. In the country-wide study of the incidence of HIB-meningitis, rather less than 10% of all patients were younger than 6 months, while epiglottitis is virtually absent in this age-group (1, 2). The costs of these cases are, however, probably compensated for by the fact that the incidence figures on which this cost-benefit analysis is based are underestimates of the true incidence. The diagnosis of HIB meningitis is not always verified, due to failure to obtain adequate cultures, or to negative cultures due to previous administration of antibiotics. Furthermore, the study on the incidence of acute epiglottitis required documentation of certain clinical criteria and many cases of probable epiglottitis were therefore not included due to poor documentation in the case records. Moreover, it is conceivable that general vaccination will reduce the carriage and spread of the organism and indirectly protect non-vaccinated infants (8).

Costs of general vaccination

During 1992–93, all counties began general vaccination with a HIB-tetanus toxoid conjugate (ACT-HIB^R, Pasteur-Mérieux, Marcy l'Étoile, France). The cost of ACT-HIB in 1993 was about SEK 125 per dose. During the time of the study, 1981–83, there were about 93,000 live births per year (11). Vaccination of these children 3 times would cost SEK 35 million per year. The birth rate has since increased to about 120,000 live births per year, which would increase vaccine costs to SEK 45 million. However, since most invasive HIB infections occur during the first years of life, the relation between disease-induced costs and vaccine costs should remain constant. Many countries recommended four doses of HIB vaccine. If future experience shows that this is necessary, vaccine costs will increase by 33%.

Since the HIB vaccine is given at the same time as vaccines against diphtheria, tetanus and polio at already existing Child Health Centres, the additional cost of vaccine administration (doctors' and nurses' time, needles, syringes) would be negligible. Costs for side effects of HIB vaccines, all of which have well documented safety records, should also be very small.

In summary, the costs generated by invasive HIB infections in children exceed the cost of the relevant vaccine and its administration. A similar conclusion was drawn in an analysis from five other industralized countries (4). The gain to society is, of course, small when set in relation to the entire budget for medical and health care. The main reason for recommending general vaccination is, therefore, not to save money, but to save human lives and alleviate suffering. The earlier-mentioned hesitancy by several authorities regarding greater cost is therefore groundless.

REFERENCES

1. Trollfors B, Claesson BA, Strangert K, Taranger J. Haemophilus influenzae meningitis in Sweden 1981–1983. Arch Dis Child 62: 1220–1223, 1987.
2. Trollfors B, Nylén O, Strangert K. Acute epiglottitis in children and adults in Sweden 1981–1983. Arch Dis Child 65: 491–494, 1990.
3. Claesson B, Trollfors B, Jodal U, Rosenhall U. Incidence and prognosis of Haemophilus influenzae meningitis in children in a Swedish region. Pediatr Infect Dis J 3: 35–39, 1984.
4. Clements DA, Booy R, Dagan R, Gilbert GL, Moxon R, Slack MPE, Takala A, Zimmermann HP, Zuber PLF, Eskola J. Comparison of the epidemiology and cost of Haemophilus influenzae type b disease in five western countries. Pediatr Infect Dis J 12: 362–367, 1993.
5. Hay JW, Daum RS. Cost-benefit analysis of haemophilus influenzae type b prevention: conjugate vaccination at eighteen months of age. Pediatr Infect Dis J 9: 246–252, 1990.
6. Hay JW, Daum RS. Cost-benefit analysis of two strategies for prevention of Haemophilus influenzae type b infection. Pediatrics 80: 319–329, 1987.
7. Statistical Yearbook of Sweden 1994. National Central Bureau of Statistics, Stockholm, Sweden.
8. Takala AK, Eskola J, Leinonen M, Käythy H, Nissinen A, Pekkanen E, Mäkelä PH. Reduction of oropharyngeal carriage of Haemophilus influenzae type b (Hib) in children immunized with an Hib conjugate vaccine. J Infect Dis 164: 982–986, 1991.
9. Eskola J, Käyhty H, Takala A, Peltola H, Rönnberg P-R, Kela E, Pekkanen E, McVerry P, Mäkelä H. A randomized prospective field trial of a conjugate vaccine in the protection of infants and young children against invasive Haemophilus influenzae type b disease. N Engl J Med 323: 1381–1387, 1990.
10. Santosham M, Wolff M, Reid R, Hohenboken M, Bateman M, Goepp J, Cortese M, Sack D, Hill J, Newcomer W, Capriotti L, Smith J, Owen M, Gahagan S, Hu D, Kling R, Lukacs L, Ellis RW, Vella PP, Calandra G, Matthews H, Ahonkhai V. The efficacy in Navajo infants of a conjugate vaccine consisting of Haemophilus influenzae type b polysaccharide and Neisseria meningitidis outer membrane protein complex. N Engl J Med 324: 1767–1772, 1991.
11. Official Statistics of Sweden. Population Changes 1981–1993. National Central Bureau of Statistics, Stockholm, Sweden.

Submitted March 16, 1994; accepted June 6, 1994

Scand J Infect Dis 26: 615–617, 1994

CASE REPORT

Pneumococcal Septicaemia and Meningitis in Vaccinated Splenectomized Adult Patients

NIELS ABILDGAARD and JOHAN LANNG NIELSEN

From the Department of Medicine and Hematology, Aarhus University Hospital, Amtssygehuset, Aarhus C, Denmark

A retrospective survey of the occurrence of pneumococcal septicaemia and meningitis in splenectomized adults was performed at a regional haematological centre after the introduction of pneumococcal vaccination in 1978. During this period 4 episodes of pneumococcal septicaemia were observed in 3 vaccinated, splenectomized patients. In all episodes the pathogenic strain was of an unusual serotype not included in the vaccine lending indirect evidence for the clinical efficacy of the pneumococcal vaccine, even in immunocompromised patients.

N. Abildgaard, MD, Department of Medicine and Hematology, Aarhus University Hospital, Amtssygehuset, DK-8000 Aarhus C, Denmark

INTRODUCTION

In 1978 a 14-valent pneumococcal polysaccharide vaccine (containing serotypes: 1, 2, 3, 4, 6A, 7F, 8, 9N, 12F, 14, 18C, 19F, 23F, 25) was introduced for routine use in Denmark in splenectomized adults and children above the age of 2 years, and in 1983 a 23-valent vaccine followed. This vaccine (Pneumovax[R], Merck, Sharp and Dohme) contains 23 different polysaccharide capsular antigens (1, 2, 3, 4, 5, 6B, 7F, 8, 9N, 9V, 10A, 11A, 12F, 14, 15B, 17F, 18C, 19A, 19F, 20, 22F, 23F, 33F) from the most frequently isolated pneumococcal serotypes (90%) in bacteraemia and meningitis in Denmark. Combined with a regime of prompt prophylactic oral penicillin treatment on the appearance of fever, the efficacy of the vaccine has apparently been high, although doubt about its efficacy in immunocompromized patients has been expressed. Impaired serological response to the vaccine has been demonstrated in B-cell malignancies and following cytostatic treatment (1–5). However, only rare cases of clinical failure of the vaccine in immunodeficient patients have been reported. Thus no cases of invasive pneumococcal infection in vaccinated splenectomized children were observed in Denmark in the period 1979–87, compared with 4% in splenectomized children in the pre-vaccine period 1969–78 (6). In adults, only sporadic cases of pneumococcal infection have been reported in vaccinated splenectomized individuals (2, 7–9), and in most of these cases the serotype of the actual pathogen, if known, was not included in the vaccine.

In the period 1979–92 we observed 4 episodes of pneumococcal septicaemia and meningitis in 3 vaccinated, splenectomized individuals (Table I). In all episodes the serotype of the isolated strain was not included in the vaccine.

CASE REPORTS

Patient A

A 56-year-old man was splenectomized in 1981 due to traumatic rupture of the spleen. Four weeks later he was vaccinated with a 14-valent pneumococcal vaccine (Pneumovax[R], Merck, Sharp and Dohme). In 1985 he was admitted to hospital with purulent meningitis and Streptococcus pneumoniae was isolated from the blood and spinal fluid. Serotyping revealed that the infecting strain was type 38, which was not a part of the vaccine.

Table I. *Four episodes of Streptococcus pneumoniae septicaemia and meningitis in vaccinated, splenectomized Danish patients*

Patients	Diagnosis	Episode	Serotype	Interval after splenectomy (months)
A	Splenic rupture	1	38	48
B	Immune thrombocytopenia (non-Hogdkin lymphoma)	2 3	24F 15F	35 41
C	Hypersplenism (sarcoidosis?)	4	38	9

Patient B

A 20-year-old man presented in May 1986 with severe idiopathic thrombocytopenia. Splenectomy was performed in February 1987. Six weeks prior to the operation he had received a 23-valent pneumococcal polysaccharide vaccination (Pneumovax[R]). In December 1987 the thrombocytopenia recurred but was successfully controlled by azathioprine (Imurel[R]). In July 1989 he got neurological symptoms. Computer tomography showed a tumour close to the 4th ventricle of the brain and biopsy gave evidence of a highly malignant non-Hodgkin lymphoma. The tumor was completely eradicated after cerebral radiation therapy, and has so far not recurred. However, azathioprine in an oral dose of 1.5–2.2 mg/kg daily has repeatedly been required to control the thrombocytopenia.

In November 1990 the patient was admitted to hospital with septic shock and disseminated intravascular coagulation. He had neglected the usual penicillin prophylaxis. Streptococcus pneumoniae type 24F was cultured from the blood. After the incident his universal antibody levels against the pneumococcal serotypes in the vaccine were examined and found acceptable at the time. The serotype 24F of the relevant pathogen is not covered by the vaccine.

In May 1991, 6 months later, the patient again experienced an attack of fever and was immediately hospitalized. On this occasion, Streptococcus pneumoniae type 15A was isolated from the blood, again a serotype not represented in 23-valent pneumococcal vaccine. In September 1991 his antibody levels were retested and found to be low, and the patient was revaccinated with the 23-valent vaccine $4\frac{1}{2}$ years after the primary immunization.

Patient C

A 45-year-old female admitted to hospital in late 1991 with a history of weight loss, nocturnal sweating, pancytopenia and enlargement of the spleen. Diagnostic procedures were not conclusive and as the pancytopenia progressed she was splenectomized in March 1992. Three weeks prior to surgery she had received a 23-valent pneumococcal vaccine (Pneumovax[R]). The spleen showed hyperplasia and extramedullary haematopoiesis. Two slightly enlarged lymph nodes along the splenic vein showed granulomatous transformation compatible with sarcoidosis. Post-operatively she recovered, gained weight and had a complete remission of the haematological disturbances.

In December 1992 the patient was hospitalized with purulent meningitis and Streptococcus pneumoniae type 38 was isolated from the spinal fluid and blood. After this episode the serum antibody levels were tested and overall found to be low, whereby she was revaccinated in February 1993.

DISCUSSION

Several studies have investigated the antibody response to pneumococcal vaccination and its persistence in different patient groups with special reference to the frequency of vaccine failure in immunocompromised patients (1–5). These studies have consistently reported that B-cell lymphomas and cytostatic treatment are associated with weakened antibody responses. Moreover the antibody levels seem to decline within 3–10 years (10–12). The clinical interpretation of these findings is, however, a subject for debate. The antibody concentration needed for protection against overwhelming pneumococcal infection has not completely been defined. In fact no cases of overwhelming pneumococcal infection have been registered in vaccinated splenectomized children in Denmark during the period 1979–87 (6). In adults, few cases of vaccine failure have been reported (2, 7–9), and in most of these cases the pneumococcal serotype, if known, has not been included in the vaccine.

During the period of 1979–92 we have in our Haematological Department, a regional centre covering approximately 1.0 million inhabitants, splenectomized more than 200 patients with haematological disorders. In this period we have witnessed 4 episodes of severe pneumococcal infection in the splenectomized individuals. In all these episodes the pathogenic strain has been of a serotype not represented in the vaccine, in our opinion lending indirect evidence of the clinical efficacy of the vaccine, even in the haematological domain. However, it should be emphasized that overwhelming pneumococcal infection as well as fulminant infection with other encapsulated bacteria is an incipient risk in splenectomized subjects. Therefore, asplenic patients must be carefully informed about the necessity of penicillin prophylaxis in the case of fever and should be given antibiotics to be used promptly whenever there is possible delay in obtaining medical help. The patients should be advised to carry either a Medic Alert disc or a card with their clinical details. Furthermore, testing of the antibody levels should be performed within a few years after the primary immunization and the need of revaccination should be considered.

ACKNOWLEDGEMENTS

We appreciate that the patients and close relatives gave us permission to publish the case stories.

REFERENCES

1. Pedersen FK, Lanng Nielsen J, Ellegaard J. Antibody response to pneumococcal vaccine in splenectomized adults and adolescents. Acta Path Microbiol Immunol Scand C 90: 257–263, 1982.
2. Grimfors G, Björkholm M, Hammarström L, Askergren J, Smith CIE, Holm G. Type-specific anti-pneumococcal antibody subclass response to vaccination after splenectomy with special reference to lymphoma patients. Eur J Haematol 43: 404–410, 1989.
3. Lindblad R, Kailser B, Magnusson B, Rödjer S, Westin J. Pneumococcal vaccination in splenectomized patients with haematological disorders. Acta Med Scand 224: 467–471, 1988.
4. Frederiksen B, Specht L, Henrichsen J, Pedersen FK, Pedersen-Bjergaard J. Antibody response to pneumococcal vaccine in patients with early stage Hodgkin's disease. Eur J Haematol 43: 45–49, 1989.
5. Siber GR, Gorham C, Martin P, Corkery JC, Schiffman G. Antibody response to pretreatment immunization and post-treatment boosting with bacterial polysaccharide vaccines in patients with Hodgkin's disease. Ann Intern Med 104: 467–475, 1986.
6. Konradsen HB, Henrichsen J. Pneumococcal infections in splenectomized children are preventable. Acta Paediatr Scand 80: 423–427, 1991.
7. Brzeski M, Smart L, Baird D, Jackson R, Sturrock R. Pneumococcal septic arthritis after splenectomy in Felty's syndrome. Ann Rheum Dis 50: 724–726, 1991.
8. Lindblad BE, Lindblad LN. Fatal pneumococcal bacteremia with disseminated intravascular coagulation and Waterhouse-Friderichsen Syndrome in a vaccinated, splenectomized adult. Acta Chir Scand 156: 487–488, 1990.
9. Zarrabi H, Rosner F, Brook S. Pneumococcal sepsis and meningitis in vaccinated subjects: A review of 55 reported cases. J Natl Med Assoc 79: 372–376, 1987.
10. Grimfors G, Söderqvist M, Holm G, Lefvert AK, Björkholm M. A longitudinal study of class and subclass antibody response to pneumococcal vaccination in splenectomized individuals with special reference to patients with Hodgkin's disease. Eur J Haematol 45: 101–108, 1990.
11. Konradsen HB, Pedersen FK, Henrichsen J. Pneumococcal revaccination of splenectomized children. Pediatr Infect Dis J 9: 258–263, 1990.
12. Konradsen HB, Henrichsen J. The need for revaccination 10 years after primary pneumococcal vaccination in splenectomized adults. Scand J Infect Dis 23: 397, 1991.

Submitted September 10, 1993; accepted May 8, 1994

Scand J Infect Dis 26: 619–621, 1994

CASE REPORT

Myonecrosis in the Leg Caused by Salmonella enteritidis

STIG JØRRING[1], HANS JØRN KOLMOS[2] and BO KLARESKOV[1]

From the Departments of [1]Orthopedics and [2]Clinical Microbiology, Hvidovre Hospital, University of Copenhagen, Denmark

Five weeks after an episode of gastroenteritis, a 65-year-old diabetic male developed an extensive myonecrosis, with gas production in the left leg caused by Salmonella enteritidis. The patient was treated with surgical revision and antibiotics. To our knowledge, this is the first case of myonecrosis with gas production in a leg caused by Salmonella enteritidis, in which the patient survived, and the limb was saved.

S. Jørring, MD, Mynstersvej 7 B, 1 TH, DK-1827 Frederiksberg C, Denmark

INTRODUCTION

Gastroenteritis is the most common form of infection caused by zoonotic Salmonella. Extra-intestinal manifestations are less frequent but have been reported in numerous locations (1). Myonecrosis caused by zoonotic Salmonella in an extremity with no relation to other foci distant to the gastrointestinal tract is very rare, and the prognosis is still dubious (2, 3).

CASE REPORT

A 65-year-old man with non-insulin dependent diabetis mellitus was admitted to the Department of Orthopedics, with a history of 6 days of fever and progressive swelling in his left leg. Five weeks earlier he had suffered from an episode of vomiting and watery diarrhea lasting 8 days. No stool cultures were performed.

On admission, the patient was moderately ill but non-toxic. Physical examination showed a body temperature of 38.0°C and swelling, tenderness, increase in heat and erythema of the medial part of the left thigh, the popliteal region and proximal part of the calf. Deep venous thrombosis was suspected. Acute phlebography revealed great masses of gas in the deep medial part of the left thigh extending down to the popliteal region. There was no sign of gas proximal to the inguinal ligament, and the bone structure was normal (Fig. 1).

Surgical revision was performed immediately, with long incisions medially and laterally on the leg. All compartments on the femur and the calf were examined. Generalized edema of the subcutaneous tissue was found, but no crepitation. After opening the fascia proximally and medially, extensive masses of gas and brown-greyish fluid were evacuated. Most of the adductor muscles and the medial part of the m. quadriceps femoris were necrotic and debrided. The peritoneum was exposed in the groin. There were no signs of infection descending from the abdomen or retroperitoneum. On the femur, v. and a. femoralis were exposed from the groin to the popliteal region. There were no arterial aneurysms, and the knee joint was not involved. Specimens taken from different sites were sent to the clinical microbiological laboratory for immediate examination, and benzylpenicillin (5×10^6 IU i.v.) and gentamicin (240 mg i.v.) were given. Microscopy of the necrotic material showed Gram-negative rods of a uniform morphology. Aerobic culture revealed growth of a Gram-negative rod in pure culture, which was identified biochemically and serologically as Salmonella enteritidis. There was no growth of anaerobic bacteriae.

After surgery the patient was treated with benzylpenicillin (2×10^6 IU/8 h i.v.) and metronidazole (500 mg/8 h i.v.), which on day 4 was changed to ciprofloxacin (400 mg/12 h i.v.) for 42 days and metronidazole (500 mg/8 h rec.) for 13 days. The wounds were inspected and revised 3 times the first day and once daily thereafter. The lateral incision was closed on the fourth day, and the medial incision was

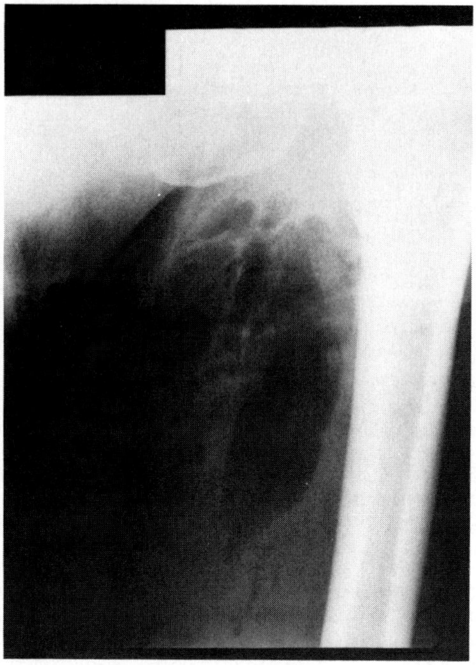

Fig. 1. X-ray of left thigh, showing gas in soft tissues.

closed with a split skin transplant on the seventh day. After 5 weeks the patient started to walk on both legs, and was discharged to his home 2 weeks later. The immediate postoperative course was complicated by paroxysmal atrial tachycardia and hypotension, which was treated with digoxin and vasopressors, and the patient needed respiratory support for 2 periods during the first 6 days. During the first 2 weeks there was virtually no gastrointestinal function, which precluded stool sampling and after this time it was considered irrelevant. The patient was free from gastrointestinal symptoms subsequently.

DISCUSSION

Microbiological investigations failed to reveal any sign of anaerobic bacteria, even though conditions for accurate diagnosis were optimal. Therefore S. enteritidis must be considered the sole cause of the patient's myonecrosis. We believe that the myonecrosis was secondary to a bacteremia following the previous episode of gastroenteritis, which presumably was caused by the same bacterium, although the myonecrosis could have been due to some other extra-intestinal focus of salmonellosis. Zoonotic Salmonella can cause arthritis and osteomyelitis and may infect pre-existing aneurysms (1), but in the present case there were no signs of such infection, and there were no signs of descending infection from the abdomen or retroperitoneum.

In the present case there was a latency of 4 weeks from the primary episode of gastroenteritis to the symptoms of myonecrosis on the femur. We find no obvious explanation for this phenomenon, but in previous cases of myonecrosis (3) and necrotizing fasciitis (4) caused by zoonotic Salmonella, a similar latency was found.

Solitary muscular infection caused by zoonotic Salmonella is very rare (2, 3, 5), and myonecrosis in an extremity with no relation to other extra-intestinal foci has been reported twice only (2, 3). In 1 case the patient underwent immediate amputation and survived (3), but in the other case the patient died within a few days (2). David et al. reported a case of myonecrosis with gas production due to zoonotic Salmonella, related to arthritis in the knee

(6), and Daus et al. reported a similar case with relation to an infected femoral aneurysm (7). Both cases proved fatal. To our knowledge, this is the first case of myonecrosis with gas production in an extremity caused by zoonotic Salmonella, in which the patient survived and the limb was saved. The severe course of this type of infection might partly be explained by the fact that all patients suffered from concomitant diseases such as diabetes mellitus or conditions with immunosuppression known to predispose for Salmonella bacteremia.

In recent years the incidence of bacteremia caused by zoonotic Salmonella has increased dramatically in the industrialized world (8), mainly due to contamination of foodstuffs. With an increasing incidence of bacteremia, more extra-intestinal infections are to be expected. The serious course of these should stimulate efforts to eliminate Salmonella from foods.

REFERENCES

1. Cohen JI, Bartlett JA, Corey GR. Extra-intestinal manifestations of salmonella infections. Medicine 66: 349–388, 1987.
2. Simeon-Aznar CP, Cuenca-Luque R, Solans-Laque R, Fernandez-Cortijo J, Bosch-Gil JA, Vilartell-Tarres M. Fulminant soft tissue infection by Salmonella enteritidis in SLE. J Rheumatol 17: 1570–1571, 1990.
3. Quale JM, Lonano F. Salmonella myonecrosis in a patient with diabetis mellitus. Am J Med Sci 301: 335–336, 1991.
4. Sanchez C, Capell S, Casanovas A, Admetella M, Sitges-Serra A. Necrotizing fasciitis caused by Salmonella enteritidis. Scand J Infect Dis 16: 321–322, 1984.
5. Tebas P, Bonilla F, Ruiz J, Diéguez B, Espana P. Non-tropical pyomyositis caused by Salmonella enterica enterica in an immunocompetent patient. Eur J Clin Microbiol Infect Dis 11: 560–561, 1992.
6. David DS, Brennan L, Grieco MH. Gas production with Salmonella thyphimurium infection. Am J Med Sci 262: 266–260, 1971.
7. Daus H, Schwarze G, Wernert N. Gasbrand und Salmonellaabcess als seltene infectiöse Komplikation bei Leukämie. Med Klin 84: 60–63, 1989.
8. Lester A, Eriksen NHR, Nielsen H, Nielsen PB, Friis-Møller A, Bruun B, Scheibel J, Gaarslev K, Kolmos HJ. Non-typhoid Salmonella bacteremia in Greater Copenhagen 1984 to 1988. Eur J Clin Microbiol Infect Dis 10: 486–490, 1991.

Submitted March 21, 1994; accepted May 16, 1994

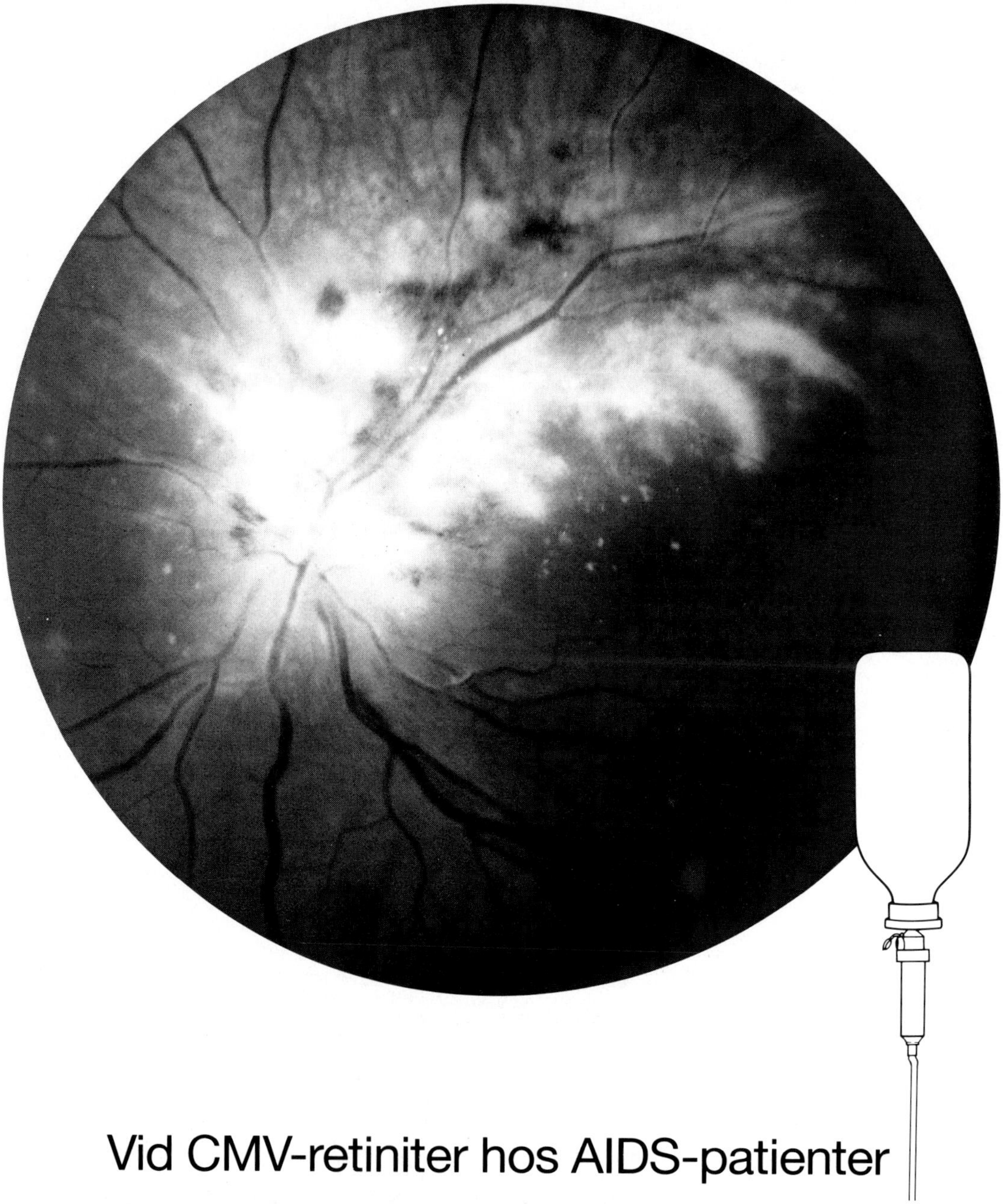

Scand J Infect Dis 26: 623–626, 1994

CASE REPORT

Cellulitis as First Clinical Presentation of Disseminated Cryptococcosis in Renal Transplant Recipients

ALPHONS M. HORREVORTS[1], FRANS T. M. HUYSMANS[2], ROLAND J. J. KOOPMAN[3] and JACQUES F. G. M. MEIS[1]

From the Departments of [1]Medical Microbiology, [2]Internal Medicine and [3]Dermatology, University Hospital Nijmegen, The Netherlands

Two renal transplant recipients with cellulitis due to Cryptococcus neoformans are described. The patients were treated empirically for a presumed bacterial erysipelas, but without response. Examination of skin biopsies revealed C. neoformans as the causative organism. In both patients the cellulitis was the presenting clinical manifestation of disseminated cryptococcosis. Therapy with antifungal agents was successful. Disseminated cryptococcal disease occurs mainly in immunocompromized patients. When left untreated, it nearly always has a fatal course. Early diagnosis and appropriate therapy are therefore essential.

A. M. Horrevorts, MD, Department of Medical Microbiology, University Hospital Nijmegen, P.O. Box 9101, 6500 HB Nijmegen, The Netherlands

INTRODUCTION

Disseminated infection by Cryptococcus neoformans is observed mainly in immunocompromized patients and cutaneous involvement occurs in 10–15% of cases (1). Primary cryptococcosis of the skin is very rare and cryptococcal skin disease should therefore be interpreted as a sign of systemic cryptococcal infection (2). Cryptococcal skin disease can manifest itself in a variety of ways, each of which is uncharacteristic for C. neoformans (3). Cellulitis is a very uncommon form (1). We describe 2 patients, both renal transplant recipients, with cellulitis caused by C. neoformans.

CASE REPORTS

Case 1

A 31-year-old woman was admitted to the hospital with fever and a lesion of the right lower leg that resembled erysipelas. The general practitioner had prescribed erythromycin, but without improvement. She had in the past had 2 unsuccessful renal transplants, followed by periods of long-term intermittent hemodialysis and peritoneal dialysis because of a terminal renal insufficiency due to an anti-GBM glomerulonephritis. She then underwent a third, successful renal transplantation. Her medication consisted of prednisone 10 mg and azathioprine 100 mg daily. Four days prior to admission she had felt feverish, without rigors, and had noticed a dry unproductive cough. On examination she appeared moderately ill with a pulse rate of 80 per min and a blood pressure of 120/90 mmHg. Her temperature was 39.0°C. Examination of heart, lungs and abdomen was unremarkable. On the skin of the right lower leg, there were a few painful, slightly elevated, erythematous patches (Fig. 1). Laboratory findings: hemoglobin 90 g/l; leukocyte count 5.2×10^9/l; platelet count 285×10^9/l; serum creatinine was stable at 86 μmol/l. The chest X-ray showed pleural fluid on the left side and 2 circular infiltrates, each with a diameter of 1.5 cm, in the right upper lobe. Because the disorder on the right lower leg resembled erysipelas, erythromycin was changed to oral penicillin. The patient became subfebrile and started to complain of headache. A broncheoalveolar lavage and a skin biopsy were performed. Microscopic examination of both showed small yeast cells and cultures yielded C. neoformans. Cerebrospinal fluid (CSF) and urine cultures both grew C. neoformans, whereas blood cultures remained sterile. The cryptococcal antigen titres in the CSF and blood were 4 and 32, respectively. Combination therapy with amphotericin B and 5-fluorocytosine was started. However, as the isolate was resistant to 5-fluorocytosine in vitro, therapy was changed to fluconazole 400 mg/day intravenously. Follow-up cultures of

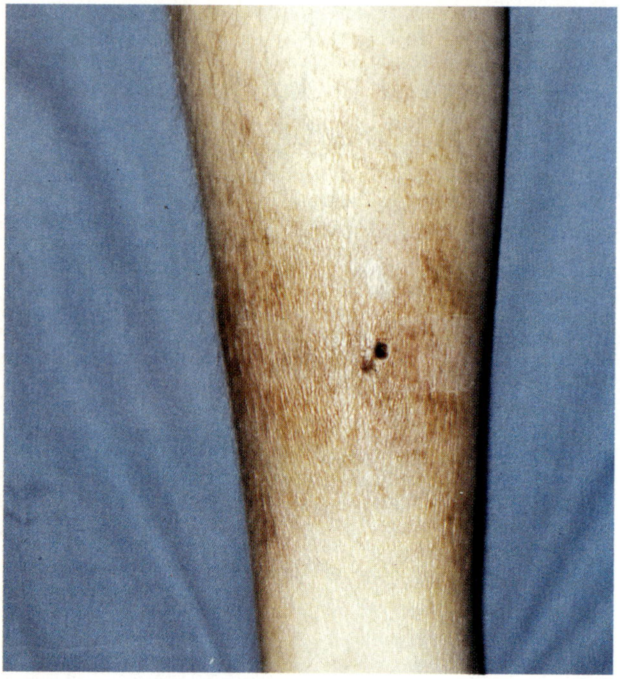

Fig. 1. Cutaneous skin lesion in a renal transplant recipient. The biopsy revealed Cryptococcus neoformans.

CSF, urine and skin biopsies remained sterile, although cryptococci were still visible in smears of skin biopsies even after 5 weeks of treatment. Combination therapy was given for 7.5 weeks after which amphotericin B was stopped (cumulative dose 1.6 g), but fluconazole was continued in a dose of 100 mg orally twice daily for 6 months. 11 weeks after admission, the patient was discharged in good condition with healed skin lesions. Cryptococcal antigen titres in CSF and blood had become negative. However, the abnormalities on the pulmonary X-ray were unchanged.

Three months after stopping medication, a control pulmonary X-ray showed that the infiltrates in the upper right side of the lung had progressed. Therefore blood CSF, urine and bronchoalveolar lavage were taken for culture, but none yielded C. neoformans. Eventually a dorsal segment of the upper lobe of the right lung was removed. Histopathological examination revealed no abnormalities other than fibrotic consolidation and cultures proved negative for C. neoformans.

Case 2

A 66-year-old woman was admitted to the hospital because of repeated episodes of high fever. A few months prior to admission she had been given antibiotics repeatedly by her general practitioner for an erysipelas-like skin lesion on the left lower leg. Several weeks prior to admission she had begun to complain of headache. During the last days, vomiting and fever >39°C developed. Her medical history recorded a double-sided hydronephrosis due to junctura stenosis for which she underwent nephrectomy in 1939 (left) and again in 1982 (right). In 1982 a period of long-term, intermittent hemodialysis followed. In 1985 she received a cadaveric renal transplant. She was receiving maintenance immunosuppressive therapy with prednisone 10 mg and azathioprine 150 mg daily. She also suffered from diabetes mellitus type II.

On physical examination, a moderately ill, slightly somnolent and dehydrated patient was seen with a temperature of 38.4°C, a pulse rate of 108 per min and a blood pressure of 140/85 mmHg. Meningeal signs were absent and fundoscopic examination showed no papilledema. The skin of the left lower leg displayed erythema (5 by 5 cm). Laboratory findings: hemoglobin 152 g/l; leukocyte count 10.6×10^9/l; platelet count 392×10^9/l; serum creatinine was stable at 84 μmol/l. The pulmonary X-ray showed no abnormalities. Blood, CSF, urine and skin biopsies were taken for culture. CSF examination revealed a leukocyte count of 800×10^6/l, an increased albumin concentration of 3 g/l, and a decreased glucose concentration of 3.8 mmol/l (blood glucose of 14.6 mmol/l). An India ink preparation of the CSF proved positive for yeasts and C. neoformans was isolated from CSF, skin biopsies and urine, while blood and sputum remained negative. Cryptococcal antigen titres in CSF and blood were 64 and 512, respectively.

Therapy was started with fluconazole 400 mg administered i.v. once a day. After 10 days, amphotericin B was added at a dose of 0.6 mg/kg/day, because the patient was deteriorating and follow-up cultures of CSF, skin biopsies and urine still yielded growth of C. neoformans. CSF and urine cultures became sterile 1 week after adding amphotericin B, and the skin biopsies after 3.5 weeks' treatment. The condition of the patient improved slowly as did the skin lesion. Amphotericin B was administered for 4 weeks to a cumulative dose 1.2 g. After 2 months of i.v. administration, fluconazole was given orally at a dose of 200 mg/day. Cryptococcal antigen titres in CSF and blood had then decreased to 0 and 256, respectively. The patient was discharged 10 weeks after admission. The administration of fluconazole was continued for 6 months and up until now, 4 years later, she is well, with no recurrence of the cryptococcosis.

DISCUSSION

Human cryptococcosis was first described by the German dermatologist Buschke in 1895 (4). It is caused by C. neoformans and is seen mainly in immunocompromized patients. Skin involvement occurs in some 10–15% of the cases and includes ulcers, acneiform papules or pustules, ecchymoses, granulomata, gummas, abscesses, vesicles. Cellulitis is the rarest presentation (3). In renal transplant recipients, infections caused by C. neoformans occurs almost exclusively in the late post-transplant period from about 4 months after transplantation and onwards (5). The reported incidence varies from 0.8 to 5.8% and use of high doses of immunosuppressive drugs leads to a higher risk of infection (6, 7). C. neoformans is considered to be the main cause of subacute or chronic meningitis in these patients. Meningitis is often preceded by several weeks of headache and fever (5, 8). In about a third of the patients a period of coughing is noted and some also suffer from pulmonary infection (5). Other predilection sites of C. neoformans include the urinary tract, bones and the skin (5, 6). Some 20–30% of transplant recipients with cryptococcal infection will have skin lesions weeks to months prior to the development of central nervous system (CNS) disease (5). Any renal transplant patient with a documented cryptococcal infection at any site should undergo lumbar puncture to exclude CNS involvement, since CNS involvement determines the intensity and duration of treatment (5). In addition to our 2 cases, 11 other recipients of renal transplant with cellulitis caused by C. neoformans have been reported (1–3, 9–12). Inclusive of our 2 patients, it concerns 10 male and 3 female patients varying in age from 31 to 66 years, all taking immunosuppressive drugs. 11 patients had received a transplant from a deceased donor. The time of manifestation of the disease varied from 1 to 10 years after transplantation. Two patients developed cellulitis after a trauma (10, 12). The cellulitis appeared to be restricted mainly to the extremities, especially the legs. One patient also suffered from cellulitis on the skin of the abdomen (12). In 8 patients C. neoformans was also recovered from more than 1 site, most commonly from CSF and sputum. Cryptococcal antigens were detected in the blood of 8 and in the CSF of 3 patients. 11 patients had been treated initially with antibacterial agents, without improvement, when specific examination revealed C. neoformans. Disseminated cryptococcosis appeared to be present in 8 patients, whereas cellulitis alone was present in 2 renal transplant recipients (2, 12). Five patients were treated with amphotericin B, 6 further in combination with 5-fluorocytosine and 2 (our 2 cases) in combination with fluconazole. The cumulative dose and duration of treatment with amphotericin B varied from 570 to 1,970 mg and from 16 days to 8 weeks, respectively. Five patients died, 1 as a direct result of the cryptococcal infection (12).

In the treatment of acute AIDS-related cryptococcal meningitis, fluconazole has been as effective as amphotericin B and, as maintenance therapy, even better than amphotericin B (13, 14). Our second case was initially treated with fluconazole alone, but because follow-up cultures of CSF still demonstrated growth of C. neoformans, amphotericin B was added. Maintenance therapy did not seem necessary, since none of our patients and none of the renal transplant patients described before (1–3, 9–12) had had a relapse of cryptococcal disease after cessation of treatment, in contrast to patients with AIDS in whom a high relapse rate is observed (3, 15). However, it is advisable to monitor the patient for at least a year after completion of the antimycotic therapy (3).

Untreated disseminated cryptococcosis is almost invariably a fatal disease. Timely diagnosis and appropriate treatment are therefore of the utmost importance. Cryptococcal cellulitis can be mistaken for a bacterial erysipelas and a delay in appropriate diagnosis can lead to high morbidity and mortality rates. As the cellulitis may be the first manifestation of a disseminated rather than a localized disease, an exhaustive examination (including a lumbar puncture) is indicated in any renal transplant recipient who presents with cellulitis.

REFERENCES

1. Shrader SK, Watts JC, Dancik JA, Band JD. Disseminated cryptococcosis presenting as cellulitis with necrotizing vasculitis. J Clin Microbiol 24: 860–862, 1986.
2. Iacobellis FW, Jacobs MI, Cohen RP. Primary cutaneous cryptococcosis. Arch Dermatol 115: 984–985, 1979.
3. Anderson DJ, Schmidt C, Goodman J, Pomeroy C. Cryptococcal disease presenting as cellulitis. Clin Infect Dis 14: 666–672, 1992.
4. Buschke A. Über eine durch Coccidiën hervorgerufen Krankheit des Menschen. Dtsch Med Wochenschr 21: 14, 1895.
5. Rubin RH. Infection in the renal and liver transplant patient. In: Rubin RH, Young LS, eds. Clinical approach to infection in the compromised host. New York: Plenum Publishing Corporation, 557–621, 1988.
6. Gallis HA, Berman RA, Cate TR, Hamilton JD, Gummells, Stickel DL. Fungal infection following renal transplantation. Arch Intern Med 135: 1163–1172, 1975.
7. Sampaio M, Ianhez LE, Sabbaga E. Protective effect of cyclosporin in human renal posttransplant cryptococcosis. Transplant Proc 24: 3091–3092, 1992.
8. Elshout van den FJJ, Huysmans FTM, Muytjens HL, Koene RAP. Cryptococcus neoformans meningitis following renal transplantation. Neth J Med 31: 183–190, 1987.
9. Mayers DL, Martone WJ, Mandell GL. Cutaneous cryptococcosis mimicking gram-positive cellulitis in a renal transplant patient. South Med J 74: 1032–1033, 1981.
10. Jennings, HS, Bradsher RW, McGee ZA, Johnson HK, Alford RH. Acute cryptococcal cellulitis in renal transplant recipients. South Med J 74: 1150–1153, 1981.
11. Perfect JR, Durack DT, Gallis HA. Cryptococcemia. Medicine 62: 98–109, 1983.
12. Carlson KC, Mehlmauer M, Evans S, Chandrasoma P. Cryptococcal cellulitis in renal transplant recipients. J Am Acad Dermatol 17: 469–472, 1987.
13. Saag MS, Powderly WG, Cloud GA, Robinson P, Grieco MH, Sharkey PK, Thompson SE, Sugar AM, Tuazon C, Fisher JF, Hyslop N, Jacobson JM, Hafner R, Dismukes WE, The NIAID Mycoses Study Group, AIDS Clinical Trials Group. Comparison of amphotericin B with fluconazole in the treatment of acute AIDS-associated cryptococcal meningitis. N Engl J Med 326: 83–89, 1992.
14. Powderly WG, Saag MS, Cloud GA, Robinson P, Meyer RD, Jacobson JM, Graybill JR, Sugar AM, McAuliffe VJ, Follansbee SE, Tuazon CU, Stern JJ, Feinberg J, Hafner R, Dismukes WE, The NIAID AIDS Clinical Trials Group, NIAID Mycoses Study Group. A controlled trial of fluconazole or amphotericin B to prevent relapse of cryptococcal meningitis in patients with the acquired immunodeficiency syndrome. N Engl J Med 326: 793–798, 1992.
15. Bozzette S, Larsen RA, Chiu J, Leal MAE, Jacobson J, Rothman P, Robinson P, Gilbert G, McCutchan JA, Tilles J, Leedom JM, Richman DD, California Collaborative Treatment Group. Placebo-controlled trial of maintenance therapy with fluconazole after treatment of cryptococcal meningitis in the acquired immunodeficiency syndrome. N Engl J Med 324: 580–584, 1991.

Submitted March 2, 1994; accepted May 1, 1994

Scand J Infect Dis 26: 627–629, 1994

CASE REPORT

Mediterranean Visceral Leishmaniasis in Pregnancy

LUIGI GRADONI[1], GIOVANNI B. GAETA[2], GIAMPIETRO PELLIZZER[3], ANGELA MAISTO[2] and ALDO SCALONE[1]

From the [1]Laboratorio di Parassitologia, Istituto Superiore di Sanità, Rome, [2]Clinica delle Malattie Infettive, Seconda Università, Naples, [3]Divisione di Malattie Infettive, Ospedale S. Bortolo, Vicenza, Italy

Visceral leishmaniasis (VL) in pregnancy is rare in Mediterranean countries. We report here 2 cases of VL in pregnant women who acquired the infection in Italy. In the first case, the disease was diagnosed and treated with liposomal amphotericin B during the pregnancy. In the second case, diagnosis was established and treatment with meglumine antimoniate both undertaken shortly after delivery. The 2 infants were followed clinically and serologically for 8–9 months after birth, but no evidence of congenital VL was observed.

L. Gradoni, MD, Laboratorio di Parassitologia, Istituto Superiore di Sanità, Viale Regina Elena 299, I-00161 Rome, Italy

INTRODUCTION

Visceral leishmaniasis (VL) acquired during pregnancy is rare in the Mediterranean countries (1), probably due to a low endemicity of the disease in the area and because Leishmania infantum affects mainly children (2). These cases may present 2 major problems: i) risk of congenital VL (3–5), and ii) theoretical risk of toxicity for the fetus of drugs administered. We report here 2 cases of VL in pregnant women who acquired the infection in the Naples province of Italy.

CASE REPORTS

Case 1

In November 1992, a 20-year-old, 5-months pregnant woman was admitted with anaemia and mild intermittent fever. On admission, her temperature was 37.3°C; splenomegaly and slight hepatomegaly were recorded. Laboratory tests showed hemoglobin 83 g/l, WBC 2.3×10^9/l and platelets 32×10^9/l. Antileishmanial IgG titre by immunofluorescent test (IFAT) was 10.240. A bone marrow aspirate showed presence of amastigotes.

The patient was treated with liposomal amphotericin B (AmBisome®, Vestar) at a daily dose of 3 mg/kg on days 0, 1, 2, 3, 4 and 10 (total dose of 18 mg/kg), as part of an ongoing multicentre clinical trial. Clinical and laboratory parameters improved very quickly and a second bone marrow aspirate, on day 21, proved negative for Leishmania on microscopy and culture. On April 2nd 1993 the patient gave birth to a normal baby with no complications.

Three serum samples were taken from the patient shortly after treatment, and one sample 8 months after delivery. Serum samples were obtained from the baby 1 week and 8 months after birth. The titre of antileishmanial IgG antibodies was determined by IFAT (Fig. 1). One week after birth, the baby showed a titre slightly lower (2560) than the one detected in his mother one month before delivery (5120). Eight months later, the child was found serologically negative, whereas his mother was still positive (2560).

Case 2

In April 1992, a 24-year-old Ghanian woman who had lived for 3 years in the Naples province gave birth to without complications a normal baby. Soon after after delivery, the woman developed severe anaemia, fever and splenomegaly, and in June she was diagnosed as having VL by microscopic examination and culture of bone marrow aspirate. The cultured parasites were identified isoenzymatically as Leishmania infantum.

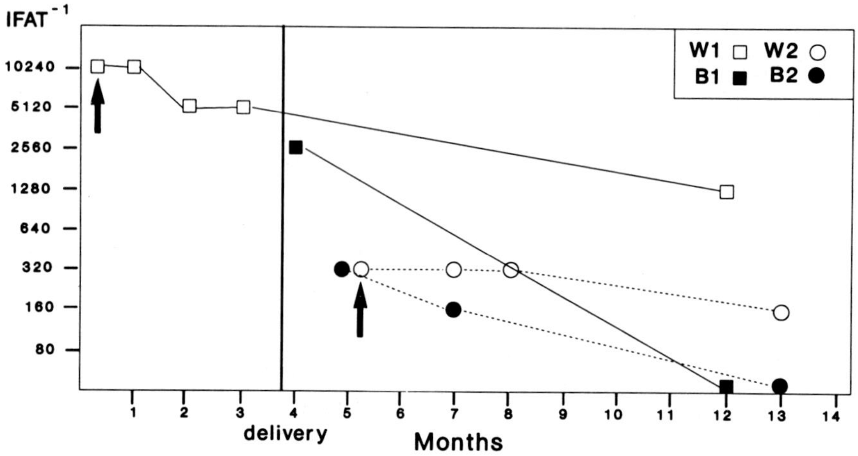

Fig. 1. Evolution of IFAT titres in 2 women suffering from visceral leishmaniasis during pregnancy (W1 and W2) and in their babies (B1 and B2). Arrows indicate when the women received drug treatment.

Treatment with meglumine antimoniate (average 18 mg Sb^V/kg/day) was administered for a total of 13 days, and then discontinued due to onset of acute pancreatitis (6). After VL had been diagnosed, her child was carefully re-examined but found in good health. Serum samples were taken from both child and mother at about 1, 3 and 9 months after birth and examined by IFAT (Fig. 1). The same antibody titre was found in samples taken in month 1 (320). Two months later, the serum titre had decreased in the boy (160) but not in his mother. In month 9 the boy was found serologically negative, whereas his mother was still positive (160).

DISCUSSION

Although rare, congenital leishmaniasis is a severe and life-threatening disease which needs prompt diagnosis (5, 7). The 2 cases we report showed that perinatal determination of specific antibodies is not diagnostic of visceral leishmaniasis, since passive IgG transmission occurs from mother to child. In these cases, absence of congenital infection was suggested by lack of clinical signs, and then confirmed by serological follow-up of the infants. Indeed, while both the mothers showed a slight decrease in antileishmanial serum antibodies during a 8–9-month period, these dropped to undetectable in the infants, during the same period. This is consistent with a physiological clearance of maternal antibodies.

Case 1 reported here is the first patient treated with liposomal amphotericin B during pregnancy. This drug has proved effective and non-toxic in immunocompetent adults and children with Mediterranean VL (8). Our patient was cured by a short course of treatment with no adverse effects on the mother or baby.

ACKNOWLEDGEMENTS

We wish to thank Vestar Inc. (San Dimas, CA, USA) for providing a free supply of AmBisome.

REFERENCES

1. Massip P, Goutner C, Dupic Y, Navarrot, P. Kala-azar chez la femme enceinte. Presse Med 15: 933, 1986.
2. World Health Organization. Control of the leishmaniases. Technical Report Series no. 793, 1990.
3. Blanc C, Robert A. Cinquième observation de kala-azar congénital. Presse Med 13: 1751, 1984.
4. Yadav TP, Gupta H, Satteya U, Kumar R, Mittal V. Congenital kala-azar. Ann Trop Med Parasitol 83: 535–537, 1989.

5. Eltoum IA, Zijlstra EE, Ali MS, Ghalib HW, Satti MMH, Eltoum B, El-Hassan AM. Congenital kala-azar and leishmaniasis in the placenta. Am J Trop Med Hyg 46: 57–62, 1992.
6. de Lalla F, Pellizzer G, Gradoni L, Vespignani M, Franzetti M. Stecca C. Acute pancreatitis associated with the administration of meglumine antimoniate for the treatment of visceral leishmaniasis. Clin Infect Dis 16: 730–731, 1993.
7. Nyakundi PM, Muigai R, Were JBO, Oster CN, Gachihi GS, Kirigi G. Congenital visceral leishmaniasis: case report. Trans R Soc Trop Med Hyg 82: 564, 1988.
8. Davidson RN, di Martino L, Gradoni L, Giacchino R, Russo R, Gaeta GB, Pempinello R, Scotti S, Raimondi F, Cascio A, Prestileo T, Caldeira L, Wilkinson RJ, Bryceson ADM. Liposomal amphotericin B (AmBisome) in Mediterranean visceral leishmaniasis: a multi-centre trial. Q J Med 87: 75–81, 1994.

Submitted May 11, 1994; accepted June 23, 1994

Scand J Infect Dis 26: 631–634, 1994

CASE REPORT

Meningeal Irritation: Possible Manifestation of Cerebral Echinococcus Infestation

ESPEN DIETRICHS[1], FRANS VAN KNAPEN[2] and SØREN J. BAKKE[3]

From the Departments of [1]Neurology and [3]Radiology, The National Hospital, Oslo, Norway and the [2]National Institute of Public Health and Environmental Protection, Bilthoven, The Netherlands

A patient with meningeal irritation and a small occipital cystic lesion is presented. Based on serological tests, the condition was diagnosed as presumably echinococcosis. To our knowledge, meningeal irritation has previously not been reported as an early symptom of cerebral Echinococcus infestation. Cysticercosis is discussed as a possible differential diagnosis.

E. Dietrichs, MD, PhD, Department of Neurology, The National Hospital, N-0027 Oslo, Norway

INTRODUCTION

Echinococcal disease has a universal distribution. It is usually caused by the tapeworm Echinococcus granulosus, often with dog as the definite host and sheep as the intermediate host. Humans may be infested as an incidental host. The liver is the organ most commonly involved (1), but the parasite may spread to form hydatid cysts in other organs such as the lungs and brain. Cerebral infestation is most common in children (2). It typically presents as a space occupying lesion (2, 3). An unusual case where an adult patient developed meningeal irritation is reported.

CASE REPORT

A 26-year-old immigrant from Bali, Indonesia had stayed in Norway for 3 years. During this period he had returned home once, and had also visited other Indonesian islands as well as several other Asian and European countries. He had a 1 year history of moderate frontal headache, but no other symptoms. Cerebral computer tomography (CT) had shown a small calcification in the right parietal cortex. He was therefore referred to the Department of Neurology, and admission was planned 2 months later. Shortly before admission, however, he developed symptoms of meningeal irritation with increasing headache, nausea and vomiting, but no fever.

On admission, examination revealed him to be in poor general condition, with neck stiffness and impaired vision from the right visual field. His general and neurological status was otherwise normal. Cerebral CT and magnetic resonance imaging (MRI) now revealed a small cystic lesion with contrast enhancement in the left occipital lobe in addition to the parietal calcification (Fig. 1). Otherwise the findings were normal. The cerebrospinal fluid (CSF) showed pleocytosis with 37×10^6 cells/l (80% lymphocytes, 19% eosinophils), an elevated protein level (0.68 g/l) and a pathological protein band on agar electrophoresis. The latter was considered indicative of infectious or inflammatory disease. Peripheral blood smear showed 1,060 eosinophils $\times 10^6$/l, but no other changes. A wide array of blood tests showed, e.g., normal electrolytes, normal liver and kidney function and normal muscle enzymes. The immunological screening was normal except for slightly elevated IgG (18 g/l). Chest X-ray and abdominal ultrasound examination showed no changes in lungs, liver or other organs.

A parasitic disease was suspected from the clinical, radiological and laboratory findings. Immunodiagnostic tests were carried out for cysticercosis and echinococcosis, but also for several other CNS-pathogenic parasites, bacteria and viruses. Since cerebral cysticercosis was considered a plausible differential diagnosis, treatment with large doses of Praziquantel (70 mg/kg/day for 2 weeks) was started before further test results could be obtained. Specific IgG antibodies against Echinococcus were later demonstrated with ELISA in serum from this patient. Therefore, immunoelectrophoresis (IEP) was carried out

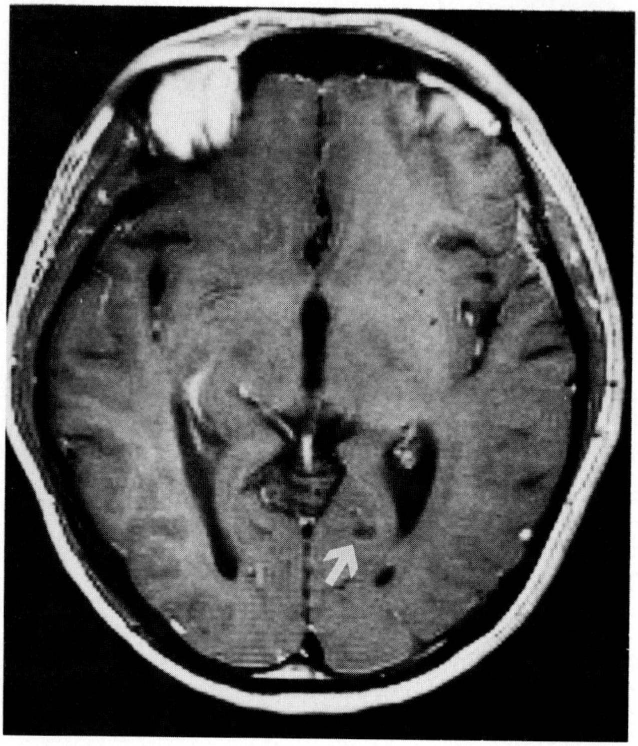

Fig. 1. Axial T1W MRI with Gadolinium contrast demonstrates a small, enhanced cyst (*arrow*) in the left occipital lobe.

as a confirmatory test. The presence of the so-called "arc 5" band is firm evidence of echinococcosis (4). Indeed, the patient reacted positively. Moreover, specific IgG antibodies to Echinococcus were found also in the CSF in a relatively high titre (Table I). Similar testing for cysticercous antibodies yielded negative results in the patient's serum, although the CSF showed a low antibody titre (see Table I).

The patient improved rapidly, and by the end of the praziquantel treatment there was a marked size reduction of the occipital cystic lesion, which no longer showed contrast enhancement. The parietal calcification was unchanged. Albendazole treatment of our patient was considered after the serological test results were received, but was found not to be indicated due to the patient's clinical and radiological improvement. The patient was followed up for 4 months, until he moved from Norway. At that time he was still symptom-free and had no radiological signs of a relapse, but control lumbar puncture showed unchanged pleocytosis, CSF protein and agar electrophoresis.

Table I. *Results of Echinococcus and cysticercus serology in serum and CSF*

Serum	CSF
Echinococcus	
ELISA 1:40	ELISA 1:16
IEP positive	
Cysticercus	
ELISA <1:40	ELISA 1:2
	ELISA antigen test: negative

DISCUSSION

Non-bacterial meningitis has been described after surgical removal of hydatid cysts (2). However, to our knowledge, meningeal irritation has not been reported as an early symptom in an unoperated patient. Presumably, in our patient, meningeal irritation occurred following spontaneous rupture of a small cyst.

The diagnosis of echinococcosis depends on the serological results. The clinical picture fits equally well with cerebral cysticercosis, which is an important differential diagnosis. The patient's native country is endemic for both echinococcosis and cysticercosis, and he had also visited other countries where both parasites occur. Meningeal irritation is well known in cysticercosis, and McCormick et al. (5) found meningismus in 8 or their 127 patients with cerebral cysticercosis. Small calcifications and cystic lesions may be found on CT-scans and MRI in both cysticercosis and echinococcosis (6, 7). Therefore, neither the size nor the site of the lesions in our patient were diagnostic of either of these conditions. However, other possible causes of meningeal irritation, such as Angiostrongylus or Gnatostoma infections, are unlikely to cause a cystic lesion which reacts to praziquantel treatment.

Our patient showed a conspicuous clinical improvement on receiving praziquantel. This could be taken as an argument against echinococcosis. However, although albendazole, rather than praziquantel, appears to be the preferred drug for echinococcosis, several in vitro and animal studies have shown that praziquantel is effective against hydatid cysts (8–11). In this context it is noteworthy that while experimental studies have shown albendazole to be a more effective drug in reducing hydatid cyst growth, praziquantel appears to be the better protoscolicidal agent (9). Theoretically, praziquantel could therefore be effective against free scolicis released by hydatid cyst rupture, as may indeed have been the case in our patient.

Hydatids and cysticerci are the larval stages of closely related Taenia species. Differences between the parasites revealed by immunodiagnostic procedures are largely dependent on the quality of the antigens applied. In our home-made ELISA assay, semi-purified (immune absorbed) sheep Echinococcus cyst fluid was used as compared with a relatively crude cysticercus antigen (home-made defatted whole cysticercus fluid). Cross-reactions were to be expected in the cysticercus immuno assay rather than in the Echinococcus immuno assay. Specific "arc 5" reaction in the immunoelectrophoresis is a typical and confirmative feature for echinococcosis. Although the immunoelectrophoresis is a test with a relatively low sensitivity (85%), its specificity is absolute for Taenia infections and in particular for Echinococcus infections (4, 12). In sheep, however, other Taenia infections may be responsible for an "arc 5" band finding when tested with Echinococcus antigen in immunoelectrophoresis (13). Also in some cases of human cysticercosis ($<5\%$) an "arc 5" band has been described (14). Nevertheless, the presence of the "arc 5" band in our patient consistutes strong evidence for echinococcosis.

Cysticercosis cannot be entirely ruled out as the cause of the meningeal irritation and cerebral cystic lesion in our patient. However, the fact that this patient showed specific serology for echinococcosis both in serum and at a relatively high titre in CSF (but not for cysticercosis) is indicative of real echinococcosis. A cross-reaction in locally (CSF) produced antibodies may warrant discussion, but in our view does not justify the diagnosis cysticercosis in preference to echinococcosis.

REFERENCES

1. Farmer PM, Chatterley S, Spier N. Echinococcal cyst of the liver: Diagnosis and surgical management. Ann Clin Lab Sci 20: 385–391, 1990.
2. Krajewski R, Stelmasiak Z. Cerebral hydatid cysts in children. Chil Nerv Syst 7: 154–155, 1991.

3. Aydin Y, Barlas O, Yolas C, Aydin IH, et al. Alveolar hydatid disease of the brain. J Neurosurg 65: 115–119, 1986.
4. Varela-Diaz VM, Guisantes JA, Ricardes MI, Yarzabal LA, Coltorti EA. Evaluation of whole and purified hydatid fluid antigens in the diagnosis of human hydatidosis by the immunoelectrophoresis test. Am J Trop Med Hyg 24: 298–303, 1975.
5. McCormick GF, Zee C-S, Heiden J. Cysticercosis cerebri. Review of 127 cases. Arch Neurol 39: 534–539, 1982.
6. Teitelbaum GP, Otto RJ, Lin M, et al. MR imaging of neurocysticercosis. AJNR Am J Neuroradiol 10: 709–718, 1989.
7. von Sinner W, te Strake L, Clark D, Sharif H. MR imaging in hydatid disease. AJR Am J Roentgenol 157: 741–745, 1991.
8. Taylor DH, Morris DL, Richards KS, Reffin D. Echinococcus multilocularis: in vivo results of therapy with albendazole and praziquantel. Trans R Soc Trop Med Hyg 82: 611–615, 1988.
9. Taylor DH, Morris DL, Reffin D, Richards KS. Comparison of albendazole, mebendazole and praziquantel chemotherapy of Echinococcus multilocularis in a gerbil model. Gut 30: 1401–1405, 1989.
10. Richards KS, Morris DL, Taylor DH. Echinococcus multilocularis: ultrastructural effect of in vivo albendazole and praziquantel therapy, singly and in combination. Ann Trop Med Parasitol 83: 479–484, 1989.
11. Xiao SH, Sun HL, Yang YQ, Jiao PY, You JQ, Guo HF. Uptake and distribution of [3H]praziquantel in Echinococcus granulosus cysts. Acta Pharmacologica Sinica 11: 176–180, 1990.
12. Varela-Diez VM, Coltorti EA, D'Alessandro A. Immunoelectrophoresis tests showing Echinococcus granulosus arc 5 in human cases of Echinococcus vogeli and cysticercosis-multiple myeloma. Am J Trop Med Hyg 27: 554–557, 1978.
13. Yong WK, Heath DD. 'Arc 5' antibodies in sera of sheep infected with Echinococcus granulosus, Taenia hydatigena and Taenia ovis. Parasite Immunol 1: 27–38, 1979.
14. Schantz PM, Shanks D, Wilson M. Serologic cross-reactions with echinococcosis and cysticercosis. Am J Trop Med Hyg 29: 609–612, 1980.

Submitted October 25, 1993; accepted May 1, 1994

Scand J Infect Dis 26: 635–642, 1994

REVIEW ARTICLE

Bacteremia in HIV-positive and AIDS Patients: Incidence, Species Distribution, Risk-factors, Outcome, and Influence of Long-term Prophylactic Antibiotic Treatment

CHRISTIAN N. MEYER[1], PETER SKINHØJ[1] and JØRGEN PRAG[2,3]

From the Departments of [1]Infectious Diseases, [2]Clinical Microbiology, Rigshospitalet, and [3]Clinical Microbiology, Statens Seruminstitut, Copenhagen, Denmark

From a cohort of 837 adult, mainly homosexual HIV-infected patients, 76 bacteremic/fungemic episodes were identified in 63 patients over a 5-year period. Compared with an age-matched reference population with an incidence of 10.3 bacteremias/10,000 person-years, the incidence was 170 among pre-AIDS ($p < 0.001$) and 3,200 among AIDS patients ($p < 0.001$). Staphylococcal infections comprised 35% of all episodes, while the HIV-related pathogens Streptococcus pneumoniae, Salmonella spp. and C. neoformans together accounted for 34%.

The overall mortality associated with clinical bacteremia was 12%, but nil for Salmonella spp. and S. pneumoniae. Predisposing factors for the infection were: low CD4 count ($< 100 \times 10^6$/l) in 71%, permanent intravenous line, 44%; neutropenia, 11% and active intravenous drug abuse, 7%. Hence, in this population, intensified hygienic precautions for intravenous lines should be the primary target for intervention. Long-term cotrimoxazole prophylaxis may prevent bacteremia with S. pneumoniae and Salmonella spp.

C. N. Meyer, MD, Department of Infectious Disease M 7721, Rigshospitalet, Tagensvej 20, DK-2200 Copenhagen, Denmark

INTRODUCTION

In addition to viral and parasitic opportunistic infections complicating HIV infection, infection with certain yeasts, Mycobacteria (including Mycobacteria avium-intracellulare complex (MAC)) and now recurrent Salmonella and Streptococcus pneumoniae are contributing to the definition of AIDS (1).

In recent articles, bacteremia in HIV-infected patients has been reported to be a substantial clinical problem (2). The HIV-positive populations described have been intravenous drug abusers (IVDU) (3) or Africans (4–6). Other HIV studies have dealt with bacteremia as part of bacterial infection in general (7), pneumococaemia (8, 9), or with community acquired bacteremia only (10). Some studies have focused on bacteremia in association with central venous catheters (CVC) (11–14).

We studied the characteristics of all bacteremic episodes in a 5-year period in a comprehensive group of Danish HIV-positive patients, focusing on incidence and on possible predisposing risk factors such as stage of HIV disease, neutropenia, CMV disease, intravenous lines, intravenous drug abuse (IVDU), as well as susceptibility to antibiotics, in search of ways to improve the treatment of this infectious complication of HIV-disease.

MATERIALS AND METHODS

The study population was a 5-year cohort of 837 adult HIV-positive patients treated and followed up at the Department of Infectious Disease, Rigshospitalet, Copenhagen. As of January 1988, 27 patients were treated for AIDS and 372 patients had earlier stages of HIV-infection. By the end of 1992 a further 439 patients had been referred. Altogether 306 developed AIDS and 220 died during this period, leaving

112 AIDS cases and 505 pre-AIDS patients under care. The total observation period was approximately 348 patient-years for AIDS cases and 2,473 patient-years for pre-AIDS patients. The HIV population comprised approximately 35% of all Danish patients, and regarding distribution of risk behaviour the AIDS cases under study were similar to all Danish AIDS patients during this period: homosexuals 73% (72%), blood product infected (mainly hemophiliacs) 5% (3.5%), IVDU 3% (7.2%), heterosexually infected 14% (14%), and unknown in 4% (2.6%). (National figures for the period are given in parentheses (15)).

All positive blood cultures from HIV-positive patients at the Department of Clinical Microbiology during the 5-year period January 1988 through December 1992 were included. The medical record of each patient was reviewed with regard to AIDS-defining events: CD4 count, neutrophil count, permanent i.v. line, HIV risk behaviour, focal infection or entrance of infection, recent medication, antibiotic therapy, clinical condition and outcome.

Blood culture sets were taken at least once during episodes of fever ≥38.5°C before the patients were given antibiotic treatment, and repeated in cases of dubious findings or persistent fever of unknown origin. The blood culture system Colorbact^R, consisted of two aerobic and one anaerobic bottle, each obtaining 5–10 ml when connected directly to the Venoject^R and Vacutainer^R blood sampling systems (16). The same blood culture systems were used in the three general hospitals serving all inhabitants in Roskilde and Bornholm counties. These counties are low incidence areas regarding HIV infection, and HIV patients are referred for care to Copenhagen. The blood culture results were available from a 22-month period in 1990–92.

The age-matched (25–59 years) incidences of bacteremia in this reference population of 139,098 persons are used here for comparison with the incidences and species distribution among the HIV-infected patients (25–57 years). Agar diffusion susceptibility tests were done with Neosensi Tabs^R (Rosco, Roskilde, DK).

Definitions

Community acquired bacteremia: a positive blood culture obtained in out-patients or at the latest 48 h after admission. Subsequent infections were considered nosocomial infections.

Neutropenia: a neutrophil count less than 0.5×10^9/l.

Septic shock: bacteremia with rectal temperature >38.5°C or <36°C, and a systolic blood pressure below 95 mmHg.

Clinically irrelevant bacteremia: a common low-pathogenic organism from skin or air such as Corynebacterium spp., S. epidermidis or Bacillus spp. grown in only one set of blood culture, considered irrelevant by physicians at the Department of Infectious Diseases and accordingly not followed by any implementation of or change in the antibiotic treatment.

Relapse: recurrence of the same microorganism later than 14 days and after attempted treatment. Recurrence within 14 days was regarded as one episode only.

Person-years: number of persons/patients multiplied with the mean time period of observation.

Statistics

Rates were compared using an analogue to Fisher's exact test valid for Poisson variables.

RESULTS

198 positive blood culture sets from 97 of 837 HIV-infected patients were found. The species distributions in blood culture sets, patients and clinical episodes are shown in Table I. Species distributions in the HIV population with and without AIDS and in the unselected age-matched general population from Roskilde and Bornholm Counties are shown in Table II. The latter 3 columns account for the total number of patients with positive blood cultures, excluding recurrent positive blood cultures. Compared with the general population, every species occurred with an increased incidence of bacteremia on average 17-fold higher among pre-AIDS patients ($p < 0.001$) and on average 310-fold higher among AIDS patients ($p < 0.001$).

Table I. *Blood-culture isolates in 837 adult HIV-infected patients, 1988–92*

Type of flora	Species	Isolates $N = 198$ (8) *n*	Patients $N = 154$ *n*	Episodes $N = 76$ (6) *n*
Skin, total		102	88	30 (5)
	S. aureus	24	19	19 (3)
	S. epidermidis	90	61	10 (1)
	Corynebacteria spp	4	6	
	C. jeikeium	2	2	1 (1)
Airway, total		20	16	16
	S. pneumoniae	15	12	12
	C. neoformans	4	3	3
	N. meningitidis	1	1	1
Intestinal, total		55	43	36
	Enterococcus spp	4	4	2
	β-haemol. strept	3	3	2 (1)
	Non-haemol. strept	4	4	1
	L. monocytogenes	1	1	1
	Peptococcus sp	1	1	
	Salmonella spp[a]	17	11	11
	E. coli	7	7	7
	Klebsiella spp	3	2	2 (1)
	P. mirabilis	1	1	1 (1)
	E. cloacae	5	3	3 (3)
	Pseudomonas spp	9	6	6 (2)
Miscellaneous, total		11	7	3
	Bacillus spp	4	4	
	Acinetobacter spp	2	1	1 (1)
	Candida spp	4	1	1
	S. cerevisiae	1	1	1

In parentheses: polymicrobial episodes.
[a] 4 S. dublin. 5 S. enterididis and 2 S. typhimurium.

Compared with data on positive blood cultures in the general population sample, the HIV-positive patients harboured a significantly higher proportion of S. epidermidis ($p < 0.01$) and Salmonella spp. ($p < 0.05$) and a significantly lower proportion of Escherichia coli ($p < 0.05$). Of the 198 strains found in positive blood culture sets in HIV-infected patients, 73 were considered clinically irrelevant. The remaining 117 samples were grouped into a total of 76 bacteremic/fungemic episodes in 63 patients, of whom 6 were females. Six episodes were polymicrobial. Staphylococcus aureus and S. epidermidis comprised 35% of all isolates, while Salmonella spp., S. pneumoniae and C. neoformans accounted for 34%. Relapses following treatment was observed in 6 cases; 4 were Salmonella spp., 1 E. coli and 1 Pseudomonas stutzeri.

Excluding relapses, the number of clinically relevant primary bacteremic episodes in pre-AIDS patients were 16, versus 54 in AIDS patients, corresponding to an incidence of 64/10,000 patient-years among pre-AIDS patients, versus 1,550 in AIDS patients. 66% of all primary episodes were community acquired, while 34% were nosocomial infections. Among pre-AIDS patients, characteristically all episodes but one (16/17) were community acquired, while a more even distribution was found in the group of AIDS patients (34/59).

Of the 6 polymicrobial episodes, the 2 among pre-AIDS patients were community acquired with mixtures of skin and intestinal flora, while the remaining 4 among AIDS patients contained skin flora in 1, gut flora in 2 and a mixture in 1.

The presumed ports of entry were: unknown in 29%, central i.v. lines in 23%, lower airways in 18%, intestines in 11%, skin in 9% (including 4 cases of localized subcutanous abscesses in IVDU), urinary tract in 5% and others in 4%. The major predisposing factors for all episodes were low CD4-count ($< 100 \times 10^6$/l) in 71% of all episodes, while median CD4 count among bacteremic pre-AIDS patients was 180 (range 8–460) and among bacteremic AIDS patients 16 (range 0–150). Central i.v. lines were present in 44%, while neutropenia (11%) and IVDU (7%) were associated with fewer episodes. No clinical risk factors were found in 9 patients, of whom 8 were pre-AIDS patients.

Compared with other microbial species, S. pneumoniae occurred at higher CD4 counts (median = 136, range 2–460) and relatively often in patients without any of the recorded predisposing risk factors, while all Salmonella and 9 of 10 episodes with other Enterobacteriaceae were seen in patients with CD4 count $< 100 \times 10^6$/l. In 20 of the 70 primary episodes, prophylactic or suppressive antibiotics were administered at the time of blood culturing: cotrimoxazole in 15 cases, clindamycin plus pyrimethamine in 3 cases, rifampicin in 2 cases and sulfadiazine in 1 case. No S. pneumoniae or Salmonella spp. were found in these patients, in contrast to 19 episodes with these 2 strains found in 54 patients not receiving any prophylactic antibiotic treatment ($p = 0.014$).

Septic shock was encountered in 8 of the 76 episodes with the following species: 2 S. aureus, 2 E. coli, 1 P. aeruginosa, 1 C. albicans, 1 C. neoformans, and 1 polymicrobial. Seven deaths were related to the episodes. The S. aureus bacteremia related mortality was 3 of 19 (16%), while the HIV-related pathogens S. pneumoniae and Salmonella spp. caused no deaths. One of 3 patients with C. neoformans died of the fungemia. Overall, bacteremia-related mortality was 12% within the AIDS group and 13% within the pre-AIDS group.

Noteworthy regarding antibiotic susceptibility patterns were netilmicin sensitivity: Enterobacteriaceae, cotrimoxazole sensitivity: Salmonella spp. and S. pneumonia, penicillin sensitivity: S. pneumoniae, methicillin sensitivity: S. aureus and penicillin sensitivity for 7 of 19 S. aureus.

DISCUSSION

Most studies have reported on AIDS related bacteremia only in special settings within the group of AIDS patients (3, 10, 17–20), while this study includes bacteremia episodes in a large group of pre-AIDS patients. Among IVDU and African patients a large proportion of Salmonella non-typhi was found (3–6). Three North-American surveys, in which the HIV patients were mainly homosexual, demonstrate a high proportion of bacteremia with staphylococci and yeasts (10, 18, 19). A study from London in which the risk behaviour was not mentioned reported a high rate of MAC, Pseudomonas spp. and S. pneumoniae (21). We did not include mycobacteremia in this study, as this AIDS-defining condition clinically manifests itself as a chronic infection different from other bactermia. Mycobacteremia with predominantly M. avium was detected in 43 out of the 333 AIDS patients studied during the 5 years, using Bactec-13A^R blood culture system in selected patients. In the group with bacteremia, 4 patients also had MAC infection. The high incidence of bacteremia with S. pneumonia, Salmonella spp., L. monocytogenes and C. neoformans in HIV patients, compared with non-HIV populations reported by other authors (8, 22–25), is supported by our findings, but the incidences of infection were higher for all species, when comparing HIV data with bacteremia rates from Danish general population patients using the same blood culture system. Incidences of Salmonella spp., Pseudomonas spp. and S. epidermidis bacteremias were 960, 720 and 560 times more frequent in AIDS patients, whereas the incidence of E. coli bacteremia was increased 108-fold (Table II).

Table II. *Incidence of positive blood-culture per 10,000 person years in the general population, and in HIV infected patients with and without AIDS*

		Reference population	Pre-AIDS patients	AIDS patients
No. person-years		250,013	2,473	348
Flora type	Species			
	Total	10.3 (258)	170 (42)**	3200 (112)**
Skin	S. aureus	1.3 (32)	36 (9)**	290 (10)**
	S. epidermidis	2.4 (61)	57 (14)**	1350 (47)**
	Corynebacteria spp	0.12 (3)	4.0 (1)	144 (5)**
	C. jeikeium	–	4.0 (1)	29 (1)
Airway	S. pneumoniae	1.1 (28)	20 (5)**	200 (7)**
	C. neoformans	–	4.0 (1)	57 (2)
	N. meningitidis	0.040 (1)	4.0 (1)*	–
Intestinal	Enterococcus spp	0.60 (15)	4.0 (1)	86 (3)*
	β-haemol. streptococci	0.44 (11)	8.1 (2)*	29 (1)
	Non. haemol. streptococci	0.28 (7)	4.0 (1)	86 (3)*
	L. monocytogenes	–	–	29 (1)
	Peptococcus sp	0.12 (3)	–	29 (1)
	Salmonella spp	0.24 (6)	12 (3)**	230 (8)**
	E. coli	1.6 (39)	4.0 (1)	173 (6)**
	Klebsiella spp	0.48 (12)	– (0)	57 (2)*
	P. mirabilis	0.040 (1)	4.0 (1)*	–
	E. cloacae	0.28 (7)	4.0 (1)	57 (2)
	Pseudomonas spp	0.24 (6)	– (0)	173 (6)**
Miscellaneous	Bacillus spp	0.080 (2)	– (0)	115 (4)**
	Acinetobacter spp	0.12 (3)	–	29 (1)
	Other bacteria	1.0 (25)	–	–
	Candida spp	0.08 (2)	–	29 (1)
	S. cerevisiae	–	–	29 (1)

In parentheses: actual numbers.
* $p < 0.02$, ** $p < 0.001$, related to the distribution in the column to the left.

The choice of comparison group may be debated as even out-patient HIV cases are being evaluated more closely than the population in general. However, rather than comparison with various high-risk referral centre patient groups (20), we believe that the data from county general hospitals provide a reasonable reflection of bacteremia in the population as a whole. This comparison did not account for the frequency of clinically irrelevant strains. The exclusion of irrelevant strains in the HIV population diminished especially the frequency of S. epidermidis (see Table I), reducing a total of 198 positive blood culture sets to 133 clinically relevant samples which were grouped into 76 clinical episodes. Relapses of bacteremia only occurred with Gram-negative rods, especially with non-typhoid Salmonella spp. Treatment of this infection during the first years of our study was intravenous ampicillin or short courses of ciprofloxacin, resulting in relapse in all 4 cases. Courses of ciprofloxacin for 4 weeks or high-dose cotrimoxazole were used subsequently and prevented further relapses, which is in accordance with previous reports (24, 26).

Salmonella spp. and S. pneumoniae episodes were predominantly community acquired. It is noteworthy that none of the patients with S. pneumoniae and Salmonella infection received cotrimoxazole as Pneumocystis carinii prophylaxis, which is otherwise recommended for immunocompromised patients, i.e. with CD4 counts $<200 \times 10^6/l$ (27, 28). S. pneumoniae bacteremia occurred in 13 cases in the age-matched reference population, corresponding to 1.1 per 10,000 person-years, while we found rates of 20 and 200 per 10,000 patient-years in pre-AIDS and AIDS patients, respectively.

11 of the 12 S. pneumoniae isolates were subtyped (3, 5, 6A, 7F, 12F, 14, 19A, 22F, 24F), and 9 belonged to types potentially covered by the presently used 23 valent vaccine. Vaccination is now being recommended for patients with HIV disease (29). 42% of all bacteremic episodes in AIDS patients were nosocomial infections, and these were caused mainly by staphylococci, emphasizing the importance of handling intravenous devices with greater care.

Denominators concerning predisposing risk factors for bacteremia were not obtainable, and the importance of risk factors could therefore not be fully elucidated. Having a low CD4 count, however, was a common predisposing risk factor studied (71%), while neutropenia was only found in few of the episodes (11%). Prophylactic use of human recombinant colony-stimulating factors in neutropenic HIV-patients has been advocated, but was not used in the present series of patients and, according to our data, this therapeutic modality could not influence the overall incidence of bacteremia in AIDS patients.

Intravenous lines, which are associated with the treatment for CMV disease were present in 44% of the episodes, and were the most common known source of infection (23%). In previous reports on HIV disease and central venous catheters (CVC) (11–14, 30), infection rates ranged between 0.13 and 0.47 per 100 catheter days, which was significantly higher than in control groups. Our data support that the overall infection rate could be reduced by intensification of aseptic CVC handling.

Retrospectively we searched for possible improvements in therapeutic intervention among these patients. In the 8 septic shock episodes, delay of relevant treatment was only found in the (fatal) Candida episode, amounting to 3 days explained by late detection. The remaining 7 episodes were treated promptly with appropriate antibiotics. The empiric regimen used consisted of intravenous cefuroxime 750 mg × 3 (or ampicillin 2 g × 4 if community acquired) and netilmicin 300 mg, and should be recommended for further use in our population as it covered 90% of the bacteremias, including all episodes with Salmonella spp. and S. pneumonia according to the susceptibility patterns observed. Methicillin-resistant S. aureus is presently very rare in Denmark (31), and 1 episode of Candida bacteremia among the HIV-infected patients during 5 years does not warrant a change in the present empiric regimen.

None of the known bacteremia studies account for the influence of prophylactic antibiotic treatment against Pneumocystis carinii, toxoplasmosis, and Mycobacteria on the outcome or species distribution of the blood cultures. Prophylaxis with cotrimoxazole has been used successfully for P. carinii pneumonia among immunocompromised high-risk patients with additionally lowered incidence of important bacterial infections as a consequence (32). Such prophylaxis could possibly reduce the incidence of infections with organisms such as Salmonella and S. pneumonia, and would have reduced morbidity – but not mortality. To clarify to what extent and in which subgroups of HIV-infected patients such an effect is obtained, prospective studies should be carried out.

In conclusion we found that bacteremia among HIV-infected patients in Denmark was acquired at a much higher frequency than in the age-matched general population; mainly during their AIDS stage, at low CD4 counts and to a high degree as nosocomial infections. A blood culture should therefore be set up whenever such infection is suspected in HIV-infected persons. The major agents found were staphylococci, associated with intravenous line infection. The increased rate of bacteremia in HIV-infected patients can thus be partly ascribed to an increased risk of nosocomial infections, but is partly due to the immunodeficiency compromising resistance, especially to encapsulated bacteria. Long-term cotrimoxazole prophylaxis may reduce the infection rate of Salmonella and S. pneumonia bacteremia.

ACKNOWLEDGEMENT

We thank Cand. Sci. Severin Olesen-Larsen for statistical advice.

REFERENCES

1. Castro KG, Ward JW, Slutsker L, Buehler JW, Jaffe HW, Berkelman RL, Curran JW. 1993 Revised Classification System for HIV Infection and Expanded Surveillance Case Definition for AIDS Among Adolescents and Adults. Clin Infect Dis 17: 802–810, 1993.
2. Northfelt DW. Bacteremia in persons with HIV infection. AIDS Clin Rev 59–79, 1991.
3. Ruiz I, Almirante B, Ocana I, Pahissa A, Capdevilla JA, Planes AM, Martinez Vazquez JM. Bacteriemias y fungemias en pacientes con SIDA. Estudio de 56 episodios. Enferm Infect Microbiol Clin 8: 548–522, 1990.
4. Gilks CF, Brindle RJ, Otieno LS, Simani PM, Newnham RS, Bhatt SM. Life threatening bacteremia in HIV-1 seropositive adults admitted to hospital in Nairobi, Kenya. Lancet 336: 545–549, 1990.
5. Lepage P, Van de Perre P, Nsengumuremyi F, van Goethem C, Bogaerts J, Hitimana DG. Bacteremia as predictor of HIV infection in African children. Acta Paediatr Scand 78: 763–766, 1989.
6. Vugia DJ, Kiehlbauch A, Yeboue K, N'Gbichi JM, Lacina D, Maran M, Gondo M. Pathogens and predictors of fatal septicemia associated with human immunodeficiency virus infection in Ivory Coast, West Africa. J Infect Dis 168: 564–570, 1993.
7. Witt DJ, Craven DE, McCabe WR. Bacterial infections in adult patients with AIDS and AIDS-related complex. Am J Med 82: 900–906, 1987.
8. Redd SC, Rutherford III GW, Sande MA, Lifson AR, Hadley WK, Facklam RR, Spika JS. The role of HIV infection in pneumococcal bacteremia in San Francisco residents. J Infect Dis 162: 1012–1017, 1990.
9. Pesola GR, Charles A. Pneumococal bacteremia with pneumonia. Mortality in AIDS. Chest 101: 150–155, 1992.
10. Krumholz HM, Sande MA, Lo B. Community-acquired bacteremia in patients with AIDS: clinical presentation, bacteriology, and outcome. Am J Med 86: 776–779, 1989.
11. Raviglione MC, Battan R, Pablos-Mendes A, Aceves-Casillas P, Mullen MP, Taranta A. Infections associated with Hickman catheters in patients with AIDS. Am J Med 86: 780–786, 1989.
12. Henry K, Thurn JR, Johnson S. Experience with central venous catheders in patients with AIDS. N Engl J Med 320: 1496, 1989.
13. Prichards JG, Nelson MJ, Burns L, Kaplowitz HJ, Caillouet BL, Sanchez MA. Infections caused by central venous catheders in patients with AIDS. South Med J 81: 1496–1498, 1988.
14. Skoutelis AT, Murphy RL, MacDonell KB, VonRoenn JH, Sterkel CD, Phair JP. Indwelling central venous catheter infections in patients with AIDS. J Acquir Immune Defic Syndr 3: 335–342, 1990.
15. Sundhedsstyrelsen AIDS-sekretariatet. Anmeldte AIDS-tilfælde i Danmark pr 31.12.92. AIDS Nyt 61: 12, 1993.
16. Prag J, Jensen J, Lebech K. Colorbact, a visually read blood culture system using darkening of haemoglobin in aerobic blood cultures as an early growth indicator compared with Bactec 6A and 7A. APMIS 99: 1089–1095, 1991.
17. Eng RH, Bishburg E, Smith SM, Geller H, Kapila R. Bacteremia and fungemia in patients with Acquired Immune Deficiency Syndrome. Am J Clin Pathol 86: 105–107, 1986.
18. Katz SJ, Wenger NS, Shapiro MF: Diagnostic value of bacterial and fungal blood cultures in patients with the acquired immunodeficiency syndrome. Am J Med 88: 28N–32N, 1990.
19. Whimbey E, Gold JWM, Polsky B, Dryjanski J, Hawkins C, Blevins A. Bacteremia and fungemia in patients with AIDS. Ann Intern Med 104: 511–514, 1986.
20. Hickey MM, Shanson DC. Septicemia in patients with and without AIDS at Westminster Hospital, London. J Infect 27: 243–250, 1993.
21. Shanson DC. Septicaemia in patients with AIDS. Trans R Soc Trop Med Hyg 84 (Suppl 1): 14–16, 1990.
22. Hawkins CC, Gold JWN, Whimbey E, Kiehn TE, Brannon P, Cammarata R, Brown AE. Mycobacterium avium complex in patients with AIDS. Ann Intern Med 105: 184–188, 1986.

23. Jurado RL, Farley MM, Pereira E, Harvey RC, Schuchat A, Wenger JD, Stephens DS. Increased risk of meningitis and bacteremia due to Listeria monocytogenes in patients with HIV infection. Clin Infect Dis 17: 224–227, 1993.
24. Sperber SJ, Schleupner CK. Salmonellosis during infection with Human Immunodeficiency Virus. Rev Infect Dis 9: 925–934, 1987.
25. Dismukes WE. Cryptococcal meningitis in patients with AIDS. J Infect Dis 157: 624–628, 1988.
26. Jacobson MA, Hahn SM, Gerberding JL, Lee B, Sande MA. Ciprofloxacin for Salmonella bacteremia in AIDS. Ann Intern Med 110: 1027–1029, 1989.
27. Schneider MME, Hoepelman AIM, Schattenkern JKMK, Nielsen TL, van der Graae Y, Frissen JPHJ, van der Ende IME. A controlled trial of aerosolized pentamidine or trimethoprim-sulfamethoxazole as primary prophylaxis against Pneumocystis carinii pneumonia in patients with human immunodeficiency virus infection. N Engl J Med 327; 1836–1841, 1992.
28. Hardy WD, Feinberg JF, Finkelstein DM, Power ME, Hk W, Kaczka C, Frame PT. A controlled trial of trimethoprim-sulfamethoxazole or aerosolized pentamidine for secondary prophylaxis of pneumocystis carinii pneumonia in patients with the acquired immunodeficiency syndrome. N Engl J Med 327: 1842–1848, 1993.
29. Filice GA, Pomeroy C. Preventing secondary infections among HIV-positive persons. Public Health Reports 106: 503–517, 1991.
30. Stanley HD, Charlebois E, Harb G, Jacobsen MA. Central venous catheter infections in AIDS patients receiving treatment for cytomegalovirus disease. J Acquir Immune Defic Syndr 7: 272–278, 1994.
31. Rosdahl VT, Knudsen AM. The decline of methicillin resistance among Danish Staphylococcus aureus strains. Infect Control Hosp Epidemiol 12: 83–88, 1991.
32. Hughes WT, Kuhn S, Chaudhary S, Feldman S, Verzosa M, Aur RJA, Pratt C, George SL. Successful chemoprophylaxis for Pneumocystis carinii pneumonitis. N Engl J Med 297: 1419–1426, 1977.

Submitted April 5, 1994; accepted July 27, 1994

Scand J Infect Dis 26: 643–651, 1994

Natural History of Asymptomatic and Symptomatic Pneumocystis carinii Infection in HIV Infected Patients

KERSTIN ELVIN[1], CHRISTER LIDMAN[2], ELSA TYNELL[3], EWERT LINDER[4] and ANDERS BJÖRKMAN[2]

From the Departments of [1]Microbiology and Tumorbiology Center, Karolinska Institute, Swedish Institute for Infectious Disease Control, [2]Division of Infectious Diseases, Karolinska Institute, Huddinge Hospital, [3]Division of Infectious Diseases, Karolinska Institute, Danderyd Hospital, and the [4]Swedish Institute for Infectious Disease Control, Stockholm, Sweden

The natural appearance of Pneumocystis carinii in induced sputum samples was studied in 60 HIV-infected patients with severe immunodeficiency and without a history of P. carinii pneumonia (PCP). The patients were prospectively evaluated for occurrence of P. carinii in induced sputum samples, PCP diagnosis and CD4+ cell counts during observation periods of 2 to 31 months. P. carinii was detected in 16 patients all of whom developed clinical PCP. In 5 patients P. carinii was detected 3 weeks to 8 months prior to clinical symptoms. Immunofluorescence using monoclonal antibody 3F6 was more sensitive than toluidine in detecting P. carinii in sputum samples ($p < 0.05$). In the patients who developed PCP a drop of the mean CD4 count to 40–50 × 10^6/l was observed 200 days before diagnosis. However, out of 13 patients with CD4 counts of 0–20 × 10^6/l only 7 developed PCP during 200 days of observation. The results do not support the suggested reactivation of a latent infection present in the vast majority of adults. PCP may instead result from exposure to the organism or presence of an unknown cofactor.

We conclude that P. carinii is present in some asymptomatic HIV patients and that the detection of the organism in sputum should be regarded as pathological and prophylaxis or treatment inserted. The risk of transmission of P. carinii to patients with severe immunodeficiency should be seriously considered.

K. Elvin, MD, Swedish Institute for Infectious Disease Control, S-105 21 Stockholm, Sweden

INTRODUCTION

Although Pneumocystis carinii pneumonia (PCP) remains the most common serious opportunistic infection among patients with HIV disease in the Western world, little is known about this organism's biologic and epidemiologic characteristics. The risk of PCP has been found to correlate to a number of circulating CD4+ cells less than 200 × 10^6/l (1, 2).

On the basis of serological studies, the infection is thought to be acquired in early childhood. The clinical manifestations in immunosuppressed patients have generally been regarded as a result of reactivation of a latent infection. However, reports of case clustering have implied that the infection may be acquired and P. carinii was not found in autopsy studies including immunocompetent as well as HIV infected patients (3, 4) nor was the organism detected in bronchoalveolar lavages (BAL) from asymptomatic HIV infected patients without a history of PCP (5, 6). In contrast, the organism has been detected at bronchoscopy for more than one month after a verified and treated P. carinii infection in AIDS patients (7) and even during prophylactic treatment in HIV infected patients (8). There is clearly a need for prospective studies on the occurrence of asymptomatic P. carinii in HIV infected individuals without a previous PCP.

Our aim was to study the occurrence and natural course of P. carinii infection in HIV infected patients in relation to the progression of immunodeficiency as measured by CD4+ cell counts.

PATIENTS AND METHODS

Patients

A total of 60 HIV antibody positive patients without previous history of PCP were followed prospectively and investigated regularly for the presence of P. carinii in induced sputum samples. Patients were enrolled during October 1989 to October 1991. Last day of follow up was June 21, 1992. The patients belonged to the control group of a multicenter randomised, primary prophylaxis versus no prophylaxis study in Stockholm, Sweden. The study was approved by the Ethics Committee Karolinska Hospital in Stockholm. Informed consent was given by all patients.

The patients entered the study if they had a confirmed HIV-infection, were 18 years or older and had CD4+ cell counts $\leq 200 \times 10^6$/l or an AIDS diagnosis based on other criteria than PCP. Patients were excluded if they had drug problems that could interfere with the study protocol. The patients had clinical check-ups and sputum examination for P. carinii detection every second month. They were also told to attend the clinic whenever any clinical symptoms occurred. CD4+ cell counts were determined every 4 months.

If P. carinii was detected in an asymptomatic patient he or she was followed up closely every second week. When there was a clinical suspicion of PCP and P. carinii was not detected in induced sputum samples, a bronchoscopy with BAL was scheduled. Confirmed PCP was defined as symptoms (cough or dyspnea or fever) in combination with detection of P. carinii in induced sputum or bronchoalveolar lavage. Clinical PCP was defined as fever and respiratory symptoms and response to treatment.

Sputum induction

Patients first brushed their teeth and gum, gargled with water or saline to clear debris from the mouth and oropharynx. They then inhaled a mist of 3% saline generated by an ultrasonic nebulizer (Omron, Model NE-U10B, Umedico AB, Roserberg, Sweden) for 10–30 min (3 ml saline nebulized/min). During this time patients were encouraged to cough and the expectorate was collected in sterile sputum containers.

P. carinii detection

Sputum samples were first liquified with 6.3 mM dithiotreitol, then 50% ethanol was added and allowed to inactivate HIV for at least 10 min. The samples were centrifuged at 1.300 g for 10 min and smears were prepared from the pellets. An indirect immunofluorescence method using monoclonal antibody 3F6 was used as previously described (9) on the smears postfixed with equal parts of methanol and acetone. To avoid confusion with fungi occasionally taking up conjugate, a control preparation incubated with conjugate only was used for each specimen. Toluidine blue O staining was performed on the smears according to Gosey et al. 1987 (10). The 2 staining procedures were performed in different laboratories and examined by 2 observers in each laboratory with no knowledge of the results of the other staining.

CD4+ cell counts

Absolute numbers of CD4+ lymphocytes were determined by flow cytometry. Until March 1990 the analyses were performed by an Ortho Spectrum III using single staining (including a non stained specimen control). From April 1990 and throughout the study a FACS scan was used (including an isotype control).

Statistical analyses

The binomial test was used to compare the sensitivity of the 2 staining methods. For PCP free survival analyses we used Kaplan–Meier life table analysis and Mantel log rank to test for group differences.

RESULTS

60 patients were enrolled in the study. Mean age was 41.4 years. Four of the 60 patients were women. Risk categories for HIV were; homosexual men ($n = 40$), intravenous drug users ($n = 12$), transfusion recipients ($n = 6$) and unknown ($n = 2$). In total, 226 induced sputum samples were obtained and analysed from 53 patients. Times and intervals of sputum sampling are illustrated by the 19 patients in fig. 1. In 7 patients no sputum sample was obtained. Two patients were unable to produce any sputum sample, and 5 patients did not attend to the scheduled clinical check-ups (2 of whom withdrew before end of study).

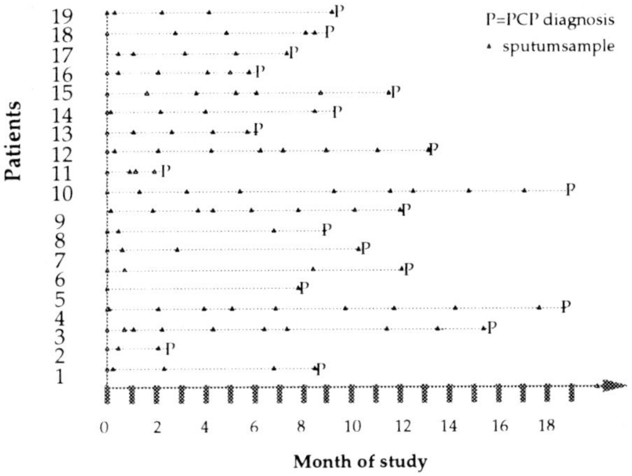

Fig. 1. Period of sputum sampling in the 19 patients receiving PCP diagnosis.

19 patients were diagnosed with PCP. 16 patients had positive findings of P. carinii in sputum (2 of these patients also underwent bronchoscopy with a confirmative positive detection of P. carinii in BAL). Three patients had their diagnosis based on clinical symptoms and response to treatment. Two of them had interstitial infiltrates on chest-X-ray. Two of the 3 patients were unable to produce a sputum sample at the time of PCP symptoms and bronchoscopy was interrupted in the third patient because of serious bleeding.

Results of the microscopical detection of P. carinii after immunofluorescence and toluidine staining respectively are presented in Table I. Immunofluorescence was significantly more sensitive than toluidine blue ($p < 0.05$).

The P. carinii positive samples were received from 16 patients all of whom developed clinical PCP. In 11 patients P. carinii was not found until the last 2 weeks before PCP diagnosis (Figs 2 and 3). In 5 patients however, P. carinii was detected in the scheduled sputum samples without accompanying symptoms 255, 189, 53, 26 and 23 days before diagnosis respectively (Fig. 4). In the 3 patients with P. carinii presenting 53 days or more before clinical PCP P. carinii was found in 5 of the 8 (62.5%) additional representative sputum samples. In all, P. carinii was detected in only 9 out of 209 (4.3%) sputum samples obtained according to the study schedule when no respiratory symptoms were present.

CD4+ cell counts ($\times 10^6$/l) were investigated every 4 months. The initial values upon entering the study were ≤ 100 in 28 patients and > 100 in 32 patients. Only 1 patient had > 200 as he entered the study with an AIDS diagnosis based on Kaposis sarcoma. The overall mean value was 107 (SEM 8.6). The range was from 10 to 280. At the time of

Table I. *Detection of Pneumocystis carinii by indirect immunofluorescence and toluidine staining of 191 induced sputum samples*

		Toluidine staining	
		+	−
IFL staining	+	12	8
	−	1	170

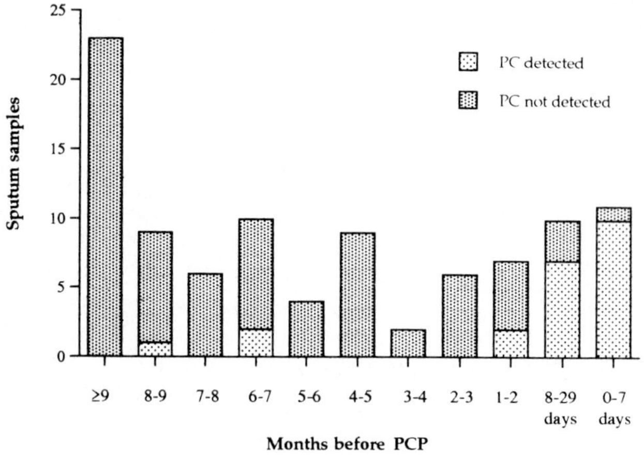

Fig. 2. Prevalence of detected P. carinii in relation to time of pneumonia diagnosis.

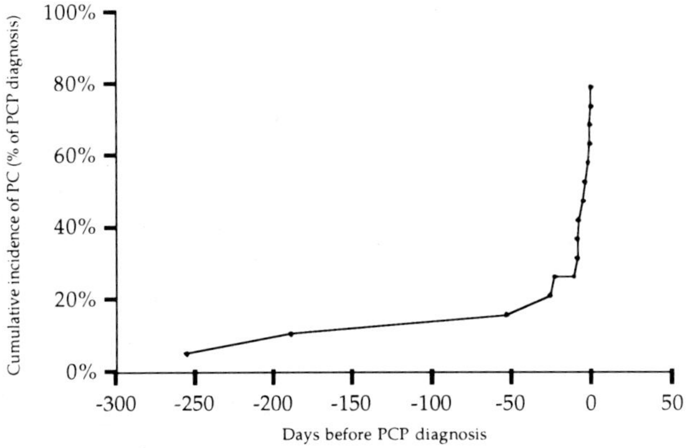

Fig. 3. Cumulative incidence of detected P. carinii in patients with clinical pneumonia.

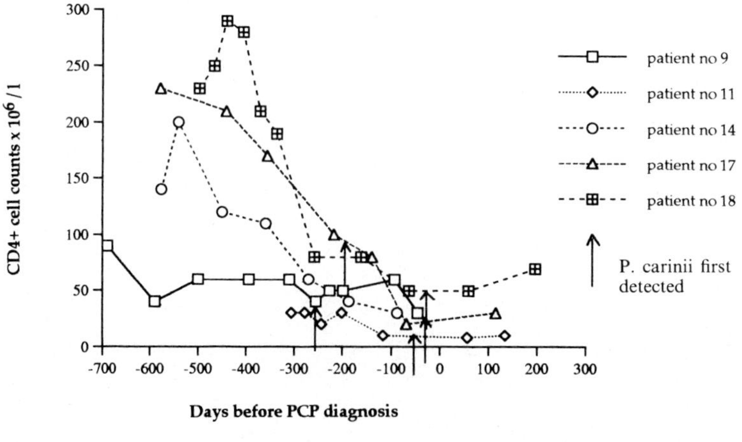

Fig. 4. Evolution of CD4+ cell counts in 5 patients with asymptomatic P. carinii before developing pneumonia.

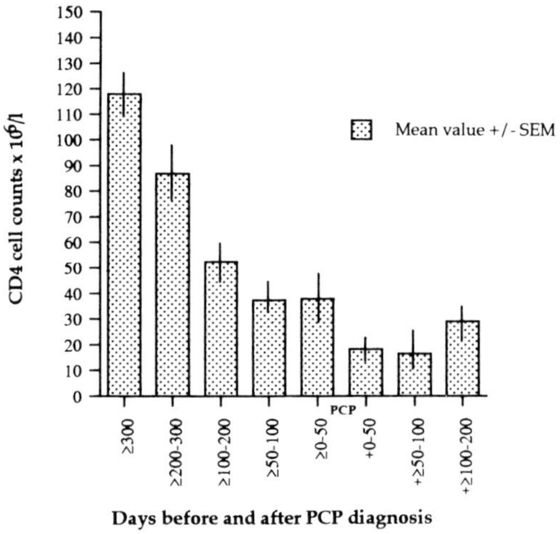

Fig. 5. Mean values of CD4 cell counts before and after PCP diagnosis in 19 patients.

asymptomatic P. carinii detection, the individual CD4+ cell counts had a mean value of 36 ranging from 8 to 80 (Fig. 4). Considering all 19 PCP patients, the CD4+ cell counts determined less than 50 days before PCP diagnosis were similar, with a mean of 38 ranging from 20 to 80. The CD4 counts apparently reached low values (about 50) already 100–200 days before the PCP diagnosis (Fig. 5).

The general incidences of PCP in relation to the CD4 counts are presented in fig. 6. At the extremely low CD4 count level of 0–20, 40% (6/15) developed PCP within 100 days and 54% (7/13) within 200 days of observation. Thus, despite this very depressed immunity 46% (6/13) did not develop signs or symptoms of PCP within 200 days of observation. Two of these eventually developed PCP within 300 days of observation. The remaining 4 patients were evaluated for risk category for HIV, age, sex and number of sputum inductions, all of which were found to be similar to the PCP patients.

The risk of PCP in the 2 subgroups of patients wtih CD4+ cell counts of ≤ 100 and > 100 respectively at study start are presented in fig. 7. There was a significant difference in PCP free survival between the 2 groups ($p < 0.05$). The groups had cumulative PCP risks of 12% and 4% respectively after 6 months and 41% and 19% respectively after 12 study months.

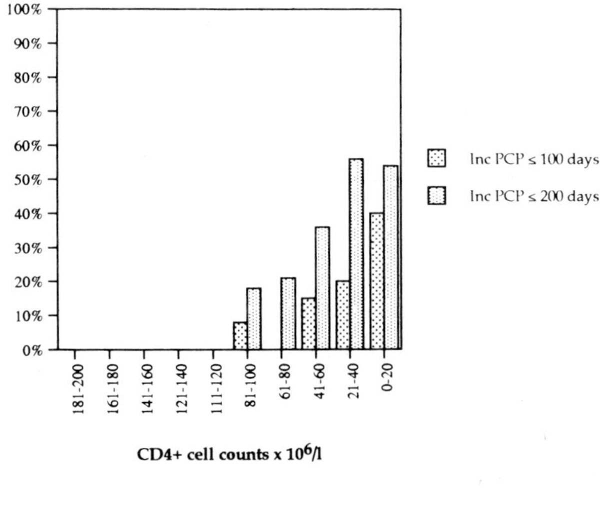

Fig. 6. The incidence of PCP within 100 and 200 days of observation respectively, after reaching various levels of CD4+ cell counts.

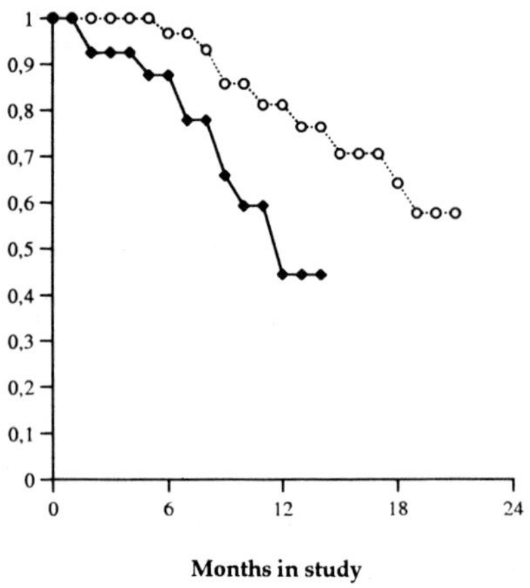

Fig. 7. The proportion of PCP free survival in 28 patients with CD4+ cell counts of $\leq 100 \times 10^6$/l —◆—, and in 31 patients with CD4+ cell counts of 101 to 200×10^6/l —○—, at study start.

After 18 months only 1 patient remained uninfected in the group with CD4+ cell counts ≤100, in contrast to 10 patients in the other group.

DISCUSSION

We have shown that P. carinii can be detected in HIV infected patients with no respiratory symptoms prior to developing PCP. Previously P. carinii was not detected in BAL samples from asymptomatic HIV infected patients in Denmark (5) or in USA (6). The BAL studies however included small numbers of patients (8 and 24 patients respectively) in whom P. carinii was screened for on one occasion only. Considering that asymptomatic P. carinii was detected in only 9 out of 209 (4.3%) scheduled sputum samples, the BAL studies may have been too small to exclude asymptomatic occurrence of P. carinii. With PCR P. carinii DNA has been amplified in a few HIV infected symptomatic patients without clinically evident PCP (11–15). Most of these patients however, have had a history of PCP and been receiving prophylaxis. The results have been interpreted as colonization. No previous study has however prospectively followed asymptomatic patients. In our PCR study (13), 1 asymptomatic HIV infected patient with positive P. carinii DNA detection in sputum did not present with PCP during 2 years of follow up before he died from other reasons.

At the time of positive P. carinii detection this patients CD4+ cell count was 350×10^6/l and remained above 200×10^6 for 1 year. Since immunocompetent rats have been shown by PCR to be transient carriers of P. carinii due to exposure (16) it is possible that the discussed HIV infected patient was a transient carrier of P. carinii.

The asymptomatically found organisms were evidently not detected by chance in patients later developing PCP since additional samples from these patients demonstrated the organism in a rate (62%) closely corresponding to the sensitivity of the IFL in sputum (74%). Since all patients in our study in whom P. carinii was detected subsequently developed clinical signs and symptoms of PCP, we conclude that asymptomatic detection is of clinical importance and treatment or prophylaxis should be instituted.

Asymptomatic P. carinii was only detected in 4.3% scheduled sputum samples. Screening of induced sputum samples with currently used detection methods in HIV infected patients at risk of developing PCP can therefore not be recommended since this would be very cost ineffective. A more practical alternative would be to routinely provide prophylactic treatment to patients with severe immunodeficiency according to CDC recommendations (17), or to provide a close clinical follow up of the patients with sputum sampling when symptoms arise, which was shown to be as efficient as primary prophylaxis with pentamidine inhalations regarding mortality and generally morbidity in our own study (unpublished results).

The combination of 2 methods for P. carinii detection and the use of a specific and sensitive immunological staining should have allowed us to reach a high level of sensitivity. With the use of a recently developed PCR (13) the sensitivity could further increase and a higher proportion of patients with asymptomatic P. carinii could possibly be identified. The immunofluorescence stain was more sensitive than the toluidine stain and the subsequent clinical evaluation also proved it to be specific. This is in contrast to a study on another monoclonal antibody (commercialised by Meridian Diagnostic Inc., Cincinnati, OH) where a subset of the positive specimens were from patients whose clinical symptoms resolved without treatment and the PCP diagnosis was questioned (18).

There was no evident correlation between conversion from asymptomatic to symptomatic disease and the number of CD4+ cells in the individual CD4+ cell count curves of the 5 patients with asymptomatic P. carinii detection (Fig. 4). However, the patients who developed PCP had a mean value of CD4 counts of about 50 for up to 200 days before diagnosis (Fig. 5). In a previous study CD4 counts done 30 to 60 days before the pulmonary diagnosis were also similar to those just before diagnosis (0–7 days) (2). The proportion of PCP free survival was as expected lower in the patients with a CD4 count ≤ 100 at study start as compared to the patients with a CD4 count of 101–200 at study start (Fig. 7).

If the infection was latent, we would have expected to see a conversion from asymptomatic to symptomatic P. carinii infection soon after the CD4 counts reached a critical low value, e.g., below 50. We would also have expected to see a relatively uniform time elapse from reaching the low CD4 value until developing PCP. In rats and mice PCP develops within 4 to 8 weeks of immunosuppression. The latency time in our patients however, varied a lot and expanded to more than 200 days in 6/13 patients with extremely low CD4 values. These results speak against the theory of latent infection. If the pneumonia results from reinfection, half of the patients were not exposed to the infection during the observed time. The exposure theory is further supported by the airborn transmission found in immunosuppressed experimental animals (19, 20) and by reports on case clustering in humans (21–25). A third possibility is that a cofactor is required, irrespective if the P. carinii infection is acquired or reactivated. In our study however, neither age, sex, risk group for HIV infection, nor the number of sputum inductions could be identified as such a cofactor.

We conclude that P. carinii is present in some asymptomatic HIV patients with severe immunodeficiency prior to the development of symptomatic PCP. Detection of the organism in sputum should be regarded as pathological and prophylaxis or treatment inserted. The occurrence of asymptomatic P. carinii infection was however not frequent enough to imply regular screening of induced sputum samples. Half of the HIV patients with CD4 cell counts at or below 20 developed PCP within 200 days possibly due to exposure to P. carinii. This possibility should be taken in consideration in the management of the PCP patients.

ACKNOWLEDGEMENTS

The authors thank Anne-Marie Karlsson, Britt-Marie Johansson, Margit Halvarsson and Theodor Capraru for their kind and efficient help in data collection.

REFERENCES

1. Phair J, Munoz A, Detels R, Kaslow R, Rinaldo C, Saah A. Group. MACS. The risk of Pneumocystis carinii pneumonia among men infected with human immunodeficiency virus type 1. N Engl J Med 322: 161–165, 1990.

2. Masur H, Ognibene FP, Yarchoan R, Shelhamer JH, Baird BF, Travis W, Suffredini AF, Deyton L, Kovacs JA, Falloon J, Davey R, Polis M, Metcalf J, Baseler M, Wesley R, Gill VJ, Fauci AS, Lane C. CD4 counts as predictors of opportunistic pneumonias in Human Immunodeficiency Virus (HIV) infection. Ann Intern Med 111: 223–231, 1989.
3. Millard PR, Heryet AR. Observations favouring Pneumocystis carinii pneumonia as a primary infection: a monoclonal antibody study on paraffin sections. J Pathol 154: 365–370, 1988.
4. Coleman DL, Luce JM, Wilber JC, Ferrer JJ, Stephens BG, Margaretten W, Wagar EA, Hadley WK, Pifer LL, Moss AR, Dodek PM, Levy JA, Murray JF. Antibody to the retrovirus associated with the acquired immunodeficiency syndrome (AIDS). Arch Intern Med 146: 713–715, 1986.
5. Lundgren JD, Orholm M, Nielsen TL, Iversen J, Hertz J, Nielsen JO. Bronchoscopy of symptom free patients infected with human immunodeficiency virus for detection of pneumocystosis. Thorax 44: 68–69, 1989.
6. Ognibene FP, Masur H, Rogers P, Travis WD, Suffredini AF, Feuerstein I, Gill VJ, Baird BF, Carrasquillo JA, Parrillo JE, Lane HC, Shelhamer JH. Nonspecific interstitial pneumonitis without evidence of Pneumocystis carinii in asymptomatic patients infected with human immunodeficiency virus (HIV). Ann Intern Med 874–879, 1988.
7. Shelhamer JH, Ognibene FP, Macher AM, Tuazon C, Steiss R, Longo D, Kovacs JA, Parker MM, Natanson C, Lane HC, Fauci AS, Parrillo JE, Masur H. Persistence of Pneumocystis carinii in lung tissue of acquired immunodeficiency syndrome patients treated for Pneumocystis pneumonia. Am Rev Respir Dis 130: 1161–1165, 1984.
8. Contini C, Romani R, Vullo V, Delia S, Sorice F. Does laboratory recovery of Pneumocystis carinii always mean clinically significant disease? AIDS 6: 1558–1559, 1992.
9. Elvin KM, Björkman A, Linder E, Heurlin N, Hjerpe A. Pneumocystis carinii pneumonia: detection of parasites in sputum and bronchoalveolar lavage fluid by monoclonal antibodies. BMJ 297: 381–384, 1988.
10. Gosey LL, Howard RM, Witebsky FG, Ognibene FP, Wu TC, Gill VJ, MacLowry JD. Advantages of a modified toluidine blue O stain and bronchoalveolar lavage for the diagnosis of Pneumocystis carinii pneumonia. J Clin Microbiol 22: 803–807, 1985.
11. Blumenfeld W, McCook O, Holodniy M, Katzenstein DA. Correlation of morphologic diagnosis of Pneumocystis carinii with the presence of pneumocystis DNA amplified by the polymerase chain reaction. Mod Pathol 5: 103–106, 1992.
12. Lipschik GY, Gill VJ, Lundgren JD, Andrawis VA, Nelson NA, Nielsen JO, Ognibene FP, Kovacs JA. Improved diagnosis of Pneumocystis carinii infection by polymerase chain reaction on induced sputum and blood. Lancet 340: 203–206, 1992.
13. Olsson M, Elvin K, Löfdahl S, Linder E. Detection of Pneumocystis carinii DNA in sputum and bronchoalveolar lavage samples by polymerase chain reaction. J Clin Microbiol 31: 221–226, 1993.
14. Tamburrini E, Mencarini P, De LA, Maiuro G, Ventura G, Antinori A, Ammassari A, Visconti E, Ortona L, Siracusano A, et al. Diagnosis of Pneumocystis carinii pneumonia: specificity and sensitivity of polymerase chain reaction in comparison with immunofluorescence in bronchoalveolar lavage specimens. J Med Microbiol 38: 449–453, 1993.
15. Wakefield AE, Guiver L, Miller RF, Hopkin JM. DNA amplification on induced sputum samples for diagnosis of Pneumocystis carinii pneumonia. Lancet 337: 1378–1379, 1991.
16. Sepkowitz K, Schluger N, Godwin T, Armstrong D, Cerami A, Bucala R. DNA amplification in experimental pneumocystosis: Characterization of serum Pneumocystis carinii DNA and potential P. carinii carrier states. J Infect Dis 168: 421–426, 1993.
17. Centers for Disease Control. Recommendations for prophylaxis against Pneumocystis carinii for adults and adolescents infected with HIV. JAMA 267: 2294–2299, 1992.
18. Ng VL, Yajko DM, McPhaul LW, Gartner I, Byford B, Goodman CD, Nassos PS, Sanders CA, Howes EL, Leoung G, et al. Evaluation of an indirect fluorescent-antibody stain for detection of Pneumocystis carinii in respiratory specimens. J Clin Microbiol 28: 975–979, 1990.
19. Hughes WT, Natural mode of acquisition for de novo infection with Pneumocystis carinii. J Infect Dis 145: 842–848, 1982.
20. Sukura A, Lindberg LA, Soveri T, Guerrero O, Chinchilla M, Elvin K, Linder E. Establishment of Pneumocystis carinii infection in a rat population. Acta Vet Scand 32: 135–137, 1991.
21. Chave J-F, David S, Wauters J-P, Van Melle G, Francioli P. Transmission of Pneumocystic carinni from AIDS patients to other immunosuppressed patients: a cluster of Pneumocystis carinii pneumonia in renal transplant recipients. AIDS 5: 927–932, 1991.

22. Bensousan T, Garo B, Islam S, Bourbigot B, Cledes J, Garre M. Possible transfer of Pneumocystic carinii between kidney transplant recipients. Lancet 336: 1066–1067, 1990.
23. Gajdusek DC. Pneumocystic carinii as the cause of human disease: Historical perspective and magnitude of the problem. Introductory remarks. Nat Cancer Inst Monogr 43: 1–10, 1976.
24. Ruebush TK, Weinstein RA, Baehner RL, et al. An outbreak of Pneumocystis pneumonia in children with acute lymphocytic leukemia. Am J Dis Child 132: 143–148, 1978.
25. Singer C, Armstrong D, Rosen PP, Schottenfeld D. Pneumocystis carinii pneumonia: a cluster of eleven cases. Ann Intern Med 82: 772–777, 1975.

Submitted August 29, 1994; accepted September 21, 1994

Scand J Infect Dis 26: 653–657, 1994

Pseudo-outbreak of Pseudomonas aeruginosa in HIV-infected Patients Undergoing Fiberoptic Bronchoscopy

HANS JØRN KOLMOS[1], AXEL LERCHE[2], KIRSTEN KRISTOFFERSEN[1] and VIBEKE THAMDRUP ROSDAHL[3]

From the Departments of [1]Clinical Microbiology and [2]Infectious Diseases, Hvidovre Hospital, University of Copenhagen, and the [3]Staphylococcus Laboratory, Statens Seruminstitut, Copenhagen, Denmark

Pseudomonas aeruginosa was isolated from bronchoalveolar lavage fluid from 8 consecutive patients undergoing bronchoscopy at an infectious diseases unit. None of the patients developed signs of respiratory tract infection that could be ascribed to the organism. The source of contamination was the suction channels of 2 fiberoptic bronchoscopes which, due to a lapse in routine procedures, were not cleansed manually prior to disinfection with glutaraldehyde. Although rarely of pathogenetic importance, the possible presence of P. aeruginosa in lavage fluids should never be discounted, as it may indicate faulty disinfection of bronchoscopy equipment and thereby point to a risk of transmission of true respiratory pathogens such as mycobacteria.

H. J. Kolmos, MD, Department of Clinical Microbiology 445, Hvidovre Hospital, DK-2650 Hvidovre, Denmark

INTRODUCTION

Bronchoalveolar lavage, using a fiberoptic bronchoscope, is a well-established procedure for obtaining material from the lower airways for microbiological examination. In HIV-infected patients this method is particularly useful, as Pneumocystis carinii and other opportunistic respiratory pathogens may be difficult to demonstrate in sputum, especially in patients receiving antipneumocystis chemoprophylaxis (1). Unfortunately, fiberoptic bronchoscopes are difficult to disinfect (2–7), and cross-infection related to their use has been described (8–11). As cross-infection can have serious consequences, particularly in patients with AIDS or other immunocompromising condition, it is of great importance to be alert to signs indicating that bronchoscopes are not adequately disinfected. In this paper we describe a pseudo-outbreak of respiratory tract infection due to Pseudomonas aeruginosa, which originated from inadequate cleansing of the suction channels of bronchoscopes prior to chemical disinfection.

MATERIALS AND METHODS

Bronchoscopy of HIV-infected patients was performed by various doctors and nurses in a dedicated room in the out-patient clinic of the infectious diseases unit at Hvidovre Hospital, using 2 fiberoptic bronchoscopes (Olympus BT-P10 and BF-1T 20D). Lavages were performed with sterile saline, and the aspirated material was examined for Pneumocystis carinii, aerobic bacteria, mycobacteria and fungi, using standard techniques. The written protocol for decontamination of bronchoscopes was based on instructions from the manufacturer. After mechanical cleansing of valves and suction channels with a neutral detergent, disinfection was to be performed in a disinfector (Horca S70), using a neutral detergent and 2% alkaline glutaraldehyde for 10 min at room temperature. After disinfection the channels of the bronchoscopes were dried by means of pressurized air. The disinfecting solution in the disinfector was changed weekly according to instructions from the manufacturer.

Serotyping and phagetyping of Ps. aeruginosa isolates was performed as described previously (12). Isolates were routinely regarded as non-identical if they differed in serotype and in phage-susceptibility by >2 strong reactions.

RESULTS

From 5 to 20 February 1991, Ps. aeruginosa was isolated from broncho-alveolar lavages of 8 consecutive patients undergoing fiberoptic bronchoscopy at the Department of Infectious Diseases at Hvidovre Hospital. Since this organism had not been isolated from lavages for the past 3 months (Table I), an outbreak was suspected and epidemiological examinations were carried out. All 8 patients had AIDS or were HIV-positive and underwent bronchoscopy for elucidation of pulmonary symptoms. None of the patients had symptoms or signs consistent with a pseudomonas infection, and the organism could not be isolated from subsequent sputum samples in any of the patients. This confirmed the impression of a pseudo-outbreak, and no antimicrobial treatment against Ps. aeruginosa was initiated.

Inspection of the bronchoscopy unit, which took place on 21 February, identified three significant problems: firstly, due to the lack of a dedicated person, the nursing staff was inexperienced with maintenance procedures for bronchoscopy equipment. Secondly, the bronchoscope disinfector had been out of operation for some weeks due to technical problems. Instead, disinfection with glutaraldehyde took place manually in a neighbouring unit, using provisional facilities. Last, but not least, mechanical cleansing of suction and biopsy channels prior to disinfection was not performed regularly, even though this was clearly recommended in the protocol.

By interviewing the staff it became clear that cleansing of suction and biopsy channels had not taken place regularly for a longer period, either when the disinfector was in use, or during the past weeks when manual disinfection had been performed. This was confirmed by inspection of the channels, which revealed deposits of organic material in both bronchoscopes. Swabs taken from the channels of both scopes and rinsing fluid from one of the scopes yielded growth of Ps. aeruginosa in pure culture. By contrast, the organism was not cultured either from the disinfector or from other environmental samples taken at the unit.

The isolates from the 8 patients belonged to 3 different types (Table II). Isolates from 4 patients belonged to the same type as the isolate from the scope-rinsing fluid (serogroup O:6, 10, $\pm$3 and phagetype 1214/col.18/col.21u). Isolates from 2 patients had the same type as the isolate found in the swab from the same scope (serogroup O:1 and phagetype 7/119x/352/1214/m4/col.2/col.11/col.18), and another patient had a very closely related

Table I. *Microbiological findings in broncho-alveolar lavages, November 1990 to May 1991*

Organism	Nov. 90 ($n = 12$)	Dec. 90 ($n = 7$)	Jan. 91 ($n = 10$)	Febr. 91 ($n = 9$)	Mar. 91 ($n = 9$)	Apr. 91 ($n = 12$)	May 91 ($n = 10$)
Pneumocystis carinii	3	1	3	3	3	6	6
Mycobacteria	0	0	2	1	0	1	0
Streptococcus pneumoniae	0	1	0	1	2	0	1
Haemolytic streptococci	0	0	0	0	0	0	1
Staphylococcus aureus	3	4	1	1	0	0	1
Haemophilus influenzae	1	0	0	1	0	0	0
Branhamella catarrhalis	0	0	0	0	1	0	0
Enterobacteriaceae	2	0	1	0	1	0	0
Pseudomonas aeruginosa	0	0	0	8	0	1	0
Acinetobacter spp.	2	1	0	0	0	0	0
Histoplasma capsulatum	0	0	0	0	1	0	0
Other yeasts	4	3	8	2	3	6	4
Entamoeba histolytica	0	0	0	0	0	0	1

Table II. *Typing of Pseudomonas aeruginosa isolates from broncho-alveolar lavages examined in February 1991 and characterization of patients*

Cases (sex/age)	Date of bronchoscopy	CD4 count ($\times 10^9$/ml)	Pseudomonas aeruginosa type: Serogroup	Pseudomonas aeruginosa type: Phage type
M/63	5 February	100	0:3,6,10	1214/col.18/col.21u
F/31	5 February	0	0:3,6,10	1214/col.18/col.21u
F/28	6 February	238	0:3,6,10	1214/col.18/col.21u
M/52	6 February	120	0:1	7/21/119x/352/1214/m4/col.2/col.11/col.18
F/29	7 February	0	0:3,6,10	1214/col.18/col.21u
M/28	15 February	60	0:1	7/109/119x/352/1214/m4/col.2/col.18/188
M/27	20 February	0	0:2,5	44/col.21
M/29	20 February	90	0:1	7/109/119x/352/1214/m4/col.2/col.11/col.18

isolate with the same serogroup, but with 3 strong reaction differences in phage reactions, compared with the other isolates. The swab isolate from the other scope was similar to the isolate from the last patient in serogroup, but had 3 strong reaction differences in phage type. The typing results thus confirmed an epidemiological relationship between the scope isolates from at least 6 patients and possibly also the last 2 patients.

Intervention consisted of a thorough mechanical cleansing of valves and suction and biopsy channels of the bronchoscopes before treatment with glutaraldehyde in the disinfector. In addition, the channels of the bronchoscopes were flushed and the exterior was wiped with 70% alcohol after treatment in the disinfector and allowed to air-dry. As shown in Table I, this stopped the pseudo-outbreak. Over the next 3 months Ps. aeruginosa was isolated from only 1 lavage specimen, which was heavily contaminated with platelet epithelial cells and bacteria from the upper airways. Unfortunately this isolate was not kept for typing.

DISCUSSION

Although all 8 patients were severely immunocompromised, judging by their low CD4 counts (Table II), they did not develop pneumonia secondary to bronchoscopy. The reason for this may be partly that Ps. aeruginosa is an organism of low pathogenicity, partly that the patients may only have been exposed to a small inoculum, since contamination was primarily localized to the suction channels of the bronchoscopes. Our results are consistent with previous studies, which indicate that the risk of infection with Ps. aeruginosa after bronchoscopy with contaminated equipment is low (2, 8, 10). Thus, the demonstration of this organism in lavages may not be so important for its role as a potential pathogen, but rather for its role as an indicator of poor hygiene in bronchoscopy units. A disinfecting procedure, which can be resisted by Ps. aeruginosa, will also be inadequate against more pathogenic and chemically more resistant organisms, such as mycobacteria. Indeed, among the relatively few well-documented cases of cross-infection following bronchoscopy, mycobacteria play a predominant role (10, 11). The risk of transmitting mycobacteria may be particularly high in bronchoscopy units serving AIDS patients, both because of the common occurrence of mycobacteria among these patients (Table I), and because of their high susceptibility to infection. The transmission of mycobacteria among AIDS patients may have serious consequences, both because they may not respond well to chemotherapy, and because multiresistant strains are now emerging that are virtually untreatable (13). In this outbreak the faulty point in decontamination was the mechanical cleansing prior to disinfection. Other investigators have reported similar experiences (3–5, 10, 11). Agents such as glutaraldehyde and alcohol act as fixatives for organic material and thereby hinder disinfection. Prior mechanical cleansing of all parts of the bronchoscope is therefore mandatory. Some authors even recommend autoclaving the valves as they are in part inaccessible to manual cleaning (11). Experimental studies indicate that disinfection with 2% alkaline glutaraldehyde for 20 min is sufficient to eradicate Mycobacterium tuberculosis, provided that the bronchoscope has been cleansed mechanically before disinfection (14). Accordingly, we have extended the disinfection time in our disinfector from 10 to 20 min.

Disinfected bronchoscopes may become contaminated with environmental mycobacteria from tap water used for rinsing after disinfection. Apart from using sterile water, ethylene oxide sterilization is the only well-documented way to eliminate this kind of contamination in bronchoscopes (6). In order to avoid transmission of environmental mycobacteria the British Thoracic Society has recommended repeating the whole decontaminating procedure immediately before bronchoscopy of immunocompromised patients and extending the disinfection time from 20 to 60 min (15). However, the efficacy of this demanding and time-consuming disinfection procedure has not been documented. Moreover it may be difficult to implement in daily clinical practice. Alcohol rinsing after disinfection with glutaraldehyde has been shown to reduce the contamination level in endoscopes (16). Consequently we recommend flushing the channels and wiping the exterior of the disinfected bronchoscope with 70% alcohol after each patient. If the bronchoscope has been out of use for >3 days we recommend repeating this procedure immediately before the next bronchoscopy. At present there are insufficient data to prove the efficacy of alcohol rinsing of bronchoscopes. Future studies should focus on this, and on the clinical significance of the presumably low level of contamination resulting.

In view of the serious consequences of transmitting mycobacterial disease, bronchoscopy units serving AIDS patients should adhere strictly to recommended guidelines and have their disinfecting procedures checked at regular intervals. Bronchoscopes should be maintained by dedicated staff. Clinical microbiologists should be alert to accumulations of Ps. aeruginosa and other water-borne organisms in lavages, since they may indicate inadequate bronchoscopy hygiene.

REFERENCES

1. Levine SJ, Masur H, Gill VJ, Feuerstein I, Suffredini AF, Brown D, Lane HC, Yarchoan R, Shelhamer JH, Ognibene FP. Effect of aerolosolized pentamidine prophylaxis on the diagnosis of Pneumocystis carinii pneumonia by induced sputum examination in patients infected with the human immunodeficiency virus. Am Rev Respir Dis 144: 760–764, 1991.
2. Surratt PM, Gruber B, Wellons HA, Wenzel RP. Absence of clinical pneumonia following bronchoscopy with contaminated and clean bronchofiberscopes. Chest 71: 52–54, 1977.
3. Goldstein B, Abrutyn E. Pseudo-outbreak of Bacillus species: related to fibreoptic bronchoscopy. J Hosp Infect 6: 194–200, 1985.
4. Prigogine T, Glupczynski Y, Van Molle P, Schmerber J. Mycobacterial cross-contamination of bronchoscopy specimens. J Hosp Infect 11: 93–95, 1988.
5. Uttley AHC, Fitch LE, Honeywell KM, Yates MD, Collins CH. Cross contamination of bronchial washings. BMJ 301: 1274, 1990.
6. Nye K, Chadha DK, Hodgkin P, Bradley C, Hancox J, Wise R. Mycobacterium chelonei isolation from broncho-alveolar lavage fluid and its practical implications. J Hosp Infect 16: 257–261, 1990.
7. Gubler JGH, Salfinger M, von Graevenitz A. Pseudoepidemic of nontuberculous mycobacteria due to a contaminated bronchoscope cleaning machine. Chest 101: 1245–1249, 1992.
8. Sammartino MT, Israel RH, Magnussen CR. Pseudomonas aeruginosa contamination of fiberoptic bronchoscopes. J Hosp Infect 3: 65–71, 1982.
9. Webb SF, Vall-Spinosa A. Outbreak of Serratia marcescens associated with the flexible fiberbronchoscope. Chest 68: 703–708, 1975.

10. Pappas SA, Schaaff DM, DiConstanzo MB, King FW, Sharp JT. Contamination of flexible fiberoptic bronchoscopes. Am Rev Respir Dis 127: 391–392, 1983.
11. Wheeler PW, Lancaster D, Kaiser AB. Bronchopulmonary cross-colonization and infection related to mycobacterial contamination of suction valves of bronchoscopes. J Infect Dis 159: 954–958, 1989.
12. Høiby N, Rosendal K. Epidemiology of Pseudomonas aeruginosa infection in patients treated at a cystic fibrosis centre. Acta Pathol Microbiol Scand Sect B 88: 125–131, 1980.
13. Frieden TR, Sterling T, Pablos-Mendez A, Kilburn JO, Cauthen GM, Dooley SW. The emergence of drug-resistant tuberculosis in New York city. N Engl J Med 328: 521–526, 1993.
14. Hanson PJV, Chadwick MV, Gaya H, Collins JV. A study of glutaraldehyde disinfection of fiberoptic bronchoscopes experimentally contaminated with Mycobacterium tuberculosis. J Hosp Infect 22: 137–142, 1992.
15. Woodcock A, Campbell I, Collins JVC, Hanson P, Harvey J, Corris P, Johnston IDA. Bronchoscopy and infection control. Lancet 2: 270–271, 1989.
16. Fraser VJ, Zuckerman G, Clouse RE, O'Rourke S, Jones M, Klasner J, Murray P. A prospective randomized trial comparing manual and automated endoscope disinfection methods. Infect Control Hosp Epidemiol 14: 383–389, 1993.

Submitted February 28, 1994; accepted July 18, 1994

Scand J Infect Dis 26: 659–666, 1994

Pneumococcal Meningitis in Adults

PETER KRAGSBJERG[1], JAN KÄLLMAN[1] and PER OLCÉN[2]

From the Departments of [1]Infectious Diseases and [2]Clinical Microbiology and Immunology, Örebro Medical Center Hospital, Örebro, Sweden

A retrospective study was conducted to examine the clinical features and outcome of 31 adult pneumococcal meningitis patients during the years 1981–92. The incidence was 1.0/100,000 adults/year. The case fatality rate was 16% (5/31), and in patients older than 70 years, 33% (3/9). Sequelae were seen in 29% (7/24), mostly otoneurologic symptoms. In 27/28 bacterial isolates the serotypes found were included in the 23-valent unconjugated polysaccharide vaccine in current use. All 28 isolates were fully sensitive to penicillin. 49/51 non-meningitis blood isolates had MIC values ≤0.06 mg/l, 2 isolates had MIC values of 0.125 mg/l and 0.25 mg/l, and 50/50 were serotypes included in the 23-valent vaccine. Pneumococcal meningitis is a disease causing considerable mortality and morbidity. The relatively low case fatality rate found in the present study may be due to the patients' good health prior to admission, rapid specific microbiological diagnosis, absence of penicillin-resistant pneumococci among the meningitis strains, and immediate institution of specific and supportive therapy.

P. Kragsbjerg, MD, Department of Infectious Diseases, Örebro Medical Center Hospital, S-701 85 Örebro, Sweden

INTRODUCTION

Pneumococcal meningitis (PM), a common bacterial infection in CNS in adults, is associated with high mortality and frequent development of neurological sequelae (1). Previous studies have reported mortality rates from 19% to 50% in PM (all ages) with the highest rates (>90%) seen among patients older than 70 years (2–5). The sequelae rate in survivors of meningitis has been reported to be 33–72%, mostly affecting patients between 15 and 50 years of age (3, 6). Increasing spread of penicillin-resistant pneumococci (PRP) has been reported from southern and eastern Europe, and recently from Iceland as the first Nordic country (7). Thus an increased awareness of antibiotic resistance is mandatory when treating invasive infections caused by pneumococci. Furthermore, continuous surveillance of pneumococcal serotypes is necessary to form a rational basis for a revision of the pneumococcal vaccines in current use.

We have conducted a retrospective study of the clinical features and outcome of PM over the last 12 years in our part of Sweden. The serotype distribution and antibiotic sensitivity of the meningitis strains were also studied. For reference, non-meningitis blood isolates from adults during the years 1987 and 1992 were compared regarding serotype distribution and penicillin sensitivity.

MATERIALS AND METHODS

The study period covered 12 years, from January 1st, 1981 through December 31st, 1992.

Patients in our county >14 years of age and with clinical signs and symptoms of meningitis requiring a diagnostic lumbar puncture were included, provided one or more of the following criteria were met: growth of S. pneumoniae in cerebrospinal fluid (CSF), growth of S. pneumoniae in blood, a positive antigen detection test for S. pneumoniae in CSF.

The standard antibiotic treatment used during the study period was intravenous benzylpenicillin 3g × 3 daily in cases of suspected PM. For patients with suspected bacterial meningitis of unknown etiology the standard regimen was intravenous ampicillin 3g × 4 plus chloramphenicol 1g × 3 daily until the pathogen was identified. In cases of penicillin allergy, chloramphenicol alone was used. Routine clinical follow-up was performed approximately 4 weeks after discharge, including in 7 cases clinical audiometric evaluation by an otologist.

To identify cases of PM we reviewed the files of patients admitted to the Department of Infectious Diseases, Örebro Medical Center Hospital (ÖMCH) diagnosed as having PM during the study period. The Department of Clinical Microbiology and Immunology, ÖMCH, is the central diagnostic laboratory for all microbiological tests in Örebro County. Since 1980, all blood and CSF bacterial isolates are stored at −70°C. Therefore, the laboratory files were also searched to identify all PM cases in the county. Furthermore, all available consecutive non-meningitis blood isolates from adults during the years 1987 and 1992 were also studied for background information.

Culture of S. pneumoniae was performed on blood agar plates and identified as S. pneumoniae by colony morphology and optochin sensitivity. Pneumococcal antigen in CSF was detected with a commercial latex- or co-agglutination method (8, 9), or an enzyme immuno assay (10). The 28/31 frozen strains available were thawed, serotyped and the penicillin sensitivity determined as described below. Serotyping of all the strains was performed at Statens Seruminstitut, Copenhagen, Denmark by the capsular reaction test using pooled sera, type and group and, when relevant, factor sera for differentiating types within groups. Oxacillin sensitivity was determined using the disc diffusion method, and MIC determinations of the meningitis strains with the E-test using Isosens agar (Oxoid) with 5% defibrinated horseblood (11). MIC values for the non-meningitis strains were obtained, using agar dilution on PDM-II + 5% horseblood performed at Smittskyddsinstitutet, Stockholm.

The study was approved by the local Ethics Committee.

RESULTS

Epidemiology

We identified 30 patients (16 females, 14 males) with 31 episodes of PM during the 12-year study period. One 67-year-old man with a previous cranial base fracture suffered 2 episodes of PM with serotype 14. Three patients had had previous episodes of meningitis. A 24-year-old man with previous multiple cranial fractures had had 4 previous episodes of meningitis, 2 due to S. pneumoniae and 2 due to Haemophilus influenzae. A 40-year-old man with previous fracture of the right orbita had had 3 episodes of meningitis, the first purulent and of unknown etiology, the second and third due to S. pneumoniae. The third patient, a 56-year-old male had had one previous episode of meningitis of unknown etiology.

The mean population older than 14 years of Örebro county during the study period was 223,040. Excluding 3 patients with PM who were visitors and fell ill during their stay in the county, the incidence rate was 1.0/100,000 adults/year. The age distribution of cases of PM in the county, in relation to the mean population during 1981–92 is depicted in Fig. 1.

There was no close geographical or temporal association between individual cases and all patients were treated at the Department of Infectious Diseases, ÖMCH.

Clinical features and treatment

The clinical and laboratory features of all patients are presented in Table I. Seven meningitis patients also had pneumonia. One patient had suspected endocarditis and one a verified endocarditis. Four patients had sinusitis and 4 acute otitis media. 24/31 patients required treatment in the intensive care unit during their stay in hospital. Four had meningitis associated with shock and 12 required mechanical ventilation.

In the present study, initial intravenous treatment was instituted with benzylpenicillin alone in 11 cases, cefotaxime in 3, cefuroxime in 6 and ampicillin in combination with chloramphenicol in 9 and alone in 3. The therapy was modified on the second or third day of treatment. In 29 patients the drug used was benzylpenicillin. In 2 cases the antibiotic treatment was changed because of suspected complicating infection. Nine patients received corticosteroid therapy in the acute stage of the disease. The mean duration of fever was 10 days (range 1–42 days).

Predisposing conditions

Predisposing and chronic diseases in the 31 adult patients with PM are shown in Table II. One of the 4 asplenic patients had been vaccinated with the current 23-valent capsular

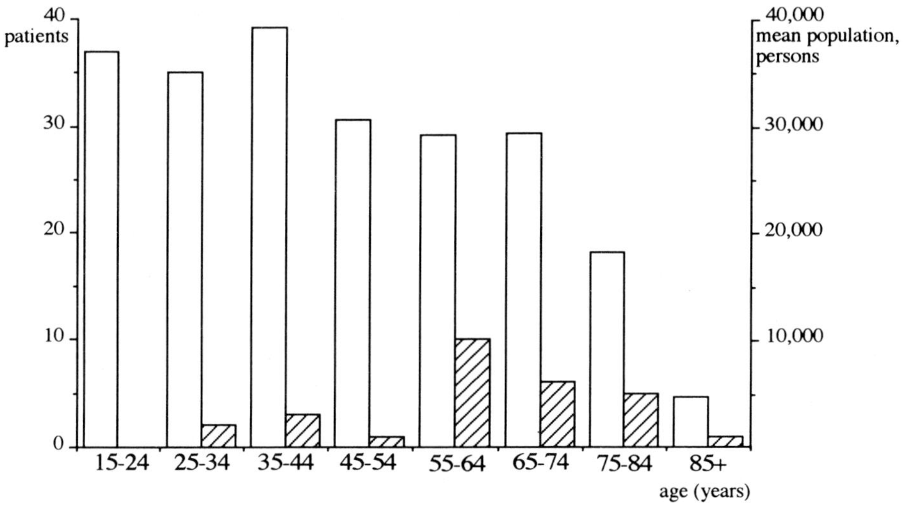

Fig. 1. Age distribution of adult cases with pneumococcal meningitis in relation to the mean population in Örebro county during the study period 1981–92. □, mean population; ▨, patients.

polysaccharide vaccine prior to the PM but none of the other patients were vaccinated prior to the meningitis.

Bacteriology

24 patients had S. pneumoniae isolated from blood and CSF or S. pneumoniae isolated from blood and a positive antigen detection test performed on CSF. Five patients had S. pneumoniae isolated from CSF or a positive antigen detection test and negative blood

Table I. *Clinical and laboratory features on admission in 31 adult cases of pneumococcal meningitis*

	n	Median	Range
Age (years)	31	64	24–89
Duration of symptoms[a] (days)	31	1	<1–8
BP systolic (mmHg)	19	145	110–210
BP diastolic (mmHg)	18	80	60–100
Heart beats/min	13	100	60–145
Level of consciousness			
Alert	11		
Confused	16		
Comatose	4		
Nuchal rigidity	22/26		
ESR (mm/h)	24	62	3–125
B-WBC ($\times 10^9$/l)	30	17.7	3–50
CSF-WBC ($\times 10^6$/l)	27	2120	1–16,000
CSF-protein (g/l)	19	2.17	0.03–6.9

[a] Time from onset of symptoms to admission.

Table II. *Predisposing and chronic diseases in 31 adult patients with pneumococcal meningitis*

	n	%
Asplenia	4	13
Cranial base fracture/ CSF leakage	6	19
Alcoholism	1	3
Malignancy	3	10
Diabetes mellitus	2	6
Arteriosclerotic heart disease, hypertension,	10	32
Rheumatoid arthritis, primary biliary cirrhosis, glomerulonephritis	1 each	3
No known predisposing disease		
<70 years	22	23
≥70 years	9	56

Some patients had more than one predisposing condition.

culture. One patient had growth of S. pneumoniae in blood, pleocytosis without bacterial growth in CSF, and a negative antigen detection test. In one patient S. pneumoniae was isolated from blood on admission and later from the meninges at autopsy. In 25 patients in whom results of both microscopy with Gram stain and culture of CSF were available, 1/22 proved negative by microscopy despite a positive culture. The 3 culture-negative samples were also negative by microscopy, but 2 of them were positive by antigen detection tests. There was no clustering in time of individual serotypes. Table III shows the serotype distribution. All isolates were sensitive to penicillin as measured with the oxacillin test. The 3 isolates with the smallest zone diameters (22, 22, and 20 mm) were tested with the E-test and all had MIC values (benzyl penicillin) < 0.06 mg/l.

Table III. *Serotype distribution in 28 cases of pneumococcal meningitis (1981–92) and in 50 non-meningitis blood isolates*

Serotype	*n*
Meningitis isolates	
23F	5
14, 19F	3 each
6A, 7F, 9V, 22F	2 each
3, 6B, 8, 11, 12F, 18C, 19F, 33, 35F	1 each
Non-meningitis isolates	
1987	
7F	3
4, 9N, 19F, 22F, 23F	2 each
3, 6B, 8, 9V, 11A, 18C, 19A	1 each
1992	
14	7
3, 9V, 18C	4 each
4, 7F, 19A, 23F	2 each
8, 11A, 22F	1 each

50/50 of the serotypes of the non-meningitis blood isolates were included in the 23-valent vaccine, but 2/51 non-meningitis blood isolates had MIC values of 0.125 mg/l and 0.25 mg/l (benzyl penicillin), the serotype of one of these isolates being unknown (Table III).

Complications

Eight patients had seizures during the acute episode. One 66-year-old woman developed an occipital cerebral infarction 2 days after admission, resulting in a left hemiparesis and recurring seizures in the left side, continuing even after discharge. Computerized tomography of the brain showed cerebral infarctions, both previous and acute. Two of the surviving patients developed disseminated intravascular coagulation, and 1 of these, a 24-year-old man, myocarditis. The other patient, a 75-year-old woman, suffered from a cerebral embolus 1 month after leaving hospital, caused by atrial fibrillation and valvular vegetations due to endocarditis. She was treated with anticoagulant therapy and developed no permanent neurological sequelae. One patient experienced cardiac decompensation progressing to pulmonary edema.

Mortality

The case fatality rate was 16% (5/31); for patients <70 years of age, 9% (2/22) and for patients >70 years of age, 33% (3/9). Patient no. 1, a previously healthy 73-year-old man, experienced a fulminant course with renal insufficiency. Dialysis was instituted but was complicated by a retroperitoneal hemorrhage resulting in hypovolemic shock. The patient died before surgery could be performed. Patient no. 2, a previously healthy 72-year-old woman had PM complicated by recurring seizures. She gradually deteriorated and died. Case no. 3, a previously healthy 66-year-old man, had a fulminant course complicated by a sinus cavernosus thrombosis. He died in a state of circulatory and respiratory collapse. Case no. 4, a 56-year-old woman with diabetes mellitus and arteriosclerotic heart disease had earlier undergone an aortocoronary bypass operation. She presented with hyperglycemic coma and had a prolonged complicated course with cardiac decompensation, seizures and subsequently a flaccid paralysis in all 4 extremities. The 5th case a 89-year-old man died on day 4 without having regained consciousness.

Sequelae

Seven patients had sequelae after the PM. Three patients suffered from vertigo, 1 from unremitting headache and asthenia, and 1 from bilateral sensorineural hearing loss. One patient had recurring seizures in the left side. One 69-year-old patient was transferred to another hospital unconscious and receiving mechanical ventilation. For 2 further patients, no information was available. In all, 17 patients were considered *not* to have sequelae due to the PM. Of the survivors for whom information was available, 29% (7/24) developed sequelae.

DISCUSSION

PM is a common acute bacterial CNS infection in adults which is still associated with a high mortality rate in older patients in spite of effective antibiotic and supportive therapy (1). In our 31 PM cases the mortality rate was 16%, which is low compared with other recent reports (2–4). One reason may be the low frequency of complicating underlying diseases and the fact that most of the patients with predisposing conditions were young and otherwise healthy. A relatively short duration from onset of disease until admission (median ≤ 24 h), rapid microbiological diagnosis, and immediate institution of effective antibiotic therapy and supportive measures are also important. A low WBC count ($<4 \times 10^9$/l) has previously been associated with a poor prognosis in pneumococcal pneumonia; accordingly, 2 of our patients, who both died, had low WBC in blood and CSF (1).

As the present report is a retrospective study, clinical evaluation of possible sequelae may be hampered; furthermore retrieval of the records was not possible in a few cases. However, most patients were followed-up either at our Department or by an otologist with clinical evaluation. In a study with 94 survivors after PM (of all ages) 24% were found to have otologic and 54% neurologic sequelae (12, 13). We found that 29% developed mostly otoneurologic sequelae, a figure corresponding to that found by Rasmussen et al. (13). Our figure may, however, be too low due to the inherent difficulties of retrospective studies regarding clinical information deduced from patients records.

Among serotypes of the pneumococci isolated from 28/31 of our patients, all except one (35F) were included in the 23-valent capsular polysaccharide vaccine, in agreement with recently published large surveys on pneumococcal serotype distribution (14, 15). In our study, the 3 most frequent isolates were 23F, 14, and 19A which is different from other larger studies where serotypes 1, 3, and 4 were found to be the most common (15, 16). We also studied the serotype distribution of the 50 non-meningitis S. pneumoniae blood isolates from adult patients during the years 1987 and 1992. All 50 belonged to serotypes included in the 23-valent vaccine. The current vaccine thus covered 77/78 of the invasive isolates in this study and if the results reflect the serotype distribution of invasive isolates in Örebro County this may be of benefit when considering the proposed extended vaccination policy.

Vaccination against meningitis caused by Haemophilus influenzae type b has been successful in the countries where it is included in the general vaccination programme for children. In Finland the disease practically disappeared after the introduction of conjugate vaccines (17). Vaccination against meningococcal meningitis is used primarily in epidemic situations. The pneumococcal 23-valent polysaccharide vaccine is generally recommended in Sweden for persons >2 years with asplenia or other diseases increasing their susceptibility to serious pneumococcal disease. In other countries general vaccination of people older than 65 years is also recommended (18). For severe pneumococcal pneumonia and invasive pneumococcal disease the protective efficacy of unconjugated polysaccharide vaccines against vaccine serotypes has been reported to be 60–70%, and the duration of adequate levels of protective antibodies has been estimated to be 5–6 years (18–20). In the present study of PM, 45% (14/31) of the patients were >65 years of age. In our region the average number of inhabitants older than 65 years during the period studied was 52,192. Thus, during the period studied, 10,000 inhabitants per year should be vaccinated, amounting to a total of 120,000 vaccine doses to prevent 9 cases of PM. To avoid 1 case of PM would require 13,300 vaccine doses, which would cost approximately 190,000 US$ to which should be added costs for transportation, use of facilities, and salary for vaccinators. This calculation applies to PM alone and the results of our study are insufficient to evaluate the overall impact of vaccination on the morbidity and mortality caused by S. pneumoniae infections. However, the incidence of PM in our region and the vaccine efficacy support vaccination of selected high-risk populations and not general vaccination of persons older than 65 years for the prevention of PM.

Since 1967, PRP have been isolated in increasing frequency all over the world and at present may constitute up to 40% of invasive isolates in countries like Spain, France and Hungary (7). As the first Nordic country, Iceland has reported an increase in resistant isolates (21). Such an increase has not occurred in Denmark so far, as shown by Nielsen (15) and the results from our material of meningitis may suggest that this was not the case in our part of Sweden up to 1993 either. However, two non-meningitis blood isolates had MIC values of 0.125 mg/l and 0.25 mg/l (PcG), indicating intermediate sensitivity. Thus, 2.5%

(2/79) of invasive isolates had reduced sensitivity to penicillin, which may be a cause for concern as such strains are more prone to cause failure in the treatment of PM (22).

In conclusion, S. pneumoniae is a bacterial pathogen causing considerable mortality and morbidity. In our region, however, the case fatality rate in PM is relatively low, which may be due to the patients' good health prior to admission, rapid specific microbiological diagnosis, absence of PRP among the meningitis strains, and immediate institution of specific and supportive therapy.

ACKNOWLEDGEMENTS

We thank Jørgen Henrichsen, Statens Serum institut, Copenhagen, Denmark, for serotyping the meningitis strains. We also thank Gunilla Källenius and Jonas Hedlund, Smittskyddsinstitutet, Stockholm, Sweden, for providing the serotypes and MIC values for the invasive non-meningitis strains.

REFERENCES

1. Musher DM. Infections caused by Streptococcus pneumoniae: Clinical spectrum, pathogenesis, immunity, and treatment. Clin Infect Dis 14: 801–809, 1992.
2. Durand ML, Calderwood SB, Weber DJ, Miller SI, Southwick FS, Caviness VS, Swartz MN. Acute bacterial meningitis in adults. N Engl J Med 328: 21–288, 1993.
3. Bruyn GAW, Kremer HPH, de Marie S, Padberg GW, Hermans J, van Furth R. Clinical evaluation of pneumococcal meningitis in adults over a twelve-year period. Eur J Microbiol Infect Dis 8: 695–700, 1989.
4. Burman LA, Norrby R, Trollfors B. Invasive pneumococcal infections: incidence, predisposing factors, and prognosis. Rev Infect Dis 7: 133–142, 1985.
5. Bohr V, Hansen B, Jessen O, Johnsen N, Kjersem H, Kristensen HS, Nyboe J, Rasmussen N. 875 cases of bacterial meningitis: Part I. Clinical data, prognosis, and the role of specialized hospital departments. J Infect 7: 21–30, 1983.
6. Bohr V, Rasmussen N, Hansen B, Gade A, Kjersem H, Johnsen N, Paulson O. Pneumococcal meningitis: an evaluation of prognostic factors in 164 cases based on mortality and on a study of lasting sequelae. J Infect 10: 143–157, 1985.
7. Appelbaum PC. Antimicrobial resistance in Streptococcus pneumoniae: An overview. Clin Infect Dis 15: 77–83, 1992.
8. Sippel JE, Prato CM, Girgis NI, Edwards EA. Detection of Neisseria meningitidis group A, Haemophilus influenzae type b, and Streptococcus pneumoniae antigens in cerebrospinal fluid specimens by antigen capture enzyme-linked immunosorbent assays. J Clin Microbiol 20: 259–265, 1984.
9. Olcén P, Danielsson D, Kjellander J. The use of protein A-containing Staphylococci sensitized with anti-meningococcal antibodies for grouping Neisseria meningitidis and demonstration of meningococcal antigen in cerebrospinal fluid. APMIS 83: 387–396, 1975.
10. Salih MAM, Ahmed HS, Hofvander Y, Danielsson D, Olcén P. Rapid diagnosis of bacterial meningitis by an enzyme immunoassay of cerebrospinal fluid. Epidemiol Infect 103: 310–310, 1989.
11. Jacobs MR. Treatment and diagnosis of infections caused by drug-resistant Streptococcus pneumoniae. Clin Infect Dis 15: 119–127, 1992.
12. Bohr V, Paulson OB, Rasmussen N. Pneumococcal meningitis. Late neurologic sequelae and features of prognostic impact. Arch Neurol 41: 1045–1049, 1984.
13. Rasmussen N, Johnsen NJ, Bohr VA. Otologic sequelae after pneumococcal meningitis: A survey of 164 consecutive cases with a follow-up of 94 survivors. Laryngoscope 101: 876–882, 1991.
14. Nielsen SV, Henrichsen J. Capsular types of Streptococcus pneumoniae isolated from blood and CSF during 1982–1987. Clin Infect Dis 15: 794–798, 1992.
15. Nielsen SV, Henrichsen J. Capsular types and susceptibility to penicillin of Pneumococci isolated from cerebrospinal fluid or blood in Denmark, 1983–1988. Scand J Infect Dis 25: 165–170, 1993.
16. Burman LÅ, Trollfors B, Norrby R, Falsen E, Haidl S, Henrichsen J. Serotype distribution of Streptococcus pneumoniae strains isolated from blood and cerebrospinal fluid in Sweden. Scand J Infect Dis 18: 45–48, 1986.
17. Peltola H, Kilpi T, Anttila M. Rapid disappearance of Haemophilus influenzae type b meningitis after routine childhood immunisation with conjugate vaccines. Lancet 340: 592–594, 1992.

18. Recommendations of the Immunization Practices Advisory Committee. Pneumococcal polysaccharide vaccine. MMWR 38: 64–76, 1989.
19. Sims RV, Steinmann WC, McConville JH, King LR, Zwick WC, Schwartz JS. The clinical effectiveness of pneumonococcal vaccine in the elderly. Ann Intern Med 108: 653–657, 1988.
20. Shapiro ED, Berg AT, Austrian R, Schroeder D, Parcellis V, Margolis A, Adair RK, Clemens JD. The protective efficacy of polyvalent pneumococcal polysaccharide vaccine. N Engl J Med 325: 1453–1460, 1991.
21. Kristinsson KG, Hjälmarsdottir MA, Steingrimsson O. Increasing penicillin resistance in pneumococci in Iceland. Lancet 339: 1606–1607, 1992.
22. Sloas MM, Barrett FF, Chesney PJ, English BK, Hill BC, Tenover FC, Leggiadro RJ. Cephalosporin treatment failure in penicillin- and cephalosporin-resistant Streptococcus pneumoniae meningitis. Pediatr Infect Dis J 11: 662–666, 1992.

Submitted May 19, 1994; accepted July 17, 1994

Scand J Infect Dis 26: 667–674, 1994

Cerebrospinal Fluid Interleukin-1β/InterLeukin-1 Receptor Antagonist Balance and Tumor Necrosis Factor-α Concentrations in Tuberculous, Viral and Acute Bacterial Meningitis

HALİS AKALIN, ALİ CEZMİ AKDİŞ, REŞİT MISTIK, SAFİYE HELVACI and KAYA KILIÇTURGAY

From the Department of Microbiology and Infectious Diseases, Uludağ University School of Medicine, Bursa, Turkey

The levels of interleukin-1β, IL-1 receptor antagonist and tumor necrosis factor-α (TNF-α) were analyzed in 19 cases of tuberculous, 14 cases of viral, and 22 cases of acute bacterial meningitis, and in 18 control subjects. 20 patients (91%) with acute bacterial and 8(42%) with tuberculous meningitis had detectable amounts of TNF-α in the initial cerebrospinal fluid (CSF) sample (mean 1044 ± 131 pg/ml, range 95–1950, and mean 61 ± 23 pg/ml, range 25–300, respectively), whereas TNF-α was not detectable in any of the patients with viral meningitis, or in any of the control subjects. IL-1β levels were 767 ± 110 pg/ml (185–2000) in acute bacterial, 345 ± 63 pg/ml (50–670) in tuberculous, 257 ± 70 pg/ml (20–700) in viral meningitis, and 37 ± 4 pg/ml (10–68) in control subjects. Il-1 receptor antagonist concentrations were significantly elevated in all meningitis groups, without significant differences between the groups. Il-1 receptor antagonist levels were 2487 ± 62 pg/ml (2250–2950) in acute bacterial, 2216 ± 82 pg/ml (1350–2550) in tuberculous and 1985 ± 92 pg/ml (650–2500) in viral meningitis, and 154 ± 26 pg/ml (20–245) in control CSF samples. A positive correlation was found between TNF and IL-1β levels ($p < 0.01$), and TNF levels and conscious state ($p < 0.05$). The ratio of concentrations of IL-1 receptor antagonist to IL-1β was 3.2 in acute bacterial meningitis, 6.9 in tuberculous meningitis and 8.3 in viral meningitis. This ratio was significantly different between the acute bacterial meningitis group and the other groups ($p < 0.01$), which indicates that the balance between cytokines and antagonists is of importance for the pathogenicity and diagnosis of central nervous system infections.

H. Akalin, MD, Department of Microbiology and Infectious Diseases, Uludağ University School of Medicine, Bursa, Turkey

INTRODUCTION

During the course of bacterial meningitis, bacterial cell wall products including peptidoglycan, teichoic acid or endotoxin, which are generated in vivo or released during antibiotic therapy, induce an intense host inflammatory response in the subarachnoid space (1–3). Tumor necrosis factor-alpha (TNF-α) and interleukin-1 beta (IL-1β) play a major role in mediating tissue injury associated with gram-negative bacterial sepsis or endotoxemia, and initiate meningeal inflammation (4–6). Their presence in the cerebrospinal fluid (CSF) of patients with acute bacterial and viral meningitis has been clearly documented (7–9).

Interleukin-1 receptor antagonist (IL-1ra), a naturally ocurring inhibitor of IL-1, occupies IL-1 receptors without inducing a biological response, and prevents IL-1 from binding to its receptors (10, 11). The balance between the production of IL-1 and IL-1ra probably influences the expression and severity of disease (12).

Mycobacterial infections of the central nervous system (CNS) constitute some 30% of the total cases of meningitis in our region. In this study, the relationship between IL-1β, IL-1ra and TNF-α in tuberculous, acute bacterial and viral meningitis was investigated.

MATERIALS AND METHODS

Patients

55 patients with meningitis and 18 control subjects were evaluated. 19 patients with newly diagnosed tuberculous meningitis (11 males and 8 females, aged 14 to 61 years, mean 31 years), 14 with non-herpes viral meningitis (10 males and 4 females, aged 14 to 52 years, mean 25 years) and 22 with acute bacterial meningitis (14 males and 8 females, aged 15 to 86 years, mean 33 years) were studied. 18 cases (11 males and 7 females, aged 1 to 8 years, mean 3 years) – in whom cerebrospinal fluid (CSF) examinations for differential diagnosis revealed no inflammation – were studied as control group. The patients were hospitalized at Uludağ University School of Medicine, Bursa (Turkey) between June 1991 and June 1993.

A diagnosis of tuberculous meningitis was based on chronic onset of meningitis, CSF findings, and good response to antituberculous therapy. Of the 19 cases of tuberculous meningitis, 4 had miliary dissemination (histopathological and radiological confirmation), 4 pulmonary tuberculosis (microbiological confirmation), 4 tuberculous lymphadenitis (histopathological confirmation), 4 intracranial tuberculoma (diagnosed with CT scans) and 3 isolated chronic meningitis. M. tuberculosis was isolated from the initial CSF culture specimens in four cases.

The following criteria were required for a diagnosis of viral meningitis: (i) CSF findings; (ii) negative bacteriological findings, including CSF and blood cultures, CSF gram-stain, and conventional antigen detection tests; (iii) no antibiotic therapy in the previous week or during hospitalization; (iv) no signs of herpes meningoencephalitis in CT scans, EEG, serological or CSF studies.

The clinical diagnosis of acute bacterial meningitis was confirmed by growth in the initial CSF sample of S. pneumoniae in 16 and N. meningitidis in 6 cases.

The mean duration between onset of symptoms and the initial CSF sample in which cytokines were measured was 2 days (range 1–4) in viral meningitis, 1 day (range 0–4) in acute bacterial meningitis and 30 days (range 7–120) in tuberculous meningitis.

Cytokine analysis

The CSF samples were collected by lumbar puncture before antibiotic treatment was started, and stored at $-80°C$ after centrifugation at $1000 \times g$ for 5 min to remove the cell pellets.

TNF-α and IL-1β were measured with a sandwich enzyme immunoassay (TNF-α ELISA kit; Cistron Biotechnologies, Pynebrook, NJ and IL-1β EIA kit; Advanced Magnetics, Inc., MA), according to the manufacturers' instructions.

IL-1ra concentrations were measured with a sandwich EIA developed by Dr. Harry Towbin, Basel (13). Briefly, microtiter plates (Maxisorb, NUNC) were coated with mouse monoclonal antibody to human IL-1ra (1384.92.17.19) 1.5 μg/ml in phosphate-buffered saline (PBS). Blocking and diluent buffer was bovine serum albumin 1% and Tween 20 0.5% in PBS, and the wash buffer was 1:3 PBS/water with Tween 20 0.05%. The plates were sequentially incubated with standards or samples for 16 h at 4°C, rabbit anti-IL-1ra for 1 h at room temperature, and peroxidase-conjugated goat anti-rabbit Ig for 1 h at room temperature. OPD was used as the substrate in citrate buffer pH 5.5, and the plates were read after 15 min at 492 nm. The samples were studied in duplicate in all ELISAs.

The lower limit of detection of the assays was 20 pg/ml for TNF-α, 10 pg/ml for IL-1β and 20 pg/ml for IL-1ra.

Statistical methods

Statistical analysis was done with Pearson's correlation test and Student's *t* test. The z test was used when comparing proportions of elevated levels. Cytokine concentrations below the lower limit of sensitivity of the assays were considered equal to zero for the purpose of statistical analysis.

RESULTS

Tuberculous meningitis

The CSF leukocyte count in tuberculous meningitis patients was $268 \pm 54 \times 10^6$/l (range $10–700 \times 10^6$), and the CSF/blood glucose ratio 0.30 ± 0.03.

The CSF TNF-α concentrations in 8 out of 19 patients (42%) with tuberculous meningitis was 61 ± 23 pg/ml (range 25–300). IL-1β and IL-1ra were detectable in all tuberculous meningitis CSF samples (mean 345 ± 63 pg/ml, range 50–670 and mean 2216 ± 82 pg/ml, range 1350–2250 respectively).

Three of 19 patients with tuberculous meningitis died, and 4 suffered various neurologic sequelae such as hydrocephalus, optic atrophy and cerebellar dysfunction.

Acute bacterial meningitis

The CSF leukocyte count in acute bacterial meningitis patients was $8037 \pm 2732 \times 10^6$/1. (range 210–49,000 × 10^6) and the CSF/blood glucose ratio was 0.21 ± 0.05. TNF-α was detectable in 20 out of 22 patients (91%) with acute bacterial meningitis at a level of 1044 ± 131 pg/ml (range 95–1950). IL-1β and IL-1ra were detectable in all acute bacterial meningitis CSF samples at a level of 767 ± 110 pg/ml (range 185–2000) and 2487 ± 62 pg/ml (range 2250–2950) respectively.

The concentrations of TNF-α were significantly higher in the acute bacterial meningitis group than in other groups ($p < 0.001$).

The degree of consciousness in the patients according to the Glasgow Coma Scale showed a significant correlation with the TNF-α levels at the time of presentation ($p < 0.05$).

IL-1β levels were significantly higher in the acute bacterial meningitis group than in other groups ($p < 0.001$), and higher levels were found in pneumococcal meningitis than in meningococcal meningitis ($p < 0.01$).

Six of 22 patients with acute bacterial meningitis died, and 1 suffered bilateral hearing loss.

Viral meningitis

The CSF leukocyte count in patients with viral meningitis was $233 \pm 49 \times 10^6$/l (range 13–480 × 10^6) and the CSF/blood glucose ratio 0.60 ± 0.06.

TNF-α was not detectable in any CSF sample from viral meningitis cases. IL-1β and IL-1ra levels were detectable in all viral meningitis samples, at 257 ± 70 pg/ml (range 20–700) and 1985 ± 92 pg/ml (range 650–2500) respectively.

All patients in this group recovered without complications.

Controls

TNF-α was not detectable in any CSF sample from control subjects. Mean IL-1β levels was 37 ± 4 pg/ml (range 10–68), and IL-1ra 154 ± 26 pg/ml (range 30–440), levels were detectable in all samples.

Correlation and statistical analysis

We found no correlation between the outcome of disease, sequelae, CSF leukocyte count, or glucose and cytokine levels.

A positive correlation between TNF-α and IL-1β levels was found ($p < 0.01$). Individual values of TNF-α and IL-1β are plotted in Fig. 1 and Fig. 2.

Sensitivity and specificity of TNF-α and IL-1β levels were calculated to compare these values with the glucose ratio and the CSF leukocyte count, which was the nonspecific parameter that best discriminated between groups of patients.

The TNF-α and IL-1β levels in CSF enabled us to discriminate acute bacterial from viral meningitis, as did the results obtained by analyzing the CSF/blood glucose ratio (Table I).

The difference in sensitivity and specificity of the CSF leukocyte count and either the CSF TNF-α or IL-1β levels was not statistically significant in distinguishing acute bacterial from tuberculous meningitis (Table II).

The presence of TNF-α in CSF from patients with meningitis appeared to distinguish acute bacterial from viral ($p < 0.001$) and tuberculous from viral meningitis ($p < 0.01$).

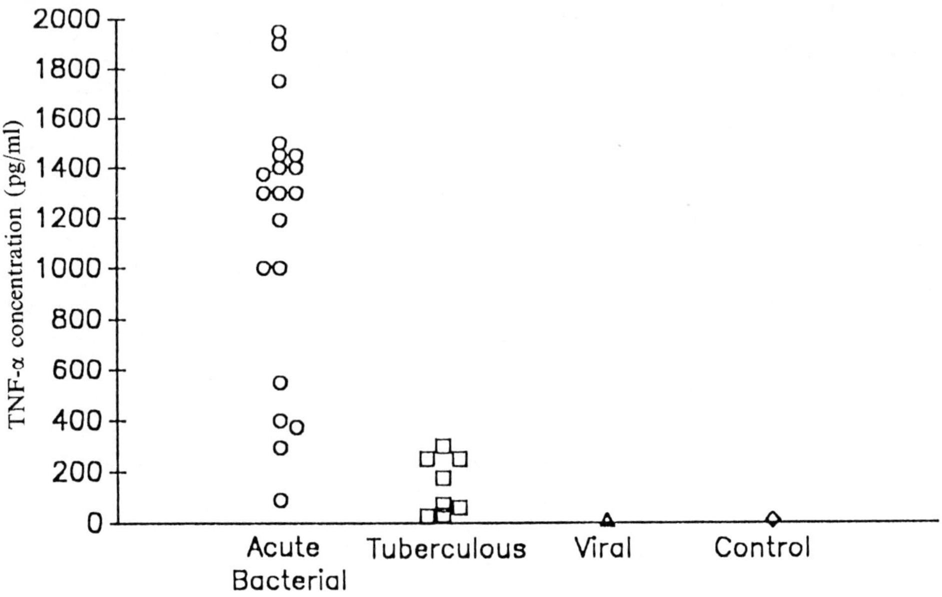

Fig. 1. Concentrations of TNF-α in the cerebrospinal fluid of 22 patients with acute bacterial, 19 patients with tuberculous and 14 with viral meningitis, and in 18 control subjects. Values below 20 pg/ml were not detected.

The CSF IL-1ra levels obtained in the 3 different meningitis groups were significantly higher than in the control group ($p < 0.001$), but did not discriminate between the meningitis groups. Individual values are plotted in Fig. 3. The ratio of Il-1ra secretion to IL-1β was 8.3 in viral meningitis and 6.9 in tuberculous meningitis. These two ratios were significantly

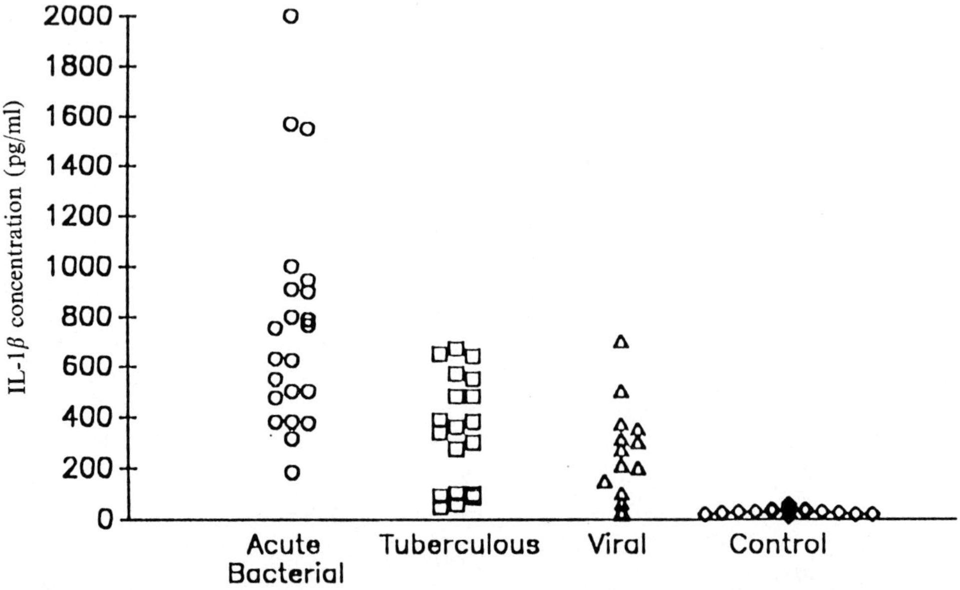

Fig. 2. Concentrations of IL-1β in the cerebrospinal fluid of 22 patients with acute bacterial, 19 with tuberculous, 14 with viral meningitis, and in 18 control subjects.

Table I. *Sensitivity and specificity of TNF-α and IL-1β levels in CSF and the CSF blood glucose ratios in distinguishing acute bacterial from viral meningitis*

	TNF-α	IL-1β	Glucose ratio[a]
Cutoff value[b]	90 pg/ml	400 pg/ml	0.45
Sensitivity	0.91	0.77	0.86
Specificity	1.0	0.86	1.0

[a] Nonspecific parameter that best discriminated between acute bacterial and viral meningitis.
[b] Cutoff value for each parameter was set at most discriminating point between acute bacterial and viral meningitis.

Table II. *Sensitivity and specificity of TNF-α levels, IL-1β levels, and leukocyte count in CSF in distinguishing acute bacterial from tuberculous meningitis*

	TNF-α	IL-1β	Leukocyte count[a]
Cutoff value[b]	300 pg/ml	400 pg/ml	500×10^6/l.
Sensitivity	0.82	0.77	0.86
Specificity	0.95[c]	0.63[c]	0.78

[a] Nonspecific parameter that best discriminated between acute bacterial and tuberculous meningitis.
[b] Cutoff value for each parameter was set at the most discriminating point between acute bacterial and tuberculous meningitis.
[c] $p < 0.05$ between values for TNF-α and IL-1β.

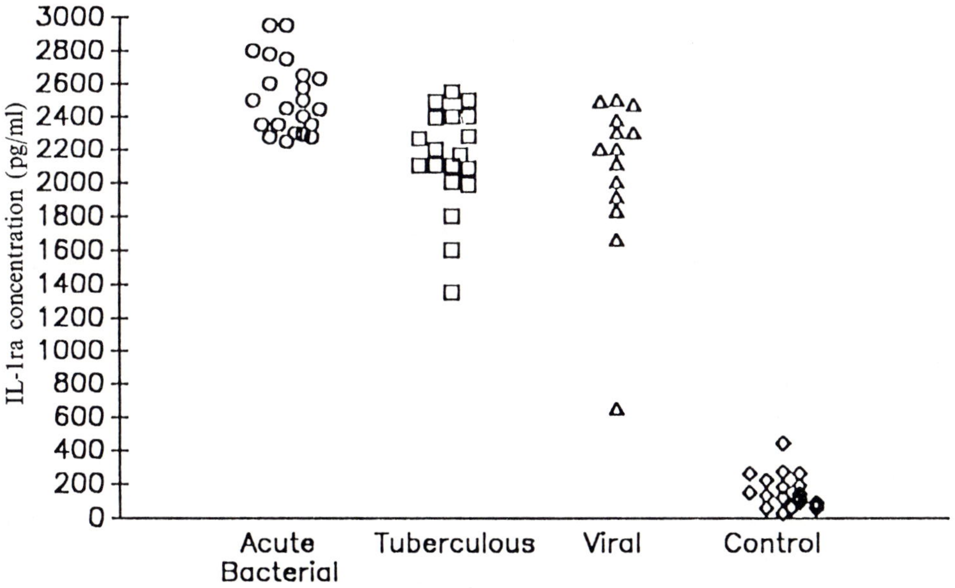

Fig. 3. Concentrations of IL-1ra in the cerebrospinal fluid of 22 patients with acute bacterial, 19 with tuberculous, 14 with viral meningitis, and in 18 control subjects.

higher than in acute bacterial meningitis (3.2 times) and parallelled overall meningeal inflammation.

DISCUSSION

The net effect of cytokines in inflammation depends on the concentration of agonist (cytokine itself) cellular receptor, and antagonists such IL-1ra (10), anti-cytokine and anti-receptor auto-antibody (14), soluble receptor (15), decoy receptor (16) and cytokines with antagonistic effects. In our study, the pro-inflammatory cytokines TNF-α and IL-1β and the antagonist IL-1ra were detected in CSF samples from meningitis patients on admission.

High levels of IL-1β and TNF-α in CSF samples from patients with acute bacterial meningitis reveals a local pro-inflammatory cytokine influx in the subarachnoid space. These two cytokines were shown to be potent inflammation inducers in the CNS in many experimental studies (2, 6). As in previous studies (8, 17, 18), TNF-α levels were markedly increased in acute bacterial meningitis, whereas all patients with viral meningitis and controls had undetectable levels. The lack of detectable TNF-α in the CSF in 2 cases (9%) of acute bacterial meningitis and 11 (58%) of tuberculous meningitis might have been due to the sensitivity of the assay. However, individual differences in the sensitivity of macrophages and endothelium in responding to bacterial components or products by synthesizing pro-inflammatory cytokines may contribute to the absence of TNF-α in the CSF from 2 cases with acute bacterial meningitis (7, 8, 17, 18).

Although there was no difference in CSF cell counts and types, relatively higher concentrations of TNF-α and IL-1β were found in tuberculous meningitis than viral meningitis. This could reflect the effect of several components of M. tuberculosis such as mycobacterium cord factor and lipoarabinomannan, which were shown to stimulate the release of cytokines in vitro (19). The effects of TNF-α and IL-1β on the formation of granulomas (20) may explain the long-term existence of tuberculomas or the paradoxical enlargement of intracranial tuberculomas with treatment, as seen in some of the cases in our clinic reported by other investigators (21).

Like other authors we found no correlation between the outcome of disease and TNF-α levels in the CSF but the level of consciousness in the patients with acute bacterial meningitis (according to the Glasgow Coma Scales) was significantly correlated with TNF-α levels at the time of presentation (7, 17). Although the exact mechanism is not known, CSF TNF-α levels may contribute to this correlation through local metabolic and vascular effects.

Experiments in rabbits demonstrated that IL-1β or TNF-α can act by altering the function of the cerebral capillary endothelium (i.e., the blood-brain barrier). Once secreted into the CSF, these cytokines might contribute to central nervous system injury by the recruitment of inflammatory cells and the subsequent release of superoxide anions, by induction of arachidonic acid metabolism, by disruption of the blood-brain barrier, or by direct cytotoxic effects (2, 6).

Compared with acute bacterial meningitis, the very low levels or absence of these two important pro-inflammatory cytokines and the relatively high levels of IL-1ra may explain why inflammation in the subarachnoid space is less aggressive in viral meningitis. The balance between the amount and secretion of IL-1 and its receptor antagonist may be critical to the severity of inflammation. Endogenously produced IL-1ra probably helps to limit the severity of the disease, but may be inadequate in overwhelming infection or acute inflammation (10–12).

IL-1 and IL-1ra gene expression and protein synthesis are regulated differently, even in the same cell (22). IL-1ra inhibits intracellular IL-1 synthesis and activity as a signal molecule (23). Other cytokines may also contribute to the balance between the production of IL-1 and that of IL-1ra in disease. IL-4, TGF-β and IL-10 increase the production of IL-1ra, but at the same time decrease the production of IL-1 (24). Also, the effective anti-viral cytokines interferon-γ (IFN-γ) and IFN-α were found to induce IL-1ra secretion (25), which could explain the high concentrations in viral meningitis.

Animal and in vitro studies have shown that high doses of IL-1ra are required to block the effects of IL-1β. In experimental endotoxemias in human volunteers, serum IL-1ra was found to be 100 times higher than IL-1β concentrations (26). In our study, concentrations of IL-1ra were 8.3-fold higher in the CSF in viral meningitis, 6.9-fold higher in tuberculous meningitis and 3.2-fold higher in acute bacterial meningitis. This difference indicates a greater inhibition of IL-1β in viral and tuberculous meningitis. Less inhibition of IL-1 and aggressive inflammation also paralleled high CSF cell counts in acute bacterial meningitis.

The detection of cytokines and antagonists in CSF may add new dimensions to current diagnostic criteria, yield additional insight into pathogenetic mechanisms, and provide new strategies for therapy. In our study, determinations of TNF-α and IL-1β from CSF samples at presentation were valuable in the differential diagnosis of acute bacterial meningitis. Determination of both IL-1 and its receptor antagonist could provide better information on the net effect of IL-1 (versus its antagonist) in the regulation of inflammation in CSF.

ACKNOWLEDGMENTS

We are grateful to Dr. Harry Towbin for providing the IL-1 receptor antagonist ELISA and for a critical review of the manuscript, and to Ferah Şengül, Raziye Ülker and Nuran Akgül for technical assistance.

REFERENCES

1. Tauber MG, Shibl AM, Hackbarth CJ, Larrick JW, Sande MA. Antibiotic therapy, endotoxin concentration in cerebrospinal fluid, and brain edema in experimental Escherichia coli meningitis in rabbits. J Infect Dis 156: 456–461, 1987.
2. Saukkonen K, Sande S, Cioffe C, Wolpe S, Sherry B, Cerami A, Tuomanen E. The role of cytokines in the generation of inflammation and tissue damage in experimental Gram-positive meningitis. J Exp Med 171: 439–448, 1990.
3. Syrogiannopoulos GA, Hansen EJ, Erwin AL, Munford RS, Rutledge J, Reisch JS, McCracken GH. Haemophilus influenzae type b lipooligosaccharide induces meningeal inflammation. J Infect Dis 157: 237–244, 1988.
4. Waage A, Halstensen A, Espevik T. Association between tumour necrosis factor in serum with fatal outcome in patients with meningococcal disease. Lancet 1: 355–357, 1987.
5. Waage A, Brandtzaeg P, Halstensen A, Kierulf P, Espevik T. The complex pattern of cytokines in serum from patients with meningococcal septic shock. J Exp Med 169: 333–338, 1989.
6. Ramilo O, Saez-Llorens X, Mertsola J, Jafari H, Olsen KD, Hansen Ej, Yoshinaga M, Ohkawara S, Nariuchi H, McCracken GH. Tumor necrosis factor α/cachectin and interleukin 1β initiate meningeal inflammation. J Exp Med 172: 497–507, 1990.
7. Mustafa MM, Lebel MH, Ramilo O, Olsen KD, Reisch JS, Beutler B, McCracken GH. Correlation of interleukin-1β and cachectin concentrations in cerebrospinal fluid and outcome from bacterial meningitis. J Pediatr 115: 208–213, 1989.
8. Nadal D, Leppert D, Frei K, Gallo P, Lamche H, Fontana A. Tumour necrosis factor-α in infectious meningitis. Arch Dis Child 64: 1274–1279, 1989.
9. Ramilo O, Mustafa MM, Porter J, Saez-Llorens X, Mertsola J, Olsen KD, Luby JP, Beutler B, McCracken GH. Detection of interleukin-1β but not tumor necrosis factor-α in cerebrospinal fluid of children with aseptic meningitis. AJDC 144: 349–352, 1990.
10. Dinarello CA, Thompson RC. Blocking IL-1: interleukin 1 receptor antagonist in vivo and in vitro. Immunol Today 12: 404–410, 1991.
11. Dinarello CA, Wolff SM. The role of interleukin-1 in disease. N Eng J Med 328: 106–112, 1993.
12. Miller LC. Lynch EA, Isa S, Logan JW, Dinarello CA, Steere AC. Balance of synovial fluid IL-1β and IL-1 receptor antagonist and recovery from Lyme arthritis. Lancet 341: 146–148, 1993.
13. Towbin H, Schmitz A, Oostrum J. van, Seitz M, Dewald B, Zingel O, Motz J, Vosbeck K, Rordorf C. A monoclonal antibody based ELISA for the human interleukin-1 receptor antagonist: its

application to measure hIL-1ra levels in monocyte cultures in synovial fluids. J Immunol Methods (in press).
14. Bendtzen K, Svenson M, Jonsson V, Hippe E. Autoantibodies to cytokines. Friends or foes? Immunol Today 11: 167–169, 1990.
15. Ozmen L, Gribaudo G, Fountoulakis M, Gentz R, Landolfo S, Garotta G. Mouse soluble IFN-γ receptor as IFN-γ inhibitor. Distribution, antigenicity, and activity after injection in mice. J Immunol. 150: 2698–2705, 1993.
16. Colotta F, Re F, Muzio M, Bertini R, Polentarutti N, Sironi M, Giri JG, Dower SK, E Sims J, Mantovani A. Interleukin 1 type II receptor: A decoy target for IL-1 that is regulated by IL-4. Science 261: 472–475, 1993.
17. Arditi M, Manogue KR, Caplan M, Yogev R. Cerebrospinal fluid cachectin/tumor necrosis factor-α and platelet-activating factor concentrations and severity of bacterial meningitis in children. J Infect Dis 162: 139–147, 1990.
18. Mustafa MM, Ramilo O, Saez-Llorens X, Olsen KD, Magness RR, McCracken GH. Cerebrospinal fluid prostaglandins, interleukin-1β, and tumor necrosis factor in bacterial meningitis. AJDC 144: 883–887, 1990.
19. Barnes PF, Chatterjee D, Abrams JS, Lu S, Wang E, Yamamura M, Brennan PJ, Modlin. L. Cytokine production induced by Mycobacterium tuberculosis lipoarabinomannan. J Immunol 149: 541–547, 1992.
20. Editorial. Granulomas and cytokines. Lancet 337: 1067–1069, 1991.
21. Chambers ST, Hendrickse WA, Record C, Rudge P, Smith H. Paradoxical expansion of intracranial tuberculomas during chemotherapy. Lancet 2: 181–183, 1984.
22. Arend WP, Smith MF, Janson RW, Joslin FG. IL-1 receptor antagonist and IL-1β production in human monocytes are regulated differently. J Immunol 147: 1530–1536, 1991.
23. Andersson J, Björk L, Dinarello CA, Towbin H, Andersson U. Lipopolysaccharide induces human interleukin-1 receptor antagonist and interleukin-1 production in the same cell. Eur J Immunol 22: 2617–2623, 1992.
24. Vannier E, Miller LC, Dinarello CA. Coordinated anti-inflammatory effects of interleukin 4: interleukin-4 suppresses interleukin 1 production but upregulates gene expression and synthesis of interleukin 1 receptor antagonist. Proc Natl Acad Sci USA 89: 4076–4080, 1992.
25. Tilg H, Mier JW, Vogel W, Aulitzky WE, Wiedermann CJ, Vannier E, Huber C, Dinarello CA. Induction of circulating IL-1 receptor antagonist by IFN treatment. J Immunol 150: 4687–4692, 1993.
26. Granowitz EV, Santos AA, Poutsiaka DD, Cannon JG, Wilmore DW, Wolff SM, Dinarello CA. Production of interleukin-1-receptor antagonist during experimental endotoxaemia. Lancet 338: 1423–1424, 1991.

Submitted April 28, 1994; accepted August 22, 1994

Scand J Infect Dis 26: 675–684, 1994

An Outbreak of Diarrhea due to Verotoxin-producing Escherichia coli in the Canadian Northwest Territories

PAMELA ORR[1,5,6], BEV LORENCZ[2], ROSEMARY BROWN[2], ROBERT KIELLY[2], BEN TAN[4], DONNA HOLTON[4], HELEN CLUGSTONE[2], LISA LUGTIG[6], CAROLYN PIM[3], SHARON MACDONALD[6], GREG HAMMOND[1,5], MICHAEL MOFFATT[6], JOHN SPIKA[4], DOUGLAS MANUEL[6], WENDY WINTHER[5], DOUGLAS MILLEY[5], HERMY LIOR[4] and NURI SINUFF[2]

From the [1]Department of Medical Microbiology, University of Manitoba, the [2]Keewatin Regional Health Board, the [3]Department of Health, Government of the Northwest Territories, the [4]Laboratory Centre for Disease Control, Ottawa, the [5]Cadham Provincial Laboratory, Winnipeg and the [6]J. A. Hildes Northern Medical Unit, University of Manitoba

In the summer of 1991 a large outbreak of Escherichia coli 0157:H7 associated diarrhea occurred in 6 Inuit communities in the Canadian Northwest Territories. The total population of these communities is 5,292. Of the 521 individuals who developed diarrhea, 152 (29%) were positive for E. coli 0157:H7 on stool culture or positive by verotoxin analysis. Median age was 6 years. The attack rate for children <1 year was 43% in the major affected community of Arviat. Hemolytic-uremic syndrome (HUS) developed in 22 cases, and 2 patients died. Asymptomatic stool carriage of verotoxin-producing E. coli (VTEC) 2–5 weeks after diarrheal illness was noted in 4/28 persons followed prospectively. Epidemic curves, case-control studies and phage type testing suggested person-to-person transmission. The original source of infection was not identified, though a food source was suspected. VTEC were detected in 6 food samples (minced beef and caribou) taken from retail outlets and homes. Primary prevention of infection through health education and promotion activities, as well as long-term follow-up of HUS survivors, are indicated in this population.

P. H. Orr, MD, Department of Medical Microbiology, Rm 503, 730 William Avenue, Winnipeg, Manitoba, Canada R3E OW3

INTRODUCTION

Over the past decade, numerous outbreaks of Escherichia coli 0157:H7 associated diarrhea have been reported in North America and Europe. The organism has been isolated from the intestinal tract of cattle, buffalo, pigs, poultry and sheep (1–4). Transmission to humans has been traced to the ingestion of contaminated water or food, including undercooked hamburger, unpasteurized milk, and vegetables grown in soil fertilized with cattle manure, as well as through person-to-person spread (5–10).

In this study we describe the clinical, microbiologic and epidemiologic features of a large outbreak of verotoxin-producing E. coli (VTEC) associated diarrhea, which occurred in the Keewatin District of the Northwest Territories, Canada in the summer of 1991. The outbreak was remarkable not only for its considerable associated morbidity and mortality, but also for the unique culture and remote location of the affected Inuit population.

MATERIALS AND METHODS

Epidemiologic investigation

The outbreak occurred from June 4 to October 31, 1991 in the settlements of Arviat, Baker Lake, Rankin Inlet, Whale Cove, Chesterfield Inlet and Sanikuluaq in the Canadian Northwest Territories (Fig. 1). The total population of these settlements is 5,292; 89% of the population are of Inuit ethnicity. Primary care was provided by nurse-practitioners and itinerant physicians at the outpatient health centre

 ISSN 0036-5548

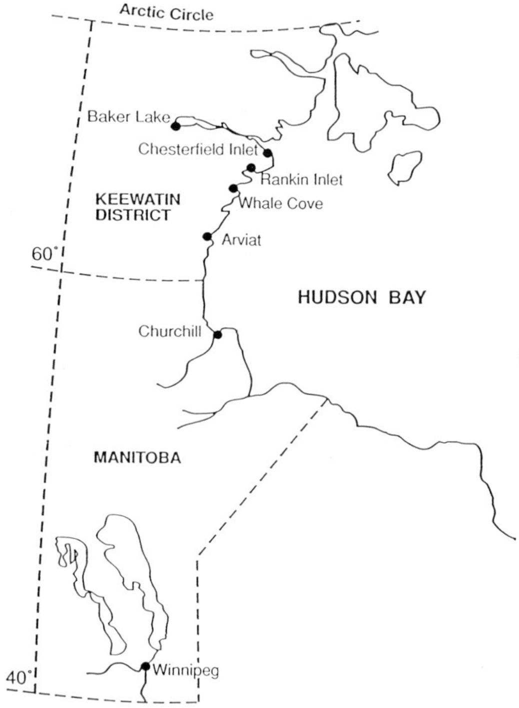

Fig. 1. Six Canadian Arctic communities of the Keewatin District, Northwest Territories.

in each community. Secondary and tertiary care were provided by referral hospitals in Churchill and Winnipeg, Manitoba.

A case of diarrhea was defined as the occurrence of ≥2 watery stools within a 24 h period. Case data were obtained prospectively, by nursing and medical staff, from patient interviews and clinical examinations. Retrospective data on the occurrence of diarrhea in previous years were collected from a review of clinical charts. Blood in the stool was detected by visual inspection of the specimen. Individuals with diarrhea who developed microangiopathic hemolytic anemia and acute renal impairment as evidenced by an active urine sediment and/or azotemia, oliguria or anuria were defined as cases of hemolytic-uremic syndrome (HUS). As thrombocytopenia may be transitory in HUS, and there were occasional delays in obtaining blood specimens, this criterion was considered strongly supportive of, but not required for, the diagnosis.

Microbiologic investigation

Stool specimens were requested from all patients with diarrhea. The specimens were collected in sterile containers and transported by commercial aircraft at room temperature to Cadham Provincial Laboratory (CPL) in Winnipeg, Manitoba. All stools were cultured on sorbitol-MacConkey agar for the presence of E. coli 0157:H7. Serotyping and phage typing of all isolates were performed at the Laboratory Centre for Disease Control (Ottawa). The E. coli 0157:H7 isolates were analysed for the presence of the verotoxin 1 (VT1) and verotoxin 2 (VT2) genes by polymerase chain reaction (11). Stool analysis for free fecal verotoxin (FVT) and verotoxin in polymyxin extracts of colony sweeps (VT:PECS) was performed using the technique of Karmali et al. (12), with confirmation through verotoxin neutralization by rabbit anti-VT1 and VT-2. A confirmed case of VTEC-associated diarrhea was defined as an individual with a positive stool culture for E. coli 0157:H7 and/or stool positive for FVT, VT:PECS, or both, in the absence of other identifiable clinical causes of diarrhea. A case was considered unconfirmed if the stool was negative for E. coli 0157:H7 and verotoxin, or if a stool specimen was not collected.

Stools were initially analysed for ova and parasites and cultured for bacterial pathogens other than VTEC, including enteropathogenic E. coli, Salmonella, Shigella, Campylobacter and Yersinia. Stools were not screened for enterotoxigenic E. coli. After July 1, 1991 routine bacterial and parasitic analyses of stools were performed only if there was strong clinical suspicion of infection due to pathogens other than VTEC. Culture and electron microscopic examinations for viral stool pathogens were not performed due to the logistics of specimen numbers and transport.

Environmental testing

Food samples obtained from the homes of diarrhea patients, and from retail outlets in Arviat and Baker Lake, were transported at the temperature at which they were collected to CPL in Winnipeg for analysis. Samples were cultured and screened for the presence of verotoxin by methods described by Sekla and Milley (13). Isolation of E. coli 0157 was attempted from all foods positive for VT, using a Rapid Hydrophobic Grid Membrane Filter-Enzyme-Labelled Antibody procedure specific for E. coli 0157:H7 (14).

Goose and caribou feces were collected from the tundra, and samples of caribou intestinal contents were collected by wildlife officers during a hunt of the local herds near Arviat. These samples were tested for E. coli by culture and verotoxin analysis. Water samples from the local natural lake reservoirs, and from post-treatment (chlorinated) sources in homes, schools and other community facilities were collected and analysed for total coliform counts according to standard methods (15); positives were subsequently screened by sorbitol fermentation. Sorbitol-negative colonies were tested for the 0157 antigen by latex agglutination (Serobact E. coli 0157, Disposable Products, Adelaide, Australia).

Statistical analysis

χ^2-analysis was used to test differences in non-continuous variables, and Fisher's exact test was used when the expected value for a cell was <5. Continuous variables were assessed using Student's t-test. The sensitivity and negative predictive value of culture, FVT and VT:PECS testing were calculated for stool specimens on which all three tests were performed. A true positive was defined as a specimen which was culture and/or FVT and/or VT:PECS positive, and a true negative specimen as culture, FVT and VT:PECS negative.

RESULTS

Between June 1 and October 31, 1991, 521 individuals from the 6 Canadian Arctic settlements (Fig. 1) of Arviat, Baker Lake, Rankin Inlet, Whale Cove, Chesterfield Inlet and Sanikiluaq developed diarrhea. The first cases occurred in Arviat, which was also the most severely affected settlement (Fig. 2). Of those affected, 270 were female and 251 were male (Table I). The median age was 6 years, with a range of 1 month to 90 years. 47% of cases were <5 years of age, and 12% were <1 year old.

Of the 521 cases, 152 (29.1%) were confirmed positive for E. coli 0157:H7 on culture, and/or were positive for verotoxin. In 369 cases, VTEC infection was unconfirmed, due to culture/toxin-negative stool specimens ($n = 197$) or unavailability of stool for testing ($n = 172$). Verotoxin-producing E. coli other than the 0157:H7 serotype were not identified in this outbreak. The sex ratio was similar for confirmed and unconfirmed cases, but confirmed cases were significantly ($p < 0.001$) more likely to be younger in age.

In Arviat the attack rates for diarrhea, and for VTEC confirmed cases, were 43% and 20% respectively for those <1 year old, increasing to 85% and 44% in those aged 1–4 years. Rates were lowest in those aged 35–64 years (12% and 3% respectively), but rose to 29% and 17% in those >65 years. Attack rates in the other settlements were lower throughout all age groups. There were no significant differences in attack rates for males vis-à-vis females.

Clinical manifestations

Of the 521 cases, 103 (19.7%) gave a history of bloody diarrhea, 328 (62.9%) had non-bloody diarrhea and 90 (17.2%) were unsure. Individuals with a history of bloody diarrhea were significantly ($p < 0.001$) more likely than those without to have VTEC-confirmed (culture and/or VT positive) stools. Clinical data were available for the first 63 cases of diarrhea initially presenting in Arviat. 34 (53.9%) of the 63 gave a history of abdominal pain, 11 (17.5%) complained of nausea, 32 (50.8%) experienced vomiting, and 13 (20.6%) fever. There was no significant difference in the frequency of these clinical symptoms between VTEC-confirmed and unconfirmed cases; data on duration of symptoms were unavailable.

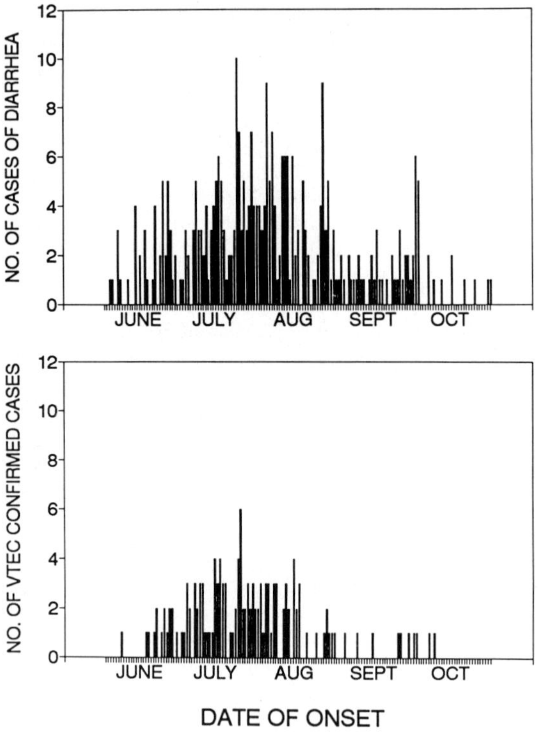

Fig. 2. Epidemic curves for all diarrhea cases, and for VTEC confirmed cases, in Arviat NWT, 1991.

Table I. *Demographic characteristics of VTEC confirmed and unconfirmed diarrhea cases, NWT outbreak 1991*

Demographic characteristic	All cases ($n = 521$)	Diarrhea cases Confirmed cases ($n = 152$)	Unconfirmed cases ($n = 369$)
Sex			
Females	270	76	194
Males	251	76	175
Age (yrs)			
<1	65	18	47
1–4	178	61	117
5–14	105	41	64*
14–64	166	29	137
65+	7	3	4
Settlement			
Arviat	319	135	184
Baker Lake	98	10	88
Rankin Inlet	96	2	94
Whale Cove	3	2	1
Chesterfield Inlet	3	2	1
Sanikiluaq	2	1	1

* $p < 0.001$

Patients were treated supportively with fluid and electrolyte management. Antibiotics and antimotility agents were not prescribed. 67 patients required hospitalization. Hemolytic uremic syndrome (HUS) developed in 22 persons, representing 4.2% of all 521 diarrhea cases or 14.4% of the 152 VTEC-confirmed cases. 14 (63.6%) of the 22 cases of HUS occurred in males, and 8 (36.4%) in females. The mean and median age were 5 and 3 years respectively; 2 cases occurred in children <1 year of age, 15 in children 1–4 years, 4 in those 5–14 years, and 1 in a 67-year-old adult. Stools were positive for VTEC in 21/22 HUS cases; in 1 case the stool was culture and verotoxin negative but a diagnosis of HUS was made on the basis of hemorrhagic colitis complicated by microangiopathic hemolytic anemia, thrombocytopenia and renal impairment with hypertension.

Transient hypertension was noted in 18 of the patients with HUS, and seizures in 2. Four patients underwent temporary peritoneal dialysis. Death occurred in 2 (9.0%) of the 22 HUS cases. The immediate cause of death was cardiac tamponade in the first case and intracranial hemorrhage in the second. Autopsy in both cases revealed acute hemorrhagic colitis associated with extensive areas of focal thrombosis and necrosis in the kidneys and myocardium, as well as pulmonary hemorrhage and effusions.

Laboratory investigations

A total of 556 stool specimens were obtained from 349 (66.9%) of the 521 individuals with diarrhea (Table II); 22 specimens were stool swabs and 534 were fecal samples. Of the 556 specimens, 204 (36.6%) were positive on culture for E. coli 0157:H7 and/or positive for verotoxin. 23 (4.3%) of the 534 stool samples were grossly bloody, and 306 (57.3%) were liquid; these specimens were significantly more likely to be VTEC-positive than stools that were non-bloody ($p < 0.001$) or solid ($p < 0.001$). The average transit time from stool collection to arrival in the laboratory was 4.3 days, and was not significantly different for VTEC-positive vs. negative specimens.

All 556 stool specimens were cultured but only 519 were analysed for FVT and 513 for verotoxin by VT:PECS method. Verotoxin testing was not possible if the specimen was a swab ($n = 22$) or if insufficient fecal material remained after culture was performed. All 3 examinations (culture, FVT and VT:PECS) were performed on 489 stool specimens. The sensitivity and negative predictive values for culture alone were 57.7% and 79.2%, for FVT alone 83.9% and 90.0%, and for VT:PECS alone 93.0% and 95.8% respectively. The combination of culture plus VT:PECS added only marginally to the sensitivity (94.1%) and

Table II. *Results of stool culture for E. coli 0157:H7 and verotoxin analysis*

	Total	Positive	Negative
No. (%) specimens	556	204 (36.7)	352 (63.3)
No. patients tested	349	152 (43.6)	197 (56.4)
Specimen characteristics			
No. (%) bloody	24	17 (70.8)	7 (29.2)*
No. (%) liquid	307	158 (51.5)	149 (48.5)*
Transit time (days)	4.3	4.2	4.3
Laboratory results			
No. cultures (%)	556	122 (21.9)	434 (78.1)
No. FVT (%)	519	167 (32.2)	352 (67.8)
No. PECS (%)	513	177 (34.5)	336 (65.5)

* $p < 0.001$

negative predictive value (96.4%) of the VT:PECS procedure alone. Culture plus FVT testing demonstrated a sensitivity of 86.0% and negative predictive value of 92.0%.

The first 99 clinical isolates of E. coli 0157:H7 were phage typed and tested by polymerase chain reaction for the presence of the genes coding for the production of verotoxin. 98 isolates were phage type 32 and positive for genes encoding both VT1 and VT2. One isolate from a 1-year-old boy from Baker Lake was phage type 34 and was positive for VT1, VT2 and a VT2 variant B subunit gene which has previously been described (16). This child fell ill in August 1991 with non-bloody diarrhea which resolved in 5 days without complications.

In order to determine the duration of excretion of E. coli 0157:H7, stool swabs for culture were obtained at approximately weekly intervals between July 15 and October 8 from 28 consecutive individuals presenting to the Arviat Health Centre with diarrhea and culture-positive stools. The age and sex distribution of these individuals did not differ significantly ($p > 0.05$) from that of culture-positive persons from either Arviat or the entire Keewatin outbreak. 24/28 (86%) were negative on their first culture. Of the remaining 4 'excretors', 3 were positive for E. coli 0157:H7 at 10–13 days after the initial positive culture and negative thereafter, and one was positive at 39 days. All 4 'excretors' were asymptomatic.

Environmental investigation

Cultures of the 64 submitted water samples were negative for E. coli 0157:H7. However coliforms were detected in 14 samples, with colony counts ranging between 2 and >1,500/100 ml. Unchlorinated water samples were taken from reservoirs, surface waters and melted snow, and accounted for the majority of coliform-positive samples. All treated (chlorinated) community water supplies compiled with the Canadian Drinking Water Guideline (17), with the exception of one sample with >1,500 coliforms/100 ml, which was collected from an open water tank in the home of 3 individuals with diarrhea.

63 food items taken from homes, local retail outlets, and from hunters on the tundra, were tested for VTEC by culture and toxin analysis. Samples included raw, frozen and dried caribou, minced beef, steak, sliced beef, chicken, pork, whale fat, cheese, and fish (char). Verotoxin was detected in 6 food specimens; 4 of these were frozen minced beef samples from retail outlets in Arviat and Baker Lake, and 2 were raw, unfrozen caribou meat samples taken from the homes of infected persons. An E. coli 0157:H7 of phage type 32 and positive by polymerase chain reaction for the genes encoding VT1 and VT2 was isolated from 1 caribou sample. The caribou meat had been handled in the home by several family members with diarrhea. It is therefore unclear whether it was originally contaminated at the time of slaughter or subsequently from handling by infected individuals. Culture of the 4 verotoxin-positive minced beef samples and the remaining verotoxin-positive caribou sample did not yield VTEC isolates of any serotype, possibly because of the large numbers of other coliform organisms also present.

Two samples of goose feces and 1 sample of caribou feces collected from the tundra were negative for E. coli 0157:H7 on culture, and negative for verotoxin. A sample of intestinal contents taken from a freshly killed caribou was also negative.

Outbreak investigation and control

The first case of bloody diarrhea occurred on June 4 in a 1-year-old female in Arviat, and the first confirmed case occurred in her 34-year-old uncle who became ill on June 8. The family of these 2 patients frequently visited each other's homes and shared meals. The second confirmed case occurred on a 4-year-old boy in Chesterfield Inlet, who fell ill on June 9. He had not had contact with any individuals from Arviat prior to the onset of his illness. The original source of infection in the index cases is unknown. The subsequent epidemic curves are consistent with person-to-person transmission, although continued exposure to a food source is also possible.

A case-control study was performed in Baker Lake. Matched for age and sex, cases were more likely than controls to have visited the local Health Centre prior to the outbreak for diarrheal illness ($p = 0.01$), and were more likely to have visited other households during the outbreak ($p = 0.008$). There were no significant differences between cases and controls in dietary history, including the consumption of cooked or raw (frozen or thawed) minced beef, caribou or other meats, methods of food preparation, handwashing, diapering practices or visits to other affected communities.

Community education programs were developed which focused on the nature of the illness and prevention of transmission by handwashing and proper food preparation. Use was made of the media (radio, TV, newspapers), and teaching took place in the home, schools, local Health Centres and at community meetings. Those involved in the education program include lay health workers, nurses, health educators, physicians, environmental specialists, teachers, health and social service committee members and elected municipal councillors.

Public health inspections were made of foodhandling practices in hotels and restaurants, and of garbage and sewage disposal areas in each community. Cultural food practices among the Keewatin Inuit include the provision of meat, including caribou and commercially prepared minced beef, in a raw (thawed or frozen) or cooked state, on plates which are then placed on tables on the kitchen floor within easy reach of young children and adults. Educational efforts during the epidemic emphasized the need to thoroughly cook meat, and to wash hands and utensils prior to and during food preparation.

Multiple cases were seen within immediate and extended families. When the epidemic failed to abate after institution of the community education program, a system of 'voluntary' isolation was initiated in an effort to reduce person-to-person transmission. Patients with diarrhea were urged to stay home until they were free from diarrhea for 3 days. There was a gradual decrease in the number of new cases seen in September and October; the onset date of the last case of diarrhea was October 31, 1991. It is unclear to what extent the control measures institute were effective in limiting disease transmission and bringing the epidemic to an end.

DISCUSSION

The salient features of this epidemic include the large number of individuals affected, as well as the need to adapt investigation and control activities to the unique culture and geography of the region. It is likely that the food practices and living conditions of the Inuit contributed to the acquisition and transmission of infection in this population. Limitations in local health care resources necessitated the mobilization and coordination of additional personnel with clinical, laboratory and public health expertise. Investigation and control efforts required knowledge of, and sensitivity to, the Inuit culture. Local health committees as well as community health representatives, who are trained as health advocates and educators, were invaluable in this regard.

The original source of infection in the index cases is unknown. Acquisition of infection through consumption of contaminated food is likely. Subsequent epidemic curves and laboratory analysis, including serotyping and phage typing, were consistent with person-to-person transmission. Interpersonal fecal-oral spread of infection in this population may have been promoted by the close physical contact which takes place between family members and friends in Inuit society.

Ingestion of undercooked contaminated minced beef appears to be the most likely source of infection in the index cases, and may also have resulted in the reintroduction of infection during the epidemic. The detection of verotoxin in 4 samples of minced beef is in keeping with previous studies demonstrating that 25–36% of Canadian retail minced beef is positive for verotoxin (2, 13). Dietary interviews conducted during the epidemic indicated that the Inuit frequently consumed raw store-bought hamburger. Hunters noted that caribou herds near Arviat were sparse during the summer of 1991, suggesting that there may have been an unusual reliance on store-bought meat during that period. However, analysis of total meat sales by the 2 retail suppliers in the communities failed to reveal a significant increase in 1991 compared with 1990.

The significance of the 2 verotoxin-positive caribou samples, 1 of which was also E. coli 0157:H7 positive with the same phage type and toxin profile as the clinical strains, is unknown. These samples were raw and had been handled by individuals with diarrhea. Samples of fresh caribou meat and intestinal contents collected by wildlife officers were negative. Previous Canadian surveys of meat for evidence of VTEC infection have not included caribou (2, 3). Such studies are recommended, particularly in view of the Inuit preference for raw caribou.

Unfortunately, due to the magnitude of the epidemic, accurate prospectively collected clinical data on symptoms were available only for the first 63 cases in Arviat. The frequency of abdominal pain (54%) was lower than that reported in previous outbreaks of hemorrhagic colitis due to confirmed E. coli 0157:H7 infection, whereas the frequencies of vomiting (51%) and fever (21%) were similar (5, 18, 19). The attack rate for individuals ≥ 65 years in Arviat was similar to that reported in an outbreak of E. coli 0157:H7 among elderly residents of a nursing home (7). However, the attack rates in children <5 years were higher than those reported in a previous day-care outbreak (5).

It is likely that the number of VTEC-positive cases was underestimated due to the lack of stool collection from all patients. The time required for specimen transport, at room temperature, to the laboratory may have resulted in false-negative cultures and/or verotoxin analysis, although the mean transit time was not significantly different for VTEC-positive and negative specimens. The high sensitivity of the VT:PECS procedure in the detection of verotoxin renders it a useful procedure in outbreak investigations (1). However, culture remains important for the epidemiologic analysis of transmission through the serotyping and phage typing of clinical isolates.

The importance of asymptomatic excretion of E. coli 0157:H7 in disease transmission within this outbreak is unknown. Stools were not collected from asymptomatic individuals during this epidemic. However, previous studies have documented asymptomatic carriage of E. coli 0157, and have suggested that these individuals may serve as sources of infection (19, 20). The prolonged excretion of E. coli 0157:H7 after resolution of diarrhea which was seen in several patients during this outbreak has been previously reported in other studies (18, 21–23), and has been reported to be of longer duration in children vis-à-vis adults (23).

Antibiotics have not proved beneficial in the treatment of VTEC infection or HUS. Retrospective studies have not shown any effect of antibiotic therapy on duration of colitis, and have yielded conflicting results regarding the risk of progression to HUS (24, 25). A small unblinded randomized trial of antibiotic therapy in children with E. coli 0157:H7 enteritis failed to demonstrate any difference in duration of symptoms, fecal carriage, or progression to HUS (26). A larger randomized, blinded, placebo-controlled trial is required, although adequate sample size may be difficult to achieve. An antibiotic trial was not performed during this outbreak because of the limited availability of health care personnel, and concerns regarding patient and community acceptance of 'blinded' placebo-controlled therapy.

Prevention of future outbreaks of E. coli 0157:H7 gastroenteritis in the Canadian arctic will depend on ongoing education and health promotion activities, coupled with improvements in housing and sanitation. Long-term follow-up of HUS survivors is indicated, as chronic renal failure requiring dialysis may eventually develop in 3–5% of affected children, and persistent hypertension in 5–14% (18, 27, 28). Clarification of the role played by host and agent factors in the clinical spectrum of VTEC-associated illness remains a research priority. If host immunity to toxin proves to be protective and longlasting, vaccines such as the synthetic Shiga toxin B-subunit peptide may prove to be an important strategy in the prevention of HUS secondary to both VTEC and Shigella.

ACKNOWLEDGEMENTS

The authors thank Dawn Colby, Anna Lutyj, and Janice Drummond for technical laboratory assistance, and Obed Anoee, the Community Health Representative from Arviat, for his invaluable assistance in the investigation and control of this outbreak.

REFERENCES

1. Karmali M. Infection by verocytotoxin-producing Escherichia coli. Clin Microbiol Rev 2: 15–38, 1989.
2. Read S, Gyles C, Clarke R, Lior H, McEwen S. Prevalence of Verocytotoxigenic E. coli in ground beef, pork, and chicken in Southwestern Ontario. Epidemiol Infect 105: 11–20, 1990.
3. Doyle M, Schoeni J. Isolation of Escherichia coli 0157:H7 from retail fresh meats and poultry. Appl Environ Microbiol 53: 2394–2396, 1987.
4. Mohammad A, Peiris J, Wijewanta E, Mahalingam S, Gunasekara G. Role of verocytotoxigenic Escherichia coli in cattle and buffalo calf diarrhea. FEMS Microbiol Lett 26: 281–283, 1985.
5. Spika J, Parsons J, Nordenberg D, Gunn R. Hemolytic uremic syndrome and diarrhea associated with Escherichia coli 0157:H7 in a day-care center. J Pediatr 109: 287–291, 1986.
6. Karmali M, Arbus G, Petric M, Patrick M, Roscoe M, Shaw J, Lior H. Hospital-acquired Escherichia coli 0157:H7-associated haemolytic uraemic syndrome in a nurse. Lancet 1: 526, 1988.
7. Carter A, Borczyk A, Carlson J, Harvey B, Hockin J, Karmali M, Krishnan C, Korn D, Lior H. A severe outbreak of Escherichia coli 0157:H7-associated hemorrhagic colitis in a nursing home. N Engl J Med 317: 1496–1500, 1987.
8. Cieslak P, Gensheimer K, Beckett J, Buffington J, Smith G, Wells J, Griffin P. A cluster of E. coli 0157:H7 infections traced to a manured vegetable garden [abstract no. 1280]. In: Program and Abstracts of 33rd Interscience Conference on Antimicrobial Agents and Chemotherapy. New Orleans: American Society for Microbiology, 354, 1993.
9. Bell B, Goldoft M, Griffin P, Lewis J, Barrett J, Wells J, Baron R, Kobayashi J. A multistate foodborne outbreak of Escherichia coli (E. coli) 0157:H7: The Washington (WA) Experience [abstract no. 1453]. In: Program and Abstracts of 33rd Interscience Conference on Antimicrobial Agents and Chemotherapy. New Orleans: American Society for Microbiology, 385, 1993.
10. Swerdlow D, Woodruff B, Brady R, Griffin P, Tippen S, Donnell D, Geldreich E, Payne B, Myer A, Wells J, Greene K, Bright M, Bean N, Blake P. A waterborne outbreak in Missouri of Escherichia coli 0157:H7 associated with bloody diarrhea and death. Ann Intern Med 117: 812–819, 1992.
11. Pollard DR, Johnson WM, Lior H, Tyler SD, Rozee K. Rapid and specific detection of verotoxin genes in Escherichia coli by the polymerase chain reaction. J Clin Microbiol 28: 540–545, 1990.
12. Karmali MA, Petric M, Lim C, Cheung R, Arbus GS. Sensitive method for detecting low numbers of verotoxin-producing Escherichia coli in mixed cultures by use of colony sweeps and polymyxin extraction of verotoxin. J Clin Microbiol 22: 614–619, 1985.
13. Sekla L, Milley D. Manitoba studies on the isolation of E. coli 0157:H7 and other verotoxigenic organisms from ground beef. In: Todd ECD, Mackenzie JM, eds. Proceedings of the Workshop on Methods to Isolate Escherichia coli 0157:H7 and other Verotoxigenic E. coli from Foods. Ottawa: Polyscience Publications Inc., 131–136, 1993.
14. Todd EC, Szabo RA, Peterkin P, Sharpe A, Parrington L, Bundle D, Gidney M, Perry M. Rapid hydrophobic grid membrane filter – enzyme-labelled antibody procedure for identification and enumeration of E. coli 1057 in foods. Appl Environ Microbiol 54: 2536–2540, 1988.

15. American Public Health Association. Standard methods for the examination of water and wastewater, 17th edn. Washington D.C.: American Public Health Association, 2005, 1989.
16. Tyler SD, Johnson WM, Lior H, Wang G, Rozee KR. Identification of verotoxin type 2 variant B subunit genes in Escherichia coli by the polymerase chain reaction and restriction fragment length polymorphism analysis. J Clin Microbiol 29: 1339–1343, 1991.
17. Health & Welfare Canada. Guidelines for Canadian Drinking Water Quality. Canadian Government Publishing Centre, Ottawa, Canada: Dept. National Health and Welfare, 1989.
18. Griffin P, Ostroff S, Tauxe R, Greene K, Wells J, Lewis J, Blake P. Illness associated with Escherichia coli 0157:H7 infections. A broad clinical spectrum. Ann Intern Med 109: 705–712, 1988.
19. Ryan CA, Tauxe RV, Hosek GW, Wells J, Stoesz P, McFadden H, Smith P, Wright G, Blake P. Escherichia coli 0157:H7 diarrhea in a nursing home: clinical, epidemiological and pathological findings. J Infect Dis 154: 631–638, 1986.
20. Ratnam S, March S, Spague W, Severs D, Sullivan R. Are humans a source of Escherichia coli 0157:H7, the agent of hemmorhagic colitis? N Engl J Med 315: 1612–1613, 1986.
21. Belongia E, Osterholm M, Soler J, Ammend D, Braun J, MacDonald K. Transmission of Escherichia coli 0157:H7 infection in Minnesota child day-care facilities. JAMA 269: 883–888, 1993.
22. Gransden W, Damm M, Anderson J, Carter J, Lior H. Hemorrhagic cystitis and balanitis associated with verotoxin-producing Escherichia coli 0157:H7. J Infect Dis 152: 775–777, 1985.
23. Pai C, Gordon R, Sims H, Bryan L. Sporadic cases of hemorrhagic colitis associated with Escherichia coli 0157:H7: clinical, epidemiologic, and bacteriologic features. Ann Intern Med 101: 738–742, 1984.
24. Robson W, Scott R, Rick G. Influence of antidiarrhea and antimicrobial medications on the hemorrhagic colitis associated with hemolytic-uremic syndrome. J Pediatr 117: 675–676, 1990.
25. Pavia A, Nichols C, Green D, Tauxe R, Mottice S, Greene K, Wells J, Siegler R, Brewer E, Hannon D, Blake P. Hemolytic-uremic syndrome during an outbreak of Escherichia coli 0157:H7 infections in institutions for mentally retarded persons: Clinical and epidemiologic observations. J Pediatr 116: 544–551, 1990.
26. Proulx F, Turgeon J, Lafleur L, Delage G, Lafleur L, Chicoine L. Randomized, controlled trial of antibiotic therapy for Escherichia coli 0157:H7 enteritis. J Pediatr 121: 299–303, 1992.
27. DeJong M, Monnens L. Haemolytic-uremic Syndrome: A 10-year follow-up study of 73 patients. Nephrol Dial Transplant 3: 379–382, 1988.
28. Siegler R, Milligen M, Burningham T, Christofferson R, Chang SY, Jorde L. Long-term outcome and prognostic indicators in the hemolytic-uremic syndrome. J Pediatr 118: 95–200, 1991.

Submitted April 18, 1994; accepted July 21, 1994

Scand J Infect Dis 26: 685–691, 1994

Increased Yields of Pathogenic Yersinia Enterocolitica Strains by Cold Enrichment

SIRKKA KONTIAINEN[1,2], AULIKKI SIVONEN[2] and OLLI-VEIKKO RENKONEN[2]

From the Departments of [1]Medical Microbiology, Aurora Hospital, and of [2]Bacteriology and Immunology, University of Helsinki, Helsinki, Finland

Yersinia strains recovered from routine stool cultures ($n = 13{,}534$) as well as clinical symptoms in the patients were analysed in order to establish whether enteric Yersinia enterocolitica strains recovered only after cold enrichment cultures shared the same pathogenicity markers and caused the same symptoms as strains from primary cultures. 93% of the 201 Yersinia isolates were Y. enterocolitica strains and 71% of these were of serotype O3. Nearly 40% of all Y. enterocolitica strains and 21% of serotype O3 strains were isolated only after 1 week's cold enrichment of stool specimens. Practically all Y. enterocolitica O3 strains, whether from primary or cold enrichment cultures, were pathogenic not only on the basis of the serotype but also on the basis of Congo-red uptake and calcium-dependent growth at 35°C (CR-MOX test). The symptoms in patients with Y. enterocolitica O3 from primary and cold enrichment cultures were similar except that abdominal pains were more frequent ($p < 0.05$) in the former. Arthropathia, mesenteric lymphadenitis and erythema nodosum were detected in 15% of the patients with Yersinia isolates and were more frequent in patients with isolates from cold enrichment or without diarrhea.

S. Kontiainen, MD, Department of Medical Microbiology, Aurora Hospital, Nordenskiöldinkatu 20, FIN-00250 Helsinki, Finland

INTRODUCTION

Enteric Yersinia enterocolitica infections cause not only acute gastroenteritis but also erythema nodosum, mesenteric lymphadenitis and reactive arthritis (1–5). Not all Yersinia strains isolated from stool specimens are pathogenic, however. Characteristics differentiating pathogenic from non-pathogenic Y. enterocolitica strains include, in addition to the serotype, Congo-red uptake and calcium-dependent growth at 35°C (6–8). Salicin fermentation, esculin hydrolysis and pyrazinamidase test are useful screening tests to identify possibly pathogenic strains (6–8). Congo-red uptake and calcium-dependent growth at 35°C measure 2 properties of the Yersinia virulence plasmid (5, 6). Pyrazinamidase test correlates to the ability of the strain to harbour this plasmid (9). Cold enrichment of stool cultures, known to increase the yields of enteric Yersinia, may also select for non-pathogenic strains (6, 10–12). Whether the prevalence of the pathogenicity markers differs in Y. entérocolitica strains recovered from primary and cold enrichment cultures is not known. Nor is it known whether the symptoms of enteric Yersinia infection differ in patients in whom Yersiniae are recovered from cold enrichment and from primary cultures.

We tested all Yersinia isolates from routine stool culture specimens during a period of 12 months for the presence of the virulence plasmid by assaying for calcium-dependent growth and Congo-red uptake at 35°C as well as for salicin fermentation and esculin hydrolysis and compared the results of these tests in strains recovered from primary and from 1-week cold enrichment cultures. The clinical history of the patients culture positive for Yersinia was also obtained.

MATERIALS AND METHODS

Stool cultures

All stool cultures performed during a period of 12 months ($n = 13{,}534$) were analysed for the presence of Yersinia (and of Salmonella, Shigella, Campylobacter, Aeromonas and Plesiomonas) species. The media used to recover Yersinia were cefsulodin-irgasan-novobiocin (CIN, Yersinia selective agar base, Difco, Detroit, MI, USA, with 4.0 mg/l of cefsulodin and 2.5 mg/l of novobiocin) and Aeromonas (Difco) media (1). Stool specimens were cultured directly of CIN and Aeromonas plates upon receipt (primary cultures) and after cold enrichment [samples inoculated in 2 ml of broth (composed of beef extract 2.4 g, peptone 10.0 g, yeast extract 0.6 g, NaCl 3.0 g and $Na_2HPO4 \times 12H_2O$ 2.0 g in 1000 ml of distilled water, prepared by Orion Diagnostica, Espoo, Finland) and kept at 4°C for 5–8 days before culture.] The plates were incubated overnight at +35°C in ambient air.

Identification of Yersinia strains

Yersinia were identified by API20E (Bio-Mérieux, Marcy-l'Etoile, France) biochemical profiles (obtained after overnight incubation at 35°C), and all isolates tested for the ability to ferment salicin (0.5% salicin; Merk, Darmstadt, Germany, in LabLemco broth, Oxoid/Unipath Ltd., Basingstoke, Hampshire, England) and to hydrolyse esculin (modified esculin agar; 1) and cultured on Congo-red magnesium oxalate (CR-MOX) agar which allows visualization of calcium-dependent growth and Congo-red uptake (6, 7). The results of salicin and esculin tests read after overnight at +35°C. Strains growing as tiny red colonies on CR-MOX agar after overnight incubation at 35°C were deemed CR-MOX positive.

Susceptibility to antimicrobial agents

Susceptibility to ampicillin, ceftriaxone, tetracycline, sulpha-trimethoprim and ciprofloxacin was tested using a disc diffusion method (tablets from Rosco, Taastrup, Denmark).

Serotyping

Biochemically defined Y. enterocolitica strains were serotyped using monoclonal anti-O3 and -O9 antibodies (Progen Biotechnik GmbH, Heidelberg, Germany), and anti-O5,27 and -O8 antisera (kindly provided by Prof. G. Wauters, Brussels, Belgium).

Patient characteristics

The clinical history of patients from whom Yersinia strains were recovered from routine stool cultures was evaluated by clinicians treating the patients. The symptoms recorded were diarrhea, fever, abdominal pains, erythema nodosum, aching joints (arthropathia) and pharyngitis. Travel history was also obtained.

Statistics

The χ^2-test was used to test the significance of the differences between frequencies.

RESULTS

Prevalence of enteric Yersinia species

Yersinia were isolated from 1.5% (201/13,534) of the stool specimens studied. In 8 specimens Aeromonas and in 2 Salmonella species were found together with Yersinia. The other isolates were Campylobacter species in 4% of the samples (574/13,534), Salmonella in 2.5% (336), Aeromonas species in 1.8% (224), Shigellae in 0.3% (38) and Plesiomonas in 0.04% (6) of the samples.

The majority of the Yersinia isolates, 93% (186/201), were Y. enterocolitica strains. The majority of these, 71% (132/186) were of the serotype O3, 7% (12) of the serotype O5,27, 1% (2) of the serotype O9, and 22% (40) not typable by the antisera available to us. The other Yersinia species found were 6 Y. pseudotuberculosis, 6 Y. kristensenii and 3 Y. frederiksenii.

Primary vs. 1-week cold enrichment cultures

41% (83/201) of all Yersinia isolates and 38% (71/186) of the Y. enterocolitica strains were found only in cold enrichment cultures. 21% (27/132) of the Y. enterocolitica serotype O3 strains were from cold, as were all O5,27, 1 of the 2 O9 and 78% (31/40) of the non-typable Y. enterocolitica strains. Four of the 6 Y.pseudotuberculosis, 5 of the 6 Y.kristensenii and all Y. frederiksenii strains were found only after cold enrichment.

CR-MOX, salicin and esculin tests

All 103 Y. enterocolitica serotype O3 strains from primary and 89% (24/27) of the O3 strains from cold enrichment cultures were salicin and esculin negative in the screening test and CR-MOX positive, i.e. pathogenic also by this test. By these criteria 33% (4/12) of the Y. enterocolitica O5,27 strains, both of the O9 strains and 25% (10/40) of the non-typable Y. enterocolitica strains were pathogenic. Of the pathogenic Y. enterocolitica serotypes (O3, O9 and O5,27), 94% from primary and 53% from enrichment cultures were pathogenic, as were 37% vs. 23%, respectively, of the strains which we could not serotype.

Susceptibility to antimicrobial agents

All Yersinia isolates were susceptible to ceftriaxone, tetracycline, sulpha-trimethoprim and ciprofloxacin, and all, except the Y. pseudo tuberculosis strains, were resistant to ampicillin.

Epidemiology

Yersinia species were recovered from all age groups, and all were sporadic cases. There was a seasonal variation in the frequency by which Y. enterocolitica serotype O3 strains were isolated. Most of the O3 strains were isolated between August and October. One-third of the Y. enterocolitica serotype O3 isolates were from children, < 15 years of age (Table I), and one-fifth from children <5 years. The numbers of non-typable Y. enterocolitica strains isolated increased with advancing age. Five of the 6 Y. pseudotuberculosis isolates were from patients <15 years. The majority of patients had not travelled outside Finland during the prededing 2 months. About 15% had visited Mediterranean or African countries.

Clinical symptoms

Diarrhea was reported by 85% of the patients with Yersinia recovered from primary and by 72% of the patients with Yersinia from cold enrichment cultures ($p < 0.05$) and fever by 65% vs. 42% ($p < 0.001$; Table II). The frequencies of other symptoms did not differ, but 50% of the patients with strains from cold enrichment culture were referred to hospitals, as opposed to 35% of those with primary isolates ($p < 0.05$).

86% of the patients with Y. enterocolitica serotype O3 had diarrhea, 67% fever and 27% abdominal pains. The prevalence of diarrhea, fever and the referral rate to hospitals did not differentiate between patients with Y. enterocolitica O3 recovered from cold enrichment, and those with primary cultures (Fig. 1) but abdominal pains were more frequent in the latter group (22% vs. 44%, $p < 0.05$). Patients with Y. enterocolitica of other serotypes than O3

Table I. *Number of Yersinia strains isolated from different age groups*

		Number of Yersinia strains isolated						
		Y. enterocolitica						
Age (yrs)	All	O3	O5	O9	NT[a]	Y. Kristen-senii	Y. pseudo-tuberculosis	Y. frede-riksenii
0–14	60	48	3	0	2	1		
15–29	44	33	1	0	8	1	0	1
30–44	39	25	4	2	6	1	1	0
45–60	29	15	2	0	10	1	0	1
>60	29	11	2	0	14	2	0	0
Total	201	132	12	2	40	6	6	3

[a] NT, not of serotypes O3; O5,27; O8; O9.

Table II. *Frequency of symptoms in patients with enteric Yersinia isolates*
$*p < 0.05$; $**p < 0.01$; $***p < 0.001$.

Symptom	% of patients with the symptom		
	All patients ($n = 201$)	Primary culture isolate ($n = 118$)	Cold enrichment isolate ($n = 83$)
Diarrhea	79.6	84.7*	72.3
Fever	55.7	65.3***	42.2
Abdominal pain	27.9	24.6	32.5
Mesenteric lymphadentitis	4.0	5.9	1.2
Erythema nodosum	2.5	2.5	2.4
Arthropathy	8.5	5.9	12.0
Pharyngitis	3.5	5.9	0
None[a]	2.5	0.9	4.8
Referred to hospital	41.8	34.8	49.8*

[a] Three patients were asymptomatic family members of an index case, 1 was a refugee (routine health check), and 1 a cirrhosis patient (in final stage of disease).

isolated from cold enrichment cultures had diarrhea and fever equally often, abdominal pains less often ($p < 0.01$) and were referred to hospital more often ($p < 0.01$) than patients with non-O3 serotype from primary cultures (Fig. 2).

19% of the patients (35/186) in whom Y. enterocolitica was recovered from stool specimens did not have diarrhea. These patients had fever less often, but abdominal pains more often than patients with diarrhea (Table III). Extra-intestinal symptoms, i.e. mesenteric lymphadenitis, erythema nodosum and arthropathia, were detected in 42% of the patients without and in 7% of the patients with diarrhea ($p < 0.001$).

About 15% of all patients had extra-intestinal symptoms (Table II). Patients with Y. enterocolitica serotype O3 from primary and cold enrichment cultures had these symptoms equally often (Fig. 1). Patients with non-O3 serotypes (Fig. 2) only had arthropathia and only if the strain was isolated form cold. Altogether 9% of the patients (17) had arthropathia. 10 of these (54%) had Y. enterocolitica serotype O3, 2 serotypes O5,27, 4

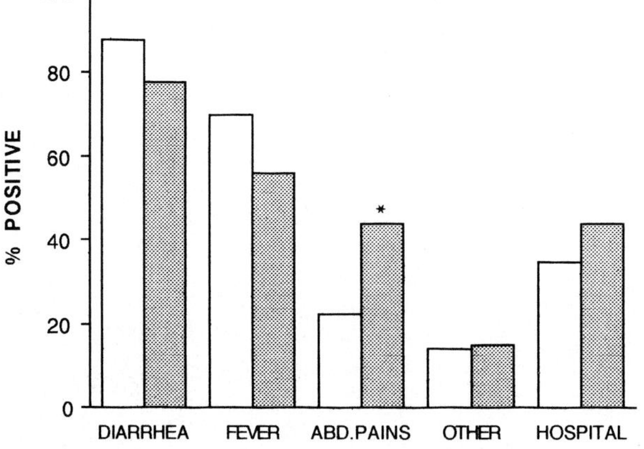

Fig. 1. Symptoms in patients in whom Y. enterocolitica serotype O3 was isolated from primary (□) or cold enrichment cultures (■). $*p < 0.05$.

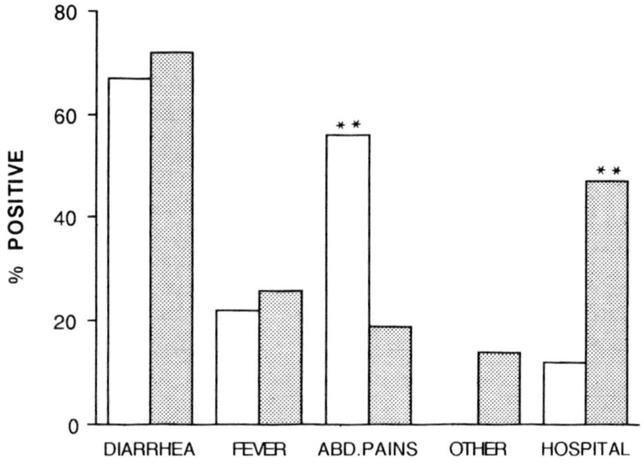

Fig 2. Symptoms in patients in whom Y. enterocolitica not of serotype O3 was isolated from primary (◇) or cold enrichment cultures (■). $^{**}p < 0.01$.

Table III. *Symptoms in Y. enterocolitica patients with or without diarrhea*

$^{*}p < 0.05$; $^{*}p < 0.01$; $^{***}p < 0.001$

Symptom	Diarrhea ($n = 149$)	No diarrhea ($n = 35$)
Fever	61.7**[a]	31.4
Abdominal pain	17.4	60.0***
Mesenteric lymphadenitis and appendecectomy	0.7	14.7***
Erythema nodosum	0.7	5.9*
Arthropathy	6.0	20.0**
Pharyngitis	4.7	0
Referred to hospital	2.0	25.7***

[a] Percentage with the given symptom.

non-typable Y. enterocolitica and 1 Y. pseudotuberculosis in the stools. About half of the Y. enterocolitica isolates in patients with arthropathia were from cold, and from patients without diarrhea. Most of these patients were >30 years of age. Four percent of the patients (8) had mesenteric lymphadenitis leading to appendecectomy. Six of these patients (75%) had Y. enterocolitica serotype O3, 1 Y. pseudotuberculosis and 1 Y. kristensenii in stool. All except Y. kristensenii were from primary cultures and 7 from patients without diarrhea. Six of these 8 patients (75%) were <15 years of age. Two percent of the patients (5) had erythema nodosum. Three had Y. enterocolitica serotype O3 and 2 Y. pseudotuberculosis in stool. Four of the isolates were from cold. Four percent of the patients (7), all with Y. enterocolitica serotype O3 from primary cultures, had pharyngitis.

35% of the patients (41/118) in whom Yersinia species were recovered from primary and 49% of the patients (41/83) in whom Yersinia species were from cold enrichment cultures were referred to hospital ($p < 0.05$; Table II). Patients without diarrhea were referred to hospital more often than patients with diarrhea. Thus, 26% of the former and 2% of the latter were referred to hospital ($p < 0.001$).

DISCUSSION

In this study, Yersinia enterocolitica comprised >90% of the enteric Yersinia species isolated. Had the cold enrichment not been performed, one-third of the Y. enterocolitica serotype O3, serotype O9 and serotype O5,27 strains as well as the majority of the other Y. enterocolitica serotypes and Yersinia species would not have been detected.

The majority of pathogenic Y. enterocolitica serotypes (O3; O9; O5,27), whether derived from primary or from cold enrichment cultures, were pathogenic also by the CR-MOX test (5–8). Thus 100% of Y. enterocolitica serotype O3 strains from primary and 90% from cold enrichment cultures were CR-MOX-positive. One-third of the non-O3, -O9, -O5,27 Y. enterocolitica serotypes from primary and one-fifth from cold enrichment cultures were likewise CR-MOX-positive.

The proportion of CR-MOX, i.e. virulence plasmid, positive Y. enterocolitica isolates in this study was greater than previously reported (8, 13). The plasmid determining CR-MOX positivity is known to be easily lost upon storage and subculture (8). We performed the CR-MOX test with freshly isolated (either primary or relatively short 1 week's cold enrichment) Y. enterocolitica strains. This may explain the higher frequency of CR-MOX-positive strains in this study.

72% of the Y. enterocolitica strains isolated were of serotype O3 and 1% of serotype O9. The prevalence of these 2 serotypes differed from that found in Finland 20 years ago when about 57% of the isolates were of O3 and 41% of O9 serotype (11). The current predominance of O3 serotype is similar to that reported for instance from Belgium and Norway (14, 15). The third-ranked pathogenic serotype in Europe, O5,27 (6, 8, 11) not found 20 years ago, comprised 7% of the isolates in this study. The proportion of the non-O3, -O9 strains was 3% 20 years ago, whereas now 20% of the strains were not of the O3, O9, O5,27 (or O8) serotypes.

Patients in whom Y. enterocolitica was isolated by cold enrichment cultures had symptoms similar to those in patients with Y. enterocolitica recovered from primary cultures. Lack of diarrhea was associated with increased number of extra-intestinal symptoms. 40% of the patients without and 7% of the patients with diarrhea had arthropathia, erythema nodosum or mesenteric lymphadenitis.

The epidemiology of Y. enterocolitica infections is poorly understood. One-fifth of the Y. enterocolitica O3 isolates were from children <5 years of age. In previous studies, Y. enterocolitica strains were also frequently isolated from young children (13, 16). Most of the patients in this study had no travel history, but most of the Y. enterocolitica isolations were made at the end of the holiday season, between August and October. The source of infection remained unknown. Local pigs are known to harbour Y. enterocolitica O3 and Y. pseudotuberculosis strains (17), but raw pork, a possible Y. enterocolitica source (14) is not consumed in Finland.

Cold enrichment increased the yields of pathogenic Y. enterocolitica strains. Most were of serotype O3, which, whether derived from primary or from cold enrichment cultures, harboured the virulence plasmid, i.e. were pathogenic also by this criterion. The symptoms were largely similar in patients with Y. enterocolitica isolated from primary and cold enrichment cultures but, judged by the referral rate to hospitals, Yersinia strains recovered from cold were associated with more serious disease. Stool specimen culture in addition to serology also seemed to be useful in establishing the etiological agent in patients with extra-intestinal symptoms but no diarrhea.

ACKNOWLEDGEMENTS

We thank Prof. G. Wauters for a kind gift of the antisera and reference stains and Leena Saraste for her patience in preparing the manuscript.

REFERENCES

1. Ahvonen P. Human Yersiniosis in Finland. II. Clinical features. Ann Clin Res 4: 39–48, 1972.
2. Leirisalo-Repo M. Yersinia arthritis. Acute clinical picture and long-term prognosis, In: Cruse JM, Lewis, Jr, RE eds. Contrib Microbiol Immunol. Basel: Karger, 145–154, 1987.

3. Carniel C, Hollaret HH. Yersiniosis. Comp Immunol. Microbiol Infec Dis 13: 15–58, 1990
4. Van Noyen R, Selderslaghs R, Bekaert J, Wauters G, Vandepitte J. Causative role of Yersinia and other enteric pathogens in the appendicular syndrome. Eur J Clin Microbiol Infect Dis 10; 735–741, 1991.
5. Cornelis G, Laroche Y, Balligand G, Sory M-P, Wauters G. Yersinia enterocolitica, a primary model for bacterial invasiveness. Rev Infect Dis 9: 64–87, 1987.
6. Balows A, Hausler WJ, Herrmann KL, Isenberg HD, Shadomy HJ, eds. Manual of clinical microbiology. Washington DC: American Society for Microbiology, 5th ed 373–375 & 1240–1241, 1991.
7. Riley G, Toma S. Detection of pathogenic Yersinia enterocolitica by using Congo-red magnesium oxalate agar medium. J Clin Microbiol 27: 213–214, 1986.
8. Farmer JJ, III, Carter GP, Miller WL, Falkow S, Wachsmuth IK, Pyrazinamidase, CR-MOX agar, salicin fermentation-esculin hydrolysis, and d-xylose fermentation for identifying pathogenic serotypes of Yersinia enterocolitica. J Clin Microbiol 30: 2589–2594, 1992.
9. Kandolo K, Wauters G. Pyrazinamidase activity in Yersinia enterocolitica and related organisms. J Clin Microbiol 10: 735–741, 1991.
10. Pai CH, Sorger S, Lafleur L, Lackman L, Marks MI. Efficacy of cold enrichment techniques for recovery of Yersinia enterocolitica from human stools. J Clin Microbiol 9: 712–715, 1979.
11. Ahvonen P. Human Yersiniosis in Finland. I. Bacteriology and serology. Ann Clin Res 4: 30–38, 1972.
12. van Noyen R, Vandepitte J, Wauters G, Selderslaghs R. Yersinia enterocolitica: its isolation by cold enrichment from patients and healthy subjects. J Clin Pathol 34: 1052–1056, 1981.
13. Morris JG Jr, Prado V, Ferreccio C, Robins-Browne RM, Bordun A-M, Cayazzo M, Kay BA, Levine MM. Yersinia enterocolitica isolated from two cohorts of young children in Santiago, Chile: incidence of and lack of correlation between illness and proposed virulence factors. J Clin Microbiol 29: 2784–2788, 1991.
14. Tauxe RV, Wauters G, Goossens V, Van Noyen R, Vandepitte J, Martin SM, De Mol P, Thiers G. Yersinia enterocolitica infections and pork: the missing link. Lancet 1: 1129–1132, 1987.
15. Ostroff SM, Kapperud G, Lassen J, Aasen S, Tauxe RV. Clinical features of sporadic Yersinia enterocolitica infections in Norway. J Infect Dis 166: 812–817, 1992.
16. Metchock B, Lonsway DR, Carter GP, Lee LA, McGowan JE Jr. Yersinia enterocolitica: A frequent seasonal stool isolate from children at an urban hospital in the southeast United States. J Clin Microbiol 29: 2868–2869, 1991.
17. Merilahti-Palo R, Lahesmaa R, Granfors K, Gripenberg-Lerche C, Toivanen P. Risk of Yersinia infection among butchers. Scand J Infect Dis 23: 55–61, 1991.

Submitted April 8, 1994; accepted August 29, 1994

Scand J Infect Dis 26: 693–696, 1994

Isolation of Nocardia sp. from Blood Cultures in a Teaching Hospital

JAIME ESTEBAN[1], JOSE-MANUEL RAMOS[1],
MANUEL L. FERNANDEZ-GUERRERO[2]
and FRANCISCO SORIANO[1]

From the [1]Department of Medical Microbiology and the [2]Division of Infectious Diseases, Fundacion Jimenez Diaz Universidad Autonoma, Madrid, Spain

To determine the clinical significance of the isolation of Nocardia sp. from blood cultures, clinical records of patients with bacteremia due to Nocardia sp. in our hospital from January 1986 to December 1990 were retrospectively reviewed. Eight patients had 9 blood cultures positive for Nocardia sp. Four of the isolates were identified as Nocardia asteroides. Only 2 of the patients had disseminated nocardiosis due to N. asteroides, and both were appropriately treated for Nocardia sp. In the other cases, isolation of Nocardia sp. was considered nonsignificant or undetermined, and all were clinically cured. Nocardia sp. may be an occasional contaminant of blood cultures. The significance of nocardemia is a matter of clinical judgment.

J. Esteban, MD, Department of Medical Microbiology, Fundacion Jimenez Diaz, Av. Reyes Catolicos 2, E-28040 Madrid, Spain

INTRODUCTION

Nocardiosis is a localized or disseminated infection caused by an aerobic actinomycete belonging to the genus Nocardia. Many species of this genus can be pathogenic for humans, N. asteroides being the most frequent. Although nocardiosis is mainly a respiratory infection, hematogenous dissemination can spread to many other sites of the body. Despite this possibility, blood isolates of Nocardia sp. are rarely reported (1, 2). We retrospectively reviewed the cases of positive blood cultures for Nocardia sp. in a university hospital during a 5 year period, with emphasis on their significance and management.

MATERIAL AND METHODS

Records from the Medical Microbiology Laboratory of the Fundación Jimenez Diaz (a 700-bed teaching hospital in Madrid, Spain) from January 1986 to December 1990 were retrospectively reviewed for isolation of Nocardia sp. from blood cultures. During this period, blood cultures were processed with the biphasic Hemoline Performance blood system (BioMerieux, France). Several blood cultures from selected patients were also processed with the lysis-centrifugation system (ISOLATOR, Merck, U.S.A.). Isolates of branched, Gram-positive rods were identified at genus and species level in accordance with common schemes (3, 4). Data were obtained for clinical follow-up for at least 1 year after the patient was discharged.

RESULTS

A total of 35,334 blood cultures were processed by the Medical Microbiology Laboratory of the Fundacion Jimenez Diaz during the study period. Nocardia sp. was isolated in 9 blood cultures from 8 patients. Clinical and microbiological data for all patients are summarized in Table I.

Table I. *Clinical and microbiological characteristics of patients with nocardiemia*

	Case no.							
	1	2	3	4	5	6	7	8
Age/Sex	52/M	66/M	29/M	59/M	2/F	76/M	78/F	60/F
Underlying diseases	Renal transplantation Immunosuppressive therapy	Chronic bronchitis Ischemic cardiopathy	None	Renal polycystosis	Acute lymphocytic leukemia	Pulmonary carcinoma	Gastrectomy	Wegener disease Renal failure
Present syndrome	Psoas abscess	Respiratory infection	Acute meningitis	UTI	Fever	Fever	Acute abdomen	Septic shock
Temperature	38.3°C	37.6°C	38°C	38.2°C	38°C	38.1°C	38.5°C	38.3°C
Chest X-ray	Normal	Interstitial chronic pattern	Normal	Normal	Normal	Pleural effusion Mediastinal mass	Normal	Normal
Treatment	IMP, DOX	None	None	E	CAZ	None	CC + Gm	SXT + TIC + GM
Evolution	Relapse	Cure	Cure	Cure	Cure	Cure	Cure	Exitus
Definitive diagnosis	Nocardia abscess	Acute respiratory infection	Viral meningitis	Urinary tract infection	Fever of unknown origin	Neoplasic fever	Cholecystitis	Pseudomonas sepsis Nocardiosis
Isolate	N. asteroides	N. asteroides	Nocardia sp.	Nocardia sp.	N. asteroides	Nocardia sp.	Nocardia sp.	N. asteroides
Number of blood cultures (Positive total)	1/1	1/2	1/2	1/2	1/1	1/2	1/4	2/4
Days for positive culture	4	7	7	7	7	5	7	4
Nocardia isolated from other sources	Psoas abscess	None	None	None	None	None	None	None

IMP: Imipenem; DOX: Doxycyclin; E: Erythromycin; CAZ: Ceftazidime; CC: Clindamycin; GM: Gentamycin; SXT: Co-trimoxazole; TIC: Ticarcillin; UTI: Urinary Tract Infection.

DISCUSSION

Nocardia, a genus of Gram positive, branched, acid-fast rods first described in 1888 (5), are ubiquitous in soil and several environmental sources (6). The isolation of Nocardia sp. from blood cultures seems to be a rare finding. Some authors have reported isolation of Nocardia sp. from blood cultures in patients with nocardiosis (4, 7–16). In almost all cases, the organism recovered is N. asteroides but other species have also been isolated from blood (17). Several authors have indicated the usefulness of biphasic fungal blood cultures for the isolation of Nocardia spp. (9, 13). All of our isolates except the one for case 1 were recovered from a biphasic blood culture system, where growth was detected on day 4–7 of incubation.

Classically, the isolation of Nocardia sp. from blood cultures has been considered as a sign of disseminated nocardiosis (9). However, only 1 of our cases had disseminated nocardiosis diagnosed by culture of the organism from a source other than blood (case 1): another case (no. 8) was diagnosed as nocardiosis despite the fact that N. asteroides was isolated only from 2 blood cultures, and no evident location of disseminated abscesses could be found. In the remaining 6 cases there was either no evidence of invasive nocardiosis, or the foci, if any, remained undiscovered. Unfortunately, the retrospective nature of our study did not allow for more exhaustive study of the patients, but the follow-up and favorable outcome in patients without specific treatment suggest that the blood isolate was not a truly significant one.

There are many reports of isolates of Nocardia sp.—mainly from the respiratory tract—in the absence of clinical disease (18–20). The significance of these isolates is doubtful; they have been interpreted as a mild form of infection (19) or colonization (18, 20). Two of our patients had underlying pulmonary disease (case nos. 2 and 6) that could represent the focus of transient bacteremia, although Nocardia sp. was not isolated from respiratory samples. In the other 4 cases (nos. 3, 4, 5, 7), no obvious focus of bacteremia could be detected, and the significance of Nocardia isolates remains unknown. In these cases, the possibility of contamination of blood cultures must be taken into account. In 6 cases, isolation of Nocardia sp. from blood cultures did not lead to a change in antimicrobial therapy, and all these patients had a favorable outcome.

In conclusion, Nocardia sp. bacteremia is a rare finding which should lead to an intensive search for the organism in sources other than blood in order to establish its true clinical significance.

REFERENCES

1. Lerner PI. Nocardia species. In: Mandell GL, Douglas RG, Bennett JE, eds. Principles and practice in infectious diseases, 3rd ed. New York : Churchill Livingstone, 1926–1932, 1990.
2. Mishra SK, Gordon R, Barnett DA. Identification of Nocardiae and Streptomycetes of medical importance. J Clin Microbiol 11: 728–736, 1980.
3. Berd D. Laboratory identification of clinically important aerobic Actinomycetes. Appl Microbiol 25: 665–681, 1973.
4. Frazier AR, Rosenow EC, Roberts GD. Nocardiosis. A review of 25 cases occurring during 24 months. Mayo Clin Proc 50: 657–663, 1975.
5. Cruz PT, Clancy CF. Nocardiosis: Nocardial osteomyelitis and septicemia. Am J Pathol 28: 607–628, 1952.
6. Goodfellow M, Lechevalier MP. Genus Nocardia. In: Sneath PHA, Mair NS, Sharpe ME, Holt JG, eds. Bergey's manual of systematic bacteriology. Baltimore: Williams & Wilkins, 1459–1471, 1986.
7. Wilson JP, Turner HR, Kirchner KA, Chapman SW. Nocardial infections in renal transplant recipients. Medicine 68: 38–57, 1989.
8. Whitmore DN, Gresham GA, Grayson MJ. Nocardiosis in anaemic patients given steroids. J Clin Pathol 14: 259–263, 1961.
9. Roberts GD, Brewer NS, Hermans PE. Diagnosis of nocardiosis by blood culture. Mayo Clin Proc 49: 293–296, 1974.

10. Fontaneda-Lopez D, Corrales-Rodriguez de Tebleque M, Fernandez-Ortega F, Sarasa-Corral JL, Gomez-Garces J, Fernandez-Guerrero M. Nocardiosis: observaciones clínicas a propósito de nueve casos. Rev Clin Esp 185: 454–458, 1989.
11. Larsen MC, Diamond HD, Collins HS. Nocardia asteroides infection. Arch Intern Med 103: 712–725, 1959.
12. Avram MM, Nair SR, Lipner HI, Cherubin CE. Persistent nocardiemia following renal transplantation. Association with pulmonary nocardiosis. JAMA 239: 2779–2780, 1978.
13. Noseda A, Serruys E, Depre G. Infection à Nocardia: problèmes diagnostiques et thérapeutiques. Presse Med 14: 2179–2182, 1985.
14. Vannier AM, Ackerman BH, Hutchins LF. Disseminated Nocardia asteroides diagnosed by blood culture in a patient with disseminated histoplasmosis. Arch Pathol Lab Med 116: 537–539, 1992.
15. Ertl G, Schaal KP, Kochsiek K. Nocardial endocarditis of an aortic valve prosthesis. Br Heart J 57: 384–386, 1987.
16. Allevato PA, Eisses JF, Mezguer E, Fisher EJ, Romig DA, Morales AR. Nocardia asteroids aortitis with perforation of the aorta. Hum Pathol 16: 743–746, 1985.
17. O'Connor PT, Dire DJ. Cutaneous nocardiosis associated with insect bites. Cutis 50: 301–302, 1992.
18. Curry WA. Human nocardiosis. A critical review with selected case reports. Arch Intern Med 140: 818–826, 1980.
19. Palmer DL, Harvey RL, Wheeler JK. Diagnostic and therapeutic considerations in Nocardia asteroides infection. Medicine 53: 391–401, 1974.
20. Rosett W, Hodges GR. Recent experiences with nocardial infections. Am J Med Sci 276: 279–285, 1978.

Submitted February 18, 1994; accepted August 18, 1994

Scand J Infect Dis 26: 697–703, 1994

Candidemia: Current Epidemiologic Characteristics and a Long-term Follow-up of the Survivors[1]

CHARLES H. DEBUSK, RONALD DAOUD, MUTHAYIPALAAM C. THIRUMOORTHI, FRANCIS M WILSON and RIAD KHATIB

From the St John Hospital and Medical Center, Detroit, Michigan, USA

All consecutive patients with positive blood culture for Candida species over a 6-year period were evaluated to define recent epidemiologic characteristics of candidemia, and to assess the prevalence of late complications. We encountered 106 cases; medical records were available for 99 of them. The rate of candidemia was increasing until 1990, after which it declined. C. albicans was the most common species, but in the last 2 years, C. tropicalis and C. parapsilosis were emerging. Overall mortality rate was 54.5% without significant variation during the study period. Antifungal therapy was withheld in 24/99 cases (24.2%). Decision to withhold treatment was taken in 19/59 cases (32.2%) before the availability of fluconazole in 1990, compared with 5/40 cases (12.5%) afterward ($p < 0.05$). Follow-up was possible in 35 instances for an average period of 17.1 months (range: 1–48 months); 7 of these individuals, all with transient candidemia, were untreated. None of the survivors developed late complications. These findings demonstrate that candidemia appears to be declining since 1990, with a noticeable decrease in the prevalence of C. albicans but an increase in that of C. tropicalis and C. parapsilosis, that fewer patients are left untreated since fluconazole became available, and that the risk of late complications among the survivors is low.

R. Khatib, MD, Medical Education Office, St John Hospital and Medical Center, 22101 Moross Road, Detroit, Michigan 48236, USA

INTRODUCTION

The incidence of candidal bloodstream infections has been increasing steadily over the last 2 decades (1, 2). Many studies have characterized the risk factors, clinical manifestations and prognostic indicators (3–14). In the past, transient candidemia was considered benign and treatment was frequently withheld because of potential amphotericin B toxicity (15, 16). Subsequently, however, treatment of all patients has been advocated regardless of underlying conditions (17, 18). These recommendations were based on several reports, primarily in immunocompromised individuals, which showed that untreated candidemia is associated with high mortality and distant foci of infection and that therapy reduces immediate mortality (4, 10, 19).

However, neither long-term outcome of infection, nor whether therapy prevents the development of late complications has yet been determined (18). In a study cited in many reviews, osteomyelitis developed in a few patients despite treatment with 200–500 mg amphotericin B (20). Whether this report reflects the result of suboptimal therapy of affected patients, or a more common but unrecognized sequela of candidemia, is not clear. We elected to study candidemia at our institution to define its recent epidemiologic characteristics and to determine the prevalence of late complications among the survivors.

---

[1] This paper was presented at the Annual Meeting of the Infectious Diseases Society of America, New Orleans, LA, USA, October 15, 1993.

 ISSN 0036-5548

METHODS

Facility: St John Hospital and Medical Center is a 607 bed community based teaching hospital on the outskirts of a major urban area.

Case findings: We reviewed the result of blood cultures in the microbiology laboratory between April 1986 and December 1991. All cases with any positive culture for Candida were selected.

Case review: The medical records of all selected cases were reviewed regarding patient demographics, underlying disease processes, source and characteristics of candidemia, type of therapy, and the outcome of infection.

Follow-up: We carried out a long-term follow-up of the survivors after discharge from the hospital by a standardized questionnaire to the attending physician about the patient's condition and by reviewing subsequent hospital admissions or outpatient visits. We looked specifically for any evidence of subsequent renal disease, hepatic dysfunction, new osseous or articular disorders, ocular complaints and whether Candida was isolated from any sterile body site in follow-up cultures.

Definitions: Source of candidemia was defined as follows:
(*a*) intravascular catheter (IVC), which implied isolating the same species from an IVC around the time of candidemia, regardless of semiquantitative culture (SQC) result (21); (*b*) unknown, which alluded to all cases with negative IVC culture or if IVC culture was not performed.

Duration of candidemia defined the interval between first and last positive blood culture. Transient candidemia implied positive blood cultures over 2 days or less, irrespective of the number of positive cultures. Sustained candidemia indicated positive blood cultures ≥ 3 days.

Culture methods: All blood cultures were done using BACTEC system (Becton Dickinson Diagnostic Instrument System, Sparks, MD). Additionally, when fungal cultures were requested, blood was cultured in Isolator 10 lysis centrifugation tubes (E.I. DuPont deNemours and Company, Wilmington, Del.). Yeasts were identified using the Vitek YBC card (Vitek Systems Inc. Hazelwood, MO) according to the manufacturer's instructions.

Statistical methods: The data were evaluated utilizing 2×2 contingency tables in conjunction with using χ^2-test or Fisher's exact test as appropriate.

RESULTS

There were 106 patients with candidemia during the study period, averaging 18.6 cases/year. The number of cases increased between 1986 and 1989, but declined thereafter (Fig. 1). The prevalence of various species of Candida changed throughout the study period. Prior to 1990, C. albicans accounted for 60–80% of the isolates, whereas non-albicans species predominated after 1990 (Table I). C. parapsilosis accounted for most of the pediatric cases (10/17; 2 of them were mixed with C. albicans). The medical records of 7 individuals were not found. Among the remaining patients, 56 were male and 43 were female. Their ages ranged between newborn and 95 years (mean 51.2 ± 28 years). Possible risk factors associated with candidemia included antibiotic therapy (77.8%), major abdominal, thoracic, cardiovascular or neurological surgery (62.6%), diabetes mellitus (27.3%), malignancy, predominantly solid tumours (25.3%), and corticosteroids (17.2%). One patient was a kidney transplant recipient, and two individuals were neutropenic briefly at the time of candidemia. 54 of the patients did not survive hospitalization (in-hospital mortality rate of 54.5%). The cause of death was Candida infection in 37 cases, based on persistent clinical signs of infection, positive blood culture, or isolating Candida from a sterile body site around the time of death (autopsies were rarely performed). Surviving patients were distinguished by younger age (mean age 39.7 ± 31 years vs. 60.8 ± 21.7 years), lower incidence of malignancy (15.6% vs. 33.3%) and higher prevalence of IVC-associated candidemia (17.7% vs. 3.7%).

The majority of patients were treated with various anti-fungal agents. Prior to 1990, amphotericin B was used with or without flucytosine in all 40 treated cases. Since 1990,

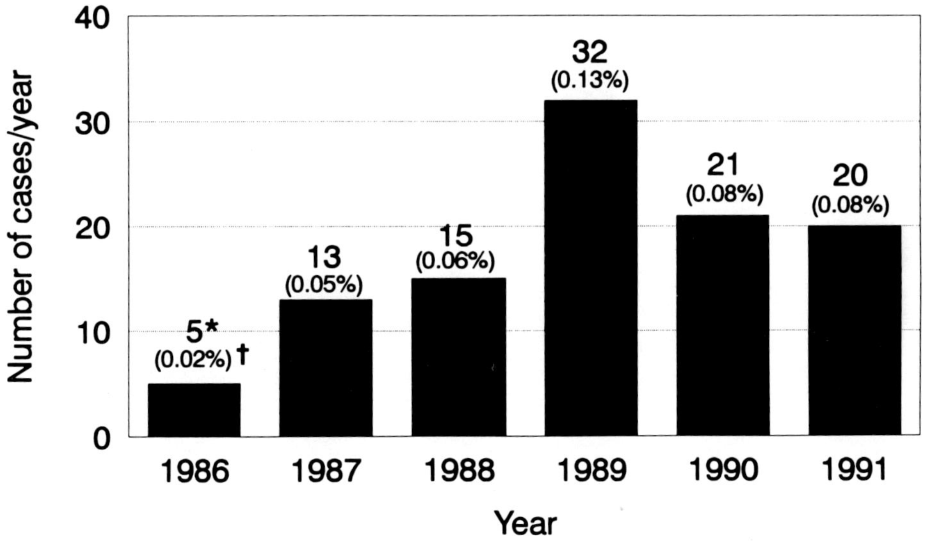

Fig. 1. Changing prevalence of candidemia during the study period. * 1986 cases represent a period of 9 months. † Based on the total number of hospital discharges.

amphotericin B usage dropped to 54.3% (19 cases; it was used with fluconazole in one of them), and fluconazole was used alone in the remaining 16 cases. Treatment was withheld in 24/99 cases (24.2%). 11 of them died and 13 individuals were discharged from the hospital. Surviving patients were well at the time of discharge; 6 of them were lost to follow-up. The decision not to treat was more frequent before 1990 (19/59 patients) than afterward (5/40) ($p < 0.05$).

Long-term follow-up of the survivors was possible in 35 cases who received various types of management (Table II). Their mean age was 37.9 ± 30.8 years (range: newborn to 84 years, median age 44 years), and male to female ratio was 1.2; none of them was neutropenic. Seven patients had underlying solid malignancy and 1 patient was a kidney transplant recipient. Yeast organisms were also present in an IVC in 6 cases and in cerebrospinal fluid

Table I. *Candida species causing blood stream invasion: changing trend*

Species	Year 1986[a]	1987	1988	1989	1990	1991	Total
C. albicans	4	7	9	24	5	9	58
C. glabrata	1	5			2	3	11
C. parapsilosis	1	1	1	3	8	3	17
C. tropicalis				1	5	5	11
C. lusitania		1		1			2
C. krusei				1	1		2
C. stellotoides				1			1
C. guillermondii				1			1
Not identified		3		1		1	5
Total	5	13	15	33[b]	21	21[b]	108[c]

[a] 1986 cases represent a period of 9 months.
[b] One case in both years represents concurrent C. parapsilosis and C. albicans fungemia.
[c] Total number of patients = 106, 2 of them with mixed candidemia.

Table II. *Survivors of candidemia: type of therapy, duration of candidemia, and length of follow-up*

Type of therapy	Duration of candidemia (days) ≤ 2	≥ 3	Total no. of cases	Length of follow-up (months): Mean ± SD (range)
Adults:				
None:	6	0	6	9.2 ± 8.2 (1–22)
Amphotericin B ≤ 200 mg:	2	0	2	22.5 ± 0.5 (22–23)
>200–500 mg:	2	1	3	22.3 ± 13.8 (4–36)
>500–1000 mg:	1	1	2	12.0 ± 2.0 (10–14)
>1000 mg:	2	1	3	31.7 ± 18.2 (6–46)
Amphotericin B & flucytosine:	0	2	2	26.5 ± 19.5 (7–46)
Fluconazole:	5	1	6	10.3 ± 6.4 (2–18)
Pediatrics:				
None:	1	0	1	14
Amphotericin B:	4	3	7	21.1 ± 15.0 (3–48)
Amphotericin B & flucytosine:	0	2	2	11.0 ± 2.0 (9–13)
Fluconazole:	0	1	1	13
All cases	23	12	35	17.1 ± 13.5 (1–48)

in 1 case. Candidemia was transient in 23 instances (65.7%): single culture was positive in 15 of them, and 2–4 cultures were positive over 1–2 days in the remaining 8 patients. It was sustained in the remaining cases, with 2–9 positive cultures over 3–18 days period. Duration of follow-up ranged between 1 and 48 (average 17.1) months; it was >6 months in 26 subjects, and >1 year in 20 of them. 20 individuals were readmitted to the hospital for various diagnoses and the remaining individuals were followed as outpatients. None of these patients developed late complications of candidemia. Eight individuals died of unrelated causes; autopsy was performed in 1 case only. Among the patients followed-up, a group of 7 individuals with transient candidemia did not receive any antifungal therapy. They were followed for an average period of 9.9 months (3 of them were followed for >1 year) without seeing any evidence of late complications (Table III).

Table III. *Characteristics of untreated survivors of transient candidemia*

Case no.	(Age[a])	Underlying condition	Species	Candidemia: No. of cultures	Candidemia: Duration (days)	Length of follow-up (months)	Diagnosis at follow-up
1	(80)	Colon carcinoma	albicans	1	1	1	Sepsis[b]
2	(58)	Ovarian sarcoma	tropicalis	1	1	2	Sepsis[c]
3	(33)	Alcoholism	albicans	1	1	2	Sepsis[d], died
4	(23)	None	guillermondii	2	1	7	Hyperventilation
5	(70)	None	albicans	1	1	22	Foot ulcer
6	(72)	Colon carcinoma	glabrata	4	2	21	Metastasis; died
7	(0.4)	None	parapsilosis	1	1	14	Viral infection[e]

[a] (year) at the time of candidemia.
[b] Intravascular catheter-associated.
[c] Neutropenia-related bacteremia.
[d] Nosocomial Staphylococcus aureus endocarditis.
[e] Emergency room visit for a presumptive viral infection.

DISCUSSION

As is well known, candidemia is associated with a high mortality and a potential for distant foci of infection (4, 10, 19, 20). Based on these observations and on a few epidemiologic studies, primarily in the immunocompromised host, treatment of all cases of candidemia is currently advocated. In a recent editorial, Edwards recommended therapy for all affected patients regardless of neutropenia or the potential of invasive disease because of lack of accurate methods to stratify patients according to the likelihood of infections of deep organs (18). Whether therapy prevents late complications has not been verified, as most previous studies did not include long-term follow-up. It is possible that such treatment improves the immediate outcome and facilitates the clearance of candidemia, but it may not completely eradicate the organisms from seeded distant target organs. Then, after discontinuing therapy, focal disease may become apparent. In support of this theory, Gathe et al. reported a few cases of osteomyelitis following therapy with amphotericin B (20). Although these complications are probably rare, their true incidence has not been determined. In addition to the treated individuals, a number of patients survive candidemia without receiving any antifungal therapy. Fraser et al. stated that 28% of their cases were not treated (1). Likewise, Komshian et al. stated that treatment was withheld in 31.1% of their cases (10). The reason for withholding antifungal therapy was not clearly defined. Among Fraser's cases, most untreated subjects were not neutropenic and they had transient candidemia. In Komshian's report, the duration of candidemia among untreated individuals was not specified. In both studies, mortality among untreated individuals was slightly higher than in treated patients but the difference was not statistically significant. Although the survivors in both studies appeared to be healthy at the time of discharge from the hospital, long-term follow-up was lacking. It is possible that complications may become evident in some of them at a later date. In support of this statement, C. albicans meningitis developed in a patient 1 year after receiving 3 days of treatment with amphotericin B for a transient candidemia that was presumed to be IVC associated (22).

Our study addresses these issues and presents recent epidemiologic characteristics of candidemia in primarily non-neutropenic patients in a community hospital. Our findings demonstrate a steady increase in the cases of candidemia prior to 1990 followed by a decrease and the incidence appears to be continuing a slight downward trend in 1992 (data not shown). It is possible that our findings reflect an outbreak of nosocomial C. albicans infection at our institution during 1989 that escaped our attention and that the rate in subsequent years represents the true and stable prevalence of candidemia after an initial rise in the late 1980s. However, we believe that this recent decline is a result of early empirical therapy of Candida infections. This approach became possible due to the availability of fluconazole which was added to the antifungal armamentarium in February, 1990. A similar decline in the incidence of candidemia was noted in several recent studies (23, 24), which suggests that this observation is not unique to our institution.

Our data also illustrate a noticeable change in Candida species causing bloodstream invasion. Prior to 1990, C. albicans was implicated in the majority of cases. Thereafter, however, C. albicans accounted for $<50\%$ of the cases, whereas non-albicans species, particularly C. tropicalis and C. parapsilosis, were more frequently encountered. It is uncertain whether this observation was due to a recent outbreak of cross-infections with C. parapsilosis and or C. tropicalis in the last 2 years of our study, or whether it represents a changing trend in the epidemiology of Candida infections. A similar decline in C. albicans and emergence of C. parapsilosis and C. tropicalis was also noted by other recent studies (23, 24). The reasons for the emergence of non-albicans species are not clear. The use of antifungal agents has been incriminated in the recent increase of C. krusei infections in immunocompromised patients (12). Whether similar or different factors are involved in the emergence of other species remains to be determined by careful epidemiological studies in various patient populations.

With regard to the treatment of candidemia, our study demonstrates that before 1990, 32.2% of patients were not treated, and that this later dropped to 12.5%. It is uncertain whether this difference was due to a fear of amphotericin B toxicity prior to 1990 and the availability of fluconazole subsequently, or whether it reflects a change in the approach to candidemia based on recent advocacy of treating of all patients (17, 18).

As to the long-term prognosis, our findings suggest that survivors of candidemia have a favourable outcome with negligible risk of late complications. This conclusion is based on the results of our follow-up of 35 cases, 12 of them with sustained candidemia. The average of follow-up was 17.1 months. Most cases were followed up >6 months and a substantial number of them for 1 year or more. Based on this observation, we believe that reported cases of metastatic foci of infection after treatment represent exceptionally rare complications of candidemia.

With respect to the untreated survivors of transient candidemia, it is tempting to state that they have a favourable outcome despite lack of therapy or that they were cured after removing an infected catheter. However, the small number of patients in this group, the short duration of follow-up in most them, and the lack of post-mortem examination to exclude delayed complications with certainty, preclude us from drawing any meaningful conclusions. Therefore, although the benefit of therapy among non-immunocompromised individuals with transient candidemia has not been substantiated, routine treatment of all candidemic patients should still be considered the standard of therapy until new data are available.

ACKNOWLEDGEMENT

The authors are grateful to Mr Frank Castronova, MA, for his assistance in statistical assessment.

REFERENCES

1. Fraser VJ, Jones M, Dunkel J, Storfer S, Medoff G, Dungan WC. Candidemia in a tertiary hospital: epidemiology, risk factors and predictors of mortality. Clin Infect Dis 15: 414–421, 1992.
2. Eppes SC, Troutman JL, Gutman LT. Outcome of treatment of candidemia in children whose central catheter were removed or retained. Pediatr Infect Dis 8: 99–104, 1989.
3. Way SB, Mori M, Pfaller MA, Woolson RF, Wenzel RP. Risk factors for hospital-acquired candidemia. A matched case-control study. Arch Intern Med 149: 2349–2353, 1989.
4. Way SB, Mori M, Pfaller MA, Woolson RF, Wenzel RP. Hospital-acquired candidemia. The attributable mortality and excess length of stay. Arch Intern Med 148: 2642–2645, 1988.
5. Wenzel RP, Pfaller MA. Candida species: emerging hospital bloodstream pathogens. Infect Contr Hosp Epidemiol 12: 524–525, 1991.
6. Prassad KJ, Feller I, Thomson PD. A ten year review of Candida sepsis and mortality in burn patients. Surgery 101: 213–216, 1987.
7. Nollas-Sallas J, Leon C, Torres-Rodrigues JM, Martin E, Sitges-Serra A. Treatment of Candidemia in critically ill surgical patients with intravenous fluconazole. Clin Infect Dis 14: 952–954, 1992.
8. Nielsen H, Stenderup J, Bruun B. Fungemia in a university hospital 1984–1988. Scand J Infect Dis 23: 275–282, 1991.
9. Leibovici L, Konisberger H, Pitlik SD, Samra Z, Drucker M. Bacteremia and fungemia of unknown origin in adults. Clin Infect Dis 14: 436–443, 1992.
10. Komshian SV, Uwaydah AK, Sobel JD, Crane LR. Fungemia caused by Candida species and Torulopsis glabrata in the hospitalized patient: frequency, characteristics, and evaluation of factors influencing outcome. Rev Infect Dis 11: 379–390, 1989.
11. Meunier F. Systemic candidal infections in neonates. Clin Infect Dis 15: 554, 1992.
12. McQuillan DP, Zingman BS, Meunier F, Levitz M. Invasive infections due to Candida krusei: report of ten cases of fungemia that include 3 cases of endophthalmitis. Clin Infect Dis 14: 472–478, 1992.

13. Meunier F, Aoun M, Bitar N. Candidemia in immunocompromised patients. Clin Infect Dis 14: S120–125, 1992.
14. Bryce EA, Roberts FJ, Sekhon AS, Coldman AJ. Yeast in blood cultures. Evaluation of factors influencing outcome. Mycology 15: 23–27, 1992.
15. Ellis CA, Spivack ML. The significance of candidemia. Ann Intern Med 67: 511–522, 1967.
16. Toala P, Schroeder SA, Daly AK, Finland M. Candida at Boston City Hospital. Clinical and epidemiological characteristics and susceptibility to eight antimicrobial agents. Arch Intern Med 126: 983–989, 1970.
17. Edwards JE Jr, Filler SG. Current strategies for treating invasive candidiasis: emphasis on infections in non-neutropenic patients. Clin Infect Dis 14: S106–113, 1992.
18. Edwards JE Jr. Should all patients with candidemia be treated with antifungal agents? Clin Infect Dis 15: 422–423, 1992.
19. Young RC, Bennett, Geelhoed GW. Fungemia with compromised host resistance: a study of 70 cases. Ann Intern Med 80: 605–612, 1974.
20. Gathe JC.Jr, Harris RL, Garland B, Bradshaw MW, Williams TW Jr. Candida osteomyelitis. Report of five cases and review of the literature. Am J Med 82: 927–936, 1987.
21. Maki DG, Weise CE, Sarafin HW. A semiquantitative culture method for identifying intravenous-catheter-related infection. N Engl J Med 296: 1305.–1309, 1977.
22. Sarmiento R, Holubka JD, Khatib R. Candida meningitis with a probable intradural fungal ball one year after candidemia. Am J Med Sci 307: 115–118, 1994.
23. Simmons BP, Gelfand MS, Gray D, Greene W, Chow S. Empiric use of amphotericin B and fluconazole for nosocomial fevers of unknown origin (NFUO) not responding to antibacterial antibiotics. Clin Infect Dis 17: 555, A145, 1993.
24. Ritter J, Molavi A, Arias K. Nosocomial blood stream infections at a tertiary care hospital, 1988–1992. Clin Infect Dis 17: 555, A146, 1993.

Submitted May 17, 1994; accepted July 22, 1994

Scand J Infect Dis 26: 706–710, 1994

Three-day Azithromycin Compared with Ten-day Roxithromycin Treatment of Atypical Pneumonia

SLAVKO SCHÖNWALD[1], BRUNO BARŠIĆ[1], IVANA KLINAR[2] and MARTA GUNJAČA[2]

From the [1]University Hospital of Infectious Diseases, "Dr. Fran Mihaljević" and [2]Pliva Pharmaceuticals, Zagreb, Croatia

An open, randomized, multicentre study compared the efficacy and safety of 3-day azithromycin with 10-day roxithromycin for the treatment of atypical pneumonia. Azithromycin was administered 500 mg once daily to 90 and roxithromycin 150 mg bid to 60 patients. Causative pathogens were identified by serological methods. In the azithromycin treatment group, Mycoplasma pneumoniae was identified in 65, Chlamydia spp. in 9 and Coxiella burnetti in 1 patient. In the roxithromycin treatment group, M. pneumoniae was identified in 39, Chlamydia spp. in 9 and C. burnetti in 3 patients. 89 azithromycin and 53 roxithromycin patients were eligible for efficacy analysis. Clinical cure rate was 98.9% in the azithromycin and 94.3% in the roxithromycin treatment group. Adverse events were observed in 3 patients in each group. Azithromycin appears to be as effective as roxithromycin for the treatment of atypical pneumonia. The 3-day azithromycin regimen may offer an additional advantage over 10-day roxithromycin by virtue of its more convenient administration.

B. Baršić, MD, University Hospital of Infectious Diseases, "Dr. Fran Mihaljević", 41000 Zagreb, Mirogojska 8, Croatia

INTRODUCTION

Azithromycin is an azalide antibiotic with specific pharmacodynamic and pharmacokinetic characteristics. It accumulates intracellularly, particularly in neutrophils and macrophages. Phagocytes deliver and maintain high azithromycin concentrations at the site of infection. Azithromycin is effective in the treatment of many respiratory infections, among them those caused by Mycoplasma pneumoniae, Chlamydia psittaci and Chlamydia pneumoniae (1). Recent studies suggest that a 3-day azithromycin regimen is useful for the treatment of respiratory infections (2, 3). That could be its additional advantage over other antimicrobials given for a longer period.

Roxithromycin is a macrolide antibiotic with antibacterial spectrum similar to that of erythromycin. It is also active against the most common pathogens that cause atypical pneumonia (5–7). Roxithromycin is usually given for 10 days.

Both drugs were tested for the treatment of community acquired pneumonia, but patients with atypical pneumonia have rarely been selectively evaluated. Their efficacy has not previously compared in comparative trials in that group of patients. The aim of our study was to compare the efficacy and the tolerability of 3-day azithromycin vs. standard, 10-day roxithromycin therapy for the treatment of atypical pneumonia. The study was multicentre, open and randomized.

PATIENTS AND METHODS

At 3 centres, 150 patients were included in the study, 90 in the azithromycin and 60 in the roxithromycin group (randomization 3:2). All patients were diagnosed as having atypical pneumonia, on the basis of history, physical examination, characteristic chest X-ray and laboratory data (low erythrocyte sedimentation rate (ESR), normal number of leukocytes and absence of neutrophilia in peripheral blood). Diagnosis of M. pneumoniae, Chlamydia spp. and Coxiella burnetti infections was made serologically (complement fixation reaction) on the basis of at least 4-fold rise in antibody titre in paired sera. At the time of the study, tests for C. pneumoniae antibodies were not performed. Diagnostic tests for Legionella spp. infections were performed routinely. Blood samples for serologic tests were taken at 2-week intervals.

All patients provided oral consent before they were included into the study. The trial was approved by ethics committees at all study centres.

Patients in whom other causes of community-acquired pneumonia were proven or where signs and symptoms and X-ray of the chest suggested the pneumonia *not* to be atypical were not included in the study. This concerned patients with purulent sputum, high ESR, or leukocytosis with neurtrophilia in peripheral blood.

Patients were randomized to receive either 500 mg azithromycin once daily for 3 days, or roxithromycin as a 150 mg tablet taken bid for 10 days. In our previous study, 3-day treatment was as effective as the 5-day regimen for patients with atypical pneumonia (4). A 10-day roxithromycin regimen was chosen because it is still the standard therapy. Both drugs were taken orally.

All patients were hospitalized and assessed clinically every day whilst hospitalized. The final evaluation of the clinical efficacy was made 14 days after commencing the therapy, on the basis of presence or disappearance of the clinical symptoms and signs of the disease, and on the regression of the infiltrate on chest X-ray. Patients discharged from the hospital before the end of the trial were given an appointment for a check-up visit on day 14. The clinical response was designated 'cure' if fever abated within 72 h of commencing treatment, and other signs and symptoms had disappeared by day 14 with complete or >50% regression of the infiltrate on control chest X-ray; or 'failure' when signs or symptoms persisted or became worse after the first 3 days of therapy and/or there was no apparent regression of the infiltrate on control chest X-ray.

All adverse events, whether observed by the investigator or reported by the patient, were recorded and classified according to their severity and causative relationship to the study drug. Laboratory tests (biochemistry, hematology) were performed at baseline and on days 11 to 14. Any patient who developed abnormal laboratory test results was followed up until the results returned to baseline or to normal.

Statistical comparisons between the treatment groups were carried out at the baseline and at the end of the study, and included comparisons of demographic data, etiologic agents, patient characteristics, frequency of adverse events and clinical response. The Fisher exact test for dichotomous and 2-way Student's t-test for continuous data were used. The level of significance was defined as $p < 0.05$.

RESULTS

Of the 150 patients included in the study, 89 in the azithromycin group (A) and 53 in the roxithromycin group (R) were eligible for efficacy analysis. 14 A patients and 9 R patients were discharged from hospital before the end of the trial, but not before 7 days after starting treatment. All were asked to come for check-up on day 14. One A patient and 5 R patients missed the check-up visit, and 2 R patients violated the protocol. Significantly more R patients were excluded from the study ($p = 0.007$). No patient was withdrawn from the study because of the missed diagnosis of atypical pneumonia.

Patients in both groups were comparable regarding the baseline demographic data (Table I). The most common cause of atypical pneumonia in both groups was M. pneumoniae (Table II). Infection with other pathogens such as Chlamydia spp. and C. burnetti was significantly less frequently proven in both groups. In a small proportion of patients from both groups, etiology could not be identified due to lack in increase of antibody titre although other parameters strongly suggested atypical pneumonia. These patients were included in the efficacy analysis.

Both drugs were equally effective in the treatment of atypical pneumonia ($p = 0.1792$) (Table III). Clinical failure was observed in 1 patient treated with azithromycin where the pathogen was Chlamydia spp. Of the 3 patients treated with roxithromycin in whom a clinical failure occurred, 1 was infected with Chlamydia spp., 1 with C. burnetti and in 1 the etiology was not proven.

Both drugs were well tolerated (Table IV). Adverse events occurred in 2 (2.2%) A- and in 3 (5.7%) R-treated patients ($p = 0.2737$), but they were mild and did not necessitate drug

Table I. *Baseline demographic characteristic of patients with atypical pneumonia*

		Azithromycin	Roxithromycin
Age (years)	mean ± SD	38 ± 14	41 ± 11
	range	14–69	16–59
Sex M/F		49/40	32/21
Height (cm)	mean ± SD	172 ± 7	178 ± 6
	range	158–195	164–193
Weight (kg)	mean ± SD	70 ± 11	81 ± 10
	range	50–100	55–94

Table II. *Etiology of atypical pneumonia based on complement fixation test*

	No. of patients (%)	
	Azithromycin	Roxithromycin
Mycoplasma pneumoniae	65 (73)	39 (73.6)
Chlamydia psittaci	9 (10.1)	9 (16.9)
Coxiella burnetti	1 (1.1)	3 (5.7)
Unknown[a]	14 (15.8)	2 (3.8)
Total	89 (100)	53 (100)

[a] $p = 0.02$, Fisher's exact test.

Table III. *Clinical response in evaluable patients at the post therapy visit (day 14 ± 1)*

	No. of patients (%)	
	Azithromycin	Roxithromycin
Clinical cure	88 (98.9)	50 (94.3)
Failure	1 (1.1)	3 (5.7)
Total	89 (100)	53 (100)

Table IV. *Adverse events in both treatment groups*

	No. of patients	
	Azithromycin (89 patients)	Roxithromycin (53 patients)
Adverse event		
Nausea	2	2
Inappetence	1	–
Abdominal pain	–	1
Possibly drug-related laboratory abnormalities		
Elevated liver enzymes	11	4
Eosinophilia	1	1

withdrawal. Possibly treatment-related laboratory abnormalities were recorded in 12 (13.5%) A- and 5 (9.4%) R-treated patients ($p = 0.2798$). The most common one was slight, reversible increase in liver enzyme levels.

DISCUSSION

Atypical pneumonia was common in our population, M. pneumoniae infections being the most frequent. In a small proportion of our patients the etiology was not proven. Their number was significantly greater in the A group. Nevertheless we included them in our final analysis because viral pneumonia is rare in adult patients and we suspect that C. pneumoniae might be the cause of the illness in some of them. During the period of the study, tests for that kind of infection were not performed in our laboratories. Legionella spp. infection was not proved in a single patient. These infections are very rare in our community.

Up to the present, doxycycline or erythromycin have usually been prescribed for the treatment of atypical pneumonia. Beside these commonly used antibiotics, good results obtained with fluoroquinolones, ciprofloxacin and ofloxacin (8), but failures in the treatment of mycoplasmal infections have been reported (9). Quinolones can be used only if a diagnosis of atypical pneumonia is firmly established. Otherwise severe, resistant pneumococcal infections can occur (10, 11). Although patients with infections of the lower respiratory tract are frequently included in clinical trials with the latest antimicrobials, results of atypical pneumonia treatment are seldom reported separately. We have already reported on azithromycin's good efficacy in the treatment of atypical pneumonia, whether with a 5-day (1) or a 3-day (5) course. Roxithromycin is a macrolide, well tolerated and active against the most common pathogens that cause atypical pneumonia. Its efficacy was demonstrated in several non-comparative trials in a very small number of patients (12–15). Hitherto, only a few comparative trials of its use in patients with atypical pneumonia have been reported (16–19); the other drugs were erythromycin and doxycycline.

Our results have confirmed the clinical efficacy and safety of both drugs in the treatment of atypical pneumonia. The 3-day azithromycin regimen may offer additional advantage over 10-day roxithromycin administration. Once daily and a 3-day course can improve compliance, compared to a 10-day drug regimen (20).

We consider azithromycin to be a good alternative for the treatment of atypical pneumonia, by virtue of its convenient 3-day dosage regimen and good efficacy.

ACKNOWLEDGEMENT

This work was supported by a grant from Pliva Pharmaceuticals, Zagreb.

REFERENCES

1. Schönwald S, Gunjača M, Kolačny-Babić L, Car V, Gošev M. Comparison of azithromycin and erythromycin in the treatment of atypical pneumonias. J Antimicrob Chemother 25 (suppl A): 123–126, 1990.
2. Hoepelman AIM, Sips AP, van Helmond JLM, van Barneveld PWC, Newe AJ, Zwinkels M, Rozenberg-Arska M, Verhoef J. A single blind comparison of a three-day azithromycin and ten-day co amoxiclav treatment of acute and lower respiratory tract infections. J Antimicrob Chemother 31 (suppl E): 147–152, 1993.
3. Myburgh J, Nagel GJ, Petschel E. The efficacy and tolerance of a three-day course of azithromycin in the treatment of community-acquired pneumonia. J Antimicrob Chemother 31 (suppl E): 163–170, 1993.
4. Schönwald S, Škerk V, Petričević I, Car V, Majerus-Mišić Lj, Gunjača M. Comparison of three-day and five-day courses of azithromycin in the treatment of atypical pneumonia. Eur J Clin Microbiol Infect Dis 10: 877–880, 1991.

5. Orfela J, Haider F, Schmit JL, Bissac E, Bryskier A. Roxithromycin in vitro activity against Chlamydia psittaci. Abstract. Book of abstracts. 18th International Congress of Chemotherapy, Stockholm, June 1993.
6. Palu G, Valisena S, Sassela D, Furneri P, Meloni GA. Antimycoplasmal activity of roxithromycin. Br J Clin Pract 48 (suppl 55): 21–23, 1988.
7. Kishimoto T, Kemura T, Kubota Y, Moyashita N, Moriya O, Okimoto N, Niki Y, Soejina R. Fundamental and clinical studies of roxithromycin for Chlamydial respiratory infection. Abstract. Book of abstracts. 18th International Congress of Chemotherapy, Stockholm, June 1993.
8. Forsberg P, Maller R, Nilsson L. Comparative study of oral ofloxacin and erythromycin in the treatment of pneumonia. Rev Infect Dis 11 (suppl 5): 1229–1230, 1989.
9. Frieden TR, Mangi RJ. Inappropriate use of oral ciprofloxacin. JAMA 264: 1438–1440, 1990.
10. Lee BL, Padula AM, Kimbrough RC, Jones SR, Chaisson RE, Mills J, Sande MA. Infectious complications with respiratory pathogens despite ciprofloxacin therapy. N Engl J Med 325: 520–521, 1991.
11. Korner RJ, Reeves DS, MacGowan AP. Lesson of the week – damage or oral fluoroquinolone treatment in community acquired upper respiratory tract infection. BMJ 308: 191–192, 1994.
12. Breux JP. Treatment of atypical pneumonia with roxithromycin. Abstract. Book of abstracts. 16th International Congress of Chemotherapy, Jerusalem, 1989.
13. Champetier de Ribes D. Roxithromycin in lower respiratory tract infections: A multicentre study. Book of abstracts. 16th International congress of Chemotherapy, Jerusalem, 1989.
14. Fernandez MacLoughlin GF, Lancel JL, Stamboulian D. Roxithromycin in the treatment of atypical pneumonia. Br J Clin Pract 42 (suppl 55): 92–93, 1988.
15. Astarloa L, Maglio F, Cangelosi D, Garcia-Messina O, Muniz FJ. Roxithromycin in the treatment of atypical pneumonia in adult patients. Br J Clin Pract 42 (suppl 55): 94–95, 1988.
16. Schönwald S, Car V, Kuzman I, Petričević I. Comparison of Rulid (roxithromycin) and erythromycin in the treatment of atypical pneumonias. Abstract. Book of abstracts. 16th International Congress of Chemotherapy, Jerusalem, 1989.
17. Gentry LO. Roxithromycin, a new macrolide antibiotic, in the treatment of infections in the lower respiratory tract: an overview. J Antimicrob Chemother 20 (suppl B): 145–152, 1987.
18. Antela A, Guerero A, Escudero R, Marti-Belda P, Mesequer M, Gonzalez J. Roxithromycin in the therapy of community-acquired pneumonie (CAP). Abstract. Book of abstracts. 18th International Congress of Chemotherapy, Stockholm, 1993.
19. Perianu M, Stamboulian D. The efficacy of roxithromycin (300 mg once daily or 150 mg bid) in the treatment of atypical pneumonia in an international multicentre study. Abstract. Book of abstracts. 17th International Congress of Chemotherapy, Berlin, 1991.
20. Bradbury F. Comparison of azithromycin versus clarithromycin in the treatment of patients with lower respiratory tract infections. J Antimicrob Chemother 31 (suppl E): 153–162, 1993.

Submitted March 16, 1994; accepted July 20, 1994

Scand J Infect Dis 26: 711–717, 1994

Health Problems and Self-medication among Swedish Travellers

CLAS AHLM, SONIA LUNDBERG, KERSTIN FESSÉ and JOHAN WISTRÖM.

Department of Infectious Diseases, University Hospital of Umeå, S-901 85 Umeå, Sweden

500 consecutive travellers seeking pre-travel health advice were issued a questionnaire before leaving Sweden to continuously record health problems and use of medication during travel. Of 442 subjects who turned in assessable questionnaires (232 male and 210 female, mean age 37 years), 81% travelled to areas at high risk for the acquisition of diarrhea. The mean duration of travel was 4 weeks. During travel 218 (49% at 95% CI 44.3 to 53.7%) of the travellers experienced some illness and 61 (14%) had symptoms of more than one illness. The mean duration of illness was 4.5 days, and 65 subjects (30% of ill travellers) were confined to bed for a mean duration of 2 days. The incidence of illness was significantly ($p < 0.01$) higher among travellers to high risk than to low risk areas (55% vs 26%), among young travellers than among elderly (65% vs 33%), and among those going on adventure tours compared with recreational tourists (74% vs 41%). Diarrhea was reported by 36% (95% CI 31.6 to 40.5%), and respiratory tract infection by 21% (95% CI 17.2 to 24.8%). Self-medication with one or several drugs was initiated by 163 (75%) travellers experiencing illness during travel. Thus, every second Swedish traveller to tropical and subtropical areas experienced some kind of travel-related, often incapacitating, health problem.

C. Ahlm, MD, Department of Infectious Diseases, University Hospital of Umeå, S-901 85 Umeå, Sweden.

INTRODUCTION

Epidemiological surveys (1–6) done in the late 1970s and early 1980s increased the awareness of travel-related health hazards and of the importance of prevention (7, 8). Recent data concerning Central European travellers to tropical and subtropical areas nevertheless indicate that the magnitude of travel-related illness is unchanged (5, 9).

This is a study of the frequency and severity of travel-related illness among Swedish travellers, and of the use of medication for the prevention or treatment of illness related to their trip.

MATERIAL AND METHODS

Travellers aged ≥ 10 years who consulted at the out patient clinic at the Deparment of Infectious Diseases, University Hospital of Umeå, Sweden (IDU) for prophylaxis before travelling abroad were included in the study. Vaccination, passive immunization and malaria chemoprophylaxis (chloroquine 300 mg base per week or chloroquine 300 mg base per week and proguanil 200 mg daily) were given according to WHO recommendations. A prescription for mefloquine for self-treatment of malaria was provided to travellers staying for more than 2 weeks in areas with known chloroquine-resistant Plasmodium falciparum. All travellers were given information concerning nutritional prophylaxis of travellers' diarrhea, and depending on destination, information was given concerning chemoprophylaxis for malaria, antimosquito measures, symptoms and signs of malaria as well as detailed instructions for self-treatment of suspected malaria.

A questionnaire was issued to 500 consecutive travellers who visited the IDU during November 1990 to May 1991. Before leaving Sweden the traveller was asked to record personal and travel details which included age, gender, destination, health status, mode and duration of travel. During travel the subjects were to record illnesses (including severity and duration), accidents and insect bites. The participants were furthermore asked to record purchase and use of medication before or during travel, and to assess compliance with anti-malarial drug prophylaxis.

Participants who did not deliver their questionnaire within 4 weeks after returning from travel were requested to do so either by mail or phone.

 ISSN 0036-5548

Asia, Africa, and South and Latin America were defined as high risk areas for the acquisition of diarrhea, whereas Central and Southern Europe (including the Canary Islands), North America, the Caribbean islands and Oceania were defined as low risk areas (3). We used the term diarrhea to characterize all forms of diarrheal illness (9), without adopting the proposed distinction (2) between "travellers' diarrhea" and "loose stools". Statistical analyses were done using the statistical package Quest™ (University of Umeå, Sweden). Chi-square tests were used for comparison of proportions. Odds ratios (OR) for the risk of acquiring travel-related health problems among different categories of travellers were calculated with 95% confidence intervals (CI). Age-adjusted ORs were analyzed with Mantel-Haentzel tests. The Student *t*-test was used to compare age and duration of travel among assessable and non-assessable subjects.

RESULTS

Of the 500 travellers enrolled in the study, 442 (232 male and 210 female subjects, mean age of 37 years, range 10 to 79 years) returned an assessable questionnaire, and were evaluated in the study. The mean duration of travel was 4 weeks (median 3 weeks, range 1 week to 26 weeks). In comparison with subjects who turned in a usable questionnaire, the 58 subjects who failed to do so were younger (mean age 30 years, $p < 0.001$) and their planned stay abroad was longer (mean 7 weeks, $p < 0.001$).

Table I. *Incidence (%) of travel-related illness, diarrhea and respiratory tract infection among different categories of travellers*

Criteria	No.	Illness (%)	Diarrhea (%)	Respiratory tract infection (%)
No. of travellers evaluated	442	49	36	21
Men	232	49	33	22
Women	210	50	39	19
Age				
10–24 years	106	65[b]	44[b]	28[c]
25–49 years	235	49[c]	37[c]	22[c]
50–80 years	101	33	25	12
Duration of travel				
1–2 weeks	215	41	31	13
3–4 weeks	117	47	36	22[d]
5–26 weeks	107	70[e]	47[d]	37[e]
Mode of travel				
Recreation	253	41	30	13
Business/educational	100	49	34	26[f]
Adventure trip	89	74[g]	55[g]	38[f]
Destination of travel				
High risk areas[a]	358	55[h]	40[h]	25[h]
Asia	197	56	40	27
South and Latin America	72	53	42	24
Africa	89	54	38	20
Low risk areas[a]	84	26	18	5

[a] For definition see Material and Methods.
[b] $p < 0.01$ compared with age groups 25–49 or 50–80 years.
[c] $p < 0.05$ compared with the age group 50–80 years.
[d] $p < 0.05$ compared with ≥ 1–2 weeks travel.
[e] $p < 0.01$ compared with ≥ 1–2 weeks travel or > 2–4 weeks travel.
[f] $p < 0.01$ compared with recreational tours.
[g] $p < 0.01$ compared with recreational or business/educational tours.
[h] $p < 0.001$ compared with travellers to low risk areas.

Most participants (81%) travelled to high risk areas (Table I), South East Asia being the most popular destination (33%). Recreational tours (57%) and adventure tours (20%) were the predominant modes of travel (Table I). Travellers to high risk areas were younger than those going to low risk areas (mean age 36 years vs 42 years, $p \leq 0.01$). They stayed abroad for longer periods of time (mean 4 weeks vs 3 weeks, $p \leq 0.01$) and were more frequently adventure tourists (23% versus 10%, $p \leq 0.01$).

Incidence and severity of travel-related illness

The incidence of travel-related illness and corresponding ORs among different categories of travellers are shown in Table I and II, respectively. During travel, 218 (49%) of the subjects experienced some kind of illness, and 61 (28% of those ill) had symptoms of more than 1 illness (Table III). The incidence of illness was significantly higher ($p < 0.001$) among travellers to high risk areas (55%, OR 3.4, when adjusted for both age and mode of travel the OR was 2.9) than among those going to low risk areas (26%) (Table I and II). Travel-related illness was furthermore significantly more common ($p < 0.01$) among younger travellers than elderly (65% vs 33%, OR 3.8), among travellers staying abroad for >4 weeks compared with short-term travellers (70% vs 41%, OR 3.2) and among those going on adventure trips than among recreational tourists (74% vs 41%, OR 4.2). The ORs for different risk factors remained essentially unaltered when adjusted for age (Table II). The incidence of illness was 83% among 23 young adventure tourists who travelled to high risk areas for >4 weeks, compared with 11% among 18 old subjects on short-term (≤2 weeks) recreational tours to low risk areas.

Table II. *Risk factors for developing illness, diarrhea or respiratory tract infection among different categories of travellers. Odds ratios (OR) in cases and references, 95% confidence interval (CI) for odds ratios, age adjusted odds ratios (AOR) and test for trend (p-value)*

	Illness			Diarrhea			Respiratory tract infection		
Variable	OR	CI	AOR	OR	CI	AOR	OR	CI	AOR
Gender									
Men	1.0			1.0			1.0		
Women	1.0	(0.7–1.5)	0.9	1.3	(0.9–2.0)	1.3	0.8	(0.5–1.3)	0.7
Age									
50–80 years	1.0			1.0		1.0	1.0		
25–49 years	2.0	(1.2–3.3)		1.8	(1.1–3.0)		2.0	(1.1–4.0)	
10–24 years	3.8[b]	(2.2–6.7)		2.3[b]	(1.3–4.2)		2.9[b]	(1.4–5.9)	
Duration of travel									
1–2 weeks	1.0			1.0			1.0		
3–4 weeks	1.3	(0.8–2.0)	1.3	1.3	(0.8–2.0)	1.3	2.0	(1.1–3.6)	2.0
5–26 weeks	3.2[b]	(2.0–5.2)	2.8	2.0[b]	(1.2–3.2)	1.8	4.2[b]	(2.4–7.1)	3.7
Mode of travel									
Recreation	1.0			1.0			1.0		
Business education	1.6	(1.0–2.6)	1.7	1.3	(0.8–2.2)	1.3	2.6	(1.4–4.5)	2.6
Adventure trip	4.2	(2.5–7.0)	3.5	3.0	(1.9–4.9)	2.6	4.1	(2.4–7.1)	3.8
Destination of travel									
Low risk areas[a]	1.0			1.0			1.0		
High risk areas[a]	3.4	(2.0–5.7)	3.4	3.0	(1.7–5.4)	2.9	6.6	(2.6–16.4)	6.7

[a] For definition see Material and Methods.
[b] Denotes statistical significance for test for trends $p \leq 0.01$.

Table III. *Incidence of illness, accidents, insect bites and (when appropriate) 95% confidence interval (CI) among 442 Swedish travellers*

Criteria	Number of travellers[a] (%) ($n = 442$)	CI
Illness	218 (49)	(44.3–53.7)
Single illness	157 (36)	
Symptoms of more than one illness	61 (14)	
Diarrhea	158 (36)	(31.6–40.5)
Diarrhea only	103 (23)	
Combined with other illness	55 (12)	
Upper respiratory tract infection	93 (21)	(17.2–24.8)
Upper respiratory tract infection only	40 (9)	
Combined with other illness	53 (12)	
Urinary tract infection	7 (2)	
Skin infection	7 (2)	
Other infection	10 (2)	
Non-infectious illness	7 (2)	
Accident or injury	29 (7)	
Insect bite	55 (12)	

[a] The same subject may appear more than once.

Diarrhea (36%) and upper respiratory infections (21%) were the 2 most frequent health problems reported (Table III). Other infections were found in 24 travellers (5%) and non-infectious illness in 2% of the travellers (Table III). Acquisition of viral hepatitis or a sexually transmitted disease was not reported by any participant. Accidents (all minor) including one traffic accident, and insect bites were recorded in 7% and 12% instances respectively (Table III). One subject received rabies vaccine after being bitten by a dog.

As shown in Tables I and II, the risk of developing diarrhea or respiratory tract infection were both significantly higher among travellers to high risk areas than to low risk areas ($p < 0.001$). Age, duration and mode of travel were other factors found to be associated with the risk for acquisition of diarrhea or respiratory tract infection (Tables I and II). When the 3 continents classified as high risk areas were compared, no difference in the incidence of diarrhea was found (Table I). As regards specific regions, the highest attack rates of diarrhea were found in travellers to Northern Africa (61%) and the Indian subcontinent (50%), whereas 34% of the subjects visiting Sub-Saharan Africa developed diarrhea.

The duration illness, degree of incapacitation and need for medical assistance caused by different illnesses are summarized in Table IV. The mean duration of illness was 4.5 days (median 3 days), and 20% experienced symptoms lasting ≥ 7 days. 65 ill travellers (30%) were confined to bed for at least 1 day (mean period of 2.0 days), and 19% required a doctor's care during their illness (Table IV). Two subjects with diarrhea were hospitalised for a short period.

Medication during travel.

No traveller used prophylactic anti-diarrheal medication. Most of the travellers (252, 57%) had anti-malarial prophylaxis. 36 (14%) of these admitted that they forgot at least 1 dose during travel and/or after travel. Self-treatment of suspected malaria was initiated by 7/182 (4%) of the subjects equipped with mefloquine as standby treatment. Adverse reactions were reported by 12% (30/252) of those taking anti-malarial drugs. All symptoms were mild and subsided spontaneously. No case of malaria was diagnosed during or after travel.

Table IV. *Duration of illness, incapacitation, and need of medical assistance in 218 travellers from Sweden*

Criteria	Outcome[a]
Mean duration of illness (days)	4.5 d
Mean duration of diarrhea (days)	3.2 d
Mean duration of respiratory tract infection (days)	5.0 d
Percentage confined to bed (% of all those ill)	30%
Due to diarrhea only	28%
Due to respiratory tract infection only	13%
Due to more than one infection	46%
Mean number of days spent in bed	2.0 d
Due to diarrhea	1.7 d
Due to respiratory tract infection	2.8 d
Due to more than one infection	2.3 d
Percentage seeking assistance of a medical doctor (% of all those ill)	19%
Due to diarrhea only	12%
Due to respiratory tract infection only	15%
Due to more than one or other infectious diseases	24%
Due to non-infectious diseases	42%

[a] The same subject may appear more than once.

Drugs other than anti-malarial drugs obtained with or without prescription were used by 163 (37%) travellers (75% of those ill). These drugs were purchased by 25% of the subjects before leaving Sweden, by another 10% at a local pharmacy during travel, and another 2% borrowed medication from fellow travellers. Drugs not prescribed by a physician were purchased by 21% of the subjects before travel, and by 5% while abroad. The following drugs were used either alone or in combination with other drugs by those suffering from diarrhea; loperamide by 47%, bacteriological anti-diarrheal preparations (containing lactobacilli, bifidobacteria or Enterococcus faecium species) by 20%, and other anti-diarrheal remedies (absorbents and herbal preparations) by 16%. Antibiotics or miscellaneous non anti-diarrheal drugs were taken by 18% and 31% respectively of those who became ill during travel.

DISCUSSION

On the basis of a response rate of up to 88%, this prospective study can be considered highly valid. It indicates that health problems are common among travellers from Sweden who visit tropical and subtropical areas. This was especially true for younger travellers and those going on adventure tours, of whom 65% and 74% reported illness. The incidence and severity of travel-related health problems in the present study are generally similar to results reported 10 to 15 years ago among Scandinavian and Central European travellers (1–6). Both in the present and in previous studies, destination, age, mode and duration of travel were identified as important risk factors for the development of illness, diarrhea or respiratory tract infection (2–5, 9, 10). The importance of these risk factors was strengthened when the present results were analyzed by calculating appropriate ORs for the factors. Although the frequencies of different illnesses were lower among older travellers than young travellers, our analyses revealed increased risk for travel-related health problems in all age groups going to high risk areas, participating in adventure tourism, or travelling for longer periods of time.

Whereas the incidence, duration and severity of diarrheal illness were similar to those observed in other studies (1–5, 9–13), the incidence of respiratory tract infection (21%) was higher than in earlier reports (1, 4). Common cold and other respiratory tract infections are probably underestimated health risks among travellers to high risk areas. Presently no specific preventive measures can be offered for these diseases.

Diarrheal illness was, despite information concerning the advantages of nutritional precaution, the predominant health problem encountered by the travellers. Purchase and use of a variety of mainly anti-diarrheal drugs was relatively common among Swedish travellers, and equalled the rates previously reported among Central European travellers (14). Loperamide, used by nearly half of those with diarrhea, seems to have gained acceptance in Sweden as the first line of self-treatment of travellers' diarrhea. Antibiotics, which have proven to be effective for the treatment of travellers' diarrhea in a large number of clinical trials (12, 15), were used by only a minority of travellers. Although absorbents and bacteriological or biological preparations, which have little or no proven effect in the treatment of infectious diarrhea (8, 15), were not recommended by the IDU, a substantial number of travellers purchased and used these remedies. They seem to be currently recommended by pharmacies visited before or during travel (16).

Self-treatment of suspected malaria infection was initiated by 4% of the travellers equipped with mefloquined for stand-by treatment, a figure similar to that previously reported in larger surveys (4, 14, 17). Based on available information (4, 14, 17–21) concerning the risk of acquisition of malaria during travel, one could estimate the actual need for self-treatment to be <1% among the participants of the present study. Although issued with detailed information regarding the symptoms and signs of malarial infection, most of the travellers who initiated self-treatment were probably unable to distinguish early malaria from other acute febrile infections. A relatively high frequency of self-treatment may be required in order to prevent a few cases of severe or fatal P. falciparum infection.

The compliance with (86%) and incidence of side effects (12%) to chloroquine or chloroquine/proguanil prophylaxis were similar to those in a previous prospective Scandinavian study (21). However, many other surveys have recorded lower compliance and higher rates of adverse reactions (14, 17, 19, 20, 22). These discrepancies might be explained by differences in study design and methods of collecting data. In contrast to most previous studies, we used prospective recording throughout the trip. Moreover, our travellers received identical detailed written information from a single source, whereas travellers investigated in other surveys usually obtained information from a variety of sources (17, 22). Beforehand knowledge of the side effects commonly experienced during chemoprophylaxis may have convinced travellers to continue prophylaxis in the presence of harmless adverse events.

According to the present study, every second Swedish traveller to tropical and subtropical areas experienced an often debilitating travel-related health problem. The high incidence of illness among certain categories of travellers, and the frequent use of drugs to treat these symptoms, emphasize the need for more detailed pre-travel information concerning health risks and possible preventive measures, as well as advice on the use of appropriate drugs for the treatment of travel-related infections.

ACKNOWLEDGEMENT

The secretarial assistance of Miss Eva Marklund is gratefully acknowledged.

REFERENCES

1. Peltola H, Kyrönseppä H, Hölsä P. Trips to the South. A health hazard. Morbidity of Finnish travellers. Scand J Infect Dis 15: 375–381, 1983.
2. MacDonald KL, Cohen ML. Epidemiology of travelers' diarrhea: current perspectives. Rev Infect Dis 8 (Suppl 2): S117–S121, 1986.

3. Steffen R. Epidemiologic studies of travelers' diarrhea, severe gastrointestinal infections, and cholera. Rev Infect Dis 8 (Suppl 2): S122-S130, 1986.
4. Steffen R. Travel medicine—prevention based on epidemiological data. Trans R Soc Trop Med Hyg 85: 156–162, 1991.
5. Black RE. Epidemiology of travelers' diarrhea and relative importance of various pathogens. Rev Infect Dis 12 (Suppl 1): S73–S79, 1990.
6. Cossar JH, Reid D, Fallon RJ, Bell EJ, Riding MH, Follett EAC, Dow BC, Mitchell S, Grist NR. A cumulative review of studies on travellers, their experience of illness and the implications of these findings. J Infect 21: 27–42, 1990.
7. Blaser MJ. Environmental interventions for the prevention of travelers' diarrhea. Rev Infect Dis 8 (Suppl 2): S142–S150, 1986.
8. Ericsson CD, DuPont HL. Travelers' diarrhea: Approaches to prevention and treatment. Clin Infect Dis 16: 616–617, 1993.
9. Kollaritsch H. Travellers' diarrhea among Austrian tourists in warm climate countries: I. Epidemiology. Eur J Epidemiol 5: 74–81, 1989.
10. Steffen R, Boppart I. Travellers' diarrhea: Baillieres Clin Gastroenterol 1: 361–376, 1987.
11. Kollaritsch H. Traveller's diarrhea among Austrian tourists to warm climate countries: II. Clinical features. Eur J Epidemiol 5: 355–362, 1989.
12. Wiström J, Jertborn M, Hedström SÅ, Alestig K, Englund G, Jellheden B, Norrby SR. Short-term self-treatment of travellers' diarrhoea with norfloxacin: a placebo-controlled study. J Antimicrob Chemother 23: 905–913, 1989.
13. Farthing MJG. Travellers' diarrhoea. Mostly due to bacteria and difficult to prevent. BMJ 306: 1425–1426, 1993.
14. Steffen R, Heusser R, Mächler R, Bruppacher R, Naef U, Chen D, Hofmann AM, Somaini B. Malaria chemoprophylaxis among European tourists in tropical Africa: Use, adverse reactions, and efficacy. Bull World Health Organ 68: 313–322, 1990.
15. DuPont HL. Travellers' diarrhea. Which antimicrobial? Drugs 45: 910–917, 1993.
16. Yudkin JS. Dispensing of inappropriate medicines for diarrhea. Lancet 335: 803, 1990.
17. Lobel HO, Phillips-Howard PA, Brandling-Bennett AD, Steffen R, Campbell CC, Huong AY, Were JBO, Moser R. Malaria incidence and prevention among European and North American travellers to Kenya. Bull World Health Organ 68: 209–215, 1990.
18. Phillips Howard PA, Radalowicz A, Mitchell J, Bradley DJ. Risk of malaria in British residents returning from malarious areas. BMJ 300: 499–503, 1990.
19. Steffen R, Fuchs E, Schildknecht J, Naef U, Funk M, Schlagenhauf P, Phillips-Howard P, Nevill C, Stürchler D. Mefloquine compared with other malaria chemoprophylactic regimens in tourists visiting East Africa. Lancet 341: 1299–1303, 1993.
20. Wetsteyn JCFM, de Geus A. Comparison of three regimens for malaria prophylaxis in travellers to east, central and southern Africa. BMJ 307: 1041–1043, 1993.
21. Fogh S, Schapira, Bygbjerg IC, Jepsen S, Mordhorst CH, Kuijlen K, Ravn P, Rønn A, Gøtzsche PC. Malaria chemoprophylaxis in travellers to east Africa; a comparative prospective study of chloroquine plus proguanil with chloroquine plus sulfadoxine-pyrimethamine. BMJ 296: 820–822, 1988.
22. Kollaritsch H, Wiedermann G. Compliance of Austrian tourists with prophylactic measures. Eur J Epidemiol 8: 243–251, 1992.

Submitted May 2, 1994; accepted August 18, 1994

Scand J Infect Dis 26: 719–723, 1994

Parental Smoking and Carriage of Neisseria meningitidis among Greek Schoolchildren

JENNY KREMASTINOU[1], CAROLINE BLACKWELL[2], GEORGINA TZANAKAKI[1], CONSTANTINA KALLERGI[3], ROBERT ELTON[4] and DONALD WEIR[2]

From the [1]National Meningitis Reference Laboratory, Athens School of Public Health and the [2]Department of Medical Microbiology and the [3]Aglaia Kyriakou Paediatric Hospital, Athens, Greece and the [4]Medical Statistics Unit, Department of Public Health Sciences, University of Edinburgh, Edinburgh, Scotland

In December 1990 and January 1991, primary (320) and secondary (697) pupils in 2 areas of Athens were screened to determine the rate of carriage of Neisseria meningitidis and to determine if the genetic and environmental factors associated with carriage of meningococci in Greece were similar to those observed for northern European populations. In 1 area, socioeconomic indicators were significantly lower than in the other ($p < 0.0005$), but the isolation rates from pupils in the areas were similar, 5.3% and 6.3%. In contrast to studies in northwest Europe, carriage was not associated with lower socioeconomic conditions, sex, numbers of individuals per household, upper respiratory tract infection, or secretor status. By univariate analysis, carriage was associated with age (15–18 years) ($p < 0.05$) and mother's or other carer's smoking habits ($p < 0.05$) – but not father's smoking. Although the proportion of fathers who smoked was greater in the area where socioeconomic indicators were lower (61%) vs. (47%) ($p < 0.0005$), the proportions of women smokers were similar (33% vs. 38%). By multiple regression analysis, the only significant factors were age ($p < 0.01$) and carer's smoking ($p < 0.05$).

C. C. Blackwell, MD, Department of Medical Microbiology, University of Edinburgh, Teviot Place, Edinburgh, Scotland EH8 9AG

INTRODUCTION

Since 1989 there has been a steady increase in the numbers of cases of disease due to Neisseria meningitidis reported to the Ministry of Health in Athens (1). In contrast to countries in northern Europe, there were no reports on carriage rates of meningococci among school children in Greece or assessment of factors associated with carriage of these bacteria among children in any country in southeast Europe. The present study had 2 objectives: to determine the carriage rate of meningococci among schoolchildren in Athens, particularly the B:2b:P1.10 phenotype frequently isolated from Greek children with meningitis (2); and to examine genetic and environmental factors associated with meningococcal disease and/or carriage in northern Europe: age (3); sex (3, 4); secretor status (5); smoking or passive exposure to cigarette smoke (5–7); lower socioeconomic conditions (3, 8); upper respiratory tract infections (9–11).

SUBJECTS AND METHODS

Children (1,038) were screened for pharyngeal carriage of meningococci during December 1990 and January 1991. Four schools were included in the study: a primary school and a secondary school in area (A) where housing costs were low; and a primary school and a secondary school in area (B) where housing costs were high.

Saliva and a throat swab were obtained from each child. Methods for culture and identification of N. meningitidis were the same as those reported previously (1, 12, 13). The saliva was frozen within 3 h of collection and secretor status determined by ELISA for H, Lewis^{a} and Lewis^{b} antigens (14, 15).

The parent or guardian of each child gave written consent for participation in the survey and provided the following information: age and sex of child; respiratory illness in the past week; number of individuals/household; smoking habits of members of the household; education level of parents. In

Greece, for epidemiological studies, socioeconomic category is assessed by the number of years of education and the highest level of school attended (16). Secondary schoolchildren were asked if they smoked.

Two-way frequency tables were anslysed by χ^2-tests with Yates' correction. Multiple logistic regression was used to examine the association between carriage and other factors adjusted for each other.

RESULTS

The 2 socioeconomic indicators used, cost of housing and educational level of the parents, were in agreement. Educational level of each parent was assigned to one of the following 5 categories based on the number of years of attendance and the type of school attended for categories 1–3: 1 = "demotico" (1–6 years); 2–"gymnasio" (6–9 years); 3 = "lykio" (9–12 years); 4 = technical college; 5 = university. Compared with area A, in area B there was a significantly lower proportion of parents in categories 1 and 2 and higher proportions of parents who had received technical training or attended university ($p < 0.0005$) (Table I).

The carriage rate was 60/1038 (5.8%), and the proportion of isolates from the 2 areas was similar: area A 30/565 (5.3%); area B 30/473 (6.3%) (Table II). Only 2 isolates, both obtained from secondary school pupils, expressed the B:2b:P1.10 phenotype (2).

Univariate analyses found no association between carriage and 2 genetic factors examined, sex or secretor status. There was no association between carriage and educational level of parents, numbers of individuals per household, area of residence, or symptoms or respiratory infection.

Among children in secondary schools, 14% of 50 smokers were carriers compared with 6.2% of 661 non-smokers ($p > 0.05$). In secondary school A, 7.6% of children were smokers, and 5/30 (17%) smokers were carriers compared with 16/352 (4.5%) non-smokers ($p < 0.025$). In secondary school B, 6% of children were smokers, but only 2/20 (10%) smokers were carriers compared with 25/305 (8.2%) non-smokers.

Compared with the proportion of carriers from households in which no adult smoked (11/311, 3.5%), the proportion of carriers was significantly higher in those in which the

Table I. *Educational level of parents in area A and area B*

		Educational category no. (%)				
	N	1	2	3	4	5
Area A	1,107	572 (52)	239 (21)	215 (19)	57 (5)	24 (2)
Area B	937	165 (18)	134 (14)	289 (31)	78 (8)	271 (29)

$p < 0.0005$.

Table II. *Isolation of meningococci from pupils in primary and secondary schools*

		Meningococci isolated	
School	*N*	*n*	(%)
Primary A	180	9	(5.0)
Primary B	144	3	(2.1)
Secondary A	385	21	(5.5)
Secondary B	328	27	(8.2)

Table III. *Sex, smoking and educational level*

	Educational category, no. (%)				
	1	2	3	4	5
Women[a]					
Smoker/total	130/395 (38)	68/177 (38)	117/299 (39)	14/47 (30)	30/109 (28)
Men[b]					
Smoker/total	222/357 (62)	115/196 (59)	113/205 (55)	47/88 (53)	71/186 (38)

Compared with non-smokers:
[a] $p > 0.05$.
[b] $p < 0.0005$.

mother or other carers smoked (33/431, 7.7%, $p < 0.05$). Father's smoking was not associated with carriage. Carriage rates in households where the mother or other carers smoked did not depend significantly on whether only the mother, only the other carers, or both smoked.

There were 15 carriers under 13 years, and in 5 cases (33%) the mothers smoked. There were 45 carriers over 12 years, and in 23 cases (51%) the mothers smoked ($p < 0.025$). When the figures were corrected for the children who were smokers, 20/38 (52.6%) carriers who were non-smokers had mothers who smoked ($p < 0.025$).

Smoking was more prevalent among fathers with fewer years of education ($p < 0.0005$), but this association was not found for mothers ($p > 0.05$) (Table III). In area B where the educational level was higher, the proportion of fathers who smoked was significantly lower 223/472 (47%) compared with area A 345/560 (61%) ($p < 0.0005$). These differences were not found for mothers in the 2 areas (A = 33% and B = 38%).

Following analysis by multiple logistic regression with reference to age, sex, school attended, respiratory infection, parental smoking and the children's smoking habits, only age ($p < 0.01$) and maternal or other carers' smoking ($p < 0.05$) remained significant. Older children and those whose carers smoked were more likely to be carriers. Although the trend with age appeared stronger in those whose carers smoked, this was not significant (interaction test in multiple logistic regression).

DISCUSSION

The proportion of carriers among children in this study did not differ from that usually found during non-epidemic periods, and the proportion of strains expressing the B : 2b : P1.10 phenotype was not high.

This was the first study to assess factors associated with carriage of meningococci in a population in southeast Europe. Several factors identified in studies of meningococcal carriage in northern Europe did not appear to influence carriage in the Greek schoolchildren: sex; secretor status; socioeconomic status; numbers of individuals per household; upper respiratory tract infections.

The isolation rate in different age bands followed a pattern similar to that found in the Stonehouse survey (3), and age was the most significant variable identified by multiple regression analysis.

In contrast to the Stonehouse survey (3) and a longitudinal survey in Belgium (8), carriage rate was no greater in the area where socioeconomic indicators were lower. For the fathers in this study and in our previous study of Greek military recruits (1), there was a significant correlation between educational level and smoking. Carriage was not, however, associated with father's smoking by either univariate or multivariate analysis. In Great Britain, the pattern for socioeconomic groups and smoking are similar for men and women (17); however, there were no differences in smoking patterns of Greek women associated with educational levels or in the percentage of mothers who smoked in the 2 areas of the city.

Among studies on exposure to cigarette smoke and infection, the strongest associations are usually with smoking habits of the mother (18, 19). If the mother's smoking is a significant factor contributing to carriage among children, this might explain the similar carriage rates for the 2 areas of Athens. The observation that carriage was also significantly associated with smoking by adults other than the father might reflect the structure of many Greek families; grandmothers often live with families with young children and are closely involved in child care. Our study suggests that in Greece, smoking by mothers or other family members traditionally involved in child care might contribute to the carriage of meningococci.

REFERENCES

1. Blackwell CC, Tzanakaki G, Kremastinou J, Weir DM, Vakalis N, Elton RA, Mentis A, Fatouros N. Factors affecting carriage of Neisseria meningitidis among Greek military recruits. Epidemiol Infect 108: 441–448, 1992.
2. Tzanakaki G, Blackwell CC, Kremastinou J, Kallergi C, Fallon RJ, Weir DM. Serogroups, serotypes and subtypes of Neisseria meningitidis isolated from patients and carriers in Greece. J Med Microbiol 38: 19–22, 1993.
3. Cartwright KAV, Stuart JM, Jones DM, Noah ND. The Stonehouse survey: nasopharyngeal carriage of meningococci and Neisseria lactamica. Epidemiol Infect 99: 591–601, 1987.
4. Olsen SF, Djurhuus B, Rasmussen K, Joensen AD, Larsen SO, Zoffman H, Lind I. Pharyngeal carriage of Neisseria meningitidis and Neisseria lactamica in households with infants within areas with high and low incidences of meningococcal diseases. Epidemiol Infect 106: 445–457, 1991.
5. Blackwell CC, Weir DM, James VS, Todd WTA, Banatvala N, Chaudhuri AKR, Gray HG, Thomson EJ, Fallon RJ. Secretor status, smoking and carriage of Neisseria meningitidis. Epidemiol Infect 104: 203–209, 1990.
6. Stuart JM, Cartwright KAV, Dawson JA, Rickard J, Noah ND. Risk factors for meningococcal disease: a case control study in south west England. Community Med 10: 139–146, 1988.
7. Stuart JM, Cartwright KAV, Robinson PM, Noah ND. Effect of smoking on meningococcal carriage. Lancet 2: 723–725, 1989.
8. de Wals P, Gilquin C, de Maeyer S, Bouckaert A, Noel A, Lechat MF, Lafontaine A. Longitudinal study of asymptomatic carriage in two Belgian populations of school children. J Infect 6: 147–156, 1983.
9. Krakinski K, Nilson JD, Butler S, Suby JP, Kusmiesz H. Possible association of mycoplasma and viral respiratory infections with bacterial meningitis. Am J Epidemiol 125: 499–508, 1987.
10. Moore PS, Hierholzer J, Dewitt W, Govan K, Djoré D, Lippeveld T, Plikayatis D, Broom CV. Respiratory viruses and mycoplasma as cofactors for epidemic groups meningococcal meningitis. JAMA 246: 1271–1275, 1990.
11. Olcén P, Kjellander J, Danielsson D, Lindquist BL. Epidemiology of Neisseria meningitidis: Prevalence and symptoms from the upper respiratory tract in family members to patients with meningococcal disease. Scand J Infect Dis 13: 105–109, 1981.
12. Young H. Cultural diagnosis of gonorrhoea with modified New York City medium (MNYC). Br J Vener Dis 54: 36–40, 1978.
13. Young H, Paterson IC, MacDonald DR. Rapid carbohydrate utilization test for identification of Neisseria gonorrhoeae. Br J Vener Dis 52: 172–175, 1979.
14. Rahat A, Stewart J, Blackwell CC, Weir DM. A semiquantative method for measurement of H type 1 and H type 2 on buccal cells and in saliva of secretors and non-secretors. Vox Sang 59: 101–105, 1990.
15. Raza MW, Blackwell CC, Molyneaux P, James VS, Ogilvie MM, Inglis JM, Weir DM. Secretor status and viral illness. BMJ 303: 815–818, 1991.

16. Trichopoulos D. Epidemiology: principles, methods, applications. Athens: R. Patisiano Publishers, 1982, 139.
17. Wald N, Kiryluk S, Darby S, Doll R, Pike M, Peto R. UK smoking statistics. Oxford: Oxford University Press, 1988.
18. Tager IB, Weiss ST, Munoz A, Rosner B, Speizer FE. Longitudinal study of the effects of maternal smoking on pulmonary function in children. N Engl J Med 309: 699–703, 1983.
19. Pershagen G. Review of epidemiology in relation to passive smoking. Arch Toxicol 9 (suppl 9): 63–73, 1986.

Submitted April 5, 1994; accepted July 21, 1994

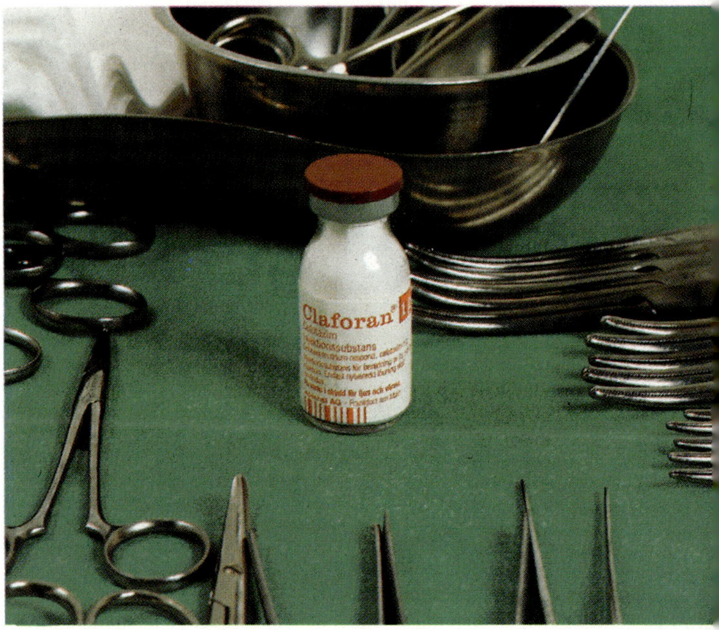
Claforan

Scand J Infect Dis 26: 725–730, 1994

Serological and Clinical Characteristics of Measles Vaccine Failure in Japan

YASUFUMI HIDAKA[1,2], TOMONOBU AOKI[1], HIDEKI AKEDA[1], CHIAKI MIYAZAKI[2] and KOHJI UEDA[2]

From the [1]Section of Pediatric Infectious Diseases, Fukuoka Children's Hospital and Medical Center for Infectious Diseases and [2]the Department of Pediatrics, Faculty of Medicine, Kyusyu University, Fukuoka, Japan

In 1991, in Fukuoka, Japan, a measles outbreak occurred in which we observed 15 cases of measles vaccine failure (MVF). We examined these patients both clinically and serologically. Seven of them, with a response pattern of an early rise in and attainment of a high hemagglutination inhibition (HI) antibody titre, were considered to be secondary vaccine failures (EH group). Eight others showed a normal (relatively late rise and low titre) HI antibody response pattern and were considered to be primary vaccine failures (LL group).

In both MVF groups, measles-specific IgM antibody was detected by enzyme immunoassay. The EH group had a milder rash than did the LL group and unvaccinated controls. We believe they had an immunological memory that modified the clinical manifestations of measles. Two cases of encephalitis were observed in the EH group; both patients recovered without sequelae.

These data suggest that the mere presence or absence of IgM antibody is not sufficient to differentiate primary from secondary MVFs. A two-dose measles vaccination scheme should be recommended to secure a booster effect, because immunity is waning in the population in which the measles vaccination rate is not high enough and in which natural measles still exists.

Y. Hidaka, MD, Department of Pediatrics, Faculty of Medicine, Kyusyu University, 3-1-1, Maidashi, Higashi-ku, Fukuoka 812, Japan

INTRODUCTION

Infection by wild measles virus is believed to afford lifelong immunity, according to observations made by Panum during an outbreak on the Faroe Islands in 1846 (1). Consequently, it has been assumed that infection with live attenuated or further attenuated measles vaccine also affords long-term, probably lifelong immunity. However, several cases of measles vaccine failure (MVF) have been reported (2–4) and the immunity conferred by measles vaccine is now considered not to be lifelong (5). In the U.S.A., a routine two-dose vaccination schedule was recommended in 1991 (6, 7). In Japan, measles vaccine was adopted for routine use in a vaccination program in 1978 and the government is attempting to increase the vaccination rate, but it is still only 70–80%.

Measles outbreaks in Japan have occurred mainly in unvaccinated populations and MVF has not been a major problem. In 1991, 13 years after the beginning of the measles vaccination program, a measles outbreak occurred in Japan and, in several districts, many cases involved individuals who had previously received attenuated live measles vaccine. This novel feature of the measles outbreak in Japan showed that secondary vaccine failure (SVF) occurred in a population whose measles vaccination rate is not high enough and in which booster effects by wild measles are believed to exist. This information is important for the measles vaccination strategy in developing countries. These MVF cases were thought to be secondary vaccine failures (SVFs), but measles-specific IgM antibody was detected in most cases. In this study, we report the serological and clinical features of cases of MVF in Japan.

MATERIALS AND METHODS

Study populations

Between January and August 1991, 303 measles patients visited Fukuoka Children's Hospital and Medical Center for Infectious Diseases, Fukuoka, Japan. Some were managed as in-patients (173 cases) and others as out-patients (130 cases). 15 patients had received a measles vaccination more than 1 month earlier. In the Fukuoka district, 2208 cases of measles were reported to the national system of surveillance of infectious diseases. Based on the rate of coverage of this surveillance, it is estimated that some 20,000 to 40,000 cases of measles occurred during this period. In this study, 15 cases of MVF were evaluated both clinically and serologically.

Case definition

The diagnosis of measles was based on the clinical course and signs. Infectious diseases specialists in our sections were consulted in all 15 cases. Typical measles cases could be diagnosed easily enough by clinical course and signs alone. Patients who did not show typical manifestations were examined serologically and thus confirmed. The criterion for serological confirmation of measles was either a significant increase in measles hemagglutination inhibition (HI) antibody titre or a positive test result for measles-specific IgM antibody.

Measles encephalitis patients in this study showed drowsiness, disorientation, signs of meningeal irritation, pleocytosis in cerebrospinal fluid, and high-voltage slow waves in the EEG.

Serological test

The HI test was performed according to standard procedure. Briefly, a test serum was heat-inactivated, treated with kaolin, and absorbed with African green monkey erythrocytes. The HI test was employed a standard microtitre method, an HI titre of 8 or higher was considered positive. To detect measles-specific IgM antibody, the sera were also tested with a commercial enzyme immunoassay (EIA) (Measles IgM-EIA [Seiken]™; Denkaseiken Co., Ltd., Tokyo) according to the manufacturer's instructions. The IgM index was scored: negative, <0.8; positive, >1.2; pending, 0.8 to 1.2. These tests were performed at the laboratory of SRL Co., Ltd., Tokyo.

History of vaccination

The vaccination history of each measles patient was checked by examining the vaccination record in the mother's maternity passbook. These descriptions constitute one of the most reliable databases in Japan confirming children's health histories.

Used vaccines were Schwartz strain, CAM strain, and AIK-C strain. These vaccines contain more than 5,000 $TCID_{50}$/0.5 ml and seroconversion rates after vaccination are more than 95%.

Statistical methods

The two-tailed Fisher's exact test was used to test for significance for dichotomous variables and the unpaired *t*-test was used for continuous variables.

RESULTS

Measles HI and IgM antibody in natural measles and MVF cases

Measles HI antibody titre was measured in cases of vaccine failure and of natural measles (Fig. 1). Cases of natural measles showed a normal pattern of rising HI antibody titre that reached levels ≤ 512-fold. Seven cases of MVF showed an early rise in HI titre and reached maximal levels $\geq 1{,}024$-fold; in 8 others, the pattern was the same as in natural measles. Cases with a pattern of an early and high rise in HI were designated EH (EH: early and high) group; cases with a pattern of a relatively late and low rise in HI, which is the natural pattern, we designated the LL (LL: late and low) group. Vaccine failures were separated into these 2 groups; the EH group was considered to retain an immunological memory of earlier vaccination, while the LL group was considered to comprise cases of primary vaccine failure (PVF) or cases of SVF with complete disappearance of immunological memory.

When IgM antibody was measured (Fig. 2), all 3 groups (EH, LL, and natural measles) showed almost the same pattern; all patients with MVF were IgM-positive. Three patients

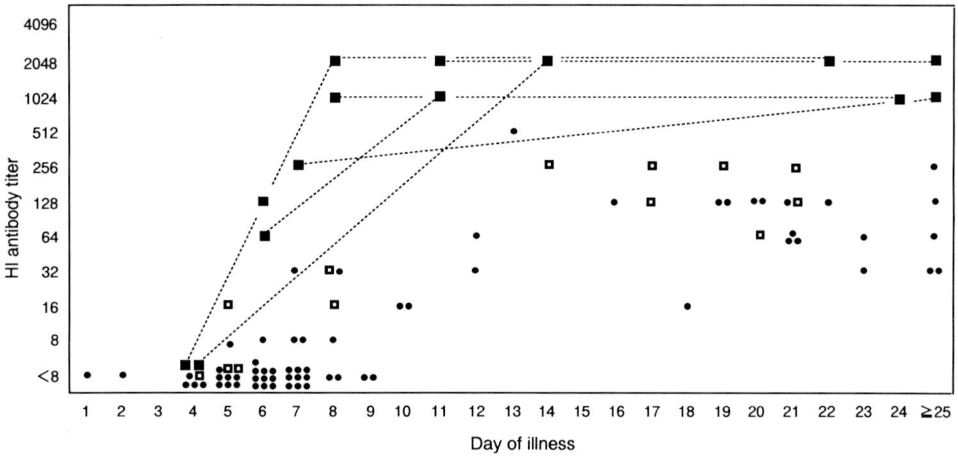

Fig. 1. Relation between measles HI antibody titre and clinical day of illness. ■ and □ indicate measles patients with a history of measles vaccination, ■, EH group; □, LL group (see text). ● indicates measles patients without a history of measles vaccination.

with MVF who showed IgM-negative results on the fourth or fifth day of illness became IgM-positive subsequently.

Clinical features in MVF cases

The characteristics of our MVF cases are shown in Table I. Unvaccinated, age-matched measles patients were selected as controls. The association between clinical and serological data was estimated in 11 natural measles patients confirmed clinically and in 15

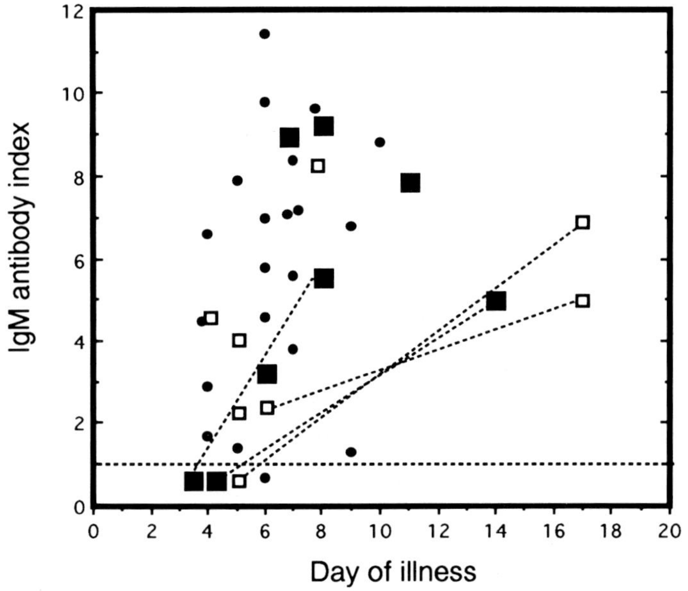

Fig. 2. Relation between measles IgM antibody and clinical day of illness. ■ and □ indicate measles patients with a history of measles vaccination, ■, EH group; □, LL group (see text). ● indicates measles patients without a history of measles vaccination.

Table I. *Characteristics of measles vaccine failure cases at Fukuoka Children's Hospital and Medical Center for Infectious Diseases, Fukuoka, 1991*

EH = early rise and high hemagglutination inhibition (HI) antibody response pattern. LL = relatively late rise and low HI antibody response pattern.

Characteristic	Unvaccinated ($n = 11$)	Vaccinated: EH group ($n = 7$)	Vaccinated: LL group ($n = 8$)
Mean age ± SD, years	10.6 ± 0.8	11.1 ± 1.4	11.1 ± 2.3
No. (%) female	4 (36)	3 (43)	2 (25)
Age at vaccination, No. (%)			
<12 months	–	0 (0)	0 (0)
12–14 months	–	0 (0)	1 (13)
≥15 months	–	6 (86)	5 (63)
unknown	–	1 (14)	2 (25)
mean ± SD	–	2.3 ± 0.5	1.9 ± 0.6
Years since vaccination, mean ± SD	–	8.4 ± 1.1	9.9 ± 2.1
Mean ± SD days from onset of fever			
First samples (4–8 days)	–	5.8 ± 1.5	5.9 ± 1.4
Second samples (11–32 days)	–	19.0 ± 7.7	17.3 ± 2.8
Maximum measured temperature (°C)	39.6 ± 0.4	39.7 ± 0.3	39.4 ± 0.6
Fever duration (days)	7.6 ± 1.3	8.1 ± 2.3	9.0 ± 4.4
Rash onset (days)	5.1 ± 1.4	3.9 ± 1.1	4.1 ± 0.8
No. (%) with typical type rash[a]	11/11 (100)	3/7 (43)	7/8 (88)
No. (%) with pigmentation	11/11 (100)	5/6 (83)	7/7 (100)
No. (%) with Koplik's spots	10/11 (91)	5/7 (71)	7/7 (100)
No. (%) with encephalitis	0/11 (0)	2/7 (29)	0/8 (0)
HI antibody titre, geometric mean			
First samples	–	56.9	7.4
Second samples[b]	–	1448.2	128.0
IgM antibody index			
First samples	–	4.63	3.69

[a] Values of unvaccinated patients differed significantly ($p < 0.05$) from those of EH group, according to Fisher's exact test.

[b] Values of EH group differed significantly ($p < 0.01$) from those of LL group according to the Welch t-test.

vaccinated patients confirmed serologically. In comparison with both the unvaccinated group and the vaccinated LL group, the vaccinated EH group showed relatively milder illness. In the EH vaccine failure group, an atypical or modified rash was observed more frequently than in the LL vaccine failure group. Two patients with encephalitis were observed in the EH vaccine failure group; both recovered completely, without any sequelae.

DISCUSSION

We compared the pattern of HI and IgM responses in cases of natural measles with those of MVF cases. MVF cases were divided into 2 groups according to the HI antibody response pattern: an EH group and an LL group. IgM antibodies were detected in both groups, rendering IgM useless for separating MVF groups. As regards clinical features, patients in the EH group had a relatively milder illness than did those in LL group.

In the U.S.A., the measles vaccination rate has nearly reached 100% and measles outbreaks are rare, though, problems of SVF are more serious than in Japan. No booster effect can be expected and a second dose of vaccine is usually recommended. In Japan, the measles vaccination rate is still only 70–80%, because there is no strict law requiring vaccination before a child is admitted to school. As a result, measles may break out anywhere. A booster effect is assumed to exist, but many of those vaccinated are thought to show waning immunity, i.e., they lack a natural booster to trigger their immunological memory. The wild measles virus differs from measles vaccine virus in the strength of initial immunological stimulation, so the level of memory cells each induces is also expected to differ. After infection with wild measles virus, immunological memory remains for life without any booster stimulation, and a rapid IgG reaction protects against secondary measles infection. Immunity from measles vaccination wanes with time and falls below a protective level in the absence of a booster. Two doses of vaccine are needed not only for instances of PVF but also for waning immunity. A two-dose vaccination should be recommended also in Japan.

In some reports, MVF is classified into primary or secondary, according to the positivity of measles-specific IgM antibody [2, 8, 9]. PVF is characterized by normal HI antibody titres, SVF by high HI antibody titres. We observed some patients who had both IgM antibody and a high HI antibody titre. Immunological memory remained in these cases, but was only partial, suggesting that they should be reclassified as SVF. As techniques for detecting IgM become more sensitive, the number of IgM-positive SVF cases will increase. There have been few studies of IgM determined by EIA in MVF. Because IgM antibody can exist in cases of SVF, a negative IgM result is insufficient to distinguish PVF from SVF. SVF must be divided according to many factors. Therefore, in this study we used the terms EH and LL groups, because PVF and SVF cannot be defined clearly unless one knows the immunological response to vaccination. In a secondary immune response, a rapid increase in IgG inhibits the production IgM derived from lymphocyte repertoires that are virgin for the measles virus. An insufficient rapid increase in IgG is unable to inhibit the IgM response completely. It is believed that the level of IgM antibody was low, but not undetectable, in SVF.

The clinical symptoms of the EH group did not differ from those of the LL group, but the rash found in EH group was milder or modified. Although the incidence of measles encephalitis is described as 1 case per thousand measles patients (10), the EH group of 7 included 2 cases of encephalitis. We cannot explain this high incidence, but we suspect that the 2 individuals have some immunological disorder. Now they have been proved to have low natural killer cell activity, and both are being examined further. Fortunately, both recovered without sequelae. Measles encephalitis is a very severe disease and we believe that the 2 vaccinated patients may owe their cure to a specific immunity to measles virus gained from vaccination, although their non-specific immunity was weak and permitted initial extensive propagation of measles virus.

ACKNOWLEDGEMENT

This study was supported in part by a Grant-in-Aid for Vaccination Research from the Ministry of Health and Welfare of Japan.

REFERENCES

1. Panum PL. Observations made during the epidemic of measles on the Faroe Islands in the year 1846. New York: American Publishing Association, 1940.
2. Edmonson MB, Addiss DG, McPherson JT, Berg JL, Circo SR, Davis JP. Mild measles and secondary vaccine failure during a sustained outbreak in a highly vaccinated population. JAMA 263: 2467–2471, 1990.
3. Mathias R, Meekison J, Arcand T, Schechter M. The role of secondary vaccine failure in measles outbreaks. Am J Public Health 79: 475–478, 1989.

4. Reyes MA, Franky De Borrero M, Roa J, Bergonzoli G, Seravia NG. Measles vaccine failure after documented seroconversion. Pediatr Infect Dis J 6: 848–851, 1987.
5. Markowitz LE, Preblud SR, Fine PE, Orenstein WA. Duration of live measles vaccine-induced immunity. Pediatr Infect Dis J 9: 101–110, 1990.
6. American Academy of Pediatrics, Committee on Infectious Diseases. Measles: reassessment of the current immunization policy. Pediatrics 84: 1110–1113, 1989.
7. Immunization Practice Advisory Committee. Measles prevention. MMWR 38 (S-9): 1–18, 1989.
8. Linnemann CC, Hegg ME, Rotte TC, Phair JP, Schiff GM. Measles IgM response during reinfection of vaccinated children. J Pediatr 82: 798–801, 1973.
9. Nagy G, Kosa S, Takatsy S, Koller M. The use of IgM test for analysis of the causes of measles vaccine failures. J Med Virol 13: 93–103, 1984.
10. Saez-Llorens X, McCracken, Jr. GH. Measles (rubeola). In: Krugman S, Katz SL, Gershon AA, Wilfert CM, eds. Infectious diseases of children. St. Louis: Mosby Year Book, 1992, 223–245.

Submitted February 7, 1994; accepted August 15, 1994

ANNOUNCEMENT

From August 27–30 the European Regional Meeting of the International Epidemiology Association (IEA) ‘Perspectives on Epidemiology in Europe’ will take place in The Hague, the Netherlands.

Mini-symposia on the topics Disease Etiology, Evidence based Medicine and Consensus Conferences, and Health in Europe will be held. In addition, the main focus will be on the presentation of abstracts on different aspects of epidemiologic research, such as chronic epidemiology, prevention programmes and community interventions etc.

The meeting will be organized jointly by the Netherlands Epidemiological Society and the National Institute of Public Health and Environmental Protection in Bilthoven.

Further details can be obtained from the organizing secretariat:

Congrex Holland
Keizersgracht 782
NL-1017 EC Amsterdam.
Tel: +31 20 6261372
Fax: +31 20 6259574

Scand J Infect Dis 26: 731–738, 1994

Comparison of Enhanced Potency Inactivated Poliovirus Vaccine (EIPV) Versus Standard Oral Poliovirus Vaccine (OPV) in Thai Infants

SRILUCK SIMASATHIEN[1], SRICHAROEN MIGASENA[2], COEN BEUVERY[3], GIJSBERT VAN STEENIS[3], RUDIWILAI SAMAKOSES[1], PUNNEE PITISUTTITHAM[1] and TIMO VESIKARI[4]

From the [1]Department of Pediatrics, Phramongkutkloa Hospital, Bangkok, Thailand, the [2]Vaccine Trial Centre, Department of Tropical Medicine, Mahidol University, Bangkok, the [3]National Institute of Public Health and Environmental Protection, Bilthoven, The Netherlands, and the [4]Department of Biomedical Sciences, University of Tampere, Tampere, Finland

Enhanced potency inactivated poliovirus vaccine (EIPV), combined with diphtheria-tetanus-pertussis (DTP) vaccine, was compared with oral poliovirus vaccine (OPV) regarding immunogenicity in Thai infants, vaccinated at 2, 4 and 6 months of age. EIPV induced significantly higher seroconversion rates than OPV to all 3 poliovirus types after the second and third immunization. After 3 doses of each vaccine, at 7 months of age, all infants receiving EIPV proved seropositive for poliovirus type 1, type 2 and type 3 neutralizing antibodies, whereas of those receiving OPV, 9% remained seronegative (titre $<1:4$) for type 1 ($p = 0.0042$) and 11% for type 3 ($p = 0.0013$). All participating children were given an additional dose of OPV at the age of 9 months and tested again at 12 months of age. At that point, virtually all infants had poliovirus neutralizing antibodies, but the geometric mean titres to each poliovirus type were significantly higher in the vaccinees who had received EIPV. It is concluded that the greater immunogenicity of EIPV vis-à-vis 3 doses of OPV may be biologically significant for protection against poliovirus types 1 and 3 in countries where cases of poliomyelitis occur in young children. These findings warrant considering EIPV, alone or in combination with OPV, for an immunization programme in Thailand and similar countries in the future.

T. Vesikari, MD, Department of Biomedical Sciences, University of Tampere, PO Box 607, FIN-33101 Tampere, Finland

INTRODUCTION

Eradication of paralytic poliomyelitis remains an elusive objective in large parts of the developing world (1–3). Oral poliovirus vaccine (OPV) is a powerful tool which has effectively eradicated paralytic poliomyelitis from the USA and other developed countries (4, 5). It is now widely recognized, however, that the immunogenicity of OPV is much lower in developing than in industrialized countries, and more immunizations than the standard 3 doses of OPV are required in order to achieve protective immunity in all or even the majority of vaccinees (1–3, 5, 6). In a recent study in Cote d'Ivoire, Africa, a fourth dose of OPV, or, alternatively, a dose of enhanced potency inactivated poliovirus vaccine (EIPV) significantly raised the prevalence of protective antibodies to critical poliovirus types 1 and 3, but did not totally eliminate a gap in protective immunity in young children (6).

EIPV is much more immunogenic than OPV (7–9), and may alone be sufficient to control poliomyelitis in countries with good immunization coverage, or, alternatively, may be considered as a component of mixed immunization programmes consisting of initial dose(s) of EIPV followed by OPV (9, 10). A major advantage of EIPV over OPV is lack of vaccine-induced poliomyelitis. This issue is becoming more important worldwide with the number of wild virus-induced cases of poliomyelitis decreasing (5).

EIPV has been regarded as too costly for developing countries, and, moreover, logistically difficult to incorporate into routine immunization programmes. However, the cost has been brought down, and EIPV can now be combined with diphtheria-tetanus-pertussis (DTP) vaccine into a single injection.

In the present study, EIPV (combined with DTP) was compared with OPV for immunogenicity in Thai infants, who received either vaccine at ages 2, 4 and 6 months, i.e. according to the standard Thai immunization schedule. A dose of OPV was administered at 9 months of age to all vaccinees, and the effect on poliovirus immunity of the fourth dose in children previously immunized with 3 doses of EIPV or OPV was studied at 12 months of age.

MATERIALS AND METHODS

Vaccinees and study design

The study was approved by the Ethics Committee of Phramongkutkloa College of Medicine, Bangkok and the Secretariat Committee for Research Involving Human Subjects of World Health Organization (WHO). Informed consent was obtained from the parents or guardians of the participating children.

The study was conducted as part of a trial of an oral rhesus-human reassortant rotavirus tetravalent vaccine (RRV-TV) given together with OPV. The total study group initially consisted of 330 infants, of whom (*a*) 110 received only OPV but no RRV-TV, (*b*) 110 received OPV with RRV- TV, and (*c*) 110 received IPV and RRV-TV. This report describes the poliovirus antibody responses in groups (*a*) and (*c*). The results of simultaneous administration of OPV and RRV-TV will be reported elsewhere (11).

The vaccinees were recruited from infants born at the Phramongkutkloa Hospital, Bangkok. Healthy full-term (≥ 37 weeks of gestation) infants with birth weight of ≥ 2500 g were recruited for the study at birth. At the time of preliminary recruitment the mothers received information about the study and the vaccines; they signed an informed consent form when the child was entering the study at 2 months of age.

The study was placebo-controlled for both EIPV and OPV, and all the vaccines were number-coded. The randomization was done by WHO in Geneva, and the manufacturers were requested to code their vaccines accordingly. The code was held in Geneva and was not made available to the investigators until completion of the study.

OPV (or the respective placebo) was given first in 2 drops. Parenteral immunization (DTP plus placebo or DTP plus EIPV) was given after the oral vaccination. The vaccines were administered at 2, 4 and 6 months of age. In addition, all children participating in the study received a dose of OPV at the age of 9 months, to ensure adequate immunization. This dosing was given at the same time with measles immunization.

Vaccines

EIPV lot number 311, prepared by the Dutch National Institute of Public Health and Environmental Protection (RIVM, Bilthoven, The Netherlands) was used. The EIPV contained 40 D-antigen units (12) of serotype 1, 8 DU of serotype 2, and 32 DU of serotype 3. EIPV was combined with DTP vaccine supplied by RIVM. Each dose contained 3 mg of aluminium phosphate as adjuvant. RIVM also supplied for the study a DTP vaccine combined with a placebo component for EIPV; the 2 injectable vaccines had an identical appearance.

A standard lot of oral poliovirus vaccine (OPV), prepared by SmithKline Beecham Biologicals (Rixensart, Belgium) for studies with the WHO Expanded Programme on Immunization (EPI), was donated by the manufacturer for the study. The vaccine was of the 10 : 1 : 3 type, and contained the following amounts of vaccine viruses: serotype 1, 10^6 $TCID_{50}$; serotype 2, 10^5 $TCID_{50}$; and serotype 3, $10^{5.5}$ $TCID_{50}$. A placebo preparation for OPV for use in the infants receiving EIPV, indistinguishable from active OPV, was also supplied by SmithKline Beecham.

Specimen collection and testing

Venous blood specimens were collected before vaccinations at 2 months of age and 1 month after each vaccination, at 3, 5 and 7 months of age, and 3 months after the third vaccination at 12 months of age. Sera were separated and stored at -70°C until shipped for testing at RIVM. All titrations were done under code.

The assay of poliovirus neutralizing antibodies was carried out as described previously, using a microneutralization test with Vero cells as substrate and type 1 Mahoney, type 2 MEF, and type 3

Saukett strains of poliovirus as challenge (13, 14). The starting dilution was 1 : 2 and the highest dilution was 1 : 4096. Sera with antibody activity ≤ 1 : 2 were regarded as negative, and sera with neutralizing antibody titre ≥ 1 : 8 as positive. Titre 1 : 4 was regarded as a borderline value. A 4-fold or greater increase in titre was considered to be a significant rise (also called seroconversion).

Statistical analysis

Data analysis was carried out using SYSTAT 5.1 (Macintosh) statistical package. Non-parametric discrete data such as seroconversion rate and prevalence of antibodies in 2 groups were compared by χ^2-test. After logarithmic transformation of the titre values, the 2-sample t-test was used for the comparison of neutralizing antibody levels between 2 groups; 95% confidence intervals for geometric mean titres (GMTs) were derived using the back-transformation of the confidence limits for logarithmically transformed data.

RESULTS

The infant groups receiving OPV and EIPV did not differ at 2 months of age from each other regarding the presence of neutralizing antibodies to poliovirus types 1, 2 and 3 (Table I). The geometric mean titres (GMTs) were low and again not different between the OPV and EIPV groups (Table II).

After the first dose of vaccine, 81% of the OPV recipients and 39% of the EIPV recipients had a significant rise in poliovirus type 2 antibodies ($p < 0.0001$). Only 25% of the infants in each group responded to poliovirus type 1, and 35% and 28% of the infants in the OPV and EIPV groups, respectively, responded to poliovirus type 3 (difference not significant). After the second and third doses of vaccine, the antibody response rates to all poliovirus types were significantly greater in the EIPV than in the OPV recipients (Table III). Altogether from the baseline at 2 months to the age of 7 months, 63/94 (67%) OPV recipients and 89/92 (96%) EIPV recipients had ≥ 4-fold rise in poliovirus type 1 antibodies ($p < 0.0001$), and 75/94 (80%) OPV recipients and 90/92 (98%) EIPV recipients had such a rise in poliovirus type 3 antibodies ($p = 0.0001$). The seroconversion rates to type 2 were 93% and 95% in the OPV and EIPV groups, respectively (difference not significant).

Acquisition of protective immunity, determined as possession of neutralizing antibodies at titre ≥ 1 : 8, followed the serological response rates (Table I). Already after the first vaccina-

Table I. *Prevalence of neutralizing antibodies at titre 1 : 8 or greater to poliovirus types 1, 2 and 3 in infants immunized at 2, 4, and 6 months of age with either OPV or EIPV and at 9 months with OPV only*

No. (%) seropositive/No. tested

	2 months baseline		3 months post 1		5 months post 2		7 months post 3		12 months post 4 (OPV)	
	OPV	EIPV	OPV	EIPV	OPV	EIPV	OPV	IPV	OPV	EIPV
Polio type 1	83/109 (76%)	87/108 (81%)	85/105 (81%)	100/103 (97%)	77/98 (79%)	94/94 (100%)	80/94 (85%)	92/92 (100%)	87/89 (98%)	84/84 (100%)
	$p = 0.4035$		$p = 0.0002$		$p < 0.0001$		$p = 0.0001$		$p = 0.1670$	
Polio type 2	90/109 (83%)	82/108 (76%)	99/103 (96%)	98/103 (95%)	94/98 (96%)	93/94 (99%)	92/94 (98%)	92/92 (100%)	(99%)	88/89 (100%)
	$p = 0.2275$		$p = 0.7332$		$p = 0.1893$		$p = 0.595$		$p = 0.3299$	
Polio type 3	46/109 (42%)	46/108 (43%)	56/104 (54%)	56/103 (63%)	72/98 (73%)	91/94 (97%)	81/94 (86%)	92/92 (100%)	82/88 (93%)	81/84 (96%)
	$p = 0.9536$		$p = 0.1764$		$p < 0.0001$		$p = 0.0002$		$p = 0.3392$	

Table II. *Geometric mean neutralizing antibodies to poliovirus types 1, 2 and 3 in infants immunized at 2, 4, and 6 months of age with OPV or EIPV and at 9 months with OPV only*

		2 months baseline		3 months post 1		5 months post 2		7 months post 3		12 months post 4 (OPV)	
		OPV	EIPV	OPV	EIPV	OPV	EIPV	OPV	EIPV	OPV	EIPV
Polio type 1	GMT	16	22	26	29	72	349	110	1696	235	1085
	95% CI	(13, 21)	(17, 29)	(18, 36)	(24, 35)	(46, 113)	(240, 507)	(71, 170)	(1365, 2108)	(165, 335)	(852, 1382)
		$p = 0.0835$		$p = 0.5543$		$p < 0.0001$		$p < 0.0001$		$p < 0.0001$	
Polio type 2	GMT	20	19	295	51	840	598	944	1709	823	1933
	95% CI	(16, 25)	(14, 25)	(209, 415)	(36, 70)	(587, 1202)	(417, 857)	(692, 1288)	(1309, 2231)	(604, 1112)	(1537, 2431)
		$p = 0.8184$		$p < 0.0001$		$p = 0.1856$		$p = 0.0045$		$p < 0.0001$	
Polio type 3	GMT	6	6	14	9	53	439	89	1236	86	561
	95% CI	(5, 7)	(5, 7)	(9, 20)	(7, 11)	(34, 83)	(289, 665)	(59, 133)	(938, 1629)	(59, 124)	(386, 814)
		$p = 0.7767$		$p = 0.0680$		$p < 0.0001$		$p < 0.0001$		$p < 0.0001$	

Table III. *Four-fold or greater rises in neutralizing antibodies to poliovirus types, 1, 2 and 3 after vaccination at 2, 4 and 6 months with either OPV or EIPV and at 9 months with OPV only*

No. (%) with ≥ 4-fold/No. tested

	2–3 months		3–5 months		5–7 months		2–7 months		7–12 months		2–12 months	
	OPV	EIPV	OPV	EIPV	OPV	EIPV	OPV	EIPV	OPV	EIPV	OPV	EIPV
Polio type 1	26/105 (25%)	26/103 (25%)	43/98 (44%)	71/94 (76%)	26/93 (28%)	49/91 (54%)	63/94 (67%)	89/92 (96%)	40/89 (45%)	14/83 (17%)	71/89 (80%)	76/84 (90%)
	$p = 0.9362$		$p < 0.0001$		$p = 0.0004$		$p < 0.0001$		0 = 0.0001		$p = 0.0490$	
Polio type 2	83/103 (81%)	40/103 (39%)	46/98 (47%)	71/94 (76%)	23/93 (25%)	36/91 (40%)	87/94 (93%)	87/92 (95%)	19/89 (21%)	16/83 (19%)	82/89 (92%)	79/84 (94%)
	$p < 0.0001$		$p < 0.0001$		$p = 0.0312$		$p = 0.5765$		$p = 0.7360$		$p = 0.6207$	
Polio type 3	36/104 (35%)	29/103 (28%)	48/98 (49%)	82/94 (87%)	27/93 (29%)	37/91 (41%)	75/94 (80%)	90/92 (98%)	18/88 (20%)	12/83 (14%)	74/88 (84%)	79/84 (94%)
	$p < 0.3167$		$p = < 0.0001$		$p = 0.0978$		$p = 0.0001$		$p = 0.3028$		$p = 0.0373$	

tion, 89% of the infants in both groups had neutralizing antibodies to poliovirus type 2, and virtually all infants had such antibodies from the second vaccination onwards. For poliovirus type 1, 77/98 (79%) OPV recipients and 94/94 (100%) EIPV recipients were seropositive after the second vaccination ($p < 0.0001$), and 80/94 (85%) OPV recipients and 92/92 (100%) EIPV recipients had neutralizing antibodies ≥ 1 : 8 after the third vaccination ($p < 0.0001$). For poliovirus type 3, 72/98 (73%) OPV recipients and 91/94 (97%) EIPV recipients were seropositive after the second ($p < 0.0001$) and 81/94 (86%) OPV recipients and 92/92 (100%) EIPV recipients after the third vaccination ($p = 0.0002$).

Infants at risk were defined as those having a neutralizing antibody titre < 1 : 4 (Table IV). Using this definition, only a few infants were seronegative to poliovirus type 2 starting from the first vaccination onwards. In contrast, about 10% of the infants in the OPV group remained seronegative to poliovirus type

Table IV. *Infants at risk, i.e. infants with neutralizing antibodies less than 1 : 4 to poliovirus types 1, 2 and 3 after immunization with OPV or EIPV at 2, 4 and 6 months of age and at 9 months with OPV*

No. (%) seronegative/No. tested

	2 months base line		3 months post 1		5 months post 2		7 months post 3		12 months post 4(OPV)	
	OPV	EIPV	OPV	EIPV	OPV	EIPV	OPV	EIPV	OPV	EIPV
Polio type 1	15/109 (14%)	8/108 (7%)	12/105 (11%)	0/103 (0)	9/98 (9%)	0/94 (0)	8/94 (9%)	0/92 (0)	2/89 (2%)	0/84 (0)
	$p = 0.1284$		$p = 0.0004$		$p = 0.0026$		$p = 0.0042$		$p = 0.1670$	
Polio type 2	9/109 (8%)	10/108 (9%)	2/103 (2%)	0/103 (0)	2/98 (2%)	1/94 (1%)	1/94 (1%)	0/92 (0)	0/89 (0)	0/84 (0)
	$p = 0.7939$		$p = 0.1553$		$p = 0.5853$		$p = 0.3212$			
Polio type 3	37/109 (34%)	31/108 (29%)	35/104 (34%)	14/103 (14%)	19/98 (19%)	2/94 (2%)	10/94 (11%)	0/92 (0)	4/88 (5%)	2/84 (2%)
	$p = 0.4053$		$p = 0.0007$		$p = 0.0001$		$p = 0.0013$		$p = 0.4393$	

1 between 3 and 7 months. For poliovirus type 3, 34% were negative at 3 months, 19% at 5, and 11% at 7 months of age, respectively. In the EIPV group, no infant was seronegative to poliovirus type 1 after the age of 3 months. For poliovirus type 3, only 2% of the infants were seronegative at 5 months and none at 7 months of age (Table IV).

EIPV induced significantly higher levels of neutralizing antibodies than OPV to poliovirus types 1 and 3, starting from the second dose of vaccine (Table II). For poliovirus type 2, the GMT of neutralizing antibodies was higher in the OPV group after the first and second dose of vaccine, but thereafter the GMT in the EIPV group was higher than in the OPV group also for type 2.

Between 7 and 12 months of age, in which time frame a fourth dose of OPV was administered at 9 months of age, 45% of the infants in the OPV group had a significant response to poliovirus type 1, as compared with 17% in the EIPV group (who also received OPV at 9 months). About 20% of the infants responded to each of poliovirus type 2 and 3. At 12 months of age, 2% of the infants in the OPV group were seronegative (titre < 1:4) to poliovirus type 1 and 5% were seronegative to poliovirus type 3. The GMTs to all 3 poliovirus types were higher in the EIPV than in the OPV group also at 12 months of age, after all vaccinees had received an additional dose of OPV (Table II).

DISCUSSION

As observed in this study, a routine immunization programme consisting of 3 doses of OPV leaves many infants in developing countries susceptible to polioviruses, particularly to serotypes 1 and 3 (1–3, 14). In poliomyelitis outbreaks in developing countries, most of the cases occur in infants <1 year of age (16).

The reason for the poor 'take' of poliovirus vaccine types 1 and 3 appears to be the dominant role of poliovirus type 2, which has a suppressing effect on other poliovirus vaccine types in OPV (14). A balanced '10:1:3' formulation of OPV increases the 'take' of poliovirus types 1 and 3, but even with this combination an immunity gap to poliovirus types 1 and 3 may persist in fully immunized infants (15).

The WHO now recommends immunization at 6, 10 and 14 weeks; this new EPI schedule may, however, be less than optimal for the 'take' of all OPV types (15). In the present study the interval between doses was 2 months, which is the standard immunization schedule in Thailand, and probably favours the 'take' of the 'sensitive' poliovirus types 1 and 3. Nevertheless, a significant proportion of infants remained susceptible to these poliovirus types after 3 doses of OPV.

Presence of immunity was defined in the study in two ways. First, possession of neutralizing antibodies at a titre 1:8 was regarded as indicative of protective immunity; this cut-off point has been previously used in many other studies on poliovirus vaccines (15). Antibody titre 1:4 was regarded as borderline, and titre levels < 1:4 were considered negative. Using this conservative definition for lack of protective antibody, 9% and 11% of the infants remained susceptible to poliovirus types 1 and 3, respectively, after a full immunization course of three doses of OPV. When a cut-off point of 1:8 was applied, the proportions of infants remaining seronegative for types 1 and 3 were 14% and 15%, respectively. Although the biological significance of this immunity gap is not clear, its presence indicates that an immunization course of 3 doses of OPV, even if spaced 2 months apart, is not fully satisfactory in Thai infants.

A fourth dose of OPV at 9 months of age significantly helped to close the immunity gap to poliovirus type 1. Antibody levels to poliovirus type 2 were already high, and a fourth dose had no effect on these. The effect on poliovirus type 3 antibodies was also minimal. The reason for preferential boosting of type 1 immunity at this stage might be previously induced immunity to types 2 and 3, which blocks the multiplication of these poliovirus types and favours multiplication of type 1. The results of giving a fourth dose of OPV were actually better in this study than in a recent study in Cote d'Ivoire (6). Administration of a fourth dose of OPV at the time of measles immunization is logistically simple and requires only a small increment in cost. Therefore, a fourth dose of OPV may be recommended to improve poliovirus immunity, particularly for type 1 in countries far from achieving complete eradication of paralytic poliomyelitis (6).

An enhanced potency IPV might form an alternative to continued use of OPV even in developing countries (2, 3, 17), provided that the cost of EIPV can be brought down to a level comparable to that of OPV. The first step in this direction is a combined EIPV plus DTP vaccine. EIPV offers the obvious advantage of stability and lack of side effects. With the decreasing incidence of wild virus-associated poliomyelitis in many developing countries, greater attention will be paid to the occurrence of cases associated with OPV. This may increase pressure to incorporate EIPV into national vaccination programmes at a stage when the number of cases of poliomyelitis becomes very small.

Considering merely protection of the individual, EIPV in its present form offers a serious alternative. In this study, with the use of EIPV a 100% protective immunity to poliovirus types 1 and 2 was achieved by 3 months and to type 3 by 7 months of age. Furthermore, the neutralizing antibody levels to all 3 poliovirus types, and particularly to types 1 and 3, were significantly higher in the EIPV than in the OPV group.

EIPV is known to induce less intestinal immunity than OPV (9, 18) and may therefore not be sufficient for eradication of poliomyelitis in endemic areas (3). However, the moment of EIPV may arrive when eradication is near completion and vaccine safety receives first priority. Furthermore, EIPV could become part of mixed immunization schedules also in developing countries (5). In the present study, 3 doses of EIPV were followed by 1 dose of OPV, and many infants had a significnat rise in their already high serum neutralizing antibody titres following this dose of OPV. It can be speculated that a dose of OPV may also have improved the intestinal immunity of the recipient children previously immunized with EIPV (8, 18). Therefore, the immunization schedule used in the present study, consisting of EIPV combined with DTP and followed by OPV at the time of measles vaccination, might also be considered for routine childhood immunization schedule in Thailand and comparable countries.

ACKNOWLEDGMENTS

We thank Ms. Tuija Poussa, M.Sc., for statistical analysis.

The study was financially supported by the Diarrhoeal Diseases Control Programme, WHO.

REFERENCES

1. Wright PF, Kim-Farley RJ, de Quadros CA, Robertson SE, Scott RM, Ward NA, Henderson RH. Strategies for the global eradication of poliomyelitis by the year 2000. N Engl J Med 335: 1774–1779, 1991.
2. Lemon SM, Robertson SE. Global eradication of poliomyelitis: recent progress, future prospects and new research priorities. In: Melnick JL, ed. Basel, Karger: Prog Med Virol 38: 42–55, 1991.
3. Hovi T. Remaining problems before eradication of poliomyelitis can be accomplished. In: Melnick JL, ed. Basel, Karger: Prog Med Virol 38: 69–95, 1991.
4. Strebel PM, Sutter RW, Cochi SL. Epidemiology of poliomyelitis in the Unites States one decade after the last reported case of indigenous wild virus-associated disease. Clin Infect Dis 14: 568–579, 1992.
5. Faden H. Poliovirus vaccination: a trilogy. J Infect Dis 168; 25–28, 1993

6. Moriniere BJ, van Loon FPL, Rhodes PH, Klein-Zappan M-L, Frank-Senat B, Herrington JE, Pallansch MA, Patriarca PA. Immunogenicity of a supplemental dose of oral versus inactivated poliovirus vaccine. Lancet 341: 1545–1550, 1993.
7. Salk D, van Wezel AL, Salle J. Induction of long term immunity to paralytic poliomyelitis by use of non-infectious vaccine. Lancet 2: 1317–1321, 1984.
8. McBean AM, Thomas ML, Albrecht P, Cuthie JC, Bernier R, The Field Staff and Coordinating Committee. Serological response to oral polio vaccine and enhanced-potency inactivated polio vaccines. Am J Epidemiol 128: 615–628, 1988.
9. Faden H, Hodlin JF, Thomas ML, McBean AM, Ferdon MB, Ogra PL. Comparative evaluation of immunization with live attenuated and enhanced potency inactivated trivalent poliovirus vaccines in childhood: systemic and local immune responses. J Infect Dis 163: 1291–1297, 1990.
10. Tulchinsky T, Abed Y, Shaheen S, Toubassi N, Sever Y, Schoenbaum N, Handsher R. A ten-year experience in control of poliomyelitis through a combination of live and killed vaccines in two developing areas. Am J Public Health 79: 1648–652, 1989.
11. Migasena S, Simasathien S, Samakoses R, Pittisuttitham P, Sangaroon P, van Steenis G, Beuvery EC, Bugg H, Bishop R, Davidson BL, Vesikari T. Simultaneous administration of oral rhesus-human reassortant tetravalent (RRV-TV) rotavirus vaccine and oral poliovirus vaccine (OPV) in Thai infants. Vaccine [in press]
12. van der Marel P, Hazendonk AG, van Wezel AL. D-antigen determination in polio vaccine production: comparison of gel diffusion and ELISA methods. Dev Biol Stand 47: 101–108, 1981.
13. Albrecht P, van Steenis G, van Wezel AL, Salk J. Standardization of poliovirus neutralizing antibody tests. Rev Infect Dis 6: S540–544, 1984.
14. Rümke HC, Schlumberger M, Flowry B, Nagel J, van Steenis B. Serological evalutation of a simplified immunization schedule using quadruple DPT-polio vaccine in Burkina Faso. Vaccine 11: 1113–1118, 1993.
15. Patriarca PA, Wright PF, John TJ. Factors affecting the immunogenicity of oral poliovirus vaccine in developing countries: review. Rev Infect Dis 13: 926–939, 1991.
16. Robertson SE, Oostvogel P. Poliomyelitis outbreaks, 1978–1988. Presented at the WHO consultation of the Eradication of poliomyelitis, Geneva, 12–14 September 1989. Document WHO/EPI/POLIO/WP89.9/SEPT.
17. Robertson SE, Traverso HP, Drucker JA, Rovira EZ, Fabre-Teste B, Sow A, N'Diaye M, Sy MTA, Diouf F. Clinical efficacy of a new, enhanced-potency, inactivated poliovirus vaccine. Lancet 1: 897–899, 1988.
18. Onorato IM, Modlin JF, McBean AM, Thoms ML, Losonsky GA, Bernier RH. Mucosal immunity induced by enhanced-potency inactivated and oral polio vaccines. J Infect Dis 163: 1–6, 1991.

Submitted July 5, 1994; accepted September 7, 1994

Scand J Infect Dis 26: 739–747, 1994

Efficacy of a Polyvalent Inactivated-virus Vaccine in Protecting Mice from Infection with Clinical Strains of Group B Coxsackieviruses

DARRYL M. SEE and JEREMIAH G. TILLES

From the Division of Infectious Diseases, Department of Medicine, U.C. Irvine Medical Center, Orange, California, USA

A polyvalent vaccine developed from formalin-inactivated prototype strains of coxsackieviruses group B1–6 was tested for its ability to protect mice from acute infection with clinical strains. Adolescent male CD1 mice received an intraperitoneal injection, repeated once or twice at 8 day intervals, containing 0.3 ml placebo or vaccine. Eight days after the final dose of vaccine, groups of 4 mice were challenged with 1×10^4 plaque-forming units of a test strain of group B coxsackievirus, and killed 3 days later. The mean neutralizing antibody titers for the 29 strains tested (4 mice/strain, $\log_2$) were 2.2 ± 0.6, 3.3 ± 0.9 or 6.4 ± 1.7 after 1, 2 or 3 doses of vaccine, respectively. In mice receiving 2 or 3 doses of vaccine, titers of virus were significantly lower in the pancreas and/or blood in 7/14 or 14/15 strains, respectively, compared to unvaccinated infected controls. Uninfected, vaccinated mice failed to develop islet cell autoantibodies, histopathological abnormalities in the pancreas, or evidence of viral RNA in the pancreas 12 weeks after 3 doses of vaccine. Thus, prophylaxis with a polyvalent, inactivated-virus vaccine reduced the severity of acute infection with clinical strains of coxsackie group B viruses. A schedule of 3 doses of vaccine was superior to 1 or 2 doses.

G. Tilles, MD, Division of Infectious Diseases, Department of Medicine, U.C. Irvine Medical Center, 101 S. City Dr. Orange, CA 92668, USA

INTRODUCTION

The enterovirus family includes the polioviruses (3 types), coxsackie group A (23 serotypes) and B (6 serotypes) viruses, echoviruses (30 serotypes), 4 unclassified serotypes (Enteroviruses 68–71) and hepatitis A virus. The enteroviruses are responsible for a variety of clinical syndromes, including exanthemas, respiratory tract infections, myopericarditis, pancreatitis, aseptic meningitis, poliomyelitis and hepatitis (1). Evidence also supports a role for these viruses in some cases of idiopathic dilated cardiomyopathy (2, 3), juvenile dermatomyositis (4), juvenile-onset diabetes mellitus (5, 6) and chronic fatigue syndrome (7).

Serological and viral isolation studies of 5–10% of the population in the US infected each year have shown that enterovirus infections in the general population are extremely common (8). Infections are especially common in children; up to 20% of the population under the age of 10 are infected with at least 1 enterovirus each month during the peak season from July through September (9). Infections are more common in the lower socioeconomic groups (10). The group B coxsackieviruses (CVB) accounted for approximately 25% of all enterovirus isolates from 1970 to 1983 in one large epidemiological study (11). Another recent study suggested that 48% of cases of aseptic meningitis in infants were caused by CVB infection (12). As with all enteroviruses, most CVB infections are benign and self limited, and up to 50–80% are asymptomatic (13). However, symptomatic disease may account for significant morbidity and loss of productivity in the normal population. In addition, mortality from disseminated or overwhelming infection can occur in newborn and immunocompromised patients (14).

To estimate the total clinical impact of CVB infections one needs to consider not only the manifestations of acute infection but also the various long term complications associated with the postulated chronic sequelae. Thus, idiopathic dilated cardiomyopathy is the most common indication for heart transplantation in the US and a leading cause of sudden death syndrome (15). Furthermore, type I diabetes mellitus has a prevalence of 0.6–2.5/1000 population in the US (16), and is associated with various complications including ketoacidosis, blindness, atherosclerotic heart disease and end-stage renal failure. In addition, a recent study of chronic fatigue syndrome revealed a prevalence of 4.6 to 11.3 per 100.000 population in the US (17). Significant morbidity and loss of productivity are also associated with this order.

Mice challenged with a myocardiotropic strain of CVB3 (RD) were protected from infection by a monovalent vaccine (18). In the present study, an inactivated-virus vaccine that was polyvalent for all 6 serotypes of CVB protected mice from acute infection with 29 clinical strains. In addition, the vaccine was not associated with subsequent autoimmune pancreatic disease.

MATERIAL AND METHODS

Virus and cells: 25 clinical isolates of coxsackieviruses groups B1–5 were obtained from David Schnurr of the California Department of Health Services. Three isolates of CVB6 were obtained from the Centers for Disease Control, Atlanta, Georgia, courtesy of Mark Pallansch. The viruses were isolated from patients of various ages presenting with symptoms such as headache, sore throat, rash and/or fever. All strains had been isolated from samples of pharyngeal wash, feces or cerebrospinal fluid. The viruses had been passaged in primary monkey kidney (MK) cells a maximum of 6 times and a median of 3 times prior to receipt. They were further passaged once or twice in our laboratory in MK cells, which were maintained through 70 to 80 serial laboratory passages. Confluent monolayers of MK cells in 75 cm^2 tissue culture flasks were inoculated with virus at a multiplicity of infection of 1 pfu per cell in Leibovitz's L15 medium supplemented with 420 μg glutamine, 420 μg arginine, 240 μg benzyl penicillin, 40 μg streptomycin and 400 μg dextrose per 1 ml (19). After adsorption of the virus for 60 min at 37°C, fetal bovine serum (FBS) was added to a final concentration of 10% and incubation continued for another 24–96 h, after which the virus-containing medium was harvested. The origin and preparation of CVB4 strain E2 has been described previously (20). Prototype strains of CVB1 (Conn), B2 (Ohio), B3 (Nancy), B4 (JVB), B5 (Faulkner) and B6 (Schmidt) were obtained from the American Type Culture Collection (Rockville, Maryland), and further passaged a maximum of 3 times in MK cells. All samples were frozen at −80°C prior to use. Virus titers were determined on monolayers of MK cells using the plaque technique (19).

Vaccine: Each prototype strain of virus was absorbed to monolayers of MK cells in 5 75 cm^2 tissue culture flasks at a multiplicity of 1 pfu per cell and incubated as described. When maximal cytopathic effect was observed, the virus-containing media for a single strain were harvested and pooled. Aliquots of 0.7 ml were frozen at −80°C for virus titer determination. The lots for the virus strains has the following titers in pfu/ml: 1.2×10^5 (CVB1), 9.6×10^4 (CVB2), 3.6×10^5 (CVB3), 9.0×10^4 (CVB4), 4.8×10^5 (CVB5) and 9.2×10^4 (CVB6). The 6 prototype lots were combined in equal proportions, incubated at 37°C for 3 days in a 1:3000 solution of formalin (pH 3.8; final concentration 3.7 mM; certified ACS grade; Fisher, Tustin, CA) and centrifuged at 1000 × g for 15 min. The supernatants were centrifuged in a Beckman L-3 ultracentrifuge at 20,000 × g for 20 min. The new supernatant was centrifuged at 105,000 × g for 7 h. The resulting pellet was resuspended in 10 ml L15 diluent, vortexed for 5 min, and stored at −80°C. An undiluted aliquot failed to form plaques on MK cell monolayers.

Mice: 4–5 week old male CD1 mice were obtained from Charles Rivers Farms, Wilmington, Mass.

Experimental design: Blood was collected from the tail vein of test mice in 250 μl heparinized hematocrit tubes, centrifuged at 8000 × g for 15 min, and the plasma frozen at −80°C. Each animal then received an intraperitoneal injection of 0.3 ml of either placebo (L15 diluent) or vaccine containing a live virus equivalent in pfu of 6×10^3 (CVB1), 4.8×10^3 (CVB2), 1.8×10^4 (CVB3), 4.5×10^3 (CVB4), 2.4×10^3 (CVB5) and 4.6×10^3 (CVB6). Eight days later (day 8), plasma samples were again collected, and the mice received a second intraperitoneal dose of placebo or vaccine. On day 16, after plasma was obtained, groups of mice were challenged intraperitoneally with either 0.1 ml containing 1×10^4 pfu of a live test virus strain or a third dose of vaccine or placebo. On day 24, those mice which had received a third dose of vaccine received their challenge with a test virus. Three days post-inoculation (p.i) of active virus, mice were anesthetized with methoxyfluorane and killed by exsanguination via cardiac puncture. Serum and tissue were collected for further studies. Groups of placebo or vaccine-treated, uninfected mice were killed 12 weeks after the third dose.

Processing of specimens

Neutralizing antibody titration: Following initial incubation of plasma samples at 56°C for 30 min, serial 2-fold dilutions of plasma in L15 diluent (0.025 ml aliquots) were incubated for 1 h at room temperature with an equal volume containing 100 $TCID_{50}$ (tissue culture infectious dose) of either prototype or test virus in L15 diluent. The solutions were then applied to 96-well microtiter plates containing confluent monolayers of MK cells grown for 48 h in supplemented L15 medium with 10% FBS. Control wells contained virus or medium only or serial 2 fold dilutions of plasma or standard antibody. Following incubation at 37°C for 1 h to permit absorption of virus, 150 μl of supplemented L15 medium was added to each well. The plates were then covered by perforated sealers and incubated at 37°C. The monolayers were observed daily for cytopathic effect (cpe) until cpe reached 4+ in the virus control. At that time the neutralizing titer was expressed as the reciprocal of the highest dilution of serum that inhibited cpe by 90%.

Virus assay: For each mouse, a portion of pancreas was weighed aseptically, homogenized in supplemented L15 diluent, and assayed for virus by the plaque technique described previously (19). Aliquots (0.1 ml) of blood were similarly processed and assayed for virus (19).

Histopathology: Portions of pancreatic tissue were fixed in 37% formalin, imbedded in paraffin, cut in 6 μm sections with a microtome, mounted and stained with hematoxylin and eosin. The severity of pancreatic inflammation was scored blindly on a scale of 1+ to 4+. A 1+ score indicated inflammation (predominately mononuclear cells with occasional granulocytes and local tissue necrosis) involving < 10% of the section, a 2+ score reflected 10–50% of the section with inflammation, a 3+ score denoted 50–90% of the section with inflammation, and a 4+ score indicated > 90% of the section with inflammation.

Islet cell autoantibody titers: Plasma from uninfected mice 12 weeks after a third dose of vaccine were assayed for autoantibody titers to islet cells from 4–5-wk-old normal CD1 mice, with an indirect immunofluorescence test using fluorescein-labelled goat anti-mouse IgG as previously described (20). Plasma from animal 7 weeks after inoculation with the diabetogenic strain CVB4 (strain E2) served as a positive control (20).

Presence of enteroviral RNA: The presence of enteroviral nucleic acid segments in pancreas tissue of uninfected animals 12 weeks after the third sequential vaccine dose was sought using polymerase chain reaction (PCR) amplification with enterovirus-specific primers as previously described (20). Pancreas tissue from mice neither vaccinated nor infected, or from unvaccinated mice 3 days after infection were used as negative and positive controls, respectively. Dot-blot hybridization with an enterovirus-specific probe was used to confirm the presence of enterovirus-specific sequences in the PCR products as previously described (20).

Statistics: Geometric means were calculated for virus and neutralizing antibody titers and compared with the Wilcoxon ranked sum test (21). The difference between histological gradings was evaluated with the Kruskal-Wallis test (21).

RESULTS

Induction of antibody (Table I)

To demonstrate the success of the vaccine in stimulating a specific antibody response in mice, serial determinations of neutralizing antibody to a specific clinical strain were made in the 4 mice to be challenged with that strain. In addition, serial determinations of neutralizing antibody to each prototype strain of virus were made in groups of 4 mice that were to be followed without viral challenge. Thus, means for each strain were calculated for neutralizing antibody titer in plasma obtained from 4 mice 8 days after each dose of vaccine. Baseline mean neutralizing antibody titer to each strain was $<3(\log_2)$. Eight days after the initial vaccine administration, a modest rise in titer to all prototype strains was recorded (mean mean

Table I. *Neutralizing antibody titers to prototype and clinical strains of coxsackie group B viruses after each dose of vaccine*

Strain	Neutalizing antibody titer mean ($\log_2 \pm$ SD) No. vaccine doses 1	2	3
Clinical			
2 vaccine doses:			
CVB1/Rog	<3	3.4 ± 0.5	
CVB1/Mas	3.5 ± 1.4	4.5 ± 1.7	
CVB2/Mart	<3	2.9 ± 0.7	
CVB2/How	<3	3.6 ± 0.9	
CVB2/Linc	<3	<3	
CVB23/Poir	<3	5.7 ± 1.9	
CVB3/Red	<3	<3	
CVB4/Mej	<3	2.8 ± 1.1	
CVB4/Ale	<3	<3	
CVB4/Mir	<3	3.1 ± 0.7	
CVB5/Bon	<3	5.1 ± 2.1	
CVB5/Greg	<3	3.7 ± 1.0	
CVB6/017	<3	<3	
CVB6/139	<3	3.4 ± 0.9	
3 vaccine doses:			
CVB1/Dix	<3	<3	7.4 ± 2.3
CVB1/Low	<3	<3	4.4 ± 1.7
CVB1/Bell	3.1 ± 1.1	5.1 ± 2.3	8.7 ± 2.7
CVB2/mal	<3	3.4 ± 0.9	6.4 ± 2.4
CVB2/Krahl	<3	2.9 ± 0.7	5.4 ± 1.7
CVB3/Oliv	3.1 ± 1.3	5.1 ± 2.9	8.8 ± 3.1
CVB3/Cole	<3	3.5 ± 1.5	4.1 ± 1.7
CVB4/Per	<3	3.7 ± 1.1	7.3 ± 1.8
CVB4/Stew	<3	<3	5.8 ± 2.1
CVB4/E2	<3	3.5 ± 1.3	7.2 ± 2.9
CVB5/Free	<3	<3	4.2 ± 1.3
CVB5/Mitch	3.6 ± 1.3	5.4 ± 1.6	9.7 ± 3.1
CVB5/May	<3	4.1 ± 1.4	8.3 ± 2.6
CVB5/Gil	<3	<3	<3
CVB6/025	<3	3.3 ± 0.8	5.9 ± 1.8
Prototype			
CVB1/Conn	3.6 ± 0.8	5.6 ± 1.2	8.9 ± 2.1
CVB2/Ohio	4.1 ± 0.9	6.4 ± 1.8	11.3 ± 3.5
CVB3/Nancy	4.5 ± 1.2	7.1 ± 2.1	10.2 ± 3.3
CVB4/JVB	3.4 ± 0.9	5.3 ± 1.8	8.9 ± 2.7
CVB5/Faulk	3.8 ± 1.1	6.0 ± 1.9	10.7 ± 3.2
CVB6/Schm	4.0 ± 1.3	6.0 ± 2.1	10.9 ± 4.3

Titers < 3 were assigned a value of 2 for purposes of calculating the mean. Values represent the mean ± SD for 4 mice. Titers were determined 8 days after each dose. Baseline titers were <3 for each strain.

titer ± SD, 3.9 ± 0.3). Although a low titer was observed for 4/29 test strains, the mean mean ± SD for all 29 strains was only 2.2 ± 0.6. One booster injection prompted approximatley a 4-fold increase in antibodies to each of the 6 prototype strains (mean mean titer ± SD, 6.2 ± 0.4). At this time, antibodies were detectable for 20/29 clinical strains, with a mean mean ± SD for all 29 strains of 3.3 ± 0.9. A third dose of vaccine produced an additional 16-

or 8-fold rise in titer for each of the 6 prototype (mean mean ± SD, 10.2 ± 1.1) or 15 test strains (mean mean ± SD, 6.4 ± 1.7), respectively. After 3 vaccine doses there was no detectable antibody response to 1 of 15 test strains (CVB/Gilbert). Comparable mean mean titers were produced for the clinical strains of each of the 6 coxsackievirus types: 6.8 ± 2.2 (CVB1), 5.9 ± 2.0 (CVB2), 6.5 ± 2.2 (CVB3), 6.8 ± 0.7 (CVB4), 6.1 ± 2.3 (CVB5) and 5.9 ± 0.0 (CVB6).

Protection from acute infection with specific strains of CVB

Viral titers (Table II): To assess the ability of vaccination to limit challenge virus infection, titers of virus were determined in the pancreas and blood of mice killed 3 days p.i. Among the 29 clinical strains evaluated, 24/29 and 27/29 had detectable virus in the pancreas or

Table II. *Titers of coxsackie group B virus in the pancreas and blood of mice 3 days after inoculation of clinical strains*

	Titer ($\log_{10}$ pfu/mg tissue or ml blood)					
	Pancreas			Blood		
Strain	No Vaccine	Vaccine	p	No Vaccine	Vaccine	p
2 vaccine doses						
CVB1/Rog	4.0 ± 0.9	2.8 ± 0.8	NS	2.7 ± 0.6	<2	< 0.5
CVB1/Mas	5.5 ± 0.8	3.1 ± 1.0	< 0.05	2.6 ± 0.9	1.3 ± 0.3	NS
CVB2/Mart	<2	<2	—	2.4 ± 0.5	<2	NS
CVB2/How	<2	<2	—	3.1 ± 0.5	1.5 ± 0.4	<0.05
CVB2/Linc	<2	<2	—	3.4 ± 0.9	3.1 ± 1.0	NS
CVB3Poir	4.8 ± 0.8	2.2 ± 0.4	<0.05	2.4 ± 0.4	<2	NS
CVB3/Red	4.1 ± 0.8	3.9 ± 0.9	NS	<2	<2	—
CVB4/Mej	3.4 ± 0.8	2.2 ± 0.5	NS	3.2 ± 0.5	3.2 ± 0.7	NS
CVB4/Ale	5.4 ± 0.9	5.0 ± 1.2	NS	2.7 ± 0.9	2.3 ± 0.5	NS
CVB4/Mir	4.1 ± 0.7	3.0 ± 1.1	NS	2.3 ± 0.4	1.9 ± 0.7	NS
CVB5/Bon	4.3 ± 0.6	1.8 ± 0.9	<0.05	2.5 ± 0.4	<2	NS
CVB5/Greg	4.8 ± 0.8	2.0 ± 0.8	<0.05	2.7 ± 0.5	1.3 ± 0.3	<0.05
CVB6/017	4.6 ± 0.4	4.9 ± 0.9	NS	<2	<2	—
CVB139	5.7 ± 0.9	3.7 ± 1.1	<0.05	2.9 ± 0.9	2.0 ± 0.9	NS
3 vaccine doses						
CVB1/Dix	4.4 ± 0.7	<2	<0.05	3.2 ± 0.6	<2	<0.05
CVB1/Low	4.8 ± 0.6	1.2 ± 0.5	<0.05	3.1 ± 0.7	1.3 ± 0.5	<0.05
CVB1/Bell	3.7 ± 0.5	<2	<0.05	2.1 ± 0.5	<2	NS
CVB2/Mal	<2	<2	—	3.3 ± 0.3	<2	<0.05
CVB2/Krahl	3.1 ± 0.6	<2	<0.05	2.4 ± 0.7	<2	NS
CVB3/Oliv	4.9 ± 0.9	<2	<0.05	2.7 ± 0.6	<2	<0.05
CVB3/Cole	4.7 ± 0.8	1.7 ± 0.9	<0.05	3.8 ± 0.7	2.1 ± 0.7	<0.05
CVB4/Per	5.2 ± 0.7	<2	<0.05	3.6 ± 0.6	<2	<0.05
CVB4/Stew	3.3 ± 0.8	<2	<0.05	2.1 ± 0.5	<2	NS
CVB4/E2	4.6 ± 0.8	1.3 ± 0.6	<0.05	2.9 ± 0.7	<2	<0.05
CVB5/Free	4.8 ± 0.7	2.3 ± 0.8	<0.05	3.2 ± 0.8	1.2 ± 0.5	<0.05
CVB5/Mitch	5.0 ± 0.6	<2	<0.05	3.1 ± 0.5	1.4 ± 0.4	<0.05
CVB5/May	4.8 ± 0.8	<2	<0.05	2.9 ± 0.7	<2	<0.05
CVB5/Gil	4.1 ± 0.4	2.8 ± 1.0	NS	1.4 ± 0.5	<2	<0.05
CVB6/025	<2	<2	—	2.7 ± 0.6	<2	<0.05

Values represent the mean ± SD for 4 mice. Titers <2 were assigned a value of 1 for purposes of calculating the mean.

blood, respectively (sensitivity, 100 pfu mg of tissue or ml blood). 4/5 CVB2 strains failed to infect the pancreas at inocula as high as 1×10^4 pfu. Detectable titers in the pancreas were significantly reduced in vaccinated mice compared to controls for 4/11 strains after 2 doses, and for 12/13 strains after 3 doses. Measureable titers in the blood were significantly reduced for 3/12 strains after 2 doses and for 12/15 strains after 3 doses.

Histology (Table III): 3 days after viral inoculation, histological sections of the pancreas of test mice revealed inflammation with a predominately mononuclear cell infiltration in evey case, except for the same glands from which no active virus had been isolated. Detectable abnormalities were significantly reduced in sections of pancreas from mice infected with 3/11 strains after 2 doses of vaccine and 9/13 strains after 3 doses of vaccine.

Table III. *Histopathologic changes in the pancreas of mice 3 days after infection with clinical strains of coxsackie group B virus*

	Histology score										
	No vaccine					Vaccine					
Strain	0	1+	2+	3+	4+	0	1+	2+	3+	4+	*p*
2 vaccine doses											
CVB1/Rog	0	1	2	1	0	1	2	1	0	0	NS
CVB1/Mas	0	0	1	2	1	0	4	0	0	0	<0.05
CVB2/Mart	4	0	0	0	0	4	0	0	0	0	—
CVB2/How	4	0	0	0	0	4	0	0	0	0	—
CVB2/Linc	4	0	0	0	0	4	0	0	0	0	—
CVB3/Poir	0	0	1	2	1	0	2	1	1	0	NS
CVB3/Red	0	0	0	2	2	0	0	2	1	1	NS
CVB4/Mej	0	1	2	1	0	0	1	1	2	0	NS
CVB4/Ale	0	0	0	0	4	0	0	0	0	4	NS
CVB4/Mir	0	0	0	2	2	0	2	2	0	0	<0.05
CVB5/Bon	0	0	1	2	1	0	1	2	1	0	NS
CVB5/Greg	0	0	3	1	0	1	2	1	0	0	NS
CVB6/017	0	0	2	2	0	0	0	1	3	0	NS
CVB6/139	0	0	0	0	4	0	2	2	0	0	<0.05
3 vaccine doses											
CVB1/Dix	0	0	2	2	0	4	0	0	0	0	<0.05
CVB1/Low	0	0	0	3	1	2	2	0	0	0	<0.05
CVB1/Bell	0	1	2	1	1	4	0	0	0	0	<0.05
CVB2/Mal	4	0	0	0	0	4	0	0	0	0	—
CVB2/Krahl	1	2	1	0	0	4	0	0	0	0	NS
CVB3/Oliv	0	0	0	1	3	3	1	0	0	0	<0.05
CVB3/Cole	0	0	0	2	2	0	1	1	1	1	NS
CVB4/Per	0	0	0	2	2	4	0	0	0	0	<0.05
CVB4/Stew	0	0	2	1	1	4	0	0	0	0	<0.05
CVB4/E2	0	0	2	2	0	3	1	0	0	0	<0.05
CVB5/Free	0	1	0	1	2	0	1	3	0	0	NS
CVB5/Mitch	0	0	0	0	4	4	0	0	0	0	<0.05
CVB5/May	0	0	1	1	2	2	2	0	0	0	<0.05
CVB5/Gil	0	0	2	1	1	0	1	2	1	0	NS
CVB6/025	4	0	0	0	0	4	0	0	0	0	—

Formalin-fixed sections of pancreas were stained with hematoxylin and eosin, and scored for inflammation (see Methods). 0: no inflammation 1+: inflammation involving < 10% of the section 2+: 10–50% of the section with inflammation 3+: 50–90% with inflammation 4+: 90% with inflammation.

Detection of long-term effects of vaccination on the pancreas

It was not possible to isolate active virus from pooled pancreata of 10 uninfected mice killed 12 weeks after inoculation with the vaccine (sensitivity 5 pfu mg). In none of the 10 mice were there histophathologic changes in the pancreas, islet cell autoantibodies in the plasma (indirect immunofluorescence test; sensitivity, 3[$\log_2$]), or evidence of viral RNA in the pancreas (PCR; sensitivity, 20 pfu/mg).

DISCUSSION

Infections with CVB are common in the general populations, particularly in the young (22). Although many cases are subclinical, symptomatic infections frequently occur. They can be associated with significant morbidity and even mortality in some groups. Many investigators have suggested associations of these viruses with chronic, life-threatening illnesses such as idiopathic dilated cardiomyopathy and juvenile-onset diabetes mellitus (23, 24). Since there are only 6 serotypes, prevention of infection with these viruses with a polyvalent vaccine may be feasible.

Like all enteroviruses, CVB are ultimately cytolytic. Host gastrointestinal mucosal cells which actively replicate and release viral particles soon lose their intregrity. The virus is then in a mandatory extracellular phase, when it is potentially vulnerable to neutralizing antibodies in the interstitial fluid and blood that could block infection of susceptible cells in other organs. Therefore, specific systemic antibodies induced by a parenteral vaccine prior to exposure to live virus might be effective in minimizing primary infection. A simple approach with inactivated whole virus may warrant a trial based upon the success of the trivalent, inactivated poliovirus vaccine (25). We have shown that inoculation of mice with a vaccine produced from formalin-inactivated prototype strains of coxsackievirus group B1–6 induced neutralizing antibodies to, and protection from challenge with, clinical strains.

In vaccinated mice, mean neutralizing antibody titers to the clinical strains were approximately 8–20-fold lower than to the prototype strains. Nevertheless, the titers generated after 3 doses were sufficient to significantly reduce acute infection, as manifested by culturable virus in blood or pancreas after challenge inoculation with 14 of the 15 clinical strains tested.

Histopathological abnormalities in the pancreas were also clearly limited by administration of the vaccine. Antibody response after 2 doses of vaccine was also sufficient to limit acute infection in animals infected with 7 of the 14 clinical strains tested.

Previous studies in humans and animals have suggested that infection with some strains of CVB may trigger autoimmune islets inflammation (26, 27). Significant amino acid homology has been reported between the P2-C protein of CVB4 and glutamate decarboxylase, an enzyme present in islet cells (28). In the present study, neither islet cell autoantibody production nor pancreatic histopathological abnormalities could be demonstrated 12 weeks after 3 sequential doses of vaccine.

Naturally occurring antigenic variants within CVB serotypes occur frequently (29). Similar variants have been demonstrated within the 3 poliovirus serotypes (30). Furthermore, clinical CVB strains vary in their capacity to infect specific cell types (18, 31). One study demonstrated that neutralizing antibody titers produced in mice after challenge with 1 CVB4 strain were 20-fold greater to the challenge strain than to the prototype CVB4 virus (JVB) (32). The results of the present study suggest significant cross-protection in mice by antibodies to the vaccine prototypes and those clinical strains of CVB tested. Different approaches to vaccine production, including the use of adjuvants, development of attenuated live viruses, preparation of purified antigens, and variations in the route of delivery, may reduce the need for multiple inoculations to stimulate protective levels of antibody. Further studies are needed to determine if cross-protection can be demonstrated for a greater number of clinical strains, and to determine the duration of protection after immunization. The results of this study support the notion that a polyvalent vaccine may also have the potential in humans to prevent infection by clinical strains of CVB.

ACKNOWLEDGEMENT

The technical assistance of Ramona Leanos is greatly appreciated.

REFERENCES

1. Pallansch MA. Epidemiology of group B coxsackieviruses. In: Bendinelli M, Friedman H, eds. Coxsackieviruses – a general update. New York: Plenum Press, 399–416, 1988
2. Kandolf R, Hofschneider PH. Viral hear disease. Springer Semin Immunopathol 11: 1–13, 1989
3. Bowles NE, Olsen EGJ, Richardson PJ, Archard LC. Detection of coxsackie-B-virus-specific RNA sequences in myocardial biopsy samples from patients with myocarditis and dilated cardiomyopathy. Lancet 1: 1120–1123, 1986
4. Christensen ML, Pachman LM, Schneiderman R, Patel DC, Friedman JM. Prevalence of coxsackie group B virus antibodies in patients with juvenile dermatomyositis. Arthritis Rheum 29: 1365–1370, 1986
5. Cudsworth AG, Gamble DR, White GBB, Lendrum R, Woodrow JC, Bloom A. Aetiology of jevenile-onset diabetes. A prospective study. Lancet 1: 385–388, 1977
6. Frisk G, Friman G, Tuvemao T, Fohlman J, Diderholm H. Coxsackie B virus IgM in children at onset of type 1 (insulin-dependent) diabetes mellitus: evidence for IgM induction by a recent or current infection. Diabetologia 35: 249–253, 1992
7. Yousef GE, Man GF, Smith DG, Bell EJ, Murugesan V, McCartney RA, Mowbray JF. Chronic enterovirus infection in patients with postviral fatigue syndrome. Lancet 1: 146–150, 1988
8. Moore M, Morens DM. Enteroviruses, including polioviruses. In: Belshe RB, ed. Textbook of Human Virology, PSG, Littleton, Massachusetts: 407–488, 1984
9. Melnick JL. Enteroviruses. In: Evans AS, ed. Viral Infections of Humans, Epidemiology and Control. New York: Plenum, 187–251, 1982
10. Melnick JL. Enteroviruses: Polioviruses, coxsackieviruses, echoviruses, and newer enteroviruses. In: Fields BN, Knipe Dm, Chanock RM, Melnick JL, Roixman B, Shope RE, eds. Virology. New York: Raven, 739–784, 1985
11. Strikas RA, Anderson LJ, Parker RA. Temporal and geographic patterns of isolates of nonpolio enteroviruses in the United States, 1970–1983. J Infect Dis 153: 346–51, 1986
12. Berlin LE. Diagnosis and etiology of aseptic meningitis in infants less than two years of age. J Infect Dis 168: 888–892, 1993
13. Kogon A, Spigland I, Frothingham TE. The virus watch program. A continuing surveillance of viral infections in metropolitan New York families. Am J Epidemiol 89: 51–65, 1969
14. Porres ER, Werthammer J, Moss N, Bernstein JM, Belshe RB. Fatal coxsackievirus B4 infection in a neonate. South Med J 78: 1254–1256, 1985
15. See DM, Tilles JG. Viral myocarditis. Rev Infect Dis 13: 951–956, 1991
16. LaPorte RE, Tajima N. Prevalence of insulin-dependent diabetes. In: National Diabetes Data group, Diabetes in America. NIH publication no. 85-1468. Washington DC: US Dept. of Health and Human Services, V-1–8, 1985
17. Gun WJ, Connell DB, Randall B. Epidemiology of chronic fatigue syndrome: The Center for Disease Control study. Ciba foundation Symposium 173: 83–93, 1993
18. Fohlman J, Pauksen K, Morein B, Bjare U, Ilbäck NG, Friman G. High yield production of an inactivated coxsackie B3 adjuvant vaccine with protective effective against experimental myocarditis. Scand J Infect Dis Suppl 88: 103–108, 1993
19. See DM, Tilles JG. Treatment of coxsackivirus A9 myocarditis in mice with WIN 54954. Antimicrob Agents Chemother 36: 425–428, 1992
20. See DM, Tilles JG. WIN 54954 treatment of mice infected with a diabetogenic strain of group B coxsackievirus. Antimicrob Agents Chemother 37: 1593–1598, 1993
21. Zar JH. Biostatistical analysis. Englewood Cliffs, NJ. Prentice-Hall, Inc., 1974.
22. Jenista JA, Powell KR, Menegus MA. Epidemiology of neonatal enterovirus infection. J Pediatr 104: 685–690, 1984

23. Abelmann WH. Myocarditis and dilated cardiomyopathy [editorial]. West J Med 150: 458–459, 1989
24. Craighead JE. The role of viruses in the pathogenesis of pancreatic disease and diabetes mellitus. Prog Med Virol 19: 161–214, 1975
25. Center for Disease Control. Poliomyelitis prevention: Enhanced-potency inactivated poliovirus vaccine – Supplementary statement. MMWR. 36: 795–798, 1987
26. Notkins AL, Onodera T, Prabhakar BS. Virus induced autoimmunity. In: Concepts in Viral Pathogenesis. Notkins AL, Oldstone MBA, eds. New York: Springer-Verlag, 210–215, 1984
27. Gerling I, Nejman C, Chatterjee NK. Effect of coxsackievirus B4 infection in mice on expression of 64,000-M autoantigen and glucose sensitivity of islets before development of hyperglycemia. Diabetes 37: 1419–1425, 1988
28. Kaufman DL, Erlander MG, Clare-Salzer M, Atkinson MA, Maclaren MK, Tobin AJ. Autoimmunity in two forms of glutamate decarboxylase in insulin-dependent diabetes mellitus. J Clin Invest 89: 283–292, 1992
29. Prabhakar BS, Haspel MV, McClintock PR, Notkins AL. High frequency of antigenic variants among naturally occurring human Coxsackie B4 isolates identified by monoclonal antibodies. Nature 300: 374–376, 1982
30. Jerzabek Z, Zabicka J, John A, Howlett J, Dunn G, Wood DJ. Application of monoclonal antibody panels in the virologic and epidemiologic review of poliomyelitis in Poland, 1981–1990. Bull World Health Organ 70: 327–333, 1992
31. Szopa TM, Ward T, Dronfield ND, Portwood ND, Taylor KW. Coxsackie B4 isolates with the potential to damage beta cells of the islets are present in clinical isolates. Diabetologia 33: 325–328, 1990
32. Yoon JW, Austin M, Onodera T, Notkins AL. Virus-induced diabetes mellitus: isolation of a virus from the pancreas of a child diabetic ketoacidosis. N Engl J Med 300: 1173–1179, 1979

Submitted March 7, 1994; accepted August 18, 1994

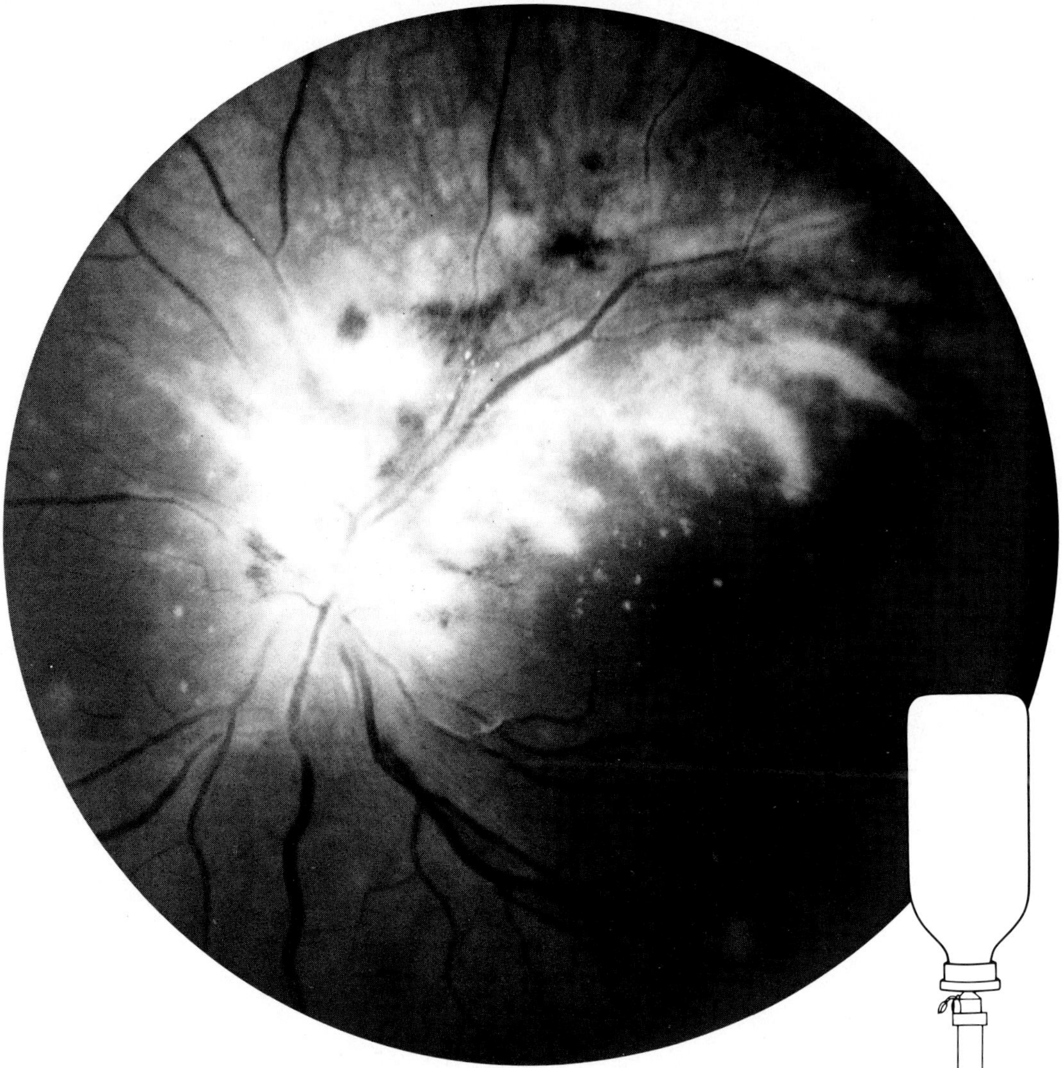

Scand J Infect Dis 26: 749–752, 1994

CASE REPORT

Long-term Remission of Kaposi's Sarcoma Following Foscarnet Treatment in HIV-infected patients

LINDA MORFELDT[1] and JAN TORSSANDER[2]

From the [1]Division of Infectious Diseases, Karolinska Institute, Danderyd Hospital, and the [2]Department of Dermatology, South Hospital, Stockholm, Sweden

Five patients with HIV-associated Kaposi's sarcoma (epidemic KS) were treated with foscarnet 180 mg/kg/day i.v. for 10 days. Four of them suffered from severe immunodeficiency with CD4 cell counts below 30 × 10⁶/l. Three of the patients went into long-term remission of KS. One patient was free of relapse for 12 months and 2 patients are still in remission after an observation period of 13 and 20 months respectively. The results suggest a possible role of foscarnet in the treatment of epidemic KS.

L. Morfeldt, MD, Department of Infectious Diseases, Karolinska Institute, Danderyd Hospital, S-182 88 Danderyd, Sweden

INTRODUCTION

Kaposi's sarcoma (KS) is the most common HIV-related neoplasia and contributes to morbidity and mortality in HIV infected patients. The majority of cases of epidemic KS is seen in homosexual males with immunodeficiency of clinical significance.

The cause of KS is not yet known. Several epidemiological studies indicate that a sexually transmissible agent is a factor of pathogenic importance (1, 2). A possible viral etiology has been proposed by several authors (3).

At present chemotherapy, interferons, radiation and different kinds of local treatment can be offered for palliation. Short remissions or considerable side-effects limit the benefit of these therapeutic regimens.

Accidentally, we noted regression of KS in 2 HIV-infected patients with CMV organ disease treated with foscarnet (an inhibitor of virus coded DNA-polymerase and reverse transcriptase). Therefore, a pilot study with foscarnet treatment of HIV infected patients with recently developed KS was performed.

PATIENTS AND METHODS

The patients were recruited from the offices of the authors. All HIV-infected patients in whom KS was diagnosed from May 1992 until May 1993 were included in the study. The 5 patients were treated with foscarnet at the Department of Infectious Diseases, Danderyd Hospital.

The KS lesions were recorded and documented before and repeatedly after treatment on a preformed templet as well as by photography. The diagnosis of KS was histologically verified in all patients.

Foscarnet was given by i.v. infusions in a dose of 180 mg/kg/day for 10 days; 60 mg/kg 3 times daily for 5 days followed by 90 mg/kg twice a day for 5 days.

CASE REPORTS

Patient 1

A 57-year old white homosexual man was admitted to the hospital because of Pneumocystis carinii pneumonia (PCP). The initial CD4 cell count was 24×10^6/l. The patient presented with 6 nodular KS skin lesions (Fig. 1a) and multiple lesions of the palate (Fig. 2a). He received a 10 days course of foscarnet. Three new skin lesions were detected 2 weeks later. One month post treatment a partial regression of some of the lesions was noted and after that all the lesions gradually diminished. After 4

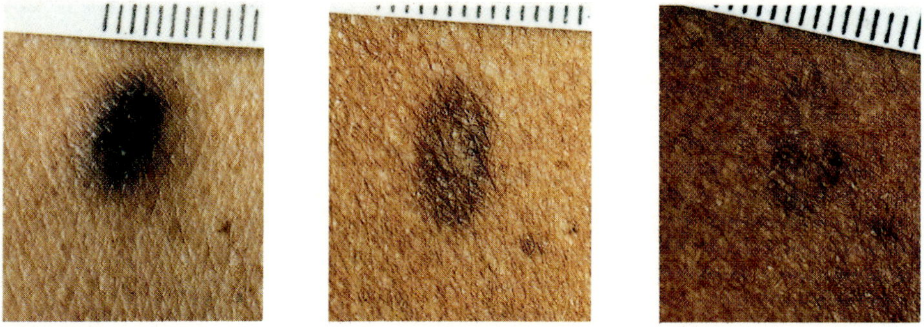

Fig. 1a, b and c

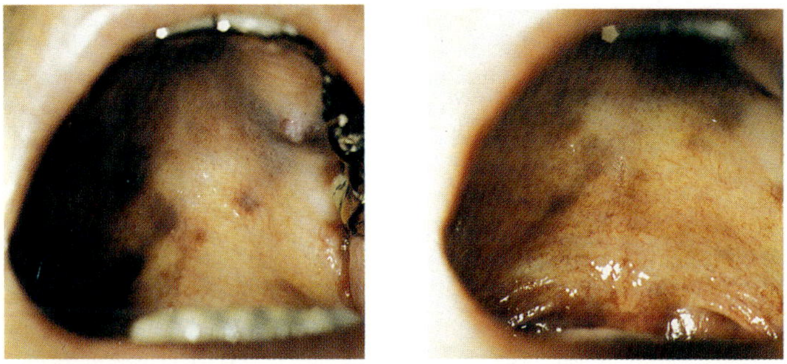

Fig. 2a and b

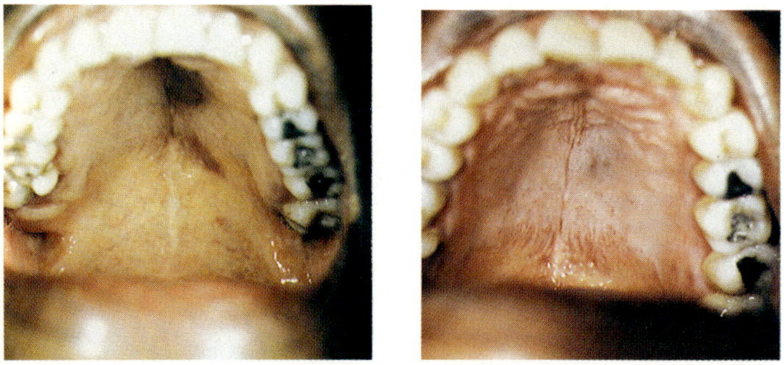

Fig. 3a and b

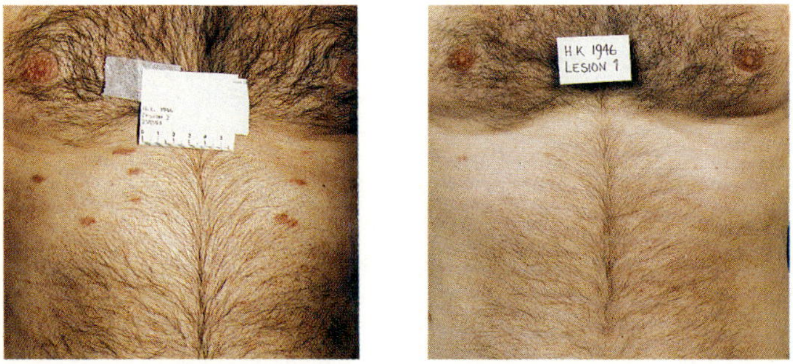

Fig. 4a and b

months of observation the nodular component of the lesions had resolved leaving brownish maculae (Fig. 1b). The lesions of the palate were hardly visible (Fig. 2b). Biopsy findings at this point indicated a parallell histological resolution. After 12 months all the skin lesions had almost completely resolved (Fig. 1c). At this time, however, the oral lesions began to recur. By month 15 the skin lesions remained unchanged but after 17 months 3 new lesions were noted and the initial ones had reappeared.

Patient 2

A 34-year old black heterosexual man from Uganda who was admitted to the hospital because of extrapulmonary tuberculosis. KS was diagnosed on admission. The CD4 cell count was 26×10^6/l. Six weeks later the patient was treated with foscarnet. At this time there were 15 KS lesions in the skin and 2 on the palate (Fig. 3a). Two weeks after completed foscarnet treatment one new KS lesion was noted. After that no more new lesions appeared. Six weeks after treatment a regression was seen in some of the lesions and subsequently all the KS lesions gradually diminished (Fig. 3b). The exception was a large KS tumor on the external ear which was treated with local radiation. At present, 20 months after foscarnet therapy, the patient is still in remission.

Patient 3

A 47-year old white homosexual man with a CD4 cell count of 270×10^6/l and no previous opportunistic infections (OI). He had a history of multiple skin lesions since 12 months. Histological examination of 2 separate lesions revealed Kaposi's sarcoma. The patient had 29 cutaneous KS lesions when foscarnet was given (Fig. 4a). Three months later one new lesion was detected. Five months after therapy there was no evidence of progression. Month 8 he received a second course of foscarnet. 13 months after the first course of foscarnet all the KS lesions had resolved (Fig. 4b). At present, 15 months after the first course of foscarnet, the patient is still in remission.

Patient 4

A 32-year old white homosexual man with a 6 months history of spiking fever. The CD4 cell count was 6×10^6/l. KS had developed over the past 2 months. At the start of foscarnet therapy there were 8 cutaneous KS lesions and one on the tongue. The fever continued and on the presumption of CMV cholitis a second course of foscarnet was given one month after the first. One month later the KS lesions had all grown in size. The general condition of the patient had deteriorated. After 3 months there was further progression of the skin lesions and extensive oesophageal KS could be demonstrated. Systemic chemotherapy was given.

Patient 5

A 33-year old white homosexual man who had a history of subfebrility since 6 months. The CD4 cell count was 24×10^6/l. Over the past 5 months this patient had developed 10 cutaneous KS lesions and 1 on the palate. Foscarnet was given but the treatment was interrupted after 6 days due to nausea and headache. One month following foscarnet therapy PCP was diagnosed and treated. A relapse of PCP occurred 2 months later. Four months after the interrupted foscarnet treatment progression of KS was noted and the lesions were subjected to local radiation therapy.

DISCUSSION

Only a few cases of spontaneous resolution of epidemic KS have been reported in the literature (4, 5, 6). One of the patients described had received foscarnet (6). In 1985, Real et

---

Fig. 1. Cutaneous Kaposi's sarcoma in **Patient 1** before (a), 4 months (b) and 12 months (c) following the foscarnet therapy (scale in mm).

Fig. 2. Kaposi's sarcoma lesions of the palate in **Patient 1** before (a) and 4 months after (b) the course of foscarnet.

Fig. 3. Kaposi's sarcoma of the palate in **Patient 2** before (a) and 5 months after (b) foscarnet therapy.

Fig. 4. Cutaneous Kaposi's sarcoma in **Patient 3** before (a) and 15 months after (b) the course of foscarnet.

al. reported 6 cases of KS with spontaneous regression constituting 3.8% of their entire KS population. None of those had a history of OI before the development of KS (5). In contrast, 2/3 patients with KS remission in our study were severely immunodeficient as defined by previous OI and low CD4 cell counts. The true incidence of spontaneous resolution of epidemic KS is not known, but according to accumulated clinical experience spontaneous recovery is a rare phenomenon.

The patients with KS resolution of this study had all received zidovudine during the observation period. Several studies have failed to show any significant anti-KS effect attributable to zidovudine (7, 8).

The 2 patients with progressive KS of this study had both other ongoing systemic complications of HIV-infection at the time when foscarnet was administered.

In the present study 3 of 5 KS patients went into long-term remission following foscarnet therapy. The findings suggest a possible anti-KS effect of foscarnet. Hypothetically, the mode of action could be antiviral, immunodulatory, cytotoxic or other. However, further investigations are required to assess the value of foscarnet as a therapeutic in Kaposi's sarcoma.

ACKNOWLEDGEMENTS

We want to thank Dr Susanne Bergdahl for inspiring clinical collaboration and the photographers at Danderyd Hospital for their excellent assistance.

REFERENCES

1. Beral V, Peterman TA, Berkelman RL, Jaffe HW. Kaposi's sarcoma among persons with AIDS: a sexually transmitted infection? Lancet 335: 123–128, 1990.
2. Elford J, McDonald A, Kaldor J, The National HIV Surveillance Committee. Kaposi's sarcoma as a sexually transmissible infection: an analysis of Australian AIDS surveillance data. AIDS 7: 1667–1671, 1993.
3. Peterman TA, Jaffe HW, Beral V. Epidemiologic clues to the etiology of Kaposi's sarcoma. AIDS 7: 605–611, 1993.
4. Janier M, Vignon MD, Cottenot F. Spontaneously healing Kaposi's sarcoma in AIDS. N Engl J Med 312: 1638–1639, 1985.
5. Real FX, Krown SE. Spontaneous regression of Kaposi's sarcoma in patients with AIDS. N Engl J Med 313: 1659, 1985.
6. O'Connell KA. Resolution of Kaposi's sarcoma. Lancet 343: 741, 1994.
7. Lane HC, Falloon J, Walker RE, Deyton L, Kovacs JA, Masur H, Banks S, Kirk LE, Baseler MW, Salzman NP, Fauci AS. Zidovudine in patients with Human Immunodeficiency Virus (HIV) infection and Kaposi sarcoma. Ann Int Med 111: 41–50, 1989.
8. de Wit R, Reiss P, Bakker PJM, Lange JMA, Danner SA, Veenhof KHN. Lack of activity of zidovudine in AIDS-associated Kaposi's sarcoma. AIDS 3: 847–850, 1989.

Submitted September 15, 1994; accepted October 3, 1994

Scand J Infect Dis 26: 753–754, 1994

CASE REPORT

Group F β-hemolytic Streptococcus, Tonsillitis and Myocarditis

OUTI MÄKI-IKOLA[1,2], REIJO PELTONEN[2] and PENTTI HÄNNINEN[2]

From the [1]National Public Health Institute, Department in Turku and the [2]Infectious Diseases Unit of Turku University Hospital, Turku, Finland

A case of tonsillitis and myocarditis is reported, where the only positive microbiological finding was a throat swab growing group F β-hemolytic streptococci. The patient made an uneventful recovery after treatment with benzylpenicillin and clindamycin.

O. Mäki-Ikola, MD, National Public Health Institute, Department in Turku, Kiinamyllynkatu 13, FIN-20520 Turku, Finland

INTRODUCTION

An acute myocarditis may arise during or after an infection caused by any one of a number of pathogens. Rheumatic fever is a classical example of reactive myocarditis and of reactive arthritis caused by infection with group A β-hemolytic streptococcus, e.g. tonsillitis. Other bacteria, including Yersinia, Salmonella and Shigella, can also cause reactive complications such as myocarditis and arthritis (1, 2). However, although non-group A β-hemolytic streptococci are known to cause reactive arthritis (3), they have not usually been associated with reactive myocarditis. Pathogenicity of non-group A β-hemolytic streptococci has recently been a topic of discussion (4–6). Here we report the case of a patient with myocarditis and tonsillitis with group F β-hemolytic streptococcus (FβHS) in his throat swab.

PATIENT RECORD

A 33-year-old usually healthy man was admitted to hospital because of a 3-day history of fever and sore throat. He had acute exudative tonsillitis with erythema. Throat culture grew β-hemolytic streptococcus with Lancefield group F carbohydrate. Routine electrocardiography showed classical signs of myocarditis and the diagnosis was confirmed by echocardiography. Cardiac auscultation revealed no abnormalities. A chest roentgenogram revealed minor heart failure. No signs of endocarditis were seen. The blood culture was negative. The serum antibody assays for Borrelia burgdorferi, Yersinia enterocolitica O:3 and O:9, Y. pseudotuberculosis I and III, Salmonellae, Corynebacterium diphtheriae, Mycoplasma pneumoniae, Chlamydia pneumoniae, Brucella, streptolysin O, deoxyribonuclease, staphylolysin and human immunodeficiency virus (and antigen detection) all proved negative. The antibody assays for the following viruses were performed for paired serum samples taken 14 days apart: Epstein Barr, cytomegalo, varicella zoster, herpes simplex 1 and 2, adeno, respiratory syncytial, para-influenza 1-3, Puumala, measles, influenza A and B, enteroviruses (pooled antigen of coxsackie A9 and B3, echo 11 and polio 1); all were negative.

Antigen detection assays for adeno, respiratory syncytial and para-influenza viruses in nasopharyngeal swab proved negative. Stool culture revealed no rota, adeno or enteroviruses, nor any bacterial pathogens. The antigen detection tests for adeno and rotaviruses in faeces proved negative. The patient was HLA B27 negative. An enzyme immunoassay for IgM, IgG and IgA class serum antibodies against FβHS (the strain used as antigen had been isolated from another patient with tonsillitis, as the original strain was lost before the following experiments and further characterization of the strain were done) revealed slight changes in antibody levels in follow-up samples in all classes: the absorbance values (optical density at a wavelength of 405 nm) were higher in the sample taken 14 days after the first sample; when the samples taken 14 and 25 days after the first sample were compared, the absorbance values were lower in the latter sample (the biggest difference in the optical density being 0.576 in the IgG

 ISSN 0036-5548

class). In immunoblotting analysis after sodium dodecyl sulphate polyacrylamide gel electrophoresis using FβHS as antigen, 2 faint bands with a molecular weight (MW) of 50–55 kD in IgM, 1 faint band of MW approx. 10 kD in IgG and bands of MW approx. 10 kD, 30 kD and 70–75 kD in IgA were visualized as either new or stronger bands in the serum samples taken 14 and 25 days after the first sample, when compared with the first sample. The patient was treated with benzyl penicillin and clindamycin and recovered from tonsillitis within a week, C-reactive protein declining from 191 to 3 mg/l (normally <10 mg/l) and lactate dehydrogenase from 617 to 317 U/l (normally <450 U/l). He did not report any symptoms of carditis during his stay in the hospital. Control echocardiography and chest roentgenogram after 11 days were normal.

DISCUSSION

To our knowledge, the possible association between FβHS and myocarditis has not been reported earlier. In our case, the vigorous search yielded no other etiological agents for tonsillitis and myocarditis besides the FβHS. Evidence supporting this association is unsubstantial, but nevertheless intriguing. The ultimate proof of an etiological association between FβHS and myocarditis must, however, come from a demonstration of direct involvement of the bacteria in the disease, as has been shown for instance in reactive arthritis (1). However, in the case of myocarditis it would require a myocardial biopsy; in our case this was not performed as it would not have been ethical in such a rather mild case of myocarditis. In view of the possible clinical significance of non-group A β-hemolytic streptococci with myocarditis, it is important that these microbes are acknowledged and reported.

REFERENCES

1. Mäki-Ikola O, Granfors K. Salmonella triggered reactive arthritis. Lancet 339: 1096–1098, 1992.
2. Laitinen O, Leirisalo M, Allander E. Rheumatic fever and Yersinia arthritis. Criteria and diagnostic problems in the changing disease pattern. Scand J Rheumatol 4: 145–157, 1975.
3. Deighton C. β haemolytic streptococci and reactive arthritis in adults. Ann Rheum Dis 52: 475–482, 1993.
4. Gossling J. Occurrence and pathogenicity of the Streptococcus milleri group. Rev Infect Dis 10: 257–285, 1988.
5. Cimolai N, Elford RW, Bryan L, Anand C, Berger P. Do the β-hemolytic non-group A streptococci cause pharyngitis? Rev Infect Dis 10: 587–601, 1988.
6. Dudley JP, Sercarz J. Pharyngeal and tonsil infections caused by non-group A streptococcus. Am J Otolaryngol 12: 292–296, 1991.

Submitted January 10, 1994; accepted July 20, 1994

Scand J Infect Dis 26: 755–757, 1994

CASE REPORT

Bilateral Pulmonary Abscesses Caused by Streptococcus Pyogenes: Diagnostic importance of fiberoptic bronchoscopy

PAUL CLEMENTSEN and NILS MILMAN

From the Department of Pulmonary Medicine, Gentofte Hospital, University of Copenhagen, Denmark

A patient with bilateral pulmonary abscesses caused by Streptococcus pyogenes is described. This bacterium is an uncommon cause of pneumonia. Metastatic foci of infection, e.g. abscess formation, may follow bacteremic spread of S. pyogenes. However, such complications are rare and the occurrence of bilateral pulmonary abscesses has not been described earlier. In the present case the diagnosis was established by fiberoptic bronchoscopy with bronchial washing.

P. Clementsen, MD, Lungemedicinsk afdeling Y, Københavns Amts Sygehus i Gentofte, DK-2900 Hellerup, Denmark

INTRODUCTION

Pneumonia caused by streptococcus pyogenes is rare (1–3) and may be difficult to diagnose, particularly in cases with development of pulmonary abscesses, which may lead to a delay in recognizing the aetiological agent. In the present case of severe pulmonary streptococcus infection, the diagnosis was obtained by fiberoptic bronchoscopy.

CASE REPORT

A 42-year-old male Pakistani was admitted to hospital with fever, coughing, a hemoptysis and dyspnea. Oral treatment with pivampicillin for 2 days had no clinical effect. He had previously been in good health apart from mild bronchial asthma and allergy to cat dander and house dust mite. He had never used intravenous drugs.

At physical examination the patient did not appear acutely ill. Auscultation of the lungs revealed rales on both sides, but no consolidation. No cardiac murmur was heard, and there were no clinical or ECG signs of endocarditis. The temperature was 37.6°C. He was not tachycardic or tachypnoic and his blood pressure was normal. His throat was not inflamed and there were no skin lesions or clubbing.

Chest X-ray revealed numerous bilateral infiltrates, up to 5 cm in diameter, some of them with cavitation and containing liquid (Fig. 1). Pulmonary scintigraphy showed matching perfusion and ventilation defects limited to areas of roentgenographic infiltration. Since microscopy of sputum revealed no pathogenic bacteria, mycobacteria or malignant cells, we performed fiberoptic bronchoscopy under local anesthesia. Due to excessive cough and lack of cooperation, bronchoalveolar lavage (BAL) could not be performed. Instead, the working channel of the bronchoscope was initially flushed with 40 ml sterile saline which was recovered by suction and discharged. Subsequently bronchial washing with 40 ml sterile saline was performed in the right middle lobe, followed by transbronchial biopsies. Protected brush for microbiological examination was not performed. Macroscopic changes consistent with bronchitis were found, but the investigation was otherwise normal.

The following day the patient's temperature rose to 40.5°C and his general condition deteriorated. He was therefore treated with intravenous benzylpenicillin two million IE, 3 times a day, whereafter he improved clinically and the temperature rapidly decreased. Treatment was continued i.v. for 5 days and then switched to oral medication. Culture of fluid obtained by bronchial washing showed heavy growth of a monoculture of group A streptococcus pyogenes sensitive to penicillin. No fungi, mycobacteria or amoebae were found. Transbronchial biopsies showed unspecific inflammatory changes. Cultures of blood, sputum and urine proved negative.

Blood tests showed IgE 835 kU/l (reference interval 0–120), IgA 4.2 g/l (0.6–3.4), IgG 19.4 g/l (5.8–14.2) and IgM 1.3 g/l (0.3–3.3). White blood cell count was slightly elevated 11.8×10^9/l on

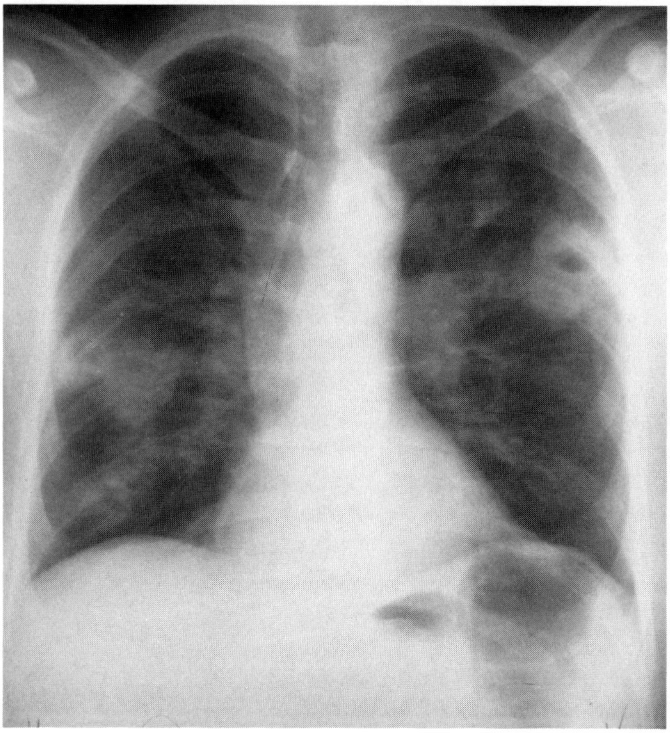

Fig. 1. Chest X-ray of a 42-year-old man with numerous bilateral pulmonary infiltrates and abscesses due to infection with Streptococcus pyogenes.

admission, and on day 3, 16.2×10^9/l with 81% neutrophils. He was seronegative for HIV 1, Mycoplasma pneumoniae and legionella.

By day 6 the pulmonary X-ray had improved considerably and during the following 3 months an almost complete regression was seen. On day 13 asymptomatic presence of cysts of Giardia lamblia in feces was demonstrated, for which the patient was treated with metronidazole. He recovered without complications and no infections were seen during the following 6 months.

DISCUSSION

Most streptococcal infections are caused by hemolytic streptococci of Lancefield's group A – Streptococcus pyogenes. Typical infections are tonsillitis, scarlet fever and erysipelas, whereas more serious infections are uncommon. However, severe group A streptococcal infections seem to be occurring with increasing frequency (4) and the bacterium may have acquired greater virulence, manifested by various severe soft-tissue infections and systemic toxicity (4). Septicemia has a high mortality (5), but has been infrequent since the introduction of penicillin. Thus Streptococcus pyogenes is found in fewer than 3% of all blood culture isolates (6).

Pneumonia is presumed to be due to hematogenous seeding of the lungs rather than a transbronchial progression of an upper respiratory tract infection (3). Bacteremia has been demonstrated in 10–15% of pneumonia cases caused by Streptococcus pyogenes (2). Blood cultures in our patient proved negative, but the radiologic appearance with multiple, bilateral abscesses nevertheless was consistent with hematogenic spread. Bacteremic spread of the streptococci may result in a variety of metastatic foci of infection, for example suppurative arthritis, brain abscess or liver abscess, but such complications are extremely rare (2). Bilateral pulmonary abscesses caused by Streptococcus pyogenes have not been described previously; only one single case of an unilateral pulmonary abscess caused by the bacterium has been reported (3).

Several risk factors have been described (e.g. advanced age, diabetes, alcoholism, compromised immunological function) (6–10), but our patient did not fit into any of these categories. This tallies with a recent study of patients with streptococcal infections (4), where host factors did not explain the emergence of the disease.

Pneumonia caused by Streptococcus pyogenes is infrequent (1) and the symptoms are indistinguishable from those of other bacterial pneumonias. The development of pulmonary abscesses may lead to confusion with other, more common causes of this condition, e.g. Staphylococcus aureus septicaemia, particularly when sputum and blood cultures are negative, as in our case. However, fiberoptic bronchoscopy is an efficient method for the diagnosis of bacterial infections in the lung (11–13). During the passage of the fiberoptic bronchoscope through the upper airways, the tip of the instrument becomes to a variable degree contaminated with bacteria from the nose and pharynx, which may be introduced into the lower respiratory tract and cause false-positive cultures. This problem can be circumvented by: 1) flushing of the working channel of the bronchoscope with 40–60 ml sterile saline, which is recovered and discharged, 2) BAL with quantitative bacterial culture, and 3) protected specimen brush.

In the present case, the working channel of the bronchoscope was flushed prior to bronchial washing, but protected specimen brushing was not performed. However, the heavy growth of a monoculture of Streptococcus pyogenes and the negative sputum culture strongly suggest that the recovered bacteria were resident in the lower respiratory tract.

REFERENCES

1. Dobson SRM. Group A streptococci revisited. Arch Dis Child 64: 977–980, 1989.
2. Bisno AL. Streptococcus pyogenes. In: Mandell GL, Douglas RG, Bennet JE, eds. Principles and practice of infectious diseases. New York: Churchill Livingstone, 1519–1528, 1990.
3. McWhinney PHM, Nathwani D. Streptococcus group A pneumonia in an intravenous drug misuser. Eur Respir J 4: 761–763, 1991.
4. Stevens DL, Tanner MH, Winship J, Swarts R, Ries KM, Schlievert PM, Kaplan E. Severe group A streptococcal infections associated with a toxic shock like syndrome and scarlet fever toxin A. N Engl J Med 321: 1–7, 1989.
5. Martin PR, Høiby EA. Streptococcal serogroup A epidemic in Norway 1987–1988. Scand J Infect Dis 22: 421–429, 1990.
6. Ispahani P, Donald FE, Aveline AJ. Streptococcus pyogenes bacteraemia: an old enemy subdued, but not defected. J Infect 16: 37–46, 1988.
7. Bibler MR, Rouan GW. Cryptogenic group A streptococcal bacteremia: experience at an urban general hospital and review of the literature. Rev Infect Dis 8: 941–951, 1986.
8. Adams EM, Gudmundsson S, Yocum DE, Haselby RC, Craig WA, Sundstrom WR. Streptococcal myositis. Arch Intern Med 145: 1020–1023, 1985.
9. Wong VK, Wright HT Jr. Group A beta-hemolytic streptococci as a cause of bacteremia in children. Am J Dis Child 142: 831–833, 1988.
10. Quintliani R, Engh GA. Overwhelming sepsis associated with group A beta hemolytic streptococci. J Bone Joint Surg (Am) 53: 1391–1399, 1971.
11. Kahn FW, Jones JM. Diagnosing bacterial respiratory infection by bronchoalveolar lavage. J Infect Dis 155: 862–869, 1987.
12. Klech H, Pohl W (eds.) Technical recommendations and guidelines for bronchoalveolar lavage (BAL). Report of the European Society of Pneumology Task Group on BAL. Eur Respir J 2: 561–585, 1989.
13. Pedersen TL, Pedersen M, Myhre J, Milman N, Johnsen H. Bronchoalveolar lavage is a safe and informative procedure in haematologic patients with nonresolving pneumonia. Eur J Haematol 49: 280–281, 1992.

Submitted March 16, 1994; accepted July 27, 1994

Scand J Infect Dis 26: 759–760, 1994

CASE REPORT

Septicaemia due to Aerococcus urinae

AINA MØLLER HEILESEN

From the Department of Clinical Microbiology, Central Hospital, Esbjerg, Denmark

In a case of septicaemia, Aerococcus urinae was isolated from the blood. The patient had undergone operation on the prostate gland. The urine was sterile.

A. M. Heilesen, MD, Department of Clinical Microbiology, Københavns Amts sygehus, Herlev Ringvej, DK-2730 Herlev, Denmark

INTRODUCTION

The genus Aerococcus was described by Williams et al. in 1953 (1). Evans (2) described Aerococcus viridans in 1986, and Aerococcus urinae was proposed in 1991 (3) as the name for a new species revealed by partial reverse transcriptase of 16 S ribosomal ribonucleic acid sequence analysis of 5 Aerococcus-like organisms isolated from patients with urinary tract infections (4, 5).

Aerococci and Aerococcuc-like organisms are generally considered apathogenic, but cases of urinary tract infections (4–6), subacute endocarditis (6–10), meningitis (11), and bacteraemia (12, 13) have been reported. However, septicaemia caused by Aerococcus urinae has not previously been reported in the literature.

CASE REPORT

The patient is an 80-year-old man, healthy to the age of 73, when he underwent an uncomplicated herniotomy. At the age of 75 he was treated with cimetidine for a peptic ulcer without complications. The now 80-year-old patient had suffered loss of weight, lower back pains, pain in the left testicle, pollakisuria and dysuria for the last 3 months, but had no complaints from other organ systems and showed no signs of infection. Cancer of the prostate gland was diagnosed, and he underwent an operation. No peroperative antibiotic prophylaxis was given. On the second postoperative day he showed signs of septicemia, with high temperature, low blood pressure, and insufficient respiration. Cultures from tracheal secretion and urine were sterile, whereas culture from blood revealed Gram-positive cocci identified as Aerococcus urinae. CRP was 106, hemoglobin was low, and there were 70% PMN leukocytes in the peripheral blood. The ECG was normal. Antibiotic treatment with Ampicillin and Gentamicin was started on day 2, and on day 5 the temperature had normalized, and the patient was referred from hospital to the outpatient clinic in good clinical condition.

MICROBIOLOGY

The identification of the Aerococcus isolated was done according to the description by Maria Aguirre and M. D. Collins (3) and confirmed by the State Serum Institute in Copenhagen. The strain was sensitive to penicillins, cephalosporins, tetracyclines, polymyxin, chloramphenicol, vancomycin and clindamycin, but resistant to gentamicin and sulfonamides.

DISCUSSION

Patients often have fever on the second day after operation, but this patient was septic, and as he was operated in the urinary tract, we suspected Aerococcus urinae to be the cause, although it was not isolated from his urine.

Aerococci are distributed world wide in the human environment, and are primarily considered airborne contaminants. The incidence of Aerococcus urinae infections is not

 ISSN 0036-5548

known. Kern and Vanek (13) described granulocytopenia as the underlying disease in 2 cases of Aerococcus bacteraemia, one of which proved fatal. Underlying diseases or special risk factors in relation to Aerococcus urinae infection are not reported, but this case shows that they may be pathogenic in immunocompetent hosts.

REFERENCES

1. Williams REO, Hirch A, Cowan ST. Aerococcus, a new bacterial genus. J Gen Microbiol 8: 475–480, 1953.
2. Evans JB. Genus Aerococcus. In: Bergey's Manual of Systematic Bacteriology 2: 1080, 1986.
3. Aguirre M, Collins MD. Phylogenetic analysis of some Aerococcus-like organisms from urinary tract infections: description of Aerococcus urinae sp. nov. J Gen Microbiol 138: 401–405, 1992.
4. Christensen JJ, Korner B, Kjærgaard H. Aerococcus-like organism – an unnoticed urinary tract pathogen. APMIS 97: 539–546, 1989.
5. Christensen JJ, Vibits H, Ursing J, Korner B. Aerococcus-like organism, a newly recognized potential urinary tract pathogen. J Clin Microbiol 29: 1049–1053, 1991.
6. Colman G. Aerococcus-like organisms isolated from human infections. J Clin Pathol 20: 294–297, 1967.
7. Janosek J, Eckert J, Hudac A. Aerococcus viridans as a causative agent of infectious endocarditis. J Clin Pathol 20: 92–96, 1980.
8. Parker MT, Ball LC. Streptococci and aerococci associated with systemic infection in man. J Med Microbiol 9: 275–302, 1976.
9. Baerwald C, Krause A, Goebel KM. Septische arthritis als erstmanifestation einer endokarditis. Z Rheumatol 49: 165–168, 1990.
10. Christensen JJ, Gutschik E, Friis-Moller A, Korner B. Urosepticemia and fatal endocarditis caused by aerococcus-like organisms.
11. Nathavitharana KA, Arseculeratne SN, Aposno HA, Vijeratnam R, Jayasena L, Navaratman C. Acute meningitis in early childhood caused by Aerococcus viridans. BMJ 286: 1248, 1983.
12. Taylor PV, Trueblood MC. Septic arthritis due to Aerococcus viridans. J Rheumatol 12: 1604–1605, 1985.
13. Kern W, Vanek E. Aerococcus bacteremia associated with granulocytopenia. Eur J Clin Microbiol 6: 670–673, 1987.

Submitted April 27, 1994; accepted July 27, 1994

Scand J Infect Dis 26: 761–764, 1994

CASE REPORT

Multifocal Musculoskeletal Cystic Tuberculosis Without Systemic Manifestations

ALAIN EID, NADEEM CHAUDRY, MOHAMED EL-GHOROURY, ABDELKADER HAWASLI, WILLIAM L. SALOT and RIAD KHATIB

From the St John Hospital and Medical Center, Detroit, Michigan, USA

A case of multifocal cystic tuberculosis is presented, affecting the clavicle and the iliac bones with considerable soft tissue involvement. It was found in a 34-year-old male, an immigrant from Yemen. The extensive cystic nature of both lesions and the lack of systemic manifestations despite multifocal disease are unusual.

R. Khatib, MD, Medical Education Office, St John Hospital and Medical Center, 22101 Moross Road, Detroit, MI 48236 USA

INTRODUCTION

Bone or joint involvement is a common presentation of extra-pulmonary tuberculosis, accounting for 2.5–19% of these cases (1–4). Ordinarily, it presents as a chronic localized destructive process at times involving adjacent structures. Systemic manifestations are uncommon without disseminated disease or associated pulmonary involvement (5).

We present a case of multifocal cystic tuberculosis affecting the iliac bone and the clavicle, with extensive involvement of adjacent soft tissues. The characteristics of these lesions and the noticeable lack of systemic manifestations were more suggestive of cystic neoplasm or echinococcosis.

CASE REPORT

A 34-year-old white male, an immigrant from Yemen, presented with a non-painful mass in the left upper chest just below mid-clavicle. It had been detected a few months earlier and thought to be a lipoma. Local excision was attempted as the mass was enlarging slowly. During surgery, the mass was noted to be necrotic and to extend to bone in the acromio-clavicular area. Histopathologic examination revealed necrotizing granulomatous inflammation with multiple Langhans' giant cells. Special stains for acid-fast organisms and for fungi were negative. Cultures were not performed. A radiologic examination, performed after excision, showed cystic changes in the lateral aspects of the clavicle (Fig. 1).

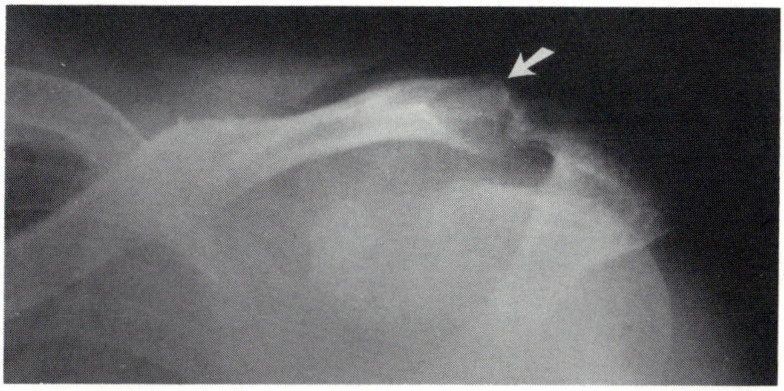

Fig. 1. A roentgenogram of the left clavicle showing a cystic lesion in the distal end of the clavicle (*arrow*).

 ISSN 0036-5548

After surgery, the wound did not heal and began to drain a serous fluid. The patient denied weight loss, fever, night sweats, pain, or any respiratory symptoms. Upon further evaluation, he was found to have an ill defined soft mass in the right iliac fossa, burrowing under the iliac crest. It was minimally tender and fixed. The chest was clear and the remainder of physical examination was unremarkable. The patient remained consistently afebrile without any signs of systemic illness.

Laboratory tests showed a hemoglobin of 131 g/l, hematocrit 39.6% and WBC count of 8.5×10^9/l with a normal differential count. Urinalysis, blood urea nitrogen, creatinine, and liver enzymes were within normal limits. A chest roentgenogram was normal. Computer-assisted tomography of the abdomen and pelvis revealed multiple multi-loculated contiguous cysts involving the psoas muscle, and extending to the iliac bone with bony erosion (Fig. 2). Plain roentgenograms showed a radiolucent lesion in the iliac bone (Fig. 3). Bone scan showed minimal increase in activity in these areas without additional lesions.

Based on the lack of systemic manifestations, we suspected that the patient might have 2 unrelated processes: chronic infection or neoplasm in the left clavicle, and an unrelated cystic neoplastic processes or echinococcosis in the abdomen. For this reason, we did not attempt diagnostic aspiration of these lesions. We proceeded to resect the distal portion of the clavicle. Four days later, an exploratory laparotomy was also performed. During surgery, the peritoneum was found free of disease but a multi-loculated cystic mass with necrosis and purulent content was noted in the right iliac fossa. It involved the right psoas muscle and all major vascular and nervous tissue with extrinsic compression and erosion of the iliac crest. It was resected *in toto*.

Histologic examination of the clavicle and the abdominal mass showed caseating granulomatous necrosis with many acid-fast bacilli. At this point, isoniazid, pyrazinamide and rifampin were started. The post-operative course was uneventful and both wounds healed satisfactorily. A tuberculin skin test

(*a*)

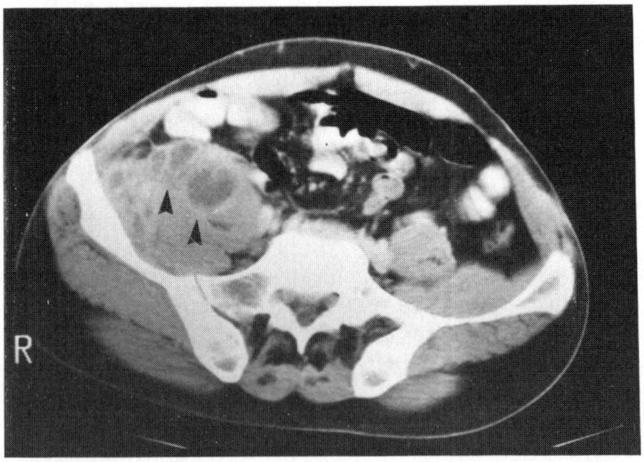

(*b*)

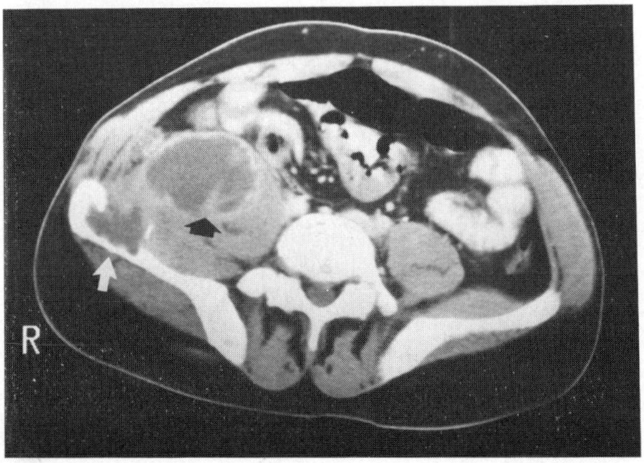

Fig. 2. Computer-assisted tomography of the pelvis with contrast enhancement. (*a*) Multiple cysts varying in size with enhancing borders, involving the psoas muscle (*arrows*); (*b*) at a different level, 2 large cystic lesions, one of them multi-loculated (*black arrow*), the other extending to the iliac bone with erosion (*white arrow*).

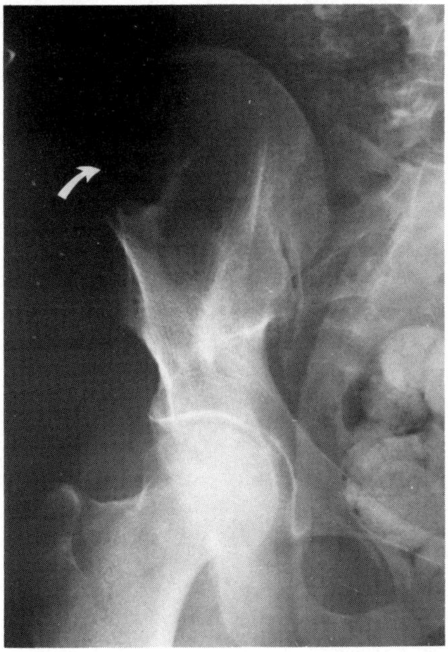

Fig. 3. Radiolucent lesion affecting the iliac bone (*arrow*).

showed 25 mm induration. Antibody test for human immune deficiency virus 1 was negative. Culture of both specimens grew Mycobacterium tuberculosis.

DISCUSSION

This patient displayed an unusual form of tuberculosis. It involved bone and surrounding soft tissues in 2 non-communicating sites in the absence of systemic manifestations and without any evidence of spread to other areas. This conclusion is based on the lack of physical findings, clear chest roentgenogram, and normal complete blood cell count, urine analysis and liver enzymes. The extensive syst formation in the involved tissues is also unusual. Although cystic disease is well described in older orthopedic literature, it remains rare and similar soft tissue involvement is unusual.

Osseous tuberculosis is a well known presentation of extra-pulmonary disease (1–4). It seems to affect predominantly immigrants from endemic countries. In a study from Great Britain, the incidence of bone tuberculosis was 85 times higher among immigrants from India than in the local population (6). It also tends to be more prevalent in the younger age groups. In a large series from Hong Kong, 70% of the patients were <10 years of age (7). Both observations, however, might be due to the prevalence of tuberculosis in these populations rather than to actual predilection for bone involvement. The vast majority of these lesions (90–95%) are localized to one site, but multifocal involvement had been described, usually in cases of disseminated disease (8).

The pathogenesis is thought to be a hematogenous spread during primary infection, with subsequent reactivation. This reactivation may originate in the bone or in the adjacent soft tissues with secondary extension to the bone (8). In our case, we suspect that coincidental simultaneous reactivation in both sites took place. The manifestations are usually due to the local process. They include pain, swelling, and, at later stages, draining sinuses. In some cases, a severe inflammatory reaction resembling a pyogenic abscess may also be present (9). Trauma frequently precedes the manifestations, probably by attracting the patient's attention to the involved area. However, trauma has been implicated in the activation of a latent focus of infection (9). Systemic manifestations such as fever, night sweats, and weight loss may occur, but are uncommon in the absence of lung involvement (1, 6, 10). The cystic form tends to be the most indolent. It is often diagnosed incidentally in patients with known visceral tuberculosis or during histopathologic examination of a suspected cystic neoplasm (5). Radiologically, the lesion appears as a well circumscribed cyst with little or no reactive sclerosis and without sequestrum formation or periosteal reaction (9, 10). Because of its chronic nature, and since differentiating it from a neoplasm based on radiologic findings alone is not possible, the diagnosis is frequently delayed (6). Hence, a high index of suspicion should be maintained during evaluation of cystic bone lesions, especially among immigrants from countries with a high prevalence of tuberculosis. In such cases, a portion of tissue should be sent for microbiologic evaluation (4, 10, 11).

In summary, our case illustrates that tuberculosis should be considered in patients with multi-loculated cystic lesions involving soft tissues and or bones. It also shows that despite multifocal involvement, systemic manifestations can be absent.

REFERENCES

1. Alvarez S, McCabe W. Extrapulmonary tuberculosis revisited: a review of experience at Boston City and other hospitals. Medicine 63: 25–55, 1984.
2. Dolberg OT, Schlaeffer F, Greene VW, Alkan ML. Extrapulmonary tuberculosis in an immigrant society: clinical and demographic aspects of 92 cases. Rev Infect Dis 13: 177–179, 1991.
3. Lachenauer C, Cosentino S, Wood R, Yousefzadeh DK, McCarthy CA. Multifocal skeletal tuberculosis presenting as osteomyelitis of the jaw. Pediatr Infect Dis J 10: 940–944, 1991.
4. Hanania N, Hoffstein V. Tuberculosis presenting with generalized lymphadenopathy, pulmonary infiltrates and bone destruction in a young man. Arch Intern Med 153: 1265–1267, 1993.
5. McTammany JR, Moser KM, Houk VN. Disseminated bone tuberculosis: review of the literature and presentation of an unusual case. Am Rev Respir Dis 87: 889–895, 1963.
6. Hodgson SP, Ormerod LP. Ten-year experience of bone and joint tuberculosis in Blackburn 1978–1987. J R Coll Surg Edinb 35: 259–262, 1990.
7. Hapman M, Murray R, Stoker D. Tuberculosis of the bones and joints. Semin Roentgenol 14: 266–282, 1979.
8. Shannon B, Moore M, Houkom J, Waeker N. Multifocal cystic tuberculosis of bone. J Bone Joint Surg Am 72: 1089–1092, 1990.
9. Edeiken J, Depalma A, Moskowitz H, Smythe V. Cystic tuberculosis of bone. Clin Orthop 28: 163–168, 1963.
10. AbdelWahab IK, Kenan S, Hermann G, Lenis M, Klein M, Rabinowitz JG. Atypical skeletal tuberculosis mimicking neoplasm. Br J Radiol 64: 551–555, 1991.
11. Sinnott JT, Gasser S, Kilgor J. A sheep in wolf's clothing. Hosp Pract 24: 153–156, 1989.

Submitted June 21, 1994; accepted July 18, 1994

Scand J Infect Dis 26: 765–766, 1994

CASE REPORT

A Case of Hydatid Cyst with Intramural Cardiac Localization

NECLA AKÇAKAYA[1], Y. SÖYLEMEZ[1], H. ÇOKUĞRAS[1], A. AYTAC[2] and F. AKALIN[1]

From the Departments of [1]Pediatrics, University of Istanbul, Cerrahpaşa Medical Faculty of Infectious Diseases, Clinical Immunology and Allergy Division, and [2]Cardiothoracic Surgery, Institute of Cardiology, University of Istanbul, Istanbul, Turkey

A 12-year-old boy with an intramural hydatid cyst of the heart is presented. In hydatid disease the incidence of cardiac cyst localization is less than 2%. The cyst was successfully excised by open heart surgery.

N. Akçakaya, MD, PhD, Department of Pediatrics, University of Istanbul, Cerrahpaşa Medical Faculty Infectious Diseases, Clinical Immunology and Allergy Division, Istanbul, Turkey

INTRODUCTION

Hydatid cyst caused by Echinococcus granulosus is widespread in almost every region of Turkey (1). The cysts are most frequently located in the liver but may occur in many different tissues (1–7).

Intracardiac localization of hydatid cyst is found in fewer than 2% of the cases (8–10). This localization of the disease is dangerous. After many asymptomatic years it may rupture into the circulation and cause anaphylactic shock, or cardiac tamponade by opening of the cyst into the pericardium (8, 9).

CASE REPORT

A 12-year-old boy was admitted with complaints of shortness of breath and palpitation. One year previously a hydatid cyst had been removed from his liver.

No abnormalities were disclosed upon physical examination of the cardiovascular system. As expected, the Casoni, Weinberg and indirect hemagglutination tests for echinococcosis proved strongly positive. X-ray examination revealed cardiomegaly and upward dislocation of the apex. There was an extremely dense area in the left lung. Electrocardiography revealed repolarization of the left ventricle.

Echocardiography and computerized axial tomography revealed a regularly shaped intramural cyst measuring 5×4.5 cm, located in the lateral wall of the left ventricle (Fig. 1). An irregularly shaped condensation in the upper anterior segment of the left lung was believed to be a ruptured old cyst, as was verified by the finding of scolices in sputum. In addition, there were five hydatid cysts in the liver. No other organ involvement was found.

The cardiac cyst was excised at the Haseki Cardiology Institute, Surgical Department, using the Cappitonnege technique and open heart surgery. For the moment the patient is in good health and waiting for another operation for the cysts in his liver. Mebendazole was given at a dosage of 10 mg/kg per day to prevent secondary hydatidosis.

DISCUSSION

Echinococcosis is frequently found in countries breeding sheep. Dogs are the main source of infection both for domestic animals and for human beings.

Infestation in humans can occur at all ages, although it is seen more frequently in childhood. The parasite is usually a slowly enlarging larval cyst which is well tolerated unless it ruptures or becomes large enough to produce symptoms of a space occupying mass. In our country, liver involvement occurs in some 50–54% and lung involvement in 35–40%. The other organs are involved in about 10%, and 15–30% of the patients have more than 1 cyst (1).

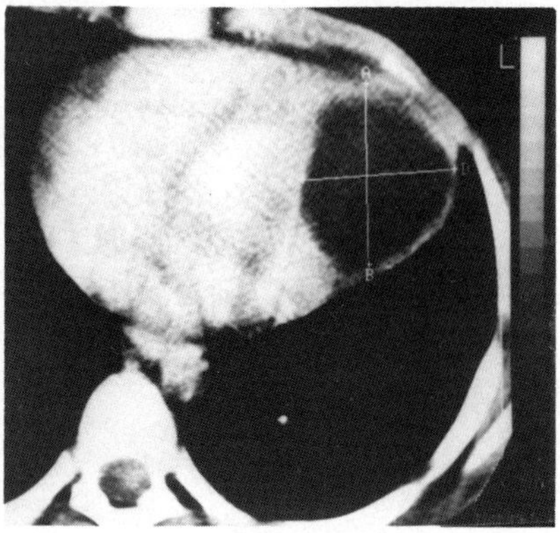

Fig. 1. Computerized axial tomography of the chest of a 12-year-old Turkish boy, showing an intramural E. granulosis cyst measuring 5 × 4.5 cm (A – B × C – D).

We have found only 1 case with cardiac (pericardial) localization among 23 cases admitted in the past decade. Cysts can be pericardial, endocardial or, in very rare cases, intramural. They can stay clincally silent for years or cause arrhythmias such as ventricular tachycardia (8–10).

In our case, despite complaints of palpitation, tachycardia and arrhythmia, we were not objectively able to confirm these. Cardiac localization of hydatid cysts is particularly dangerous, as the cyst may rupture into the pericardial sac, causing cardiac tamponade or into the circulation, causing massive pulmonary embolism, pulmonary hypertension, obstruction of the cardiac values, atrioventricular conduction defects and pulmonary or systemic metastases.

Recently, albendazole 10 mg/kg per day for 3 months has been recommended for the treatment of hydatid cyst (3–6). We, however, administered mebendazole 10 mg/kg per day as albendazole is not commercially available in our country.

REFERENCES

1. Merdivenci A. Türkiyede Hidatik Kist Hastalığı, Hilal matbaası, İstanbul, 1976.
2. Oliver JM, Benito LP. Cardiac hydatid cyst diagnosed by two-dimensional echo-cardiography. Am Heart J 104: 164–165, 1982.
3. Morris DL, Clarkson MS, Stallbaumer MF, Pritchard J, Jones RO, Cninnery JB. Albendazole treatment of pulmonary hydatid cysts in naturally infected sheep, a study with relevance to the treatment of hydatid cysts in naturally infected sheep; a study with relevance to the treatment of hydatid cysts in man. Thorax 40: 453–458, 1985.
4. Morris DL, Dykes PW, Marriner S, Bogan J, Burrows F, Skeene, Smith, H, Clarkson MJ. Albendazole-objective evidence of response in human hydatid disease. JAMA 253: 14; 2053–2057, 1985.
5. Keystone JS. Larval tapeworm infections: echinococcosis. In: Kaplan SL, ed. Current therapy in pediatric infectious disease. St. Louis: Mosby Year Book, 326–329, 1993.
6. Turner JA, Cestodes: echinococcosis. In: Feigin RD, Cherry JD eds. Textbook of Pediatric Infectious Diseases. W. B. Saunders Company, 2118–2121, 1987.
7. Yamaguchi, T. Hepatosplenomegaly: echinococcosis. A Colour Atlas of Clinical Parasitology. Wolfe Medical Publications Ltd., 1981, 62–63.
8. Frauquet T, Lecumberri F, Joly M. Hydatid heart disease. Br J Radiol 57; 171–173, 1984.
9. Byard WR, Bourne YA. Cardiac echinococcosis with fatal intracerebral embolism. Arch Dis Child 66: 155–156, 1991.
10. Sirinelli A, Le Guludec D, Laine JF, Sebag C, Bourguignon M, Slama M, Davy JM, Motte G. Ventricular tachycardia revealing a hydatid cyst. Am Heart J 114: 656–659, 1987.

Submitted April 27, 1994; accepted August 6, 1994

Scand J Infect Dis 26: 767–770, 1994

CASE REPORT

Isolated Kidney Localization of Invasive Aspergillosis in a Patient with AIDS

PIERLUIGI VIALE[1], ANGELA DI MATTEO[1], MARZIO SISTI[1], FRANCO VOLTOLINI[2], CARLO PATIES[3], and FRANCESCO ALBERICI[1]

From the [1]Division of Infectious Diseases, [2]Second Division of Surgery, and the [3]Pathology Service, Ospedale Civile di Piacenza, Piacenza, Italy

Although the importance of Aspergillus in AIDS is now increasing, extra-pulmonary disease is still an unusual event, especially when a single localization occurs. A case of isolated renal aspergilloma in an AIDS patient is described. At onset, no recognized risk factors were present in our patient. An early surgical approach combined with antifungal chemotherapy (amphotericin B, Itraconazole) led to a good control of the disease, with no evidence of recrudescence at 8 months' follow-up.

P. Viale, MD, Division of Infectious Diseases, Ospedale Civile di Piacenza, via Taverna 49, I-29100 Piacenza, Italy

INTRODUCTION

Aspergillus spp. is considered unusual as an agent of opportunistic infections in AIDS. Nevertheless its role as a pathogen in this disease is now increasing, probably due to prolonged survival and frequent occurrence of neutropenia and impaired macrophage function. Invasive disease is the Aspergillus infection most frequently reported, with prevalent localization to the lungs. Extrapulmonary disease is still rare, especially as a single, deep localization. We report a case of isolated renal aspergilloma, an extremely uncommon feature of invasive aspergillosis in AIDS patients.

CASE REPORT

A 28-year-old male, former intravenous drug user was admitted to the Division with a 2-week history of left lower back pain unresponsive to ketoprofen and with intermittent temperature up to 38°C, nocturnal sweating and a 5 kg weight loss over 1 month.

AIDS had been diagnosed 3 months earlier, due to Pneumocystis carinii pneumonia (PCP), which had been successfully treated with Co-trimoxazole plus prednisone. During the ensuing 2 months he had been well except for an ALT elevation detected 1 month after the onset of PCP which was ascribed to Co-trimoxazole toxicity. Abdominal ultrasound scanning revealed liver and spleen enlargement but the kidneys were normal. He was treated with zidovudine (250 mg b.i.d.) and aerosolized pentamidine once a month. On admission to hospital his temperature was 37.8°C, pulse 80 and blood pressure 130/80. The patient complained of severe pain in his left flank. On physical examination the abdomen was soft, not distended but tender in the left upper quadrant. Hepatomegaly and mild splenomegaly were noted.

Laboratory data showed a WBC count of 4.3×10^9/l, neutrophil count of 2.83×10^9/l, an absolute CD4 lymphocyte count of 8×10^6/l and normal values of serum creatinine and electrolytes. The urinalysis revealed 20–30 WBCs per high-power field. Radiographs of the chest were normal.

A 60×57 mm round mass in the lower pole of the left kidney was detected by means of abdominal sonography. The lesion was surrounded by a thick hyperechoic wall with a complex, partly anechoic centre, consistent with a loculated abscess. A computer-steered tomographic (CT) scan confirmed the presence of a large heterogeneous mass in the lower pole of the left kidney with suspected extension to the perinephric fat and thickening of the ipsilateral psoas, quadratus lumborum and iliacus muscles.

There was no evidence of renal vein or inferior vena cava involvement (Fig. 1). A renal abscess was diagnosed. On the second day of hospitalization a needle aspiration of the mass yielded 7 cc of grey-yellow pus. Microscopic examination of the aspirate showed necrotic material, polymorphonuclear

 ISSN 0036-5548

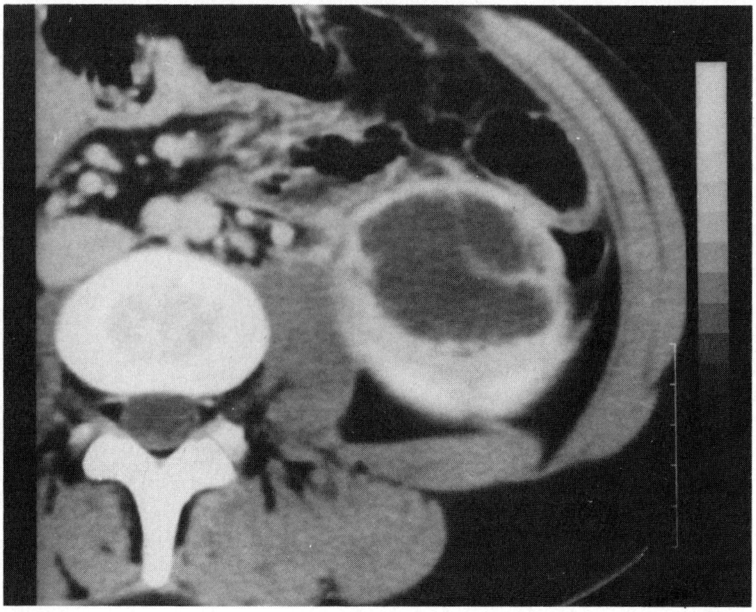

Fig. 1. CT scan appearance: Multiloculated, dishomogeneous renal mass with a strong ring enhancement. Involvement of ipsilateral iliopsoas muscle and perinephric fat.

leukocytes and hyphae consistent with Aspergillus species. Itraconazole 200 mg orally twice daily was instituted. Two days later, Aspergillus fumigatus was grown from the aspirate, while sputum, urine and blood cultures remained negative. Two additional percutaneous aspirations were performed on days 5 and 7, both yielding 50 ml of yellow purulent material. A drainage tube was left in situ and amphotericin B (25 mg diluted in 25 ml of 5% glucose solution) was administered daily by local instillation. On the following days the patient remained febrile, with progressive deterioration of the general status, increasing abdominal and left flank discomfort, anorexia, weight loss and occurrence of leukopenia. All blood and urine cultures, and an Aspergillus serum antigen test were negative.

After 2 weeks of treatment the patient underwent a left nephrectomy. A bulging, variegated renal mass with a polycyclic outline, 5 × 5 cm in size, was found in the lower pole. There was no macroscopical evidence of extension to the perirenal tissues, ureter or vasa. Following nephrectomy a thorough debridement of the perinephric fat and several biopsies and cultures from muscle tissue were performed. Microscopic examination showed a single large abscess with central necrosis and cavitation and a convoluted profile. A peripheral granulomatous reaction with histiocytes and a few multinucleated giant cells was present. Some smaller abscesses in the surrounding renal parenchyma most probably represented transverse sections of digitiform projections of the main abscess. The central necrosis contained nuclear debris and abundant dichotomous branching septatae hyphae, most of them with similar radial orientation, consistent with Aspergillus spp. (Fig. 2). The inflammatory process with necrosis, fungi and granulomatous reaction also involved the perirenal adipose tissue. Cultures of the necrotic material, perinephric fat and muscle biopsies subsequently grew Aspergillus fumigatus.

The patient had a normal postoperative course. On day 2 after surgery, intravenous amphotericin B was started (total dose 1.5 g in 3 weeks) and on day 7, when a normal oral intake was restored, Itraconazole 200 mg twice daily was readministered.

The patient's general status improved dramatically with the resolution of symptoms, afebrility and gradual weight gain, although cultures from postoperative drainage still grew Aspergillus fumigatus. 15 days after the operation he was discharged from hospital. A week later, dehiscence of the surgical wound occurred, with purulent discharge giving cultures positive for Aspergillus fumigatus. A CT-scan revealed multiple fluid collections in the left perinephric space, the largest 32 × 40 mm. Despite this rather discouraging complication, no surgical revision was required, as repeated local drainage and treatment with Itraconazole 200 mg twice daily achieved a complete recovery in 2 months. At follow-up, 8 months

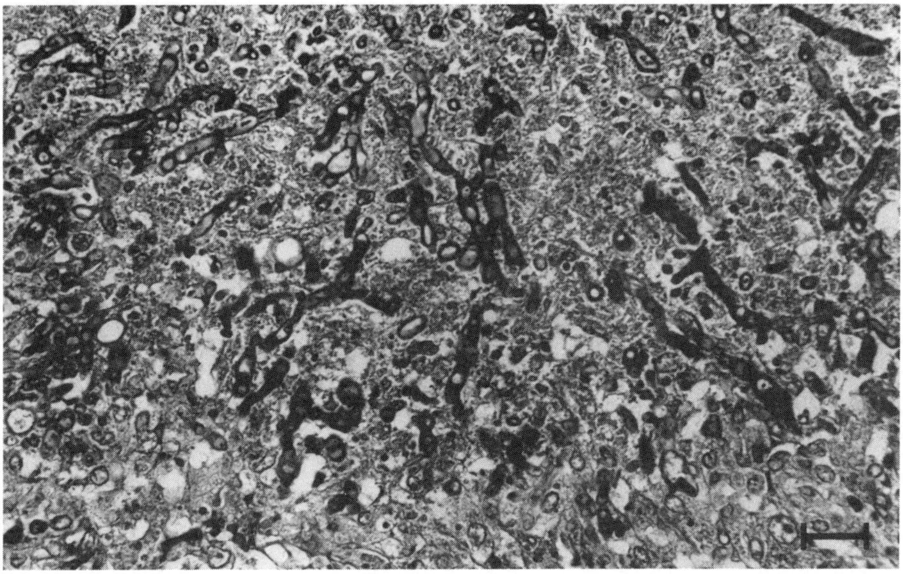

Fig. 2. Microscopic examination (magnification 40×): Dichotomous branching (with acute angle) septatae hyphae within the abscess.

later, the patient felt well. Suppressive treatment with Itraconazole 200 mg daily, was continued without side effects.

DISCUSSION

Kidney localization of Aspergillus infection occurred in 8% and 12% of patients respectively in 2 large series of non-AIDS patients (1–2), but it is an unusual finding when isolated (3–4). In AIDS patients, infection with Aspergillus species remains a rare occurrence. Nevertheless cases of invasive aspergillosis have been reported with rising frequency in recent years (5–7). Most of the case reports include at least one of the risk factors associated with this disease: neutropenia, use of corticosteroids, antineoplastic agents, broad-spectrum antibiotics, alcoholism, intravenous drug and marijuana use and underlying lung disease (5–7). In AIDS patients, as in others, the majority of cases reported had their aspergillosis localized to the lung, isolated or with concomitant involvement of brain, heart, kidney, sinuses, muscles or bones (8–11). In the English literature, only 2 cases of isolated renal aspergillosis in AIDS have been reported (12, 13).

In our case the isolated kidney localization of invasive Aspergillosis without specific risk factors was especially noteworthy. Firstly our patient was not taking illicit drugs, nor steroids, nor any drugs other than zidovudine and aerosolized pentamidine at the onset. Furthermore there was no history of alcoholism or leukopenia before the onset. Recently, however, the absence of risk factors has been increasingly reported (14).

The early surgical intervention was probably of importance for the favourable outcome. Early surgery, in our experience, is the treatment of choice even when severe immunodeficiency is present. Lastly, high dosage Itraconazole seems to be efficacious in sterilising the site of infection and preventing relapses.

ACKNOWLEDGEMENT

This study was supported by the Centro Studi AIDS e Malattie Infettive, Piacenza, Italy.

REFERENCES

1. Young RC, Benett JE, Vogel CL, Carbone PP, Devita VT. Aspergillosis: the spectrum of the disease in 98 patients. Medicine (Baltimore) 49: 147–173, 1970.
2. Meyer RD, Young LS, Armstrong D, Yu B. Aspergillosis complicating neoplastic disease. Am J Med 54: 6–15, 1973.
3. Melchior J, Mebust WK, Valk WL. Ureteral colic from a fungus ball: unusual presentation of systemic aspergillosis. J Urol 108: 698–699, 1972.
4. Baird RW, Lancaster DJ. Diabetic ketoacidosis as the presentation of renal aspergilloma. Am J Med 85: 453–454, 1988.
5. Pursell KJ, Telzak EE, Armstrong D. Aspergillus species colonization and invasive disease in patients with AIDS. Clin Infect Dis 14: 141–148, 1992.
6. Minamoto GY, Barlam TF, Vander Els N. Invasive aspergillosis in patients with AIDS. Clin Infect Dis 14: 66–74, 1992.
7. Dennig DW, Stephen BS, Follansbee E, Scolaro M, Norris S, Edelstein H, Stevens DA. Pulmonary aspergillosis in the Acquired Immunodeficiency Syndrome. N Engl J Med 324: 654–662, 1991.
8. Woods GL, Goldsmith JC. Aspergillus infection in the central nervous system in patient with AIDS. Arch Neurol 47: 181–184, 1990.
9. Schonheyder H, Hoffmann S, Jensen HL, Hansen BF, Franzmann MB. Aspergillus fumigatus fungaemia and myocarditis in a patient with AIDS. APMIS 100: 605–608, 1992.
10. Cox JN, di Dió F, Pizzolato P, Lerch R, Pochon N. Aspergillus endocarditis and myocarditis in a patient with AIDS. A review of the literature. Virchows Arch A Pathol Anat Histopathol 417: 255–259, 1990.
11. Decker CF, Perenti DM. Invasive aspergillosis in patients with HIV infection: report of two patients and review of the literature. J Acquir Immuno Defic Syndr 4: 603–606, 1992.
12. Halpern M, Szabo S, Hochberg E, Hammer GS, Lin J, Gurtman AC, Sacks H, Shapiro RS, Hirschmann SZ. Renal aspergilloma: an unusual cause of infection in a patient with AIDS. Am J Med 92: 437–440, 1992.
13. Weiss L, Piketty C, George F, Lavardre V, Kazatchkine MD. An unusual isolated kidney localization of invasive aspergillosis in an AIDS. Abstract PuB 7585 – VIII International Conference on AIDS. Amsterdam, The Netherlands, 19–24 July, 1992.
14. Lortholary O, Meyohas MC, Dupont B, Cadranel J, Salmon-Ceron D, Peyramond D, Simonin D and Centre d'informations et de Soins de l'Immunodéficience Humaine de l'est Parisien, for the French Cooperative Study Group on Aspergillosis in AIDS. Invasive aspergillosis in patients with acquired immunodeficiency syndrome: report of 33 cases. Am J Med 95: 177–187, 1992.

Submitted March 30, 1994; accepted July 17, 1994

Scand J Infect Dis 26: 771–773, 1994

SHORT COMMUNICATION

Group B Meningococcal Meningitis in India

MOHNISH SURI[1], MADHULIKA KABRA[1], SARMAN SINGH[2], ASHOK RATTAN[3] and ISHWAR C. VERMA[1]

From the Departments of [1]Pediatrics, [2]Laboratory Medicine and [3]Microbiology, All India Institute of Medical Sciences, New Delhi, India

The first case of infection with Group B meningococcus in India is reported. The patient was a 4-month-old boy who presented with meningitis and died within 6 h of admission. Gram stain of CSF showed meningococci and latex particle agglutination test on CSF was strongly positive for Neisseria meningitidis serogroup B. The CSF was also positive for meningococcus by polymerase chain reaction using primers NM1 and NM6, which amplify a 650 bp region of the dihydropteroate synthase (dhps) gene of N. meningitidis.

I. C. Verma, MD, Genetics Unit, Department of Pediatrics, Old Operation Theatre Building, All India Institute of Medical Sciences, Ansari Nagar, New Delhi-110 029, India

INTRODUCTION

Pyogenic meningitis is a worldwide common medical emergency. There are several causative organisms, of which Neisseria meningitidis (Grp. A, C, Y, W135) and Streptococcus pneumoniae (pneumococcus) are the commonest etiological agents in children older than 3 months, in India (1, 2). Other organisms less often reported include Haemophilus influenzae type "b", Staphylococcus aureus, and Enterobacteria (1, 3). Meningococcal disease is endemo-epidemic in India (4). In the last 2 reported epidemics of meningococcal meningitis in India, the causative serotype was Group A (4–6), as also in sporadic cases. To the best of our knowledge, there is no previous report of N. meningitidis group B causing meningitis in India. We therefore wish to report the first case of fatal meningitis, in an infant, caused by this rare strain of N. meningitidis.

CASE REPORT

A 4-month-old boy was brought to the hospital with complaints of drowsiness, refusal to feed and extreme irritability. On examination he was febrile (temperature 38.9°C), drowsy and distressed. He had no skin rash, and systemic examination was normal. A lumbar puncture showed turbid cerebrospinal fluid containing 0.96×10^9/l white cells, of which 70% were polymorphs. Glucose content of the fluid was 0.6 mmol/l (concomitant blood sugar 2.3 mmol/l) and protein content 2.33 g/l. Gram stain revealed numerous meningococci. The latex particle agglutination test (Wellcozyme, U.K.) was strongly positive for N. meningitidis serogroup B. The child was treated with intravenous ampicillin (300 mg/kg/day) and chloramphenicol (100 mg/kg/day) and supportive care, but he died within 6 h of hospitalization.

MATERIALS AND METHODS

Polymerase chain reaction (PCR)

As the organism failed to grow in culture from blood and cerebrospinal fluid, we performed the polymerase chain reaction (PCR) on the patient's CSF, using the oligonucleotide primers NM1 (5′-GGG TCG ACG GTT TCA GAC GGC ATA TAA-3′) and NM6 (5′-GTA AAC GGG CTT AAC TAC CGC-3′). These primers are designed to amplify a 650 bp fragment of the dihydropteroate synthase (dhps) gene of N. meningitidis (Dr Björn E. Kristiansen, personal communication).

The PCR was done by the method described by Kristiansen et al. (7). 250 μl CSF was mixed with 750 μl TE buffer (10 mM Tris-HCl, 1 mM EDTA, pH 8.0) and centrifuged. The pellet was resuspended in 20 μl of TE buffer. To 10 μl of this solution, 2 μl 10% Triton X-100 and 3 μl proteinase K were added,

Fig. 1. Photograph of electrophoresed PCR products. *Lane 2*, Positive (control) CSF sample; *Lane 3*, Negative (control) sample; *Lane 4*, CSF sample from patient.

and the suspension incubated at 55°C for 45 min. 10 μl of this mixture was used for PCR after heating it to 100°C in a waterbath for 10 min.

The PCR mixture (100 μl) consisted of 10 μl target DNA (CSF as treated above), 50 mM KCl, 10 mM Tris-HCl (pH 8.3), 1.5 mM $MgCl_2$, 0.01% gelatin, 200 μM each dNTP, 500 ng of each primer and 1.25 units of Taq polymerase. 40 cycles of amplification were carried out on an automated thermal cycler. Each cycle consisted of 1 min denaturation at 94°C, 1 min annealing at 55°C and 2 min extension at 72°C.

10 μl of the PCR product was electrophoresed on 2% agarose gel and the amplified DNA bands visualized under ultraviolet light after ethidium bromide staining. A positive and negative control sample was run with every batch of CSF samples processed. The positive control consisted of CSF from a culture-positive patient with meningococcal meningitis and the negative control consisted of sterile double-distilled water, both of which were processed in parallel with the test CSF samples.

The patient's CSF proved positive for meningococcus by PCR (Fig. 1).

DISCUSSION

The parents of the infant described had employed a maid-servant for the care of the child, only 1 week prior to his illness. She had recently come to India from Nepal. It is possible that this exotic serotype of meningococcus was imported into India by this Nepali girl, who infected the child. However, the only reported outbreaks of meningococcal meningitis in Nepal (in 1983–84 and 1984–85) were caused by N. meningitidis Group A (4, 8).

Epidemics of meningococcal meningitis have been recorded in India in 1935, 1933–39, 1966–67 and 1985–89 (4). Serotyping of the causative meningococcus in the last two outbreaks demonstrated that the organisms were serogroup A (5, 6). In contrast, serogroup B seems to be the predominant disease producing organism in countries of northwest Europe, including Norway, Iceland, Denmark, Britain and The Netherlands (9).

The occurrence of Group B meningococcal disease in India has extremely important public health implications. Specifically, no effective vaccine exists to prevent Group B meningococcal disease, unlike Group A and C meningococcal disease, where vaccines are available (10). Since this is the first report of Group B meningococcal disease from India, close surveillance is warranted to document any further cases of Group B disease, whether sporadic or epidemic. In this regard it is important to remember the example of Norway, where in the early 1970s the prevailing serogroup A and C meningococci almost disappeared, to be replaced by the new serogroup B meningococcus (9, 11, 12).

Recent publications (13, 14) suggest that patients with suspected meningococcal septicemia or meningitis should be given a single dose of intravenous benzylpenicillin by their general practitioner before transfer to a hospital. Although this is associated with a reduction in mortality, it also reduces the chance of isolating the organism from blood and CSF culture. Under these circumstances PCR, using primers NM1 and NM6, is a useful technique to document the presence of meningococcus in the CSF of such patients. It is both sensitive and specific (unpublished observations), and not affected by prior antibiotic treatment of the patient, since the target for the PCR is bacterial DNA which is present even in the killed organisms. Detection of meningococci in the CSF of patients with suspected meningitis, by PCR, will confirm the diagnosis and allow chemoprophylaxis to be given to household contacts. It will also provide useful epidemiological data on meningococcal meningitis.

ACKNOWLEDGEMENTS

The authors wish to thank Dr Björn E. Kristiansen of Telelab A/S, Skein, Norway for providing us the primers NM1 and NM6, and Ms Mette Olsen, also of Telelab A/S, for helping us standardize the PCR for detection of meningococcus in the Genetics Unit, Department of Pediatrics. Dr Suri also acknowledges the Pool Scheme of the Council of Scientific and Industrial Research, Government of India.

REFERENCES

1. Kabra SK, Kumar P, Verma IC, et al. Bacterial meningitis in India: an IJP survey. Indian J Pediatr 58: 505–511, 1991.
2. Kumar P, Verma IC. Antibiotic therapy for bacterial meningitis in children in developing countries. Bull World Health Organ 71: 183–188, 1993.
3. Singh H, Sarkar R, Sachdev HPS, Lata S. Immunological tests in acute bacterial meningitis. Indian Pediatr 25: 323–328, 1988.
4. Verghese T, Kumari S, Ichhpujani RL. Meningococcal meningitis. Delhi: National Institute of Communicable Diseases, 13–20, 1990.
5. Bhatia SL, Sharma KB, Natarajan R. An outbreak of meningococcal meningitis in Delhi. Indian J Med Res 56: 259–263, 1968.
6. Deorari AK, Verma IC, Maheswari MC, Bhujwala RA, Paul VK. Prognostic factors related to mortality in meningococcal disease. Indian J Med Res 86: 212–217, 1987.
7. Kristiansen BE, Ask E, Jenkins A, Fermer C, Radström P, Sköld O. Rapid diagnosis of meningococcal meningitis by polymerase chain reaction. Lancet 337: 1568–1569, 1991.
8. Epidemic meningococcal disease: recommendations for travelers to Nepal. MMWR 34: 119–120, 125, 1985.
9. Poolman JT, Lind I, Jonsdottir K, Fröholm LO, Jones DM, Zanen HC. Meningococcal serotypes and serogroup B disease in North-West Europe. Lancet 2: 555–558, 1986.
10. Jones DM. Current and future trends in immunization against meningitis. J Antimicrob Chemother 31 (suppl B): 93–99, 1993.
11. Bovre J, Gedde-Dahl TW. Epidemiological patterns of meningococcal disease in Norway 1975–79. NIPH Ann 3: 9–23, 1980.
12. Bovre K, Fröholm LO, Gaustad P, Holten E, Høiby EA. Some agent characteristics and their coexistence related to occurrence and severity of systemic meningococcal disease in Norway, winter 1981–82. NIPH Ann 6: 75–84, 1983.
13. Strang JR, Pugh EJ. Meningococcal infections: reducing the case fatality rate by giving penicillin before admission to hospital. BMJ 305: 141–143, 1992.
14. Cartwright K, Reilly S, White D, Stuart J. Early treatment with parenteral penicillin in meningococcal disease. BMJ 305: 143–147, 1992.

Submitted April 11, 1994; accepted July 29, 1994

Scand J Infect Dis 26: 777–778, 1994

SHORT COMMUNICATION

Legionella Urinary Antigen in Early Disease

SVERKER BERNANDER[1], BENGT GÄSTRIN[2], STURE LÖFGREN[3], and ANNE-MARIE OLINDER-NIELSEN[4]

From the [1]Department of Clinical Microbiology, Karolinska Hospital, and the [2]Department of Bacteriology, National Bacteriological Laboratory, the [3]Department of Clinical Bacteriology, and [4]Infectious Diseases, Ryhov County Hospital Jönköping, Sweden

The results of Legionella urinary antigen testing were correlated to the interval between onset of disease and sampling of urine in 134 patients in connection with a large outbreak of Legionnaires' disease at a Swedish hospital. In 17 patients with the disease, 5/7 sampled during the first 5 days of illness proved negative in the urinary antigen test. The risk of obtaining negative results during the first days of the disease is emphasized.

S. Bernander, MD, Department of Clinical Microbiology, Karolinska Hospital, S-171 76 Stockholm, Sweden

INTRODUCTION

Radioimmunossay (RIA) and enzyme immunoassay (EIA) methods have been developed for the detection of Legionella antigen in urine and have been successfully used in several studies (1–6). Generally speaking specificity is high, near 1.0, whereas sensitivity is lower. In connection with an outbreak of Legionnaires' disease in a hospital in southern Sweden (7), we attempted to evaluate a commercial kit for testing Legionella antigen in urine. The results of the urinary antigen test were correlated to the time of onset of the disease.

MATERIALS AND METHODS

In 31 patients affected by the outbreak, the causative organism was Legionella pneumophila serogroup 1. During the latter part of the outbreak, urine specimens were obtained from 134 consecutive and evaluable patients who had been admitted to the hospital on suspicion of pneumonia or lower respiratory tract disease. 10 patients were samples twice, in which cases only the first urine sample was included. The time of disease onset was carefully recorded by the physician in charge of the ward. Acute and convalescent sera were collected and tested for antibodies against Legionella. Lung tissue from 1 patient and sputum from only 7 patients were cultured and studied with DFA. Antigen of L. pneumophila serogroup 1 in urine specimens was detected with RIA (EquateLegionella Urinary Antigen, Binax Inc., Portland, ME, USA). The degree of antigenuria is calculated as a ratio of $CPM_{\text{patient specimen}}/CPM_{\text{negative control}}$. Values ≥ 3 were considered positive in accordance with the manufacturer's recommendations.

Antibodies were detected using the indirect immunofluorescence antibody test with a heat-killed antigen of L. pneumophila serogroups 1–8, L. micdadei, L. bozemanii and L. longbeachae. A 4-fold titre change (rise or decline) or single titre of ≥ 128 were considered positive.

Lung tissue or sputum was acid-treated and cultured on buffered charcoal yeast extract agar with α-ketoglutarate and on the same agar with addition of cefamandole and polymyxin B for 7 days at 37°C (8). FITC-conjugated monoclonal reagents (Genetic Systems, USA) were used for DFA.

RESULTS

16 patients proved positive in serology for L. pneumophila serogroup 1. One of these was also culture positive in sputum. Another patient was positive with DFA in lung tissue from the autopsy. This patient was seronegative in an early sample taken before he died. Of these 17 patients, 9 proved positive in the urinary antigen test and 8 were negative. Five of 7

 ISSN 0036-5548

samples (71%) obtained during the first 5 days of disease proved negative and 4/7 (57%) obtained during days 30–60. All 3 samples obtained during days 6–14 were positive. The overall sensitivity was 0.53 and specificity 0.98.

DISCUSSION

In 1 study, RIA for L. pneumophila serogroup 1 urinary antigen was found to be positive in at least 80% of proven clinical cases, including those tested during the first 3 days of disease (5). In another study, using culture-confirmed cases as a 'gold standard', sensitivity was 0.93 and specificity 1.0 (9). In our study, with almost only serological confirmation, sensitivity was much lower, and seems to have been associated with early specimen collection after disease onset. This has not been stressed earlier, though in 1 report a case with a negative value after 4 days became positive on the fifth day (10). Since our patients were nosocomially infected we were able to determine the disease onset accurately. In earlier reports, these data may have been acquired retrospectively (5, 10). In our study no negative tests were found among the patients sampled between days 6 and 14. Though these were few in number, earlier studies have shown a high sensitivity. Specimens collected a month or more after disease onset showed, as can be expected, some negative results. As has been shown earlier, antigenuria can persist for at least 2 months (4, 5).

In summary, we have observed that negative tests for Legionella urinary antigen occur during the first 5 days of Legionnaires' disease. Thus clinicians should repeat the test if suspicion of the disease persists.

REFERENCES

1. Berdal BP, Forshy CE, Feeley JC. Detection of Legionella pneumophila antigen in urine by enzyme-linked immunospecific assay. J Clin Microbiol 9: 575–578, 1979.
2. Kohler RB, Zimmerman SE, Wilson E, Allen SD, Edelstein PH, Wheat LJ, White A. Rapid radiommunoassay diagnoisis of Legionnaires disease. Detection and partial characterization of urinary antigen. Ann Intern Med 94: 601–605, 1981.
3. Fehrenbach FJ, Horbach I, Ruf B, Schurmann D, Pohle HD. Rapid detection of Legionella antigen in tissue and body fluids. Isr J Med Sci 22: 706–710, 1986.
4. Ruf B, Schurman D, Horbach I, Fehrenbach FJ, Pohle HD. Prevalence and diagnosis of Legionella pneumonia: a 3-year prospective study with emphasis on application of urinary antigen detection. J Infect Dis 162: 1341–1348, 1990.
5. Kohler RB, Winn CW Jr, Wheat LJ. Onset and duration of urinary antigen-excretion in Legionnaires disease. J Clin Microbiol 20: 605–607, 1984.
6. Samuel D, Harrison TG, and Taylor AG. Detection of Legionella pneumophila serogroup 1 urinary antigen using an enhanced chemoluminescence ELISA. J Biolumin Chemilumin 5: 183–185, 1990.
7. Darelid J, Bengtsson L, Gästrin B, Hallander H, Löfgren S, Malmvall BE, Olinder-Nielsen AM, Thelin AC. An outbreak of Legionnaires' disease in a Swedish hospital. Scand J Infect Dis 26: 417–425, 1994.
8. Edelstein PH. Improved semiselective medium for isolation of Legionella pneumophila from contaminated clinical and environmental specimens. J Clin Microbiol 14: 298–303, 1981.
9. Aguero-Rosenfeld ME, Edelstein PH. Retrospective evaluation of the Du Pont radioimmunossay kit for detection of Legionella pneumophila serogroup 1 antigenuria in humans. J Clin Microbiol 26: 1775–1778, 1988.
10. Birtles RJ, Harrison TG, Samuel D, Taylor AG. Evaluation of urinary antigen ELISA for diagnosing Legionella pneumophila serogroup 1 infection. J Clin Pathol 43: 685–690, 1990.

Submitted April 27, 1994; accepted September 7, 1994

LETTER TO THE EDITORS

Chlamydia pneumoniae (TWAR): A Common Agent in Acute Bronchitis

Dear Sir,

Interest in Chlamydia pneumoniae (TWAR) as a respiratory tract pathogen is steadily increasing. It is important to gather more data concerning the prevalence of this pathogen, and its importance in various clinical entities such as bronchitis and pneumonia. In an article in Scand J Infect Dis 26: 179–187, 1994, Falck and co-workers conclude "that C. pneumoniae can be a major cause of acute bronchitis". The objective of their study was to investigate the prevalence of infections associated with C. pneumoniae, and the authors state that evidence for such infection was found in approximately 25% of 114 patients with various respiratory tract diseases. The data presented certainly indicate that a C. pneumoniae infection probably was the cause of the disease in several patients. However, I do not believe that the main objective of the study was answered. My reasons are the following;

1) Patient selection. Patients were included if they had symptoms of respiratory tract infection for >1 week. Thus, it is still not known whether C. pneumoniae is a common cause of acute bronchitis, since the number of patients with symptoms for <1 week was not reported. Furthermore, 20% of the originally enrolled patients were not included because they did not meet the inclusion criteria. If these patients did not have respiratory tract symptoms, why were they enrolled? If they had respiratory tract symptoms, what then was the definition of "no ongoing infection"?

2) Serologic diagnosis. There is no consensus concerning the definition of a serological diagnosis of C. pneumoniae (1). In this paper, according to Table I, a "confirmed" C. pneumoniae infection was defined as an IgM titer of ≥16, or a 4-fold rise in the titer of IgG. However, the pattern of serological reactions among the 15 patients reported to have a confirmed infection seems confusing to me. A 4-fold increase in IgG titers was seen in only 6/15 patients, and in 3 of them, the IgG titer rose to not more than 64 (and no IgM). One patient (no. 37) had a 4-fold decrease in IgG titer, and no IgM reaction, and thus did not meet the criteria for a confirmed infection. In 8 patients the diagnosis was based on IgM. Two of these had an increase (2-fold) and 2 had a decrease in IgG titers. Another patient had an IgM titer of 32 only in the second test, whereas IgG was 1024 both after 2 and 8 weeks of illness.

3) Other infections. The authors state in "Results" that "a number of additional patients were found to have IgG titers of 512 and were most likely infected with C. pneumoniae according to their clinical histories". However, later on in the same section they continue that "no specific symptom signifying infection with C. pneumoniae could be defined". M. pneumoniae was the only other etiologic agent that was tested for (positive in 2 patients). In patients with a history of respiratory tract symptoms for weeks and months (up to 48 weeks) there is of course a possibility of several different etiologic agents, mixed infections, or of C. pneumoniae with a secondary infection. Most of the antibiotics given were also effective for the treatment of S. pneumoniae, M. catharralis and, to a somewhat lesser extent, H. influenzae. Without the knowledge of the prevalence of these bacterial pathogens, and of respiratory tract viruses, in the population studied, it is difficult to assess the importance of the serological findings of C. pneumoniae.

Finally, I agree with the authors in that there is a need for continuous surveillance of the spectrum of causative agents in lower respiratory tract infections as a basis for the choice of antibiotic treatment. However, such studies should include a wide spectrum of agents. As for the authors conclusion, I believe this should state only that C. pneumoniae can cause acute bronchitis and other respiratory infections.

REFERENCES

1. Ekman MR, Leinonen M, Syrjälä, H, Linnanmäki E, Kujala P, Saikku P. Evaluation of serological methods in the diagnosis of Chlamydia pneumoniae pneumonia during an epidemic in Finland. Eur J Clin Microbiol Infect Dis 12: 756–760, 1993.

Address for correspondence: **Åke Örtqvist**, Department of infectious diseases, Danderyd Hospital, S-188 88 Danderyd, Sweden

REPLY

Dear Sir,

Dr Örtqvist has written a letter to the Editor regarding our paper, Chlamydia pneumoniae (TWAR): a common agent in acute bronchitis. The background for our investigation was as follows:

Several cases of sudden, unexpected death (SUD) occurred among elite orienteers during the years 1989–92. Some of these originated from our geographical area. A report published in August 1992 (1) implicated an association between Chlamydia pneumoniae and a case of SUD.

During the autumn of 1992 we observed an increased number of longstanding respiratory tract infections in our area. Among others, a team of bandy players in the highest division was infected. Case 79 in our report was one of them (2). Two other athletes were observed for suspected myocarditis.

Another elite orienteer died suddenly in early November. The general anxiety in our area increased when a 16-year-old girl died shortly after this while jogging.

At this point we decided to investigate whether exposure to C. pneumoniae was common in the area, and if C. pneumoniae was associated with respiratory infections. We agree with Örtqvist that it would have been ideal to direct our investigation toward most established respiratory pathogens, including viral agents. The epidemiological situation and the available economic resources made this impossible. We therefore decided to study the prevalence of infections associated with C. pneumoniae.

Some of the patients in the original material had to be excluded later, i.e., all players from the infected bandy team who had recovered before the start of the study. Another reason for exclusion was that consecutive specimens were not obtained from all children under 10 years of age.

We are well aware of the apparent lack of consensus regarding the criteria for a diagnosis based on serological findings. This is also further complicated by technical problems due to the technique used (3), and by the primary or recurrent nature of the infection. We defined a "confirmed" infection as a patient with an inverted IgM titer of ≥ 16 or a 4-fold change in IgG or IgA titer. We agree with Örtqvist that the line in Table I "Confirmed C. pneumoniae infection: 4-fold IgG rise . . ." should instead have been . . . 4-fold IgG change. We believe that determinations of specific IgA antibodies may often provide valuable information for the evaluation of serological findings, as stated by Saikku (4) and Ekman et al. (5).

Since our paper was accepted for publication, Garyston et al. (6) have published a report of an outbreak of respiratory infections in university students. Their findings are similar to ours. We maintain C. pneumoniae may be a common agent in acute bronchitis.

REFERENCES

1. Wesslén L, Påhlsson C, Friman G, Fohlman J, Lindqvist O, Johansson, C. Myocarditis caused by Chlamydia pneumoniae (TWAR) and sudden unexpected death in a Swedish elite orienteer. Lancet 340: 427–8, 1992.
2. Falck G, Heyman L, Gnarpe J, Gnarpe H. Chlamydia pneumoniae (TWAR): a common agent in acute bronchitis. Scand J Infect Dis 26: 179–187, 1994.
3. Grayston JT, Campbell LA, Kuo C-C, Mordhorst CH, Saikku P, Thom DH, Wang S-P. A new respiratory tract pathogen: Chlamydia pneumoniae strain TWAR. J Infect Dis 161: 618–625, 1990.
4. Saikku P, Leinonen M, Tenkanen L, Linnanmäki E, Ekman MR, Manninen V, Mänitäri M, Frick MH, Huttunen JK. Chronic Chlamydia pneumoniae infection as a risk factor for coronary heart disease in the Helsinki heart study. Ann Intern Med 116: 273–278, 1992.
5. Ekman MR, Leinonen M, Syrjälä H, Linnanmäki E, Kujala P, Saikku P. Evaluation of serological methods in the diagnosis of Chlamydia pneumoniae pneumonia during an epidemic in Finland. Eur J Clin Microbiol Infect Dis 12: 756–760, 1993.
6. Grayston T, Aldous MB, Easton A, Wang S-P, Kuo C-C, Campbell LA, Altman J. Evidence that Chlamydia pneumoniae causes pneumonia and bronchitis. J Infect Dis 1993: 168: 1231–1235.

Göran Falck, Lena Heyman, Håkan Gnarpe and Judy Gnarpe

Address for correspondence: G. Falck, MD, Apoteksgårdens Vårdcentrum, S-714 22 Kopparberg, Sweden

No. 1

Review Article

H. Hemila: Does vitamin C alleviate the symptoms of the common cold? – a review of current evidence 1

Articles

J. Mustonen, M. Brummer-Korvenkontio, K. Hedman, A. Pasternack, K. Pietilä and A. Vaheri: Nephropathia epidemica in Finland: a retrospective study of 126 cases 7
M. García-Bengoechea, A. Cortés, P. López, J. L. Vega, J. I. Emparanza, A. Sarriugarte, E. Santos and J. I. Arenas: Intrafamilial spread of hepatitis C virus infection 15
S. Iwarson, W. Jilg and T. Stroffolini: Substantial decline of notified hepatitis B in Europe after 1985 19
J. Blomberg, T. Moestrup, J. Frimand, B-G Hansson, K. Krogsgaard, L. Grillner and E. Nordenfelt: HTLV-I and -II in intravenous drug users from Sweden and Denmark 23
H. L. Hansen, L. Brandt, J. Jensen, U. Balslev, S. Skarphedinsson, A. F. Jørgensen, K. David and F. T. Black: HIV infection among seafarers in Denmark 27
K. Elvin, A. Björkman, N. Heurlin, B-M. Eriksson, L. Barkholt and E. Linder: Seroreactivity to Pneumocystis carinii in patients with AIDS versus other immunosuppressed patients 33
D. Gabrilovich, L. Ivanova, L. Serebrovskaya, G. Shepeleva and V. Pokrovsky: Clinical significance of neutrophil functional activity in HIV infection 41
M. Peters, D. Schürmann, F. Bergmann, T. Grünewald, H. Timm, H. D. Pohle and B. Ruf: Safety of alternating ganciclovir and foscarnet maintenance therapy in human immunodeficiency virus (HIV)-related cytomegalovirus infections. An open-labeled pilot study 49
R. Manfredi, P. Vezzadini, M. P. Fanti and F. Chiodo: Vasoactive intestinal polypeptide (VIP) secretion and refractory diarrhea in patients with AIDS or AIDS-related complex (ARC) 55
H. Portier, P. Chavanet, A. Waldner-Combernoux, J. P. Kisterman, P. C. Grey, F. Ichou and C. Safran: Five versus ten days treatment of streptococcal pharyngotonsillitis: a randomized controlled trial comparing cefpodoxime proxetil and phenoxymethyl penicillin 59
M. Walder, E. Karlsson and B. Nilsson: Sensitivity of 880 blood culture isolates to 24 antibiotics 67
E. Rintala: Incidence and clinical significance of positive blood cultures in febrile episodes of patients with hematological malignancies 77
M. Studahl, B. Bergman, P. Kälebo and J. Lindberg: Septic arthritis of the knee. A 10-year review and long-term follow-up using a new scoring system 85
L-M. Tang and S-T. Chen: Klebsiella pneumoniae meningitis: prognostic factors 95

Case Reports

H. Lecour, L. Santos, M. Oliveira, A. Pereira and J. Simões: Salmonella typhi meningitis 103
M. Vadillo, X. Corbella and J. Carratala: AIDS presenting as septic shock caused by Mycobacterium tuberculosis 105
M. Okano, K. Kishiyama, N. Satake, S. Kubo and N. Ishikawa: A case of fulminant ecthyma gangrenosum associated with Pseudomonas aeruginosa infection in a patient with methylmalonic acidemia 107
T. Tantawichien, K. Tungsanga and D. Swasdikul: Reversible severe neutropenia after ceftriaxone 109
L. M. Lagging, C. M. Breland, D. J. Kennedy, T. W. Milligan, M. L. Sokol-Anderson and T. U. Westblom: Delayed treatment of pulmonary blastomycosis causing vertebral osteomyelitis, paraspinal abscess, and spinal cord compression 111
N. Obel and F. T. Black: Microscopic examination of sperm as the diagnostic clue in a case of Schistosoma haematobium infection 117

Letters to the Editors

F. Messina, P. Del Bravo, S. Luchi, D. Aquilini and A. Scasso: Abdominal lymphonodal enlargement in HIV patients detected by ultrasonography 119

Reply

F. Cassani, P. Costigliola, M. Zoli, L. Baffoni, N. Dentale, E. Ricchi, F. Chiodo, G. Pilati, F. B. Bianchi and E. Pisi 120

No. 2

Articles

A. Krook and J. Blomberg: HTLV-II among injecting drug users in Stockholm 129
E. Perez-Trallero, G. Cilla, M. Urbieta, M. Dorronsoro, F. Otero and J. M. Marimon: Falling incidence and prevalence of hepatitis A in northern Spain 133
K. Skaug, I. J. Hagen and B. von der Lippe: Three cases of acute hepatitis E virus infection imported into Norway 137
M. Glimåker, P. Olcén and B. Andersson: Interferon-γ in cerebrospinal fluid from patients with viral and bacterial meningitis 141
L. Motiejunas, J. Bunikis, A. G. Barbour and A. Sadziene: Lyme borreliosis in Lithuania 149
M. Arpi, M. A. Victor, J. K. Møller, V. Jønsson, M. Mørk Hansen, N. A. Peterslund and B. Bruun: Changing etiology of bacteremia in patients with hematological malignancies in Denmark 157
M. A. Victor, M. Arpi, B. Bruun, V. Jønsson and M. Mørk Hansen: Xanthomonas maltophilia bacteremia in immunocompromised hematological patients 163
A. Jensen, W. Frederiksen and P. Gerner-Smidt: Risk factors for listeriosis in Denmark, 1989–1990 171
G. Falck, L. Heyman, J. Gnarpe and H. Gnarpe: Chlamydia pneumoniae (TWAR): a common agent in acute bronchitis 179
M. Floor, F. van Akkeren, M. Rozenberg-Arska, M. Visser, A. Kolsters, H. Beumer and J. Verhoef: Effect of loracarbef and amoxicillin on the oropharyngeal and intestinal microflora of patients with bronchitis 191
A. Persson and L. Rombo: Intestinal parasites in refugees and asylum seekers entering the Stockholm area, 1987–88: evaluation of routine stool screening 199

Case Reports
E. Andström, S. Bygdeman, S. Ahlén. A. Heimdal and B. Nyström: Stomatococcus mucilaginosus septicemia in two bone marrow transplanted patients 209
K. Gillet-Juvin, M. Stern, D. Israël-Biet, D. Penaud and F. Carnot: A highly unusual combination of pulmonary pathogens in an HIV infected patient 215
P. Chan, J. J. Huang and Y. J. Yang: Left vocal cord palsy: an unusual presentation of a mycotic aneurysm of the aorta caused by Salmonella cholerasuis 219
A. Møller Heilesen and P.-H. Christensen: Abscess of the submandibular gland caused by Salmonella typhimurium biotype 10 223
M. E. Ellis, H. Clink, D. Younge and B. Hainau: Successful combined surgical and medical treatment of fusarium infection after bone marrow transplantation 225

No. 3

Historical Review
U. Högberg: Effect of introduction of sulphonamides on the incidence of and mortality from puerperal sepsis in a Swedish county hospital 233

Articles
K. Krogsgaard, S. Boesgaard, J. Aldershvile, H. Arendrup, S. A. Mortensen, G. Petterson and The Copenhagen Heart Transplant Group: Cytomegalovirus infection rate among heart transplant patients in relation to the anti-thymocyte immunoglobulin induction therapy 239
A. Thorén and A. Widell: PCR for the diagnosis of enteroviral meningitis 249
B. Johansson, Z.-B. Yun and A. Sönnerborg: Variability of the E2/NS1 region of Swedish hepatitis C virus strains and its correlation to genotypes 255
Z. B. Yun, O. Reichard, M. Chen, J. Lundeberg, G. Norkrans, A. Fryden, A. Sönnerborg and O. Weiland: Serum hepatitis C virus RNA levels in chronic hepatitis C – importance for outcome of interferon alfa-2b treatment 263
J. Lundeberg, L. Bondesson, A. Hedrum, L. Grillner, M. Stark, G. von Krogh and M. Uhlén: Microtiter assay for colorimetric detection of in vitro amplified Chlamydia trachomatis sequences 275
P. Carlson, O.-V. Renkonen and S. Kontiainen: Arcanobacterium haemolyticum and streptococcal pharyngitis 283
R. Ikäheimo, A. Siitonen, U. Kärkkäinen, J. Mustonen, T. Heiskanen and P. H. Mäkelä: Community-acquired pyelonephritis in adults: characteristics of E. coli isolates in bacteremic and non-bacteremic patients 289
L.-B. B. Jeng, J.-D. Lin and M.-F. Chen: Acute suppurative thyroiditis: a ten-year review in a Taiwanese hospital 297
K. Ekdahl and C. Kamme: Increasing resistance to penicillin in Streptococcus pneumoniae in southern Sweden 301
The Swedish CDAD Study Group: Treatment of Clostridium difficile associated diarrhea and colitis with an oral preparation of teicoplanin; a dose finding study 309
J. Rydberg, C. Larsson and H. Miörner: Resistance to fluoroquinolones in Pseudomonas aeruginosa and Klebsiella pneumoniae 317
L. A. Noach, W. L. Langenberg, M. A. Bertola, J. Dankert and G. N. J. Tytgat: Impact of metronidazole resistance on the eradication of Helicobacter pylori 321
R. Achí, L. Mata and A. A. Lindberg: Serum antibody titres to Shigella lipopolysaccharides and invasion plasmid antigens in healthy Costa Rican and Swedish women 329
S. Hammers-Berggren, A.-M. Lebech, M. Karlsson, U. Andersson, K. Hansen and G. Stiernstedt: Serological follow-up after treatment of Borrelia arthritis and acrodermatitis chronica atrophicans 339
J. Junttila, R. Tanskanen and J. Tuomi: Prevalence of Borrelia burgdorferi in selected tick populations in Finland 349

Short Communication
N. Cimolai: Mycoplasma pneumoniae lacks immunologically-active eukaryotic actin-like antigens 358

No. 4

Review Article
C. Watanakunakorn and S. C. Perni: Proteus mirabilis bacteremia: a review of 176 cases during 1980–1992 361

Articles
A. Boehler, A. Schaffner, F. Salomon and G. Keusch: Cytomegalovirus disease of late onset following renal transplantation: a potentially fatal entity 369
S. Panhani and K. M. Heinonen: Screening for congenital cytomegalovirus infection among preterm infants born before the 34th gestational week in Finland 375
K. Ritter, A. Uy, S. Ritter and R. Thomssen: Hemolysis and autoantibodies to triosephosphate isomerase in a patient with acute hepatitis A virus infection 379
O. Reichard, H. Glaumann and O. Weiland: Long-term histological outcome in patients with chronic hepatitis C treated repeatedly with interferon alpha-2b without sustained response 383
S. Einarsson, H. K. Sigurdsson, S. D. Magnusdottir, H. Erlendsdottir, H. Briem and S. Gudmundsson: Age specific prevalence of antibodies against Chlamydia pneumoniae in Iceland 393
B. A. Claesson and M. Leinonen: Moraxella catarrhalis – an uncommon cause of community-acquired pneumonia in Swedish children 399
J. Kavaliotis, A. Tsiaousi, D. Papavasiliou and A. Kansouzidou: Non-typhoid salmonella meningitis 403
B. Olesen, H. J. Kolmos, F. Ørskov and I. Ørskov: Cluster of multiresistant Escherichia coli O78:H10 in Greater Cophenhagen 406
M. Kristjánsson, B. Viner and J. N. Maslow: Polymicrobial and recurrent bactermia with Shigella in a patient with AIDS 411
J. Darelid, L. Bengtsson, B. Gästrin, H. Hallander, S. Löfgren, B.-E. Malmvall, A.-M. Olinder-Nielsen an

A.-C. Thelin: An outbreak of Legionnaires' disease in a Swedish hospital 417
K. Vos, A. P. van Dam, H. Kuiper, H. Bruins, L. Spanjaard and J. Dankert: Seroconversion for Lyme borreliosis among Dutch military 427
A. Li, C. R. Zhao, E. Ekwall and A. A. Lindberg: Serum IgG antibody responses to Shigella invasion plasmid-coded antigens detected by immunoblot 435
B. Barry, P. Gehanno, M. Blumen and I. Boucot: Clinical outcome of acute otitis media caused by pneumococci with decreased susceptibility to penicillin 446
G. Granström and M. Granström: Effect of erythromycin treatment on antibody responses in pertussis 453
B. Andreassen Rix, A. Zhobakas, C. H. Wachmann, V. Bakasenas and T. Rønne: Immunity from diphtheria, tetanus, poliomyelitis, measles, mumps and rubella among adults in Lithuania 459
J. Struve, B. Aronsson, B. Frenning, M. Forsgren and O. Weiland: Seroconversion after additional vaccine doses to non-responders to three doses of intradermally or intramuscularly administered recombinant hepatitis B vaccine 468
B. Björkholm, M. Wahl, M. Granström and L. Hagberg: Immune status and booster effects of low doses of tetanus toxoid in Swedish medical personnel 471
E. Chryssanthou, B. Andersson, B. Petrini, S. Löfdahl, J. Tollemar: Detection of Candida albicans DNA in serum by polymerase chain reaction 479

Case Reports
K. Martin, M. Sharland and E. G. Davies: Encephalopathy associated with Salmonella enteritidis infection 486
G. J. Stranks and M. I. McLaren: Salmonella paratyphi – an unusual cause of primary septic arthritis of the hip 489
O. A. Alexeyev, V. G. Morozov, A. G. Efremov and B. Settergren: A case of haemorrhagic fever with renal syndrome complicated by spleen haemorrhage 491
H. Hardardóttir, K. Vikenes, A. Digranes, J. Lassen and A. Halstensen: Mixed bacteremia with Vibrio metschnikovii in an 83-year-old female patient 493
K. Konstantopoulos, A. Avlami, K. Demarongona, G. Sideris, L. Rekoumi, J. Stefanou, E. Voskaridou and D. Loukopoulos: Bacteroides fragilis arthritis in a sickle cell-thalassaemia patient 495
R. S. Dykhuizen, K. N. Kerr and R. L. Soutar: Air crescent sign and fatal haemoptysis in pulmonary mucormycosis 498

No. 5

Review Article
I. Brook: Peptostreptococcal infection in children 503

Articles
K.-S. Tveit, A. Nyfors and A. Nilsen: HIV-seropositive rate and HIV test activity among STD clinic attendees in Bergen, Norway 511
E. Smith and MK Orholm: Danish AIDS patients 1988–1993: a recent decline in Pneumocystis carinii pneumonia as AIDS-defining disease related to the period of known HIV positivity 517
M. Gisslén, F. Chiodi, D. Fuchs, G. Norkrans, B. Svennerholm, H. Wachter and L. Hagberg: Markers of immune stimulation in the cerebro-spinal fluid during HIV infection: a longitudinal study 523
A. Orrling, A. Stjernquist-Desatnik, C. Schalén and C. Kamme: Clindamycin in persisting streptococcal pharyngotonsillitis after penicillin treatment 535
P. Gottfarb and A. Brauner: Children with persistent cough – outcome with treatment and role of Moraxella catarrhalis 545
I. Jönsson, T. Holme and A. Krook: Significance of isolation of Moraxella catarrhalis in routine cultures from the respiratory tract in adults: antibody response studied in a whole cell EIA 553
M. Roberg, P. Forsberg, A. Frydén, B. Hederstedt, D. Hydén and L. Ödkvist: Long-term findings in patients with facial palsy and antibodies against Borrelia burgdorferi 559
K. Hjelt, N. Højlyng, P. Howitz, N. Illum, E. Munk, N. H. Valerius, K. Fursted, K. N. Hansen, I. Heltberg and C. Koch: The role of mycobacteria other than tuberculosis (MOTT) in patients with cystic fibrosis 569
P. Gehanno, B. Barry, S. Bobin and C. Safran: Twice daily cefpodoxime proxetil compared with thrice daily amoxicillin/clavulanic acid for treatment of acute otitis media in children 577
Z. Erjavec, H. G. de Vries-Hospers, H. van Kamp, D. van der Waaij, M. R. Halie and S. M. G. J. Daenen: Comparison of imipenem versus cefuroxim plus tobramycin as empirical therapy for febrile granulocytopenic patients and efficacy of vancomycin and aztreonam in case of failure 585
T. Ejlertsen, A. Jensen, A. Lester and V. T. Rosdahl: Epidemiology of toxic shock syndrome toxin-1 production in Staphylococcus aureus strains isolated in Denmark between 1959 and 1990 599
M. Amit, S. D. Pitlik, Z. Samra, H. Konisberger, M. Drucker and L. Leibovici: Bacteremia in patients without known underlying disorders 605
B. Trollfors: Cost-benefit analysis of general vaccination against Haemophilus influenzae type b in Sweden 611

Case Reports
N. Abildgaard and J. L. Nielsen: Pneumococcal septicaemia and meningitis in vaccinated splenectomized adult patients 615
Myonecrosis in the leg caused by Salmonella enteritidis 619
A. M. Horrevorts, F. T. M. Huysmans, R. J. J. Koopman and J. F. G. M. Meis: Cellulitis as first clinical presentation of disseminated cryptococcosis in renal transplant recipients 623
L. Gradoni, G. B. Gaeta, G. Pellizzer, A. Maisto and A. Scalone: Mediterranean visceral leishmaniasis in pregnancy 627
E. Dietrichs, F. van Knapen and S. J. Bakke: Meningeal irritation: possible manifestation of cerebral Echinococcus infestation 631

Review Article

C. N. Meyer, P. Skinhøj and J. Prag: Bacteremia in HIV-positive and AIDS patients: incidence, species distribution, risk-factors, outcome, and influence of long-term prophylactic antibiotic treatment 635

Articles

K. Elvin, C. Lidman, E. Tynell, E. Linder and A. Björkman: Natural history of asymptomatic and symptomatic Pneumocystis carinii infection in HIV infected patients 643

H. J. Kolmos, A. Lerche, K. Kristoffersen and V. T. Rosdahl: Pseudo-outbreak of Pseudomonas aeruginosa in HIV-infected patients undergoing fiberoptic bronchoscopy 653

P. Kragsbjerg, J. Källman and P. Olcén: Pneumococcal meningitis in adults 659

H. Akalin, A. C. Akdiş, R. Mistik, S. Helvaci and K. Kiliçturgay: Cerebrospinal fluid interleukin-1β/Interleukin-1 receptor antagonist balance and tumor necrosis factor-α concentrations in tuberculous, viral and acute bacterial meningitis 667

P. Orr, B. Lorencz, R. Brown, R. Kielly, B. Tan, D, Holton, H. Clugstone, L. Lugtig, C. Pim, S. Macdonald, G. Hammond, M. Moffatt, J. Spika, D. Manuel, W. Winther, D. Milley, H. Lior and N. Sinuff: An outbreak of diarrhea due to verotoxin-producing Escherichia coli in the Canadian Northwest Territories 675

S. Kontiainen, A. Sivonen and O.-V. Renkonen: Increased yields of pathogenic Yersinia enterocolitica strains by cold enrichment 685

J. Esteban, J.-M. Ramos, M. L. Fernandez-Guerrero and F. Soriano: Isolation of Nocardia sp. from blood cultures in a teaching hospital 693

C. H. DeBusk, R. Daoud, M. C. Thirumoorthi, F. M. Wilson and R. Khatib: Candidemia: current epidemiologic characteristics and a long-term follow-up of the survivors 697

S. Schönwald, B. Baršić, I. Klinar and M. Gunjača: Three-day azithromycin compared with ten-day roxithromycin treatment of atypical pneumonia 706

C. Ahlm, S. Lundberg, K. Fessé and J. Wikström: Health problems and self-medication among Swedish travellers 711

J. Kremastinou, C. Blackwell, G. Tzanakaki, C. Kallergi, R. Elton and D. Weir: Parental smoking and carriage of Neisseria meningitidis among Greek schoolchildren 719

Y. Hidaka, T. Aoki, H. Akeda, C. Miyazaki and K. Ueda: Serological and clinical charcteristics of measles vaccine failure in Japan 725

S. Simasathien, S. Migasena, C. Beuvery, G. van Steenis, R. Samakoses, P. Pitisuttitham and T. Vesikari: Comparison of enhanced potency inactivated poliovirus vaccine (EIPV) versus standard oral poliovirus vaccine (OPV) in Thai infants 731

D. M. See and J. G. Tilles: Efficacy of a polyvalent inactivated-virus vaccine in protecting mice from infection with clinical strains of group B coxsackieviruses 739

Case Reports

L. Morfeldt and J. Torssander: Long-term remission of Kaposi's sarcoma following foscarnet treatment in HIV-infected patients 749

O. Mäki-Ikola, R. Peltonen and P. Hänninen: Group F β-hemolytic streptococcus, tonsillitis and myocarditis 753

P. Clementsen and N. Milman: Bilateral pulmonary abscesses caused by Streptococcus pyogenes: diagnostic importance of fiberoptic bronchoscopy 755

A. M. Heilesen: Septicaemia due to Aerococcus urinae 759

A. Eid, N. Chaudry, M. El-Ghoroury, A. Hawasli, W. L. Salot and R. Khatib: Multifocal musculoskeletal cystic tuberculosis without systemic manifestations 761

N. Akçakaya, Y. Söylemez, H. Çokuğras, A. Aytac and F. Akalin: A case of hydatid cyst with intramural cardiac localization 765

P. Viale, A di Matteo, M. Sisti, F. Voltolini, C. Paties and F. Alberici: Isolated kidney localization of invasive Aspergillosis in a patient with AIDS 767

Short Communications

M. Suri, M. Kabra, S. Singh, A. Rattan and I. C. Verma: Group B meningococcal meningitis in India 771

S. Bernander, B. Gästrin, S. Löfgren, A.-M. Olinder-Nielsen: Legionella urinary antigen in early disease 777

Letters to the Editors

Å. Örtqvist: Chlamydia pneumoniae (TWAR): a common agent in acute bronchitis 779

Reply

G. Falck, L. Heyman, H. Gnarpe and J. Gnarpe 780

LIST OF AUTHORS

For Å and Ä see A, for Ö and Ø see O

Abildgaard N. 615
Achí R. 329
Ahlén S. 209
Ahlm C. 711
Akalin F. 765
Akalin H. 667
Akçakaya N. 765
Akdiş A. C. 667
Akeda H. 725
Akkeren F. van 191
Alberici F. 767
Aldershvile J. 239
Alexeyev O. A. 491
Amit M. 605
Andersson B. 141, 479
Andersson U. 339
Andreassen Rix B. 459
Andström E. 209
Aoki T. 725
Aquilili D. 119
Arenas J. I. 15
Arendrup H. 239
Aronsson B. 468
Arpi M. 157, 163
Avlami A. 495
Aytac A. 765

Bakasenas V. 459
Bakke S. J. 631
Balslev U. 27
Barbour A. G. 149
Barkholt L. 33
Barry B. 446, 577
Baršić B. 706
Bengtsson L. 417
Bergman B. 85
Bergmann F. 49
Bernander S. 777
Bertola M. A. 321
Beumer H. 191
Beuvery C. 731
Björkholm B. 471
Björkman A. 33, 643
Black F. T. 27, 117
Blackwell C. 719
Blomberg J. 23, 129
Blumen M. 446
Bobin S. 577
Boehler A. 369
Boesgaard S. 239
Bondesson L. 275
Boucot I. 446
Brandt L. 27
Brauner A. 545
Bravo P. Del 119
Breland C. M. 111
Briem H. 393
Brook I. 503
Brown R. 675
Bruins H. 427
Brummer-Korvenkonti M. 7
Bruun B. 157, 163
Bunikis J. 149
Bygdeman S. 209

Carlson P. 283
Carnot F. 215
Carratala J. 105
Chan P. 219
Chaudry N. 761
Chavanet P. 59
Chen M.-F. 297
Chen M. 263
Chen S.-T. 95
Chiodi F. 523
Chiodo F. 55
Christensen P.-H. 223
Chryssanthou E. 479
Cilla G. 133
Cimolai N. 358
Claesson B. A. 399
Clementsen P. 755
Clink H. 225
Clugstone H. 675
Çokuğras H. 765
Corbella X. 105
Cortés A. 15

Daenen S. M. G. J. 585
Dam A. P. van. 427
Dankert J. 321, 427
Daoud R. 697
Darelid J. 417
David K. 27
Davies E. G. 486
DeBusk C. H. 697
Demarongona K. 495
Dietrichs E. 631
Digranes A. 493
Dorronsoro M. 133
Drucker M. 605
Dykhuizen R. S. 498

Efremov A. G. 491
Eid A. 761
Einarsson S. 393
Ejlertsen T. 599
Ekdahl K. 301
Ekwall E. 435
Ellis M. E. 225
Elton R. 719
Elvin K. 33, 643
El-Ghoroury M. 761
Emparanza J. I. 15
Eriksson B.-M. 33
Erjavec Z. 585
Erlendsdottir H. 393
Esteban J. 693

Falck G. 179
Fanti M. P. 55
Fernandez-Guerrero M. L. 693
Fessé K. 711
Floor M. 191
Forsberg P. 559
Forsgren M. 468
Frederiksen W. 171
Frenning B. 468
Friman J. 23
Fryden A. 263, 559
Fuchs D. 523
Fursted K. 569

Gabrilovich D. 41
Gaeta G. B. 627
García-Bengoechea M. 15
Gästrin B, 417, 777
Gehanno P. 446
Gehanno P. 577
Gerner-Smidt P. 171
Gillet-Juvin K. 215
Gisslén M. 523
Glaumann H. 383
Glimåker M. 141
Gnarpe H. 179
Gnarpe J. 179
Gottfarb P. 545
Gradoni L. 627
Granström G. 453
Granström M. 453, 471
Grey P. C. 59
Grillner L. 23, 275
Grünewald T. 49
Gudmundsson S. 393
Gunjača M. 706

Hagberg L. 471, 523
Hagen I. J. 137
Hainau B. 225
Halie M. R. 585
Hallander H. 417
Halstensen A. 493
Hammers-Berggren S. 339
Hammond G. 675
Hänninen P. 753
Hansen H. 27
Hansen K. N. 569
Hansen K. 339
Hansen M. M. 157, 163
Hansson B.-G. 23
Hardardóttir H. 493
Hawasli A. 761
Hederstedt B. 559
Hedman K. 7
Hedrum A. 275
Heilesen A. M. 223, 759
Heimdal A. 209
Heinonen K. M. 375
Heiskanen T. 289
Heltberg I. 569
Helvaci S. 667
Hemilä H. 1
Heurlin N. 33
Heyman L. 179
Hidaka Y. 725
Hjelt K. 569
Högberg U. 233
Højlyng N. 569
Holme T. 553
Holton D. 675
Horrevorts A. M. 623
Howitz P. 569
Huang J. J. 219
Huysmans F. T. M. 623
Hydén D. 559

Ichou F. 59
Ikäheimo R. 289
Illum N. 569
Ishikawa N. 107
Israël-Biet D. 215
Ivanova L. 41
Iwarson S. 19

Jeng L.-B. B. 297
Jensen A. 171, 599
Jensen J. 27
Jilg W. 19
Johansson B. 255
Jönsson I. 553
Jønsson V. 157, 163
Jørgensen A. F. 27
Jørring S. 619
Junttila J. 349

Kabra M. 771
Kälebo P. 85
Kallergi C. 719
Källman J. 659
Kamme C. 301, 535
Kamp H. van 585
Kansouzidou A. 403

Kärkkäinen U. 289
Karlsson E. 67
Karlsson M. 339
Kavaliotis J. 403
Kennedy D. J. 111
Kerr K. N. 498
Keusch G. 369
Khatib R. 697, 761
Kielly R. 675
Kiliçturgay K. 667
Kishiyama K. 107
Kisterman J. P. 59
Klareskov B. 619
Klinar I. 706
Knapen F. van 631
Koch C. 569
Kolmos H. J. 406, 619, 653
Kolsters A. 191
Konisberger H. 605
Konstantopoulos K. 495
Kontiainen S. 283, 685
Koopman R. J. J. 623
Kragsbjerg P. 659
Kremastinou J. 719
Kristjánsson M. 411
Kristoffersen K. 653
Krogh G. von 275
Krogsgaard K. 23, 239
Krook A. 129, 553
Kubo S, 107
Kuiper H. 427

Lagging L. M. 111
Langenberg W. L. 321
Larsson C. 317
Lassen J. 493
Lebech A.-M. 339
Lecour H. 103
Leibovici L. 605
Leinonen M. 399
Lerche A. 653
Lester A. 599
Li A. 435
Lidman C. 643
Lin J.-D. 297
Lindberg A. A. 329, 435
Lindberg J. 85
Linder E. 33, 643
Lior H. 675
Lippe B. von der 137
Löfdahl S. 479
Löfgren S. 417, 777
López P. 15
Lorencz B. 675
Loukopoulos D. 495
Luchi S. 119
Lugtig L. 675
Lundberg S. 711
Lundeberg J. 263, 275

Macdonald S. 675
Magnusdottir S. D. 393
Maisto A. 627
Mäkelä P. H. 289
Mäki-Ikola O. 753
Malmvall B.-E. 417
Manfredi R. 55
Manuel D. 675
Marimon J. M. 133
Martin K. 486
Maslow J. N. 411
Mata L. 329
Matteo A. di 767
McLaren M. I. 489
Meis J. F. G. M. 623
Messina F. 119
Meyer C. N. 635
Migasena S. 731
Milley D. 675
Milligan T. W. 111
Milman N. 755
Miörner H. 317
Mistik R. 667
Miyazaki C. 725
Moestrup T. 23
Moffatt M. 675
Møller J. K. 157
Morfeldt L. 749
Morozov V. G. 491
Mortensen S. A. 239
Motiejunas L. 149
Munk E. 569
Mustonen J. 7, 289

Nielsen J. L. 615
Nilsen A. 511
Nilsson B. 67
Noach L. A. 321
Nordenfelt E. 23
Norkrans G. 263, 523
Nyfors A. 511
Nyström B. 209
Obel N. 117
Ödkvist L. 559
Okano M. 107
Olcén P. 141, 659
Olesen B. 406
Olinder-Nielsen A.-M. 417, 777
Oliveira M. 103
Orholm M. K. 517
Orr P. 675
Orrling A. 535
Ørskov F. 406
Ørskov I. 406
Otero F. 133
Örtqvist Å. 779

Panhani S. 375
Papavasiliou D. 403
Pasternack A. 7
Paties C. 767
Pellizzer G. 627
Peltonen R. 753
Penaud D. 215
Pereira A. 103
Perez-Trallero E. 133
Perni S. C. 361
Persson A. 199
Peters M. 49
Peterslund N. A. 157
Petrini B. 479
Petterson G. 239
Pietilä K. 7
Pim C. 675
Pitisuttitham P. 731
Pitlik S. D. 605
Pohle H. D. 49
Pokrovsky V. 41
Portier H. 59
Prag J. 635

Ramos J.-M. 693
Rattan A. 771
Reichard O. 263, 383
Rekoumi L. 495
Renkonen O.-V. 283, 685
Rintala E. 77
Ritter K. 379
Ritter S. 379
Roberg M. 559
Rombo L. 199
Rønne T. 459
Rosdahl V. T. 599, 653
Rozenberg-Arska M. 191
Ruf B. 49
Rydberg J. 317

Sadziene A. 149
Safran C. 59, 577
Salomon F. 369
Salot W. L. 761
Samakoses R. 731
Samra Z. 605
Santos E. 15
Santos L. 103
Sarriugarte A. 15
Satake N. 107
Scalone A. 627
Scasso A. 119
Schaffner A. 369
Schalén C. 535
Schönwald S. 706
Schürmann D. 49
See D. M. 739
Serebrovskaya L. 41
Settergren B. 491
Sharland M. 486
Shepeleva G. 41
Sideris G. 495
Sigurdsson H. K. 393
Siitonen A. 289
Simasathien S. 731
Simões J. 103
Singh S. 771
Sinuff N. 675
Sisti M. 767
Sivonen A. 685
Skarphedinsson S. 27
Skaug K. 137
Skinhøj P. 635
Smith E. 517
Sokol-Anderson M. L. 111
Sönnerborg A. 255, 263
Soriano F. 693
Soutar R. L. 498
Söylemez Y. 765
Spanjaard L. 427
Spika J. 675
Stark M. 275
Steenis van G. 731
Stefanou J. 495
Stern M. 215
Stiernstedt G. 339
Stjernquist-Desatnik A. 535
Stranks G. J. 489
Stroffolini T. 19
Struve J. 468
Studahl M. 85
Suri M. 771
Svennerholm B. 523
Swasdikul D. 109

Tan B. 675
Tang L.-M. 95
Tanskanen R. 349
Tantawichien T. 109
The Copenhagen Heart Transplant Group 239
The Swedish CDAD Study Group 309
Thelin A.-C. 417
Thirumoorthi M. C. 697
Thomssen R. 379
Thorén A. 249
Tilles J. G. 739
Timm H. 49
Tollemar J. 479
Torssander J. 749
Trollfors B. 611
Tsiaousi A. 403
Tungsanga K. 109
Tuomi J. 349
Tviet K.-S. 511
Tynell E. 643
Tytgat G. N. J. 321
Tzanakaki G. 719

Ueda K. 725
Uhlén M. 275
Urbieta M. 133
Uy Z. 379

Vadillo M. 105
Vaheri A. 7

'alerius N. H. 569
'ega J. L. 15
'erhoef J. 191
'erma I. C. 771
'esikari T. 731
'ezzadini P. 55
'iale P. 767
'ictor M. A. 157, 163
'ikenes K. 493
'iner B. 411

Visser M. 191
Voltolini F. 767
Vos K. 427
Voskaridou E. 495
Vries-Hosapers H. G. de 585

Waaij D. van der 585
Wachmann C. H. 459
Wachter H. 523
Wahl M. 471
Walder M. 67
Waldner-Combernoux A. 59
Watankunakorn C. 361
Weiland O. 263, 383, 468
Weir D. 719
Westblom T. U. 111
Widell A. 249
Wikström J. 711
Wilson F. M. 697
Winther W. 675

Yang Y. J. 219
Younge D. 225
Yun Z.-B. 255, 263

Zhao C. R. 435
Zhobakas A. 459

ACKNOWLEDGEMENTS

The Editors of Scandinavian Journal of Infectious Diseases wish to express their sincere gratitude to the following persons outside the Editorial Board who have acted as referees during the past year. The standard of the journal depends to a very large extent on the skill and interest of these reviewers.

Alestig K.
Andersson J.
Aronsson B.
Aust-Kettis A.

Banck G.
Berglund O.
Blomberg J.
Boman G.
Braconier J. H.
Burman L. G.

Carlsson J.
Castor B.
Christenson B.
Claesson B.
Cronberg S.

Danielsson D.
Danielsson Å.
Dornbusch K.

Eklund A.
Ekwall E.
Elvin K.
Engstrand L.
Eriksson M.
Ernst A.
Evengård B.

Forsgren A.
Forsgren M.
Frederiksen W.
Friman G.

Gamstorp I.
Gebre-Medhin M.
Giesecke J.
Gnarpe H.
Gnarpe J.
Gothefors L.
Granström M.
Grillner L.
Gustavson K.-H.
Gustavsson R.

Hagberg L.
Hambraeus A.
Hansson B. G.
Hedström S.-Å.
Hemmingson A.
Hjelm E.
Hofvander Y.
Hovelius B.
Højlyng N.

Iversen J.
Iwarson S.

Johansson S.
Julander I.
Juto P.

Kahlmeter G.
Kalin M.
Kame C.
Kollberg H.
Kronvall G.
Källenius G.

Lebech M.
Lidman K.
Lindberg J.
Linde A.
Lindquist L.
Ljungberg B.
Ljungman P.
Lönnerholm G.

Mattsson L.

Nihlén B.
Niklasson B.
Nilsson U.
Nord C. E.
Norkrans G.
Nyrén O.
Nyström B.

Odlind-Thornquist I.
Olin P.
Olsson R.

Palmblad J.
Peltola H.
Petrini B.

Ringertz S.
Ripa T.
Rombo L.

Salmi A.
Samuelsson A.
Sandberg T.
Sandström E.
Schvarez R.
Schwan A.
Simonson B.
Sköld M.
Sokal-Andersen M.
Stiernstedt G.
Strandvik B.
Struwe J.
Svenungsson B.
Sönnerborg A.

Taube A.
Thyresson N.
Trollfors B.

Wadström T.
Walder M.
Wejstål R.
Widell A.
Widerström O.
Wiström J.
Wretlind B.

Örtqvist Å.